PEDIATRIC SURGERY

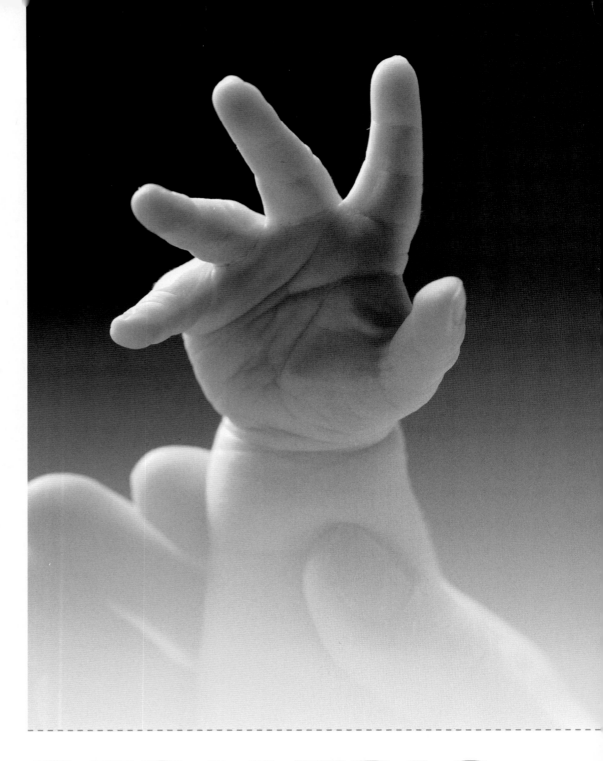

PEDIATRIC SURGERY

SEVENTH EDITION

VOLUME ONE

EDITOR IN CHIEF

Arnold G. Coran, MD

Emeritus Professor of Surgery
Section of Pediatric Surgery
University of Michigan Medical School and
    C. S. Mott Children's Hospital
Ann Arbor, Michigan
Professor of Surgery
Division of Pediatric Surgery
New York University Medical School
New York, New York

ASSOCIATE EDITORS

N. Scott Adzick, MD

Surgeon-in-Chief
The Children's Hospital of Philadelphia
C. Everett Koop Professor of Pediatric Surgery
University of Pennsylvania School of Medicine
Philadelphia, Pennsylvania

Thomas M. Krummel, MD

Emile Holman Professor and Chair
Department of Surgery
Stanford University School of Medicine
Susan B. Ford Surgeon-in-Chief
Lucile Packard Children's Hospital
Stanford, California

Jean-Martin Laberge, MD

Professor of Surgery
McGill University
Attending Pediatric Surgeon
Montreal Children's Hospital of the McGill University
    Health Centre
Montreal, Quebec, Canada

Robert C. Shamberger, MD

Chief of Surgery
Children's Hospital Boston
Robert E. Gross Professor of Surgery
Harvard Medical School
Boston, Massachusetts

Anthony A. Caldamone, MD

Professor of Surgery (Urology) and Pediatrics
Brown University School of Medicine
Chief of Pediatric Urology
Hasbro Children's Hospital
Providence, Rhode Island

ELSEVIER
SAUNDERS

1600 John F. Kennedy Blvd.
Ste 1800
Philadelphia, PA 19103–2899

PEDIATRIC SURGERY

ISBN: 978-0-323-07255-7
Volume 1 9996085473
Volume 2 9996085538

Notices

Knowledge and best practice in this field are constantly changing. As new research and experience broaden our understanding, changes in research methods, professional practices, or medical treatment may become necessary.

Practitioners and researchers must always rely on their own experience and knowledge in evaluating and using any information, methods, compounds, or experiments described herein. In using such information or methods they should be mindful of their own safety and the safety of others, including parties for whom they have a professional responsibility.

With respect to any drug or pharmaceutical products identified, readers are advised to check the most current information provided (i) on procedures featured or (ii) by the manufacturer of each product to be administered, to verify the recommended dose or formula, the method and duration of administration, and contraindications. It is the responsibility of practitioners, relying on their own experience and knowledge of their patients, to make diagnoses, to determine dosages and the best treatment for each individual patient, and to take all appropriate safety precautions.

To the fullest extent of the law, neither the Publisher nor the authors, contributors, or editors, assume any liability for any injury and/or damage to persons or property as a matter of products liability, negligence or otherwise, or from any use or operation of any methods, products, instructions, or ideas contained in the material herein.

Library of Congress Cataloging-in-Publication Data

Pediatric surgery. —7th ed. / editor in chief, Arnold G. Coran ; associate editors, N.
    Scott Adzick ... [et al.].
        p. ; cm.
    Includes bibliographical references and index.
    ISBN 978-0-323-07255-7 (2 vol. set : hardcover : alk. paper)
    I. Coran, Arnold G., 1938- II. Adzick, N. Scott.
    [DNLM: 1. Surgical Procedures, Operative. 2. Child. 3. Infant. WO 925]

    617.9'8—dc23

                                2011045740

Editor: Judith Fletcher
Developmental Editor: Lisa Barnes
Publishing Services Manager: Patricia Tannian
Senior Project Manager: Claire Kramer
Designer: Ellen Zanolle

Printed in the United States of America

Last digit is the print number: 9   8   7   6   5   4   3   2   1

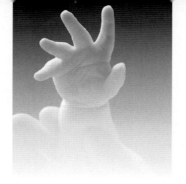

About the Editors

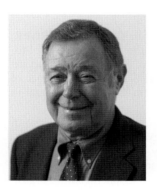

ARNOLD G. CORAN, MD, is Emeritus Professor of Surgery at the C. S. Mott Children's Hospital and the University of Michigan Medical School. He was the Chief of Pediatric Surgery and the Surgeon-in-Chief at the C. S. Mott Children's Hospital and Professor of Pediatric Surgery at the University of Michigan Medical School from 1974 to 2006. He is also currently Professor of Surgery in the Division of Pediatric Surgery at New York University School of Medicine. He was one of the editors of the fifth and sixth editions of *Pediatric Surgery* and is the current Editor in Chief of this seventh edition. His expertise in pediatric surgery centers on complex esophageal and colorectal diseases in infants and children. He is the past President of the American Pediatric Surgical Association and the past Chairman of the Surgical Section of the American Academy of Pediatrics. He has been married to Susan Coran for 50 years and has three children and nine grandchildren.

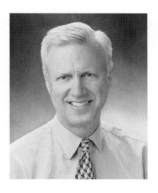

N. SCOTT ADZICK, MD, has served as the Surgeon-in-Chief and Director of The Center for Fetal Diagnosis and Treatment at The Children's Hospital of Philadelphia since 1995. He is the C. Everett Koop Professor of Pediatric Surgery at the University of Pennsylvania School of Medicine. Dr. Adzick was raised in St. Louis, received his undergraduate and medical degrees from Harvard, and has a Master of Medical Management degree from Carnegie Mellon University. He was a surgical resident at the Massachusetts General Hospital and a pediatric surgery fellow at Boston Children's Hospital. His pediatric surgical expertise is centered on neonatal general and thoracic surgery, with a particular focus on clinical applications of fetal diagnosis and therapy. He has received grant support from the National Institutes of Health for more than 20 years and has authored more than 550 publications. He was elected to the Institute of Medicine of the National Academy of Science in 1998. Scott and Sandy Adzick have one son.

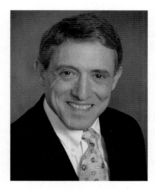

ANTHONY A. CALDAMONE, MD, graduated from Brown University and Brown School of Medicine. He was the first graduate of the medical school to become full professor at the institution. He did his residency at the University of Rochester and completed his fellowship under Dr. John W. Duckett at The Children's Hospital of Philadelphia. He is currently Professor of Surgery (Urology) and Pediatrics and Program Director for the Urology Residency at Brown University School of Medicine and Chief of Pediatric Urology at Hasbro Children's Hospital in Providence.

Dr. Caldamone has served as President of the New England Section of the American Urological Association (AUA). He has also served as Secretary-Treasurer and President of the Society for Pediatric Urology. He has been on several committees of the AUA including the Socio-Economic Committee, Publications Committee, and Nominating Committee. He is currently Executive Secretary of the Pediatric Urology Advisory Council. Locally he has served as President of the Rhode Island Urological Society, as President of the Brown Medical Alumni Association, as Chairman of the Board of Directors of Komedyplast Foundation, and as a member of the Board of Regents of La Salle Academy.

Dr. Caldamone has been on several medical missions to the Middle East, South America, and Bangladesh and has been on the Board of Directors of Physicians for Peace.

He was one of the editors of the sixth edition of *Pediatric Surgery*. He is currently an Editor for the *Journal of Pediatric Urology* and is Editor in Chief of the *Dialogues in Pediatric Urology*.

Dr. Caldamone is married to Barbara Caldamone and has two children, Amy and Matthew.

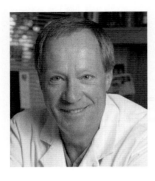

THOMAS M. KRUMMEL, MD, is the Emile Holman Professor and Chair of the Department of Surgery at Stanford University and the Susan B. Ford Surgeon-in-Chief at Lucile Packard Children's Hospital. Dr. Krummel has served in leadership positions in the American College of Surgeons, the American Pediatric Surgical Association, the American Surgical Association, the American Board of Surgery, and the American Board of Pediatric Surgery. He has mentored more than 150 students, residents, and postdoctoral scholars. He and his wife, Susie, have three children.

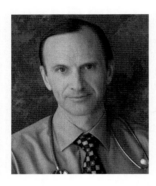

JEAN-MARTIN LABERGE, MD, is Professor of Surgery at McGill University and surgeon at the Montreal Children's Hospital of the McGill University Health Centre. He was the Director of Pediatric Surgery at the Montreal Children's Hospital from 1996 to 2008 and Program Director from 1994 to 2008. He is editorial consultant for the *Journal of Pediatric Surgery* and *Pediatric Surgery International* and was guest editor of two issues of *Seminars in Pediatric Surgery*. He has contributed chapters to several textbooks, including previous editions of *Pediatric Surgery,* Holcomb and Murphy's *Ashcraft's Pediatric Surgery,* Taussig and Landau's *Pediatric Respiratory Medicine,* and *Paediatric Surgery: A Comprehensive Text for Africa.* His research has focused on the effects of fetal tracheal occlusion to promote lung growth. His clinical interests include fetal diagnosis and treatment, congenital lung lesions, and anorectal malformations. He was President of the International Fetal Medicine and Surgery Society and is the immediate past President of the Canadian Association of Paediatric Surgeons (2009–2011). He has been married to Louise Caouette-Laberge, a pediatric plastic surgeon, for 34 years and has four children and three grandchildren.

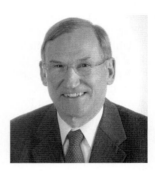

ROBERT C. SHAMBERGER, MD, is the Robert E. Gross Professor of Surgery at Harvard Medical School and is Chief of Surgery at Children's Hospital in Boston.

Dr. Shamberger's expertise in pediatric surgery centers on oncology, inflammatory bowel disease, and chest wall deformities. He was Chair of the Surgical Committee for the Pediatric Oncology Group and Children's Oncology Group, as well as a member of the National Wilms' Tumor Study Group. He is the current President of the American Pediatric Surgical Association and Chairman of the Section on Surgery of the American Academy of Pediatrics. He has been married to Kathy Shamberger for 39 years and has three children and one grandchild.

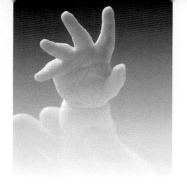

Contributors

Mark C. Adams, MD, FAAP
Professor of Urology and Pediatrics
Vanderbilt University School of Medicine
Pediatric Urologist
Monroe Carell Jr. Children's Hospital at Vanderbilt
Nashville, Tennesee

Obinna O. Adibe, MD
Assistant Professor of Surgery
Assistant Professor in Pediatrics
Duke University School of Medicine
Durham, North Carolina

Jeremy Adler, MD, MSc
Assistant Professor
Pediatrics and Communicable Diseases
University of Michigan
C. S. Mott Children's Hospital
Ann Arbor, Michigan

N. Scott Adzick, MD
Surgeon-in-Chief
The Children's Hospital of Philadelphia
C. Everett Koop Professor of Pediatric Surgery
University of Pennsylvania School of Medicine
Philadelphia, Pennsylvania

Craig T. Albanese, MD
Professor of Surgery
Pediatrics and Obstetrics and Gynecology
Chief, Division of Pediatric Surgery
Department of Surgery
Stanford Hospital and Clinics, Stanford Medicine
John A. and Cynthia Fry Gunn
    Director of Surgical Services
Lucile Packard Children's Hospital at Stanford
Palo Alto, California

Walter S. Andrews, MD
Professor of Pediatric Surgery
Department of Surgery
University of Missouri at Kansas City
Director of Renal Liver Intestinal Pediatric Transplantation
    Programs
Department of General Surgery
Children's Mercy Hospital
Kansas City, Missouri

Harry Applebaum, MD
Attending Pediatric Surgeon
Southern California Permanente Medical Group
Clinical Professor of Surgery
David Geffen School of Medicine
University of California, Los Angeles
Los Angeles, California

Marjorie J. Arca, MD
Associate Professor
Division of Pediatric Surgery
Medical College of Wisconsin
Clinical Director
Pediatric Surgical Critical Care
Children's Hospital of Wisconsin
Milwaukee, Wisconsin

Daniel C. Aronson, MD, PhD
President
International Society of Paediatric Surgical Oncology
Department of Surgery/Pediatric Surgery
Radboud University Nijmegen Medical Center
Nijmegen, The Netherlands

Richard G. Azizkhan, MD, PhD
Surgeon-in-Chief
Lester Martin Chair of Pediatric Surgery
Pediatric Surgical Services
Cincinnati Children's Hospital Medical Center
Professor of Surgery and Pediatrics
University of Cincinnati College of Medicine
Cincinnati, Ohio

Robert Baird, MD CM, MSc, FRCSC
Assistant Professor of Surgery
Pediatric General Surgery
Montreal Children's Hospital
McGill University
Montreal, Quebec, Canada

Sean Barnett, MD, MS
Assistant Professor of Surgery
Division of Pediatric General and Thoracic Surgery
Cincinnati Children's Hospital Medical Center
Cincinnati, Ohio

Douglas C. Barnhart, MD, MSPH
Associate Professor
Department of Surgery and Pediatrics
University of Utah
Attending Surgeon
Primary Children's Medical Center
Salt Lake City, Utah

Katherine A. Barsness, MD
Assistant Professor of Surgery
Division of Pediatric Surgery
Northwestern University
Feinberg School of Medicine
Attending Physician
Division of Pediatric Surgery
Children's Memorial Hospital
Chicago, Illinois

Robert H. Bartlett, MD
Professor Emeritus of Surgery
University of Michigan Medical School
Ann Arbor, Michigan

Laurence S. Baskin, MD
Professor and Chief, Pediatric Urology
Departments of Urology and Pediatrics
University of California, San Francisco
San Francisco, California

Spencer W. Beasley, MB ChB, MS, FRACS
Professor and Clinical Director
Department of Pediatric Surgery
Christchurch Hospital
Professor
Department of Surgery
Christchurch School of Medicine and Health Sciences
University of Otago
Christchurch, New Zealand

Michael L. Bentz, MD
Professor and Chairman
University of Wisconsin Plastic Surgery
University of Wisconsin-Madison
Madison, Wisconsin

Deborah F. Billmire, MD
Professor
Department of Surgery
Section of Pediatric Surgery
Indiana University
Indianapolis, Indiana

Scott C. Boulanger, MD, PhD
Assistant Professor of Surgery
Division of Pediatric Surgery
Case Western Reserve University School of Medicine
Cleveland, Ohio

Mary L. Brandt, MD
Professor and Vice Chair
Michael E. DeBakey Department of Surgery
Baylor College of Medicine
Houston, Texas

John W. Brock III, MD
Professor and Director
Division of Pediatric Urology
Vanderbilt University
Surgeon-in-Chief
Monroe Carell Jr. Children's Hospital at Vanderbilt
Nashville, Tennesee

Rebeccah L. Brown, MD
Associate Professor of Clincal Surgery and Pediatrics
Department of Pediatric Surgery
Cincinnati Children's Hospital Medical Center
Associate Director of Trauma Services
Department of Trauma Services
Associate Professor of Surgery
Department of Surgery
University of Cincinnati Hospital
Cincinnati, Ohio

Imad F. Btaiche, PhD, BCNSP
Clinical Associate Professor
Department of Clinical Social and Administrative Sciences
University of Michigan College of Pharmacy
Clinical Pharmacist, Surgery and Nutrition Support
Program Director, Critical Care Residency
University of Michigan Hospitals and Health Centers
Ann Arbor, Michigan

Ronald W. Busuttil, MD, PhD
Distinguished Professor and Executive Chairman
UCLA Department of Surgery
David Geffen School of Medicine
University of California, Los Angeles
Los Angeles, California

Anthony A. Caldamone, MD
Professor of Surgery (Urology) and Pediatrics
Brown University School of Medicine
Chief of Pediatric Urology
Hasbro Children's Hospital
Providence, Rhode Island

Donna A. Caniano, MD
Professor of Surgery and Pediatrics
Department of Surgery
Ohio State University College of Medicine
Surgeon-in-Chief
Nationwide Children's Hospital
Columbus, Ohio

Michael G. Caty, MD
John E. Fisher Professor of Pediatric Surgery
Department of Pediatric Surgical Services
Women and Children's Hospital of Buffalo
Professor of Surgery and Pediatrics
Department of Surgery
State University of New York at Buffalo
Buffalo, New York

Christophe Chardot, MD, PhD
Professor
Universite Rene Descartes
Pediatric Surgery Unit
Hopital Necker Enfants Malades
Paris, France

Dai H. Chung, MD
Professor and Chairman
Janie Robinson and John Moore Lee Endowed Chair
Pediatric Surgery
Vanderbilt University Medical Center
Nashville, Tennessee

Robert E. Cilley, MD
Professor of Surgery and Pediatrics
Department of Surgery
Penn State College of Medicine
Hershey, Pennsylvania

Nadja C. Colon, MD
Surgical Research Fellow
Pediatric Surgery
Vanderbilt University Medical Center
Nashville, Tennesee

Paul M. Columbani, MD
Robert Garrett Professor of Surgery
Department of Surgery
The Johns Hopkins University School of Medicine
Pediatric Surgeon in Charge
The Johns Hopkins Hospital
Baltimore, Maryland

Arnold G. Coran, MD
Emeritus Professor of Surgery
Section of Pediatric Surgery
University of Michigan Medical School and C. S. Mott
  Children's Hospital
Ann Arbor, Michigan
Professor of Surgery
Division of Pediatric Surgery
New York University Medical School
New York, New York

Robin T. Cotton, MD, FACS, FRCS(C)
Director
Pediatric Otolaryngology–Head and Neck Surgery
Cincinnati Children's Hospital
Professor
Department of Otolaryngology
University of Cincinnati College of Medicine
Cincinnati, Ohio

Robert A. Cowles, MD
Assistant Professor
Department of Surgery
Columbia University College of Physicians and Surgeons
Assistant Attending Surgeon
Department of Surgery
Morgan Stanley Children's Hospital of New York–Presbyterian
New York, New York

Charles S. Cox, Jr., MD
The Children's Fund Distinguished Professor of Pediatric Surgery
Pediatric Surgery
University of Texas Medical School at Houston
Houston, Texas

Melvin S. Dassinger III, MD
Assistant Professor of Surgery
Department of Pediatric Surgery
University of Arkansas for Medical Sciences
Little Rock, Arkansas

Andrew M. Davidoff, MD
Chairman
Department of Surgery
St. Jude Children's Research Hospital
Memphis, Tennessee

Richard S. Davidson, MD
Division of Orthopedics
The Children's Hospital of Philadelphia
Philadelphia, Pennsylvania

Paolo De Coppi, MD, PhD
Clinical Senior Lecturer
Surgery Unit
University College of London Institute of Child Health
London, United Kingdom

Bryan J. Dicken, MD, MSc, FRCSC
Assistant Professor of Surgery
Pediatric Surgery
University of Alberta
Stollery Children's Hospital
Alberta, British Columbia, Canada

William Didelot, MD
Vice Chairman, Orthopedic Section
Pediatric Orthopedics
Peyton Manning Children's Hospital
Indianapolis, Indiana

John W. DiFiore, MD
Clinical Assistant Professor of Surgery
Case School of Medicine
Staff Pediatric Surgeon
Children's Hospital at Cleveland Clinic
Cleveland, Ohio

Patrick A. Dillon, MD
Associate Professor of Surgery
Department of Surgery
Division of Pediatric Surgery
Washington University School of Medicine
St. Louis, Missouri

Peter W. Dillon, MD
Chair, Department of Surgery
John A. and Marian T. Waldhausen Professor of Surgery
The Pennsylvania State University College of Medicine
Hershey, Pennsylvania

Patricia K. Donahoe, MD
Marshall K. Bartlett Professor of Surgery
Harvard Medical School
Director, Pediatric Surgical Research Laboratories
Massachusetts General Hospital
Boston, Massachusettes

Gina P. Duchossois, MS
Injury Prevention Coordinator
Trauma Program
The Children's Hospital of Philadelphia
Philadelphia, Pennsylvania

James C. Y. Dunn, MD, PhD
Associate Professor
Surgery
University of California, Los Angeles School of Medicine
Los Angeles, California

Sanjeev Dutta, MD, MA
Associate Professor of Surgery and Pediatrics
Department of Surgery
Stanford University
Surgical Director
Multidisciplinary Initiative for Surgical Technology Research
Stanford University
SRI International
Stanford, California

Simon Eaton, BSc, PhD
Senior Lecturer
Surgery Unit
University College London Institute of Child Health
London, United Kingdom

Peter F. Ehrlich, MD, MSc
Associate Professor
Pediatric Surgery
University of Michigan C. S. Mott Children's Hospital
Ann Arbor, Michigan

Martin R. Eichelberger, MD
Professor of Surgery and Pediatrics
George Washington University
Children's National Medical Center
Washington, District of Columbia

Lisa M. Elden, MD, MS
Assistant Professor
Otorhinolaryngology
Head and Neck Surgery
University of Pennsylvania School of Medicine
Attending
Division of Otolaryngology
Department of Surgery
The Children's Hospital of Philadelphia
Philadelphia, Pennsylvania

Jonathan L. Eliason, MD
Assistant Professor of Vascular Surgery
Department of Surgery
University of Michigan
Ann Arbor, Michigan

Sherif Emil, MD, CM
Associate Professor and Director
Division of Pediatric General Surgery
Department of Surgery
Montreal Children's Hospital
McGill University Health Centre
Montreal, Quebec, Canada

Mauricio A. Escobar, Jr., MD
Pediatric Surgeon
Pediatric Surgical Services
Mary Bridge Children's Hospital and Health Center
Clinical Instructor
Department of Surgery
University of Washington
Tacoma, Washington

Richard A. Falcone, Jr., MD, MPH
Associate Professor of Surgery
Division of Pediatric and Thoracic Surgery
Department of Surgery
Cincinnati Children's Hospital Medical Center
University of Cincinnati College of Medicine
Cincinnati, Ohio

Mary E. Fallat, MD, FACS, FAAP
Hirikati S. Nagaraj Professor and Chief, Pediatric Surgery
Division Director, Pediatric Surgery
University of Louisville
Surgeon-in-Chief
Kosair Children's Hospital
Louisville, Kentucky

Diana L. Farmer, MD
Professor and Chair
Surgery School of Medicine
University of California Davis
Surgeon-in-Chief
University of California Davis Children's Hospital
Sacramento, California

Douglas G. Farmer, MD, FACS
Director, Intestinal Transplant Program
Co-Director, Intestinal Failure Center
University of California Los Angeles Medical Center
Los Angeles, California

Albert Faro, MD
Associate Professor of Pediatrics
Associate Medical Director
Pediatric Transplant Program
Pediatrics
Washington University
St. Louis Children's Hospital
St. Louis, Missouri

Michael J. Fisher, MD
Assistant Professor of Pediatrics
Department of Pediatrics
University of Pennsylvania School of Medicine
Attending Physician
Division of Oncology and Center for
 Childhood Cancer Research
Children's Hospital of Philadelphia
Philadelphia, Pennsylvania

Steven J. Fishman, MD
Associate Professor of Surgery
Children's Hospital Boston
Boston, Massachusettes

Tamara N. Fitzgerald, MD, PhD
Senior Resident, Department of Surgery
Yale University
New Haven, Connecticuit

Alan W. Flake, MD
Professor of Surgery
Director, Children's Center for Fetal Research
General, Thoracic, and Fetal Surgery
Children's Hospital of Philadelphia
Philadelphia, Pennsylvania

Robert P. Foglia, MD
Professor, Division Chief, Pediatric Surgery
Hellen J. and Robert S. Strauss and Diana K. and Richard
 C. Strauss Chair in Pediatric Surgery
Department of Surgery
University of Texas Southwestern
Surgeon-in-Chief
Children's Medical Center
Dallas, Texas

Henri R. Ford, MD, MHA
Vice President and Chief of Surgery
Pediatric Surgery
Children's Hospital Los Angeles
Professor and Vice Chair
Vice Dean of Medical Education
Department of Surgery
Keck School of Medicine
University of Southern California
Los Angeles, California

Andrew Franklin, MD
Clinical Fellow
Pediatric Anesthesiology
Monroe Carell Jr. Children's Hospital at Vanderbilt
Nashville, Tennesee

Jason S. Frischer, MD
Assistant Professor of Surgery
Pediatric General and Thoracic Surgery
University of Cincinnati School of Medicine
Cincinnati Children's Hospital Medical Center
Cincinnati, Ohio

Stephanie M. P. Fuller, MD
Assistant Professor
Surgery
University of Pennsylvania School of Medicine
Attending Surgeon
Division of Cardiothoracic Surgery
The Children's Hospital of Philadelphia
Philadelphia, Pennsylvania

Sanjiv K. Gandhi, MD
Associate Professor of Surgery
Surgery
British Columbia Children's Hospital
Vancouver, British Columbia, Canada

Victor F. Garcia, MD, FACS, FAAP
Founding Trauma Director, Professor of Surgery
Trauma Service, Pediatric Surgery
Cincinnati Children's Hospital
Courtesy Staff Surgery
University Hospital
Cincinnati, Ohio

John M. Gatti, MD
Associate Professor and Director of
 Minimally Invasive Urology
Surgery and Urology
University of Missouri, Kansas City
Children's Mercy Hospital
Surgery and Urology
Associate Clinical Professor
Urology
University of Kansas School of Medicine
Kansas City, Missouri

Michael W. L. Gauderer, MD
Professor of Surgery and Pediatrics
Division of Pediatric Surgery
Children's Hospital
Greenville Hospital System University Medical Center
Greenville, South Carolina

James D. Geiger, MD
Professor of Surgery
Pediatric Surgery
University of Michigan
Ann Arbor, Michigan

Keith E. Georgeson, MD
Joseph M. Farley Professor of Surgery
Department of Surgery
Division of Pediatric Surgery
The University of Alabama School of Medicine
Birmingham, Alabama

Cynthia A. Gingalewski, MD
Assistant Professor of Surgery and Pediatrics
Department of Surgery
Children's National Medical Center
Washington, District of Columbia

Kenneth I. Glassberg, MD, FAAP, FACS
Director of Pediatric Urology
Professor of Urology
Columbia University Medical Center
New York, New York

Philip L. Glick, MD, MBA, FACS, FAAP, FRCS(Eng)
Vice Chairman
Department of Surgery
Professor of Surgery
Pediatrics and Obstetrics/Gynecology
State University of New York at Buffalo
Buffalo, New York

Kelly D. Gonzales, MD
Research Fellow
Division of Pediatric Surgery
University of California, San Francisco School of Medicine
San Francisco, California

Tracy C. Grikscheit, MD
Assistant Professor of Surgery
Department of Surgery
Division of Pediatric Surgery
University of Southern California, Los Angeles
Assistant Professor of Surgery
Department of Pediatric Surgery
Children's Hospital Los Angeles
Los Angeles, California

Jay L. Grosfeld, MD
Lafayette Page Professor of Pediatric Surgery and Chair, Emeritus
Section of Pediatric Surgery
Indiana University School of Medicine
Surgeon-in-Chief, Emeritus
Pediatric Surgery
Riley Children's Hospital
Indianapolis, Indiana

Travis W. Groth, MD
Pediatric Urology Fellow
Department of Pediatric Urology
Children's Hospital of Wisconsin
Milwaukee, Wisconsin

Angelika C. Gruessner, MS, PhD
Professor
Mel and Enid Zuckerman College of Public Health/
 Epidemiology and Biostatistics
University of Arizona
Tucson, Arizona

Rainer W. G. Gruessner, MD
Professor, Chief of Surgery
Department of Surgery
University of Arizona College of Medicine
Surgery Clinical Service Chief
Surgery
University Medical Center
Tucson, Arizona

Ivan M. Gutierrez, MD
Pediatric Surgery Research Fellow
General Surgery
Children's Hospital Boston
Boston, Massachusettes

Philip C. Guzzetta, Jr., MD
Professor
Surgery and Pediatrics
George Washington University Medical Center
Pediatric Surgeon
Division of Pediatric Surgery
Children's National Medical Center
Washington, District of Columbia

Jason J. Hall, MD
Houston Plastic and Craniofacial Surgery
Houston, Texas

Thomas E. Hamilton, MD
Instructor in Surgery
Pediatric Surgery
Harvard Medical School
Adjunct Assistant Professor of Surgery and Pediatrics
Chief, Division of Pediatric Surgery
Boston University School of Medicine
Boston, Masachussettes

Carroll M. Harmon, MD, PhD
Professor of Surgery
Surgery
University of Alabama at Birmingham
Children's Hospital of Alabama
Birmingham, Alabama

Michael R. Harrison, MD
Professor of Surgery, Pediatrics, Obstetrics-Gynecology,
 and Reproductive Sciences, Emeritus
University of California, San Francisco
Attending
Surgery, Pediatrics, Obstetrics-Gynecology
University of California San Francisco Medical Center
San Francisco, California

Andrea Hayes-Jordan, MD, FACS, FAAP
Director
Pediatric Surgical Oncology
Surgical Oncology and Pediatrics
University of Texas MD Anderson Cancer Center
Houston, Texas

Stephen R. Hays, MD, MS, BS
Associate Professor
Anesthesiology and Pediatrics
Vanderbilt University Medical Center
Director
Pediatric Pain Services
Monroe Carell Jr. Children's Hospital at Vanderbilt
Nashville, Tennessee

John H. Healey, MD
Chief of Orthopaedic Surgery
Department of Surgery
Memorial Sloan-Kettering Cancer Center
Professor of Orthopaedic Surgery
Orthopaedic Surgery
Weill Cornell Medical College
Attending Orthopaedic Surgeon
Department of Orthopedic Surgery
Hospital for Special Surgery
New York, New York

W. Hardy Hendren III, MD
Chief, Emeritus
Robert E. Gross Distinguished Professor of Surgery
Children's Hospital Boston
Boston, Massachusetts

Bernhard J. Hering, MD
Professor of Surgery and Medicine
Surgery
University of Minnesota
Director, Islet Transplantation
University of Minnesota Medical Center
Scientific Director
Schulze Diabetes Institute
Minneapolis, Minnesota

David N. Herndon, MD
Professor, Jesse H. Jones Distinguished Chair in Burn Surgery
Surgery
University of Texas Medical Branch
Chief of Staff and Director of Research
Medical Staff
Shriner's Hospitals for Children
Galveston, Texas

Shinjiro Hirose, MD
Assistant Professor
Department of Surgery
University of California, San Francisco
San Francisco, California

Jennifer C. Hirsch, MD, MS
Assistant Professor of Surgery and Pediatrics
Pediatric Cardiac Surgery
University of Michigan Hospital
Ann Arbor, Michigan

Ronald B. Hirschl, MD
Head, Section of Pediatric Surgery
Surgeon-in-Chief
C. S. Mott Children's Hospital
Ann Arbor, Michigan

David M. Hoganson, MD
Department of Surgery
Children's Hospital Boston
Boston, Massachusetts

George W. Holcomb III, MD, MBA
Surgeon-in-Chief
Pediatric Surgery
Children's Mercy Hospital
Kansas City, Missouri

Michael E. Höllwarth, MD
University Professor
Head
Department of Pediatric Surgery
Medical University of Graz
Graz, Austria

B. David Horn, MD
Assistant Professor
Clinical Orthopaedic Surgery
University of Pennsylvania
Philadelphia, Pennsylvania

Charles B. Huddleston, MD
Professor of Surgery
Department of Cardiothoracic Surgery
Washington University School of Medicine
Professor of Surgery
Cardiothoracic Surgery
St. Louis Children's Hospital
St. Louis, Missouri

Raymond J. Hutchinson, MD, MS
Professor
Pediatrics
Associate Dean, Regulatory Affairs
University of Michigan
Ann Arbor, Michigan

John M. Hutson, DSc, MS, BS, FRACS, FAAP
Professor of Paediatric Surgery
Department of Pediatrics
University of Melbourne
Professor
Surgical Research
Murdoch Children's Research Institute
Melbourne, Austrailia

Grace Hyun, MD
Assistant Professor
Urology
Mount Sinai Medical School
Associate Director
Pediatric Urology
Urology
Mount Sinai Medical Center
New York, New York

Thomas H. Inge, MD, PhD
Associate Professor of Surgery
Department of Surgery
University of Cincinnati
Associate Professor of Surgery and Pediatrics
Division of Pediatric General and Thoracic Surgery
Cincinnati Children's Hospital Medical Center
Cincinnati, Ohio

Tom Jaksic, MD
W. Hardy Hendren Professor
Surgery
Harvard Medical School
Vice Chairman
Department of Pediatric General Surgery
Children's Hospital Boston
Boston, Massachusetts

Andrew Jea, MD
Assistant Professor
Department of Neurological Surgery
Baylor College of Medicine
Houston, Texas
Director of Neuro-Spine Program
Department of Surgery
Division of Pediatric Neurosurgery
Texas Children's Hospital
Houston, Texas

Martin Kaefer, MD
Associate Professor
Indiana University
Riley Hospital for Children
Indianapolis, Indiana

Kuang Horng Kang, MD
Research Fellow
Department of Surgery
Harvard Medical School
Research Fellow
Department of Surgery
Children's Hospital Boston
Boston, Massachusettes

Christopher J. Karsanac, MD
Assistant Professor
Pediatrics and Anesthesiology
Monroe Carell Jr. Children's Hospital at Vanderbilt
Nashville, Tennessee

Kosmas Kayes, MD
Pediatric Orthopedics
Peyton Manning Children's Hospital
Volunter Clinical Faculty
Orthopedics
Indiana University School of Medicine
Indianapolis, Indiana
Medical Director
Biomechanics Laboratory
Ball State University
Muncie, Indiana

Robert E. Kelly, Jr., MD
Pediatric Surgeon
Children's Surgical Specialty Group
Children's Hospital of the King's Daughter
Sentara Norfolk General Hospital
Norfolk, Virginia

Edward M. Kiely, FRCS(I), FRCS(Eng), FRCPCH
Consultant Pediatric Surgeon
Great Ormond Street Hospital for Children
London, United Kingdom

Michael D. Klein, MD
Arvin I. Philippart Chair and Professor of Surgery
Wayne State University School of Medicine
Children's Hospital of Michigan
Detroit, Michigan

Matthew J. Krasin, MD
Associate Member
Radiological Sciences
St. Jude Children's Research Hospital
Memphis, Tennessee

Thomas M. Krummel, MD
Emile Holman Professor and Chair
Department of Surgery
Stanford University School of Medicine
Susan B. Ford Surgeon-in-Chief
Lucile Packard Children's Hospital
Stanford, California

Ann M. Kulungowski, MD
Department of Surgery
Children's Hospital Boston
Boston, Massachusettes

Jean-Martin Laberge, MD
Professor of Surgery
McGill University
Attending Pediatric Surgeon
Montreal Children's Hospital of the McGill University
    Health Centre
Montreal, Quebec, Canada

Ira S. Landsman, MD
Chief
Division of Pediatric Anesthesiology
Vanderbilt Hospital
Nashville, Tennessee

Jacob C. Langer, MD
Professor of Surgery
Department of Surgery
University of Toronto
Chief and Robert M. Filler Chair
Division of General and Thoracic Surgery
Hospital for Sick Children
Toronto, Ontario, Canada

Michael P. La Quaglia, MD
Chief
Pediatric Surgery
Memorial Sloan-Kettering Cancer Center
Professor of Surgery
Weill Medical College of Cornell University
New York, New York

Marc R. Laufer, MD
Chief of Gynecology
Department of Surgery
Children's Hospital Boston
Center for Infertility and Reproductive Surgery
Brigham and Women's Hospital
Boston, Massachusettes

Hanmin Lee, MD
Associate Professor
Department of Surgery
University of California, San Francisco
Director
Fetal Treatment Center
University of California, San Francisco
San Francisco, California

Joseph L. Lelli, Jr., MD
Chief
Pediatric Surgery
Children's Hospital of Michigan
Detroit, Michigan

Marc A. Levitt, MD
Associate Professor
Cincinnati Children's Hospital Medical Center
Department of Surgery
Division of Pediatric Surgery
University of Cincinnati
Cincinnati, Ohio

James Y. Liau, MD
Craniofacial Fellow
Division of Plastic Surgery
Chapel Hill, North Carolina

Craig Lillehei, MD
Surgeon
Department of General Surgery
Children's Hospital Boston
Boston, Massachusettes

Harry Lindahl, MD, PhD
Associate Professor
Paediatric Surgery
Helsinki University Central Hospital Children's Hospital
Helinski, Finland

Gigi Y. Liu, MD, MSc
Research Assistant
Department of Surgery and Pediatrics
Stanford University
PGY-1
Department of Internal Medicine
Johns Hopkins University
Baltimore, Maryland

H. Peter Lorenz, MD
Professor of Plastic Surgery
Department of Surgery
Stanford University School of Medicine
Stanford, California
Service Chief
Plastic Surgery
Director
Craniofacial Anomalies Program
Plastic Surgery
Lucile Packard Children's Hospital
Palo Alto, California

Thomas G. Luerssen, MD, FACS, FAAP
Professor of Neurological Surgery
Department of Neurological Surgery
Baylor College of Medicine
Chief, Division of Pediatric Neurosurgery
Chief Quality Officer
Department of Surgery
Texas Children's Hospital
Houston, Texas

Jeffrey R. Lukish, MD
Associate Professor of Surgery
Surgery
Johns Hopkins University
Baltimore, Maryland

Dennis P. Lund, MD
Professor of Surgery
Surgery
University of Wisconsin School of Medicine and Public Health
Surgeon-in-Chief
American Family Children's Hospital
University of Wisconsin Hospital and Clinics
Chairman, Division of General Surgery
Surgery
University of Wisconsin School of Medicine and Public Health
Madison, Wisconsin

John C. Magee, MD
Associate Professor of Surgery
Department of Surgery
University of Michigan
Ann Arbor, Michigan

Eugene D. McGahren III, MD, BA
Professor of Pediatric Surgery and Pediatrics
Division of Pediatric Surgery
University of Virginia Health System
Charlottesville, Virginia

Eamon J. McLaughlin, MD
Medical Student
Department of Neurosurgery
University of Pennsylvania Medical Center
Medical Student
Department of Neurosurgery
The Children's Hospital of Philadelphia
Philadelphia, Pennsylvania

Leslie T. McQuiston, MD
Assistant Professor of Surgery
Urology and Pediatrics
Department of Surgery
Division of Pediatric Surgery
Dartmouth-Hitchcock Medical Center/Dartmouth Medical
    School
Lebanon, New Hampshire

Rebecka L. Meyers, MD
Chief of Pediatric Surgery
Division of Pediatric Surgery
University of Utah
Chief of Pediatric Surgery
Pediatric Surgery
Primary Children's Medical Center
Salt Lake City, Utah

Alastair J. W. Millar, DCH, MBChB, FRCS, FRACS, FCS(SA)
Charles F. M. Saint Professor of Pediatric Surgery
Institute of Child Health
University of Cape Town
Red Cross War Memorial Children's Hospital
Cape Town, South Africa

Eugene Minevich, MD, FAAP, FACS
Associate Professor
Pediatric Urology
Cincinnati Children's Hospital Medical Center
Cincinnati, Ohio

Edward P. Miranda, MD
Department of Plastic Surgery
California Pacific Medical Center
San Francisco, California

Michael E. Mitchell, MD
Professor and Chief
Pediatric Urology
Medical College of Wisconsin
Children's Hospital of Wisconsin
Milwaukee, Wisconsin

Kevin P. Mollen, MD
Assistant Professor of Surgery
Department of Surgery
University of Pittsburgh School of Medicine
Division of Pediatric General and Thoracic Surgery
Children's Hospital of Pittsburgh
Pittsburgh, Pennsylvania

R. Lawrence Moss, MD
Robert Pritzker Professor and Chief
Pediatric Surgery
Yale University School of Medicine
Surgeon-in-Chief
Yale New Haven Children's Hospital
New Haven, Connecticuit

Pierre Mouriquand, MD, FRCS(Eng), FEAPU
Professor, Directeur of Pediatric Urology
Pediatric Urology
Hôpital Mère-Enfants
Université Claude-Bernard
Lyon, France

Noriko Murase, MD
Associate Professor
Department of Surgery
University of Pittsburgh
Pittsburgh, Pennsylvania

J. Patrick Murphy, MD
Chief of Section of Urology
Department of Surgery
Children's Mercy Hospital
Professor of Surgery
Department of Surgery
University of Missouri at Kansas City
Kansas City, Missouri

Joseph T. Murphy, MD
Associate Professor
Division of Pediatric Surgery
University of Texas Southwestern Medical Center
Dallas, Texas

Michael L. Nance, MD
Director, Pediatric Trauma Program
The Children's Hospital of Philadelphia
Professor of Surgery
Surgery
University of Pennsylvania
Philadelphia, Pennsylvania

Saminathan S. Nathan, MBBS, Mmed, FRCS, FAMS
Associate Professor
Orthopedic Surgery
Yong Loo Lin School of Medicine
National University of Singapore
Head, Division of Musculoskeletal Oncology
Clinical Director
Department of Orthopaedic Surgery
Senior Consultant, Division of Hip and Knee Surgery
Principal Investigator
Musculoskeletal Oncology Research Laboratory
University Orthopaedics, Hand, and Reconstructive Microsurgery Cluster
National University Health System
Singapore

Kurt D. Newman, MD
Professor of Surgery and Pediatrics
Department of Surgery
The George Washington University Medical Center
President and Chief Executive Officer
Children's National Medical Center
Washington, District of Columbia

Alp Numanoglu, MD
Associate Professor
Department of Pediatric Surgery
Red Cross War Memorial Children's Hospital and University of Cape Town
Cape Town, South Africa

Benedict C. Nwomeh, MD, FACS, FAAP
Director of Surgical Education
Department of Pediatric Surgery
Nationwide Children's Hospital
Associate Professor of Surgery
Department of Surgery
The Ohio State University
Columbus, Ohio

Richard G. Ohye, MD
Associate Professor
Cardiac Surgery
University of Michigan
Section Head, Pediatric Cardiovascular Surgery
Cardiac Surgery
University of Michigan Health Systems
Ann Arbor, Michigan

Keith T. Oldham, MD
Professor and Chief
Division of Pediatric Surgery
Medical College of Wisconsin
Milwaukee, Wisconsin

James A. O'Neill, Jr., MD
J. C. Foshee Distinguished Professor and Chairman, Emeritus
Section of Surgical Sciences
Vanderbilt University School of Medicine
Nashville, Tennessee

Mikko P. Pakarinen, MD, PhD
Associate Professor in Pediatric Surgery
Pediatric Surgery
University of Helsinki
Consultant in Pediatric Surgery
Pediatric Surgery
Children's Hospital
University Central Hospital
Helsinki, Finland

Nicoleta Panait, MD
Chief Resident
Department of Pediatric Urology
Hôpital Mère-Enfants
Université Claude-Bernard
Lyon, France

Richard H. Pearl, MD, FACS, FAAP, FRCS
Surgeon-in-Chief
Children's Hospital of Illinois
Professor of Surgery and Pediatrics
University of Illinois College of Medicine at Peoria
Peoria, Illinois

Alberto Peña, MD
Director
Colorectal Center for Children
Pediatric Surgery
Cincinnati Children's Hosptial Medical Center
Cincinnati, Ohio

Rafael V. Pieretti, MD
Assistant Professor of Surgery
Harvard Medical School
Chief Section of Pediatric Urology
Massachusetts General Hospital
Boston, Massachusetts

Agostino Pierro, MD, FRCS(Engl), FRCS(Ed), FAAP
Nuffield Professor of Pediatric Surgery and
    Head of Surgery Unit
University College London Institute of Child Health
Great Ormond Street Hospital for Children
London, United Kingdom

Hannah G. Piper, MD
Fellow Pediatric Surgery
Pediatric Surgery
University of Texas Southwestern
Fellow in Pediatric Surgery
Pediatric Surgery
Children's Medical Center
Dallas, Texas

William P. Potsic, MD, MMM
Professor of Otorhinolaryngology–Head and Neck Surgery
University of Pennsylvania Medical Center
Vice Chair for Clinical Affairs
Director of Ambulatory Surgical Services
Department of Surgery
The Children's Hospital of Philadelphia
Philadelphia, Pennsylvania

Howard I. Pryor II, MD
General Surgery Resident
Department of Surgery
George Washington University
Washington, District of Columbia
Surgical Research Fellow
Department of Surgery
Massachusetts General Hospital
Boston, Massachusettes

Pramod S. Puligandla, MD, MSc, FRCSC, FACS
Associate Professor of Surgery and Pediatrics
Departments of Surgery and Pediatrics
The McGill University Health Centre
Program Director
Division of Pediatric General Surgery
The Montreal Children's Hospital
Departments of Pediatric Surgery and Pediatric Critical Care
    Medicine
The Montreal Children's Hospital
Montreal, Quebec, Canada

Prem Puri, MS, FRCS, FRCS(ED), FACS, FAAP(Hon.)
Newman Clinical Research Professor
University of Dublin
President
National Children's Research Centre
Our Lady's Children's Hospital
Crumlin, Dublin, Ireland
Consultant Pediatrician Surgeon/Pediatric Urologist
Beacon Hospital
Sandyford, Dublin, Ireland

Faisal G. Qureshi, MD
Assistant Professor Surgery and Pediatrics
Department of Pediatric Surgery
Children's National Medical Center
Washington, District of Columbia

Frederick J. Rescorla, MD
Professor of Surgery
Department of Surgery
Indiana University School of Medicine
Surgeon-in-Chief
Riley Hospital for Children
Clarian Health Partners
Indianapolis, Indiana

Yann Révillon, MD
Professor
Université René Descartes
Pediatric Surgery Unit
Hôpital Necker Enfants Malades
Paris, France

Jorge Reyes, MD
Director of Pediatric Solid Organ Transplant Services
Surgery
Seattle Children's Hospital
Chief
Division of Transplant Surgery
Surgery
University of Washington
Seattle, Washington
Medical Director
LifeCenter Northwest Organ Donation Network
Bellevue, Washington

Marleta Reynolds, MD
Lydia J. Fredrickson Professor of Pediatric Surgery
Department of Surgery
Northwestern University's Feinberg School of Medicine
Surgeon-in-Chief and Head
Department of Surgery
Children's Memorial Hospital
Chicago, Illnois
Department of Surgery
Northwestern Lake Forest Hospital
Lake Forest, Illinois
Attending
Department of Surgery
Northwestern Community Hospital
Arlington Heights, Illinois

Audrey C. Rhee, MD
Indiana University
Department of Urology
Riley Hospital for Children
Indianapolis, Indiana

Barrie S. Rich, MD
Clinical Research Fellow
Memorial Sloan-Kettering Cancer Center
New York, New York

Richard R. Ricketts, MD
Professor of Surgery
Chief
Department of Surgery
Division of Pediatric Surgery
Emory University
Atlanta, Georgia

Richard C. Rink, MD, FAAP, FACS
Professor and Chief
Pediatric Urology
Riley Hospital for Children
Robert A. Garrett Professor of Pediatric Urologic Research
Pediatric Urology
Indiana University School of Medicine
Indianapolis, Indiana

Risto J. Rintala, MD, PhD
Professor of Pediatric Surgery
Department of Pediatric Surgery
Hospital for Children and Adolescents
University of Helsinki
Helsinki, Finland

Albert P. Rocchini, MD
Professor of Pediatrics
Pediatrics
University of Michigan
Ann Arbor, Michigan

David A. Rodeberg, MD
Co-Director and Surgeon-in-Chief of the
   Maynard Children's Hospital
The Verneda and Clifford Kiehn Professor of Pediatric Surgery
Chief, Division of Pediatric Surgery
Department of Surgery
Brody School of Medicine
East Carolina University
Greenville, North Carolina

A. Michael Sadove, MD, FACS, FAAP
James Harbaugh Endowed Professor of Surgery, Retired
Indiana University School of Medicine
Professor of Oral and Maxillofacial Surgery
Indiana University School of Dentistry
Indiana University North Hospital
President of the Medical Staff
Director of Cleft Program
Peyton Manning Children's Hospital
St. Vincent Medical Center
Indianapolis, Indiana

Bob H. Saggi, MD, FACS
Associate Professor of Surgery
Clinical Professor of Pediatrics
Tulane University School of Medicine
Associate Program Director
Liver Transplantation and Hepatobiliary Surgery
Tulane University Medical Center
Abdominal Transplant Institute
New Orleans, Louisiana

L. R. Scherer III, MD, BS
Professor
Surgery
Director
Trauma Services
Riley Hospital for Children
Indianapolis, Indiana

Daniel B. Schmid, MD, BA
Resident Physician
Plastic and Reconstructive Surgery
University of Wisconsin
Madison, Wisconsin

Stefan Scholz, MD, PhD
Chief Resident in Pediatric Surgery
Department of Surgery
Division of Pediatric Surgery
Johns Hopkins University
Baltimore, Maryland

Marshall Z. Schwartz, MD
Professor of Surgery and Pediatrics
Drexel University College of Medicine
Surgeon-in-Chief
Chief, Pediatric Surgery
St. Christopher's Hospital for Children
Philadelphia, Pennsylvania

Robert C. Shamberger, MD
Chief of Surgery
Children's Hospital Boston
Robert E. Gross Professor of Surgery
Harvard Medical School
Boston, Massachusetts

Nina L. Shapiro, MD
Associate Professor
Surgery/Division of Head and Neck Surgery
University of California, Los Angeles School of Medicine
Los Angeles, California

Curtis A. Sheldon, MD
Director
Urogenital Center
Professor
Division of Pediatric Surgery
Cincinnati Children's Hospital Medical Center
Cincinnati, Ohio

Stephen J. Shochat, MD
Professor
Department of Surgery
St. Jude Children's Research Hospital
Memphis, Tennessee

Douglas Sidell, MD
Resident Physician
Department of Surgery
Division of Head and Neck Surgery
University of California, Los Angeles
Los Angeles, California

Michael A. Skinner, MD
Professor
Department of Pediatric Surgery and General Surgery
The University of Texas Southwestern Medical School
Dallas, Texas

Jodi L. Smith, MD, PhD
John E. Kalsbeck Professor and Director of Pediatric
  Neurosurgery
Neurological Surgery
Riley Hospital for Children
Indiana University School of Medicine
Indianapolis, Indiana

Samuel D. Smith, MD
Chief of Pediatric Surgery
Division of Pediatric Surgery
Arkansas Children's Hospital
Boyd Family Professor of Pediatric Surgery
Surgery
University of Arkansas for Medical Sciences
Little Rock, Arkansas

Charles L. Snyder, MD
Professor of Surgery
Department of Surgery
University of Missouri at Kansas City
Kansas City, Missouri

Allison L. Speer, MD
General Surgery Resident
Department of Surgery
University of Southern California, Los Angeles
Research Fellow
Department of Pediatric Surgery
Children's Hospital, Los Angeles
Los Angeles, California

**Lewis Spitz, MD(Hon.), PhD, FRCS, FAAP(Hon.),
FRCPCH(Hon.), FCS(SA)(Hon.)**
Emeritus Nuffield Professor of Paediatric Surgery
Institute of Child Health
University College, London
Great Ormond Street Hospital for Children
London, United Kingdom

Thomas L. Spray, MD
Chief and Alice Langdon Warner Endowed Chair in
  Pediatric Cardiothoracic Surgery
Division of Cardiothoracic Surgery
The Children's Hospital of Philadelphia
Professor of Surgery
Department of Surgery
University of Pennsylvania School of Medicine
Philadelphia, Pennsylvania

James C. Stanley, MD
Handleman Professor of Surgery
Department of Surgery
University of Michigan, Ann Arbor
Director, Cardiovascular Center
University of Michigan
Ann Arbor, Michigan

Thomas E. Starzl, MD, PhD
Professor of Surgery
University of Pittsburgh
Montefiore Hospital
Professor of Surgery
Director Emeritus Thomas E. Starzl Transplantation Institute
VA Distinguished Service Professor
Pittsburgh, Pennsylvania

Wolfgang Stehr, MD
Attending Surgeon
Pediatric Surgical Associates of the East Bay, Children's
    Hospital and Research Institute
Oakland, California

Charles J. H. Stolar, MD
Professor of Surgery and Pediatrics
Surgery
Columbia University
College of Physicians and Surgeons
New York, New York

Phillip B. Storm, MD
Assistant Professor of Neurosurgery
Department of Neurosurgery
The Children's Hospital of Philadelphia
Philadelphia, Pennsylvania

Steven Stylianos, MD
Professor of Surgery and Pediatrics
Hofstra University North Shore–LIJ School of Medicine
Hempstead, New York
Chief, Division of Pediatric Surgery
Associate Surgeon-in-Chief
Cohen Children's Medical Center of New York
New Hyde Park, New York

**Ramnath Subramaniam, MBBS, MS(Gen Surg), MCh
(Paed), FRCSI, FRCS(Paed), FEAPU, PG Cl Edn**
Pediatric Surgery and Urology
Leeds Teaching Hospitals NHS Trust
Leeds, United Kingdom

Riccardo Superina, MD
Professor
Department of Surgery
Feinberg School of Medicine
Northwestern University
Director, Transplant Surgery
Department of Surgery
The Children's Memorial Hospital
Chicago, Illinois

David E. R. Sutherland, MD, PhD
Professor of Surgery
Schulze Diabetes Institute and Department of Surgery
University of Minnesota
Minneapolis, Minnesota

Leslie N. Sutton, MD
Professor
University of Pennsylvania School of Medicine
Chief, Division of Neurosurgery
Director, Neurosurgery Fellowship Program
The Children's Hospital of Philadelphia
Philadelphia, Pennsylvania

Roman Sydorak, MD
Pediatric Surgeon
Kaiser Los Angeles Medical Center
Division of Pediatric Surgery
Los Angeles, California

Karl G. Sylvester, MD
Associate Professor
Department of Surgery and Pediatrics
Stanford University School of Medicine
Stanford, California
Lucile Packard Children's Hospital
Palo Alto, California

Daniel H. Teitelbaum, MD
Professor of Surgery
Surgery
University of Michigan
Ann Arbor, Michigan

Joseph J. Tepas III, MD, FACS, FAAP
Professor of Surgery and Pediatrics
Surgery
University of Florida College of Medicine
Jacksonville, Florida

John C. Thomas, MD, FAAP
Assistant Professor of Urologic Surgery
Division of Pediatric Urology
Monroe Carell Jr. Children's Hospital at Vanderbilt
Nashville, Tennessee

Dana Mara Thompson, MD, MS
Chair, Division of Pediatric Otolaryngology
Department of Otorhinolaryngology
Head and Neck Surgery
Mayo Clinic
Associate Professor of Otolaryngology
Mayo Clinic College of Medicine
Rochester, Minnesota

Juan A. Tovar, MD, PhD, FAAP(Hon.), FEBPS
Professor and Chief Surgeon
Pediatric Surgery
Hospital Universitario La Paz
Madrid, Spain

Jeffrey S. Upperman, MD
Director
Trauma Program
Associate Professor of Surgery
Pediatric Surgery
Children's Hospital, Los Angeles
Los Angeles, California

Joseph P. Vacanti, MD
Surgeon-in-Chief
Department of Pediatric Surgery
Director
Pediatric Transplantation Center
Massachusetts General Hospital
Boston, Massachusetts

John A. van Aalst, MD, MA
Director of Pediatric and Craniofacial Plastic Surgery
Department of Surgery
Division of Plastic Surgery
University of North Carolina
Chapel Hill, North Carolina

Dennis W. Vane, MD, MBA
J. Eugene Lewis Jr., MD, Professor and Chair of Pediatric Surgery
Department of Surgery
St. Louis University
Surgeon-in-Chief
Cardinal Glennon Children's Medical Center
St. Louis, Missouri

Daniel Von Allmen, MD
Professor of Surgery
Department of Surgery
University of Cincinnati College of Medicine
Director
Division of Pediatric Surgery
Department of Surgery
Cincinnati Children's Hospital
Cincinnati, Ohio

Kelly Walkovich, MD
Clinical Lecturer
Pediatrics and Communicable Diseases
University of Michigan
Clinical Lecturer
Pediatrics and Communicable Diseases
University of Michigan Medical School
Ann Arbor, Michigan

Danielle S. Walsh, MD, FACS, FAAP
Associate Professor
Surgery
East Carolina University
Surgery
Pitt County Memorial Hospital
Maynard Children's Hospital
Greenville, North Carolina

Brad W. Warner, MD
Jessie L. Ternberg, MD, PhD, Distinguished Professor
   of Pediatric Surgery
Department of Surgery
Washington University School of Medicine
Surgeon-in-Chief
Director
Division of Pediatric General Surgery
St. Louis Children's Hospital
St. Louis, Missouri

Thomas R. Weber, MD
Director
Pediatric General Surgery
Advocate Hope Children's Hospital
Professor
Pediatric Surgery
University of Illinois
Chicago, Illinois

Christopher B. Weldon, MD, PhD
Instructor in Surgery
Department of Surgery
Harvard Medical School
Assistant in Surgery
Department of Surgery
Children's Hospital Boston
Boston, Massachusetts

David E. Wesson, MD
Professor
Department of Surgery
Baylor College of Medicine
Houston, Texas

Ralph F. Wetmore, MD
E. Mortimer Newlin Professor of Pediatric Otolaryngology
The Children's Hospital of Philadelphia
University of Pennsylvania School of Medicine
Philadelphia, Pennsylvania
Chief
Division of Pediatric Otolaryngology
The Children's Hospital of Philadelphia
Philadelphia, Pennsylvania

J. Paul Willging, MD
Professor
Otolaryngology–Head and Neck Surgery
University of Cincinnati College of Medicine
Cincinnati Children's Hospital Medical Center
Cincinnati, Ohio

Jay M. Wilson, MD, MS
Associate Professor of Surgery
Department of Surgery
Harvard Medical School
Senior Associate in Surgery
Department of Surgery
Children's Hospital Boston
Boston, Massachusettes

Lynn L. Woo, MD
Assistant Professor
Pediatric Urology
Case Western Reserve University College of Medicine
Pediatric Urology
Rainbow Babies and Children's Hospital
University Hospitals of Cleveland
Cleveland, Ohio

Russell K. Woo, MD
Assistant Clinical Professor of Surgery
Department of Surgery
University of Hawaii
Honolulu, Hawaii

Elizabeth B. Yerkes, MD
Associate Professor
Department of Urology
Northwestern University Feinberg School of Medicine
Attending Pediatric Urologist
Division of Pediatric Urology
Children's Memorial Hospital
Chicago, Illinois

Moritz M. Ziegler, MD, MA(Hon.), MA(Hon.), BS
Surgeon-in-Chief, Retired
Ponzio Family Chair, Retired
Department of Surgery
The Children's Hospital, Denver, Colorado
Professor of Surgery, Retired
Department of Surgery
University of Colorado
Denver School of Medicine
Denver, Colorado

Arthur Zimmermann, MD
Professor of Pathology, Emeritus
Director
Institute of Pathology
University of Bern
Bern, Switzerland

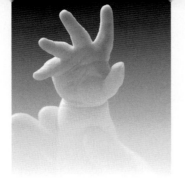

Preface

In June 1959, a group of five distinguished pediatric surgeons from the United States and Canada formed an editorial board to investigate the possibility of writing an authoritative, comprehensive textbook of pediatric surgery. The five individuals assembled were Kenneth Welch, who served as chairman of the board from Boston Children's Hospital (the original name); Mark Ravitch from The Johns Hopkins Hospital; Clifford Benson from Detroit Children's Hospital (the original name); William Snyder from Los Angeles Children's Hospital; and William Mustard from The Hospital for Sick Children in Toronto, Canada. From 1953 to 1962, the most comprehensive textbook of pediatric surgery was *The Surgery of Infancy and Childhood* by Robert E. Gross. At that time, Dr. Gross had no plans to write a second edition of his book. He was the sole author of the first edition of his book and did not wish to carry out such a monumental task with a second edition. The five editors thought that an updated textbook of pediatric surgery was needed. The first edition was published in 1962 and quickly became recognized as the most definitive and comprehensive textbook in the field. Between 1962 and 2006, six editions of the book were published. During this period, this textbook has been considered the bible of pediatric surgery. The editors and authors have changed during the 44 years that elapsed from the first to the sixth editions. In most cases, the editorial board changed gradually with the deletion and addition of two to three pediatric surgeons with each edition. The editors of the fifth edition also continued as the editors of the sixth edition. In the current seventh edition, the editorial board has been replaced except for Arnold Coran, who has functioned as the Chief Editor of this edition, and Anthony Caldamone, who continues to be the editor for the urology section. A new generation of pediatric surgical leaders has emerged since the last edition, and the editorial board reflects that change. Robert Shamberger from Children's Hospital Boston, Scott Adzick from The Children's Hospital of Philadelphia, Thomas Krummel from the Lucile Packard Children's Hospital and Stanford University Medical Center, and Jean-Martin Laberge from the Montreal Children's Hospital of the McGill University Health Centre represent the new members of the editorial board.

The seventh edition continues its international representation, with authors from several countries contributing chapters. Most of the previous chapters have been retained, but, in several cases, new authors have been assigned to these chapters. Of special interest is the addition of a new chapter (Chapter 16) on patient- and family-centered pediatric surgical care, a relatively new concept in the management of the pediatric surgical patient. Two chapters from the sixth edition, "Bone and Joint Infections" and "Congenital Defects of Skin, Connective Tissues, Muscles, Tendons, and Joints," have been deleted because currently, most pediatric surgeons do not deal with these problems. A few of the urology chapters have been merged, but all the material from the previous edition is included in these chapters. The chapter "Congenital Heart Disease and Anomalies of the Great Vessels" (Chapter 127) was kept comprehensive because so many of these patients have co-existent pediatric surgical problems or have surgical problems after cardiac surgery. Overall, there are 131 chapters in this edition, all of which are written by experts in the field and represent a comprehensive treatise of the subject with an exhaustive bibliography. In addition, each chapter provides a complete discussion of both open and closed techniques, when appropriate, for the management of the surgical problem.

One of the remarkable things about this edition is that not a single sheet of paper was used by the authors or editors in the creation of the book. Everything from the writing of the chapter to its editing was done electronically. This entire process was overseen by Lisa Barnes, the developmental editor at Elsevier. All the editors wish to thank her for her patience, availability, and efficiency in completing this textbook. Finally, we want to thank all the authors for their outstanding chapters, which will provide definitive and comprehensive information on the various pediatric surgical problems to pediatric surgeons throughout the world and thus improve the surgical care of infants and children worldwide.

THE EDITORS

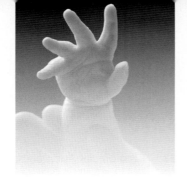

Contents

Part IX • SPECIAL AREAS

PEDIATRIC SURGERY

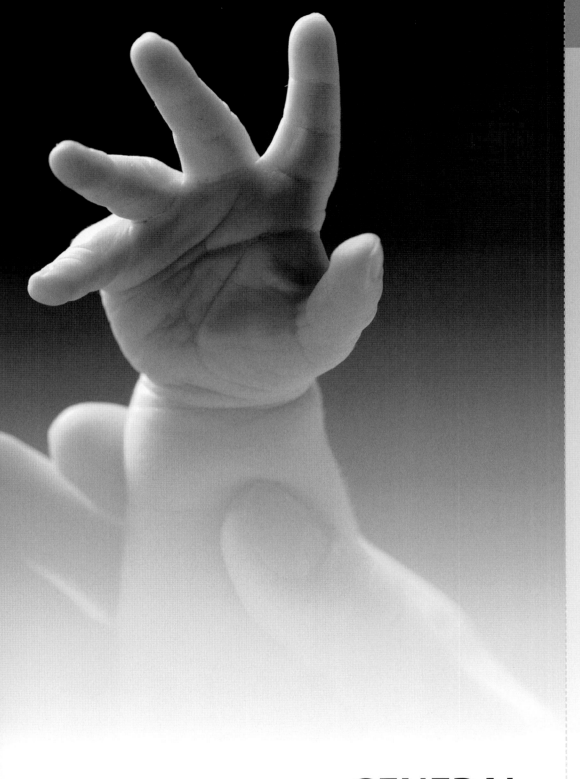

Part I

GENERAL

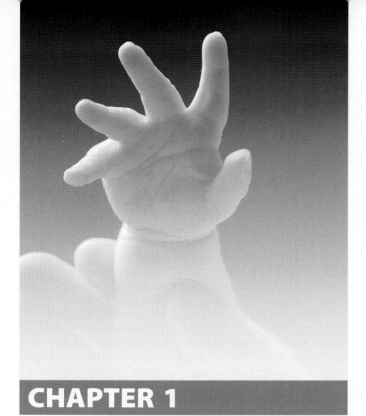

CHAPTER 1

History of Pediatric Surgery: A Brief Overview

Jay L. Grosfeld and James A. O'Neill, Jr.

The history of pediatric surgery is rich, but only the major contributions and accounts of the leaders in the field can be summarized here.

Early Years

The development of pediatric surgery has been tightly bound to that of surgery in adults, and in general, surgical information was based on simple observations of obvious deformities, such as cleft lip and palate, skeletal deformities, and imperforate anus. The only basic science of the 2nd through 16th centuries, until the 19th, was anatomy, mostly developed by surgeons; so, technical care was based on this, regardless of the patient's age. The fate of affected infants with a defect was frequently related to the cultural and societal attitudes of the time, and most did not survive long. A better understanding of the human body was influenced by Galen's study of muscles, nerves, and blood vessels in the 2nd century.[1] Albucasis described circumcision, use of urethral sounds, and cleft lip in Cordoba in the 9th century.[2] Little progress was made during the Middle Ages. In the 15th and 16th centuries, Da Vinci provided anatomic drawings; Vesalius touched on physiology; and Ambrose Paré, better known for his expertise in war injuries, wrote about club foot and described an omphalocele and conjoined twins.[3] The 17th and 18th centuries were the era of the barber surgeon. Johannes Fatio, a surgeon in Basel, was the first to systematically study and treat surgical conditions in children, and he attempted separation of conjoined twins in 1689.[4] Other congenital malformations were identified as a result of autopsy studies, including descriptions of esophageal atresia in one of thoracopagus conjoined twins by Durston in 1670,[5] intestinal atresia by Goeller in 1674,[6] an instance of probable megacolon by Ruysch in 1691,[7] and a more precise description of esophageal atresia by Gibson in 1697,[8] but there were no attempts at operative correction. Surgery for children was usually limited to orthopedic procedures, management of wounds, ritual circumcision, and drainage of superficial abscesses. In 1793, Calder[9] was the first to describe duodenal atresia. In France, Duret[10] performed the initial colostomy for a baby with imperforate anus in 1793, Amussat[11] performed the first formal perineal anoplasty in 1834, and in the United States, Jacobi[12] performed the first colostomy for probable megacolon in 1869. Up to this point, no surgeon devoted his practice exclusively to children. Despite this fact, a movement began to develop hospitals for children, led mainly by women in various communities, who felt that adult hospitals were inappropriate environments for children.

In Europe, the major landmark in the development of children's hospitals was the establishment of the Hôpital des Enfants Malades in Paris in 1802, which provided treatment for children with both medical and surgical disorders.[13] Children younger than 7 years of age were not admitted to other hospitals in Paris. Subsequently, similar children's hospitals were established in major European cities, including Princess Lovisa Hospital in Stockholm in 1854, and other facilities followed in St. Petersburg, Budapest, East London, and Great Ormond Street, London.[14] Children's hospitals in the United States opened in Philadelphia (1855), Boston (1869), Washington, DC (1870), Chicago (1882), and Columbus, Ohio (1892).[15] The Hospital for Sick Children in Toronto was established in 1885. Some of these facilities started out as foundling homes and then mainly cared for orthopedic problems and medical illnesses. Few had full-time staff, because it was difficult to earn a living caring for children exclusively.

Major advances in the 19th century that would eventually influence surgical care were William T.G. Morton's introduction of anesthesia in 1864, antisepsis using carbolic acid championed by Joseph Lister and Ignaz Semelweiss in 1865, and Wilhelm Roentgen's discovery of the x-ray in 1895. Harald Hirschsprung of Copenhagen wrote a classical treatise on two infants with congenital megacolon in 1886,[16] and Max Wilms, then in Leipzig, described eight children with renal tumors in 1899.[17] Fockens accomplished the first successful anastomosis for intestinal atresia in 1911[18]; Pierre Fredet (1907)[19] and Conrad Ramstedt (1912)[20] documented effective operative procedures (pyloromyotomy) for hypertrophic pyloric stenosis; and N.P. Ernst did the first successful repair of duodenal atresia in 1914, which was published 2 years later.[21]

20th Century: The Formative Years

UNITED STATES

There was little further progress in the early 20th century because of World War I and the Great Depression. It was during this time that a few individuals emerged who would devote their total attention to the surgical care of children. William E. Ladd of Boston, Herbert Coe of Seattle, and Oswald S. Wyatt of Minneapolis, the pioneers, set the stage for the future of pediatric surgery in the United States.[14,15,22]

Ladd, a Harvard medical graduate in 1906, trained in general surgery and gynecology and was on the visiting staff at the Boston Children's Hospital. After World War I, he spent more time there and subsequently devoted his career to the surgical care of infants and children and became surgeon-in-chief in 1927. His staff included Thomas Lanman, who attempted repair of esophageal atresia in more than 30 patients unsuccessfully, but the report of his experience set the stage for further success. Ladd recruited Robert E. Gross, first as a resident and then as a colleague. Ladd developed techniques for management of intussusception, pyloric stenosis, and bowel atresia; did the first successful repair of a correctable form of biliary atresia in 1928; and described the Ladd procedure for intestinal malrotation in 1936 (Fig. 1-1, *A* and *B*).[23–26] While Ladd was out of Boston, and against his wishes, Gross, then 33 years old and still a resident, performed the first ligation of a patent ductus arteriosus in 1938. One can imagine how this influenced their relationship. Nonetheless, in 1941, Ladd and Gross published their seminal textbook, *Abdominal Surgery of Infants and Children.*[27] 1941 was of importance not only because of the entry of the United States into WW II, but that was the year that Cameron Haight,[28] a thoracic surgeon in Ann Arbor, Michigan, and Rollin Daniel, in Nashville, Tennessee, independently performed the first successful primary repairs of esophageal atresia.

In addition to his landmark ductus procedure, Gross' surgical innovations, involving the great vessels around the heart, coarctation of the aorta, management of vascular ring deformities, and early use of allografts for aortic replacement, were major contributions to the development of vascular surgery (Fig. 1-2).[14] The training program in Boston grew and recruited future standouts in the field, such as Alexander Bill, Orvar Swenson, Tague Chisholm, and H. William Clatworthy. Ladd retired in 1945 and was succeeded by Gross as surgeon-in-chief. Gross was a very skillful pediatric surgeon and cardiovascular surgical pioneer who continued to attract bright young trainees to his department. In 1946, C. Everett Koop and Willis Potts spent a few months observing at the Boston Children's Hospital and then returned to the Children's Hospital of Philadelphia and Children's Memorial Hospital in Chicago, respectively. Luther Longino, Judson Randolph, Morton Wooley, Daniel Hays, Thomas Holder, W. Hardy Hendren, Lester Martin, Theodore Jewett, Ide Smith, Samuel Schuster, Arnold Colodny, Robert Filler, Arvin Phillipart, and Arnold Coran were just a few of the outstanding individuals attracted to the Boston program. Many became leaders in the field, developed their own training programs and, like disciples, spread the new gospel of pediatric surgery across the country. After Gross retired, Judah Folkman, a brilliant surgeon-scientist, became the third surgeon-in-chief in Boston in 1968. W. Hardy Hendren, Moritz Ziegler, and, currently, Robert Shamberger followed in the leadership role at the Children's Hospital, Boston.[15,25]

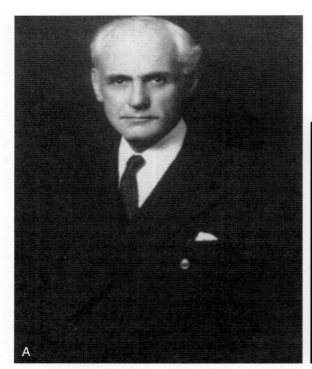

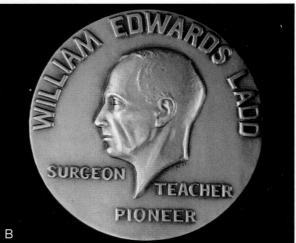

FIGURE 1-1 **A,** William E. Ladd. **B,** To honor Dr. Ladd's pioneering achievements, the Ladd Medal was established by the Surgical Section of the American Academy of Pediatrics to award individuals for outstanding achievement in pediatric surgery.

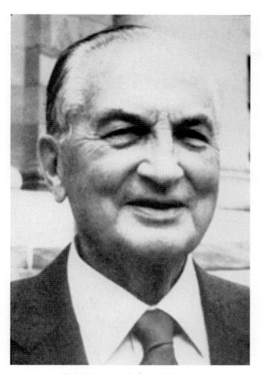

FIGURE 1-2   Robert E. Gross.

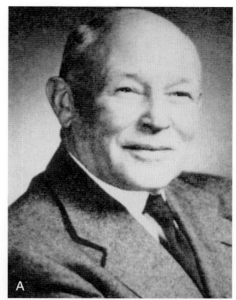

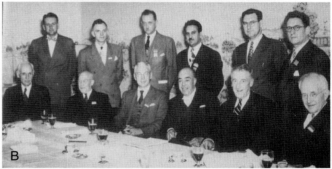

FIGURE 1-3   **A,** Herbert Coe, Seattle, Washington. **B,** Photograph of the first meeting of the Section on Surgery, American Academy of Pediatrics, November 12, 1948. Seated, from *left to right,* are Drs. William E. Ladd, Herbert Coe, Frank Ingraham, Oswald Wyatt, Thomas Lanman, and Clifford Sweet. Standing, from *left to right,* are Drs. Henry Swan, J. Robert Bowman, Willis Potts, Jesus Lozoya-Solis (of Mexico), C. Everett Koop, and Professor Fontana.

Herbert Coe was raised in Seattle, Washington, and attended medical school at the University of Michigan. After training in general surgery, he returned to Seattle in 1908 and was on staff at the Children's Orthopedic Hospital. After WWI, he spent time at the Boston Children's Hospital as an observer, gaining experience in pediatric surgical care. When he returned to Seattle in 1919, he was the first to exclusively limit his practice to pediatric surgery. He initiated the first children's outpatient surgical program in the country. He was a strong advocate for children and, in 1948, helped to persuade the leadership of the American Academy of Pediatrics (AAP) to form its surgery section, which he saw as a forum for pediatric surgeons to gather, share knowledge, and gain recognition for their new specialty (Fig. 1-3). Alexander Bill joined Coe in practice following his training in Boston and subsequently became surgeon-in-chief at the Children's Orthopedic Hospital.[14,15]

Oswald Wyatt, a Canadian by birth, attended both undergraduate school and medical school at the University of Minnesota. He trained in general surgery in Minneapolis. After serving in the military in WWI, Wyatt returned to Minneapolis and entered surgical practice. In 1927, he spent time with Edwin Miller at the Children's Memorial Hospital in Chicago. When he returned to Minneapolis, he then limited his surgical practice to children. When Tague Chishom completed his training with Ladd and Gross in 1946, he joined Wyatt's practice. Together they developed one of the largest and most successful pediatric surgery community practice groups in the country.[14,15]

In 1948, C. Everett Koop became the first surgeon-in-chief at the Children's Hospital in Philadelphia and served until 1981. He was followed by James A. O'Neill and subsequently Scott Adzick. Prominent trainees from this program include

William Kiesewetter, Louise Schnaufer, Dale Johnson, John Campbell, Hugh Lynn, Judah Folkman, Howard Filston, John Templeton, Moritz Ziegler, Don Nakayama, Ron Hirschl, and others. Dr. Koop was the second president of the American Pediatric Surgical Association (APSA) and also served as Surgeon General of the United States from 1981 to 1989 (Fig. 1-4).

Also in 1948, Orvar Swenson performed the first successful rectosigmoidectomy operation for Hirschsprung disease at Boston Children's Hospital (Fig. 1-5).[29] In 1950, he became surgeon-in-chief of the Boston Floating Hospital and subsequently succeeded Potts as surgeon-in-chief at the Children's Memorial Hospital in Chicago.

H. William Clatworthy, the last resident trained by Ladd and Gross' first resident, continued his distinguished career as surgeon-in-chief at the Columbus Children's Hospital, (now Nationwide Children's Hospital) at Ohio State University in 1950 (Fig. 1-6). Clatworthy was a gifted teacher and developed a high-quality training program that produced numerous graduates who became leaders in the field and professors of pediatric surgery at major universities, including

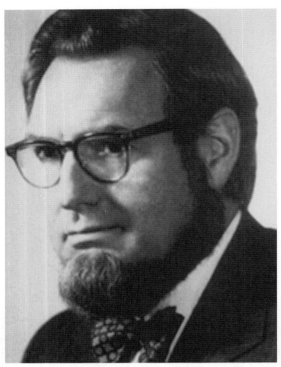

FIGURE 1-4   C. Everett Koop.

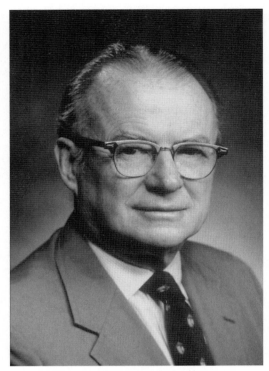

FIGURE 1-6   H. William Clatworthy, Jr.

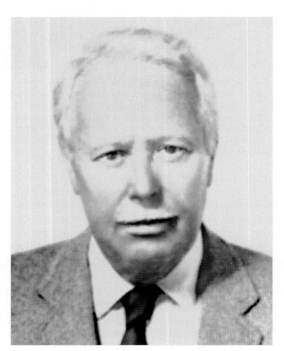

FIGURE 1-5   Orvar Swenson.

Nashville, and Philadelphia), Jay Grosfeld (Indianapolis), Neil Feins (Boston), Arnold Leonard (Minneapolis), and Medad Schiller (Jerusalem).[25] E. Thomas Boles succeeded Dr. Clatworthy as surgeon-in-chief in 1970.

EDUCATION, ORGANIZATIONAL CHANGES, AND RELATED ACTIVITIES

Following World War II, a glut of military physicians returned to civilian life and sought specialty training. A spirit of academic renewal and adventure then pervaded an environment influenced by the advent of antibiotics, designation of anesthesia as a specialty, and the start of structured residency training programs in general surgery across the country. By 1950, one could acquire training in children's surgery as a preceptor or as a 1- or 2-year fellow at Boston Children's Hospital (Gross), Children's Memorial Hospital in Chicago (Potts), Children's Hospital of Philadelphia (Koop), Boston Floating Hospital (Swenson), Babies' Hospital in New York (Thomas Santulli), or the Children's Hospital of Los Angeles (William Snyder). There were two established Canadian programs in Toronto and Montreal. The training program at the Columbus Children's Hospital (Clatworthy) started in 1952. Other programs followed in Detroit (C. Benson), Cincinnati (L. Martin), Pittsburgh (Kiesewetter), and Washington, DC (Randolph). The output of training programs was sporadic, and some graduates had varied experience in cardiac surgery and urology, but all had broad experience in general and thoracic pediatric surgery. Gross published his renowned textbook, *The Surgery of Infancy and Childhood,* in 1953.[30] This extraordinary text, the "Bible" of the fledgling field, described in detail the experience at Boston Children's Hospital in general pediatric surgery, cardiothoracic

Peter Kottmeier (Brooklyn), Jacques Ducharme (Montreal,) Lloyd Schulz (Omaha), James Allen (Buffalo), Beimann Othersen (Charleston), Dick Ellis (Ft. Worth), Alfred de Lorimier (San Francisco), Eric Fonkalsrud (Los Angeles), Marc Rowe (Miami and Pittsburgh), James A. O'Neill (New Orleans, surgery, and urology and became the major reference source for all involved in the care of children. The successor to this book, *Pediatric Surgery,* originally edited by Clifford Benson, William Mustard, Mark Ravitch, William Snyder, and Kenneth Welch was first published in two volumes in 1962 and has now gone through seven editions. It continues to be international and encyclopedic in scope, covering virtually every aspect of children's surgery. Over time, Judson Randolph, E. Aberdeen, James O'Neill, Marc Rowe, Eric Fonkalsrud, Jay Grosfeld, and Arnold Coran were added as editors through the sixth edition. As the field has grown, several other excellent texts have been published, adding to the rich literature in pediatric surgery and its subspecialties.

The 1950s saw an increasing number of children's surgeons graduating from a variety of training programs in the United States and Canada. Many entered community practice. A number of children's hospitals sought trained pediatric surgeons to direct their surgical departments, and medical schools began to recognize the importance of adding trained pediatric surgeons to their faculties. In 1965, Clatworthy requested that the surgical section of the AAP form an education committee whose mandate was to evaluate existing training programs and make recommendations for the essential requirements for educating pediatric surgeons. Originally, 11 programs in the United States and 2 in Canada met the standards set forth by the Clatworthy committee. In short order, additional training programs, which had been carefully evaluated by the committee, implemented a standard curriculum for pediatric surgical education.[14,15,31,32]

In the 1960s, a number of important events occurred that influenced the recognition of pediatric surgery as a bona fide specialty in North America.[33] Lawrence Pickett, then secretary of the AAP Surgical Section, and Stephen Gans were strong proponents of the concept that the specialty needed its own journal. Gans was instrumental in starting the *Journal of Pediatric Surgery* in 1966, with Koop serving as the first editor-in-chief.[34] Eleven years later, Gans succeeded Koop as editor-in-chief, a position he held until his death in 1994. Jay Grosfeld then assumed the role and continues to serve as editor-in-chief of the *Journal of Pediatric Surgery* and the *Seminars of Pediatric Surgery,* which was started in 1992.

Lucian Leape, Thomas Boles, and Robert Izant promoted the concept of a new independent surgical society, in addition to the surgical section of the AAP. The idea was quickly embraced by the pediatric surgical community, and the American Pediatric Surgical Association (APSA) was launched in 1970, with Gross serving as its first president.[35,36]

In the 1950s and 1960s, three requests to the American Board of Surgery (ABS) to establish a separate board in Pediatric Surgery were unsuccessful. However, with the backing of a new independent surgical organization, established training programs, a journal devoted to the specialty, and inclusion of children's surgery into the curricula of medical schools and general surgical residency programs, another attempt was made to approach the Board for certification.[35] Harvey Beardmore of Montreal (Fig. 1-7), a congenial, diplomatic, and persuasive individual, was chosen as spokesperson. He succeeded where others had failed. In 1973, the ABS approved a new Certificate of Special Competence in Pediatric Surgery to be awarded to all qualified applicants. There was no grandfathering of certification, because all applicants for the certificate had to pass a secured examination administered by the

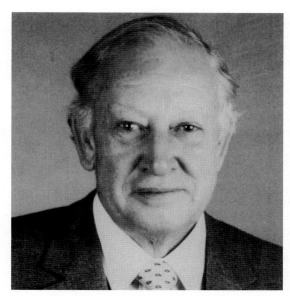

FIGURE 1-7 Harvey Beardmore, distinguished Canadian pediatric surgeon from Montreal.

ABS. The first examination was given in 1975 and, for the first time in any specialty, diplomats were required to recertify every 10 years. The accreditation of training programs was moved from the Clatworthy Committee of the AAP, initially, to the APSA Education Committee, and, following Board approval of certification for the specialty, to the Accreditation Council for Graduate Medical Education (ACGME) Residency Review Committee (RRC) for Surgery in 1977.

In 1989, the Association of Pediatric Surgery Training Program Directors was formed and developed as a liaison group with the RRC. Prospective residents applied for postgraduate training in pediatric surgery, initially through a matching process overseen by APSA and, in 1992, through the National Residency Matching Program (NRMP). In 1992, the ABS developed an in-training examination to be given annually to all pediatric surgical residents. In 2000, the ABS approved a separate pediatric surgery sub-board to govern the certification process. By 2010, there were 49 accredited training programs in the United States and Canada. The American College of Surgeons (ACS) recognized pediatric surgery as a separate specialty and developed focused programs at its annual congress devoted to the specialty, including a pediatric surgery research forum. Pediatric surgeons have an advisory committee at the College and have served in leadership positions on numerous committees, the Board of Governors, Board of Regents and as vice-president and president of the College (Kathryn Anderson). At this point pediatric surgery had come of age in North America and the world.

Research

Early research in pediatric surgery was clinical in nature and involved clinical advances in the 1930s and 1940s.[14] Ladd's operation for malrotation in 1936 was a signal event based on anatomical studies.[26] In addition to Gross' work on patent ductus arteriosus and coarctation, Alfred Blalock's systemic-to-pulmonary shunt for babies with tetralogy of Fallot was another landmark. Potts' direct aortic-to-pulmonary artery shunt accomplished similar physiologic results but required a special clamp. When Potts and Smith developed a clamp with many delicate teeth to gently hold a pulsatile vessel securely, they implemented a major technical advance that enabled the development of vascular surgery.[14] To bridge the gap in long, narrow coarctations of the aorta, Gross devised the use of freeze-dried, radiated aortic allografts and demonstrated their initial effectiveness, further promoting the use of interposition grafts in vascular surgery.[14]

Research in surgical physiology affecting adult surgical patients began to be integrated with research adapted to children. Studies of body composition in injured and postoperative patients by Francis D. Moore in adults were adapted to infants by Rowe in the United States, Peter Rickham and Andrew Wilkinson in the United Kingdom, and Ola Knutrud in Norway. Curtis Artz, John Moncrief, and Basil Pruitt were leaders in adult burn care management, and they stimulated O'Neill's interest in burn and injury research, in children.[14] In 1965, Stanley Dudrick and Douglas Wilmore, working with Jonathan Rhodes in Philadelphia, introduced the use of total parenteral nutrition, first studied in dogs, to sustain surgical patients chronically unable to tolerate enteral feedings, saving countless patients of all ages.[37] Shortly thereafter, Ola Knutrud and colleagues in Norway introduced the use of intravenous lipids. In the 1960s following extensive laboratory studies, Robert Bartlett and Alan Gazzaniga instituted extracorporeal membrane oxygenation (ECMO) for infants with temporarily inadequate heart and lung function, including those with congenital diaphragmatic hernia, certain congenital heart anomalies, meconium aspiration, and sepsis.[38] The technique was subsequently expanded for use in older children and adults. ECMO has been used successfully in thousands of infants and children worldwide.

The field of organ transplantation led by Joseph Murray, Thomas E. Starzl, and Norman Shumway in the United States, Peter Morris and Roy Y. Calne in the United Kingdom, Henri Bismuth and Yann Revillion in France, Jean-Bernard Otte in Belgium, as well as others, provided new options for the treatment of end-stage organ failure in patients of all ages. Renal, liver, and bowel transplantation have significantly altered the outcomes of infants with uncorrectable biliary atresia, end-stage renal disease, short bowel syndrome, and intestinal pseudo-obstruction. The use of split liver grafts and living-related donors to offset the problems with organ shortage, has added to the availability of kidneys, liver, and bowel for transplantation, but shortages still exist. Joseph Vacanti and colleagues in Boston and Anthony Atala in Winston Salem have laid the preliminary groundwork for the development of the field of tissue engineering. Using a matrix for select stem cells to grow into various organs, these investigators have successfully grown skin, bone, bladder, and some other tubular organs.

Ben Jackson of Richmond, J. Alex Haller in Baltimore, and Alfred de Lorimier in San Francisco, began experimenting with fetal surgery in the late 1960s and early 1970s.[15] De Lorimier's young associate, Michael Harrison and his colleagues (Scott Adzick, Alan Flake, and others) have provided new insights into fetal physiology and prenatal diagnosis and pursued clinical investigations into the practicalities of intrauterine surgery. Fetal intervention has been attempted for obstructive uropathy related to urethral valves, repair of congenital diaphragmatic hernia, twin–twin transfusion syndrome, arteriovenous shunting for sacrococcygeal teratoma, cystic lung disease, a few cardiac defects, large tumors of the neck, and myelomeningocele repair. Some of these initiatives have been abandoned, but limited protocol-driven investigation continues for fetal myelomeningocele repair in Nashville, Philadelphia, and San Francisco, and fetoscopically placed balloon tracheal occlusion in selected fetuses with diaphragmatic hernia in San Francisco, Providence, and Leuven, Belgium in an attempt to avoid pulmonary hypoplasia.

Patricia Donohoe has carried out fundamental fetal research investigating growth factors that influence embryologic development. Her seminal work defined müllerian inhibitory substance, which influences sexual development and tumor induction. Judah Folkman's discovery of the new field of angiogenesis and antiangiogenesis led him to postulate and search for antiangiogenic agents for use as cancer inhibitors. Antiangiogenic agents are currently being used clinically in a number of cancer protocols for breast and colon cancer, neuroblastoma, gastrointestinal stromal tumors, and others.

Clinical Advances Related to Research

Although many clinical and research accomplishments have occurred in the United States, many related ones have occurred in other parts of the world as more collaborations have developed. However, the United States got a head start on many of these researches, because medical developments were not as hampered during WWII in the United States as in Europe and Asia.

In the late 1960s and early 1970s, the advent of neonatal intensive care units (NICUs) and the evolving subspecialty of neonatology had a major impact on the survival of premature infants and the activities of pediatric surgeons. The first pediatric surgical ICU was established at Children's Hospital of Philadelphia in 1962. Prior to the availability of infant ventilators, monitoring systems, other life support technologies, and microtechniques, most premature infants succumbed. Most infants weighing greater than 1000 g and 75% to 80% weighing greater than 750 g now survive with satisfactory outcomes. With these advances came new challenges in dealing with premature and micropremature surgical patients with immature physiology and conditions previously rarely encountered, such as necrotizing enterocolitis. This led to a universal emphasis on pediatric surgical critical care.

Sophisticated advances in imaging, including computerized tomography (CT), and use of prenatal ultrasound and magnetic resonance imaging to detect anomalies prior to birth and portable sonography for evaluation of cardiac defects, renal abnormalities, and intracranial hemorrhage in the NICU advanced patient care and survival.

The introduction of nitric oxide, surfactant, and newer ventilator technologies, such as oscillating and jet ventilators, have markedly diminished complications and improved outcomes for infants with respiratory distress. Exogenous administration of indomethacin to induce ductus closure and reduce the need for operative intervention has also enhanced survival.

The evolution of comprehensive children's hospitals capable of providing tertiary care to high-risk patients enabled the activities of pediatric surgeons, and this was further amplified by the expansion of specialists in the critical support services of pediatric anesthesia, pathology, and radiology. Other surgical disciplines began to focus their efforts on children, which eventually led to pediatric subspecialization in orthopedics, urology, plastic surgery, otolaryngology, ophthalmology, cardiac surgery, and neurosurgery.

Because it was recognized that trauma was the leading cause of death in children, trauma systems, including prehospital care, emergency transport, and development of assessment and management protocols, were developed by J. Alex Haller, Martin Eichelberger, James O'Neill, Joseph Tepas, and others, dramatically improving the survival of injured children. The implementation of the Glasgow Coma and Pediatric Injury Severity scores aided in triage and outcome research studies. After the initial favorable experience with nonoperative management of splenic injury in children reported by James Simpson and colleagues in Toronto in the 1970s,[39] nonoperative management protocols were applied to blunt injuries of other solid organs, and the availability of modern ultrasound and CT imaging dramatically changed the paradigm of clinical care. A national pediatric trauma database was subsequently developed, which has provided a vital data research base that has influenced trauma care. Criteria for accreditation of level 1 pediatric trauma centers were established through the Committee on Trauma of the ACS to standardize trauma systems and ideal methods of management.

Pediatric surgeons have been intimately involved in collaborative multidisciplinary cancer care for children with solid tumors since the early 1960s. Cooperative cancer studies in children antedated similar efforts in adults by more than 2 decades. In the United States, the National Wilms' Tumor Study, Intergroup Rhabdomyosarcoma Study, Children's Cancer Group, Pediatric Oncology Group and, more recently, Children's Oncology Group are examples. Tremendous strides have been achieved by having access to many children with a specific tumor managed with a standard protocol on a national basis. C. Everett Koop, Judson Randolph, H. William Clatworthy, Alfred de Lorimier, Daniel Hays, Phillip Exelby, Robert Filler, Jay Grosfeld, Gerald Haase, Beimann Othersen, Eugene Weiner, Richard Andrassy, and others represented pediatric surgery on many of the early solid tumor committees. They influenced the concepts of delayed primary resection, second-look procedures, primary reexcision, selective metastectomy, staging procedures, and organ-sparing procedures. Antonio Gentils-Martins in Portugal and Denis Cozzi in Rome have been the leading proponents of renal-sparing surgery for Wilms' tumors.[40] Currently, 80% of children with cancer now survive. The elucidation of the human genome has led to an understanding of genetic alterations in cancer cells and has changed the paradigm of care. Individualized risk-based management, depending on the molecular biology and genetic information obtained from tumor tissue, often determines the treatment protocol and the intensity of treatment for children with cancer.

In addition to the accomplishments noted above, major advances in clinical pediatric surgery, education, and research continue to unfold, and some of these contributions have been extended to adult surgery as well. Examples include the nonoperative management of blunt abdominal trauma, Clatworthy's mesocaval (Clatworthy-Marion) shunt for portal hypertension, and Lester Martin's successful sphincter-saving pull-through procedures for children with ulcerative colitis and polyposis in 1978, all techniques which have been adapted to adults. Jan Louw of Cape Town clarified the etiology of jejunoileal atresia and its management in 1955, and Morio Kasai of Sendai revolutionized the care of babies with biliary atresia by implementing hepatoportoenterostomy in 1955. The latter procedure was implemented in the United States by John Lilly and Peter Altman and in the United Kingdom by Edward Howard, Mark Davenport, and Mark Stringer. Samuel Schuster's introduction of temporary prosthetic coverage for abdominal wall defects; Donald Nuss' minimally invasive repair of pectus excavatum; Hardy Hendren's contributions in managing obstructive uropathy and repair of patients with complex cloaca; Barry O'Donnell and Prem Puri's endoscopic treatment (sting procedure) for vesicoureteral reflux; Mitrofanoff's use of the appendix as a continent catheterizable stoma for the bladder; Joseph Cohen's ureteral reimplantation technique; Malone's institution of the antegrade continent enema (MACE procedure) for fecal incontinence; Douglas Stephen's introduction of the sacroabdominal perineal pull-through for imperforate anus in 1953; Alberto Peña and DeVries' posterior sagittal anorectoplasty in the 1970s; Luis de la Torre's introduction of the transanal pull-through for Hirschsprung disease in the 1990s; laparoscopic-assisted pull-through for Hirschsprung disease and anorectal malformations by Keith Georgeson, Jacob Langer, Craig Albanese, Atsayuki Yamataka, and others; the longitudinal intestinal lengthening procedure by Adrian Bianchi and introduction of the serial transverse enteroplasty (STEP) procedure by H. B. Kim and Tom Jaksic for infants with short bowel syndrome; and use of the gastric pull up for esophageal replacement by Spitz and later Arnold Coran all represent some of the innovative advances in the specialty that have improved the care of children. Early use of peritoneoscopy by Stephen Gans and thoracoscopy by Bradley Rodgers in the 1970s influenced the development of minimally invasive surgery (MIS) in children. Bax, George Holcomb, Craig Albanese, Thom Lobe, Frederick Rescorla, Azad Najmaldin, Gordon MacKinlay, Keith Georgeson, Steven Rothenberg, C. K. Yeung, Jean-Luc Alain, Jean-Stephane Valla, Nguyen Thanh Liem, Felix Schier, Benno Ure, Marcelo Martinez-Ferro, and others have been the early international leaders in pediatric MIS.

CANADA

As events in children's surgery were unfolding in the United States, Canadian pediatric surgery was experiencing a parallel evolution. References have already been made above to some of the clinical and research contributions made in Canada. Alexander Forbes, an orthopedic surgeon, played a leading role at the Montreal Children's Hospital from 1904 to 1929. Dudley Ross was chief-of-surgery at Montreal Children's Hospital from 1937 to 1954 and established the first modern children's surgical unit in Quebec. In 1948, he performed the first successful repair of esophageal atresia in Canada.[41] David Murphy served as chief of pediatric surgery and director of the pediatric surgical training program from 1954 to 1974. He was assisted by Herbert Owen and Gordon Karn, and his first trainee in 1954 was Harvey Beardmore.[42] Beardmore served as chief-of-surgery from 1974 to 1981 and was followed by Frank Guttman from 1981 to 1994 and Jean-Martin Laberge after that. The Sainte-Justine Hospital in Montreal, was founded in 1907. The hospital was combined with the Francophone Obstetrical Unit of Montreal, creating one of the largest maternal/child care centers in North America. Pierre-Paul Collin arrived at the hospital in 1954 after training in thoracic surgery in St. Louis, bringing a commitment to child care. He recruited Jacques Ducharme, who had trained in pediatric surgery in Columbus, Ohio, to join him in 1960. They trained a number of leaders in pediatric surgery in

Canada, including Frank Guttman, Hervé Blanchard, Salam Yazbeck, Jean-Martin Laberge, and Dickens St.-Vil. Jean Desjardins became chief in 1986.

The Hospital for Sick Children in Toronto was established in 1875 by Mrs. Samuel McMaster, whose husband founded McMaster University in Ontario.[42] As was the case in the United States, adult surgeons operated on children in Toronto at the end of the 19th and beginning of the 20th centuries. Clarence Starr, an orthopedic surgeon, was the first chief-of-surgery from 1913 to 1921. W. Edward Gallie served as chief surgeon at the Hospital for Sick Children from 1921 to 1929 and was named chair of surgery at the University of Toronto, where he established the Gallie surgical training program. The Gallie School of Surgery in Canada was compared with that of Halsted at Johns Hopkins in the United States.[42] Because of increasing responsibilities as chair, Gallie relinquished his role as chief of pediatric surgery to Donald Robertson, a thoracic surgeon who held the post until 1944. Arthur Lemesurer, a plastic and orthopedic surgeon became chief and in 1949 began a general pediatric surgical training program that produced Clinton Stephens, James Simpson, Robert Salter, Phillip Ashmore, Donald Marshall, and Stanley Mercer, to name some of the illustrious graduates who became leaders in the field of pediatric surgery in Canada.[14,42] In 1956, Alfred Farmer became surgeon-in-chief at the Hospital for Sick Children and developed several specialty surgical divisions, including one for general pediatric surgery. This allowed for separate specialty leadership under direction of Stewart Thomson from 1956 to 1966. Clinton Stephens was chief from 1966 to 1976 and was ably supported by James Simpson and Barry Shandling. During these 2 decades there was an impressive roster of graduates, including Phillip Ashmore, Gordon Cameron, Samuel Kling, Russell Marshall, Geoffrey Seagram, and Sigmund Ein. The tradition of excellence in pediatric surgery was continued with the appointment of Robert Filler, who arrived from Boston in 1977. Jacob Langer is the current chief of pediatric surgery in Toronto. From the latter three key surgical centers, leadership and progress in pediatric surgery spread across the Canadian provinces with the same comprehensive effect seen in the United States. Colin Ferguson, who trained with Gross in Boston, became chief-of-surgery in Winnipeg. Stanley Mercer began the pediatric surgery effort in Ottawa; there was also Samuel Kling, in Edmonton, where he was joined by Gordon Lees and James Fischer, and Geoffrey Seagram in Calgary. In 1957, Phillip Ashmore was the first trained pediatric surgeon in Vancouver, and he was joined by Marshall and Kliman, who trained at Great Ormond Street. In 1967, Graham Fraser, who also trained at Great Ormond Street joined the Vancouver group and became director of the training program. He was succeeded by Geoffrey Blair. Alexander Gillis trained with Potts and Swenson in Chicago and, in 1961, was the first pediatric surgeon in Halifax, Nova Scotia. He started the training program there in 1988. Gordon Cameron, a Toronto graduate, was the first chief of pediatric surgery at McMasters University in Hamilton. Currently, Peter Fitzgerald is head of the training program in Hamilton, which was approved in 2008.[42] The Canadian Association of Pediatric Surgeons (CAPS) was formed in 1967, three years before APSA, with Beardmore serving as the first president and Barry Shandling as secretary.[43] There are currently eight accredited pediatric surgery training programs in Canada: Halifax, Montreal Children's Hospital, Sainte-Justine Hospital in Montreal, Children's Hospital of Eastern Ontario

in Ottawa, Hospital for Sick Children in Toronto, Hamilton, Calgary, Alberta, and Vancouver. All these programs are approved by the Royal College of Surgeons of Canada, and candidates for training match along with the U.S. programs through the NRMP.

UNITED KINGDOM AND IRELAND

In 1852, the Hospital for Sick Children at Great Ormond Street (HSC) opened its doors in a converted house in London.[44] The hospital was the brainchild of Charles West, whose philosophy was that children with medical diseases required special facilities and attention, but those with surgical disorders at the time, mostly trauma related, could be treated in general hospitals.[44] West opposed the appointment of a surgeon to the staff, but the board disagreed and appointed G.D. Pollock. Pollock soon resigned and was replaced by Athol Johnson in 1853. T. Holmes, who followed Johnson, published his 37-chapter book, *Surgical Treatment of the Diseases of Infancy and Childhood,* in 1868.[45] Pediatric care in the 19th century either followed the pattern established in Paris, where all children were treated in hospitals specially oriented toward child care, or the Charles West approach, common in Britain,[46] such as those in Birmingham and Edinburgh, established to provide medical treatment but not surgery for children. In contrast, the Board at the Royal Hospital for Sick Children in Glasgow (RHSC) appointed equal numbers of medical and surgical specialists.[14,47] A major expansion in children's surgery in the latter part of the 19th century followed the development of ether and chloroform anesthesia and the gradual acceptance of antiseptic surgery. Joseph Lister provided the main impetus for antiseptic surgery, which he developed in Glasgow before moving to Edinburgh and then to King's College, London. One of Lister's young assistants in Glasgow was William Macewen, known as the father of neurosurgery, and one of the original surgeons appointed to the RHSC.[14] In Scotland, where pediatric care was generally ahead of the rest of Britain, the Royal Edinburgh Hospital for Sick Children (REHSC) opened in 1860 but did not provide a surgical unit until 1887. The sewing room was used as an operating theater.[48] Joseph Bell, President of the Royal College of Surgeons of Edinburgh, Harold Styles, John Fraser, and James J. Mason Brown, also a president of the Royal College of Surgeons of Edinburgh were the senior surgeons from 1887 to 1964. Gertrude Hertzfeld held a surgical appointment at the REHSC from 1919 to 1947, one of the few women surgeons of that era.[46] In the 19th century, training in pediatric surgery, independent of general surgery in the United Kingdom, occurred in Glasgow. Soon after these hospitals opened, their boards recognized the need for developing dispensaries or outpatient departments. In Manchester, the dispensary actually preceded the hospital. Dispensaries handled many surgical patients, and much of the pediatric surgery of the day was done there. One of the outstanding surgeons of that generation was James Nicoll, who reported 10 years of his work in 1909,[49] one of more than 100 of his publications. He was the "father of day surgery," although only part of his time was devoted to children's surgery because he had a substantial adult practice.[50] He performed pyloromyotomy with success in the late 19th century in a somewhat different fashion from Ramstedt. The Board of the RHSC decided that both physicians or surgeons appointed to the hospital must devote all their professional time to the treatment of children. In 1919, the University of Glasgow received funding to establish both medical and surgical lectureships, the first academic appointments in Britain. Alex MacLennan was appointed Barclay lecturer in surgical and orthopedic diseases of children at the University of Glasgow from 1919 to 1938. His successor, Matthew White, the Barclay lecturer in 1938, was a thoracic and abdominal surgeon. Mr. Wallace Dennison and Dan Young were among the other surgeons who later filled these posts. In Edinburgh, the children's surgical services and the adult services remained closely associated until Mason Brown became the chief.[14]

Modern pediatric surgery was a development that had to wait until after World War II. Introduction of the National Health Service in Britain, which provided access to care for all citizens, the development of the plastics industry, and many other technical innovations in the mid-20th century, allowed great strides, particularly in neonatal surgery and critical care.[14] In London, and elsewhere in England, general surgeons who were interested in pediatric surgery carried on their pediatric practices in conjunction with their adult practices. Financial considerations influenced their activities, because few were able to earn a living in pediatric surgical practice alone. However, further developments in the specialty were closely related to committed individuals.

Denis Browne, an Australian who stayed in London after serving in WWI, was appointed to the HSC in London in 1924. Browne was the first surgeon in London to confine his practice to pediatric surgery, and he is recognized as the pioneer of the specialty in the United Kingdom.[51-53] He was a tall impressive figure with a somewhat domineering, authoritative manner (Fig. 1-8). Browne's longtime colleague James Crooks called him an "intellectual adventurer, a rebel and a cynic."[51] After World War II, many surgeons from overseas spent time in the United Kingdom; the majority visited the HSC, where they were influenced by Browne. Some subsequently established internationally recognized centers such as Louw in South Africa, and Stephens and Smith in Australia. Browne's major interest was structural orthopedic anomalies, and as an original thinker, he achieved widespread recognition for promoting intrauterine position and pressure as a cause of these deformities.[53] He developed instruments, retractors, and splints to assist in his work, all named after himself. His early contemporaries were L. Barrington-Ward and T. Twistington Higgins, surgeons of considerable stature. It was Higgins who initially held discussions in London that led to the formation of the British Association of Pediatric Surgeons (BAPS) in 1953. Browne became the association's first and longest-serving president. The Denis Browne Gold Medal, an award given by the BAPS, remains a symbol of his presence and demonstrates his views (Fig. 1-9). In his later years in the National Health Service, his colleagues included George McNab, introducer of the Holter valve for hydrocephalus; David Waterston, an early pediatric cardiothoracic surgeon; and David Innes Williams, doyen pediatric urologist of Britain.[14] Each of these outstanding men made major contributions to the development of pediatric surgery. Many young surgeons continued to flock to HSC in London for training in pediatric surgery, including Nate Myers, Barry O'Donnell, H.H. Nixon and others. Andrew Wilkinson replaced Browne as surgeon-in-chief. Many other developments were also taking place. Wilkinson in London and Knutrud in Oslo were studying infant metabolism. Isabella Forshall, later joined by Peter Rickham, established an excellent clinical service in Liverpool. She was one of the few female pediatric surgeons of the time and was president of the BAPS in 1959. Pediatric surgery services were established in Sheffield by Robert Zachary, and in Manchester, Newcastle, Birmingham, Southampton, Bristol, Nottingham, and Leeds. Lewis Spitz from South Africa trained at Alder Hey Hospital in Liverpool with Peter Rickham in 1970. After a brief stay in Johannesburg, he immigrated to the United Kingdom to work with Zachary in Sheffield in 1974. He was then named the Nuffield Professor and head at Great Ormond Street, London and provided excellent leadership and strong surgical discipline at the HSC, leading by example for many years, until 2004 when he retired. His main areas of expertise included esophageal surgery, congenital hyperinsulinism, and separation of conjoined twins.[54,55] His colleagues included Kiely, Brereton, Drake, and Pierro. The latter established a strong research base at the institution and succeeded Spitz as the Nuffield Professor.

IRELAND

In 1922, Ireland was divided into six northern counties under British rule and 26 southern counties that became the Republic of Ireland. The first children's hospital in Ireland was in the south, the National Children's Hospital, opening on Harcourt Street in Dublin in 1821.[56] The Children's University Hospital in Dublin was founded on Temple Street in 1872. John Shanley, a general surgeon, was appointed to the Temple Street facility and devoted all his surgical activities to children. Another general surgeon, Stanley McCollum, worked at the National Hospital and did pediatric surgery at the Rotunda at the Maternity Hospital. A third children's hospital, Our Lady's Hospital for

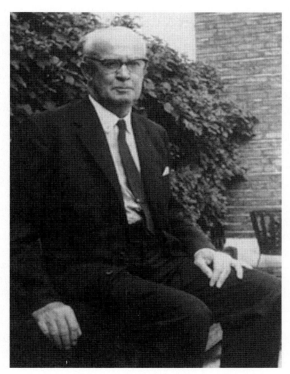

FIGURE 1-8   Sir Denis Browne, London, United Kingdom.

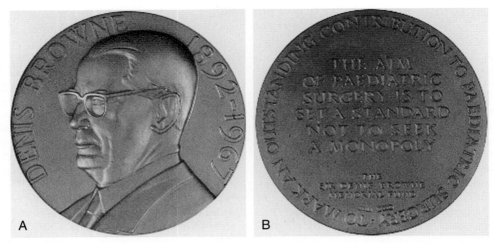

FIGURE 1-9   Denis Browne Gold Medal. **A,** Front of the medal. **B,** Back of the medal, which reads, "The aim of paediatric surgery is to set a standard not to seek a monopoly."

Sick Children, managed by the Daughters of Charity of St. Vincent De Paul, opened in 1956 in Crumlin. Barry O'Donnell was the first full-time, fully trained pediatric surgeon at this facility. Each of the children's hospitals had an academic affiliation, the National Hospital with Trinity College, and Temple Street and Our Lady's with The Royal College of Surgeons University College. Edward Guiney was added to the consultant staff of Our Lady's in 1966 and also was appointed to Temple Street and assisted McCollum at the National Children's Hospital, Dublin. From 1979 to 1993, Ray Fitzgerald, Prem Puri, and Martin Corbally were added as consultant pediatric surgeons. Following Barry O'Donnell's retirement in 1991 and Guiney stepping down in 1993, Fergal Quinn was eventually named to replace him. The Children's Research Center was developed in 1971, with Guiney appointed as director in 1976. He was replaced by Prem Puri, who has mentored numerous overseas research fellows and provided outstanding research concerning many neonatal and childhood conditions. O'Donnell conceived and Puri developed the innovative sting procedure to endoscopically treat vesicoureteral reflux, initially by Teflon injection and subsequently with Deflux. O'Donnell, Guiney, and Fitzgerald have served as presidents of the BAPS. Both O'Donnell and Puri are Denis Browne Gold Medal recipients and achieved international stature. Fitzgerald was president of European Pediatric Surgeons Association (EUPSA) and IPSO, and O'Donnell was president of the Royal College of Surgeons of Ireland. Puri served as president of EUPSA and the WOFAPS (World Federation of Associations of Pediatric Surgeons)

Pediatric surgery in Northern Ireland developed more slowly. Brian Smyth, who trained at Great Ormond Street and Alder Hey Hospitals, was appointed the first specialist pediatric surgeon consultant in 1959. He was joined by a Scotsman, William Cochran, who trained in Edinburgh. Following training in Newcastle and Cape Town, Victor Boston was added as a pediatric surgery consultant in 1975. Political unrest and economic constraints placed some limitations on growth in the north. Cochran returned to Scotland, and in 1995, McCallion was added as a consultant. Today they have similar standards to the southern centers in Ireland.

EUROPE

Europe served as the cradle of pediatric surgery, but because of space limitations, only the major developments and leading figures can be discussed. In France, the Hôpital des Enfants Malades has a long and storied history, starting with the contributions of Guersant, Giraldes, and de Saint-Germain from 1840 to 1898.[57] Most of their work involved orthopedic conditions and the management of infectious problems. Kirmisson, also well-versed in orthopedic disorders, was appointed the first professor of pediatric surgery in 1899 and published a pediatric surgical textbook in 1906 that contained radiologic information and discussed osteomyelitis and some congenital anomalies. In 1914, Broca described the management of intussusception, instances of megacolon, and experience with Ramstedt's operation for pyloric stenosis. He was succeeded by Ombredanne, a self-taught pediatric surgeon whose works were published by Fevre in 1944.[58] Petit performed the first successful repair of type C esophageal atresia in France in 1949. Because of two world wars, intervals of foreign occupation, and long periods of recovery in all of Europe, it was some time after WWII before modern pediatric surgery could develop in this part of the world. Following WWII, Bernard Duhamel was at the Hôpital des Enfantes Malades but moved to St. Denis, where he devised the retrorectal pull-through for Hirschsprung disease, an alternative procedure to the Swenson operation in 1956 (Fig. 1-10).[59] He was the first editor of *Chirurgie Pediatrique,* started in 1960. Denys Pellerin became chief-of-surgery at the Hôpital des Enfantes Malades and developed a strong department at the institution until he retired in 1990. His successor was Claire Nihoul-Fekete, the first female professor of pediatric surgery in France. Fekete was recognized for her stylish demeanor and expertise in intersex surgery, esophageal anomalies, and congenital hyperinsulinism. She was succeeded by Yann Revillion, an international leader in intestinal transplantation. Yves Aigran plays a leadership role as well. Elsewhere, Michel Carcassone, who developed pediatric surgery in Marseille, had expertise in treating portal hypertension and was an early advocate of a primary pull-through procedure for Hirschsprung disease. He also served as the

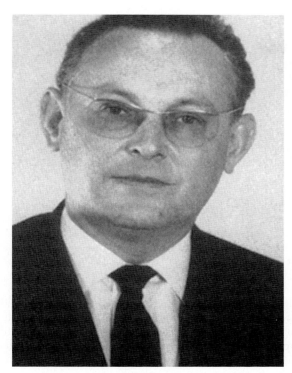

FIGURE 1-10   Bernard Duhamel, Paris, France.

editor-for-Europe for the *Journal of Pediatric Surgery*. J.M. Guys is currently chief in Marseilles. Prevot was the first leader in Nancy. The Société Francaise de Chirurgie Infantile was established in 1959, with Fevre as the first president. The group changed its name to the French Society of Pediatric Surgery in 1983. A strong pediatric oncology presence has existed in Villejuif for many years, initially under the direction of Mme. Odile Schwiesgut.

Pediatric surgical development in Scandinavia also has a rich history. In Sweden, The Princess Lovisa Hospital in Stockholm opened in 1854, but it was not until 1885 that a surgical unit was added under the direction of a general surgeon.[60,61] The first pediatric surgery unit was actually started at the Karolinska Hospital in 1952 and was transferred to St. Gorans Hospital in 1982. In 1998, all pediatric surgery in Stockholm was moved to the newly constructed Astrid Lindgren Children's Hospital at Karolinska University. Three other major pediatric surgery centers were developed in Gothenberg, Uppsala, and Lund. Philip Sandblom was appointed chief-of-surgery at Lovisa from 1945 to 1950, and then he moved to Lund and, later, Lausanne as chief-of-surgery. He was succeeded by Theodor Ehrenpreis, who moved to the Karolinska Pediatric Clinic in 1952. He had a strong interest in research in Hirschsprung disease. Gunnar Ekstrom took his place, and he was succeeded by Nils Ericsson, whose major interest was pediatric urology. Bjorn Thomasson became chief at St. Gorans in 1976. Tomas Wester is the current chief in Stockholm. Gustav Peterson was the initial chief of pediatric surgery in Gothenberg. Ludvig Okmian became the chief of pediatric surgery in Lund in 1969 and helped develop the infant variant of the Engstrom ventilator, and along with Livaditis, employed circular myotomy for long gap esophageal atresia. In 1960, Gunnar Grotte was appointed the first chief of pediatric surgery in Uppsala. He was joined by Leif Olsen, and their major

interests included pediatric urology, Hirschsprung disease, and metabolism. The Swedish Pediatric Surgical Association was formed in 1952, and Swedes also participate in the Scandinavian Association of Pediatric Surgeons, founded in 1964.

In Finland, pediatric surgery developed after WWII. Mattie Sulamaa, the pioneer in Finland, was the first to work in the new children's hospital in Helsinki, which opened in 1946. He was instrumental in introducing pediatric anesthesiology. He trained young students, who later started programs at children's hospitals in Turku and Oulu, and university centers in Tampere and Kuopio. He retired in 1973 and was succeeded by Ilmo Louhimo, who specialized in cardiothoracic surgery. He trained Harry Lindahl and Risto Rintala. Rintala is the current chief at Helsinki Children's Hospital and is well recognized for his expertise in pediatric colorectal surgery. Lindahl is a leader in upper gastrointestinal surgery, endoscopy, and the management of esophageal atresia.

There were no children's hospitals in Norway. However, pediatric surgery was strongly influenced by Ola Knutrud of Oslo, beginning in 1962 when he was appointed chief of pediatric surgery at the University Rikshospital. He was an early leader in the field, with interest in pediatric fluid and electrolyte balance, metabolism, fat nutrition, and congenital diaphragmatic hernia. In 1975, Torbjorn Kufaas was named chief of pediatric surgery at the University Hospital in Trondheim.

In Denmark, the first children's hospital opened in1850 and moved to a new facility named after Queen Louise in 1879, with Harald Hirschsprung, a pediatrician appointed as chief physician. Hirschsprung's interests centered on surgical problems, including esophageal atresia, intussusception, ileal atresia, pyloric stenosis, and congenital megacolon.[62] C. Winkel Smith and Tyge Gertz initiated pediatric surgery at University Hospital in Copenhagen, with the latter performing the first successful repair of esophageal atresia in Denmark in 1949. Smith mysteriously disappeared in 1962 but was not declared deceased until 1968.[63] Knud Mauritzen was named his successor as director of pediatric surgery in Copenhagen. Ole Nielsen, a urologic surgeon, succeeded him. Carl Madsen became consultant surgeon at Odense University Hospital; however, there is no department of pediatric surgery there or in Arhus, where pediatric urology and children's surgery are performed in the Department of Urology or Surgery. The only Danish department of pediatric surgery exists in Copenhagen. Although the Danish governmental specialty rules listed pediatric surgery as a specialty in 1958, this was rescinded in 1971 and has not been restored.[63]

Modern pediatric surgery in Switzerland starts with the pioneer in that country, Max Grob. A native of Zurich, he trained in general surgery with Clairmont in Zurich in 1936 and then spent 6 months in Paris at the Hôpital des Enfantes Malades under Ombredanne. He returned to Zurich and entered private practice. It was during WWII that he was appointed to replace Monnier, a general surgeon in charge at the Children's Hospital, whom he met during training. His pediatric surgical practice was quite varied and included plastic surgery and cardiac surgery.[64] He modified Duhamel's operation for Hirschsprung disease and did the first hiatal hernia repair in a child in Switzerland. He trained a new generation of pediatric surgeons in Zurich, including Marcel Bettex, Noel Genton, and Margrit Stockman. The Swiss Society of Pediatric Surgery was formed in 1969, with Grob as its first president.[65] Peter Paul Rickham moved from Liverpool to succeed Grob in Zurich in 1971. Marcel Bettex developed a separate department of pediatric surgery in Bern, as did Noel Genton in Lausanne, Alois Scharli in Luzern, Anton Cuendet in Geneva, and Nicole in Basel. Urs Stauffer replaced Professor Rickham as chief in Zurich in 1983. Martin Meuli is the current chief in Zurich. Claude Lecoutre succeeded Cuendet in Geneva. The current chief there is Barbara Wildhaber. Peter Herzog is presently chief in Basel, Marcus Schwoebel in Lausanne, and Zachariah Zachariou in Bern. Alois Scharli began the journal *Pediatric Surgery International* in 1985 and served as editor-in-chief for 18 years, followed by Puri and Coran as the current co–editors-in-chief.

In Germany, pediatric care began with the development of children's hospital facilities in various cities across the country, most notably, in Munich, Cologne, and Berlin. Early contributions from Max Wilms in Liepzig and Conrad Ramstedt in Münster have been previously noted.[17,20] Progress was somewhat hampered by war, political and social unrest, and the separation of the country into East Germany and West Germany during the occupation following WW II. Children's surgical units developed either in university settings within adult hospitals or in independent children's hospitals. The contributions of Anton Oberniedermayr and Waldemar Hecker in Munich, who was the first professor of pediatric surgery in the Federal Republic of Germany, Fritz Rehbein in Bremen, and Wolfgang Maier in Kahrlsruhe are well recognized.[66] Fritz Rehbein's clinic in Bremen attracted many young men to train there. He was a thoughtful and resourceful pediatric surgical leader who contributed much to patient care, including the Rehbein strut for pectus excavatum, modifications in esophageal surgery, low pelvic anterior resection for Hirschsprung disease (the Rehbein procedure),[67,68] and a sacral approach with rectomucosectomy of the atretic rectum with abdominoperineal pull-through for high imperforate

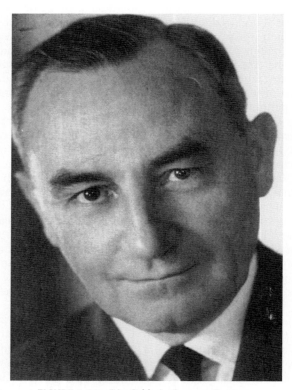

FIGURE 1-11 Fritz Rehbein, Bremen, Germany.

anus (Fig. 1-11). He was a founding editor of *Zeitschrift Kinderchirurgie* in 1964, which was the precursor of the *European Journal of Pediatric Surgery* following merger with the French journal *Chirurgie Pedaitrique* in 1990. Alex Holschneider was editor from 1980 to 2007, and Benno Ure of Hannover has been the editor-in-chief since 2007. Many of Rehbein's trainees went on to leadership roles in other European cities, including Michael Hoellwarth (Graz), Alex Holschneider (Cologne), Pepe Boix-Ochoa (Barcelona), and others. He was recognized throughout Europe as a leader in the field and was a recipient of the Denis Browne Gold Medal from the BAPS and many other awards. His contributions to European pediatric surgery are recognized by the establishment of the Rehbein Medal, awarded each year by the EUPSA, representing 28 countries in Europe. In West Germany, pediatric surgery was not recognized as an independent specialty until 1984. Following the fall of the Berlin Wall and the reunification of Germany in 1990, the 33 East German pediatric surgery programs joined those of the West from the Federal Republic of Germany and formed a joint German Society of Pediatric Surgery.

In Italy, early evidence of a hospital devoted to children dates back to the 15th century with the Hospital of the Innocents in Florence, which was more of a foundling home than a hospital. Other facilities for sick children were documented in the 1800s in many Italian cities. The first hospital dedicated to children's surgery was in Naples in 1880. In Milan in 1897, Formiggini was the surgeon-in-charge, and he eventually started the first Italian pediatric surgical journal, *Archivio di Chirurgia Infantile,* in 1934. It was a short-lived effort, however. Once again WW II delayed progress. Carlo Montagnani spent 18 months in Boston in 1949 and returned to Florence, where he translated Gross' textbook into Italian. He had a productive career as a pioneer pediatric surgeon. He organized the Italian Society of Pediatric Surgery in 1964, with Pasquale Romualdi of Rome serving as the first president. That was the same year Franco Soave of Genoa described the endorectal pull-through for Hirschsprung disease (Fig. 1-12). In 1992, the Italian journal ceased to publish, and the *European Journal of Pediatric Surgery* became the official journal of the Italian Society. Major advances in the management of neonatal conditions, childhood tumors, Hirschsprung disease, esophageal disorders, and pediatric urology have emanated from Italy in the past 2 decades from centers in Rome, Milan, Genoa, Naples, Pavia, Florence, Bologna, Turin, and others.

In the Netherlands, the first children's hospital was opened in Rotterdam in 1863, with eight beds located in a first-floor apartment. The children's hospital in Amsterdam followed in 1865 in an old orphanage. In 1899, the name of the facility was changed to Emma Children's Hospital, after the Queen. Volunteer adult surgeons did whatever children's surgical work that presented. Throughout the rest of the 19th century, additional children's facilities sprung up in other cities. R.J. Harrenstein was the first full-time surgeon appointed at the Emma Children's Hospital. In the 1970s, Born at The Hague and David Vervat in Rotterdam dedicated themselves to children's care. Vervat was also an early editorial consultant for the *Journal of Pediatric Surgery.* Jan Molenaar trained with Vervat and eventually replaced him at Erasmus University in Rotterdam in 1972. Molenaar served as the editor-for-Europe for the *Journal of Pediatric Surgery.* Franz Hazebroeck replaced Molenaar as chief in 1998, and Klaas Bax subsequently succeeded Hazebroeck. The Rotterdam school focused on basic

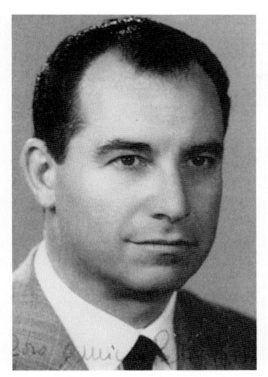

FIGURE 1-12 Franco Soave, Genoa, Italy.

science research and a high level of clinical care. Anton Vos spent time in Boston with Gross and Folkman and later returned to Amsterdam as an associate of Professor Mak Schoorl. In 1991, he was appointed professor of pediatric surgery at the University of Amsterdam with a strong focus on pediatric oncology. Hugo Heij succeeded Vos as chief in 1999. Currently there are five pediatric surgery training programs in the Netherlands located in Rotterdam, Amsterdam, Utrecht, Nijmegen, and Groningen. Trainees are certified by the European Board of Pediatric Surgery (EBPS), sponsored by the Union of European Medical Specialties (EUMS).

In Spain, the modern day pioneers included Julio Monoreo, who was appointed the first head of pediatric surgery at the Hospital of the University of La Paz, Madrid in 1965. Pepe Boix-Ochoa filled the same role at Hospital Valle de Hebron in Barcelona. Juan Tovar succeeded Monoreo after his passing. In the 1970s and 1980s, major regional pediatric surgical centers were located in numerous cities around the country. The Spanish Pediatric Surgical Association was formed as an independent group for pediatrics in 1984. Tovar is the current editor-for-Europe for the *Journal of Pediatric Surgery* and served as president of EUPSA.

Other leaders in Europe included Aurel Koos, Imre Pilaszanovich, and Andras Pinter in Hungary; Petropoulos, Voyatzis, Moutsouris Pappis, and Keramidis in Greece; Kafka, Tosovsky, and Skaba in the Czech Republic; Kossakowski, Kalicinski, Lodzinski, and Czernik in Poland; and Ivan Fattorini in Croatia. In Austria, the leaders in the field included Sauer and Hoellwarth in Graz, Rokitansky and Horcher in Vienna, Menardi in Innsbruck, Oesch in Salzburg, and Brandesky in Klangenfurt. In Turkey, Ihsan Numanoglu developed the first pediatric surgery service in Izmir in 1961. Akgun Hiksonmez started the program at Hacettepe

University in Ankara in 1963. Acun Gokdemir was an early pediatric urologist in Istanbul. Daver Yeker, Cenk Buyukunal, Nebil Buyukpamukcu, and Tolga Dagli are major contributors to contemporary Turkish pediatric surgery and urology. The Turkish Association of Pediatric Surgeons (TAPS) formed in 1977, with Hicsonmez elected the first president.

AUSTRALIA AND NEW ZEALAND

The first children's hospital opened in Melbourne, Australia in 1870.[69] In 1897, Clubbe performed a successful bowel resection for intussusception in Sydney. In 1899, Russell published the method of high ligation of an inguinal hernia sac. Hipsley described successful saline enema reduction of intussusception in 1927. As was the case elsewhere, pediatric surgery did not experience significant growth until after WW II. Howard performed the first successful repair of esophageal atresia in Melbourne in 1949. He was joined there by F. Douglas Stephens, who had spent time with Denis Browne in London, and he directed the research program at the Royal Melbourne Children's Hospital for many years. Bob Fowler and Durham Smith later joined the Melbourne group. They set a standard for investigation of malformations of the urinary tract and anorectum. Stephens developed the sacroperineal pull-through operation for high anorectal malformations. The pediatric surgery staff in Melbourne was exemplary and added Nate Myers, Peter Jones, Alex Auldist, Justin Kelley, Helen Noblett, and Max Kent to the group. Archie Middleton, Douglas Cohen, and Toby Bowring led the way in Sydney, Geoff Wylie in Adelaide, Alastair MacKellar in Perth, and Fred Leditschke in Brisbane.

Pediatric surgical contributions from Australia were considerable. Myers was an expert in esophageal atresia and provided the first long-term outcome studies.[70] Noblett promoted nonoperative gastrografin enema for simple meconium ileus and devised the first forceps for submucosal rectal biopsy for Hirschsprung disease.[71,72] Jones spearheaded the nonoperative management of torticollis and management of surgical infections. Fowler devised the long-loop vas operation for high undescended testis[73]; MacKellar instituted the first trauma prevention program; Kelly developed a scoring system for fecal incontinence and total repair of bladder exstrophy; and Smith and Stephens developed the Wingspread classification for anorectal malformations. Hutson's studies on the influence of hormones and the genitofemoral nerve on testicular descent and colonic motility, Cass' insights into the genetics of Hirschsprung disease, and Borzi and Tan's leadership in pediatric MIS are more recent examples of Australian contributions to the field. Pediatric surgery in New Zealand took longer to develop. There are now four major training centers in Auckland, Hamilton, and Wellington on the North Island and Christchurch on the South Island. Leaders include Morreau in Auckland, supported by Stuart Ferguson and others; Brown in Hamilton; Pringle in Wellington; and Beasley in Christchurch. A significant outreach program for the islands of the South Pacific is in place.

ASIA

There have been significant contributions to pediatric surgery from Japan, China, Taiwan, and other Asian countries following WW II. In China, Jin-Zhe Zhang in Beijing survived war, national turmoil, and the Cultural Revolution to emerge as that nation's father figure in children's surgery. Other early leaders included She Yan-Xiong and Ma in Shanghai and Tong in Wuhan. The latter was the first editor of the *Chinese Journal of Pediatric Surgery*. The first pediatric surgery congress in China was held in 1980, and the China Society of Pediatric Surgeons was formed in 1987. There is a new generation of pediatric surgeons, including Long Li, G-D Wang, and others. Major children's hospitals are now located in Beijing, Shanghai, Fudan, Shenyang, Wuhan, and many other mainland cities. The use of saline enemas under ultrasound guidance, as well as the introduction of the air-enema for reduction of intussusception, are examples of significant Chinese contributions. Paul Yue started the first pediatric surgery unit in Hong Kong in 1967. H. Thut Saing was appointed the first chair of pediatric surgery at the University of Hong Kong in 1979.[74] Paul Tam and CK Yeung trained with Saing and went on to have very productive careers. Tam spent time at Oxford in the United Kingdom and returned to become chair of pediatric surgery at the University of Hong Kong in 1996. Yeung succeeded Kelvin Liu as chief of pediatric surgery at the Chinese University Prince of Wales Hospital. Both Tam and Yeung provided pediatric surgery leadership in Hong Kong and have been productive in the study of the genetic implications of many surgical disorders, including Hirschsprung disease and neuroblastoma (Tam) and application of MIS, particularly in pediatric urology (Yeung).

V.T. Joseph was the first director of pediatric surgery in Singapore in 1981. Following his departure, Anette Jacobsen has been influential in further developing the specialty and providing strong leadership in children's surgery in Singapore.[74] Sootiporn Chittmittrapap, Sriwongse Havananda, and Niramis have been strong advocates in establishing a high level of pediatric surgical care in Thailand. In Vietnam, years of political strife and conflict delayed progress in children's surgery. Nguyen Thanh Liem has emerged as a leading contributor from Hanoi, with extensive experience in the use of MIS for managing a myriad of pediatric surgical conditions. There are now 13 pediatric surgical centers in Vietnam.[74]

In Japan, the first generation of pediatric surgeons appeared in the early 1950s: Ueda in Osaka, Suruga at Juntendo University in Tokyo, Kasai at Tohoku University in Sendai, and Ikeda at Kyushu University in Fukuoka. Suruga performed the first operation for intestinal atresia in 1952. Kasai performed the first hepatoportoenterostomy for uncorrectable biliary atresia in 1955 (Fig. 1-13), and Ueda performed the first successful repair of esophageal atresia in 1959.[14] The first children's hospital in the country was the National Children's Hospital in Tokyo, opened in 1965. The first department of pediatric surgery was established at Juntendo University in Tokyo in 1968 by Suruga (Fig. 1-14); today, training programs exist in nearly all the major university centers. The Japanese Society of Pediatric Surgeons and its journal were established in 1964, paralleling developments in other parts of the world. The second generation of pediatric surgeons include Okamoto and Okada in Osaka; Nakajo, Akiyama, Tsuchida, and Miyano in Tokyo; Ohi and Nio in Sendai; Suita in Fukuoka and Ken Kimura in Kobe and later in Iowa and Honolulu. These individuals made seminal contributions in the fields of nutrition, biliary and pancreatic disease, management of choledochal cyst, oncology, and intestinal disorders, including Hirschsprung

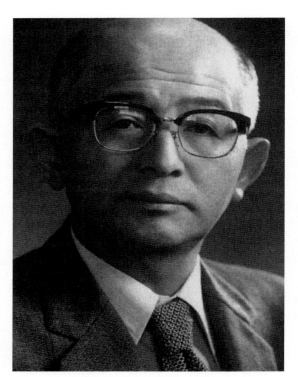

FIGURE 1-13 Morio Kasai, Sendai, Japan.

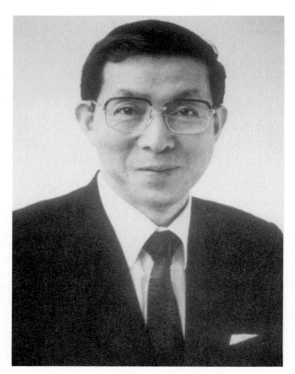

FIGURE 1-14 Keijiro Suruga, Tokyo, Japan.

disease, esophageal atresia, duodenal atresia, and tracheal reconstruction. In recent decades, laboratories and clinical centers in Asia, particularly in Japan and Hong Kong, have generated exciting new information in the clinical and basic biological sciences that continues to enrich the field of children's surgery.

DEVELOPING COUNTRIES

Nowhere in the world is the global burden of surgical disease more evident than in Africa. Pediatric surgery in underdeveloped areas of the world suffers from a lack of infrastructure, financial resources, and governmental support. In Africa, hepatitis B, malaria, malnutrition, human immunodeficiency virus–acquired immune deficiency virus (HIV-AIDS), and the ravages of political unrest and conflict play a major role in the higher childhood mortality noted on the continent. There are some exceptions, such as South Africa, where pediatric surgery is an established specialty with major children's centers in Cape Town, Johannesburg, Durban, Pretoria, and Bloemfontein; in Egypt with centers in Cairo and Alexandria; and in Nairobi, Kenya. The pioneer pediatric surgeon in South Africa was Jan Louw of Cape Town (Fig. 1-15). Collaborating with Christian Barnard in 1955, they demonstrated, in a fetal dog model, that most jejunoileal atresias were related to late intrauterine vascular accidents to the bowel and/or mesentery. Sidney Cywes succeeded Louw at the Red Cross Memorial Children's Hospital in 1975. He was the first surgeon in the country to limit his practice to children.

Cywes was joined in Cape Town by Michael Davies, Heinz Rode, Alastair Millar, Rob Brown, and Sam Moore. Millar is the current surgeon-in-chief. Michael Dinner was the first professor of pediatric surgery at Witwatersrand University in Johannesburg. Derksen and Jacobs started the pediatric surgery service in Pretoria and were succeeded by Jan Becker in 1980. R. Mikel was the first professor of pediatric surgery at

the University of Natal in Durban; he was succeeded by Larry Hadley. The South African Association of Pediatric Surgeons was formed in 1975, with Louw serving as its first president.[75] Major contributions to pediatric surgical care from South Africa include management of intersex, separation of conjoined twins, childhood burn care, pediatric surgical oncology, treatment of jejunoileal atresia, caustic esophageal injury, Hirschsprung disease, and liver transplantation. In 1994 in Nairobi, where pediatric surgery was pioneered by Julius Kyambi, the Pan African Pediatric Surgical Association (PAPSA) was established with pediatric surgeons from all the nations on the continent joining as members.

In India, the Association of Indian Surgeons first recognized pediatric surgery as a separate section in 1964. This organization subsequently became independent as the Indian Association of Pediatric Surgeons (IAPS) and met for the first time in New Delhi in 1966. Facilities for pediatric surgical care were limited to a few centers in metropolitan areas. Early leaders in the field included S. Chatterjee, R.K. Ghandi, P. Upadhaya, R.M. Ramakrishnan, V. Talwalker, and S. Dalal. Ms. Mridula Rohatgi was the first female professor of pediatric surgery. Professor Ghandi served as president of the WOFAPS, and presently, Professor Devendra Gupta of New Delhi is the president-elect of that organization. There are currently 24 pediatric surgery teaching centers in the country, all located in major cities. Rural care is still less than desirable, and there are only 710 pediatric surgeons to care for a population of 1.2 billion people.

Space limitations prevent individual mention of some other countries and deserving physicians who have made contributions to the field of pediatric surgery.

The discipline of pediatric surgery around the world is mature at this point and as sophisticated as any medical field. It has become a science-based enterprise in a high-technology environment. In the developed world, children with surgical problems have never been as fortunate as now. Pediatric surgery has truly become internationalized, with various countries developing national societies and striving to improve the surgical care of infants and children. The availability of the Internet to rapidly disseminate information has provided a method to share knowledge and information regarding patient care. The World Federation of Associations of Pediatric Surgeons (WOFAPS), which originated in 1974 and under the leadership of Professor Boix-Ochoa, the organization's secretary general, has grown and matured as an organization that now comprises more than 100 national associations.[76] It is an international voice for the specialty and sponsors a world congress of pediatric surgery every 3 years in a host country and provides education, support, and assistance to underdeveloped countries to improve the surgical care of infants and children. With children representing a higher percentage of the population in the developing world, this becomes an increasingly important factor in enhancing the global effort to provide better surgical care for children.

The complete reference list is available online at www.expertconsult.com.

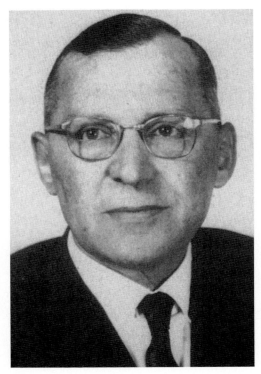

FIGURE 1-15   Professor Jan Louw, Cape Town, South Africa.

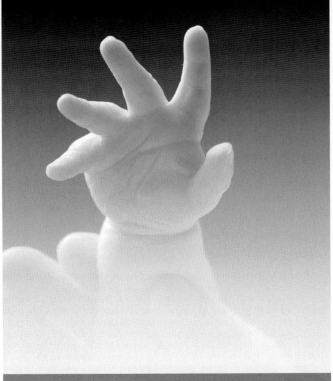

CHAPTER 2

Molecular Clinical Genetics and Gene Therapy

Alan W. Flake

The topics of this chapter are broad in scope and outside the realm of a classic core education in pediatric surgery. However both molecular genetics and gene therapy will be of increasing clinical importance in all medical specialties, including pediatric surgery, in the near future. A few conservative predictions include improvements in the diagnostic accuracy and prediction of phenotype, the development of new therapeutic options for many disorders, and the optimization of pharmacotherapy based on patient genotype, but there are many other possible uses. The goal here is to provide an overview of recent developments that are relevant or potentially relevant to pediatric surgery.

Molecular Clinical Genetics

Although hereditary disease has been recognized for centuries, only relatively recently has heredity become the prevailing explanation for numerous human diseases. Before the 1970s, physicians considered genetic diseases to be relatively rare and irrelevant to clinical care. With the advent of rapid advances in molecular genetics, we currently recognize that genes are critical factors in virtually all human diseases. Although an incomplete indicator, McKusick's *Mendelian Inheritance in Man* has grown from about 1500 entries in 1965[1] to 12,000 in 2010, documenting the acceleration of knowledge of human genetics. Even disorders that were once considered to be purely acquired, such as infectious diseases, are now recognized to be influenced by genetic mechanisms of inherent vulnerability and genetically driven immune system responses.

Despite this phenomenal increase in genetic information and the associated insight into human disease, until recently there was a wide gap between the identification of genotypic abnormalities that are linked to phenotypic manifestations in humans and any practical application to patient treatment. With the notable exceptions of genetic counseling and prenatal diagnosis, molecular genetics had little impact on the daily practice of medicine or more specifically on the practice of pediatric surgery. The promise of molecular genetics cannot be denied however. Identifying the fundamental basis of human disorders and of individual responses to environmental, pharmacologic, and disease-induced perturbations is the first step toward understanding the downstream pathways that may have a profound impact on clinical therapy. The ultimate application of genetics would be the correction of germline defects for affected individuals and their progeny. Although germline correction remains a future fantasy fraught with ethical controversy,[2] there is no question that molecular genetics will begin to impact clinical practice in myriad ways within the next decade. A comprehensive discussion of the field of molecular genetics is beyond the scope of this chapter, and there are many sources of information on the clinical genetics of pediatric surgical disorders.

HUMAN MOLECULAR GENETICS AND PEDIATRIC SURGICAL DISEASE

The rapid identification of genes associated with human disease has revolutionized the field of medical genetics, providing more accurate diagnostic, prognostic, and potentially therapeutic tools. However, increased knowledge is always associated with increased complexity. The classic model assumed that the spread of certain traits in families is associated with the transmission of a single molecular defect, with individual alleles segregating into families according to Mendel's laws, whereas today's model recognizes that very few phenotypes can be satisfactorily explained by a mutation at a single gene locus. The phenotypic diversity recognized in disorders that were once considered monogenic has led to a reconceptualization of genetic disease. Although mendelian models are useful for identifying the primary cause of familial disorders, they appear to be incomplete as models of the true physiologic and cellular nature of defects.[3-5] Numerous disorders that were initially characterized as monogenic are proving to be either caused or modulated by the action of a small number of loci. These disorders are described as oligogenic disorders, an evolving concept that encompasses a large spectrum of phenotypes that are neither monogenic nor polygenic. In contrast to polygenic or complex traits, which are thought to result from poorly understood interactions between many genes and the environment, oligogenic disorders are primarily genetic in cause but require the synergistic action of mutant alleles at

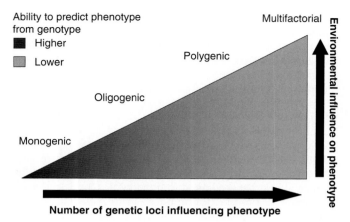

FIGURE 2-1 Conceptual continuum of modern molecular genetics. The genetic characterization of a disorder depends on (1) whether a major locus makes a dominant contribution to the phenotype, (2) the number of loci that influence the phenotype, and (3) the presence and extent of environmental influence on phenotype. The farther toward the right a disorder lies, the greater the complexity of the genetic analysis and the less predictive genotype is of phenotype.

a small number of loci. One can look at modern molecular genetics as a conceptual continuum between classic mendelian and complex traits (Fig. 2-1). The position of any given disorder along this continuum depends on three main variables: (1) whether a major locus makes a dominant contribution to the phenotype, (2) the number of loci that influence the phenotype, and (3) the presence and extent of environmental influence on the phenotype.

DISEASE-SPECIFIC EXAMPLES OF CHANGING CONCEPTS IN MOLECULAR GENETICS

Monogenic Disorders

Cystic fibrosis (CF) is an example of a disorder close to the monogenic end of the continuum, but it also illustrates the complexity of the genetics of some disorders, even when a mutation of a major locus is the primary determinant of phenotype. On the basis of the observed autosomal recessive inheritance in families, the gene *CFTR* (cystic fibrosis transmembrane conductance regulator) was first mapped in humans to chromosome 7q31.2.[6] Once the *CFTR* gene was cloned,[7] it was widely anticipated that mutation analyses might be sufficient to predict the clinical outcome of patients. However analyses of *CFTR* mutations in large and ethnically diverse cohorts indicated that this assumption was an oversimplification of the true genetic nature of this phenotype, particularly with respect to the substantial phenotypic variability observed in some patients with CF. For instance, although *CFTR* mutations show a degree of correlation with the severity of pancreatic disease, the severity of the pulmonary phenotype, which is the main cause of mortality, is difficult to predict.[8–10] Realization of the limitations of a pure monogenic model prompted an evaluation of more complex inheritance schemes. This led to the mapping of a modifier locus for the intestinal component of CF in both human and mouse.[11,12] Further phenotypic analysis led to the discovery of several other loci linked to phenotype, including (1) the association of low-expressing mannose-binding lectin (*MBL2*; previously known as *MBL*) alleles, human leukocyte antigen

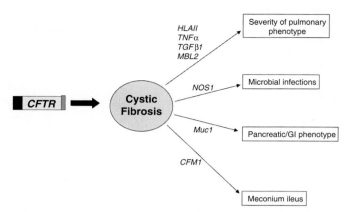

FIGURE 2-2 Complexity in monogenic diseases. Mutations in the *cystic fibrosis transmembrane conductance regulator* (*CFTR*) almost always cause the cystic fibrosis (CF) phenotype. Owing to modification effects by other genetic factors, the presence and nature of mutations at the *CFTR* locus cannot predict the phenotypic manifestation of the disease. Therefore, although CF is considered a mendelian recessive disease, the phenotype in each patient depends on a discrete number of alleles at different loci. *CFM1*, cystic fibrosis modifier 1; *GI*, gastrointestinal; *HLAII*, major histocompatibility complex class II antigen; *MBL2*, mannose-binding lectin (protein C) 2; *Muc1*, mucin 1; *NOS1*, nitric oxide synthase 1; *TGFB1*, transforming growth factor-β1; *TNF*, tumor necrosis factor encoding gene.

(HLA) class II polymorphisms, and variants in tumor necrosis factor-α (*TNFA*) and transforming growth factor-β1 (*TGFB1*) with pulmonary aspects of the disease;[13–16] (2) the correlation of intronic nitric oxide synthase 1 (*NOS1*) polymorphisms with variability in the frequency and severity of microbial infections[17]; and (3) the contribution of mucin 1 (*Muc1*) to the gastrointestinal aspects of the CF phenotype in mice (Fig. 2-2).[18] Further layers of complexity have been discovered for both *CFTR* and its associated phenotype. First, heterozygous CF mutations have been associated with susceptibility to rhinosinusitis, an established polygenic trait.[19] Second, and perhaps more surprising, a study group reported that some patients with a milder CF phenotype do not have any mutations in *CFTR*. This indicates that the hypothesis that *CFTR* gene dysfunction is a requisite for the development of CF might not be true.[20] Identification of these and many other gene modifiers and appreciation of their importance in this and other diseases is a major step forward. Although at the present time, the effects of these polymorphisms are incompletely understood, such findings could lead to potential therapeutic targets for CF or identification of risk factors early in life.

Oligogenic Disorders

Recent developments in defining the molecular genetics of Hirschsprung disease (HD) exemplify a relatively new concept in genetics—the oligogenic disorder. Although mathematic analyses of oligogenicity are beyond the scope of this discussion,[21,22] it is important to recognize that modifications of traditional linkage approaches are useful tools for the study of oligogenic diseases, especially if a major locus that contributes greatly to the phenotype is known. In the case of HD, two main phenotypic groups can be distinguished on the basis of the extent of aganglionosis: short-segment HD (S-HD) and the more severe long-segment HD (L-HD). Autosomal dominant inheritance with incomplete penetrance has been proposed for L-HD, whereas complex inheritance that involves an autosomal recessive trait has been observed in S-HD. Oligogenicity has been established in both HD variants by virtue of several factors: a recurrence risk that varies from 3% to 25%, depending on the length of aganglionosis and the sex of the patient; heritability values close to 100%, which indicates an exclusively genetic basis; significant clinical variability and reduced penetrance; and nonrandom association of hypomorphic changes in the endothelin receptor type B (EDNRB) with rearranged during transfection (RET) polymorphisms and HD.[23,24] So far a combination of linkage, positional cloning studies, and functional candidate gene analyses has identified eight HD genes (Table 2-1),[25] of which the proto-oncogene RET is thought to be the main predisposing locus,[26,27] particularly in families with a high incidence of L-HD.[28]

The non-mendelian transmission of HD has hindered the identification of predisposing modifier loci by conventional linkage approaches. When these approaches (parametric and nonparametric linkage studies) were carried out on a group of 12 L-HD families, very weak linkage was observed on chromosome 9q31. However based on the hypothesis that only milder RET mutations could be associated with another locus, families were categorized according to the RET mutational data. Significant linkage on chromosome 9q31 was detected when families with potentially weak RET mutations were analyzed independently,[27] indicating that mild RET alleles, in conjunction with alleles at an unknown gene on chromosome 9, might be required for pathogenesis. The mode of inheritance in S-HD has proved to be more complex than that in L-HD, requiring further adjustments to the linkage strategies. Recently the application of model-free linkage, without assumptions about the number and inheritance mode of segregating factors, showed that a three-locus segregation was both necessary and sufficient to manifest S-HD, with RET being the main locus, and that the transmission of susceptibility alleles was additive.[28]

The inheritance patterns observed in disorders such as HD illustrate the power of both expanded models of disease inheritance that account for reduced penetrance and phenotypic variability and the ability of these models to genetically map loci involved in oligogenic diseases, which is a first step toward identifying their underlying genes. More important, the establishment of non-mendelian models caused a change of perception in human genetics, which in turn accelerated the discovery of oligogenic traits.

Polygenic or Complex Disorders

Polygenic or complex disorders are thought to result from poorly understood interactions between many genes and the environment. An example of a polygenic disorder relevant to pediatric surgery is hypertrophic pyloric stenosis (HPS). The genetic cause of HPS has long been recognized, with frequent familial aggregation, a concordance rate of 25% to 40% in monogenetic twins, a recurrence rate of 10% for males and 2% for females born after an affected child, and a ratio of risk of 18 for first-degree relatives compared with the general population.[29] However this risk is considerably less than would be predicted based on mendelian patterns of inheritance.[30] In addition, HPS has been reported as an associated feature in multiple defined genetic syndromes[31–35] and chromosomal abnormalities[36–40] and anecdotally with many other defects,[41–45] suggesting a polygenic basis. Although the molecular genetic basis of HPS remains poorly defined, a likely common final pathway causing the disorder is altered expression of neural nitric oxide synthase (NOS1) within the pyloric muscle.[46] A detailed analysis of the molecular mechanisms of this alteration has been published, describing a reduction of messenger RNA (mRNA) expression of NOS1 exon 1c, with a compensatory up-regulation of NOS1 exon 1f variant mRNA in HPS.[46] DNA samples of 16 HPS patients and 81 controls were analyzed for NOS1 exon 1c promoter mutations and single nucleotide polymorphism (SNP). Sequencing of the 5′-flanking region of exon 1c revealed mutations in 3 of 16 HPS tissues, whereas 81 controls showed the wild-type sequence exclusively. Carriers of the A allele of a previously

---

TABLE 2-1

Genes Associated with Hirschsprung Disease and Relationship to Associated Anomalies

Gene	Gene Locus	Gene Product	Inheritance	Population Frequency (%)	Associated Anomalies	Incidence in Gene HD (%)
RET	10q11.2	Coreceptor for GDNF	AD	17-38 (S-HD) 70-80 (L-HD) 50 (familial) 15-35 (sporadic)	CCHS MEN2A MEN2B	1.8-1.9 2.5-5.0 Unknown
GDNF	5p12-13.1	Ligand for RET and GFRα-1	AD	<1*	CCHS	1.8-1.9
NRTN	19p13.3	Ligand for RET and GFRα-2	AD	<1*	Unknown	—
GFRA1	10q26	Coreceptor for GDNF	Unknown	†	Unknown	—
EDNRB	13q22	Receptor for EDN3	AD/AR	3-7	Waardenburg syndrome	Unknown
EDN3	20q13.2-13.3	Ligand for EDNRB	AD/AR	5	CCHS Waardenburg syndrome	1.8-1.9 Unknown
ECE1	1p36.1	EDN3 processing gene	AD	<1	Unknown	—
SOX10	22q13.1	Transcription factor	AD	<1	Waardenburg syndrome type 4	Unknown

*Limited data available.
†No mutations detected thus far in humans, but associated with HD in mice.
AD, autosomal dominant; AR, autosomal recessive; CCHS, congenital central hypoventilation syndrome (Ondine's curse); ECE1, endothelin-converting enzyme-1; EDNRB, endothelin receptor type B; EDN3, endothelin 3; GDNF, glial cell line–derived neurotrophic factor; GFRA1, GDNF family receptor α-1; HD, Hirschsprung disease; L-HD, long-segment HD; MEN, multiple endocrine neoplasia; NRTN, neurturin; RET, rearranged during transfection; S-HD, short-segment HD; SOX, SRY (sex determining region Y)-box 10.

uncharacterized *NOS1* exon 1c promoter SNP (-84G/A SNP) had an increased risk of HPS developing (odds ratio, 8.0; 95% confidence interval, 2.5 to 25.6), which could indicate that the -84G/A promoter SNP alters expression of *NOS1* exon 1c or is in linkage dysequilibrium with a functionally important sequence variant elsewhere in the *NOS1* transcription unit and therefore may serve as an informative marker for a functionally important genetic alteration. The observed correlation of the -84G/A SNP with an increased risk for the development of HPS is consistent with a report showing a strong correlation of a microsatellite polymorphism in the *NOS1* gene with a familial form of HPS.[47] However the -84G/A SNP does not account for all HPS cases; therefore other components of the nitric oxide–dependent signal transduction pathway or additional mechanisms and genes may be involved in the pathogenesis of HPS. This is in accordance with other observations suggesting a multifactorial cause of HPS.[29] In summary, genetic alterations in the *NOS1* exon 1c regulatory region influence expression of the *NOS1* gene and may contribute to the pathogenesis of HPS, but there are likely numerous other genes that contribute to the development of HPS as well as predispose to environmental influences in this disorder.

These examples provide insight into the complexity of current models of molecular genetics and illustrate the inadequacy of current methods of analysis to fully define genetic causes of disease, particularly polygenic disorders. The majority of pediatric surgical disorders currently fall into the category of undefined multifactorial inheritance, which is even less well understood than the genetic categories described. In these disorders, no causative, predisposing, or influencing gene loci have been identified. Isolated regional malformations are presumed to result from interactions between the environment and the actions of multiple genes. Multifactorial inheritance is characterized by the presence of a greater number of risk genes within a family. The presumption of a genetic basis for the anomalies is based on recurrence risk. The recurrence risks in multifactorial inheritance disorders, although generally low, are higher than in the general population; they are increased further if more than one family member is affected, if there are more severe malformations in the proband, or if the parents are closely related. Beyond these generalizations, genetics can provide little specific information about this category of disorder.

UTILITY OF MOLECULAR GENETICS IN CLINICAL PEDIATRIC SURGERY

Genetic Counseling and Prenatal Diagnosis

As mentioned earlier there is still a gap between genotypic understanding of a disorder and direct application to clinical treatment. The exceptions are in the areas of genetic counseling and prenatal diagnosis. Pediatric surgeons are likely to require some knowledge of molecular genetics as their role in prenatal counseling of parents continues to increase. Molecular genetics can supply specific information about an affected fetus by providing genotypic confirmation of a phenotypic abnormality, a phenotypic correlate for a confirmed genotype, and in many instances the recurrence risk for subsequent pregnancies and the need for concern (or lack thereof) about other family members. Once again HD is an example of how

molecular genetics can be valuable in genetic counseling.[48,49] The generalized risk to siblings is 4% and increases as the length of involved segment increases. In HD associated with known syndromes, genetic counseling may focus more on prognosis related to the syndrome than on recurrence risk. In isolated HD a more precise risk table can be created. Risk of recurrence of the disease is greater in relatives of an affected female than of an affected male. Risk of recurrence is also greater in relatives of an individual with long-segment compared with short-segment disease. For example the recurrence risk in a sibling of a female with aganglionosis beginning proximal to the splenic flexure is approximately 23% for a male and 18% for a female, whereas the recurrence risk in a sibling of a male with aganglionosis beginning proximal to the splenic flexure is approximately 11% for a male and 8% for a female. These risks fall to 6% and lower for siblings of an individual with short-segment disease. Prenatal diagnosis is possible if the mutation within the family is known. However because the penetrance of single gene mutations is low (except for *SOX10* mutations in Waardenburg syndrome), the clinical usefulness of prenatal diagnosis is limited.

More commonly, a general knowledge of genetics can allow accurate counseling of recurrence risk and reassurance for parents of an affected fetus diagnosed with a multifactorial inheritance defect, the most common circumstance involving prenatal consultation with a pediatric surgeon. Pediatric surgeons should also be aware of the value of genetic evaluation of abortus tissue in cases of multiple anomalies when after counseling the parents choose to terminate the pregnancy. It is a disservice to the family not to send the fetus to an appropriate center for a detailed gross examination and a state-of-the-art molecular genetic assessment when appropriate.

As molecular genetics increasingly characterizes the genes responsible for specific disorders, their predisposing and modifier loci, and other genetic interactions, a better ability to predict the presence and severity of specific phenotypes will inevitably follow. This will allow prenatal counseling to be tailored to the specific fetus and lead to improved prognostic accuracy, giving parents the opportunity to make more informed prenatal choices.

Postnatal Treatment

In the future molecular genetics will allow specific therapies to be optimized for individual patients. This may range from specific pharmacologic treatments for individual patients based on genotype and predicted pharmacologic response to anticipation of propensities for specific postoperative complications, such as infection or postoperative stress response. Of course the ultimate treatment for an affected individual and his or her progeny would be to correct the germline genetic alteration responsible for a specific phenotype. Although there are many scientific and ethical obstacles to overcome before considering such therapy, it is conceivable that a combination of molecular genetics and gene transfer technologies could correct a germline mutation, replacing an abnormal gene by the integration of a normal gene and providing the ultimate preventive therapy. Although the state of gene transfer technology is far from this level of sophistication, progress in the past 3 decades can only be described as astounding. The next section provides an overview of the current state of gene transfer and its potential application for therapy.

Gene Therapy

Gene therapy remains controversial; however its tremendous potential cannot be denied, and significant strides in safety have been made in the past few years. The year 2000 brought the first clinical gene therapy success—treatment of X-linked severe combined immune deficiency (XSCID)[50]—only to have this dramatic achievement undermined by the induction of leukemia by a mechanism of insertional oncogenesis in four of the nine successfully treated patients.[51] This and other adverse events[52,53] threatened to overshadow the substantial progress made in gene transfer technology in recent years. The adversity has accelerated progress in our understanding of the mechanisms of insertional oncogenesis and in the design of vectors with much lower propensity to induce malignancies.[54] Methods for gene transfer are being developed that have greater safety, specificity, and efficacy than ever before. With improved understanding of the risks and better vector design, several recent trials of gene therapy for immunodeficiency disorders[55] and for ocular disease[56] have demonstrated early success. The technology of gene transfer can be divided into viral vector–based gene transfer and nonviral gene transfer. Because of the limited scope of this chapter and the limited efficiency of non-viral-based gene transfer thus far, only the current state of viral-based gene transfer is reviewed.

VIRAL VECTORS FOR GENE TRANSFER

Viruses are highly evolved biologic machines that efficiently penetrate hostile host cells and exploit the host's cellular machinery to facilitate their replication. Ideally viral vectors harness the viral infection pathway but avoid the subsequent replicative expression of viral genes that causes toxicity. This is traditionally achieved by deleting some or all of the coding regions from the viral genome but leaving intact those sequences that are needed for the vector function, such as elements required for the packaging of viral DNA into virus capsid or the integration of vector DNA into host chromatin. The chosen expression cassette is then cloned into the viral backbone in place of those sequences that were deleted. The deleted genes encoding proteins involved in replication or capsid or envelope proteins are included in a separate packaging construct. The vector genome and packaging construct are then cotransfected into packaging cells to produce recombinant vector particles (Fig. 2-3).

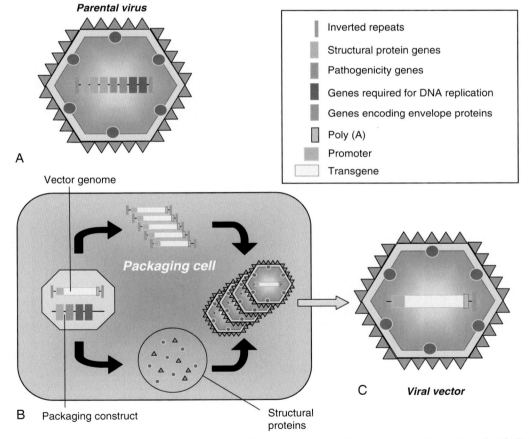

FIGURE 2-3   Requirements for the creation of a generic viral vector. **A,** The basic machinery of a chosen parental virus is used, including genes encoding specific structural protein genes, envelope proteins, and proteins required for DNA replication, but not genes encoding proteins conferring pathogenicity. **B,** The vector is assembled in a packaging cell. A packaging (helper) construct, containing genes derived from the parent virus, can be delivered as a plasmid or helper virus or stably integrated into the chromatin of the packaging cell. Pathogenicity functions and sequences required for encapsidation are eliminated from the helper construct so that it cannot be packaged into a viral particle. In contrast, the vector genome contains the transgenic expression cassette flanked by inverted terminal repeats and *cis*-acting sequences that are required for genome encapsidation. Viral structural proteins and proteins required for replication of the vector DNA are expressed from the packaging construct, and the replicated vector genomes are packaged into the virus particles. **C,** The viral vector particles are released from the packaging cell and contain only the vector genome.

TABLE 2-2
Five Main Viral Vector Groups

Vector	Coding	Packaging Capacity (kb)	Tissue Tropism	Vector Genome	Type Advantages	Material Disadvantages
Retrovirus	RNA	8	Dividing cells only	Integrated	Persistent gene transfer in dividing cells	Requires cell division; may induce oncogenesis
Lentivirus	RNA	8	Broad, including stem cells	Integrated	Integrates into nondividing cells; persistent gene transfer	Potential for oncogenesis
HSV-1	dsDNA	40	Neural	Episomal	Inflammatory response; limited tropism	Large packaging capacity; strong tropism for neurons
AAV	ssDNA	<5	Broad	Episomal (90%) Integrated (<10%)	Noninflammatory; nonpathogenic	Small packaging capacity
Adenovirus	dsDNA	8 30*	Broad	Episomal	Extremely efficient gene transfer in most tissues	Capsid-mediated potent immune response; transient expression in dividing cells

*Helper dependent.
AAV, adeno-associated vector; ds, double-strand; HSV-1; herpes simplex virus-1; ss, single-strand.

Given the diversity of therapeutic strategies and disease targets involving gene transfer, it is not surprising that a large number of vector systems have been devised. Although there is no single vector suitable for all applications, certain characteristics are desirable for all vectors if they are to be clinically useful: (1) the ability to be reproducibly and stably propagated, (2) the ability to be purified to high titers, (3) the ability to mediate targeted delivery (i.e., to avoid widespread vector dissemination), and (4) the ability to achieve gene delivery and expression without harmful side effects. There are currently five main classes of vectors that, at least under specific circumstances, satisfy these requirements: oncoretroviruses, lentiviruses, adeno-associated viruses (AAVs), adenoviruses, and herpesviruses. Table 2-2 compares the general characteristics of these vectors.

Oncoretroviruses and lentiviruses are "integrating," that is, they insert their genomes into the host cellular chromatin. Thus they share the advantage of persistent gene expression. Nonintegrating viruses can achieve persistent gene expression in nondividing cells, but integrating vectors are the tools of choice if stable genetic alteration must be maintained in dividing cells. It is important to note, however, that stable transcription is not guaranteed by integration and that transgene expression from integrated viral genomes can be silenced over time.[57] Oncoretroviruses and lentiviruses differ in their ability to penetrate an intact nuclear membrane. Retroviruses can transduce only dividing cells, whereas lentiviruses can naturally penetrate nuclear membranes and can transduce nondividing cells, making them particularly useful for stem cell targeting applications.[58,59] Because of this difference, lentivirus vectors are superseding retrovirus vectors for most applications. Because of their ability to integrate, both types of vector share the potential hazard of alteration of the host cell genome. This could lead to the undesirable complications of human germline alteration or insertional mutagenesis, particularly important considerations for pediatric or fetal gene therapy.[2] Nevertheless these vectors have proved most efficient for long-term gene transfer into cells in rapidly proliferative tissues and for stem cell directed gene transfer.

Nonintegrating vectors include adenovirus, AAV, and herpesvirus vectors. Adenovirus vectors have the advantages of broad tropism, moderate packaging capacity, and high efficiency, but they carry the usually undesirable properties of high immunogenicity and consequent short duration of gene expression. Modifications of adenovirus vectors to reduce immunogenicity and further increase the transgene capacity have consisted primarily of deletion of "early" (E1-E4) viral genes that encode immunogenic viral proteins responsible for the cytotoxic immune response.[60,61] The most important advance, however, has been the development of helper-dependent adenoviruses (HD-Ads) from which all viral genes are deleted, thus eliminating the immune response to adenoviral-associated proteins.[62] These vectors may ultimately be most valuable for long-term gene transfer in tissues with very low rates of cell division, such as muscle or brain. AAV is a helper-dependent parvovirus that in the presence of adenovirus or herpesvirus infection undergoes a productive replication cycle. AAV vectors are single-strand DNA vectors and represent one of the most promising vector systems for safe long-term gene transfer and expression in nonproliferating tissues. AAV is the only vector system for which the wild-type virus has no known human pathogenicity, adding to its safety profile. In addition the small size and simplicity of the vector particle make systemic administration of high doses of vector possible without eliciting an acute inflammatory response or other toxicity. Although the majority of the AAV vector genome after transduction remains episomal, an approximately 10% rate of integration has been observed.[63] There are two primary limitations of AAV vectors. The first is the need to convert a single-strand DNA genome into a double strand, limiting the efficiency of transduction. This obstacle has been overcome by the development of double-strand vectors that exploit a hairpin intermediate of the AAV replication cycle.[64] Although these vectors can mediate a 10- to 100-fold increase in transgene expression in vitro and in vivo, they can package only 2.4 kb of double-strand DNA, limiting their therapeutic usefulness. This relates to the second primary limitation of AAV vectors, which is limited packaging capacity (4.8 kb of single-strand DNA). One approach to address this limitation is to split the expression cassette across two vectors, exploiting the in vivo concatemerization of rAAV genomes. This results in reconstitution of a functional cassette after concatemerization in the cell nucleus.[65,66] Finally, an approach that has become common for enhancing or redirecting the tissue tropism of AAV vectors is to pseudotype the vectors with capsid proteins from alternative serotypes of AAV.[67] Although most rAAV vectors have been derived from AAV2, nine distinct AAV serotypes have been identified thus far, all of which differ in efficiency for transduction of specific cell types. AAV vectors have proved particularly useful for muscle, liver, and central nervous system directed gene transfer.

Herpes simplex virus (HSV-1) vectors are the largest and most complex of all currently used vector systems. Their primary advantages are a very large packaging capacity (up to 40 kb) and their strong neurotropism, allowing lifelong expression in sensory neurons. This has made neuropathologic disorders a primary target for HSV-1–mediated gene transfer.

CLINICALLY RELEVANT CHALLENGES IN GENE TRANSFER

The adverse events described previously demonstrate the potential for disaster when using vector-based gene transfer. Major initiatives must be undertaken to delineate the potential complications of gene transfer with specific vectors to convince physicians and the public of their safety for future clinical trials. Nevertheless because of the potential benefit, continued efforts to develop safe and efficacious strategies for clinical gene transfer are warranted.

One of the primary obstacles to successful gene therapy continues to be the host immune response. The intact immune system is highly capable of activation against viral vectors using the same defense systems that combat wild-type infections. Viral products or new transgene encoded proteins are recognized as foreign and are capable of activating an immune response of variable intensity. Adenovirus vectors are the most immunogenic of all the viral vector types and induce multiple components of the immune response, including cytotoxic T-lymphocyte responses, humoral virus–neutralizing responses, and potent cytokine-mediated inflammatory responses.[68] Great progress has been made in reducing T-cell responses against adenoviral antigens by the development of HD-Ad vectors from which all adenoviral genes are deleted. These vectors have demonstrated reduced immunogenicity with long-term phenotypic correction of mouse models and negligible toxicity.[69,70] However even HD-Ad vectors or less immunogenic vector systems such as AAV or lentivirus vectors can induce an immunologic response to capsid proteins[71] or to novel transgene encoded proteins,[72] a potentially limiting problem in a large number of human protein deficiency disorders caused by a null mutation. Thus the application of gene transfer technology to many human disorders may require the development of effective and nontoxic strategies for tolerance induction.[73]

Another major area of interest that may improve the safety profile of future viral vector–based gene transfer is specific targeting to affected tissues or organs. Wild-type virus infections are generally restricted to those tissues that are accessible through the route of transmission, whereas recombinant vectors are not subject to the same physical limitations. The promiscuity of viral vectors is a significant liability, because systemic or even local administration of a vector may lead to unwanted vector uptake by many different cell types in multiple organs. For instance, lack of adenovirus vector specificity was directly linked to the induction of a massive systemic immune response that resulted in a gene therapy–

related death in 1999.[68] Because many of the toxic effects of viral vector–based gene transfer are directly related to dose, increasing the efficiency with which viral vectors infect specific cell populations should reduce viral load and improve safety.

There are a variety of promising methods to achieve the targeting of viral vectors for specific organs or cell types. Perhaps the simplest approach is vector pseudotyping, which has been performed for retrovirus, lentivirus, and AAV vectors. By changing the capsid envelope proteins to alternative viral types or serotypes, a portfolio of vectors with different tropisms can be generated.[74] Another approach is the conjugation of capsid proteins to molecular adapters such as bispecific antibodies with specific receptor binding properties.[75,76] A third approach is to genetically engineer the capsid proteins themselves to alter their receptor binding (i.e., to abolish their normal receptor binding) or to encode a small peptide ligand for an alternative receptor.[77] These and other approaches, when combined with the appropriate use of tissue-specific promoters, may significantly reduce the likelihood of toxicity from viral-based gene therapy.

Another important obstacle to human gene therapy— particularly fetal gene therapy—is the potential for insertional mutagenesis when using integrating vectors. Until recently this risk was considered extremely low to negligible, based on the assumption that oncogenesis requires multiple genetic lesions and the fact that induced cancer had not been observed in any of the hundreds of patients treated with retrovirus vectors in the many gene therapy trials. However in two trials of retroviral gene therapy for XSCID[50,78] leukemia developed in 5 of 20 patients treated.[51,79] Evidence suggests that this was caused by retroviral genome insertion in or near the oncogene *LM02*. These concerns have been further heightened by evidence that retroviral genes are not randomly inserted, as previously believed; rather, they preferentially integrate into transcriptionally active genes.[80] Although such events may be more likely to occur under the unique selective influences of XSCID, it is clear that the risk of insertional mutagenesis can no longer be ignored. Approaches designed to neutralize cells expressing transgene if and when an adverse event occurs, such as engineering suicide genes into the vector, are one option, but this would also neutralize any therapeutic effect. More exciting approaches are based on site-specific integration—for instance, taking advantage of site-integration machinery of bacteriophage ϕX31.[81] This is undoubtedly only one of many approaches that will use site-specific integration in the future and should, if successful, negate the risk of insertional mutagenesis. Even without site-specific integration, vector design, such as inclusion of a self-inactivating long terminal repeat in lentiviral vector design, can markedly reduce the likelihood of insertional mutagenesis.[54]

Finally, a critical issue for in vivo gene transfer with integrating vectors in individuals of reproductive age is the potential for germline transmission, with alteration of the human genome. The risk of this event is poorly defined at present and is most likely extremely low, although in some circumstances (e.g., fetal gene transfer), it could be increased.[2] Although still not technically possible, the intentional site-specific correction of defects in the germline would be the ultimate in gene therapy. However even if the technology becomes available, the intentional alteration of the human genome raises profound ethical and societal questions that will need to be thoroughly addressed before its application. The considerations are similar to those for insertional mutagenesis, so many of the approaches mentioned earlier for gene targeting and reduction of the potential for insertional mutagenesis are applicable here as well.

OVERVIEW OF THE CURRENT STATUS OF GENE TRANSFER

At present it is clear that viral vectors are the best available vehicle for efficient gene transfer into most tissues. Several gene therapy applications have shown promise in early-phase clinical trials. Although the adverse events noted in the XSCID trial have dampened enthusiasm, this still represents the first successful treatment of a disease by gene therapy. The treatment of hemophilia B using rAAV is promising,[82] as are the successful trials for ocular disease[56] and adenosine deaminase SCID[55] mentioned previously. The next few years are likely to bring advances in the treatment of certain types of cancer using conditionally replicating oncolytic viruses and in the treatment of vascular and coronary artery disease using viral vectors that express angiogenic factors. In the future new disease targets are likely to become approachable through the fusion of viral vector–mediated gene transfer with other technologies such as RNA interference, a powerful tool to achieve gene silencing. Such vectors could be useful in developing therapy for a range of diseases, such as dominantly inherited genetic disorders, infectious diseases, and cancer. Advances in the understanding of viral vector technology and DNA entry into cells and nuclei will likely lead to the development of more efficient nonviral vector systems that may rival viral vectors in efficiency and have superior safety. Gene vector systems of the future may be very different from those in use today and will ultimately provide efficient delivery of target-specific regulated transgene expression for an appropriate length of time.

The complete reference list is available online at www. expertconsult.com.

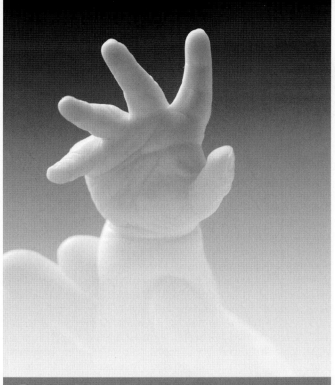

CHAPTER 3

Impact of Tissue Engineering in Pediatric Surgery

Howard I. Pryor II, David M. Hoganson, and Joseph P. Vacanti

Tissue engineering is a rapidly developing interdisciplinary field at the intersection of clinical medicine, cellular biology, and engineering. The goal of tissue engineering is to create living replacement organs and tissues to provide, restore, maintain, or improve lost or congenitally absent function.[1] Early attempts by surgeons to restore function include various wooden and metal prostheses mentioned in the Talmud and a description of a rhinoplasty using a forehead flap detailed in the *Sushruta Samhita* from around 6 BC. Modern medicine has embraced both the use of manufactured substitutes (such as Dacron aortic grafts) to repair abdominal aortic aneurysms and the approach of redirecting autologous tissue for a new function, as in the transfer of a toe to replace a finger. In the past half-century, the development of immunosuppressive medication has allowed for allogeneic substitution of tissues, as in organ transplantation, demonstrating that functional replacement can be lifesaving.

Unfortunately, all these approaches have significant limitations. In pediatric surgery, prosthetic material poses several problems, including material failure, increased rates of infection, and immunodestruction of foreign material. In addition, nonliving material does not grow with the patient nor does it adapt to changing circumstances, so pediatric patients may need to undergo multiple operations with increasing levels of complexity. Native substitutions of tissue are limited by the dilemma of prioritizing the value of various tissues and accepting the functional tradeoff that must be made when redirecting tissue to new functions. The effectiveness of organ transplantation is limited by a short supply of donor organs and a long list of associated morbidities related to lifelong immunosuppression. None of these approaches has permanently solved the need to replace composite tissues.

The field of tissue engineering evolved from the collaboration of Dr. Joseph Vacanti, a pediatric surgeon, and Robert Langer, Ph.D., a chemical engineer, in the laboratory of Dr. Judah Folkman at Children's Hospital Boston as a response to the need for replacement composite tissues. In a white paper published by the National Science Foundation, it was observed that "most lead authors in Tissue Engineering have worked at least once with Langer and Vacanti."[2] Tissue engineering is considered specifically applicable to pediatric surgery because the durability of surgical therapy must be greatest in children. The outcome may be measured over decades, and the surgical reconstruction is subjected to higher levels of growth and physiologic change. This can be especially challenging for congenital defects in which the amount of available donor tissue may be insufficient and prosthetic material may not approximate the functional, cosmetic, and growth requirements of the missing tissue. Satisfying this ongoing medical need is the focus of tissue engineering.

Interdisciplinary Approach

Engineering is fundamentally different from science. The goal of science is to understand and define natural relationships. In contrast, the goal of engineering is to take advantage of relationships defined by science to address problems with solutions that do not exist in nature.[3] Engineering has been defined as the creative application of "scientific principles to design or develop structures, machines, apparatus, or processes" to solve a specific problem.[4] An engineer's invention must be communicated in concrete terms, and it must have defined geometry, dimensions, and characteristics. Engineers usually do not have all the information needed for their designs, and they are typically limited by insufficient scientific knowledge.[3] Traditionally, engineering has been based on physics, chemistry, and mathematics and their extensions into *materials science*, solid and *fluid mechanics*, thermodynamics, transfer phenomena, and systems analysis.[5] Tissue engineering is an approach that attempts to combine these traditional engineering principles with the biologic sciences to produce viable structures that replace diseased or deficient native structures.[6] As of 2004, aggregate development costs in tissue engineering exceeded $4.5 billion, and the field has encountered the kinds of challenges converting bench-top science into clinically marketable tools that were experienced during the development of other breakthrough medical technologies.[7]

Unlike biologic scientists, tissue engineers are not free to select the problems that interest them. Instead, tissue engineers must tackle the problems that present clinical dilemmas. Frequently, the solutions must satisfy conflicting requirements; for instance, safety improvements increase complexity, but increased efficiency increases costs.[5] Problem solving is common to all engineering work. Although the problems may vary in scope and complexity, a common engineering design approach is applicable (Fig. 3-1). First, the problem is thoroughly analyzed, and a preliminary solution is selected. The preliminary solution is further subdefined by the identification of design variables that must be addressed. The preliminary solution is then refined by accounting for as many variables as possible and creatively synthesizing a new preliminary design. The preliminary design is checked for accuracy and adequacy. Finally, the results are interpreted in terms of the original problem. If the results are satisfactory, the engineering design process is complete. If the results do not adequately resolve the original problem, the design is analyzed for failure points, and the process is repeated until the original problem is solved.[5]

The short history of tissue engineering is replete with examples of this approach. For instance, monolayer cell culture has been used in the biologic sciences for decades, but this culture system typically supports only small numbers

of cells in poorly organized sheets. Early attempts to organize these sheets into more clinically relevant constructs focused on the addition of an underlying support or scaffold for the cells as a substitute for the extracellular matrix (ECM).[8–11] Although these innovative approaches improved the handling characteristics and achievable cell mass of these constructs, new problems were identified in terms of poor clinical function, and the iterative process was begun anew, leading to the development of bioreactors. Early bioreactors were dynamic tissue culture devices with simple mechanical designs meant to provide oxygen exchange, defined nutrient flow rates, and electrical and mechanical stimulation that more closely approximated physiologic conditions. The results of these studies revealed further improvements in cell morphologic features, growth characteristics, and metabolic activity.[12–14] As the field of tissue engineering matures, the design variables that must be addressed for each construct will be expanded and refined accordingly.

Several fundamental biology-limited design variables of tissue engineering have been identified, including cell source, ECM, co-culture cell populations, and culture environment (Fig. 3-2). Many initial studies focused on the use of

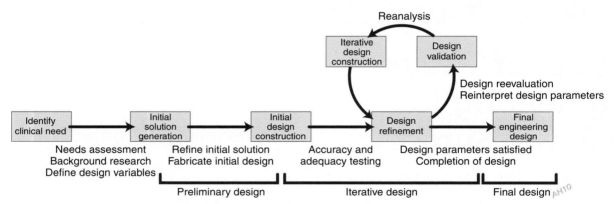

FIGURE 3-1 The iterative engineering design process. The engineering design process begins with the identification of a problem. The problem is analyzed to assess the minimum solution requirements, research the background of previous work, and define the variables that must be addressed. The preliminary design phase begins with an initial solution design and ends when the preliminary design is constructed. The iterative design phase begins with testing of the preliminary design and proceeds through design refinement, validation, and creation of subsequent designs. If a secondary design fails to satisfy initial requirements, the iterative process is undertaken repeatedly until the criteria are met. The final design phase is characterized by the formal definition of the satisfactory design through mathematic equations, drawings, and operating parameters.

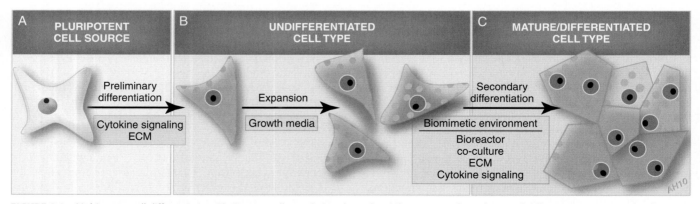

FIGURE 3-2 Multipotent cell differentiation. Pluripotent cell populations have the ability to expand in culture and differentiate into a variety of mature cell types. **A,** The process begins with expansion of the pluripotent cell type in the presence of ECM and cytokines that preserve their expandability while focusing their differentiation down the desired lineage. **B,** The partially differentiated cells are then expanded in growth media to clinically significant quantities. **C,** Using biomimetic culture techniques—including ECM, cytokine signaling, co-culture, and bioreactors—the cells are differentiated into the desired mature cell type.

autologous organ-derived, fully differentiated parenchymal, or primary, cells. Because primary cells are typically in short supply and do not naturally replicate in large quantities, several other cell sources have been investigated, including autologous bone marrow and adipose-derived mesenchymal stem cells, umbilical cord blood cells, Wharton jelly–derived cells, amniotic fluid cells, and allogeneic embryonic stem cells.[15–21] These cell populations have the ability to expand in culture and have demonstrated adequate plasticity to differentiate into a variety of cells, including the epithelium of liver, lung, and gut, as well as the cells of both hematopoietic and endothelial systems.[16,17,22–25] As the differentiation scheme for each of these cellular populations becomes clarified, it has been suggested that cell banks for tissue-engineering applications be developed to respond more rapidly to the clinical need for tissue-engineered constructs.[26]

As more immature cell populations have been investigated, the essential role of ECM in differentiation and maintenance of organ structure has become apparent. For structural tissue constructs such as bone, merely providing the cell population with a polymer scaffold with properties similar to type I collagen has proved less satisfactory than adding elements commonly found in forming bone, such as hydroxyapatite or calcium phosphate.[26–29] Similarly, in liver tissue constructs that use collagen, Matrigel and PuraMatrix hydrogel sandwiches have resulted in greater hepatocyte longevity.[30,31] Work in liver tissue engineering also demonstrated the benefit of co-culturing primary cells with tissue-specific supporting cells.[32] The adult liver requires many complex cell-cell interactions for coordinated organ function, and in vitro investigations have shown that co-cultured hepatocytes and nonparenchymal cells were more tolerant of the culture environment.[33] Co-culture of embryonic stem cells with adipose-derived mesenchymal stem cells (ADSCs) or fibroblasts resulted in enhanced culture viability and formation of vascular tubelike structures.[12,22,34] Even with the correct combinations of cells and ECM, the culture environment must mimic the in vivo environment for the tissue construct to demonstrate clinical function. A fundamental limitation of the field to date has been the adequate mass transfer of nutrients and oxygen to meet the metabolic needs of tissue constructs. The driving force for mass transfer is a concentration gradient that must be kept in perfect balance with the supply of depleted resources precisely as they are used, perpetuating the net transfer of mass from an area of high concentration to an area of low concentration.[35] In addition to a precisely tuned nutrient supply, the mechanical and anatomic in vivo environment must also be mimicked. For cardiac tissue engineering, this has been shown to be important, because constructs cultured without electrical and mechanical stimulation fail to meet critical design criteria when compared with constructs in a biomimetic environment.[6] Highly complex flow bioreactors have been designed to systematically quantify the independent and coupled effects of cyclic flexure, stretch, and flow on engineered heart valve tissue formation in vitro.[36] Researchers have evaluated tissue-engineered heart valves using a bioreactor that automatically controls mean pressure, mean flow rate, beat frequency (heart rate), stroke volume, and the shape of the driving pressure waveform.[37] In addition, researchers studying the liver have developed a biomimetic flat-plate bioreactor system housing phenotypically stabilized

hepatocyte-fibroblast co-cultures in an effort to recapture the zonal features of the liver.[38]

However, the nascent field of biomimetic bioreactors has only recently begun to bring the entire weight of the field of engineering to bear. Three critical advancements that the broad field of engineering will lend to the field of tissue engineering are computational fluid dynamics, advanced modeling, and real-time culture monitoring. Computational fluid dynamics is a technique of design analysis that allows for the accurate prediction of shear stress, culture medium dynamic velocity, and mass transfer of nutrients and oxygen.[36] This technique can be applied as a modeling method in which a virtual design is created and tested by simulation. The virtual design can then be refined and retested several times before the expense of building a real prototype.[6,36,37] This modeling strategy has been applied in a few instances to predict the production of collagenous ECM in engineered tissues, to accurately reproduce scaffold mechanical properties, and to mathematically model oxygen transport in a bioreactor.[6,36,38,39] This type of modeling in the field of tissue engineering will allow for the development of theoretical frameworks to model complex biologic phenomena that can be used to guide sound, hypothesis-driven examinations of new problems and analyze engineered implant performance in vitro and after implantation.[6] The broad field of engineering will also provide the monitoring strategies required to define success in the development of tissue-engineered constructs. One example is the use of nondestructive, high-resolution, nonlinear optical microscopic imaging to observe the development of collagen in tissue-engineered constructs over time.[40] Another example of advanced monitoring is the use of a computer-controlled closed-loop feedback bioreactor to study the effects of highly controlled pulsatile pressure and flow waveforms on biologically active heart valves.[37] As the field of tissue engineering evolves, the need for thoughtfully designed, well-monitored biomimetic culture systems that emulate physiologic conditions will be required to understand the complex culture protocols necessary to yield functional tissue grafts.[14,41]

Cartilage and Bone Tissue Engineering

Pediatric surgeons encounter many congenital and acquired problems that are characterized by structural bone and cartilage defects. These defects may range from cleft palates and craniofacial abnormalities to significant long bone defects after cancer surgery. The current standard of care for most of these lesions includes bone grafting, but donor site morbidity after bone graft harvest remains a recognized limitation to this technique.[42] Grafting in children is also complicated by the fact that the pediatric skeletal system is still developing and the thickness of the nascent bone is thinner compared with adult bone.[43] To supplement the grafting approach, tissue engineers have sought to generate greater quantities of bone and cartilage. One of the earliest successes in bone and cartilage tissue engineering stemmed from the observation that chondrocytes harvested from articular surfaces differentiated in culture to cartilage, whereas chondrocytes from periosteum initially resembled cartilage but progressed in culture to form new bone.[44] In the ensuing 15 years, the tissue engineering of bone and cartilage has evolved into a complex interaction of osteoinductive factors, osteoprogenitor cells, advanced scaffold technology, and an adequate blood supply.[25]

Cartilage is a relatively simple tissue with limited spontaneous regenerative capacity and a low metabolic rate.[45,46] However, early studies with polymer constructs of polyglycolic acid and polylactic acid molded into predetermined shapes led to the formation of cartilage in the shape of a human ear, a temporomandibular joint disk, and articular cartilage for meniscus replacement (Fig. 3-3).[47–50] Since these early studies, an entire research and industrial complex has evolved to develop adequate cartilage replacements for clinical use; a summary of the entire body of work would be beyond the scope of this book. The two principal limitations to the use of most of the resulting constructs are (1) the low replication rate of primary chondrocytes and (2) the relatively low construct strength compared with native tissue.[51] Several groups have addressed the cell source issue through the evaluation of stem cells focusing primarily on bone marrow–derived and adipose-derived mesenchymal stem cells. Both cell types are easily isolated and can be induced to secrete myriad cartilaginous ECM components after differentiation in chondrogenic culture conditions.[52,53] However, increasing construct cell density through the use of a stem cell source is not enough to address the issue of low construct strength. Several groups have shown that cartilaginous ECM secretion and subsequent construct strength are increased when

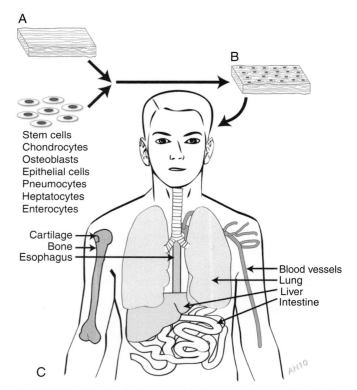

Stem cells
Chondrocytes
Osteoblasts
Epithelial cells
Pneumocytes
Heptatocytes
Enterocytes

Cartilage
Bone
Esophagus

Blood vessels
Lung
Liver
Intestine

FIGURE 3-3 The classic tissue-engineering paradigm. **A,** The classic tissue-engineering paradigm is based on the expansion of pluripotent or primary parenchymal cells in static culture and the creation of a biocompatible polymer scaffold. **B,** The expanded cellular population is seeded onto the scaffold and allowed to expand further in culture. **C** The tissue-engineered construct can then be implanted in a variety of positions to replace absent or lost tissue.

constructs are cultured under dynamic conditions. Such conditions include constant media perfusion, biaxial loading, and rolling media bottle bioreactors.[41,52,54] In each case, the histologic presence of cartilage ECM was markedly increased, and the compressive force sustained by each construct was significantly increased compared with controls. However the optimum culture conditions remain undefined and will likely be unique for each cartilage type applied in the clinical setting.

The tissue engineering of bone evolved from early studies in cartilage tissue engineering in which bovine periosteal cells were seeded onto polyglycolic acid scaffolds to repair cranial bone defects in nude rats.[55] Since these first steps, bone tissue engineering has been approached in many ways. Several methods have been tried, including the implantation of collagen scaffolds containing stem cells transfected with a virus for BMP-2 (a bone forming protein), which demonstrated accelerated osteogenesis.[25,56] Cellular implantation studies have demonstrated that biomimetic scaffolds with porosity greater than 90% and a pore size ranging from 300 to 500 μm improve bone tissue regeneration.[57,58] Ultrastructural evaluation has shown that when bone scaffolds contain nanometer surface features, bone regeneration can be further optimized.[59] As a tissue, bone is significantly more vascular than cartilage, and a principal limitation to bone construct size has been the diffusion distance from surface to center of the construct. One recent approach to this problem is the technique of co-culturing mesenchymal stem cells with endothelial cells in a fibronectin-collagen gel to induce spontaneous angiogenesis within the construct.[60] The use of vascular endothelial growth factor–releasing ADSCs and endothelial cells to more closely mimic the environment of developing bone and direct the growth of blood vessels into 3D PLAGA scaffolds has also been reported.[61] Applying typical engineering analytic tools, a mathematic framework for predicting the development of engineered collagenous matrix has been developed.[40] Some groups have taken advantage of the bone's natural regenerative capacity to use the periosteal space as a bioreactor to develop autologous bone grafts between the surface of a long bone and its periosteum.[13] Given the pace at which this field of tissue engineering is advancing, bone and cartilage tissue engineering will likely provide the most short-term clinically useful products, including constructs to address joint reconstruction and complex congenital anomalies with which pediatric orthopedic surgeons must contend.

CARDIAC TISSUE ENGINEERING

Approximately 1% of all newborns are diagnosed with cardiac defects, including valvular disorders, making heart malformations the most common pathologic congenital condition in humans.[26] Limited options exist for the successful treatment of these patients and include mechanical valve replacement, biologic valve replacement, and ultimately, heart transplantation. Mechanical valves are an imperfect solution because they require lifelong anticoagulation and can spawn systemic thromboembolism.[62] Biologic valves do not require systemic anticoagulation but often calcify, and they must be replaced after several years.[59] Although heart transplantation is the ultimate therapeutic option, this modality is limited by the scarcity of suitable donor organs, requires lifelong immunosuppression, and is associated with serious complications, such as kidney failure and malignancies.[26] The perfect solution to this clinical dilemma would be the development of a nonthrombotic, self-repairing tissue valve replacement that grows with the patient and remodels in response to in vivo stimuli.[59,63]

Over the past decade, an enormous amount of research has been focused on developing a tissue-engineered heart valve meeting these criteria. Although a thorough review would be outside the scope of this book, highlights from such research illustrating tissue engineering's interdisciplinary approach follow.

Initial studies evaluated single-cell populations grown on biocompatible scaffolds in static culture conditions and clearly demonstrated short-term hemodynamic functionality with minimal calcification when implanted in sheep.[64,65] Valves co-cultured with autologous medial and endothelial cells before implantation were shown to function in vivo for up to 5 months and resemble native valves in terms of matrix formation, histologic characteristics, and biomechanics.[66] It was hypothesized that further improvement in valve performance could be obtained by culturing valves under pulsatile flow to generate a biomimetic environment resembling in vivo conditions.[6] Valves cultured under these conditions have demonstrated increased mechanical strength and improved cellular function within the construct.

Although a great deal of progress has been made in the pursuit of a tissue-engineered heart valve, these valves still need to be tested and succeed in the aortic position, where they are needed most.[63] Furthermore, the critical ability of these tissue-engineered constructs to grow with the patient must be clearly demonstrated and will be the focus of the next decade of research.

Vascular Tissue Engineering

In addition to valvular repair, children with complex *congenital heart defects* often require a new vascular conduit to reroute blood flow due to an anomaly. One such example is the Fontan procedure, in which *venous blood* is directed to the *pulmonary arteries* without passing through the *right ventricle*.[67] A host of synthetic and biologic conduits have been deployed in this location, but none of them has provided perfect results. Synthetic conduits incite a foreign body reaction and are a significant cause of thromboembolic complications.[68] Biologic grafts have significantly lower thromboembolic complication rates compared with synthetic grafts but become stenotic and calcify over time because of an immune-mediated process found to be more aggressive in younger patients.[69,70] Moreover, both graft types lack significant growth potential, and it is assumed that all such conduits will eventually need to be replaced.[69,71] Given the morbidity of repeated open-heart procedures on a child, investigators have looked to tissue engineering as an alternative to the use of synthetic and biologic conduits.[72]

As the most successful example of applied tissue engineering to date, Shin'oka and colleagues reported the first human use of a tissue-engineered blood vessel in a 4-year-old girl to replace an occluded pulmonary artery after a Fontan procedure (Fig. 3-4).[72] The conduit used was a 1:1 polycaprolactone, polylactic acid copolymer scaffold seeded with autologous peripheral venous endothelial cells. After 7 months of follow-up, no complications were noted. This successful experience has launched a clinical trial of 42 patients receiving similar scaffolds seeded with autologous bone marrow–derived cells.[73] At 16 months of follow-up, the group reported no significant complications, although one patient died from unrelated causes. The harvest of bone marrow–derived cells is associated with several morbidities, including pain and infection, so several alternative cells sources have been sought. Two such cell sources include adipose-derived endothelial progenitor cells and umbilical cord–derived cells.[23,74]

As the interdisciplinary approach of tissue engineering has been applied to the development of the tissue-engineered vascular graft (TEVG), several areas for improvement have been identified. Using a bioreactor that provided physiologic stimulation similar to the pulmonary artery, physiologically

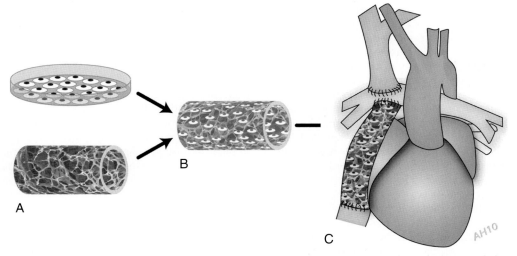

FIGURE 3-4   Tissue-engineered vascular graft. **A,** Tissue-engineered vascular grafts are constructed from a host of cells expanded in culture (autologous peripheral venous endothelial cells, bone marrow–derived cells, adipose-derived endothelial progenitor cells, and umbilical cord–derived cells) and a conduit composed of 1:1 polycaprolactone and polylactic acid copolymer scaffold. **B,** The expanded cellular population is seeded onto the construct and allowed to attach in culture before implantation. **C,** The tissue-engineered vascular graft has been used as an extracardiac conduit in the Fontan procedure.

dynamic conditions up-regulated collagen production by fourfold over the static controls in an in vitro TEVG.[37] Sophisticated monitoring techniques have been developed to evaluate TEVG for the development of normal vascular architecture. Qualitative immunohistochemical and quantitative biochemical analyses demonstrate that the ECM of the TEVG resembled the ECM of the native inferior vena cava after explantation in animal studies.[75]

This type of successful translation of cardiovascular tissue-engineering principles from the bench to the clinic could lead to improved vascular grafts for other cardiovascular surgical applications.[68] Two obvious applications of this developing field are small-diameter vascular grafts and new vascular stent materials.[59] The development of a small-diameter tissue-engineered graft could fill a significant void in the field of vascular surgery, because grafts smaller than 6 mm cannot be satisfactorily constructed from textile or polytetrafluoroethylene (PTFE) and must be bypassed with autologous arteries and veins, with a limited supply for multiple operations.[76] Further, the development of an inexhaustible supply of vascular constructs for in vitro use could lead to the rapid advancement of stenting technologies by eliminating the expense and time expended in animal trials. The pursuit of these near-term goals would result in a dramatic expansion of the field of tissue engineering over the next 10 years.

Gastrointestinal Tissue Engineering

Gastrointestinal tissue engineering has the potential to improve outcomes in two clinical settings for pediatric surgeons: esophageal atresia and short-bowel syndrome. Long-gap esophageal atresia is a daunting clinical problem requiring delayed repair and transposition of a remote portion of bowel.[77–79] Complications from these procedures abound, including stricture, leakage, and malnutrition secondary to shortening of the gastrointestinal tract.[80,81] Moreover, synthetic conduits are unavailable and would lack the critical ability to grow with the patient throughout childhood. As a result, many groups have sought to develop a tissue-engineered esophageal construct that could be used to treat long-gap atresia. Initially, it was demonstrated that organoid units transplanted from adult autologous esophagus onto a biodegradable scaffold form complex tissue indistinguishable from native esophagus.[82] Tissue-engineered esophagus has been used both as a patch and as an interposition graft in rats in preliminary studies.[82] However, these organoid units required resection of significant esophageal length. Recent studies have revealed that isolated esophageal cells could be seeded under low density on collagen polymers and could be expanded in vitro, leading to a potential autologous tissue–engineered esophageal construct.[83]

Of the morbid conditions associated with bowel resection, short-bowel syndrome is the most devastating. It is characterized by progressive weight loss, malnutrition, vitamin deficiency, and infections associated with the vascular access commonly used to support patients with this syndrome.[84,85] This clinical condition develops when less than one third of normal jejunal-ileal length remains, a distance of 25 to 100 cm in neonates.[86] Pediatric surgeons influence the morbidity and mortality of patients with pediatric gastrointestinal disorders such as inflammatory bowel disease and necrotizing enterocolitis because these disorders can require resection of large portions of small bowel.[20,87] Despite efforts to maximize bowel preservation at the time of surgery and the use of gut lengthening procedures to extend the remaining small bowel's functional surface area, many patients become dependent on total parenteral nutrition.[88] These patients are at risk for liver dysfunction as a result of impaired enterohepatic bile salt circulation and abnormal bile acid metabolism, resulting in overt liver failure. This liver dysfunction is recognized as an indication for small intestine transplantation, a procedure fraught with poor survival and lifelong morbidities.[89]

The generation of a composite tissue resembling small intestine from intestinal cells heterotopically transplanted as organoid units was first reported in 1998.[86] Organoid units were derived from full-thickness harvests of intestine and loaded on 2-mm cylindric bioresorbable polymers before implantation in the omentum. The resulting engineered bowel demonstrated polarization of the epithelial cells, which faced the lumen of the cyst. The other layers of the intestinal wall were histologically present with substantial vascularization.[86] Subsequent studies have evaluated a variety of scaffold and cellular combinations that further improve the clinical potential of this therapy.

These evaluations revealed that the ability of intestinal organoid units to recapitulate full-thickness bowel was based on the presence of a mesenchymal core surrounded by a polarized intestinal epithelium, representing all the cells within a full-thickness section of bowel.[90,91] The neomucosa generated by this method in rats demonstrated epithelial barrier function and active transepithelial electrolyte movement equal to that of native adult tissue.[86] Additional studies have supported the finding that the neointestine is not merely anatomically intact but is able to absorb energy-dense nutrients, suggesting a future human application for tissue-engineered intestine.[20] Unfortunately, the use of organoid units requires invasive procedures for harvest, and a more ideal cell source is needed. Such a source would possess the ability to differentiate into all aspects of the intestine, including absorptive and secretory cells as well as vasculature and physical support structures.[20]

The ideal scaffold material has similarly not yet been identified. Initial work on the topic evaluated several options, including AlloDerm and small intestinal submucosa (SIS).[92,93] The latter has been used to support mucosal regeneration across a gap in resected bowel in experimental models.[94] It has also been shown to degrade within 3 months after operative implantation replaced by host-derived tissue.[95] In one large animal study, a commonly used human biomaterial, polyglycolic acid, was used as the scaffold for the first engineered intestine implanted during a single anesthetic administration. It was seeded with autologous tissue arising from organ-specific stem cells.[96] Although all these results point to a future tissue-engineered construct that increases absorptive surface area, a future challenge will focus on the recovery of peristaltic activity of the regenerated bowel. This will require advances in both smooth muscle incorporation and reinnervation of the regenerated bowel.[95] Tissue-engineered gastrointestinal replacement with peristalsis would provide a critical advancement in the treatment of many pediatric surgical diseases and may significantly affect patient care, with improved surface area, transporter function, immune characteristics, and architecture.

Liver Replacement and Tissue Engineering

The liver is a complex vital organ that supports homeostasis through metabolism, excretion, detoxification, storage, and phagocytosis of nutrients and toxins. Acute or chronic liver dysfunction accounts for the death of 29,000 Americans each year, with acute failure mortality rates exceeding 80%.[97,98] In children, liver dysfunction can be caused by biliary atresia–related liver cirrhosis and metabolic diseases such as alpha-1 antitrypsin deficiency, Wilson disease, tyrosinemia, and others.[99] Despite investigation into a wide array of liver support protocols, orthotopic liver transplantation remains the only definitive treatment for severe hepatic failure. Three thousand of these procedures are performed annually, leaving thousands of patients on waiting lists in need of an alternative option. The field of hepatic tissue engineering developed as an attempt to solve this problem.

Initial studies in the field of hepatic tissue engineering were based on the injection of isolated hepatocytes into the portal vein, peritoneal cavity, spleen, and pancreas.[100–102] These cells engrafted and corrected both isolated and global metabolic deficiencies, but these successes were time-limited because the mass of the injected cells was small, and the functional capacity of the cells decreased over time. Methods to increase the tissue-engineered liver mass included concurrent hepatotropic stimulation through partial hepatectomy, portacaval shunting, and injection of liver toxins.[103–106] Even with maximal hepatotropic stimulation, these methods failed to yield adequate hepatocellular function to detoxify a patient in fulminant hepatic failure. A more advanced tissue-engineered liver construct was sought to provide temporary liver function replacement based on the concept of kidney dialysis therapy and was referred to as an extracorporeal bioartificial liver device (BAL).[107] The goal of such a device is to support patients in acute liver failure while liver regeneration occurs and, if that fails, to serve as a bridge to transplantation.[108] Unfortunately, despite a wide array of devices tested, none has delivered the desired results.[107] Most BALs tested to date contain a singular hepatocyte cell population without associated nonparenchymal cells. Such a device's lifetime is limited because hepatocytes degenerate within hours to days in such an environment.

The cellular physiology of the liver is complex. Hepatocytes are anchorage-dependent cells and require an insoluble ECM for survival and proliferation.[85] The adult liver also requires a complex cell-cell interplay between hepatocytes and the nonparenchymal cell populations, including biliary epithelium, Kupffer cells, stellate cells, and sinusoidal endothelial cells. These interactions are essential for proper organ function, and hepatocytes dedifferentiate within 2 weeks when these communications are severed.[109] To preserve and encourage these necessary interactions in future BALs, several groups have proposed to organize the underlying scaffold to serve as a template to guide cell organization and growth.[85] Given the high metabolic requirements of liver tissue, this organized structure would allow more efficient diffusion of oxygen and nutrients and removal of waste. A further advance of this concept, being refined at the Massachusetts General Hospital Tissue Engineering and Organ Fabrication Laboratory, is the development of a polymer device with an integrated vascular network to provide immediate access to the blood supply after implantation (see the discussion on future directions in the next section).[18] This de novo vascular system could be used as a template for any complex tissue such as liver or lung. Future designs are based on a modular concept that allows for the fabrication of implantable devices containing a large mass of cells within a structured environment, complete with de novo blood supply.

One significant challenge that remains entirely unaddressed in the field of hepatic tissue engineering is the development of an artificial biliary system. One solution may lie in the use of multipotent cells that can differentiate down both the hepatocytic and biliary lineages during postimplantation remodeling.[99]

Future Directions: Vascular Networks

The advances of tissue engineering have occurred primarily through interdisciplinary efforts of electrical, chemical, and mechanical engineers; scientists, in fields such as developmental biology, biomaterials science, and stem cell biology; and clinicians from surgical and medical fields.[110] This approach has been successful in the initial development of avascular or thin tissues with low metabolic activity and functions limited to mechanical activity, such as skin, bone, cartilage, and heart valves (Table 3-1).[12,18,59] Engineering more complex tissues with a significant homeostatic contribution and high metabolic activity necessitates the development of a vasculature within the construct that promotes cell survival, tissue organization, and rapid nutrient supply immediately after implantation.[12,18]

Native tissues are supplied by capillaries that are spaced a maximum of 200 μm from one another, permitting a natural diffusion limit for nutrients and gases.[111,112] Two approaches have been investigated to address this goal of providing nutrients to every cell in a tissue construct within the tissue's natural diffusion limit (Fig. 3-5).[12,113] One strategy relies on the tissue construct's natural ability to sprout new or bridging vessels or to invite ingrowth of existing vessels.[12] Despite numerous attempts, it has been difficult to develop a de novo angiogenesis-based vasculature within a tissue construct because of the challenges involved in the differentiation and sustenance of multiple (i.e., vascular progenitor and parenchymal) cell types in a concomitant fashion.[13] To date, only one group has had success in a tissue-engineered bone construct.[60] Several previous attempts to invite ingrowth after implantation have revealed that blood vessel invasion from the host tissue is limited to a depth of several hundred micrometers from the surface of the implant.[61] This results in a central zone of necrosis because only the periphery of the graft is efficiently vascularized.[60,114] The difficulties with in vitro vascularization have led to the development of an alternative solution: preformed vascular networks.[26]

The design of preformed vascular networks is only beginning to be defined as a natural extension of previously identified axioms of vascular biology. Such networks will have to be designed individually for the intended tissue based on the tissue's inherent resistance to flow, nutrient transfer requirements, and waste removal needs.[113] Such control of the microenvironmental niche within each tissue will be

TABLE 3-1

Existing Tissue Engineered Products

Brand Name	Application	Manufacturer	Cells	Matrix
Bioseed Oral Bone	Bone	BioTissue Technologies	Autologous osteocytes	Fibrin gel
Osteotransplant	Bone	Co.Don AG	Autologous osteocytes	Fibrin gel
Carticel	Cartilage	Genzyme Biosurgery	Autologous chondrocytes	
Hyalograft C	Cartilage	Fidia Advanced Biopolymers	Autologous chondrocytes	Hyaluronic acid
MACI	Cartilage	Verigen AG	Autologous chondrocytes	Collagen
Chondrotransplant	Cartilage	Co.Don AG	Autologous chondrocytes	
Bioseed-C	Cartilage	BioTissue Technologies	Autologous chondrocytes	3D fibrin matrix
NOVOCART	Cartilage	TETEC AG	Autologous chondrocytes	
Chondrotec	Cartilage	CellTec GmbH	Autologous chondrocytes	Fibrin gel
Cartilink-1 Cartilink-2	Cartilage Cartilage	Interface Biotech A/S	Autologous chondrocytes Autologous chondrocytes	Periosteum Bovine collagen
Bioseed-M	Oral mucosa	BioTissue Technologies	Oral mucosal cells	Fibrin gel
Integra	Skin	Integra LifeSciences	Dermal fibroblasts	Bovine collagen
Dermagraft	Skin	Advanced Tissue Sciences, Inc.	Neonatal fibroblast	Polyglactin mesh
Apligraf	Skin	Organogenesis Inc.	Allogenic fibroblasts and epidermal cells	Bovine collagen
Epicel	Skin	Genzyme Biosurgery	Autologous keratinocytes	
Transcyte	Skin	Smith & Nephew	Human fibroblast	Polymer membrane
Hyalograft 3D Laserskin	Skin	Fidia Advanced Biomaterials	Autologous fibroblasts Autologous keratinocytes	Hyaluronic acid Hyaluronic acid
Bioseed-S Melanoseed	Skin	BioTissue Technologies	Keratinocytes Melanocytes	Gel-like fibrin Gel-like fibrin
Autoderm Cryoceal	Skin	XCELLentis	Human Keratinocytes	None
Epibase	Skin	Laboratoire Genevrier	Autologous keratinocytes	Collagen
Orcell	Skin	Ortec Inc.	Allogeneic fibroblasts Allogenic keratinocytes	Collagen
Vivoderm	Skin	ER Squibb & Sons Inc	Autologous keratinocytes	Hyaluronic acid
Acudress	Skin	Iso Tis SA	Keratinocyte precursors	Fibrin
Vascugel	Vascular	Pervasis	Allogenic endothelial cells	Gelatin sponge

Data from references 115–119.

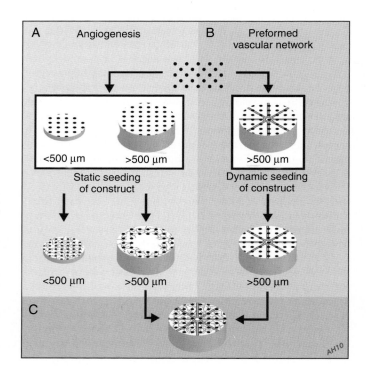

FIGURE 3-5 Angiogenesis versus preformed vascular networks. **A,** The angiogenesis approach to vascularized tissue constructs relies on the natural ability of a construct to form new vessels or invite ingrowth of existing vessels. For constructs less than 500 μm in every dimension, cells can survive on diffusion alone as new vessel ingrowth reaches the entire cellular population. For constructs larger than 500 μm, a necrotic core develops because cells greater than 500 μm from nutrients cannot survive on diffusion long enough to allow vessel ingrowth. **B,** Using tissue-specific design criteria, preformed vascular networks can provide nutrients to within 150 μm of each cell in a construct with dimensions greater than 500 μm, thereby preventing a necrotic core. **C,** Using a resorbable scaffold to manufacture the preformed vascular network will allow the network to serve as a starting point for angiogenesis in the construct while providing the required nutrients during the ingrowth process.

key to successful tissue regeneration and has only been possible because of recent manufacturing advancements in the field of mechanical engineering, such as electrical discharge machining and micromilling.[113] Such networks can serve as the "vascular scaffold" for subsequent post-implantation remodeling.[12] As solutions to these near-term limitations evolve, more problems will be identified that will require an interdisciplinary approach to tissue engineering.

The future of tissue engineering is dependent on a robust blend of fundamental iterative engineering design, developmental and cellular biology, and surgical expertise to optimize the clinical use of new engineered constructs. The initial efforts to develop clinically useful tissues have succeeded in thin tissues supplied by diffusion. Future successful efforts in the design of vascularized structures and the evolution of autologous cell sources for tissues will eventually result in the development of clinically useful tissue-engineered organs.

The complete reference list is available online at www. expertconsult.com.

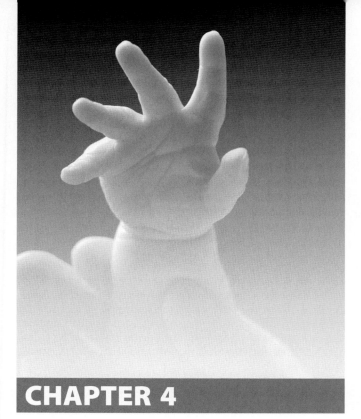

CHAPTER 4

Advanced and Emerging Surgical Technologies and the Process of Innovation

Sanjeev Dutta, Russell K. Woo, and
Thomas M. Krummel

"Change is inevitable. Change is constant."

—Benjamin Disraeli

From the eons of evolutionary change that gifted *Homo sapiens* with an opposable thumb, to the minute-to-minute changes of the neonatal surgical patient, change and the adaptive response to change defines either success or failure.

The development and use of tools and technologies remains a distinguishing characteristic of mankind. The first hunter-gatherers created, built, and modified tools to the demands of a specific task. In much the same fashion, the relentless development and use of surgical tools and technologies has defined both our craft and our care since the first bone needles were used in prehistoric times.

This chapter attempts to highlight those advanced and emerging surgical technologies that shape the present and direct future changes. A framework to facilitate both thought and action about those innovations to come is presented. Finally, the surgeon's role in the ethical process of innovation is discussed. The authors remain acutely attuned to Yogi Berra's admonition, "Predictions are difficult, especially about the future."

As advances in surgical technologies have occurred, our field has moved forward, often in quantum leaps. A thoughtful look around our operating rooms, interventional suites, critical care units, and even teaching facilities is cause to reflect on our use of and even dependence on tools and technologies. Clamps, catheters, retractors, energy sources, and monitors fill these spaces; they facilitate and enhance surgeons' capabilities in the process of diagnosis, imaging, physiologic care, molecular triage, and in the performance of surgical procedures. Surgeons constantly function as users of technology; thus a fundamental understanding underpins their thoughtful use. The use of a drug without understanding the mechanism and side effects would be regarded as malpractice. A similar case must be made for surgical tools and technologies.

New technologies result from an endless cycle through which innovation occurs. Such a cycle may begin with a fundamental research discovery or begin at the bedside with an unsolved patient problem. Frequently, innovation requires a complex interplay of both. Surgeons are uniquely positioned and privileged to contribute to and even define this cycle. The face of a patient with the unsolvable problem is a constant reminder of our responsibility to advance our field. Theodore Kocher's success in thyroid surgery was enabled by his toothed modification of existing clamps to facilitate thyroid operations. Tom Fogarty's development of the balloon catheter began as a surgical assistant witnessing both the failures and disastrous consequences of extensive arteriotomies for extraction of emboli. His simple, brilliant concept has arguably created the entire field of catheter-based manipulation. John Gibbon's successful construction of a heart-lung machine was initially motivated by the patient with the unsolved problem of pulmonary emboli and the need for surgical extraction. Although his original intention has been eclipsed by Lazar Greenfield's suction embolectomy catheter and venacaval filter, and dwarfed by the utility of the heart-lung machine in cardiac surgery, the story remains the same. Unresolved problems and a surgeon determined to find a solution have led to countless innovations that have changed our field forever. The surgeon's role must extend outside the operating room. Surgeons must remain aware and connected to the tools and techniques of diagnosis, monitoring, and education. Mark M. Ravitch, an extraordinary pediatric surgeon, innovator, and one of the most literate surgeons of the twentieth century, described surgery as an intellectual discipline characterized not only by operative procedures but also by the attitude or responsibility toward care of the sick. Dr. Ravitch's contribution to the development of stapling devices deserves enormous credit.[1]

A surgical operation can be defined as "an act performed with instruments or by the hands of a surgeon." This implies an image and a manipulation; the manipulation implies an energy source. Historically, we have regarded the "image" to be that of a direct visual image and "manipulation" performed with the direct contact of two hands or surgical tools.

TABLE 4-1

Surgical Operation: Image and Manipulation

Image	Manipulation
Direct visual	Two hands direct
Video image	Two hands, long tools robots
Ultrasonography (US)	Cold, thermal
Computed tomography	Radiofrequency
Magnetic resonance imaging	Photodynamic energy
	Focused US energy

The laparoscopic revolution has taught us that the image can be a video image and the manipulation performed by two hands using long tools. Now those long tools are occasionally attached to surgical robots. Our notion about the image has come to include ultrasonography/ultrasound (US), computed tomography (CT), or magnetic resonance imaging (MRI), and the manipulation can include such energy sources as cold, heat, radiofrequency, photodynamic, or chemical energy. Extracorporeal shock wave lithotripsy is an important example of this principle, when applied to renal calculi. How will the "image" and "manipulation" exist in the future (Table 4-1)?

Current and Future Diagnostic Technologies

Accurate evaluation of surgical disease has always been a vital aspect of surgical practice, always preceding operation. Whether in the clinic, the emergency room, or a hospital bed, precise assessment to correctly guide operative or nonoperative therapy defines surgical judgment and care. A thorough history and detailed physical examination will forever remain the foundation of assessment; however, the thoughtful addition of adjunctive imaging studies has added considerably to the evaluation of surgical patients. Driven by advancements in medicine, engineering, and biology, these studies use increasingly sophisticated technologies. These technologies promise to arm surgeons with more detailed anatomic, functional, and even molecular information in the coming years.

During the last 3 decades, the introduction and improvement of US, CT, and MRI techniques have revolutionized the clinical evaluation of surgical disease. The fine anatomic data that these imaging modalities provide has facilitated the accurate diagnosis of a wide variety of conditions. Functional imaging techniques, such as positron emission tomography (PET) and functional MRI, have been developed to provide accurate and often real-time biologic or physiologic information. In the field of pediatric surgery, these imaging modalities may be used in the diagnosis and characterization of disease, for preoperative surgical planning, and for postoperative follow-up and evaluation. This section will provide an overview of the imaging modalities used in pediatric surgery, focusing on emerging techniques and systems.

ULTRASONOGRAPHY

Ultrasound imaging has become a truly invaluable tool in the evaluation of the pediatric surgical patient. Providing anatomic as well as real-time functional information, US imaging has several unique advantages that have made it particularly useful in the care of children. These include their relatively low cost, their portability and flexibility (seamless movement from the operating room, intensive care unit, or emergency room), and their safety in children and fetuses because they do not rely on ionizing radiation. For these reasons, this section will pay particular attention to US imaging, highlighting emerging advances in its technology and practice including three-dimensional (3D) US imaging, US contrast imaging, and US harmonic imaging.

Ultrasonography uses the emission and reflection of sound waves to construct images of body structures. In essence, medical US operates on the same principle as active sound navigation and ranging (SONAR): a sound beam is projected by the US probe into the body, and based on the time to "hear" the echo, the distance to a target structure can be calculated.[2] In the body, the sound waves are primarily reflected at tissue interfaces, with the strength of the returning echoes mainly correlating with the properties of the tissues being examined. The advantages of US imaging include lack of ionizing radiation, real-time imaging with motion, and relatively fast procedure times.[3]

In modern US imagers, numerous transducer elements are placed side by side in the transducer probe. The majority of US imaging devices currently use linear or sector scan transducers. These consist of 64 to 256 piezoelectric elements arranged in a single row. With this arrangement, the transducer can interrogate a single slice of tissue whose thickness is correlated to the thickness of the transducer elements.[2] This information is then used to construct real-time, dynamic, two-dimensional images. Color, power, and pulsed wave Doppler imaging are variations of this technology that allow color or graphical visualization of motion.[3] Specifically, conventional Doppler imaging provides information of flow velocity and direction of flow by tracking scattering objects in a region of interest.[4] In contrast, power Doppler displays the power of the Doppler signal and has proven to be a more sensitive method in terms of signal-to-noise ratio and low flow detectability.[5]

In pediatric surgery, US imaging is widely used in the evaluation of multiple pathologies, including appendicitis, testicular torsion, intussusception, and hypertrophic pyloric stenosis.[6,7] In addition, US is a powerful and relatively safe tool for the prenatal diagnosis of congenital diseases. Prenatal US evaluation is useful in facilitating the prenatal diagnosis of abdominal wall defects, congenital diaphragmatic hernias, sacrococcygeal teratomas, cystic adenomatoid malformation, pulmonary sequestration, neural tube defects, obstructive uropathy, facial clefting, and twin-twin syndromes.[8] Furthermore, sonographic guidance is vital to accomplishing more invasive prenatal diagnostic techniques such as amniocentesis and fetal blood sampling.[8]

Three-Dimensional Ultrasonography

Although two-dimensional (2D) US systems have improved dramatically over the last 30 years, the two-dimensional images produced by these systems continue to require a relatively large amount of experience to effectively interpret. This stems from the fact that the images represent one cross section, or slice, of the target anatomy, requiring users to reconstruct the three-dimensional picture in their mind. Given these limitations, 3D US systems, which provide volumetric instead of cross-sectional images, have recently been developed and have seen increased use for many applications.

The first reported clinical use of a 3D US system occurred in 1986 when Kazunori Baba at the Institute of Medical Electronics, University of Tokyo, Japan, succeeded in obtaining 3D fetal images by processing 2D images on a mini-computer.[9] Since then, multiple 3D US systems have been developed with the purpose of providing more detailed and user-friendly anatomic information. These multislice, or volumetric, images are generally acquired by one of the following techniques:

1. Use of a two-dimensional array where a transducer with multiple element rows is used to capture multiple slices at once and render a volume from real 3D data.
2. Use of a one-dimensional phased array to acquire several 2D slices over time. The resultant images are then fused by the US computer's reconstruction algorithm.

The three-dimensional information acquired by these techniques is then used to reconstruct and display a 3D image by either maximum signal intensity processing, volume rendering, or surface rendering. Currently, 3D US systems are available from several manufacturers, including General Electric, Phillips, and Siemens. When these three-dimensional images are displayed in a real-time fashion; they have the ability to provide functional information on the physiology of a patient. An example of this is the evaluation of cardiac function using real-time US. Real-time, 3D US is sometimes referred to as 4D US, though it is still essentially providing a three-dimensional image. Figure 4-1 represents a 3D US view of a fetus in utero.

In the field of pediatric surgery, 3D US systems have not yet seen routine clinical application. However, their utility in perinatal medicine has been increasingly investigated. Specifically, 3D US systems have been used for detailed prenatal evaluation of congenital anomalies. In a study published in 2000, Dyson

and colleagues[10] prospectively scanned 63 patients with 103 anomalies with both 2D and 3D US techniques. Each anomaly was reviewed to determine whether 3D US data were either advantageous, equivalent, or disadvantageous compared with 2D US images. They found that the 3D US images provided additional information in 51% of the anomalies, provided equivalent information in 45% of the anomalies, and were disadvantageous in 4% of the anomalies. Specifically, they found that 3D US techniques were most helpful in evaluating fetuses with facial anomalies, hand and foot abnormalities, and axial spine and neural tube defects. 3D ultrasonography offered diagnostic advantages in about one half of the selected cases studied and affected patient management in 5% of cases. They concluded that 3D US was therefore a powerful adjunctive tool to 2D US in the prenatal evaluation of congenital anomalies.[10]

Similarly, Chang and colleagues reported several series where 3D US techniques were used to effectively evaluate fetal organ volumes, estimating fetal lung volume for the evaluation of pulmonary hypoplasia,[11] cerebellar volume,[13,14] heart volume,[15] adrenal gland volume,[16] and liver volume.[17] In all of these studies, 3D US images provided more accurate data than 2D images.[11]

In 2007, Kurjak and colleagues reviewed, in *Perinatology,* the published experience with 3D and 4D US.[18] Their analysis highlighted reports detailing the use of 3D US to more accurately evaluate fetal craniofacial anomalies. In one study, 4D US was used to measure external ear length, a parameter that is classically difficult to accurately determine using 2D US. Short external ear length is one of the most consistent anthropomorphic characteristics found in neonates with Down syndrome (see Fig. 4-1). In another report, 3D US evaluation of the fetal central nervous system was found to improve the diagnosis of malformations with a sensitivity of up to 80%. More relevant to pediatric surgery, 3D US systems combined with the use of high-frequency transvaginal US probes enhanced the detection rate of cystic hygromas, with earlier and more frequent detection of these lesions. The use of 3D US to evaluate the fetal heart has also shown promise. A recently introduced US technique, tomographic US imaging (TUI), allows the examiner to review multiple parallel images of the beating heart. Using the known advantages of multislice imaging commonly used in computed tomography and magnetic resonance imaging, TUI can provide a more precise determination of the relationships between adjacent cardiac structures.

In addition to prenatal evaluation, 3D US systems have been used to image the ventricular system in neonates and infants to aid in the preoperative planning of neuroendoscopic interventions.[19,20] Similarly, these systems have seen relatively extensive use in the area of transthoracic echocardiographic imaging for the evaluation of congenital cardiac anomalies.[21,22] From an experimental standpoint, Cannon and colleagues studied the ability of 3D US to guide basic surgical tasks in a simulated endoscopic environment.[23] They found that 3D US imaging guided these tasks more efficiently and more accurately than 2D US imaging.[23] Overall, 3D US systems appear to allow the visualization of complex structures in a more intuitive manner compared with 2D systems. In addition, they appear to enable more precise measurements of volume and the relative orientation of structures.[24] As technology improves, the use of such systems in the field of pediatric surgery is likely to increase.

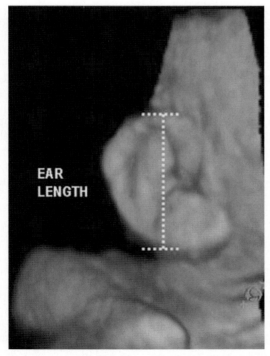

FIGURE 4-1   Three-dimensional ultrasound image of a fetal ear. (From Kurjak A, Miskovic B, Andonotopo W, et al: How useful is 3D and 4D US in perinatal medicine? J Perinat Med, 2007;35:10-27.) *(See Expert Consult site for color version.)*

Ultrasound Contrast Imaging and Ultrasound Harmonic Imaging

In addition to 3D US, significant advances have recently been made with respect to US contrast imaging and harmonic imaging, which may serve to improve the quality of information obtained by US techniques and may expand the clinical use of US as an imaging modality.

Ultrasound contrast imaging techniques are currently used for the visualization of intracardiac blood flow to evaluate structural anomalies of the heart.[25] In general, US contrast agents are classified as free gas bubbles or encapsulated gas bubbles. Simply stated, these gas bubbles exhibit a unique resonance phenomenon when isonified by an US wave, resulting in a frequency-dependent volume pulsation that makes the resonating bubble behave as a source of sound, not just a reflector of it.[4] Currently, new methods are being developed to enhance the contrast effect, including harmonic imaging, harmonic power Doppler imaging, pulse inversion imaging, release-burst imaging, and subharmonic imaging.[4] As these methods improve, US contrast imaging may serve to provide clinicians with more detailed perfusion imaging of the heart as well as tumors and other anatomic structures. Figure 4-2 depicts an US image of the left ventricle using microbubble contrast.

Interest in US harmonic imaging occurred in 1996 after Burns observed harmonics generated by US contrast agents.[26] Since then, significant developments have occurred in the use of the harmonic properties of sound waves to improve the quality of US images. In brief, sound waves are the sum of different component frequencies, the fundamental frequency (first harmonic) and harmonics, which are integral multiples of the fundamental frequency. The combination of the fundamental frequency and its specific harmonics gives a signal its unique characteristics. When US contrast agents are used, harmonics are generated by reflections from the injected agent and not by reflections from tissue. When no contrast is used, harmonics are generated by the tissue itself.[27]

Although the fundamental frequency consists of echoes produced by tissue interfaces and differences in tissue properties, the harmonics are generated by the tissue itself. In this manner, harmonic intensity increases with depth until natural tissue attenuation overcomes this effect. In contrast, the intensity of the fundamental frequency is attenuated linearly with depth.[27] Tissue harmonic imaging takes advantage of these properties by using the harmonic signals that are generated by tissue and by filtering out the fundamental echo signals that are generated by the transmitted acoustic energy.[28] This theoretically leads to an improved signal-to-noise ratio and contrast-to-noise ratio. Additional benefits of US harmonic imaging include improved spatial resolution, better visualization of deep structures, and a reduction in artifacts produced by US contrast agents.[27] Figure 4-3 compares an image obtained by US harmonic imaging and one obtained by standard 2D US.

Ultrasonography and Fetal Surgery

With the advent of fetal surgery in 1980, US evaluation became an increasingly important noninvasive modality for diagnosing and characterizing diseases that are amenable to fetal surgical intervention.[29] Today, fetal surgical techniques are used in selected centers to perform a variety of procedures, including surgical repair of myelomeningocele, resection of sacrococcygeal teratoma in fetuses with nonimmune hydrops, resection of an enlarging congenital cystic adenomatoid malformation that is not amenable to thoracoamniotic shunting, and tracheal balloon occlusion for severe left congenital diaphragmatic hernia.[30,31] In all of these procedures, sonography currently remains the modality of choice for fetal diagnosis and treatment because of its safety and real-time capabilities. Specifically, fetal US can be used to characterize the severity of the congenital anomaly and to determine its appropriateness for intervention. During open hysterotomy, US is used to determine an appropriate location for the uterine incision away from the placenta and to monitor fetal heart rate and contractility. During procedures that do not use open hysterotomy, such as radiofrequency ablation for twin-reversed arterial perfusion sequence, laser ablation for twin-twin transfusion syndrome, and shunt placements for large pleural effusions, and bladder outlet obstruction, fetal US is used to directly guide the intervention. In addition, US imaging is vital to the postoperative care and follow-up of fetal surgical patients, because they remain in utero after their surgical procedure.

COMPUTED TOMOGRAPHY

Computed tomography was invented in 1972 by British engineer Godfrey Hounsfield of EMI Laboratories, England, and independently by South African–born physicist Allan Cormack of Tufts University, Massachusetts. Since then, the use of CT imaging has become widespread in multiple fields of medicine and surgery. Currently, advances in technology have improved the speed, comfort, and image quality of modern CT scanners. In addition, recent advances, such as multidetector CT computed tomography (MDCT) and volumetric reconstruction, or 3D CT, may be particularly valuable in

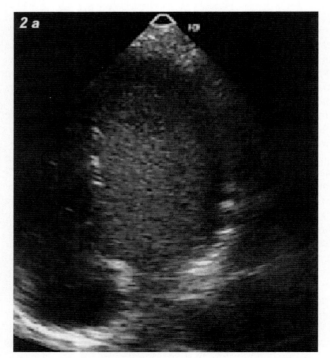

FIGURE 4-2 Ultrasound contrast image of the left ventricle. (From Frinking PJ, Bouakaz A, Kirkhorn J, et al: US contrast imaging: Current and new potential methods. US Med Biol 2000;26:965-975.)

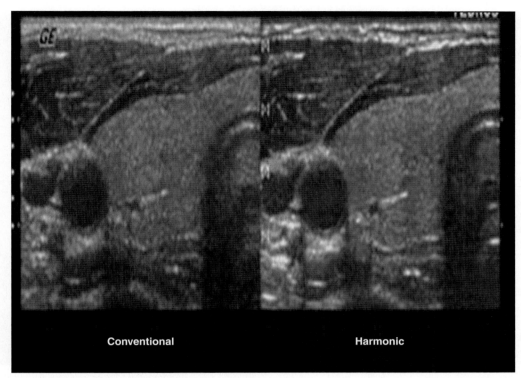

FIGURE 4-3   Conventional versus ultrasound harmonic imaging. (From Tranquart F, Grener N, Eder V, Pourcelot L, et al: Clinical use of US tissue harmonic imaging. US Med Biol 1999;25:889-894.)

the care of pediatric surgical patients. This section will provide a brief overview of CT imaging, focusing on MDCT and volumetric imaging and their implications in pediatric surgery.

Multidetector Computed Tomography

Computed tomography uses a tightly arranged strip of radiation emitters and detectors that circles around a patient to obtain a two-dimensional map of x-ray attenuation values. Numerical regression techniques are then used to turn this list of attenuation values into a two-dimensional slice image. CT has undergone several major developments since its introduction.

Introduced in the early 1990s, single-detector helical or spiral CT scanning revolutionized diagnostic CT imaging by using slip rings to allow for continuous image acquisition.[32] Before this development, the table and patient were moved in a stepwise fashion after the acquisition of each image slice, resulting in relatively long scanning times. Helical CT scanners use slip ring technology that allows the tube and detector to continually rotate around the patient. Combined with continuous table motion through the rotating gantry, this significantly improves the speed of CT studies. The improved speed of helical CT scanners enables the acquisition of large volumes of data in a single breath hold.

Helical CT has improved during the past 15 years, with faster gantry rotation, more powerful x-ray tubes, and improved interpolation algorithms.[33] However, the greatest advance has been the recent introduction of multidetector-row CT (MDCT) scanners.[32] In contrast to single-detector–row CT, MDCT uses multiple parallel rows of detectors that spiral around the patient simultaneously. Currently capable of acquiring four channels of helical data at the same time, MDCT scanners are significantly faster than single-detector helical CT scanners. This has profound implications for the clinical application of CT imaging, especially in the pediatric patient where the issues of radiation exposure and patient cooperation are magnified. Fundamental advantages of MDCT compared with earlier modalities include substantially shorter acquisition times, retrospective creation of thinner or thicker sections from the same raw data, and improved 3D rendering with diminished helical artifacts.[33]

In the pediatric population, MDCT provides a number of advantages compared with standard helical CT. Because of the increased speed of MDCT, there may be a decreased need for sedation in some pediatric studies. There is also a reduction in patient movement artifact as well as a potential for more optimal contrast enhancement over a greater portion of the anatomy of interest. The volumetric data acquired also provides for the ability of multiplanar reconstruction, which can be an important problem-solving tool. MDCT has been increasingly used for pediatric trauma, pediatric tumors, evaluation of solid abdominal parenchymal organ masses, suspected abscess, or inflammatory disorders.[34] Specifically, MDCT is increasingly used in the evaluation of children with abdominal pain, particularly in patients with suspected appendicitis.[35] Callahan and colleagues used MDCT in the evaluation of children with appendicitis and reduced the total number of hospital days, negative laparotomy rate, and cost per patient.[36] In addition, MDCT may be useful in identifying alternative diagnoses, including other bowel pathologies, ovarian pathologies, and urinary tract pathologies (Fig. 4-4).[35]

Similarly, MDCT may be valuable in the evaluation of urolithiasis and inflammatory bowel disease (IBD). MDCT has gained acceptance as a primary modality for the evaluation of children with abdominal pain and hematuria in which urolithiasis is suspected.[35] CT findings of urolithiasis include visualization of the radiopaque stone, dilatation of the ureter

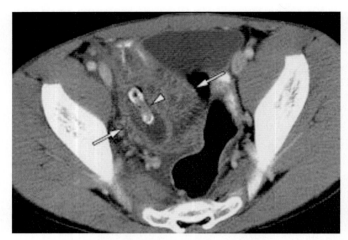

FIGURE 4-4 Multidetector computed tomography of an 8-year-old boy with appendicitis. The *arrows* point to an inflammatory mass in the right lower quadrant with a possible appendicolith *(arrowhead)*. (From Donnelly LF, Frush DP: Pediatric multidetector body CT. Radiol Clin North Am 2003;41:637–655.)

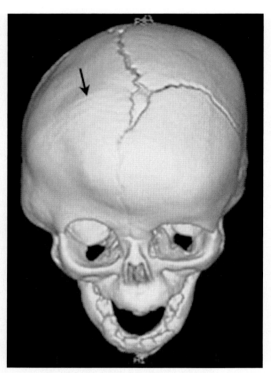

FIGURE 4-5 3D computed tomography reconstruction of an infant skull showing premature closure of the right coronal suture. (From Rubin GD: 3-D imaging with MDCT. Eur J Radiol 2003;45(Suppl 1):S37–S41.)

or collecting system, asymmetric enlargement of the kidney, and perinephric stranding.[35] Of note, MDCT evaluation of these patients usually requires a noncontrast study. Another area in which CT is showing increased use is for the evaluation of children with IBD.[35] In these patients, CT may be superior to fluoroscopy for demonstrating inflammatory changes within the bowel as well as extraluminal manifestations of IBD, such as peribowel inflammatory change or abscess.[35]

In the chest, MDCT is used for the evaluation of infection and complication of infections, as well as cancer detection and surveillance. Evaluation of congenital abnormalities of the lung, mediastinum, and heart are also indications. In particular, MDCT may be useful in the assessment of bronchopulmonary foregut malformations in which sequestration is a consideration.[34] Similarly, the use of MDCT in the evaluation of the pediatric cardiovascular system has been particularly valuable.[37] Assessment of cardiovascular conditions, such as aortic aneurysms, dissections, and vascular rings, may be significantly better than with echocardiography. Finally, MDCT is advantageous in the evaluation of patients with pectus malformations, because it allows for lower doses of radiation.[35]

Three-Dimensional Computed Tomography

The advent of helical CT and MDCT has enabled the postacquisition processing of individual studies for the creation of three-dimensional CT image reconstructions. These 3D reconstructions are valuable in the preoperative planning of complex surgical procedures. Although 3D CT imaging has been possible for almost 25 years, the quality, speed, and affordability of these techniques have only recently improved enough to result in their incorporation into routine clinical practice.[38] Currently, four main visualization techniques are used in CT reconstruction labs to create 3D CT images. These include multiplanar reformation, maximum intensity projections, shaded surface displays, and volume rendering. Multiplanar reformation and maximum intensity projections are limited to external visualization, while shaded surface displays and volume rendering allow immersive or internal visualization, such as virtual endoscopy.[33]

Three-dimensional CT has been beneficial in the preoperative planning of pediatric craniofacial, vascular, and spinal operations. Specifically, 3D CT has been used to evaluate maxillofacial fractures[39] and craniofacial abnormalities, as well as vascular malformations. Figure 4-5 illustrates a 3D CT reconstruction of an infant with craniosynostosis. Similarly, 3D CT has been reported useful in the planning of hemivertebra excision procedures for thoracic and thoracolumbar congenital deformities.[40] A particularly interesting application of 3D CT is the creation of "virtual endoscopy" images for the interior surface of luminal structures, such as the bowel, airways, blood vessels, and urinary tract.[33] In particular, virtual endoscopy using 3D CT may be useful in the diagnosis of small bowel tumors, lesions that are often difficult to detect using standard modalities (Fig. 4-6).[38]

Electron Beam Computed Tomography

Introduced clinically in the 1980s, electron beam computed tomography (EBCT) scanners are primarily used in adult cardiology to image the beating heart. As opposed to traditional CT scanners, EBCT systems do not use a rotating assembly consisting of an x-ray source directly opposite an x-ray detector. Instead, EBCT scanners use a large, stationary x-ray tube that partially surrounds the imaging field. The x-ray source is moved by electromagnetically sweeping the electron beam focal point along an array of tungsten anodes positioned around the patient. The anodes that are hit emit x-rays that are collimated in a similar fashion to standard CT scanners. Because this is not mechanically driven, the movement can be very fast. In fact, EBCT scanners can acquire images up to 10 times faster than helical CT scanners. Current EBCT systems are capable of performing an image sweep in 0.025 seconds compared with the 0.33

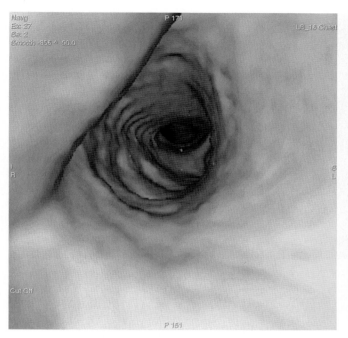

FIGURE 4-6 Virtual colonoscopy.

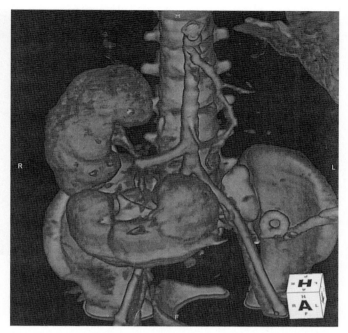

FIGURE 4-7 Electron beam computed tomography of transplanted kidney. (From Talisetti A, Jelnin V, Ruiz C, et al: Electron beam CT scan is a valuable and safe imaging tool for the pediatric surgical patient. J Pediatr Surg 2004;39:1859–1862.)

seconds for the fastest mechanically swept CT systems. This rapid acquisition speed minimizes motion artifacts, enabling the use of EBCT scanners for imaging the beating heart. In addition to faster image acquisition times resulting in decreased motion artifacts, EBCT scanners generally result in a 6- to 10-fold decrease in radiation exposure compared with traditional CT scanners.

To date, EBCT scanners have not yet seen widespread adoption. The systems are necessarily larger and more expensive than helical CT scanners. Advances in multidetector helical CT scan designs have enabled cardiac imaging using standard, mechanically driven systems.

The use of EBCT in the pediatric population has primarily been reported for the imaging of cardiac anomalies.[41,42] However, as we increasingly understand the risks associated with ionizing radiation exposure in children, the decreased exposure associated with EBCT systems appears attractive. In addition, the faster acquisition times and minimization of motion artifact could theoretically result in decreased sedation requirements in young patients. Talisetti and colleagues reported the use of EBCT to evaluate several pediatric surgical patients—one patient with thoracic dystrophy and an abdominal wall hernia, one patient with ascites status postrenal transplant (Fig. 4-7), and several patients with renal and pelvic tumors.[43] In their report, they highlighted the potential advantages of decreased radiation exposure and sedation requirements associated with EBCT systems.

MAGNETIC RESONANCE IMAGING

The first MRI examination on a human was performed in 1977 by Dr. Raymond Damadian, with colleagues Dr. Larry Minkoff and Dr. Michael Goldsmith. This initial exam took 5 hours to produce one, relatively poor quality image. Since then, technological improvements have increased the resolution and speed of MRI. Today, MRI is able to provide unparalleled

noninvasive images of the human body. In addition, newer MRI systems now allow images to be obtained at subsecond intervals, facilitating fast, near real-time MRI. Similarly, new MRI techniques are now being developed to provide functional information on the physiologic state of the body. This section will provide a brief overview of MRI, focusing on recent technologic advances, such as *ultrafast MRI, higher field strength MRI systems, motion artifact reduction techniques,* and *functional MRI.*

MRI creates images by using a strong, uniform magnetic field to align the spinning hydrogen protons of the human body. A radiofrequency (RF) pulse is then applied, causing some of the protons to absorb the energy and spin in a different direction. When the RF pulse is turned off, these protons realign and release their stored energy. This release of energy gives off a signal that is detected, quantified, and sent to a computer. Because different tissues respond to the magnetic field and RF pulse in a different manner, they give off variable energy signals. These signals are then used to create an image using mathematical algorithms.

Higher Field Strength MRI Systems

Over the last decade, MRI has advanced significantly with the transition from 1.5 Tesla (T) to 3.0 T field strength systems (Fig. 4-8). Using higher magnetic field strength, 3.0 T systems demonstrate improved image resolution, faster image acquisition speeds, and improved fat suppression.[44] In addition, 3.0 T systems theoretically enable a twofold increase in signal-to-noise ratio (SNR) compared with 1.5 T systems as SNR increases linearly with field strength. This is particularly important for imaging smaller patients with anatomical structures. Although 3.0 T systems are rapidly becoming the standard in pediatric MRI imaging, ultrahigh field strength 7.0 T systems are currently being evaluated. These systems

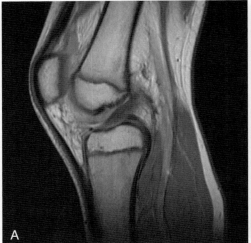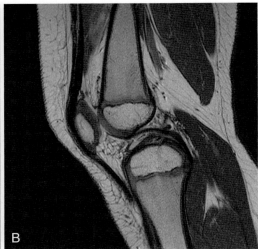

FIGURE 4-8 Comparison of image quality between 1.5 T (**A**) and 3.0 T (**B**). (From MacKenzie JD, Vasanawala SS: Advances in pediatric MR imaging. Magn Reson Imaging Clin N Am 2008;16:385–402.)

potentially provide the same advantages listed above but to a higher degree. Disadvantages include higher deposition of radiofrequency energy, magnification of artifacts, and more challenging hardware and software design. Although still under investigation, ultrahigh field strength MRI may enable unique studies such as sodium imaging, which can be used to monitor renal physiology and function, myocardial viability, and phosphorous imaging, which has been suggested as a method of evaluating organ pH and cancer metabolism.[44]

Ultrafast MRI

The first major development in high speed MRI occurred in 1986 with the introduction of the gradient-echo pulse sequence technique (GRE). This technique decreased practical scan times to as little as 10 seconds. In addition to increasing the patient throughput of MRI scanners, the faster scan times significantly increased the application of MR imaging in body regions (e.g., the abdomen) where suspended respiration could eliminate most motion-related image distortions.[45,46] Since then, GRE techniques have undergone iterations and further developments, such as balanced steady-state imaging, achieving subsecond level scan times.

More recently, parallel imaging (or parallel MRI) has emerged as a method of increasing MRI imaging speed. Parallel imaging techniques are able to construct images using reduced data sets by combining the signals of several coil elements in a phased array. In this manner, higher imaging speeds are achievable, generally allowing speed increases of two- to threefold.[44] In addition, MRI parallel imaging results in improved signal-to-noise ratio, thereby decreasing artifact and improving image quality.

The high speed of ultrafast MRI represents a significant advantage in the care of children. Most traditional MR protocols require 30 to 40 minutes of table occupancy. During this time the patient must remain still to avoid motion artifact.[47] For many children, this often requires sedation, general anesthesia, and even muscular blockade to enable them to remain motionless long enough for a quality study to be completed. This is obviously a significant impediment toward the widespread use of MRI in children. Ultrafast MRI significantly reduces this requirement, not only minimizing the potential side effects of

sedation during routine MRI studies but also allowing the use of MRI to study high-risk infants who cannot be adequately sedated or paralyzed.[48]

Ultrafast MRI also significantly reduces the motion artifacts that occur in the abdomen and thorax resulting from normal respiratory and peristaltic movements. In particular, the smearing artifact associated with the use of oral contrast agents during MR imaging of the intestinal tract had previously decreased image quality.[49] Using GRE and parallel imaging techniques, modern MRI can achieve scan times that are fast enough to be completed during a breath hold and are fast relative to normal abdominal motion.[44] In addition, by decreasing motion artifact and enabling fast image acquisition, ultrafast MRI protocols enable the practical application of cardiac MRI and fetal MRI.[50] Similarly, volumetric or 3D MRI has become practically feasible in children with ultrafast MRI techniques that decrease the acquisition time required for these data intensive studies.[44]

Motion Artifact Reduction Techniques

Motion artifacts may be secondary to physiologic movement (cardiac, respiratory, and peristaltic) as well as voluntary movement. This is particularly significant in pediatric patients. Recently, several techniques have been used to minimize motion artifacts. One broad method employs high-speed image acquisition as detailed above. Another method is navigation imaging where extra navigator echoes are used to detect image displacements. These displacements are used to reject or correct data reducing artifacts.[44] Currently, navigation imaging has been applied to cardiac imaging and hepatobiliary imaging to reduce motion artifacts caused by respiratory movement. Similarly, PROPELLER (periodically rotated overlapping parallel lines with enhanced reconstruction) imaging is a method for reducing motion artifacts by signal averaging successive rotating samples of data.

Functional Magnetic Resonance Imaging

Functional magnetic resonance imaging (fMRI) is a rapidly evolving imaging technique that uses blood flow differences in the brain to provide in vivo images of neuronal activity. First described just more than 15 years ago, fMRI has seen widespread clinical and research application in the adult population. Functional MRI is founded on two basic physiologic assumptions regarding neuronal activity and metabolism. Specifically, fMRI assumes that neuronal activation induces an increase in local glucose metabolism, and that this increased metabolic demand is answered by an increase in local cerebral blood flow.[51] By detecting small changes in local blood flow, fMRI techniques are able to provide a "functional" image of brain activity. Currently, the most commonly used technique is known as "blood oxygen level–dependent" (BOLD) contrast, which uses blood as an internal contrast medium.[52] BOLD imaging takes advantage of small differences in the magnetic properties of oxygenated and deoxygenated hemoglobin. Since neuronal activation is followed by increased and relatively excessive local cerebral blood flow, more oxygenated hemoglobin appears in the venous capillaries of activated regions of the brain. These differences are detected as minute distortions in the magnetic field by fMRI and can be used to create a functional image of brain activity.[51]

Functional magnetic resonance imaging requires significant subject preparation in order to prepare the child to lie still in the scanner for the duration of the study. Various preparation techniques have been described that decrease the anxiety and uncertainty that a child might experience regarding the study. These include presession educational videos, presession tours with members of the radiology staff, and presession practice runs. Optimally, fMRI studies require a nonsedated, cooperative patient to assess functional neuronal activity. However, it has been recently shown that passive range of motion may activate the sensorimotor complex in sedated patients. This may enable functional motor mapping in patients who are unable to cooperate with active tasks.[53]

At this time, the use of fMRI in the pediatric population is still at the earliest stages. However, fMRI holds tremendous promise in the evaluation of central nervous system (CNS) organization and development, characterization of brain plasticity, and the evaluation and understanding of neurobehavioral disorders.[51] In addition, current clinical applications of fMRI include the delineation of eloquent cortex near a space-occupying lesion and the determination of the dominant hemisphere for language. fMRI is also used to map the motor cortex. These clinical applications are designed to provide preoperative functional information for patients undergoing epilepsy or tumor surgery.[53] This information can be used to guide resection and to predict postoperative deficits.[53]

Fetal Magnetic Resonance Imaging

Magnetic resonance imaging has become an increasingly used imaging modality for the evaluation of fetal abnormalities. Rapid image acquisition times and motion artifact reduction techniques allow for effective imaging studies despite fetal movement. Although US remains the primary modality for imaging the unborn fetus, fetal MRI has demonstrated several distinct advantages. In addition to providing fine anatomic detail, fetal MRI is not limited by maternal obesity, fetal position, or oligohydramnios—all factors that can limit the effectiveness of US evaluation.[54] The use of fetal MRI to characterize fetal CNS, thoracic, abdominal, genitourinary, and extremity anomalies has been well described. Particularly relevant to the field of pediatric surgery, fetal MRI has been used to assist in the prenatal differentiation between enteric cysts and meconium pseudocysts. Similarly, fetal MRI is used to characterize the nature and origin of abdominal masses and to evaluate

fetal tumors.[54] Such information may be valuable for prenatal counseling and decision making as well as for preoperative planning. As the field of fetal surgery matures, fetal MRI may become increasingly useful in the evaluation of abnormalities amenable to fetal intervention.

POSITRON EMISSION TOMOGRAPHY IMAGING

Positron emission tomography, or PET, is an increasingly used imaging technology that provides information on the functional status of the human body. First developed in 1973 by Edward Hoffman, Michael Ter-Pogossian, and Michael Phelps at Washington University, PET imaging is now one of the most commonly performed nuclear medicine studies in the United States.[55] Although CT, MRI, and US imaging techniques provide detailed information regarding the anatomic state of a patient, PET imaging provides information on the current metabolic state of the patient's tissues. In this manner, PET imaging is often able to detect metabolic changes indicative of a pathologic state before anatomic changes can be visualized.

PET imaging is based on the detection of photons released when positron emitting radionuclides undergo annihilation with electrons.[56] These radionuclides are created by bombarding target material with protons that have been accelerated in a cyclotron.[56] These positron-emitting radionuclides are then used to synthesize radiopharmaceuticals that are part of biochemical pathways in the human body.[56] The most commonly used example of this is the use of the fluorinated analog of glucose, 2-deoxy-2-(18)F-fluoro-D-deoxyglucose (FDG).[57] Like glucose, FDG is phosphorylated by the intracellular enzyme hexokinase. In its phosphorylated form, FDG does not cross cell membranes and therefore accumulates within metabolically active cells. In this manner, PET imaging using FDG provides information about the glucose use in different body tissues.[57]

In order to be detected, FDG is synthesized using ^{18}F, a radioisotope with a half-life of 110 minutes.[57] The synthesis process begins by accelerating negatively charged hydrogen ions in a cyclotron until they gain approximately 8 MeV of energy. The orbital electrons from these hydrogen ions are then removed by passing through a carbon foil. The resultant high-energy protons are then directed toward a target chamber that contains stable ^{18}O enriched water.[56] The protons undergo a nuclear reaction with the ^{18}O enriched water to form hydrogen ^{18}F fluoride. The reaction is detailed in the equation that follows.[56]

$$H_2(^{18}O) + {}^1H + \text{ energy} \rightarrow H_2(^{18}F)$$

^{18}F is an unstable radioisotope that decays by beta-plus emission or electron capture and emits a neutrino (v) and a positron (β^+).[56] The emitted positrons are then annihilated with electrons to release energy in the form of photons, which are detected by modern PET scanners and are the basis of PET imaging. The detectors in PET scanners are scintillation crystals coupled to photomultiplier tubes. Currently, most PET scanners use crystals composed of bismuth germinate, cerium-doped lutetium oxyorthosilicate, or cerium-doped gadolinium silicate.[56] Because PET scanning uses unstable radioisotopes, PET probes must be synthesized immediately prior to a PET study. This limits the immediate and widespread availability of PET imaging, because the studies must therefore be scheduled in advance. FDG is a convenient probe because its half-life of 110 minutes allows it to be transported from a remote cyclotron to a PET scanner in enough time to perform a typical whole-body PET imaging study ($\geq$30 minutes).[57]

In a typical PET study, the radiopharmaceutical agent is systemically administered to the patient by intravenous injection. The patient is then imaged by the PET scanner, which measures the radioactivity (photon emission as above) throughout the body and creates 3D pictures or images of tissue function. Currently, PET imaging is used extensively for the accurate evaluation and monitoring of tumors of the lung, colon, breast, lymph nodes, and skin.[58] PET imaging is used to facilitate tumor diagnosis, localization, and staging; monitoring of antitumor therapy; tumor tissue characterization; radionuclide therapy; and screening for tumor recurrence.[59] Though nonspecific, FDG is often used because malignant cells generally display increased glucose use with up-regulation of hexokinase activity.[56]

PET imaging has also been used to assess the activity of noncancerous tissues to provide information on their viability or metabolic activity. In adults, PET scans are used to determine the viability of cardiac tissue in order to decide whether a patient would benefit from coronary bypass grafting.[60,61] Recently, this application was extended to the pediatric population in order to assess cardiac function after arterial switch operations with suspected myocardial infarction.[62] Similarly, PET scans can be used to visualize viability of brain tissue in order to make prognostic determinations after stroke.[63] Finally, PET imaging is used to identify regions of abnormal activity in brain tissue, helping to localize seizure foci or diagnose functional disorders, such as Parkinson disease and Alzheimer disease.[64,65]

Though PET imaging provides important functional information regarding the metabolic activity of human tissues, it often provides relatively imprecise images compared with traditional anatomic imaging modalities. This is in large part because of the physics of PET as an imaging modality. Specifically, the positrons emitted by radionuclides, such as FDG, generally have enough kinetic energy to travel a small distance before annihilating with an electron.[56] This distance is called the *mean positron range* and varies depending on tissue density. The difference in position between the initial location of the positron and its site of annihilation results in positron range blurring. This limits the spatial resolution of PET imaging, which is typically considered to be approximately 5 mm using current scanners.[56] *Noncollinearity* or variation in the path of emitted photons other than the expected 180 degrees, also contributes to decreased spatial resolution in PET imaging. Because of these limitations, PET imaging is often useful for highlighting areas suspicious for malignancy but may be difficult to use during preoperative planning, because it does not accurately correlate the area of suspicion with detailed anatomic information.[58]

Recently, combined PET/CT scanners have been developed that simultaneously perform PET scans and high resolution CT scans. Introduced 10 years ago, these scanners provide functional information obtained from the PET scan and accurately map it to the fine anatomic detail of the CT scan (Fig. 4-9).[57] Prior to the availability of PET/CT scanners, CT and PET scans of the same patient acquired on different scanners at different times were often aligned using complex, labor-intensive algorithms.[57] However, other than for brain imaging, these algorithms often failed to adequately fuse the studies. In contrast, combined PET/CT scanners rely on hardware fusion and not solely software manipulation and do not suffer these limitations.

In the field of pediatric surgery, PET/CT scanning represents a new imaging modality with tremendous potential in regard to preoperative planning and postoperative follow-up. However, several issues specific to the pediatric population make the implementation of PET imaging challenging, including the need for fasting, intravenous access, bladder catheterization, sedation, and clearance from the urinary tract.[66,67] Currently, the clinical application of combined PET/CT imaging in the pediatric population has not been extensively studied. However, the combination of functional information with fine anatomic data provides obvious advantages with regard to surgical planning and will therefore likely play a large role in surgical practice.

MOLECULAR IMAGING

Ultrasonography, CT, MRI, and PET imaging represent established technologies that are commonly used in the care of pediatric patients around the world. Although these technologies provide detailed anatomic and even functional information, their clinical application has yet to provide information at the cellular/molecular level. In contrast to these classical imaging modalities, a new field termed "molecular imaging" sets forth to probe the molecular abnormalities that are the basis of disease rather than to image the end effects of these alterations.[68] Molecular imaging is a rapidly growing research discipline that combines the modern tools of molecular and cell biology with noninvasive imaging technologies. The goal of this new field is to develop techniques and assays for imaging physiologic events and pathways in living organisms at the cellular/molecular level, particularly those pathways that are key targets in specific disease processes. The development and application of molecular imaging will someday directly affect patient care by elucidating the molecular processes underlying disease and lead to the early detection of molecular changes that represent "predisease" states.[69]

Molecular imaging can be defined as "the in vivo characterization and measurement of biologic processes at the cellular and molecular level."[68] From a simplistic standpoint, molecular imaging consists of two basic elements:

1. Molecular probes whose concentration, activity and/or luminescent properties are changed by the specific biologic process under investigation[69]
2. A means by which to monitor these probes[69]

Currently, most molecular probes are either radioisotopes that emit detectable radioactive signals or light- or near-infrared (NIR)–emitting molecules.[69] These probes are considered either direct binding probes or indirect binding probes.[70] Radiolabeled antibodies designed to facilitate the imaging of cell-specific surface antigens or epitopes are commonly used examples of direct binding probes.[70] Similarly, radiolabeled oligonucleotide antisense probes developed to specifically hybridize with target messenger RNA (mRNA) or proteins for the purpose of direct, in vivo imaging are more recent examples.[70] Radiolabeled oligonucleotides represent complimentary sequences to a small segment of target mRNA or DNA, allowing for the direct imaging of endogenous gene

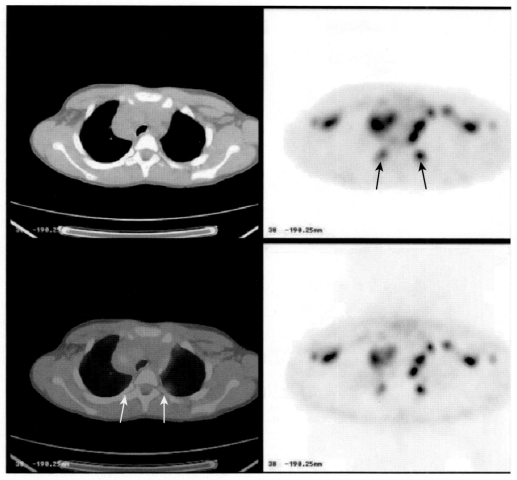

FIGURE 4-9   Combined positron emission tomography (PET)-CT images (axial) through the upper chest of a 7-year-old girl with a mediastinal mass found to be a necrotizing granuloma. Multiple sites of 2-deoxy-2-(18)F-fluoro-D-deoxyglucose (FDG)–avid axillary lymph nodes and multiple foci within the mediastinal mass are visualized. Arrows highlight the symmetric avidity of the costovertebral junctions for FDG that can be seen in children. (From Kaste SC: Issues specific to implementing PET-CT for pediatric oncology: What we have learned along the way? Pediatr Radiol 2004;34:205-213.) *(See Expert Consult site for color version.)*

expression at the transcriptional level.[70] Finally, positron-emitting analogs of dopamine, used to image the dopamine receptors of the brain, are other examples of direct binding probes.[69]

Although direct binding probes assist in the imaging of the amount or concentration of their targets, indirect probes reflect the activities of their macromolecular targets. Perhaps the most widely used example of an indirect binding probe is the hexokinase substrate FDG. The most common probe used in clinical PET imaging, FDG is used for neurologic, cardiovascular, and oncology investigations.[69] Systemically administered FDG is accessible to essentially all tissues.[69]

The use of reporter transgene technology is another powerful example of molecular imaging with indirect binding probes. Reporter genes are nucleic acid sequences encoding easily assayed proteins. Such reporter genes have been long used in molecular biology and genetics studies to investigate intracellular properties and events, such as promoter function/strength, protein trafficking, and gene delivery. Using molecular imaging techniques, reporter genes have now been used to analyze gene delivery, immune cell therapies, and the in vivo efficacy of inhibitory mRNAs in animal models.[71] In vivo bioluminescent imaging using the firefly or *Rinella*

luciferase or fluorescent optical imaging using green fluorescent protein (GFP) or DsRed are optical imaging examples of this technique (Fig. 4-10).[72,73] Recently, semiconductor quantum dots have been used in fluorescent optical imaging studies. Although fluorescent proteins are limited in their number of available colors, quantum dots can fluoresce at different colors over a broad region of the spectrum by altering their size and surface coating. To date, the quantum dots that have been tested with in vivo experimental models include amphiphilicpoly (acrylic acid), short-chain (750 D) methoxy-PEG and long-chain (3400 D) carboxy-PEG quantum dots, and long-chain (5000 D) methoxy-PEG quantum dots.[74]

In the field of immunology and immunotherapy research, Costa and colleagues transduced the autoantigen-reactive CD4+ T-cell population specific for myelin basic protein (MBP) with a retrovirus that encoded a dual reporter protein composed of GFP and luciferase, along with a 40 kD monomer of interleukin-12 as a therapeutic protein.[75] Bioluminescent imaging (BLI) techniques were then used to monitor the migratory patterns of the cells in an animal model of multiple sclerosis. BLI demonstrated that the immune cells that would typically cause destruction of myelin trafficked to the central nervous system in symptomatic animals. Furthermore, they

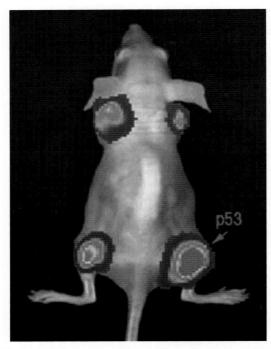

FIGURE 4-10   Nude mouse carrying a wild-type *TP53*-expressing human colon xenograft with a stably integrated *TP53*-responsive luciferase reporter gene. Injection of exogenous *TP53* expressed by an adenovirus vector led to detectable increase in luciferase activity within an established tumor *(arrow)*. (From Schnepp R, Hua X: A tumor-suppressing duo: TGFbeta and activin modulate a similar transcriptome. Cancer Biol Ther 2003;2:171-172.) *(See Expert Consult site for color version.)*

found that CD4 T-cell expression of the IL-12 immune modulator resulted in a clinical reduction in disease severity.[75]

Similarly, Vooijs and colleagues generated transgenic mice in which activation of luciferase expression was coupled to deletion of the retinoblastoma (*Rb*) tumor suppressor gene.[76] Loss of *Rb* triggered the development of pituitary tumors in their animal model, allowing them to monitor tumor onset, progression, and response to therapy in individual animals by repeated CCD (charged coupled device) imaging of luciferase activity.[76] Although optical imaging techniques are commonly used, reporter genes can also encode for extracellular or intracellular receptors or transporters that bind or transport a radiolabeled or paramagnetic probe, allowing for PET-, SPECT- (single-photon emission tomography), or MRI-based molecular imaging.[70]

The second major element of molecular imaging is the imaging modality/technology itself. Direct and indirect binding probes can be radiolabeled to allow nuclear-based in vivo imaging of a desired cellular/molecular event or process using PET or SPECT imaging. In fact, micro-PET and micro-SPECT systems have been developed specifically for molecular imaging studies in animal models.[68] Similarly, optical imaging techniques, such as bioluminescent imaging, near-infrared spectroscopy, and visible light imaging using sensitive CCDs can be used with optically active probes to visualize desired cellular events. Finally, anatomic imaging modalities, such as MRI, CT, and US, have all been adopted for use in animal-based molecular imaging studies.[68]

At this time, the field of molecular imaging is largely an experimental one, with significant activity in the laboratory and little current clinical application. Molecular imaging research is largely focused on investigating the molecular basis of clinical disease states and their potential treatments, including mechanisms surrounding apoptosis, angiogenesis, tumor growth and development, and gene therapy.[68]

DNA MICROARRAYS

The descriptive term *genomics* acknowledges the shift from a desire to understand the actions of single genes and their individual functions to a more integrated understanding of the simultaneous actions of multiple genes and the subsequent effect exerted on cellular behavior. DNA microarrays, or gene chips, are a recent advancement that allows the simultaneous assay of thousands of genes.[77] Microarray technology has been applied to redefine biologic behavior of tumors, cross-species genomic comparisons, and large scale analyses of gene expression in a variety of conditions. In essence, it represents a new form of patient and disease triage, *molecular triage*.

Innovative Therapeutics: Technologies and Techniques

A surgical operation requires two key elements: an "image," or more broadly, information regarding the anatomy of interest, and a "manipulation" of the patient's tissue with the goal of a therapeutic effect. Classically, the "image" is obtained through the eyes of the surgeon and the "manipulation" is performed using the surgeon's hands and simple, traditional surgical instruments. During the last several decades, this paradigm has been broadened by technologies that enhance these two fundamental elements.

As opposed to standard, line-of-sight vision, an "image" may now be obtained through an operating microscope or through a flexible endoscope or laparoscope. This endoscope may be monocular or binocular, providing 2D or 3D visualization. These technologies provide the surgeon with high-quality, magnified images of anatomical areas that may be inaccessible to the naked eye. Similarly, a surgical "manipulation" of tissue and organs may be accomplished using a catheter, flexible endoscope, or longer laparoscopic instruments. Furthermore, devices such as staplers, electrocautery, ultrasonic energy tools, and radiofrequency emitters are all used to manipulate and affect tissue with a therapeutic goal. These technologies have changed the way surgical procedures are performed, enabling and even creating fields such as laparoscopic surgery, interventional endoscopy, and catheter-based intervention. In addition to these advances, several emerging technology platforms promise to further broaden this definition of surgery. These include stereotactic radiosurgery and surgical robotics. This section presents a review of several of these technologies with a focus on the current status of hemostatic and tissue ablative instruments, stereotactic radiosurgery, and surgical robotics.

HEMOSTATIC AND TISSUE ABLATIVE INSTRUMENTS

Handheld energy devices designed to provide hemostasis and ablate tissue are some of the most widely used surgical technologies throughout the world. Since the first reports of electrosurgery in the 1920s,[78] multiple devices and forms of energy have been developed to minimize blood loss during tissue dissection. These instruments, including monopolar and bipolar electrocautery, ultrasonic dissectors, argon beam coagulators, cryotherapy, and infrared coagulators, are used in operating rooms on a daily basis. In addition, improvements to these tools and their techniques or use are continually being developed.

Electrocautery

The application of high-frequency alternating current is now known variously as electrocautery, electrosurgery, or simply "the Bovie." Although the concept of applying an electrical current to living tissue was reported as far back as the late sixteenth century, the practical application of electrocautery in surgery did not begin to develop until the early 1900s. In 1908, Lee de Forest developed a high-frequency generator that was capable of delivering a controlled cutting current. However, this device used expensive vacuum tubes and therefore saw very limited clinical application. In the 1920s, W.T. Bovie developed a low-cost spark-gap generator. The potential for using this device in surgery was recognized by Harvey Cushing during a demonstration in 1926, and the first practical electrosurgery units were in use soon thereafter.[78]

Monopolar electrocautery devices deliver the current through an application electrode through the patient's body returning to a grounding pad. Without a grounding pad, the patient would suffer a thermal burn injury wherever the current sought reentry. The area of contact is critical, because heat is inversely related to the size of the application device. Accordingly, the tip of the device is typically small, in order to generate heat efficiently, and the returning electrode is large, to broadly disperse energy. There are three other settings that are pertinent: the frequency of the current (power setting), the activation time, and the characteristics of the waveform produced by the generator (intermittent or continuous).

In the "cut" mode, heat is generated quickly with minimal lateral spread. As a result, the device separates tissue without significant coagulation of underlying vessels. In the "coag" mode, the device generates less heat at a slower frequency with larger lateral thermal spread. Consequently, tissue is desiccated and vessels become thrombosed.

Bipolar cautery creates a short circuit between the grasping tips of the instruments; thus the circuit is completed through the grasped tissue between the tips. Because heat develops only within the short-circuited tissue, there is less lateral thermal spread and the mechanical advantage of tissue compression, as well as thermal coagulation.

Recently, advanced bipolar devices use a combination of pressure and bipolar electrocautery to seal tissues. These devices then use a feedback-controlled system that automatically stops the energy delivery when the seal cycle is complete. The tissues are then divided sharply within the sealed zone. Advanced bipolar devices are capable of sealing blood vessels up to 7 mm in diameter, with the seal reportedly capable of withstanding 3 times normal systolic blood pressure. Examples of this class of device include the LigaSure distributed by Covidien (Mansfield, Mass.) and the ENSEAL device distributed by Ethicon Endosurgery (Cincinnati, Ohio).

Argon Beam Coagulator

The argon beam coagulator creates an electric circuit between the tip of the probe and the target tissue through a flowing stream of ionized argon gas. The electrical current is conducted to the tissue through the argon gas and produces thermal coagulation. The flow of the argon gas improves visibility and disperses any surface blood, enhancing coagulation. Its applications in hepatic surgery are unparalleled.

Surgical Lasers

Lasers (*L*ight *A*mplification by *S*timulated *E*mission of *R*adiation) are devices that produce an extremely intense and nearly nondivergent beam of monochromic radiation, usually in the visible region. When focused at close range, laser light is capable of producing intense heat with resultant coagulation. Lateral spread tends to be minimal, and critically, the laser can be delivered through a fiber optic system.

Based on power setting and the photon chosen, depth can be controlled. Penetration depth within the tissue is most shallow with the argon laser, intermediate with the carbon dioxide laser, and of greatest depth with the neodymium-yttrium aluminum garnet (Nd-YAG) laser. Photosensitizing agents provide an additional targeting advantage. The degree of absorption, and thus destruction, depends upon the wavelength selected and the absorptive properties of the tissue based on density, fibrosis, and vascularity.

Photodynamic Therapy

A novel use of light energy is used in photodynamic therapy. A photosensitizer that is target cell–specific is administered and subsequently concentrated in the tissue to be eradicated. The photosensitizing agent may then be activated with a light energy source, leading to tissue destruction. Applications have been widespread.[79] Metaplastic cells, in particular in Barrett esophagus, may also be susceptible.[80]

Ultrasonography

In addition to the diagnostic use of US at low frequency, the delivery of high-frequency US can be used to separate and coagulate tissue. Focused acoustic waves are now used extensively in the treatment of renal calculi as extracorporeal shock wave lithotripsy (ESWL). The focused energy produces a shock wave resulting in fragmentation of the stones to a size that can be spontaneously passed.

When high-intensity focused US (HIFU) energy from multiple beams is focused at a point on a target tissue, heating and thermal necrosis results. None of the individual ultrasonic beams is of sufficient magnitude to cause injury, only at the focus point does thermal injury result. Thus subcutaneous nodules may be targeted without injury to the skin, or nodules within the parenchyma of a solid organ may be destroyed without penetrating the surface. Thus far, however, the focal point is extremely small, thus limiting utility.

Harmonic Scalpel

When US energy at very-high frequency (55,000 Hz) is used, tissue can be separated with minimal peripheral damage. Such high-frequency energy creates vibration, friction, heat, and ultimately, tissue destruction.

Cavitation Devices

The CUSA, a cavitation ultrasonic aspirator, uses lower-frequency US energy with concomitant aspiration. Fragmentation of high-water–content tissue allows for parenchymal destruction, while highlighting vascular structures and permitting their precise coagulation.

Radiofrequency Energy

High-frequency alternating current (350 to 500 kHz) may be used for tissue division, vessel sealing, or tissue ablation. The application of this energy source heats the target tissue, causing protein denaturization and necrosis. A feedback loop sensor discontinues the current at a selected point, minimizing collateral damage. Its targeted use in modulating the lower esophageal sphincter for the treatment of reflux has been reported.[81]

Microwave Energy

Microwave energy (2,450 MHz) can be delivered by a probe to a target tissue. This rapidly alternating electrical signal produces heat and thus coagulation necrosis.

Cryotherapy

At the other end of the temperature spectrum, cold temperatures destroy tissue with a cycle of freezing and thawing with ice crystal formation in the freezing phase and disruption during the thawing phase. Thus far this modality has less utility because high vascular flow, especially in tumors, tends to siphon off the cold.

IMAGE-GUIDED THERAPY

In recent years, ultrasonography, computerized tomography, and magnetic resonance imaging have expanded beyond their role as mere diagnostic modalities, and are now the foundation of sophisticated interactive computer applications that directly guide surgical procedures.[3,82,83] Recent developments in computation technology have fundamentally enhanced the role of medical imaging, from diagnostics described previously to computer-assisted surgery (CAS). During the last decade, medical imaging methods have grown from their initial use as physically based models of human anatomy to applied computer vision and graphical techniques for planning and analyzing surgical procedures. With rapid advances in high-speed computation, the task of assembling and visualizing clinical data has been greatly facilitated, creating new opportunities for real-time, interactive computer applications during surgical procedures.[77–80] This area of development, termed image-guided surgery, has slowly evolved into a field best called *information-guided therapy* (IGT), reflecting the use of a variety of data sources to implement the best therapeutic intervention. Such therapeutic interventions could conceivably range from biopsy to simulation of tissue to direct implantation of medication to radiotherapy. Common to all these highly technical interventions is the need to precisely intervene with the therapeutic modality at a specific point.

However, the effective use of biomedical engineering, computation, and imaging concepts for IGT has not reached its full potential. Significant challenges remain in the development of basic scientific and mathematical frameworks that form the foundation for improving therapeutic interventions through application of relevant information sources.

Significance

As stated in the National Institutes of Health 1995 *Support for Bioengineering Research Report* (http://grants.nih.gov/grants/becon/externalreport.html), an appropriate use of technology would be to replace traditional invasive procedures with non-invasive techniques. The current interest in research in CAS, or IGT, can be attributed in part to the considerable clinical interest in the well-recognized benefits of minimal access surgery (MAS), remaining cognizant of its limitations.

Image-based surgical guidance, on the other hand, addresses these limitations. Image-guided surgical navigational systems have now become the standard of care for cranial neurosurgical procedures in which precise localization within and movement through the brain is of utmost importance.

Patient-specific image data sets such as CT or MRI, when correlated with fixed anatomic reference points (fiducials), can provide surgeons with detailed spatial information about the region of interest. Surgeons can then use these images to precisely target and localize pathologies. Intraoperative computer-assisted imaging improves the surgeon's ability to follow preoperative plans by showing location and optimal directionality. Thus the addition of CAS provides the advantages of MAS with the added benefits of greater precision and the increased likelihood of complete and accurate resections. The junction between CAS and MAS presents research opportunities and challenges for both imaging scientists and surgeons.

General Requirements

Patient-Specific Models   Unlike simulation, IGT requires that modeling data be matched specifically to the patient being treated, since standard fabricated models based upon typical anatomy are inadequate during actual surgical procedures upon a specific patient. Patient-specific images can be generated preoperatively (e.g., by CT or MRI) or intraoperatively (e.g., by US or x-ray).

High Image Quality   IGT depends on spatially accurate models. Images require exceptional resolution in order to portray realistic and consistent information.

Real-Time Feedback   Current systems make the surgeon wait while new images are being segmented and updated. Thus fast dynamic feedback is needed, and the latencies associated with visualization segmentation and registration should be minimized.

High Accuracy and Precision   An American Association of Neurosurgeons survey of 250 neurosurgeons[57] disclosed that surgeons had little tolerance for error (102-mm accuracy in general, and 2 to 3 mm for spinal and orthopedic applications). All elements of visualization, registration, and tracking must be accurate and precise, with special attention given to errors associated with intraoperative tissue deformation.

Repeatability and Robustness   Image-guided therapy systems must be able to automatically incorporate a variety of data so that algorithms work consistently and reliably in any situation.

Correlation of Intraoperative Information with Preoperative Images This requirement is a critical area of interest to biomedical engineers and is especially critical for compensation of tissue deformation. Whether produced by microscopes, endoscopes, fluoroscopes, electrical recordings, physiological simulation, or other imaging techniques, preoperative and intraoperative images and information need to be incorporated into and correlated by the surgical guidance system.

Intuitive Machine and User Interfaces The most important part of any IGT system is its usability. The surgeon's attention must be focused on the patient and not the details of the computational model.

Ultrasound Image-Guided Therapy

Compared with adults, children have excellent US image resolution because of minimal subcutaneous tissue. Furthermore, the lack of ionizing radiation, fast procedure times, relatively low cost, as well as its real-time and multiplanar imaging capabilities, make US especially attractive in the pediatric population. US is the most accessible advanced imaging tool that surgeons can currently use independently. Intraoperative applications include using it as an aid to vascular access, intraoperative tumor localization and resection, and drainage procedures.[84–87]

Computed Tomography and Magnetic Resonance Image-Guided Therapy

Computed tomography and magnetic resonance imaging are not widely used by surgeons without the involvement of radiologists. Although CT-based IGT offers excellent visualization that is not limited by the presence of air or bone, its use in the pediatric population has been limited by concern for the downstream effects of ionizing radiation.[88,89] In addition, there are limited imaging planes, poor differentiation of some lesions related to less fat in babies and children, as well as longer procedure times and greater costs than for US intervention. Nonetheless, CT-guided therapeutic interventions, such as lung and bone biopsies or drainage of deep fluid collections, are routinely done, particularly now that radiation exposure can be reduced with pulsed or intermittent fluoroscopic techniques and dedicated pediatric CT parameters.[82]

The advantages of MRI as a guiding tool include exquisite soft tissue detail, multiplanar real-time imaging, and the ability to assess physiologic and functional parameters (temperature, flow, perfusion).[82,90] Traditional interventional MRI units include an opening that allows easy access to the patient. These units have relatively low field strength, however, which results in poorer image resolution. Higher field strength magnets are now preferred, albeit at the cost of decreased patient accessibility and the requirement of nonferromagnetic instruments. To date, the majority of pediatric applications of MRI-guided therapy have been in the field of neurosurgery. Common applications include tumor ablation/resection or biopsy.[90,91] Currently, there are no data on MRI-guided abdominal interventions in the pediatric population. In 2005, Schulz and colleagues[90] reviewed indications for MR-guided interventions in children. They determined that MR-guided imaging is not a reliable method for chest interventions. They also suggested that the primary use of intraoperative MRI will be for lesions in particularly difficult-to-access areas with nonpalpable findings, such as intracranial and skull base tumors. Future potential applications of MRI include endovascular procedures[91] and thermal ablation of tumors.

Navigational systems establish the relationship between the surgeon's movements and image-based information. They enable the use of preoperative imaging for precise intraoperative localization and resection of lesions using an exact navigation pathway. Neuronavigation systems provide this precise surgical guidance by referencing a coordinate system of the brain with a parallel coordinate system of the three-dimensional image data of the patient.[92,93] These data are displayed on the console of the computer workstation so that the medical images become point-to-point maps of the corresponding actual locations within the brain. The spatial accuracy of these systems is further enhanced by the use of intraoperative MRI that provides real-time images to document the residual lesion and to assess for brain shift during surgery.[94] The precision (error rates of 0.1 to 0.6 mm) provided by neuronavigation systems enables minimal access neurosurgical procedures, significantly reducing morbidity for both adult and pediatric patients.[95] Neuronavigation has not yet been successfully deployed for abdominal surgery. The inability to simply transfer the methodology from neurosurgery is mainly a result of intraoperative organ shifting and corresponding technical difficulties in the online applicability of presurgical cross-sectional imaging data. Furthermore, it remains unclear whether 3D planning and interactive planning tools will increase precision and safety of abdominal surgery.

Radiotherapy and Fractionation

The field of radiation oncology represents perhaps the most mature example of IGT. Radiation therapy, or *radiotherapy*, refers to the use of ionizing radiation for the treatment of pathologic disorders. The use of radiation to cure cancer was first reported in 1899, very soon after Roentgen's discovery of x-rays in 1895.[96] In the 1930s, Coutard described the practice of "fractionation,"[96] which refers to the division of a total dose of radiation into multiple smaller doses, typically given on a daily basis. Fractionation is a bedrock principle that underlies the entire field of radiotherapy.[97,98] By administering radiation in multiple daily fractions over the course of several weeks, it is possible to irradiate a tumor with a higher total dose while relatively sparing the surrounding normal tissue from the most injurious effects of treatment. By fractionating the therapy, normal tissue should be allowed to recover while pathologic tissue is destroyed. Though fractionation regimens differ depending on specific pathology, current regimens often involve up to 30 treatments.[96]

Stereotactic Radiosurgery

Stereotactic radiosurgery refers to the method and corresponding technology for delivering a single high dose of ablative radiation to target tissue using precision targeting and large numbers of cross-fired highly collimated beams of high-energy ionizing radiation. Conceptualized in the 1950s by Swedish neurosurgeon Lars Leksell, this technology has been used to treat/ablate a variety of benign and malignant intracranial lesions without any incision.[99] Leksell showed that there was an exponential relation between dose and the time during which necrosis developed.[96]

Most recently, radiosurgical techniques are being applied toward the treatment of extracranial diseases, including spinal tumors and lesions of the thoracic and abdominal cavities.[100,101] Many of the newest applications of stereotactic radiosurgery fall under the traditional realm of general surgery, including lung, liver, and pancreatic cancers. The lesioning of normal brain tissue, such as the trigeminal nerve (trigeminal neuralgia), thalamus (tremor), and epileptic foci (intractable seizures) is also an important clinical application of this technology.[102] Numerous studies have demonstrated radiosurgery to be an important treatment option for many otolaryngologic conditions, such as skull base and neck tumors.[103–106] As the scientific understanding and clinical practice of radiosurgery develops, such technology may become an increasingly valuable, minimally invasive option for treating a range of pediatric general surgical diseases.

Stereotactic radiosurgery has the potential advantage of delivering a much larger radiation dose to a pathologic lesion without exceeding the radiation tolerance of the surrounding normal tissue. This single, or limited, dose treatment of a small volume of tissue is achieved by targeting the tissue with large numbers of intersecting beams of radiation. "Stereotactic" refers to the fact that radiosurgery uses computer algorithms to coordinate the patient's real-time anatomy in the treatment suite with a preoperative image to allow precise targeting of a desired tissue area. To achieve this, the patient's anatomy must usually be fixed using a stereotactic frame.[96] The preoperative images are then taken with the frame in place, and the patient's anatomy is mapped in relation to the frame. This stereotactic frame is rigidly fixed to the patient's skull, thereby limiting movement of the target anatomy. In addition, the frame serves as an external fiducial system that correlates the coordinates of the target tissues, determined during preoperative imaging and planning, to the treatment room. Radiosurgical treatment is then delivered to the appropriate tissue using this coordinate system.

Stereotactic Radiosurgical Platforms

Currently, there are several classes of stereotactic radiosurgery systems in use. These include heavy-particle radiosurgery systems, Gamma Knife radiosurgery, and linear accelerator radiosurgery. Currently, heavy particle radiosurgery systems and Gamma Knife radiosurgery systems are only used to treat intracranial lesions. In contrast, linear accelerator systems have been adapted to treat both cranial and extracranial lesions.

Linear Accelerator Radiosurgery

Linear accelerators, or linacs, have long been a mainstay of standard fractionated radiotherapy and were modified for radiosurgery in 1982.[96] Linac radiosurgery has become a cost effective and widely used alternative to Gamma Knife radiosurgery. When used for radiosurgery, linacs crossfire a photon beam by moving in multiple arc-shaped paths around the patient's head. The area of crossfire where the multiple fired beams intersect receives a high amount of radiation, with minimal exposure to the surrounding normal tissue.[96] Patients treated with linac radiosurgery must also wear a stereotactic frame fixed to the skull for preoperative imaging and therapy. Currently, linac radiosurgery is the predominant modality in the United States, with approximately 6 times more active centers than Gamma Knife facilities.[96]

Frameless Image-Guided Radiosurgery

Recently, novel systems have been developed that use linear accelerators with innovative hardware and software systems capable of performing frameless image-guided radiosurgery. One such system, the CyberKnife (Accuray, Sunnyvale, Calif.), uses a lightweight linac unit, designed for radiosurgery, mounted on a highly maneuverable robotic arm.[107] The robotic arm can position and point the linear accelerator with 6 degrees of freedom and 0.3-mm precision. In addition, the CyberKnife system features image guidance, which eliminates the need to use skeletal fixation.[102,108] The CyberKnife acquires a series of stereoscopic radiographs that identify a preoperatively placed gold fiducial. This fiducial is placed under local anesthetic during the preoperative imaging and planning sessions to allow the system to correlate the patient's target anatomy with the preoperative image for treatment. By actively acquiring radiographs during the treatment session, the system is able to track and follow the patient's target anatomy in near real-time during treatment.[102,108] With this image guidance system, the CyberKnife is able to function without a fixed stereotactic frame, enabling fractionation (often termed hypofractionated radiosurgery or radiotherapy) of treatments as well as extracorporeal stereotactic radiosurgery. In pediatric surgery, this may represent a significant technical advantage, because it may enable the use of radiosurgery for the treatment of intrathoracic and intraabdominal pathologies (Fig. 4-11). Similarly, the Novalis Tx (Varian Medical Systems, Palo Alto, Calif.) uses an integrated cone beam CT scan system to provide volumetric imaging as well as fluoroscopic imaging to compensate for respiratory motion to enable frameless, image-guided radiosurgery. In contrast, the Trilogy system (Varian Medical Systems, Palo Alto, Calif.) uses real-time optical guidance to direct radiation delivery to the target lesion (Fig. 4-12). Both of these systems use a multileaf collimator that adapts radiation treatment to complex shapes. In addition, they use intensity modulation to help limit toxicity to surrounding tissue. Both systems deliver treatments in sessions of less than 30 minutes, which may decrease the need for sedation in pediatric patients.[109] Furthermore, the Trilogy system minimizes radiation exposure further by using an optically based guidance system.[109]

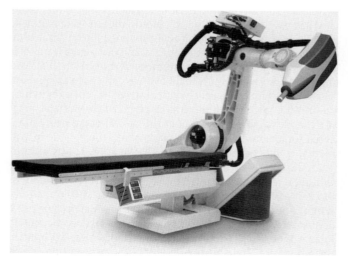

FIGURE 4-11 Cyberknife System (Courtesy Accuray, Sunnyvale, Calif.) *(See Expert Consult site for color version.)*

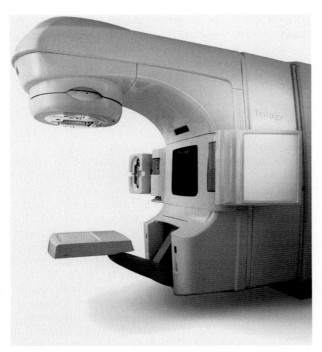

FIGURE 4-12 Trilogy Radiosurgery System (Courtesy Varian Medical Systems, Palo Alto, Calif.) *(See Expert Consult site for color version.)*

CLINICAL APPLICATION OF STEREOTACTIC RADIOSURGERY IN CHILDREN

To date, pediatric radiosurgery has primarily been used to treat intracranial pathologies. Hadjipanavis and colleagues reported a series of 37 patients (mean age 14) with unresectable pylocytic astrocytomas treated with stereotactic radiosurgery.[110] They found radiosurgery to be a valuable adjunctive strategy in patients whose disease was not amenable to surgical therapy.[110] Somaza and colleagues reported their experience with the use of stereotactic radiosurgery for the treatment of growing and unresectable deep-seated pilocytic astrocytomas in 9 pediatric patients.[111] Two of the patients had already failed fractionated radiotherapy, and 7 patients were considered to be at high risk for adverse radiation effects given their young age. After 19 months follow-up, there was a marked decrease in tumor size in 5 patients, while the remaining 4 patients displayed no further tumor growth. Overall, the authors felt that stereotactic radiosurgery offered a safe and effective therapy in the management of children with deep, small-volume pilocytic astrocytomas.[111]

The use of stereotactic radiosurgery for the treatment of nonmalignant intracranial lesions in children has also been described. Specifically, the use of radiosurgery for the treatment of cerebral arteriovenous malformations (AVMs) has been reported. Although microsurgical resection remains the treatment of choice for most accessible AVMs, lesions located in critical cortical areas or in deep portions of the brain are increasingly treated with radiosurgery because of the risk of surgical resection.[112] Foy and colleagues reported a series of 60 pediatric patients with AVMs treated with radiosurgery. Nidus obliteration was reported at 52% after a single radiosurgery session, increasing to 63% with repeated sessions.[112] Similarly Nicolato and colleagues reported a cohort of 62 children with AVMs treated with radiosurgery. They reported an obliteration rate of 85.5%.[113] Overall, these authors conclude that stereotactic radiosurgery is a safe and effective option for properly selected children with AVMs. In particular, it may benefit children with AVMs located in critical portions of the brain where surgical resection may pose a large risk.[112]

Compared with the adult population, the experience with stereotactic radiosurgery in children is still limited. The early reports described above all highlight the safety and efficacy of radiosurgery as a treatment modality, but clinical follow-up is still early, with many of the reports limiting the use of radiosurgery to the treatment of surgically unresectable disease. Despite relatively limited experience, the use of stereotactic radiosurgery in children may offer several theoretical advantages specific to the pediatric population. Compared with standard, fractionated radiotherapy, stereotactic radiosurgical techniques deliver conformal radiation treatment with millimeter versus centimeter accuracy. All radiation treatments are a balance between providing enough radiation to effectively treat pathologic tissues while minimizing harmful exposure to adjacent normal tissues. In pediatric patients, the distances between normal and pathologic tissues may be very small. In addition, the developing brains of children may be more sensitive to the effects of ionizing radiation than adult brains. In particular, potential cognitive and endocrine disabilities have been described in children after radiotherapy to the brain.[111,114,115] These concerns have largely limited the use of radiation for the treatment of intracranial tumors in infants. Therefore the improved accuracy provided by stereotactic radiosurgery may be particularly important in the pediatric population.

In addition to accuracy, stereotactic radiosurgical techniques differ from radiotherapy in that they use only one or few treatment sessions. As detailed above, standard, fractionated radiotherapy often uses tens of treatment sessions to maximize the beneficial effects of the treatment while minimizing the harmful effects to normal tissues. In children, these multiple treatment sessions may represent a significant challenge. In smaller children, sedation, or even anesthesia, may be necessary to avoid movement. Such interventions are not without risk, and limiting the number of treatment sessions may serve to minimize the overall risk to the child.

Although the advantages of stereotactic radiosurgery in the pediatric population appear promising, it should be noted that there also exist specific disadvantages and limitations that must be overcome. Radiosurgical techniques generally use a stereotactic frame to coordinate preoperative imaging with actual radiation delivery. However, these frames must be secured to the skull using pins and screws. In adults, this can often be performed using only local anesthetic agents. In children, this likely requires significant sedation and possibly general anesthesia. Furthermore, the skulls of infants are soft and less rigid, because their cranial sutures have not yet fused. Because of this, standard stereotactic frames often cannot be applied. Similarly, radiosurgery treatment sessions require the patient to remain still in order for the systems to accurately deliver the radiation treatment. Adults are able to cooperate with the therapy and do not require sedation, whereas younger children and infants may require conscious sedation or general anesthesia. Although this drawback is limited by the relatively few sessions necessary with radiosurgery, it still diminishes the minimally invasive nature of the therapy compared with its application in the adults.

Recently, frameless, image-guided stereotactic radiosurgery has been reported in children. Giller and colleagues described the use of the CyberKnife system in 21 patients, ages ranging from 8 months to 16 years, with tumors considered unresectable. Diagnoses included pilocytic astrocytomas, anaplastic astrocytomas, ependymomas, medulloblastomas, atypical teratoid/rhabdoid tumors, and craniopharyngiomas. Local control was achieved in the patients with pilocytic and anaplastic astrocytoma, three of the patients with medulloblastoma, and the three with craniopharyngioma, but not for those with ependymoma. There were no procedure-related mortalities or complications, and local control was achieved in more than half of the patients. Seventy-one percent of patients received only one treatment session, and 38% of patients did not require general anesthesia. No patients required rigid skull fixation.[115] In an additional report, the same group highlighted the use of the CyberKnife system to perform radiosurgery in five infants.[114] Although standard stereotactic frames were not required, patient immobilization was aided by general anesthesia, form-fitting head supports, face masks, and body molds. No treatment-related toxicity was encountered, and the authors concluded that "radiosurgery with minimal toxicity can be delivered to infants by use of a robotically controlled system that does not require rigid fixation."[114]

Whereas the use of stereotactic radiosurgery for intracranial lesions is well established, its use for treatment of extracranial lesions, specifically intrathoracic and intraabdominal pathologies is still developing. Intracranial contents can be easily immobilized using stereotactic frames, while abdominal and thoracic organs show significant movement resulting from respiration, peristalsis, and so on. As a result, only a small body of literature exists regarding the application of stereotactic radiosurgery for extracranial lesions. Recently, several reports have described the efficacy of stereotactic radiosurgery in adults for the treatment of lesions in the liver,[117,118] pancreas,[119,120] lung,[118,121] and kidney[122,123]—anatomical areas that have traditionally been under the watch of general surgeons. Novel image guidance technologies as well as soft tissue immobilization devices are used to make these therapies possible.

At this time, the majority of the literature represents case reports and series detailing the safety and feasibility of extracranial radiosurgery. In addition, many of the reports focus on the technical and engineering aspects of applying radiosurgical techniques to extracranial targets, with little data on patient outcomes. All of these reports have focused on the adult patient population with no significant reports in children. Despite this inexperience, the technology surrounding stereotactic radiosurgery is rapidly developing and shows significant promise toward the minimally invasive treatment of potentially poorly accessible lesions. Newer, frameless, image-guided systems may some day enable the minimally invasive treatment of a variety of pediatric malignancies.

Radioimmunoguided Surgery

Antibodies labeled with radionuclides, when injected systemically, may bind specifically to tumors, thus allowing gamma probe detection.[124–126] For the most part, nonspecific binding and systemic persistence has minimized the signal-to-noise ratio, thus limiting this approach. The Food and Drug Administration (FDA) approved several new radiolabeled antibodies for the identification of occult metastases in patients. Beyond imaging, the theoretical opportunity to use a gamma probe to identify "hot spots" adds a new source of information to the surgeon. Full exploitation of this methodology beyond specific functioning endocrine tumors and draining nodal basins in breast cancer and melanoma shows real promise.

NEXT-GENERATION MINIMAL ACCESS SURGERY

Minimal access surgery (MAS) forms the cornerstone of clinical innovation in present day pediatric surgery. Most pediatric general surgical procedures are now performed using some minimal access approach, and in many cases, these approaches are now considered standard of care. The next evolution in pediatric MAS involves further implementation of laparoscopic, endoscopic, and imaging techniques, with the ultimate goal of achieving scarless and painless surgery. Termed *stealth surgery*, this is an emerging surgical paradigm that encompasses a variety of techniques, each with the goal of performing complex operations without leaving visible evidence that they occurred.[127] This is achieved by placing incisions in inconspicuous or camouflaged locations and using MAS technologies to perform the operation. Examples of stealth surgery include subcutaneous endoscopy, single-incision laparoscopy, and natural orifice translumenal surgery (NOTES).

Traditionally, surgical culture has discounted the importance of scarring caused by surgical procedures. Scarring has been seen as either an unfortunate necessity or a minor outcome issue. This is interesting considering that the surgical scar is often the only collateral outcome of an operation that lasts a lifetime. At best, incisions have been placed in skin creases in an effort to camouflage the scar. Despite this, scarring is unpredictable, particularly if the scar is hypertrophic, keloid, or stretched, or if it becomes infected. There is evidence to suggest that visible scarring in children can result in reduced self-esteem, impaired socialization skills, and lower self-ratings of problem-solving ability.[128,129] Furthermore, other children judge children with facial deformities more negatively than those without facial deformities. Scarring of the chest and abdominal wall has not been as extensively studied, but it is likely that, at least in some circumstances, it can also have psychological implications. Stealth surgery aims to address surgical scarring, and collectively reflects a greater responsibility of surgeons toward the collateral damage of surgical procedures.

Subcutaneous Endoscopy

Subcutaneous endoscopy involves tunneling under the skin from inconspicuous locations to target removal of lesions at more conspicuous locations. Many surgical subspecialties, including plastic surgery,[130] otolaryngology,[131] and maxillofacial surgery,[132] have used subcutaneous endoscopic techniques, typically through hidden incisions on the scalp, for management of a variety of benign forehead lesions. Endoscopic removal of such lesions through scalp incisions using browlift equipment is also described in the pediatric general surgery literature,[133] as is removal of neck lesions through two or three small incisions placed in the axilla. This latter approach, called transaxillary subcutaneous endoscopy, has been used to address torticollis,[134] and also to remove lesions, such as thyroglossal cysts, cervical lymph nodes, parathyroid adenomas,[135] and thyroid nodules.[136] Transaxillary access has also been used for subcutaneous lesions of the chest wall, such as dermoid cysts and lipomas.[137]

Subcutaneous endoscopy for forehead lesions is performed through a 1.5- to 2.0-cm scalp incision using standard browlift equipment (Fig. 4-13). Dissecting instruments of 2- to 3-mm diameter are passed inline through the same incision as the endoscope. The subperiosteal plane is most commonly used to approach the lesion, but the subgaleal plane can also be used. The approach is ideal for lateral brow dermoid cysts or those found between the eyebrows (nasoglabellar cyst). The approach is not used for lesions that have intracranial extension.

Transaxillary subcutaneous endoscopic excision of neck lesions is performed by placing two or three endoscopic ports in the ipsilateral axilla, posterior to the lateral border of the pectoralis major muscle (Fig. 4-14). A subcutaneous workspace is then created, extending to the neck. The platysma muscle is traversed superior to the clavicle, and the target lesion is then dissected free. Recognition of landmarks and accurate anatomical orientation is subject to a learning curve, but visualization of all structures, including recurrent laryngeal nerves, is excellent. It is important to avoid extensive use of thermal energy sources in the neck, especially monopolar cautery, because of the thermal spread of such instruments. It is preferable to use bipolar cautery when possible, or else a thermal sealing/cutting device such as the Ligasure (Valleylab, Boulder, Colo.). The cosmetic benefits of this approach are apparent, because the patient is left with no scar on the face or neck. Pain is controlled with non-narcotic analgesics, and patients can typically be discharged the same day.

Single Incision Laparoscopy

Single incision laparoscopy is an evolution of minimal access surgery that promises virtually scarless abdominal operations. Various acronyms, including SILS (single-incision laparoscopic surgery; Covidien), LESS (laparoendoscopic single-site surgery), SPA (single-port access surgery),[138] OPUS (one-port umbilical surgery), and SAS (single-access site surgery) have been applied to this technique. The essential element is the use of a single small incision, usually placed at the umbilicus through which multiple laparoscopic instruments are passed either through a single-port device with multiple conduits or through multiple closely spaced ports (Fig. 4-15). Single incision approaches have been described in the adult literature for appendectomy, nephrectomy,[139] adrenalectomy,[140] cholecystectomy,[141] and colectomy,[142] and in the pediatric general surgical literature for appendectomy,[143] varicocelectomy,[144] cholecystectomy, and splenectomy.[145]

Cosmesis is the most apparent benefit of single-incision laparoscopy, because the single scar produced can be effectively hidden in the existing umbilical scar. The cosmetic benefit, including psychosocial factors, has not been objectively demonstrated, but the complete absence of a visible scar is achievable with this method. The procedures are feasible in equivalent operative times to standard laparoscopy,

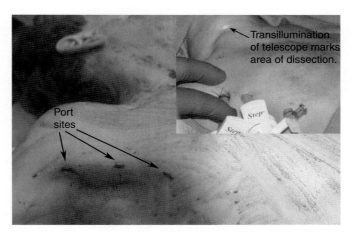

FIGURE 4-14 Transaxillary subcutaneous access can be used to access lesions in the neck and chest wall. A cavernous subcutaneous workspace is created to facilitate dissection. In this image, the light at the tip of the telescope can be seen transilluminating the skin. *(See Expert Consult site for color version.)*

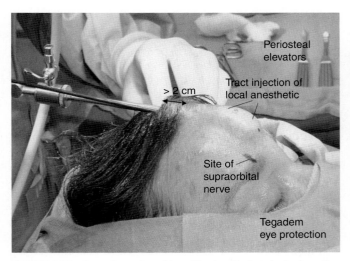

FIGURE 4-13 For endoscopic excision of forehead lesions, hydrodissection with local anesthetic is used to create a path toward the lesion in the subperiosteal or subgaleal plane, starting about 2 centimeters posterior to the hairline. The telescope and dissecting instruments are placed through a 1 to 2 cm V-shaped incision on the scalp. *(See Expert Consult site for color version.)*

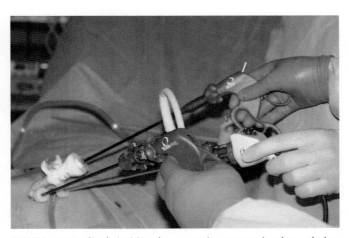

FIGURE 4-15 Single-incision laparoscopic surgery involves placing multiple ports, or a commercially available single-port device, at the umbilicus. Instruments with dexterous end effectors can be exploited to achieve triangulation around the target tissue, which is otherwise difficult to achieve with standard rigid laparoscopic instruments in this setting. *(See Expert Consult site for color version.)*

without additional safety concerns. Although clinical trials are underway, outcomes in terms of pain, recovery, and hospital stay have not been assessed—anecdotally these outcomes mirror those of standard laparoscopy.

A number of critical challenges in performing single-incision laparoscopy have led to some innovative solutions. (1) Close co-location of the instruments can result in bothersome instrument backend, hand, and camera collisions that impair mobility. This is addressed with the use of ports and instruments of varying lengths to offset backends, angled light-cord adapters for rigid telescopes, or flexible tip telescopes with low-profile backends. (2) When using standard rigid laparoscopic instruments, it is difficult or impossible to achieve an equal degree of triangulation around the target tissues (ideally 60 degrees) as can be achieved in standard laparoscopy and that is necessary for safe, precise, and efficient dissection. Instruments with an additional joint near their tip that gives two additional degrees of freedom (Realhand, Novare Surgical, Cupertino, Calif.; Autonomy Laparo-Angle, Cambridge Endo, Framingham, Mass.; Roticulator, Covidien, Norwalk, Conn.) have been applied to single-incision laparoscopy for this reason. With these "dexterous" instruments, triangulation can be achieved by first crossing the instrument shafts at or just below the level of the fascia, then deflecting the tips inward to create triangulation. (3) The maneuvers necessary to work with instruments in this configuration can be confusing and counterintuitive, because the instrument tips are frequently opposite the hand configuration, or the surgeon's hands are sometimes crossed. Developers of surgical telemanipulation platforms have taken advantage of computer algorithms used in their existing telemanipulation platforms (e.g., da Vinci Si, Intuitive Surgical, Sunnyvale, Calif.) to provide a single-incision laparoscopy platform that can correct for paradoxical movements and give the surgeon the perception that their hand movements are being mirrored by the robotic instruments.[146]

Single-incision laparoscopy will likely play a role in pediatric surgical procedures for larger children and adolescents, primarily because of the avoidance of visible scarring. Its role in neonatal surgery is less clear. Existing instrumentation is too large for neonatal anatomy. Furthermore, proponents of umbilical laparotomy show that most abdominal procedures can be performed in neonates through umbilical incisions that can be camouflaged with an umbilicoplasty.[147] When possible, this approach offers a cheaper alternative to single-incision laparoscopy. Cost continues to be a consideration when adopting these novel minimal access procedures, because they generate the need for more complex technologies, but a cost assessment is difficult to perform in the early stages of adoption because of the dynamic nature of the technologies used and the costs they incur.

NATURAL ORIFICE TRANSLUMENAL ENDOSURGERY

Perhaps a more extreme evolution of scarless surgery is natural orifice translumenal endosurgery (NOTES), which aims to perform abdominal or thoracic procedures by way of transoral, transgastric/transesophageal, transrectal or transvaginal access. Some surgeons consider single-incision laparoscopy a bridge to NOTES, while others see at as a more palatable alternative to NOTES. In adults, the potential advantages of

NOTES include decreased or no postoperative pain, no requirement of general anesthetic, the performance of procedures in an outpatient setting, and possibility of reducing costs. In children, NOTES remains uncharted, and its application in this population seems not only conceptually unappealing (transvaginal access is unlikely to be considered in a young girl), but also currently fraught with undue risk (leakage and infection risk with transgastric or transrectal access). Adult subjects asked to rate their preference of technique in the absence of safety profile data preferred single-incision laparoscopy and standard laparoscopy versus NOTES and open surgery.[148] However, there are unique pediatric surgical conditions described below that are intriguing targets for this approach, and research in this area allows an opportunity to discover novel techniques and technologies that may be more generally applicable to pediatric minimal access surgery.

The development of NOTES is an interesting case study in surgical innovation because of the way it has progressed, in contrast to conventional laparoscopy. The rapid adoption of laparoscopy into mainstream surgical practice without oversight or appropriate training heralded increased complication rates, such as that of bile duct injury during laparoscopic cholecystectomy[149] and complications not previously seen, such as intestinal and vascular injury from port placement. To avoid a similar scenario with NOTES, delegates from the American Society of Gastrointestinal Endoscopy (ASGE) and the Society of American Gastrointestinal and Endoscopic Surgeons (SAGES) established the Natural Orifice Surgery Consortium for Assessment and Research (NOSCAR),[150] with the purpose of defining guidelines for the safe, ethical, and evidence-based development of NOTES. The technical challenges, and hence areas of research focus, they identified included (1) creation and secure closure of the defect created in the hollow viscus for peritoneal access, (2) prevention of peritoneal contamination and maintenance of sterility, (3) adequate visualization and orientation in the peritoneal cavity, and (4) effective instrument triangulation around target tissues and adequate retraction of adjacent tissues.

A second unique feature of NOTES is the early involvement of industry in device development, in close collaboration with both surgeons and gastroenterologists with an interest in therapeutic endoscopy. Both specialties have recognized the need to collaborate on NOTES development because of its hybrid use of endoscopic and laparoscopic techniques. The medical device industry, in turn, has engaged early in this effort to remain competitive and obtain market share in this potentially large market. Although widespread use of NOTES has not materialized, research and development in this area has resulted in the development of a host of novel technologies ranging from dexterous flexible endoscopic surgical tools to intraluminal suturing devices.

In pediatric surgery, the adoption of NOTES for common pediatric conditions in the near future seems improbable because of small markets, the persistent need for general anesthetic, and a lack of any clear significant benefit versus single-incision laparoscopy. There are, however, some interesting possibilities for the use of NOTES in neonatal surgery, such as for duodenal atresia, urologic anomalies, and esophageal atresia. The latter is perhaps the most compelling. Although a thoracoscopic approach to esophageal atresia is well described, there has been slow adoption of this approach because of its technical difficulty, particularly with respect to thoracoscopic suturing of the anastomosis, which requires very precise movements in a limited workspace with highly fragile tissues that are under tension. The possibility of performing some or all of the operation transorally using flexible tools with purpose-specific attachments that allow fistula closure and/or esophageal anastomosis may allow a wider adoption of a minimal access approach to this condition by trivializing the technical difficulty of creating the anastomosis. Unfortunately, market sizes for diseases such as esophageal atresia do not support investment in purpose-specific technology, but development of dual-purpose tools that can also be applied to larger (adult) markets may provide the basis for their development.

Endolumenal Therapies

Innovations in intraluminal endoscopic therapies have centered mainly on totally endoscopic antireflux procedures, some of which have been applied to children. Some of these procedures (Enteryx, Gatekeeper) have fallen out of favor because of safety concerns or lack of efficacy. Use of Enteryx came to a halt in 2005 when the FDA requested a recall by Boston Scientific of all Enteryx systems following reports of adverse effects (and cases of fatality) resulting from inadvertent Enteryx injection into the mediastinum, pleural space, and aorta (with consequent arterial embolism). The Enteryx system is mentioned here only to exemplify the potential for serious complications with novel technologies, and reinforce the need for proper efficacy and safety trials before their widespread application, particularly in the pediatric population.

Use of other devices, such as Endocinch (Bard, Warwick, RI), Stretta (Curon Medical, Sunnyvale, Calif.), NDO Plicator (NDO Surgical, Mansfield, Mass.), have shown short-term improvements in gastroesophageal reflux disease (GERD) symptoms but without objective evidence of reduced lower esophageal acid exposure or long-term durability.[151] The Stretta procedure was the first interventional endoscopic GERD therapy to gain FDA approval in 2000. Consisting of a catheter, soft guidewire tip, balloon basket assembly, and four electrode delivery sheaths positioned radially, the Stretta device uses radiofrequency (RF) energy to increase the tone of the lower esophageal sphincter (LES). Its mechanism of action is unclear, but it is believed that the RF energy results in shrinkage of collagen fibers, resulting in elevation of postprandial LES pressure[152] and reduction of transient lower esophageal sphincter relaxations. Islam and colleagues studied the effects of the Stretta procedure on a small series of six pediatric patients (mean age 12 +/− 4 years), concluding that the procedure was safe and effective.[153] Five of the six patients were asymptomatic at 3 months, and three were able to discontinue antisecretory medication. Mean reflux score improved significantly after 6 months; however, pH studies were not done. Without significant improvements in acid exposure, the benefit of this procedure in children is questionable, because common indications for surgical management of pediatric GERD consist mainly of complications of esophageal acid exposure, such as esophagitis, pharyngitis, or aspiration, as opposed to minor GERD symptoms.

Also approved for use by the FDA in 2000, the EndoCinch system aims to reduce gastric reflux by pleating the gastroesophageal junction (GEJ). The 30- to 60-minute procedure begins with insertion of the Endocinch device through an overtube. Suction applied 1 to 2 cm below the squamocolumnar junction facilitates full-thickness placement of two adjacent sutures. The sutures are then "cinched" together or brought into approximation, to create a pleat. Usually several pleats are created, significantly narrowing the lumen at the GEJ. The resulting rosette of tissue (gastroplication) is intended to prevent reflux of gastric contents into the esophagus. Only one pediatric study describes the effects of the Endocinch system for treating GERD.[154] Seventeen patients with median age 12.4 years (range, 6.1 to 15.9 years) underwent gastroplication. All patients showed significant improvement in early postoperative assessments of symptom severity, symptom frequency, and quality of life. These effects persisted at 1-year follow-up in the majority of patients and were reflected in reduced pH indices. In adult patients, lack of long-term durability has been attributed to suture degradation and loss, both demonstrated on follow-up endoscopy.[155,156] The reason for the longer durability of this procedure in children compared with adults is unclear but may be a consequence of a greater ability to achieve full-thickness esophageal bites in the smaller patients.

The latest transoral endoscopic device on the market is the EsophyX (Endogastric Solutions, Redmond, Wash.), which is designed to achieve transoral incisionless fundoplication (TIF). The goal of this antireflux procedure is to endoluminally create an anteriorly placed 3- to 5-cm, 200- to 270-degree valve at the distal esophagus secured by special fasteners. The end result is creation of an antireflux barrier and reestablishment of the angle of His. The device does not have to be inserted and removed for each stitch, and its function allows reduction of a small hiatal hernia, although the crura remains unapproximated. Although adult studies have shown long-term reductions in proton pump inhibitor use, improved quality of life, and reduced esophageal acid exposure, data for the pediatric population is forthcoming.[157] Use of the device is limited only to larger children whose esophagi can accommodate a device that is 18 mm in diameter.

SURGICAL ROBOTICS

Innovations in endoscopic technique and equipment continue to broaden the range of applications in minimal access surgery. However, many minimal access procedures have yet to replace the traditional open approach. Difficulties remain in achieving dexterity and precision of instrument control within the confines of a limited operating space. These difficulties are further compounded by the need to operate from a 2D video image. Robotic surgical systems have evolved to address these limitations.

Since their introduction in the late 1990s, the use of computer-enhanced robotic surgical systems has grown rapidly. Originally conceived to facilitate battlefield surgery, these systems are now used to enable complex minimal access surgical (MAS) procedures. In children, early reports described the feasibility of using surgical robots to complete common and relatively simple pediatric general surgical procedures.[158–160] More recently, the use of robotic surgical systems in human patients has been described in multiple surgical disciplines, including pediatric general surgery, pediatric urology, and pediatric cardiothoracic surgery.[161–163] In addition, the feasibility of complex, technically challenging procedures, such as robotic-assisted fetal surgery, has been reported in animal models.[164,165]

Robotic Technology in Surgery

For several decades, robots have served in a variety of applications, such as manufacturing, deep-sea exploration, munitions detonation, military surveillance, and entertainment. In contrast, the use of robotic technology in surgery is still a relatively young field. Improvements in mechanical design, kinematics, and control algorithms originally created for industrial robots are directly applicable to surgical robotics.

The first recorded application of surgical robotics was for CT-guided stereotactic brain biopsy in 1987.[166] Since then, technologic advancements have led to the development of several different robotic systems. These systems vary significantly in complexity and function.

Classification of Robotic Surgical Systems

One method of classifying robots is by their level of autonomy. Under this classification, there are currently three types of robots used in surgery: autonomous robots, surgical-assist devices, and teleoperators (Table 4-2).

An autonomously operating robot carries out a preoperative plan without any immediate control from the surgeon. The tasks performed are typically focused or repetitive but require a degree of precision not attainable by human hands. An example is the ROBODOC system (Curexo Technology, Fremont, Calif.) that is used in orthopedic surgery to accurately mill out the femoral canal for hip implants.[167] Another example is the CyberKnife system, previously referenced, which consists of a linac mounted on a robotic arm to precisely deliver radiotherapy to intracranial and spinal tumors.[168,169]

The second class of robot is the surgical-assist devices, where the surgeon and robot share control. The most well-known example of this group is the AESOP (*Automatic Endoscopic System for Optimal Positioning*; formerly produced by Computer Motion, Goleta, Calif.). This system allows a surgeon to attach an endoscope to a robotic arm that provides a steady image by eliminating the natural movements inherent in a live camera holder. The surgeon is then able to reposition the camera by voice commands.

The final class consists of robots whose every function is explicitly controlled by the surgeon. The hand motions of the surgeon at a control console are tracked by the electronic controller and then relayed to the slave robot in such a manner that the instrument tips perfectly mirror every movement of the surgeon. Because the control console is physically separated from the slave robot, these systems are referred to as teleoperators. All the recent advances in robotic-assisted surgery have involved this class of machines.

Current Status of Robotic Technology Used in Pediatric Surgery

Currently, there is only one commercially available robotic surgical system—the da Vinci Surgical System (Intuitive Surgical, Sunnyvale, Calif.). Though the da Vinci is popularly referred to as a surgical robot, this is a misnomer, because "robot" implies autonomous movement. The da Vinci does not operate without the immediate control of a surgeon. A better term may be "computer-enhanced telemanipulators." However, for the sake of consistency with published literature, this chapter will continue to refer to such systems as robots.

The da Vinci Surgical System   The da Vinci system is made up of two major components (Figs. 4-16 and 4-17).[162] The first component is the surgeon's console, which houses the visual display system, the surgeon's control handles, and the user interface panels. The second component is the patient side cart, which consists of two to three arms that control the operative instruments and another arm that controls the video endoscope.

The operative surgeon is seated at the surgeon's console, which can be located up to 10 meters away from the operating table. Within the console are located the surgeon's control handles, or masters, which act as high-resolution input devices that read the position, orientation, and grip commands from the surgeon's finger tips. This control system also allows for computer enhancement of functions, such as motion scaling and tremor reduction. The image of the operative site is projected to the surgeon through a high-resolution stereo display that uses two medical-grade cathode ray tube (CRT) monitors to display a separate image to each of the surgeon's eyes.

The standard da Vinci instrument platform consists of an array of 8.5-mm diameter instruments. These instruments provide 7 degrees of freedom through a cable-driven system.

TABLE 4-2		
Classification of Robotic Surgical Systems		
Type of System	***Definition***	***Example***
Autonomous	System carries out treatment without immediate input from the surgeon	CyberKnife ROBODOC
Surgical-Assist	Surgeon and robot share control	Aesop
Teleoperators	Input from the surgeon directs movement of instruments	da Vinci System

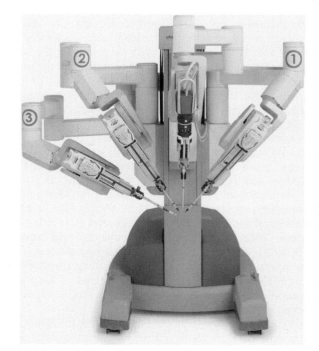

FIGURE 4-16 The Intuitive Surgical da Vinci Si robotic surgical system (Courtesy Intuitive Surgical, Sunnyvale, Calif.) *(See Expert Consult site for color version.)*

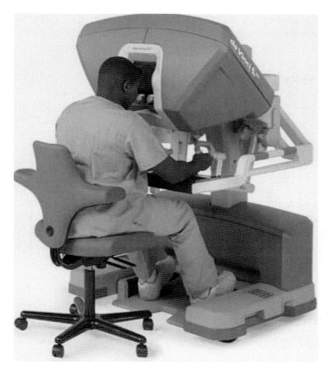

FIGURE 4-17 The Intuitive Surgical da Vinci Si robotic surgical system. (Courtesy Intuitive Surgical, Sunnyvale, Calif.) *(See Expert Consult site for color version.)*

A set of 5-mm instruments are also available. These instruments use a "snake wrist" design and also provide 7 degrees of freedom (Fig. 4-18).

Since its inception in 1995, the da Vinci system has undergone several iterations. The current system, called the da Vinci Si, features high-definition optics and display as well as smaller and more maneuverable robotic arms. Other features include dual console capability for training purposes.

Current Advantages and Limitations of Robotic Pediatric Surgery

The utility of the different robotic surgical systems is highly influenced by the smaller size of pediatric patients and the reconstructive nature of many pediatric surgical procedures. Overall, the advantages of the robotic systems stem from technical features and capabilities that directly address many of the limitations of standard endoscopic techniques and equipment. Unlike conventional laparoscopic instrumentation, which requires manipulation in reverse, the movement of the robotic device allows the instruments to directly track the movement of the surgeon's hands. Intuitive nonreversed instrument control is therefore restored, while preserving the minimal access nature of the approach. The intuitive control of the instruments is particularly advantageous for the novice laparoscopist.

In infants and neonates, the use of a magnified image via operating loupes or endoscopes is often necessary to provide more accurate visualization of tiny structures.[170,171] This enhanced visualization is taken a step further with robotic systems, because they are capable of providing a highly magnified, 3D image. The 3D vision system adds an additional measure of accuracy by enhancing depth perception and magnifying images by a factor of ten. The alignment of the visual

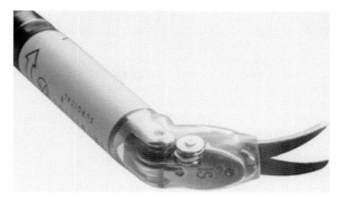

FIGURE 4-18 Articulated robotic instrument. (Courtesy Intuitive Surgical, Sunnyvale, Calif.) *(See Expert Consult site for color version.)*

axis with the surgeon's hands in the console further enhances hand–eye coordination to a degree uncommon in traditional laparoscopic surgery.

Similarly, the presence of a computer control system enables electronic tremor filtration, which makes the motion of the endoscope and the instrument tips steadier than with the unassisted hand. The system also allows for variable motion scaling from the surgeon's hand to the instrument tips. For instance, a 3:1 scale factor maps 3 cm of movement of the surgeon's hand into 1 cm of motion at the instrument tip. In combination with image magnification from the video endoscope, motion scaling makes delicate motions in smaller anatomic areas easier and more precise.[160]

The da Vinci system uses instruments that are engineered with articulations at the distal end that increase their dexterity compared with traditional MAS tools. This technology permits a larger range of motion and rotation, similar to the natural range of articulation of the human wrist, and may be particularly helpful when working space is limited. The da Vinci instruments feature 7 degrees of freedom (including grip), while standard laparoscopic instruments are only capable of 5 degrees of freedom, including grip. This increased dexterity may be particularly advantageous during complex, reconstructive operations that require fine dissection and intracorporeal suturing.

Finally, by separating the surgeon from the patient, teleoperator systems feature ergonomically designed consoles that may decrease the fatigue often associated with long MAS procedures. This may become a more significant issue as the field of pediatric bariatric surgery develops because of the larger size and thicker body walls of bariatric patients.

Although robotic surgical systems provide several key advantages versus standard minimal access surgery, there are a number of technological limitations specific to pediatric surgery. First and foremost is the size of the robotic system. Compared with many pediatric surgical patients, the size of the da Vinci surgical cart may be overwhelming. This size discrepancy may restrict a bedside surgical assistant's access to the patient while the arms are in use, and may require the anesthesiology team to make special preparations to ensure prompt access to the patient's airway.[170]

The size and variety of available robotic instruments is limited compared with those offered for standard laparoscopy. Currently, the da Vinci system is the only platform undergoing further development at the industry level. A suite of 5-mm instruments with 7 degrees of freedom has been introduced for use with this system. Although these instruments represent a significant improvement compared with the original 8.5-mm instruments regarding diameter, the number of instruments offered is still somewhat limited. Furthermore, these instruments use a new "snakewrist" architecture that requires a slightly larger amount of intracorporeal working room to take full advantage of their enhanced dexterity. Specifically, the instruments are limited by a greater than 10-mm distance from the distal articulating joint or wrist and the instrument tip.

There are a number of general limitations inherent to the available robotic surgical system that must be overcome before they are universally accepted in pediatric as well as adult surgery. These include the high initial cost of the robotic systems as well as the relatively high recurring costs of the instruments and maintenance.[162] In addition, this system does not offer true haptic feedback.[170] Even though such feedback is reduced in standard minimal access surgery compared with open surgery, it is further reduced or absent with a robotic interface. This disadvantage is partially compensated for by the improved visualization offered by the robotic systems, but it remains a potential drawback when precise surgical dissection is required.

The robotic systems require additional, specialized training for the entire operating room team. This translates into robotic procedure times that are predictably longer when compared with the conventional laparoscopic approach, at least until the surgical team becomes facile with the use of the new technology. Even with an experienced team, setup times have been reported to require an additional 10 to 35 minutes at the beginning of each robotic-assisted case.[170]

Applications of Robotic Technology to Pediatric Surgery

To date, only a small body of literature regarding the application of robotic technology for pediatric surgical procedures has shown the feasibility of robotic-assisted surgery. A wide variety of abdominal and thoracic procedures have been reported in the fields of pediatric general, cardiothoracic, and urologic surgery. The bulk of the literature represents class IV evidence, consisting of case reports and case series with no class I evidence. In 2009, van Haasteren and colleagues[172] reviewed the literature and found a total of eight peer-reviewed case series and five studies comparing robotic surgery with open or conventional laparoscopic surgery. Several of the studies had a retrospective design, and there were no randomized studies. From their review, they concluded that the published literature demonstrates that robotic surgical systems can be safely used to perform a variety of abdominal and thoracic operations. They were not able to identify evidence that robotic-assisted surgery provided any improvement in clinical outcomes compared with conventional open or laparoscopic surgery.[172]

The first reports describing the use of robotic surgical systems for abdominal procedures in children were published in 2002,[158,160] and robotic-assisted surgery has only seen modest adoption in the field of pediatric general surgery. The cause of this is likely multifactorial and in many ways mirrors the adoption curve seen in adult general surgery. To date, robotic-assisted surgery has found the most widespread adoption in the field of adult urology, specifically for prostatectomies. This operation takes advantage of the strengths of the current robot, namely articulated instruments and

3D visualization that assist in the complex dissection and reconstruction required in a narrow space. It is also a single quadrant operation that does not require significant repositioning of either the patient or the robotic system once the procedure begins. Lastly, prostatectomies are a relatively high-volume operation that is reproducible. This leads to improved efficiency, because the operating room team has only one setup to master. In contrast, the field of pediatric general surgery is characterized by a wide variety of complex but low-volume operations performed in small children. There is no high-volume operation in pediatric general surgery that takes advantage of robotic assistance. In addition, the instrument size and haptic limitations of the current robotic system are not ideal for use in many of our smaller patients.[173] These issues will likely be addressed by further advancement of the technology, with evolved incarnations of robotic surgery possibly playing a larger role in pediatric general surgery in the future.

Microtechnologies and Nanotechnologies—Size Matters

An arsenal of technology will emerge from material science and its application principles to microelectromechanical systems (MEMS)[174,175] and nanoelectromechanical systems (NEMS). Just as the electronics industry was transformed by the ability to manipulate electronic properties of silicon, the manipulation of biomaterials at a similar scale is now possible. For the last 40 years the common materials of stainless steel, polypropylene, polyester, and polytetrafluroethylene have been unchanged. A recent example of this potential is the use of nitinol (equiatomic nickel-titanium), a metal alloy with the property of shape memory.

An important concept and distinction in device manufacturing is that of the "top down" versus "bottom up" assembly. Top down refers to the concept of starting with a raw material and shaping it into a device. In a typical MEMS device, silicon is etched, heated, and manipulated to its final form. In the nascent field of nanotechnology, the underlying conceptual principle is that of self-assembly. Here component ingredients are placed together under optimal conditions and self assemble into materials. This process is much more one of biologic assembly.

Microelectromechanical Systems

The evolution of surgical technology has followed the trends of most industries—the use of technology that is smaller, more efficient, and more powerful. This trend, which has application in the medical and surgical world, is embodied in MEMS devices.

Most MEMS devices are less than the size of a human hair, and although they are scaled on the micron level, they may be used singly or in groups. MEMS devices have been used for years in automobile airbag systems and in inkjet printers.

Because the medical community relies increasingly on computers to enhance treatment plans, it requires instruments that are functional and diagnostic. Such a level of efficiency lies at the heart of MEMS design technology, which is based on creating devices that can actuate, sense, and modify the outside world on the micron scale. The basic design and fabrication of most MEMS devices resemble the fabrication of the standard integrated circuit, which includes crystal growth, patterning, and etching.[176]

MEMS devices have a particular usefulness in biologic applications because of their small volumes, low energy, and nominal forces.[177] Increased efficacy of instruments and new areas of application are also emerging from specific and successful biomedical applications of MEMS.[178] There are two basic types of MEMS devices: sensors and actuators. Sensors transduce one type of energy (such as mechanical, optical, thermal, or otherwise) into electrical energy or signals. Actuators take energy and transform it into an action.

Sensors

Sensors transduce or transform energy into an electrical signal. The incoming energy may be mechanical, thermal, optical, or magnetic. Sensors may be active or passive systems. Active sensors can derive their own energy from an input signal, whereas passive sensors require an outside energy source to function. Almost all of these devices are in their developmental stage but give form to the concept.

Data Knife and H-Probe Surgical Instruments   MEMS devices are particularly suited to surgical applications, because their small dimensions naturally integrate onto the tips of surgical tools. One example is the "Data Knife" (Verimetra, Pittsburgh, Penn.), which uses microfabricated pressure sensors that are attached to the blade of a scalpel (Fig. 4-19). While cutting, the Data Knife pressure sensors cross reference with previously gathered ex vivo data to inform the surgeon about the type of tissue that is being divided. This information becomes particularly useful during endoscopic cases in which a sense of tactile feedback is reduced or lost entirely.

Verimetra's H-probe uses similar sensors to "palpate" calcified plaques transmurally during coronary bypass surgery. The intention is to eliminate poor positioning of the bypass graft conduit by more precisely targeting an ideal anastomotic site before arteriotomy.

Arterial Blood Gas Analyzer   MEMS technology can be applied to the analysis of arterial blood gases. This MEMS-based analyzer was founded on established methods in infrared spectroscopy. It consists of an infrared light source, an infrared sensor, and an optical filter. The infrared light is passed through the filter, which is designed to monitor the infrared spectrums of oxygen, carbon dioxide, and other associated blood gases. Because most gases have a known infrared absorption, the sensor can be designed with specific values for infrared signatures.

Once again, because of microscaling techniques and because of the relatively small sample size, the test can be performed in less time than conventional arterial blood gas analysis. One specific example is an arterial blood gas catheter for monitoring blood in preterm infants, in which real-time data can be gathered by way of oxygen and carbon dioxide–specific sensors.

Blood Pressure Sensor   The biggest success story in medical MEMS technology is the disposable blood pressure sensor. Disposable blood pressure sensors replace reusable silicon-beam or quartz-capacitive pressure transducers that can cost as much as $600 and have to be sterilized and recalibrated for reuse. These expensive devices measure blood pressure with a saline solution–filled tube-and-diaphragm arrangement that must be connected directly to the arterial lumen. In the silicon MEMS blood pressure transducer, pressure corresponds to deflection of a micromachined diaphragm. A resistive element, a strain gauge, is ion implanted on the thin silicon diaphragm. The piezo-resistor changes output voltage with variations in pressure. Temperature compensation and calibration can be integrated in one sensor.

Other MEMS Sensors in Medicine   The Wheatstone bridge piezo-resistive silicon pressure sensor is a prime example of a MEMS device that is used commonly in medical applications. Able to measure pressures that range from less than 0.1 to more than 10,000 psi, this sensor combines resistors and an etched diaphragm structure to provide an electrical signal that changes with pressure. These types of sensors are used primarily in blood pressure monitoring equipment, but their use in the medical field extends to respiratory monitors, dialysis machines, infusion pumps, and medical drilling equipment. They are also used in inflatable hospital bed mattresses to signal an alarm upon detection of a lack of motion over a significant period of time.

Actuators

An actuator is a fluid-powered or electrically powered device that supplies force and motion. There are several kinds of actuators used in MEMS devices. These include electrostatic, piezoelectric, thermal, magnetic, and phase recovery. Actuators in medicine are used in valves, accelerometers, and drug delivery systems. Future use to produce muscle activation or "artificial muscles" is predicted.

Drug Delivery Systems

MEMS devices are used in drug delivery systems in the form of micropumps. A typical drug pump consists of a pump chamber, an inlet valve, an outlet valve, a deformable diaphragm, and an electrode. When a charge is applied to the electrode, the diaphragm deforms, which increases the volume in the pump chamber. The change in volume induces a decrease in pressure in the pump chamber. This opens the inlet valve. When the charge is terminated, the pressure returns to normal, by closing the inlet valve, opening the outlet valve, and allowing the fluid to exit. Other micropumps incorporate pistons or pressurized gas to open the outlet valves.

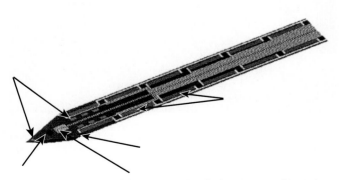

FIGURE 4-19   Data Knife MEMS-based scalpel. (Courtesy of Verimetra, Pittsburgh, Penn.)

One of the more attractive applications for implantable pumps is insulin delivery. There are disadvantages of current insulin micropumps, most notably their expense. The drug supply must be refilled once every 3 months, and each pump costs between $10,000 and $12,000. Furthermore, insulin is unstable at core body temperature. Therefore an insulin analogue must be synthesized that would be stable at physiologic temperatures. Thinking forward, a biomechanical pancreas, which senses glucose and insulin levels and titrates insulin delivery, would be an interesting MEMS combination of a sensor and an actuator.

Next Steps for MEMS

MEMS devices are in the same state today as the semiconductor industry was in the 1960s. Like the first semiconductors, MEMS devices are now largely funded by government agencies, such as the Defense Advanced Research Projects Agency (DARPA). Relatively few commercial companies have taken on MEMS devices as a principal product. However, no one could have predicted in 1960 that, 40 years later, a conglomerate of semiconductors would be on virtually every desktop in the United States. It is then not unreasonable to predict potential value, including surgical applications, for MEMS devices.

Indwelling microsensors for hormone and peptide growth factors might replace episodic examinations, lab determinations, or CT scans to monitor tumor recurrence. As more devices are fabricated, the design process becomes easier, and the next technology can be based on what was learned from the last. At some point in the future, we will view MEMS devices as common surgical modalities, smart instruments, inline laboratories, surveillance devices, and perhaps for cellular or even DNA insertion.

NANOELECTROMECHANICAL SYSTEMS

Applications of nanotechnology and nanoelectromechanical systems in medicine and surgery have been recently reviewed.[175] Size does matter. In medicine and biology, the major advantage of decreasing size scale is the ability to enable materials or particles to find places in body compartments to which they could otherwise not be delivered. Current and future applications of surgical interest include coating and surface manipulation, the self-assembly or biomimicry of existing biologic systems, and targeted therapy in oncology.

Coating and Surface Manipulation

Although most medical devices are composed of a bulk material, biologic incorporation or interaction occurs only at the thinnest of surfaces. To optimize this surface interaction, sintered orthopedic biomaterials have been developed. A thin layer of beads are welded or "sintered" by heat treatment on top of the bulk material.[179] This bead layer optimizes bone ingrowth, while the bulk material is responsible for the mechanical stability of the device. Hydroxyapatite-coated implants represent a biologically advanced coating of the device with ceramic hydroxyapatite,[180] thereby inducing bony ingrowth by mimicking the crystalline nature of bone (biomimicry). Future attempts involve coating with the RGD peptide, the major cell attachment site in many structural proteins.

Cardiovascular stents, and now drug-eluting stents, provide a similar example. The current generation of drug eluting stents has a micron-thick coating made of a single polymer that releases a drug beginning at the time of implantation.[181] The drug coating of rapamycin or paclitaxel diffuses slowly into the tissue microenvironment to prevent a fibrotic reaction. The future ideal stent will likely be engineered to optimize the bulk material and the coating. Indeed, the perfectly biocompatible material may be one in which a bulk material is artificial and the surface is seeded with the patient's own cells, for example, an endothelialized Goretex vascular stent.[182]

Self Assembly

NEMS materials are produced from a self-directed or self-assembly process in which mixtures of materials are allowed to condense into particles, materials, or composites.[183] Thus NEMS processing starts with a nonsolid phase, typically a solution, and by manipulating the environment, materials are created.

Recently, biologic molecules such as proteins and DNA have been used to stabilize nanoparticle crystals and create materials with unique properties, opening the door to unlimited diversity in the next generation of nanoparticles and materials.[184,185] Such processes mimic nature's ability to produce materials such as pearls, coral, and collagen.

NEMS in Oncology

More than in any other field, microscale and nanoscale technologies will provide the field of oncology with critical therapeutic advances. In considering the perverse biologic process of malignant transformation and spread, our current therapies are gross and nontargeted. Figure 4-20 depicts a complex nanoparticle[186] composed of an iron oxide core surrounded by silicon oxide shells. Ligands may be attached to the silicon oxide coating that may then target the iron oxide to a specific site. Such technology can be used for diagnostic purposes based on tumor permeability and therapeutic options.

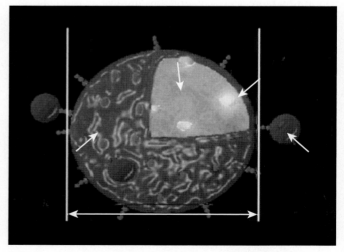

FIGURE 4-20 A schematic of a nanoparticle. An iron oxide core is surrounded by a silicon oxide shelf. Ligands attached to the silicon oxide can target the iron oxide to a specific site or potentially a tumor. The iron oxide can be heated in a magnetic field. Alternatively, the iron oxide may carry a toxin, a gene, or a pharmaceutical. Surface arrows highlight customized ligands while inner arrows point out therapeutic materials that can be placed in the iron oxide core.

Harisinghani and colleagues[186] used iron oxide nanoparticles to identify tumor metastases in lymph nodes of patients with prostate cancer. The authors demonstrated increased sensitivity and specificity in identifying nodes that ultimately contained tumor. Further work with magnetic nanoparticles functionalized with tumor-specific antibodies will enhance a specific uptake by tumors.

Surgical Innovator

Most clinical innovations in surgery relate to a novel operation, a novel device, or both. Occasionally, the novel procedure or device is of the surgeon's own development. In all cases, the surgeon holds the responsibility of ensuring that the implementation of these innovations is done in an ethical fashion. There are guidelines that surgeons can follow to help them safely and ethically introduce innovative solutions to their practice.

INNOVATIVE DEVICES

In the United States, pediatric research falls under the regulation of institutional review boards (IRBs), which serve the purpose of upholding the guidelines set forth by state and federal legislative bodies. The FDA regulates the use of all surgical devices.[187] Although the majority of pediatric surgeons will not design large clinical trials or novel devices, it is helpful to understand the regulatory processes when implementing new techniques or devices into one's practice.

The FDA categorizes new devices into three classes based on the potential risk incurred by using the device in humans. Class I devices pose minimal harm to the recipient and do not typically require premarket notification or approval (i.e., clinical data supporting safety and efficacy). Class II devices pose an intermediate level of potential harm but have demonstrated clinical efficacy comparable to similar existing devices. Class III devices pose significant potential harm to the recipient and require premarket approval with clinical data supporting safety and efficacy.

If a surgeon intends to study a novel device as part of a clinical trial in humans, the collection of preliminary data for non-FDA–approved devices is regulated by IRBs. If an IRB determines that the device provides insignificant risk to the study participants, the study may proceed. However, if an IRB concludes that the proposed study exposes the participants to significant risk, the FDA must approve an investigational device exemption prior to commencement of the study.[187]

If a device treats a condition that affects less than 4000 people per year in the United States, which applies to most pediatric conditions, it may qualify for humanitarian device exemptions (HDE). This allows approval of such devices when safety has been demonstrated and the probable benefits outweigh the risks of using the device.[187] HDE aids in disseminating high-impact technologies designed for rare conditions, technologies that would otherwise have delayed time to market because of the inability to properly power premarket clinical trials.

The pediatric surgeon using a novel non-FDA–approved device should obtain IRB approval. If there is sufficient patient risk associated with the use of the novel device, the investigator must obtain investigational device exemption from the FDA. Once clinical safety and efficacy are established, one can apply for FDA approval. If the device has significant potential benefit for an uncommon disease, the investigator has the option to apply for an HDE.

INNOVATIVE PROCEDURES

An innovative procedure may be composed of a new way of surgically correcting a condition, with or without the use of a device not approved for that use. Minor modifications to existing procedures would not be included in this category. The off-label use of an adult device in children may or may not be seen as innovative, depending on the circumstances surrounding its use. In all cases, a reasoned approach, such as that outlined in Table 4-3, can help to ensure safe and effective implementation of the innovation.

The Department of Health and Human Services (DHHS) categorizes pediatric research into four successive categories based on the degree of risk and the potential benefit to the study participant.[188] The first three of these codes encompass studies with potential for benefit to the participant with relatively low levels of risk exposure. The fourth code includes research that exposes participants to the potential risk in the *absence* of direct or indirect benefit but that has the potential to benefit children in general. A study that falls under this category may not be approved solely by an IRB but must have the authorization of the Secretary of the DHHS.

All pediatric research proposals, regardless of which DHHS code they fall under, must demonstrate an appropriate process for obtaining both patient *assent* and parent/guardian *consent* as defined by The American Academy of Pediatrics Committee on Bioethics.[189] The currently accepted standard of care is to obtain patient assent prior to enrollment in a study when feasible (i.e., when the patient is developmentally capable of affirming participation after receiving a cognitive age-appropriate explanation of the study/procedure, risks, benefits, and alternative options). Parental permission/consent is required whenever possible (i.e., nonemergent settings) if the patient is a nonemancipated minor. Practically speaking, parental permission/consent involves all of the components of informed consent in an adult population.

PEDIATRIC DEVICE DEVELOPMENT

The medical device industry has shown little interest in pediatric device development because of small market sizes and regulatory hurdles.[190] Similarly, entrepreneurs trying to promote medical device concepts have had little success in getting their ideas funded through typical funding channels, such as venture capital, for these same reasons. The consequence is that pediatric surgeons and others performing pediatric procedures are left to use adult devices off-label in children, "jerry-rig" their own devices, or simply do without. All of these approaches potentially result in a substandard level of care for pediatric patients.

Recognizing the dire need for pediatric-specific devices and the lack of interest from medical device companies, medical practitioners have in recent years taken a more active role in pediatric device development. More focused efforts at pediatric specific medical device innovation have emerged, in response to the dearth of innovation for this population.

TABLE 4-3

Approach to Introducing Innovative Procedures into Pediatric Surgical Practice

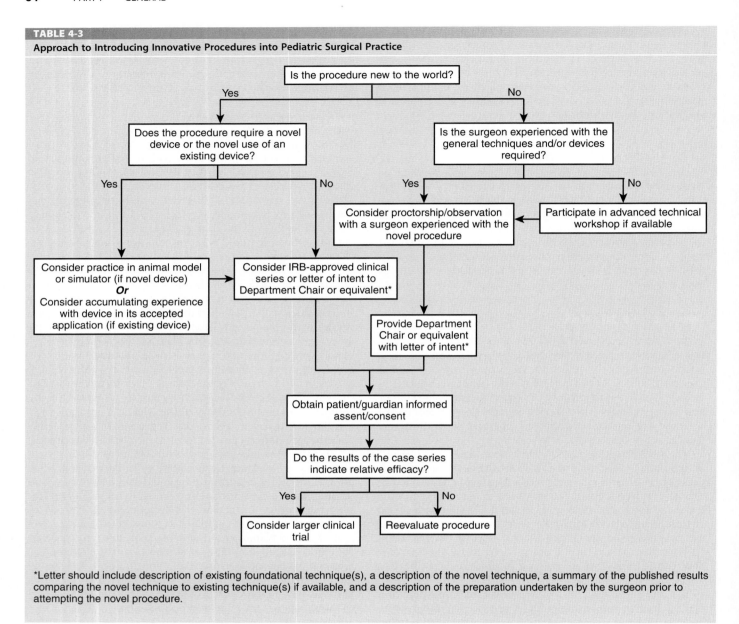

*Letter should include description of existing foundational technique(s), a description of the novel technique, a summary of the published results comparing the novel technique to existing technique(s) if available, and a description of the preparation undertaken by the surgeon prior to attempting the novel procedure.

From Kastenberg Z, Dutta S: Guidelines for innovation in pediatric surgery. J Laparoendosc Adv Surg Tech A 2011;21:371–374.

In September 2007, President George W. Bush signed into law the *FDA Amendments Act of 2007*, which included *Title III: Pediatric Medical Device Safety and Improvement Act*. This Act, which was designed to improve the research, manufacture, and regulatory processes for pediatric medical devices, also aimed to establish nonprofit consortia to stimulate development of pediatric devices. As a consequence, the United States Congress charged the FDA with dispersing grant funds for the creation of pediatric device consortia (PDC), organizations devoted to creating a national platform for the development of pediatric-specific medical devices, and demonstrating the timely creation of such devices. The first of these consortia include the PDC at University of California, San Francisco (http://www.pediatricdeviceconsortium.org) led by Dr. Michael Harrison, the University of Michigan PDC (http://peddev.org) led by Dr. James Geiger, the Pediatric Cardiovascular Device

Consortium at Boston Children's Hospital led by Dr. Pedro Del Nido, and the Multidisciplinary Initiative for Surgical Technology Research (MISTRAL; www.mistralpediatric.org), a collaborative effort between one of the authors (SD) representing Stanford University and SRI International, an engineering firm based in Menlo Park, Calif. Notably, three of these four consortia are led by pediatric general surgeons, attesting to the pioneering role our specialty can play in the advancement of pediatric medical technologies. These consortia have taken the lead in establishing formalized collaborative ventures that engage clinical and technical expertise in needs identification, foundational science research, and device design and prototyping. Going beyond the typical role of the academic institution, these collaborative groups are also identifying paths to market for the devices they develop through such strategies as spin-off companies or partnerships with commercialization entities.

Furthermore, the consortia provide pediatric surgeons-in-training an opportunity to immerse themselves in the innovation process, focusing specifically on the unique challenges of developing devices for children.

The market strategy for pediatric devices depends on the nature of the device. For example, many pediatric applications may require a device to be miniaturized for use in children. The technical solutions used to achieve this can then be applied in much larger adult markets. In areas such as minimal access surgery, smaller devices are also seen as beneficial for adult applications. This "trickle up" effect of the technology to adult applications can justify production of the device for pediatric markets because of the potential to also use it in much larger adult markets. Licensing to commercialization entities interested in applying the technology to adult markets may come with the caveat that they also address the pediatric need. In some circumstances where the device is quite specific to a rare pediatric condition, philanthropic support may be necessary to help it get to market, such as that by an individual or a foundation with particular interest in child health or the specific disease.

Device development can be seen as a form of translational science, where the basic research, design, prototyping, and testing of novel devices comprise unique intellectual contributions. Some institutions are beginning to recognize the scholarly potential for device innovation and crediting the researchers engaged in it, thus making it a potential basis for academic promotion. The measures of scholarly productivity may be different than traditional research tracks but nevertheless hold value for the academic institution. For example, device innovators may not be able to publish extensively because of concerns about protection of intellectual property (at least in the initial stages of device development), but the generation of grants, patents, and usable devices that positively impact healthcare can have great value for the institution.

Innovative Surgical Training

The practice of surgery is a visual, cognitive, and manual art and science that requires the physician to process increasingly large amounts of information. Techniques are becoming more specific and complex, and decisions are often made with great speed and under urgent circumstances, even when rare problems are being addressed. Simulation and virtual reality (VR)[191,192] are two concepts that may reshape the way we think about surgical education, rehearsal, and practice.

SURGICAL SIMULATION

Simulation is a device or exercise that enables the participant to reproduce or represent, under test conditions, phenomena that are likely to occur in actual performance. There must be sufficient realism to suspend the disbelief of the participant. Simulation is firmly established in the commercial airline business as the most cost-effective method of training pilots. Pilots must achieve a certain level of proficiency in the simulator before they are allowed to fly a particular aircraft and must pass regular proficiency testing in the simulator to keep their licenses. Military organizations use a similar method for training in basic flying skills and find simulation useful in teaching combat skills in complex tactical situations. Surgical simulation therefore has roots in the techniques and experiences that have been validated in other high-performance, high-risk organizations.

The expense and risk of learning to fly motivated Edward Link to construct a mechanical device he called "the pilot maker" (Link, http://www.link.com/history.html). The addition of instrument sophistication enables the training of individuals to fly in bad weather. At the onset of World War II, with an unprecedented demand for pilot trainees, tens of thousands were trained in Link simulators.[193]

The medical community is beginning to use simulation in several areas for training medical personnel, notably surgeons, anesthesiologists, phlebotomists, paramedics, and nurses. The ability of the simulator to drill rehearsed pattern recognition repetitively in clinical practice makes just as much sense for the surgical disciplines as it does for aviators. Surgical care entails a human risk factor, which is related to both the underlying disease and the therapeutic modality. Risk can be reduced through training. One of the ways to accomplish both of these goals is through simulation.

Simulation is loosely defined as the act of assuming the outward qualities or appearances of a given object or series of processes.[194] It is commonly assumed that the simulation will be coupled with a computer, but this is not requisite. Simulation is a technique, not a technology, used to replace or amplify real experiences with guided experiences that evolve substantial aspects of the real world in a fully interactive manner.[195] To perform a simulation, it is only necessary to involve the user in a task or environment that is sufficiently "immersive" so that the user is able to suspend reality to learn or visualize a surgical teaching point. The knowledge that is gained is then put to use in education or in the live performance of a similar task. Just as one can simulate a National Football League football game with a console gaming system, surgeons can learn to tie knots using computer-generated virtual reality, or simulate the actions of a laparoscopic appendectomy with the use of a cardboard box painted to resemble a draped abdomen.

Visual Display Systems in Simulation

Simulator technology involves the design of training systems that are safe, efficient, and effective for orienting new trainees or providing advanced training to established clinicians. This involves teaching specific skills and generating scenarios for the simulation of critical or emergent situations. The entertainment industry is by far the main user and developer of visual displays. So much headway has been made in the advancement of visual technologies by the entertainment industry that many visual devices that are used in simulation are borrowed from these foundations. Considering that the graphic computing power of a $100,000 supercomputer in 1990 was essentially matched by the graphic capability of a $150.00 video game system in 1998, the available technology today is more than capable of representing a useful surgical simulation faithfully.[196]

Props are a key component of the visual act of simulation. Although laparoscopic surgical procedures can be represented on a desktop computer, a much more immersive experience can be carried out by involving monitors and the equipment used in an actual operating room. For example, mannequin simulators, although internally complex, can serve to complement the simulation environment. Simulation of procedures, such as laparoscopic operations, should use displays similar to those used in the actual operating room.

Simulation of open procedures, on the other hand, requires systems that are presently in the developmental stages. The level of interaction between the surgeon and the simulated patient requires an immersive visualization system, such as a head-mounted display. The best approach for a developer of a simulator for open procedures would be to choose a system with good optical qualities and concentrate on developing a clear, stable image. Designs for this type of visualization include "see-through displays" in which a synthetic image is superimposed on an actual model.[176] These systems involve the use of a high-resolution monitor screen at the level of the operating table. The characteristics of the displayed image must be defined in great detail.

Human/Simulator Interface and Tactile Feedback

Force feedback is the simulation of weight or resistance in a virtual world. Tactile feedback is the perception of a sensation applied to the skin, typically in response to contact. Both tactile and force feedback were necessary developments, because the user needs the sensation of touching the involved virtual objects. This so-called **haptic loop**, or the human-device interface, was originally developed with remote surgical procedures in mind and has much to lend to the evolution of surgical simulation.

Technologies that can address haptic feedback are maturing, as noted by rapid development of haptic design industries in the United States, Europe, and Japan and in many university-based centers.[197] Haptic technologies are used in simulations of laparoscopic surgical procedures, but extending this technology to open procedures in which a surgeon can, at will, select various instruments will require a critical innovation.

Image Generation

The generation of 3D, interactive, graphic images of a surgical field is the next level in surgical simulation. Seeing and manipulating an object in the real world is altogether different from manipulating the same object in virtual space. Most objects that are modeled for simulations are assumed to be solids. In human tissue, with the possible exception of bone, this is not the case. Many organs are deformable semisolids, with potential spaces. Virtual objects must mirror the characteristics of objects in the real world. Even with today's computing power, the task of creating a workable surgical surface (whether skin, organ, or vessel) is extremely difficult.

A major challenge in the creation of interactive surgical objects is the reality that surgeons change the structural aspects of the field through dissection. On a simulator, performing an incision or excising a problem produces such drastic changes that the computer program supporting the simulation is frequently incapable of handling such complexity. This also does not include the issue of blood flow, which would cause additional changes to the appearance of the simulated organ. Furthermore, the simulation would have to be represented in real time, which means that changes must appear instantaneously.

To be physically realistic, simulated surgical surfaces and internal organs must be compressible in response to pressure applied on the surface, either bluntly or by incision. Several methods of creating deformable, compressible objects exist in computer graphic design.

Frequently, simulator graphic design is based on voxel graphics. A voxel is an approximation of volume, much in the same way a pixel is an approximation of area. Imagine a voxel as a cube in space, with length, width, and depth. Just as pixels have a fixed length and width, voxels have a fixed length, width, and depth. The use of volume as the sole modality to define a "deformable object," however, does not incorporate the physics of pressure, stress, or strain. Therefore the graphic image will not reflect an accurate response to manipulation. The voxel method does not provide a realistic representation of real-time changes in the organ's architecture, which would occur after a simulated incision.

A more distinct approach to the solution for this problem is with the use of finite elements. Finite elements allow the programmer to use volume, pressure, stress, strain, and density as bulk variables. This creates a more detailed image, which can be manipulated through blunt pressure or incision. Real-time topologic changes are also supported.

For the moment, a good alternate solution to the problem is to avoid computational models. Some groups have used hollow mannequins with instruments linked to tracking devices that record position. Task trainers allow one to practice laparoscopic skills directly by the use of the equivalent of a cardboard box with ports to insert endoscopic tools. These tools are used to complete certain tasks, such as knot tying or object manipulation.

Simulation in Education, Training, and Practice

Historically, surgical training has been likened to an apprenticeship. Residents learn by participating, taking more active roles in patient care or the operative procedure as their experience increases. Despite potential flaws, this model has successfully trained generations of surgeons throughout the world. Error and risk to patients are inherent in this traditional method of education, despite honest attempts at mitigation, and will always be a factor in the field of surgery, no matter how it is taught. New methods of surgical training exist, however, that can help to reduce error and risk to the patient.[198,199]

Training in simulated environments has many advantages. The first advantage is truly the crux of simulation: It provides an environment for consequence-free error, or freedom to fail. Simulator-based training incurs no real harm, injury, or death to the virtual patient. If a student transects the common duct during a simulated cholecystectomy, the student simply notes the technical error and learns from the mistake. Furthermore, simulations can be self directed and led by a virtual instructor or can be monitored and proctored by a real instructor. This means that the student can learn on his or her own time, outside of the operating room.[200]

Simulators are pliable tools. Depending on the assessment goals of a particular simulator, tasks can be modified to suit the educational target. For example, self-contained "box trainers," which are used to teach a particular dexterous skill, can be modified to be less or more difficult or to teach grasping skills versus tying skills. In more complex computer-based simulations, variables can be changed automatically by the computer or manually by the instructor, even during the simulation. These variables range from changes in the graphic overlay to the introduction of an unexpected medical emergency. Approaches to learning laparoscopic navigational skills within the human body have benefited considerably from such techniques. A prime objective of surgical education is to learn how to function mentally and dexterously in a 3D environment. Surgical "fly-through" programs can be invaluable resources to learn this kind of special orientation inside the human body.[201]

Perhaps one of the greatest benefits of surgical simulation is the ability of early learners to become skilled in basic tasks that have not been previously presented in formal training. The orientation of medical students, now frequently excluded from patient care tasks, may aid in their engagement, education, and recruitment to surgical careers. Therefore the most consistent success has been the discovery that simulators are most beneficial to individuals with little or no previous experience in the simulated task.[202]

Looking Forward

Simulation successes, particularly in the aviation industry, strongly suggest utility to medical and surgical applications. As with any form of new technology, advances depend on many factors. A product made solely for the sake of technology is doomed to fail; therefore the simulation market must be driven by clinical and educational need. In these early stages of surgical simulation, simpler, mannequin-based trainers have proven to be more useful. However, as graphic design and human interface technology evolve, simulations become more realistic, and equipment prices fall, more immersive computer-generated models will lead the way for this unique form of continuing medical education.

VIRTUAL REALITY

Virtual reality (VR), although closely related to simulation, has many unique aspects. Simulation is the method for education and training; VR is the modality for making simulation look more real. VR, simply stated, is the creation of a 3D artificial environment with which a user in the real world may interact. VR, in contrast to simulation, almost always relies on computers and computer software to generate a virtual environment. Furthermore, an interface device is required to immerse the user.[203] This device could be as simple as a mouse or keyboard or as complex as VR-based goggles or headsets. The basic intention of VR is to divert the user's attention from the outside world to a manufactured, virtual world with detailed, interactive content based on visuals, sound, and touch. When optimized, such an experience would immerse the participants such that reality becomes this virtual environment.

Although the term *virtual reality* was introduced by Jaron Lanier in 1989, the concept as we currently know it emerged long before that time. In 1963, funding from the Advanced Research Projects Agency (ARPA) gave Ivan Sutherland the opportunity to create Sketchpad, one of the first graphics design tools. By this time, Sutherland was developing the head-mounted display (HMD), which heralded the theories and themes of modern immersive science (Fig. 4-21).

Sutherland used what he learned in his research with HMDs to create scene generators for Bell Helicopter Laboratories. With scene generation, computer graphics would replace the standard video camera–generated display used in the flight simulators manufactured by Bell Laboratories (Fig. 4-22). With his partner, David Evans, Sutherland founded Evans & Sutherland, Inc., which is currently based in Salt Lake City

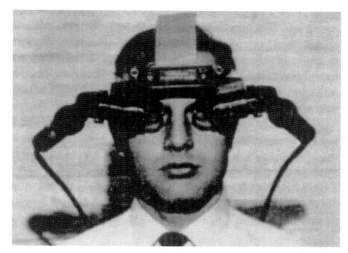

FIGURE 4-21 Sutherland's head-mounted display. (From National Systems Contractors Association Multimedia Online Expo, "Science for the New Millenium.")

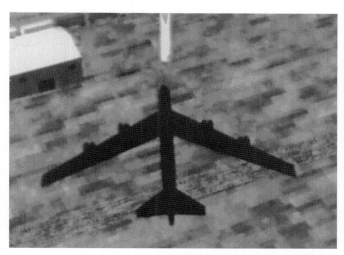

FIGURE 4-22 Scene Generation Software, Evans & Sutherland. (From National Systems Contractors Association Multimedia Online Expo, "Science for the New Millenium.")

and designs several VR-based products. Sutherland's foray into medicine occurred in 1971, when he developed the first arterial anastomosis simulation. With the simultaneous development of computer interface tools, such as the mouse, VR immersion became possible, because the ordinary user could now interact easily with the computer in a manner that was more intuitive than a keyboard.

By the early 1970s, ARPA was forced to concentrate its research and development on weapons for the Vietnam conflict. This led to an exodus of talent from ARPA to Xerox, which had established the Palo Alto Research Center (PARC). During the 1970s, major advances in technology meant that computers were becoming more powerful, smaller, and cheaper. The personal computer, laser printer, and desktop architecture were all developed at Xerox PARC.[204]

After the Vietnam conflict, the technologies advanced in war were directed towards other industries. Science and, even more so, entertainment began to look at VR as a way to enhance their respective businesses. VR has had obvious application in making blockbuster films with dazzling special effects (e.g., *Star Wars*, *The Terminator*, and *The Perfect Storm*). It was during the 1970s that many different industries began to see the applications and implications of VR. Three-dimensional mapping of genomes in DNA research led VR into medicine. For the first time, real-time modification of computer-aided design models became available. Thomas Zimmerman designed a "data glove," a type of human interface device, out of the desire to convert gestures into music by feeding these gestures directly into a computer, which could interpret the movements as sound. He patented the glove in 1982. The glove could interpret the wearer's hand movements and finger flexion, allowing them to interact with a 3D environment.

Jaron Lanier first combined the HMD and data glove in 1986, giving the world a more realistic version of immersive VR. This step meant that users could not only see the 3D environment but could also interact with it, feeling the objects and seeing themselves interacting in VR at the same time. Since these forefathers of VR presented their ideas and concepts to the world, there have been many groups, organizations, and individuals that have been interested in exploring and adding to the general knowledge of this field.

The evolution of VR for surgery began in the 1980s. It was quickly realized that simulation and VR for surgical procedures did not have to rely on an especially detailed graphic terrain, which was the case for complex professional flight simulators. In fact, even moderately detailed surgical VR systems could accomplish the purpose of "task training." This reinforced the fact that, for surgeons, one of the primary goals of training was to establish technical skills. Therefore simple graphic representations of two hollow tubes with an interface for needle holders and forceps would be enough to teach someone about the principles of bowel anastomosis. In the late 1980s, Scott Delp of Stanford University developed one of the first surgical VR-based simulators for lower extremity tendon transfers. In 1991, Richard Satava and Jaron Lanier designed the world's first intra-abdominal interactive simulation.

These seminal events in surgical VR were followed by more improved versions based on similar computer-assisted digitizing and rendering techniques. Although these early iterations lacked the computing power to combine maximum detail with surgical flexibility and dynamic change, they proved to be more than enough to establish the concept.

Components of Virtual Reality

Construction of a virtual environment requires a computer system, a display monitor, an interface device, and compiler software. Surgical simulations and artificial environments are based on the same types of programming methods. Computational speed must be sufficient to power the graphics to deliver a minimum frame rate so that the user does not experience flicker or the perception of frames changing on the monitor. To accomplish this, the simulation should be delivered to the user's eye at no less than 30 Hz, or 30 frames per second. This is equivalent to most televisions. Five years ago, this kind of graphic generation required high-end graphics (Silicon Graphics, Mountain View, Calif.) or a workstation (SUN, Mountain View, Calif.). Now, dual-processor or single-processor personal computers can render graphics at this speed.

The software required to produce virtual worlds has specific requirements. First, the programmer must design the software to match the physical constraints of the real world. The heart, for example, cannot be allowed to float in thin air during a coronary bypass graft simulation. It must have some representation of gravity, compressibility, volume, and mass. These constraints, and more, must be considered for the virtual world to approach reality. Second, the software must be designed so that user interaction will be compiled and processed efficiently and accurately, so as not to become unstable to the user who is dynamically changing the simulation. Forceps pulling on tissue must appropriately deform the graphic representation of that tissue, for example. The software also must be able to communicate force feedback, through external devices, to the user in real time.

Patient-Specific Virtual Reality

Surgical dissection, although second nature to a surgeon, is difficult to program into a computer system. The thousands of anatomic interactions can easily exceed the processor power; therefore digital rendering of patient data must be performed as efficiently as possible.

Patient-specific data for VR can come from several sources. MRI, magnetic resonance angiography, CT imaging, PET scanning, US scanning, and single photon emission CT imaging are among the common modalities. Traditionally, a physician mentally organizes these two-dimensional stacks of data, compiles it in his or her brain, and visualizes a 3D representation of the patient, not unlike the Visible Human data set (Fig. 4-23). With VR, these image stacks are meshed by the computer to realize the data in three dimensions automatically; this was previously a mental task, performed by the surgeon before an operation.[197]

Using different types of data sources, such as MRI or CT scanning, allows VR programmers to take advantage of the unique properties of each scanning method. CT scanning, for example, is particularly useful for scanning bones. MRI is more useful for soft tissue scanning. These properties can be combined to create a realistic VR image.

The manner in which these 3D images are represented within the system has a profound impact on the overall performance of the simulation. Patient data sets from CT scans, MRI, and other methods originate as voxels.[205,206] Voxel graphics are based on volume and result in an image that contains an infinite amount of data points. To compute changes in each point would put a tremendous strain on any computer. Other forms of VR rendering exist, however, to ease the strain on the system and to speed up the simulation.

Surface Rendering

Rendering is the process of digitizing data into a computerized image by applying parameters to the data. To reduce the number of data points that require computation, surface rendering converts volume-based images into geometric primitives, which have far fewer data points.[207] This could be a patchwork of polygons that are based on the boundaries of different regions in the image. Boundary regions could be between fascia and fat or gray matter and white matter. Such separation requires knowledge of the properties of each region, because some blurring occurs in voxel images, such as CT scans. Shading algorithms can blend layers or regions so that the final product has a smooth appearance (Fig. 4-24). The number

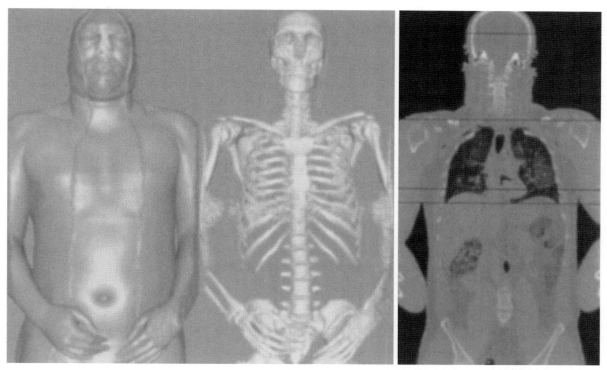

FIGURE 4-23   Visible Human Project. Reconstruction of a 3D model based on MRI and CT data. (Courtesy the National Library of Medicine Dataset.)

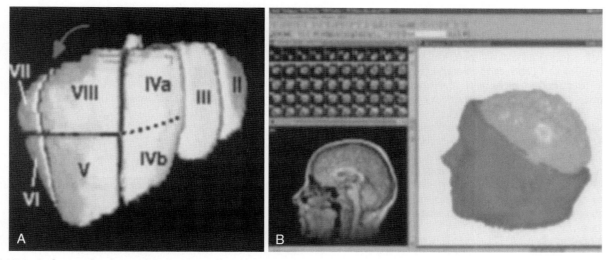

FIGURE 4-24   Surface-rendered view of the liver (**A**) and brain (**B**). (Courtesy 3-D Doctor: 3-D Imaging, Rendering, and Measurement Software for Medical Images, Lexington, Mass.)

of geometric elements is extremely important in the surface method of VR. One must remember that each movement of the simulation by the user in virtual space requires a recalculation of each geometric object by the computer in real time. If there are too many polygons to reproduce quickly, then the simulation will "jerk," making it less real and perhaps unusable. When compared with voxel-based imagery, surface-rendered objects run unequivocally faster.

Volume Rendering

Volume rendering requires special equipment to handle the immense amounts of data that must be compiled. This method works explicitly with volumetric data and renders them each

time the data set is manipulated by the user. This is different from surface rendering in that surface rendering splits the volume into groups of polygonal surfaces. Surface-rendered objects are adequate when the surgeon wants to limit the inspection to the surface of an object, but as its name implies, surface rendering only displays the surface part of the data set. Currently, higher-end computer equipment, such as a graphics workstation, is necessary to render volume-based graphics.

Finite Elements

Finite elements are based on geometric networks that are placed under the constraints of physics. Forces of pressure, elasticity, stress, and strain affect the shape and nature of the object being manipulated. Such manipulation will affect not only the surface of the model but also the volume. When combined with a detailed graphic overlay, finite element models can provide the most accurate simulation to date.[206]

Visual Displays

In a perfect world, VR can incorporate any, or all, of our five senses, but it usually relies most heavily on our most critical visual sense. The basics of our visual system can be categorized in three groups: depth perception, field of view, and critical fusion frequency.

Depth perception in humans is limited to approximately 30 meters, because the eyes are close together in relation to the distance being seen. VR systems must allow the user to reproduce these mechanisms, or proper depth cannot be achieved. The eye needs only a limited field of view to feel as though it is part of a virtual environment. Critical fusion frequency is the frequency at which static images, in rapid succession, appear to be a seamless stream of moving data. This is much like the old methods of animation in which shuffled flash cards gave the appearance of an animated cartoon. The approximate frequency for smooth video is approximately 30 to 40 Hz. Such displays must be capable of delivering a 3D image. The most dynamic form of VR visual display is the head mounted display. Although VR can be, and often is, represented on desktop monitors, the sense of immersion is not as complete when the participant is not in a closed system like an HMD. On a desktop monitor, a 3D environment is being projected on a 2D screen.

There are two basic methods of 3D visualization. The first method uses two separate displays, one to each eye, giving a stereoscopic effect. The second method uses a head-mounted tracking system that changes the perspective of the system to match the direction in which the user is looking. This tracking method must coordinate the movement of the user's head and hands.

Many different types of HMDs are available. The capabilities of a particular HMD depend on its final purpose. HMDs exist for personal video gaming, architecture, and missile guidance alike. There are also many modes of HMD instrumentation. Opaque displays, for example, completely occlude any visual contact with the outside world. Any visual input comes solely from the head-mounted video display.

Fakespace, Inc. (Menlo Park, Calif.) offers a binocular omni-orientation monitor (BOOM). This is a head-coupled display that is externally supported by a counterbalanced stand. Because this is not worn by the user and is supported by an external platform, the BOOM system can allow for additional hardware technology to be added to the system, thereby creating a very high-fidelity visual. Resolutions of 1280 × 1024, which are better than most computer monitors, are standard on the Fakespace system. The BOOM device is, of course, weightless to the user and relies on a motion-tracking system to keep face-forward perspective. The swivel stand allows for a superior degree of freedom (DOF) and field of view.

One of the more novel and immersive visual display systems is the Cave Automatic Virtual Environment (CAVE; Fakespace/Electronic Visualization Laboratories), which is a room-sized multiuser system. Graphics are projected stereoscopically onto the walls and the floor and are viewed with shutter glasses. Users wear position trackers that monitor the user's position within the CAVE by way of a

supercomputer. Changes in perspective are constantly updated as the user moves around this "confined" space. Monocular head-mounted systems allow the wearer to have contact with the outside environment while data are delivered (Fig. 4-25). Surgical applications include the ability to perform an operation while simultaneously processing data about the patient's vital signs and imaging studies.

Virtual retinal displays scan light directly onto the viewer's retina. Because of this feature, the viewer perceives an especially wide field of view. Although still in development, retinal displays have so far been able to deliver resolutions close to human vision, while encased in a lightweight, portable system.[208] Virtual retinal displays have been developed at the University of Washington's Human Interface Technology laboratory.

Input Devices

The best way to interact with the virtual world is with one's hands. It is both natural and intuitive. The DataGlove system (VPL Research, Redwood City, Calif.) (Fig. 4-26) is the archetypical system.

The DataGlove System frees up the user's hands from a keyboard. Commands are simplified, and tasks are carried out by rudimentary pointing or grasping in the virtual environment. Since the conception of the DataGlove, many manufacturers

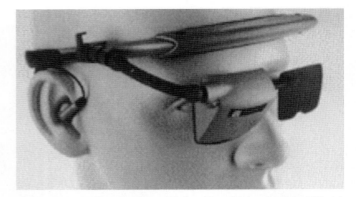

FIGURE 4-25 eGlass II, with eye Blocker. (VirtualVision, Redmond, Wash.)

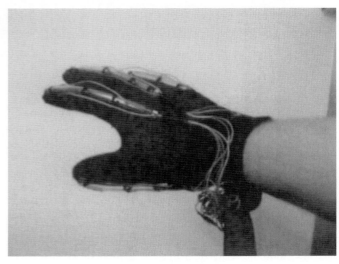

FIGURE 4-26 Generic dataglove.

have developed similar interface products. Data gloves process information by many different methods. Some gloves use mechanical sensors or strain gauges over the joints of the hand to determine position. Other gloves use fiberoptic circuits to measure the change in light intensity and angle of the fiberoptic band as the hand flexes and extends. Trackers are also positioned on some gloves to monitor their position in free space. In any configuration, the data glove remains an intuitive solution to a complex problem.

Force and Tactile Feedback

Force (resistance) and tactile (contact or touch) feedback could be the two most important goals of surgical VR, yet they are also among the most difficult to achieve. Surgeons rely on a keen sense of touch and resistance with the human environment, and without these senses, fidelity suffers. Laparoscopy is one example of how touch sense is displaced from the surgeon's hands.[209]

The tangible senses are very hard to generate artificially. Humans can easily judge the force with which to pick up a glass of water to bring it smoothly to the mouth. A computer, if incorrectly programmed, may mistake the picking up of a glass to the hoisting of a cinderblock, causing the virtual glass of water to be thrown completely across the room. Until recently, the one major component that was lacking in VR simulations was the sense of touch, or haptics.

Haptic feedback requires two basic features to render the sense of touch back to the user. First, the system needs a computer that is capable of calculating the interaction between the 3D graphics of the simulation and the user's hand, all in real time. Second, the loop requires some form of interface device (whether a joystick, a glove, or other device) for the user to be able to interact with the computer. The computer systems that support haptics are typically 3D graphics workstations with hardware video acceleration.[197,210] These systems are connected to an interface device, such as the popular PhanTOM joystick (SenseAble Technologies, Woburn, Mass.) (Fig. 4-27). Such joystick-based devices can function to provide up to six DOF. Again, the computer's visuals must refresh at a rate approximately 30 times per second to create a smooth simulation.

Like muscle linkages to bone, since all forces must be generated in relation to a point of fixation and an axis of motion, current force feedback systems require an exoskeleton of mechanical linkages. Force feedback systems currently use one of two approaches to this exoskeleton. The first system uses an exoskeleton that is mounted on the outside of the hand, similar to the ones used for electromechanical tracking. The linkages consist of several pulleys that are attached to small motors that use long cables. The motors are mounted away from the hand to reduce weight but can exert a force on various points of the fingers by pulling the appropriate cable. The second system consists of a set of small pneumatic pistons between the fingertips and a base plate on the palm of the hand. Forces can be applied to the fingertips only, by applying pressure to the pistons.

Because these systems reflect all their forces back to somewhere on the hand or wrist, they can allow you to grasp a virtual object and feel its shape but cannot stop you from passing your hand through that object. To prevent this, the exoskeleton must be extended to a base that is mounted on the floor through more linkages along the arm and body or an external system similar to a robot arm.

Multiple methods of generating force or tactile feedback have been developed. Piezoelectric vibration systems generate slight vibrations onto the user's fingertips when simulated contact is made. Electrotactile feedback works on the same principle of fingertip sensation, although there are no moving parts. A small current is passed over the skin surface in the case of virtual contact. Micropin arrays consist of a bed of fine pins that extend onto a fingertip to produce extremely fine details. Micropins can recreate the feeling of edges. Pneumatic feedback uses gloves with air pockets placed within the glove. These pockets inflate at the desired time to represent the sense of touching a surface. Temperature feedback uses heating coils on the hand to represent temperature change.

Tracking in Virtual Reality

Virtual reality is based on spacial relationships. Even though the user is presented with a virtual representation of certain objects, the computer must know where the user is in relation to such objects. Otherwise, the user's hand, for example, would pass through a virtual glass rather than grasping it. Some VR systems solve this problem by following, or tracking, the critical interface points between the user and the computer. Tracking systems are placed on helmets and gloves so that the computer knows when to react. Several tracking methods exist.[202]

Mechanical tracking systems are physically in connection with the user's interface. The user's helmet is tethered at one end and interfaced with the computer at the other. This direct connection is fast, but the subject is always attached to the system, which limits movement.

Cameras in conjunction with small flashing beacons placed on the body can be used as a method for optical tracking. Multiple cameras taking pictures from different perspectives can analyze the configuration of the flashing light-emitting diodes on the body. These pieces of 2D data are compiled into a single 3D image. Such processing takes time, a critical drawback of optical tracking. Magnetic-field signals can be used; source elements placed on the hand can be tracked with a sensor. Disadvantages include interference from nearby magnetic sources and a maximum useable distance.

Acoustic trackers use high-frequency sound to triangulate to a source within the work area. These systems rely on line-of-sight between the source and the microphones and can suffer from acoustic reflections if they are surrounded by hard walls or other acoustically reflective surfaces. If multiple

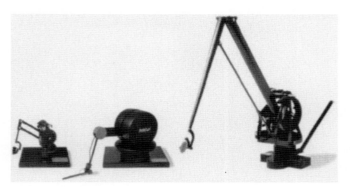

FIGURE 4-27 PhanTOM interfaces. (SenseAble Technologies, Woburn, Mass.)

acoustic trackers are used together, they must operate at non-conflicting frequencies, a strategy also used in magnetic tracking.

Challenges of Virtual Reality

As with any emerging technology, there is an ebb and flow of hype and hope.[210] VR is no exception. In order to exceed the hype, areas that have the greatest room for improvement are graphics and haptic feedback. Because of the massive processing power that is required to create a full VR production, one must currently trade off graphic detail for performance. Currently, this means VR is defined by the phrase, "It can be good, fast, and cheap; pick two." This results in simulations that have a cartoon quality, so that they may have a reasonable run time. Even with a forced reduction in graphic detail, there is still a slight perception of delay, or lag, in the time between user interface and VR reaction. The visual representation of an incision is still very difficult to achieve accurately.

Haptic feedback requires equal computing power (if not more) and can cause instabilities or inaccuracies in the system. Many VR forced feedback systems can be forced to fail, by "pushing through" the force feedback and ruining the illusion.

Virtual Reality Preoperative Planning

Beyond simple task training, one of the great advantages and goals of VR is the ability to plan and perform an operation on patient-specific data before actually performing the operation on the same human being. This goes far beyond early learning on a generic task or human. Surgeons, when planning an operation, traditionally compile data such as CT scans or MRIs, along with patient examinations and charts, into a solution envisioned in their head. It takes years of experience and training to master such visualization, especially when it comes to translating multiple 2D images into a 3D paradigm.

For many surgical specialties, VR techniques can assemble patient-specific data into graphic "before and after" images, which can be manipulated by the surgeon before the operation so that the outcome of the case may be predicted. These outcomes would be based on decisions that the surgeon would make during the operation. Furthermore, as more procedures are developed, VR preplanning can be used as a research model based on actual patient data that would be used to predict the outcome of a novel surgical application. VR enhancement also preemptively speeds up decision processes for complicated cases by providing the surgeon with a preplanned outline of the procedure, thereby making the hospital system more efficient. VR preoperative planning is available for general surgery, vascular surgery, plastic surgery, neurosurgery, and orthopedic surgery.

Craniofacial reconstructive surgery is a difficult task. The surgeon who is asked to handle a difficult or even routine operation of this kind reconstructs 3D data from 2D CT or MRI scans. No matter how experienced the surgeon, the predictions of outcomes in plastic reconstructions are limited, at best, with the use of this traditional method. As a result, the preoperative plan is often modified in the operating room during the operation. For these reasons, rehearsal and preparation with VR have been applied with increasing frequency in this area.[211,212]

There are many methods of computer-assisted planning for craniofacial surgery, but most produce a 3D interactive image that can predict the outcome of the case based on what the surgeon does on a workstation ahead of time. This process starts with a patient-specific CT or MRI scan that is cut in transverse sections, as is the case in facial reconstruction for trauma or malformation.[213] Once the images are scanned from the patient, they are segmented and specified into bone and soft tissue windows. This results in a mass of 2D cuts that must be rendered into a 3D environment. Patient-specific CT images are typically processed on a graphics workstation.

The University of Erlangen in Germany has demonstrated a method with "marching cubes" for 2D to 3D reconstruction from CT scans.[214] In this process, a CyberWare (Cyberware, Monterey, Calif.) scanner is used to scan the patient's skin surface features, which are compressed to reduce the volume of data. The skin and bone windows are compiled similarly into a 3D image. This image may be cut at any plane to focus on a particular area of interest. Keeve and colleagues[211] simulated a Dal-Pont osteotomy of the mandible using this technique. After the 3D image is rendered, any number of cutting, moving, and manipulating steps may be performed, which will predict the reconstructive outcome in the operating room (Fig. 4-28). "Before and after" pictures of actual patients with this type of computer-aided design models for facial reconstruction yield positive results.

The National Biocomputational Center at Stanford University uses a slightly different rendering paradigm that is based on CT images, called virtual environment for surgical planning and analysis (VESPA). Montgomery and colleagues[213] developed VESPA for use in craniofacial reconstruction, as well as breast

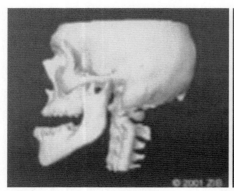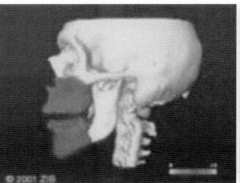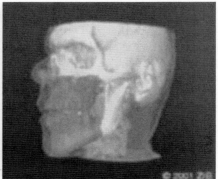

FIGURE 4-28 3D planning of a high Le Fort I-Osteotomy (Konrad-Zue-Zentrum for Informationstechnik, Berlin, Germany). (Courtesy SenseAble Technologies, Woburn, Mass.)

surgery, soft tissue reconstruction, and repair of congenital defects. Once CT images are acquired, voxel-based or volume-based images are focused down the area of interest, which results in very specific, segmented data. 3D images are broadcast onto a high-definition CRT monitor, and the user, who is wearing tracked CrystalEyes (StereoGraphics, San Rafael, Calif.) shutter glasses and a FasTrak (Polhemus, Colchester, Vt.) stylus for user input, can view and manipulate the virtual object.

The complexity of facial reconstructive surgery almost demands this kind of preoperative power, because conventionally there is only so much planning and prediction that can be performed by the surgeon who uses 2D conventions. Preplanning will allow the physician and the patient to view precise outcomes; this not only reassures both parties but also allows for reduced anesthesia times.

Virtual Reality–Based Three-Dimensional Surgical Simulators

The actual practice of surgical procedures is a highly visual and, subsequently, manual task with constant visual and haptic feedback and modification.[215] This represents a formidable challenge. To create a VR surgical simulator for education or practice, the programmers must develop a system that adequately represents the surgical environment; it must react to the surgical changes (e.g., incision, dissection, resection) that the surgeon imparts to the operative field and must give the surgeon appropriate forced feedback. These prerequisites must be accomplished in a manner that is transparent to the surgeon (i.e., the virtual operation room should mimic a real operating room). Depending on the target audience and application, many surgical simulators have been developed. VR surgical simulators have been applied to open surgical procedures, laparoscopic surgery, and remote telepresent surgery.

The Karlsruhe "VEST" Endoscopic Surgery Trainer (IT VEST Systems AG, Bremen, Germany) is likely the most developed surgical endoscopic simulator (Fig. 4-29). This device mimics the surgically draped human abdomen and allows for the insertion of multiple laparoscopic instruments and an endoscopic camera. Force feedback is provided and applied to the laparoscopic instruments. Visual displays are generated with proprietary KISMET (Kinematic Simulation, Monitoring, and Off-Line Programming Environment for

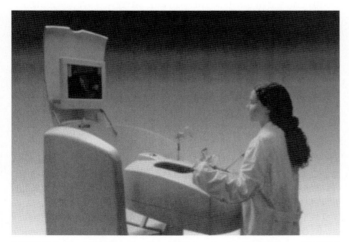

FIGURE 4-29   VEST/LapSim One endoscopic surgical trainer. (IT VEST Systems AG, Bremen, Germany). (Courtesy of IT VEST Systems AG.)

Telerobotics) 3D generation surgical environments.[216] This software affords the user high-fidelity immersion into a virtual laparoscopic scenario of a minimally invasive cholecystectomy, complete with real-time tissue dynamics and kinematic tissue response to user interaction. The laparoscopic instruments are tracked with sensors, to mimic the same DOF of actual endoscopic tools that are placed into a human abdominal cavity. This system is processed by a graphics workstation and has the ability to support total immersion goggles and telepresence training. As computing and graphic power become more developed, the graphic representations will become more detailed and hopefully approach that of the video monitors in an actual operating room.

Other surgical simulation systems are also available. Boston Dynamics (Cambridge, Mass.) has developed an anastomosis simulation with Pennsylvania State University based on force feedback surgical instruments and 3D vision with shutter goggles. This system allows the user to place sutures in a bowel or vessels to simulate the delicate nature of anastomosis. A "surgical report card" is a unique implementation in this system, which analyzes the surgeon's performance in real time. Comments on performance include time, accuracy, angle of needle insertion, and tissue damage.[217]

Virtual reality simulators for bronchoscopy, catheter insertion, and endoscopy are so real that residents and fellows use these to get exposure to procedures not already in their arsenal of experience. Stanford University has used the BronchSim and CathSim devices (Immersion Medical Technologies, Gaithersburg, Md.) and the VR Med Upper GI simulator (Fifth Dimension Technologies, Pretoria, South Africa) to evaluate surgical procedure training. A study that involved the BronchSim device that was conducted at Stanford University consisted of three sections: practice, navigation and visualization, and diagnosis and therapy. The subject was introduced to the bronchoscope and the simulation by a narrative from the training staff, which was supplemented by four videos on basic bronchoscopy, which were supplied with the Immersion Medical Technologies software. One of the tasks involved diagnosing an intraluminal bronchial wall tumor from CT scans and plain radiographs of the chest, then using the provided biopsy tool to safely take a sample of the tumor and control hemorrhage. The BronchSim device was able to distinguish between experts and novices, and subjective data from Likert questionnaires suggested an increase in procedural ability and familiarity in bronchoscopy. Similar educational studies were completed with the same internal structure for evaluation. These studies returned equally encouraging results.

With the advent of computer-assisted medicine, VR training tools have never been so accessible to medical educational programs as they are today. Our results, and the results of many others, suggest that surgical education that incorporates VR systems can be used in a training program, for both medical students and residents entering careers for which this procedure might be performed. Experience suggests that many VR simulator interfaces are realistic enough to serve not only as a teaching tool but also as a method for honing present skills.

SIMULATION IN SURGICAL EDUCATION

Current training in surgery is focused on core knowledge, patient care, team training, and procedural skills. Surgical simulators can be used to enhance each of these components.

Simulation can be used for skills training, patient treatment, and crisis training in primary and continuing education for both residents and practicing surgeons.

Surgical simulation has been adopted by several surgical centers and residency programs through the formation of "simulation centers." Mannequin simulators are being used to train surgical interns and residents in crisis treatment, and as a formal credentialing method for certain aspects of advanced cardiac life support (ACLS) and advanced trauma life support (ATLS).

As an example of mannequin-based core knowledge training, a simulation of initial burn surgical treatment has been developed. Treatment of acute burn injury is a core surgical skill, and proper treatment ranks in urgency with the care of a myocardial infarction. Despite the expertise needed to treat burns, only 20% of surgical residencies have a formal burn rotation.

The METI (Medical Education Technologies, Incorporated, Sarasota, Fla.) human patient simulator (HPS), a life-sized male mannequin model that is linked to a customizable computer system, was used. The HPS has been proven to simulate normal and pathologic states reliably and is certified for ATLS and ACLS credentialing. Simulated output is through standard bedside monitoring equipment, spontaneous respiration, eye opening, pulses, voice response, and robotic limb motion. The test scenario demonstrated a 40%, third-degree burn. Initially, expert intensive care and burn surgeons were asked to validate the scenario for accuracy and relevancy. Next, senior surgery residents were exposed to the 30-minute simulation. Lickert scale questionnaires and expert debriefings were provided to each of the subjects. Each resident's performance was filmed for expert review by an attending physician. The computer-driven response of the HPS was based on the residents' ability to perform ATLS, while simultaneously treating the burned patient with fluids, intubation, and escharotomy.

Attending physicians responded that the proposed scenario accurately reflected the key treatment points for ATLS protocols and burn treatment. These experts also perceived that residents who were exposed to the simulation could function as a physician responder in a similar situation. After being debriefed, each subject was more confident with burn treatment, fluid calculation, intubation and ventilator management, and thoracic and extremity escharotomies. Burn treatment simulation can teach residents to process situations that are not experienced in training and can function as a credentialing platform for new faculty. This first validation of simulated burn training with the HPS suggests a feasible solution to a serious educational dilemma.

Also popular are surgical "fly-through" VR-based tools that are designed to provide a medical student or resident with a first exposure to surgical anatomic relationships in three dimensions. Projects that involve the virtual human male have taken advantage of the data sets that were acquired from this model to create a virtual human anatomy resource in which the student may approach any anatomic structure from any angle or route. The Visible Human Project data sets can be rendered in three dimensions to create virtual detailed fly-through movies. These fly-throughs can be modified to demonstrate the before and after effects of many common surgical procedures and to provide an "endoscopic" view of the abdominal cavity. As more surgical procedures are developed that require more detailed and specific knowledge of surgical relationships, and as the time for surgical education continues to decrease, VR fly-throughs will provide an efficient solution to the education problem.

TRAINING THE MINIMAL ACCESS THERAPIST

Because of the overlap between IGT, endoscopy, and surgery, interspecialty battles over the control of this field are to some extent inevitable. There is, however, a move toward the concept of a "minimal access therapist," an individual with training in minimal access surgery, endoscopy, and imaging, and one who can independently deliver complex minimal access care.[82,218] How such a minimal access therapist will be trained and credentialed remains to be seen, but the development of this field will require the cooperation of surgeons, endoscopists, and radiologists. Simulation and the use of virtual reality will likely play a role. Pediatric surgery is already seeing a move in this direction as minimal access pediatric surgeons embrace the use of intraoperative US, fluoroscopy, and therapeutic endoscopy.

The vision for the integrated environment in which the minimal access therapist will work is radically different from the conventional operating room. Most notably, the surgeon's view of the operative field will be complemented by augmented reality visualization in which the surgeon is aided by images showing what is beyond the visible surface. Instrumentation combining features of laparoscopic tools with endoscopic tools will be used, potentially with robotic guidance. The overall goal is to integrate preoperative and intraoperative imaging data with a robotic-assisted platform into a unified surgical delivery system.

TRAINING THE SURGICAL INNOVATOR

Technology continues to advance rapidly, becoming more complex and interdisciplinary; at the same time, clinical surgery has become increasingly demanding, requiring intense focus. As a result, the gap between technical advances and creative surgeons is growing. This chapter is an attempt to narrow that gap.

If, indeed, change is constant, and that constant cycling has advanced our field, then it is incumbent upon us as a specialty to understand, thoughtfully incorporate, and even direct the useful change of surgical innovation. Surgeons are undeniably uniquely positioned and privileged to contribute to this cycle, but the growing gap creates a special field of knowledge perhaps requiring a specialized education program.

Formal education programs that teach the process of innovation to young surgeons are appearing across the country. One example is the Biodesign Program at Stanford University, a 2-year fellowship in surgical innovation offered to graduate level engineering students and residents. In the first year, fellows participate in didactic courses that teach the practical issues in needs assessment, technology solutions, intellectual property, ownership, the FDA approval process, and the underpinning economics of this process. A team-based project course is a large component of the first year. A second year is spent further developing an identified project. At the completion of the program the fellow has the requisite skills to become a significant contributor to the next cycle of surgical innovation in children and in adults. Depending on the prior background of the fellow, a Masters degree in bioengineering is also achievable. Now in its 10th year, more than 80 graduates are now dispersed around the world, including one of the authors (RKW).

The Biodesign Program is part of a campus-wide interdisciplinary program entitled "Stanford's Bio-X Initiative" involving over 500 scientists from the life sciences, engineering, chemistry, and physics, with broad research themes in biocomputation, biophysics, genomics and proteomics, regenerative medicine, and chemical biology. Networks such as Bio-X focus explicitly on technology transfer to bring innovations bidirectionally to the bedside-to-bench cycle. This represents a unique academic program focused on the invention and implementation of new health-care technologies through interdisciplinary research and education at the emerging frontiers of engineering and the biomedical sciences.

Conclusion

If pediatric surgery is to remain an active participant in the endless cycle of change, then an acknowledgement of the role of technology in advancing our care and a desire to actively embrace and drive the process forward in an ethical fashion is essential. To sit on the sideline is to invite a slow and agonizing death of us as individuals and, more critically, of our field and our responsibility to it. This two-volume text is a tribute to those who came before us and, in the space of less than 50 years, defined our specialty. We, as stewards of this generation, must be architects of the next 50 years.

The complete reference list is available online at www. expertconsult.com.

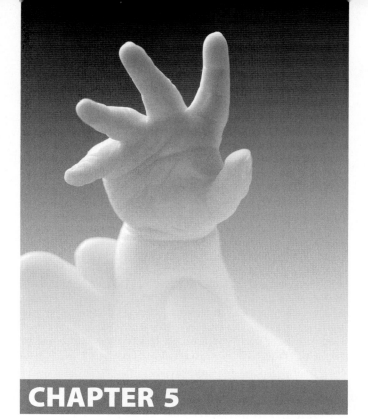

CHAPTER 5

Prenatal Diagnosis and Fetal Therapy

Hanmin Lee, Shinjiro Hirose, and Michael R. Harrison

As the field of fetal diagnosis and therapy expands, pediatric surgeons are increasingly involved in the management of surgical anomalies before birth. Advances in imaging and sampling of the fetus have increased the accuracy of the diagnosis of many anomalies and improved stratification of disease severity. These advances in prenatal diagnosis have led to improved perinatal care. Severe lesions detected early enough may lead to counseling and termination of pregnancy. Most correctable defects are best managed by optimizing location, mode and timing of delivery, and postnatal care of the infant (Table 5-1). Some prenatally diagnosed conditions have progressive and severe sequelae and may be treated with fetal intervention. Some attempts at fetal therapy have resulted in tremendous success, whereas many others have resulted in unclear or no improvement.

Finally, serial study of affected fetuses may help unravel the developmental pathophysiology of some surgically correctable lesions and thus lead to improved treatment before or after birth. It is important that surgeons familiar with the management of lesions after birth be involved in management decisions and family counseling.[1]

In this chapter we review the current techniques of fetal diagnosis and intervention and specific fetal anomalies that have particular interest to pediatric surgeons.

Fetal Diagnosis

Over the past 4 decades, fetal diagnosis has improved tremendously. Obstetricians are now able to accurately detect many genetic anomalies prenatally and are able to detect many anatomic abnormalities by fetal ultrasonography (US), echocardiography, and magnetic resonance imaging (MRI). In this section we discuss invasive and noninvasive methods of diagnosis of fetal anomalies.

BIOCHEMICAL SCREENING

An elevated alpha fetoprotein (AFP) level in maternal serum and amniotic fluid is a reliable indicator of a fetal abnormality. Although used to screen for neural tube defects, AFP is also elevated in defects such as omphalocele, gastroschisis, and sacrococcygeal teratoma, in which transudation of fetal serum is increased. AFP is the major glycoprotein of fetal serum and resembles albumin in molecular weight, amino acid sequence, and immunologic characteristics. The AFP level in fetal serum reaches a peak of 3 mg/mL at 13 to 15 weeks of gestation. AFP concentration in amniotic fluid follows a curve similar to that of fetal serum, but at a 150-fold dilution. Maternal serum levels continue to rise throughout pregnancy until the middle of the third trimester. Typically AFP is measured in the second trimester at 15 to 18 weeks. Measuring other markers—inhibin, estriol, and human chorionic gonadotropin—enhances aneuploidy screening. Testing of these four markers is referred to as a *quad screen*.

Increasingly screening for aneuploidy is being performed in the first trimester because of the results of the First and Second Trimester Evaluation of Risk (FASTER) trial. The FASTER trial compared the accuracy of second-trimester serum quad screening to first-trimester triple screening consisting of maternal serum testing for pregnancy-associated plasma protein A (PAPP-A) and free beta-human chorionic gonadotropin (beta-hCG) combined with an ultrasonographic examination to determine the fetal nuchal translucency. The sensitivity and specificity of detecting trisomy 21 in this study by noninvasive first-trimester screening were found to be comparable to noninvasive quad screening performed in the second trimester.[2]

FETAL SAMPLING

Cells can be obtained for karyotyping and DNA-based diagnosis of many genetic defects and inherited metabolic abnormalities. Amniocentesis in the middle of the second trimester has been the most common method of fetal sampling. Chorionic villus sampling (transvaginal or transabdominal) as early as 10 weeks of gestation has become used increasingly because complication rates for the procedure are now comparable to those of amniocentesis.[3] Thus current first-trimester noninvasive screening or chorionic villus sampling, or both, give women earlier information with which to make decisions concerning their pregnancies.

Powerful new sorting techniques now allow isolation of fetal cells and free fetal DNA in the maternal circulation, allowing noninvasive genetic testing for fetal diseases by maternal blood sampling.[4,5] Increased access to fetal genetic

TABLE 5-1

Prenatal Diagnosis and Management

Defects Usually Managed by Pregnancy Termination

Anencephaly, hydranencephaly, alobar holoprosencephaly

Severe anomalies associated with chromosomal abnormalities (e.g., trisomy 13)

Bilateral renal agenesis, infantile polycystic kidney disease

Severe untreatable inherited metabolic disorders (e.g., Tay-Sachs disease)

Lethal bone dysplasias (e.g., thanatophoric dysplasia, recessive osteogenesis imperfecta)

Defects Detectable In Utero but Best Corrected After Delivery Near Term

Esophageal, duodenal, jejunoileal, and anorectal atresias

Meconium ileus (cystic fibrosis)

Enteric cysts and duplications

Small intact omphalocele and gastroschisis

Unilateral multicystic dysplastic kidney, hydronephrosis

Craniofacial, limb, and chest wall deformities

Simple cystic hygroma

Small sacrococcygeal teratoma, mesoblastic nephroma, neuroblastoma

Benign cysts (e.g., ovarian, mesenteric, choledochal)

Defects That May Lead to Cesarean Delivery

Conjoined twins

Giant or ruptured omphalocele, gastroschisis

Severe hydrocephalus; large or ruptured meningomyelocele

Large sacrococcygeal teratoma or cervical cystic hygroma

Malformations requiring preterm delivery in the presence of inadequate labor or fetal distress

Defects That May Lead to Induced Preterm Delivery

Progressively enlarging hydrocephalus, hydrothorax

Gastroschisis or ruptured omphalocele with damaged bowel

Intestinal ischemia and necrosis secondary to volvulus or meconium ileus

Progressive hydrops fetalis

Intrauterine growth retardation

Arrhythmias (e.g., supraventricular tachycardia with failure)

Defects That May Require EXIT Procedure

Congenital high airway obstruction syndrome (CHAOS)

Large cervical tumors (e.g., teratoma)

Masses obstructing trachea or mouth (e.g., cystic hygroma)

Conditions requiring immediate ECMO cannulation

Chest mass preventing lung expansion

ECMO, extracorporeal membrane oxygenation.

material, combined with advances in the human genome project, has led to testing of greater numbers of genetic abnormalities prenatally. Increasingly, single nucleotide polymorphism arrays are being developed to genetically characterize diseases further and will clearly augment testing for aneuploidy in the future.[6]

FETAL IMAGING

Ultrasonography

Fetal anatomy, normal and abnormal, can be accurately delineated by US. This noninvasive technique appears to be safe for both the fetus and the mother and is now routinely applied in most pregnancies. Most anatomic surveys are performed in the middle of the second trimester between 18 and 20 weeks' gestation. The scope and reliability of the information obtained are directly proportional to the skill and experience of the ultrasonographer and ultrasonologist. For example management of a fetal defect requires a thorough evaluation of the fetus for other abnormalities because malformations often occur as part of a syndrome.

Real-time US may yield important information on fetal movement and fetal vital functions (heart rate, breathing movements) that reflect fetal well-being. Serial US evaluation is particularly useful in defining the natural history and progression of fetal disease. Further, US can stratify the severity of a disease. For instance details of the ultrasonogram that correlate with outcome include presence or absence of associated anomalies, presence or absence of hydrops fetalis, presence or absence of liver herniation into the chest, and relative lung size. The details of a complete anatomic survey are extensive and are covered elsewhere.[1] Finally, real-time US is critical for guidance during fetal interventions. It may be the only method of guidance in some procedures such as needle aspiration for fetal fluid or tissue sampling. For fetal endoscopic or open fetal procedures, US not only gives valuable information about the fetus but also gives information about the uterus, particularly placental location.

Echocardiography

The field of echocardiography has seen rapid growth in the past 10 years because of advances in ultrasound technology and increasing experience with the assessment of the normal and abnormal fetal heart. Most structural cardiac anomalies can be detected prenatally.[7–9] Many abnormalities of interest to pediatric surgeons, such as congenital diaphragmatic hernia (CDH) and omphalocele, have a high incidence of associated structural cardiac anomalies, and the identification of these anomalies can affect postnatal outcome and prenatal counseling. The determination of cardiac function has played a significant role in predicting outcome for fetal anomalies that may cause cardiac dysfunction, such as sacrococcygeal teratoma and congenital pulmonary adenomatoid malformations, as well as twin anomalies that are less familiar to pediatric surgeons such as twin-twin transfusion syndrome (TTTS) and twin reversed arterial perfusion (TRAP) sequence. Further, fetal cardiac monitoring by perioperative echocardiography has been used to monitor the fetal response to surgery.[10] Finally, because the natural history of cardiac anomalies are now better understood,[9] ameliorating or reversing their progressive effects with fetal intervention by echocardiographic guidance has been attempted.[11–13]

Magnetic Resonance Imaging

Although US remains the primary mode of imaging the fetus, magnetic resonance imaging (MRI) is used increasingly for a variety of abnormalities to evaluate the fetal spine, brain, and body. MRI has proved to be a valuable imaging technique because of the high resolution capabilities that are complementary to US, which is less costly and more accessible, and as a real-time modality that can show motion and changes over time. There are no known adverse effects of MRI on the fetus when it is performed with MRI scanners that are 1.5 T or less.[14] Figure 5-1 shows an ultrasonographic image of a CDH, and Figure 5-2 shows an MRI image of a CDH.

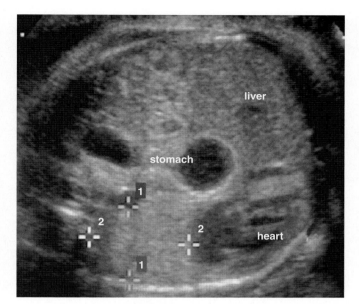

FIGURE 5-1 Transaxial ultrasonographic image of the chest in a fetus with a left diaphragmatic hernia (liver, stomach, and heart labeled). Measurements of the right lung (*1* and *2*) are made using electronic calipers to calculate the LHR.

Fetal Access

Although most prenatally diagnosed anatomic malformations are best managed by appropriate medical and surgical therapy after maternal transport and delivery, a few simple anatomic abnormalities that have predictable devastating developmental consequences may require correction before birth.[15] In the 1980s the developmental pathophysiology of several potentially correctable lesions was worked out in animal models; the natural history was determined by serial observation of human fetuses; selection criteria for intervention were developed; and anesthetic, tocolytic, and surgical techniques for hysterotomy and fetal surgery were refined.[1,15–20]

This investment in basic and clinical research has benefited an increasing number of fetal patients with a few relatively rare defects and will benefit many more as new forms of therapy—including stem cell transplantation, tissue engineering, and gene therapy—are applied to a wide variety of anatomic and biochemical defects. Some milestones in this development of fetal therapy appear in Table 5-2.

The technical aspects of hysterotomy for open fetal surgery that evolved over 30 years of experimental and clinical work are presented in Figure 5-3.[1] Because the morbidity of hysterotomy (particularly preterm labor) is significant, videoendoscopic fetal surgery (FETENDO) techniques that obviate the need for a uterine incision were developed (Fig. 5-4).[21] Percutaneous fetoscopic intervention has been applied clinically for diagnostic biopsies, laser ablation of

TABLE 5-2

Fetal Conditions That May Require Prenatal Medical Treatment

Defects	Treatment
Erythroblastosis fetalis (erythrocyte deficiency)	Erythrocytes—intraperitoneal or intravenous
Pulmonary immaturity (surfactant deficiency)	Glucocorticoids—transplacental
Metabolic block (e.g., methylmalonic acidemia, multiple carboxylase deficiency)	Vitamin B_{12}—transplacental Biotin—transplacental
Cardiac arrhythmia (supraventricular tachycardia)	Digitalis—transplacental Propranolol—transplacental Procainamide—transplacental
Endocrine deficiency (e.g., hypothyroidism, adrenal hyperplasia)	Thyroid—transamniotic Corticosteroids—transplacental
Nutritional deficiency (e.g., intrauterine growth retardation)	Protein-calories—transamniotic or intravenous

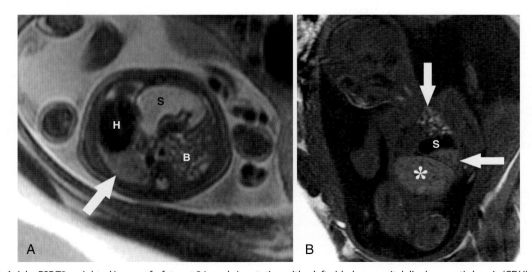

FIGURE 5-2 **A,** Axial ssFSE T2-weighted image of a fetus at 24 weeks' gestation with a left-sided congenital diaphragmatic hernia (CDH). The heart *(H)* and right lung *(arrow)* are displaced to the right. The left lung is not visible, and instead the left side of the chest contains herniated stomach *(S)* and bowel *(B)*. **B,** Sagittal spoiled gradient-echo T1-weighted magnetic resonance image shows the stomach *(s)* in the left side of the chest. Note the liver *(asterisk)* is of relatively high signal intensity, facilitating the identification of the herniated left lobe *(horizontal arrow)* in the left side of the chest. The herniated bowel loops *(vertical arrow)* in the left side of the chest are also of relatively high signal intensity.

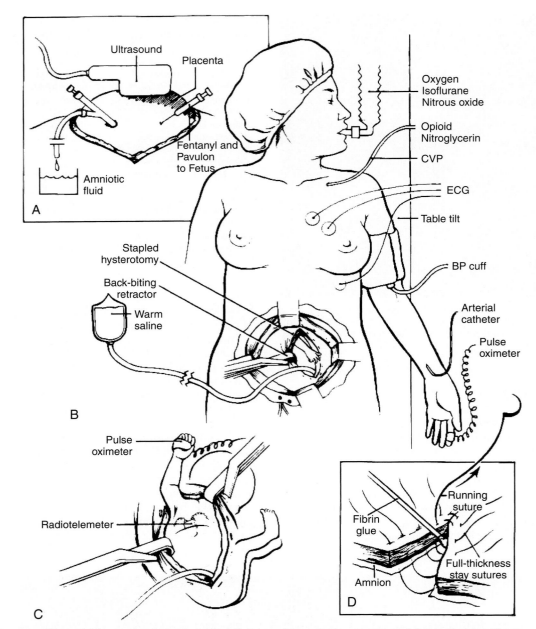

FIGURE 5-3   Summary of open fetal surgery techniques. **A,** Uterus is exposed through a low transverse abdominal incision. Ultrasonography is used to localize the placenta, inject the fetus with narcotic and muscle relaxant, and aspirate amniotic fluid. **B,** The uterus is opened with staples that provide hemostasis and seal the membranes. Warm saline solution is continuously infused around the fetus. Maternal anesthesia, tocolysis, and monitoring are shown. **C,** Absorbable staples and back-biting clamps facilitate hysterotomy exposure of the pertinent fetal part. A miniaturized pulse oximeter records pulse rate and oxygen saturation intraoperatively. A radiotelemeter monitors fetal electrocardiogram *(ECG)* and amniotic pressure during and after operation. **D,** After fetal repair the uterine incision is closed with absorbable sutures and fibrin glue. Amniotic fluid is restored with warm lactated Ringer solution. BP, blood pressure; CVP, central venous pressure.

placental vessels in twin-twin transfusion syndrome,[22] fetal cystoscopy and urinary tract decompression,[23,24] cord ligature or division in anomalous twins,[25,26] division of amniotic bands, and tracheal occlusion for CDH.[27] Percutaneous ultrasonographically guided intervention has been applied to placement of catheter shunts (bladder, chest),[24,28] vascular access (heart,[29] umbilical vessels), radiofrequency ablation of large tumors or anomalous twins,[30] aspiration of fluid from fetal body cavities,[28] and administration of drugs or cells directly to the fetus.[31]

Management of Mother and Fetus

Breaching the uterus, whether by puncture or incision, incites uterine contractions. Despite technical advances, disruption of membranes and preterm labor are the Achilles' heel of fetal therapy. Although halogenated inhalation agents provide satisfactory anesthesia for mother and fetus, the depth of anesthesia necessary to achieve intraoperative uterine relaxation

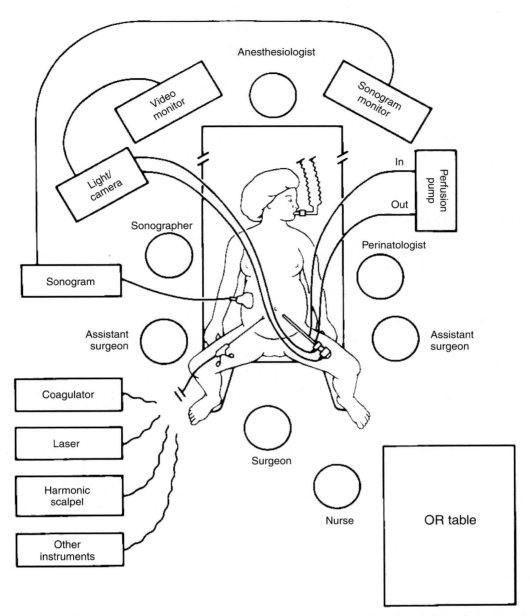

FIGURE 5-4   Drawing of the operating room set-up. Note that there are two monitors at the head of the table: one for the fetoscopic picture and the other for the real-time ultrasonographic image.

can produce fetal and maternal myocardial depression and affect placental perfusion.[10] Indomethacin can constrict the fetal ductus arteriosus and the combination of magnesium sulfate and betamimetics can produce maternal pulmonary edema. The search for a more effective and less toxic tocolytic regimen led to the demonstration in monkeys that exogenous nitric oxide ablates preterm labor induced by hysterotomy.[32] Intravenous nitroglycerin is a potent tocolytic but requires careful control to avoid serious complications.[1]

Postoperative management is dictated by the degree of intervention. Open fetal surgery by maternal laparotomy and hysterotomy is usually performed with the patient under general anesthesia. Fetal well-being and uterine activity are recorded externally by tocodynamometer. Extensive monitoring, both fetal and maternal, continues postoperatively. Patient-controlled analgesia or continuous epidural

analgesia, or both, ease maternal stress and aid tocolysis. After contractions are controlled, monitoring and tocolysis continue and fetal sonograms are obtained at least weekly. Open hysterotomy requires cesarean delivery in this and future pregnancies because of the potential for uterine rupture.[33,34] The most common immediate maternal complication is pulmonary edema due to the administration of perioperative tocolytic agents and intravenous fluids. The incidence was as high as 28% in previous experiences, but with refinement of surgical techniques and tocolytic management the incidence is now approximately 5%.[35] Bleeding that requires transfusion is an infrequent but significant complication of open fetal surgery. Preterm labor and membrane rupture are the most significant complications throughout the remainder of the pregnancy. Close monitoring for contractions, amount of amniotic fluid, membrane disruption, and cervical shape and length must be performed throughout pregnancy.

Patients who undergo percutaneous procedures, performed either with fetoscopic guidance or with image guidance using 1- to 3-mm-diameter devices, usually receive regional or local anesthesia. The requirement for tocolytic therapy is significantly less than for open fetal surgery, and most patients can be safely discharged from the hospital within 24 to 48 hours after the procedure.[35] Maternal bleeding and pulmonary edema are rare. However membrane rupture and preterm labor remain significant complications,[22] and close monitoring is required throughout the remainder of pregnancy.

Risks of Maternal-Fetal Surgery

The risk of the procedure for the fetus is weighed against the benefit of correction of a fatal or debilitating defect. The risks and benefits for the mother are more difficult to assess. Most fetal malformations do not directly threaten the mother's health, yet she must bear significant risk and discomfort from the procedure. She may choose to accept the risk for the sake of the unborn fetus and to alleviate the burden of raising a child with a severe malformation.

There is a paucity of published data on the maternal impact of fetal surgical interventions.[34] We analyzed maternal morbidity and mortality associated with different types of fetal intervention (open hysterotomy, different endoscopic procedures, and percutaneous techniques) to quantify this risk. We performed a retrospective evaluation of a continuous series of 187 procedures performed between July 1989 and May 2003 at the University of California, San Francisco (UCSF) Fetal Treatment Center.

Fetal surgery was performed in 87 patients by open hysterotomy, 69 patients underwent endoscopic techniques, and 31 patients underwent percutaneous techniques. There was no maternal mortality. Endoscopic procedures, even with laparotomy, showed statistically significantly less morbidity compared with the open hysterotomy group regarding cesarean section as the mode of delivery (94.8% versus 58.8%; $P < 0.001$), requirement for intensive care unit (ICU) stay (1.4% versus 26.4%; $P < 0.001$), length of hospital stay (7.9 days versus 11.9 days; $P = 0.001$), and requirement for blood transfusions (2.9% versus 12.6%; $P = 0.022$). It was not significant for premature rupture of membranes, pulmonary edema, abruptio placentae, postoperative vaginal bleeding, uncontrollable preterm labor leading to preterm delivery, or interval from fetal surgery to delivery. In more recent series, however, the incidence of pulmonary edema after percutaneous fetal endoscopic surgery has been low.[22] The group that had percutaneous procedures had the least morbidity.[35]

Our study of maternal outcome confirmed that fetal surgery can be performed without maternal mortality. Short-term morbidity can be serious, with impact on maternal health, length of pregnancy, and survival of the fetus.

Because midgestation hysterotomy is not performed in the lower uterine segment, delivery after fetal surgery and all future deliveries should be by cesarean section. In our series uterine disruptions occurred in subsequent pregnancies; uterine closure and neonatal outcome were excellent in both cases. Finally, the ability to carry and deliver subsequent infants does not appear to be jeopardized by fetal surgery.[33]

PRENATAL DIAGNOSIS DICTATES PERINATAL MANAGEMENT

The nature of the defect determines perinatal management (see Table 5-1).[1] When serious malformations that are incompatible with postnatal life are diagnosed early enough, the family has the option of terminating the pregnancy. Most correctable malformations that can be diagnosed in utero are best managed by appropriate medical and surgical therapy after delivery near term; prenatal diagnosis allows delivery at a center where a neonatal surgical team is prepared. Elective cesarean delivery rather than a trial at vaginal delivery may be indicated for fetal malformations that cause dystocia or that will benefit from immediate surgical repair in a sterile environment.

Early delivery may be indicated for fetal conditions that require treatment as soon as possible after diagnosis, but the risk of prematurity itself must be carefully considered. The rationale for early delivery is unique to each anomaly but the principle remains the same: continued gestation will have progressive ill effects on the fetus. In some cases the function of a specific organ system is compromised by the lesion (e.g., hydronephrosis) and will continue to deteriorate until the lesion is corrected. In some malformations, the progressive ill effects on the fetus result directly from being in utero (e.g., the bowel damage in gastroschisis from exposure to amniotic fluid).

Some fetal deficiency states may be alleviated by treatment before birth (Table 5-3). For example blood can be transfused into the fetal peritoneal cavity or directly into the umbilical artery, and antiarrhythmic drugs can be given transplacentally to convert fetal supraventricular tachycardia. When the necessary substrate, medication, or nutrient cannot be delivered across the placenta, it may be injected into the amniotic fluid from which it can be swallowed and absorbed by the fetus. In the future it is possible that deficiencies in cellular function will be corrected by providing the appropriate stem cell graft or the appropriately engineered gene.[31,36]

Fetal Anomalies

The only anatomic malformations that warrant consideration are those that interfere with fetal organ development and that if alleviated would allow normal development to proceed (Table 5-4). Initially a few life-threatening malformations were studied intensively and successfully corrected. Over the past two decades an increasing number of fetal defects have been defined and new treatments devised.[1,18] As less invasive interventional techniques are developed and proved safe, a few nonlethal anomalies (e.g., myelomeningocele) have become candidates for fetal surgical correction.[37–39] Finally, stem cell transplantation, gene therapy, and tissue engineering should open the door to treatment of a variety of inherited disorders.[31,36,40,41] In the next section of this chapter, we give an overview of fetal anomalies that may be amenable to fetal intervention as well as fetal anomalies that are of specific interest to pediatric surgeons.

URINARY TRACT OBSTRUCTION

Fetal urethral obstruction produces pulmonary hypoplasia and renal dysplasia, and these often-fatal consequences can be ameliorated by urinary tract decompression before birth.[24]

The natural history of untreated fetal urinary tract obstruction is well documented, and selection criteria based on fetal urine electrolyte and ß$_2$-microglobulin levels and the ultrasonographic appearance of fetal kidneys have proved reliable.[24] Of all fetuses with urinary tract dilatation, as many as 90% do not require intervention. However fetuses with bilateral hydronephrosis due to urethral obstruction in whom oligohydramnios subsequently develops require treatment. If the lungs are mature the fetus can be delivered early for postnatal decompression. If the lungs are immature the bladder can be decompressed in utero by a vesicoamniotic shunt placed percutaneously using ultrasonographic guidance or by fetoscopic vesicostomy.[24,28] Fetal cystoscopic ablation of posterior urethral valves has also been reported, with the potential benefit of maintenance of the normal physiologic state of fetal bladder filling and emptying.[23,42]

Experience treating several hundred fetuses in many institutions suggests that selection is good enough to avoid inappropriate intervention and that restoration of amniotic fluid can prevent the development of fatal pulmonary hypoplasia. It is not yet clear how much renal function damage can be reversed by decompression. In one retrospective series of fetuses treated with vesicoamniotic shunting for lower urinary tract obstruction, survival at 1 year was 91%, with two neonatal deaths from pulmonary hypoplasia. There was a 39% incidence of prune belly syndrome, more than 50% demonstrated some renal dysfunction, and 33% required renal replacement. Approximately half of the children had persistent respiratory problems, musculoskeletal problems, and frequent urinary tract infections. Nearly two thirds of them had poor growth.[43] Identifying fetuses who may consistently have renal benefit from fetal intervention is likely contingent on the development of more sensitive biomarkers for early fetal renal dysfunction.

AIRWAY OBSTRUCTION

The tracheal occlusion strategy for fetal CDH required development of techniques to safely reverse the obstruction at birth. The ex utero intrapartum treatment (EXIT) procedure is a technique in which the principles of fetal surgery (anesthesia for mother and fetus, complete uterine relaxation, and maintenance of umbilical circulation to support the fetus) are used during cesarean delivery to allow the airway to be secured while the fetus remains on maternal bypass. The EXIT procedure has been used successfully to reverse tracheal occlusion, repair the trachea, secure the airway by tracheotomy, resect large cervical tumors, place vascular cannulas for immediate extracorporeal membrane oxygenation (ECMO) (EXIT to ECMO), and manage laryngeal obstruction in congenital high airway obstruction syndrome (CHAOS).[44–46]

The EXIT procedure provides a wonderful opportunity for surgeons, perinatologists, neonatologists, and anesthesiologists to learn to work together, and this should be one of the first procedures done in developing a fetal treatment center.

CONGENITAL PULMONARY AIRWAY MALFORMATION

Although congenital pulmonary airway malformation (CPAM), traditionally referred to as congenital cystic adenomatoid malformation (CCAM), often presents as a benign pulmonary mass

TABLE 5-3		
Milestones		
Intrauterine transfusion (IUT) for Rh disease	Women's National Hospital, Auckland, NZ	1961
Hysterotomy for fetal vascular access—IUT	University of Puerto Rico	1964
Fetoscopy—diagnostic	Yale	1974
Experimental pathophysiology (sheep model)	UCSF	1980
Hysterotomy and maternal safety (monkey model)	UCSF	1981
Vesicoamniotic shunt for uropathy	UCSF	1982
Open fetal surgery for uropathy	UCSF	1983
International Fetal Medicine and Surgery Society founded	Santa Barbara	1982
CCAM resection	UCSF	1984
First edition of *Unborn Patient: Prenatal Diagnosis and Treatment*	UCSF	1984
Intravascular transfusion	King's College, London University	1985
CDH open repair	UCSF	1989
Anomalous twin—cord ligation, RFA, and so on	King's College, London University	1990
NIH Trial: Open repair CDH	UCSF	1990
Aortic balloon valvuloplasty	King's College, London University	1991
SCT resection	UCSF	1992
Laser ablation of placental vessels	St Joseph's Hospital, Milwaukee; King's College, London University	1995
EXIT procedure for airway obstruction	UCSF	1995
Stem cell treatment for SCIDS	Detroit	1996
EXIT for CHAOS	CHOP	1996
Eurofetus founded	University Hospital Leuven, Belgium	1997
Myelomeningocele—open repair	Vanderbilt	1997
NIH Trial: FETENDO balloon CDH	UCSF	1998
Mediastinal teratoma resection	CHOP	2000
Eurofetus trial for twin-twin transfusion syndrome	University Hospital Gasthuisberg, Belgium; Universite Paris-Ouest Versailles, France	2001
NIH Trial: open repair myelomeningocele	UCSF, CHOP, Vanderbilt	2002
Balloon dilation for hypoplastic heart	Harvard	2003
NAFTNet founded	North America	2005
Percutaneous temporary tracheal occlusion for CDH	University Hospital Leuven, Belgium	2006

CCAM, cystic adenomatoid malformation; CDH, congenital diaphragmatic hernia; CHAOS, congenital high airway obstruction syndrome; CHOP, Children's Hospital of Philadelphia; EXIT, ex utero intrapartum treatment; NIH, National Institutes of Health; RFA, radiofrequency ablation; SCIDS, severe combined immunodeficiency disease; SCT, sacrococcygeal teratoma; UCSF, University of California, San Francisco.

in infants and children, some fetuses with large lesions die in utero or at birth from hydrops and pulmonary hypoplasia. The pathophysiologic characteristics of hydrops and the feasibility of resecting the fetal lung have been studied in animals. Experience managing more than 200 patients suggests that

TABLE 5-4

Fetal Conditions That May Benefit from Treatment Before Birth

Effect on Development

	Rationale for Treatment	Result Without Treatment	Recommended Treatment
Life-threatening defects			
Urinary obstruction (urethral valves)	Hydronephrosis	Renal failure	Percutaneous vesicoamniotic shunt
	Lung hypoplasia	Pulmonary failure	Fetoscopic ablation of valves
			Open vesicostomy
Cystic adenomatoid malformation	Lung hypoplasia-hydrops	Hydrops, death	Open pulmonary lobectomy
			Ablation (laser/RFA)
			Steroids
Congenital diaphragmatic hernia			Open complete repair
	Lung hypoplasia	Pulmonary failure	Temporary tracheal occlusion
			Tracheal clip (open and fetoscopic)
			Fetoscopic balloon (percutaneous/reversible)
Sacrococcygeal teratoma	High-output failure	Hydrops, death	Open resection of tumor
			Vascular occlusion—RFA, alcohol
			RFA
Twin-twin transfusion syndrome	Donor-recipient steal through placenta	Fetal hydrops, death, neurologic damage to survivor	Fetoscopic laser ablation of placental vessels
			Amnioreduction
			Selective reduction
Acardiac/anomalous twin (TRAP)	Vascular steal	Death/damage to surviving twin	Selective reduction
	Embolization		Cord occlusion/division
			RFA
Aqueductal stenosis	Hydrocephalus	Brain damage	Ventriculoamniotic shunt
Valvular obstruction	Hypoplastic heart	Cardiac failure	Balloon valvuloplasty
Congenital high airway obstruction (CHAOS)	Overdistention by lung fluid		Fetoscopic tracheostomy
		Hydrops, death	EXIT
Cervical teratoma	Airway obstruction	Hydrops, death	Open resection
	High-output failure		EXIT
			Vascular occlusion—alcohol/RFA
Non-life-threatening defects			
Myelomeningocele	Spinal cord damage	Paralysis, neurogenic bladder/bowel, hydrocephalus	Open repair (NIH trial)
			Fetoscopic coverage
Gastroschisis	Bowel damage	Malnutrition/short bowel	Serial amnioexchange
Cleft lip and palate	Facial defect	Persistent deformity	Fetoscopic repair*
			Open repair
Metabolic and cellular defects			
Stem cell enzyme defects	Hemoglobinopathy	Anemia, hydrops	Fetal stem cell transplant
	Immunodeficiency	Infection/death	Fetal gene therapy*
	Storage diseases	Retardation/death	
Predictable organ	Agenesis/hypoplasia heart/lung/kidney	Neonatal heart/lung/kidney failure	Induce tolerance for postnatal organ transplant*
			Tissue engineering*

*Not yet attempted in human fetuses.
CHAOS, congenital high airway obstruction syndrome; EXIT, ex utero intrapartum treatment; NIH, National Institutes of Health; RFA, radiofrequency ablation; TRAP, twin reversed arterial perfusion.

most lesions can be successfully treated after birth and that some lesions resolve before birth. Although only a few fetuses with very large lesions experience hydrops before 26 weeks of gestation, these lesions may progress rapidly and the fetuses die in utero.[47]

Careful ultrasonographic surveillance of large lesions is necessary to detect the first signs of hydrops because fetuses in whom hydrops develops can be successfully treated by emergency resection of the cystic lobe in utero.[48] Size of the CPAM is an important determinant of outcome and the most commonly used metric is the CCAM volume ratio (CVR). CVR is a ratio of the volume of CPAM/fetal head circumference, and higher CVR has been shown to produce a higher incidence of the development of hydrops fetalis and perinatal mortality.[49] That study also found that microcystic CPAMs tend to plateau in size at 26 to 28 weeks of gestation, whereas macrocystic CPAMs may grow rapidly throughout gestation. Fetal pulmonary lobectomy for fetuses with microcystic CPAM and hydrops fetalis has proved surprisingly simple and quite successful at two large fetal surgery centers, although there is a high likelihood for preterm labor and premature delivery.[44] In 2003, we reported our initial experience with maternal corticosteroid administration for fetuses with microcystic CPAM lesions and hydrops, showing reversal of hydrops and survival in patients.[50] The cumulative data for treatment of 37 fetuses with large microcystic CPAMs at three centers showed 87% overall survival and 80% survival for those with hydrops (16/20 patients).[51] The effect of the steroids on the CPAM is unclear and difficult to elucidate as there is no sufficient animal model for microcystic CPAM. However some have speculated that CPAM represents an arrested state of normal lung development that has been characterized by increased cell proliferation and decreased apoptosis.[52]

We hypothesized that administration of maternal corticosteroids may drive maturation of microcystic CPAM tissue into more mature pulmonary tissue, decreasing proliferation of the lesions. The experience of treating large fetal macrocystic CPAM with maternal steroid administration has not been successful.[53] For lesions with single large cysts thoracoamniotic shunting has been the best option.[54]

CONGENITAL DIAPHRAGMATIC HERNIA

The history of the evolution of fetal diagnosis and therapy for CDH outlines many of the successes and disappointments of the field. Prenatal diagnosis is now made routinely for CDH.

CDH can now be diagnosed accurately by midgestation, and the severity can be reasonably stratified by fetal US, MRI, and echocardiography. The diagnosis of fetal CDH is usually made by second-trimester anatomic ultrasonographic survey. Typical findings include mediastinal shift with abdominal viscera in the thorax. Careful attention is paid to the presence of other anomalies that can significantly affect the outcome for patients with CDH, including cardiac anomalies, aneuploidy, and other genetic syndromes such as Fryns syndrome. The most consistent prognostic factor for isolated CDH is presence or absence of liver herniation into the chest.[55] For prenatally diagnosed CDH, the presence of liver herniated into the chest is correlated with decreased survival compared with patients without liver herniation. Attempts at further stratifying the severity of CDH by determining relative lung size have met with variable success. The primary ultrasonographic measurement is lung/head ratio (LHR). To determine LHR a two-dimensional measurement of the lung is made at the level of the four-chambered view of the heart (numerator) and is compared with the head circumference to control for differences in gestational age and fetal size. LHR in the presence of liver herniated into the chest has been shown to have close correlation to survival in several single-institution series as well several multi-institutional series.[55,56] LHR shows substantial variability among ultrasonologists and requires an ultrasonologist with extensive experience in evaluating fetuses with CDH. LHR without liver herniation has not been shown to correlate with outcome.

Lung volume on MRI is the other primary measurement to determine severity of fetal CDH. Three-dimensional interpretation of fetal MRI data is performed and compared with nomograms for fetal lung volume to calculate the percentage of expected lung volume.[57] Some centers have found ultrasonographic measurements to be more predictive of outcome, whereas others have found MRI measurements to be more predictive.

Fetuses without liver herniation and with a favorable LHR (>1.4) have low mortality after term delivery at tertiary centers. However fetuses with liver herniation and a low LHR have high mortality and morbidity despite recent advances in intensive neonatal care, including ECMO, nitric oxide inhalation, high-frequency ventilation, and delayed operative repair of the diaphragmatic hernia.[19,58–63] The fundamental problem in newborns with CDH is pulmonary hypoplasia. Research in experimental animal models and later in human patients over 2 decades has aimed to improve growth of the hypoplastic lungs before they are needed for gas exchange at birth. Anatomic repair of the hernia by open hysterotomy proved feasible but did not decrease mortality and was abandoned.[64,65] Fetal tracheal occlusion was developed as an alternative strategy to promote fetal lung growth by preventing normal egress of lung fluid. Occlusion of the fetal trachea was shown to stimulate fetal lung growth in a variety of animal models.[66–68] Techniques to achieve reversible fetal tracheal occlusion were explored in animal models and then applied clinically, evolving from external metal clips placed on the trachea by open hysterotomy or fetoscopic neck dissection to internal tracheal occlusion with a detachable silicone balloon placed by fetal bronchoscopy through a single 5-mm uterine port.[69–71]

Our initial experience suggested that fetal endoscopic tracheal occlusion improved survival in human fetuses with severe CDH.[71–73] To evaluate this novel therapy we conducted a randomized controlled trial comparing tracheal occlusion with standard care.[74] Survival with fetal endoscopic tracheal occlusion (73%) met expectations (predicted 75%) and appeared better than that of historical controls (37%) but proved no better than that of concurrent randomized controls. The higher than expected survival in the standard care group may be because the study design mandated that patients in both treatment groups be delivered, resuscitated, and intensively managed in a unit experienced in caring for critically ill newborns with pulmonary hypoplasia.[74]

Attempts to improve outcome for severe CDH by treatments either before or after birth have proved double-edged swords. Intensive care after birth has improved survival but has increased long-term sequelae in survivors and is expensive.[19,59–61,63] Intervention before birth may increase lung size but prematurity caused by the intervention itself can be detrimental.[65,72,75–77] In our study newborns with severe CDH who had tracheal occlusion before birth were born on average at 31 weeks as a consequence of the intervention. The observation that their rates of survival and respiratory outcomes (including duration of oxygen requirement) were comparable to infants without tracheal occlusion who were born at 37 weeks suggests that tracheal occlusion improved pulmonary hypoplasia, but the improvement in lung growth was affected by pulmonary immaturity related to earlier delivery.[74]

The current results underscore the role of randomized trials in evaluating promising new therapies. This is the second National Institutes of Health (NIH)-sponsored trial studying a new prenatal intervention for severe fetal CDH. The first trial showed that complete surgical repair of the anatomic defect (which required hysterotomy), although feasible, was no better than postnatal repair in improving survival and was ineffective when the liver as well as the bowel were herniated.[65] That trial led to the abandonment of open complete repair at our institution and subsequently around the world. Information derived from that trial regarding measures of severity of pulmonary hypoplasia (including liver herniation and the development of the LHR) led to the development of an alternative physiologic strategy to enlarge the hypoplastic fetal lung by temporary tracheal occlusion[73,76,77] and to the development of less invasive fetal endoscopic techniques that did not require hysterotomy to achieve temporary reversible tracheal occlusion.[21,69,71]

Our ability to accurately diagnose and assess severity of CDH before birth has improved dramatically. Fetuses with CDH who have associated anomalies do poorly, whereas fetuses with isolated CDH, no liver herniation, and an LHR greater than 1.4 have an excellent prognosis (100% in our experience). In this study fetuses with an LHR between 0.9 and 1.4 had a chance of survival greater than 80% when delivered at a tertiary care center. The small number of fetuses with an LRH less than 0.9 had a poor prognosis in both treatment groups and should be the focus of ongoing study.[74] Further, animal models have shown that reversal of tracheal occlusion before delivery may minimize the damage to type II pneumocytes and surfactant production that prolonged tracheal occlusion may cause.[78]

With the advent of further miniaturized fetoscopic equipment, the group in Leuven, Belgium has led efforts to perform percutaneous temporary fetoscopic tracheal occlusion for isolated severe (liver herniation into chest, LHR <1.) CDH. They have reported 50% survival with gestational age at delivery of 34 weeks in fetuses undergoing temporary tracheal occlusion compared with survival of less than 15% in a cohort of fetuses with similar prenatal variables.[79] The European experience now consists of more than 200 patients with temporary tracheal occlusion, and a prospective randomized trial comparing that strategy to standard postnatal care is under way in Europe.[80] The low survival of patients with standard postnatal care in Europe has been criticized, as survival in that cohort in the United States at certain tertiary centers has been significantly higher. UCSF currently is conducting a safety and feasibility trial for temporary percutaneous fetoscopic tracheal occlusion for severe CDH with oversight by the US Food and Drug Administration (FDA).

Myelomeningocele

Myelomeningocele is a devastating birth defect with sequelae that affect both the central and peripheral nervous systems. Altered cerebrospinal fluid dynamics result in the Chiari II malformation and hydrocephalus. Damage to the exposed spinal cord results in lifelong lower extremity neurologic deficiency, fetal and urinary incontinence, sexual dysfunction, and skeletal deformities. This defect carries enormous personal, familial, and societal costs, as the near-normal life span of the affected child is characterized by hospitalization, multiple operations, disability, and institutionalization. Although it has been assumed that the spinal cord itself is intrinsically malformed in children with this defect, recent work suggests that the neurologic impairment after birth may be due to exposure and trauma to the spinal cord in utero and that covering the exposed cord may prevent the development of the Chiari malformation.[37,39,81]

Since 1997 more than 200 fetuses have undergone in utero closure of myelomeningocele by open fetal surgery. Preliminary clinical evidence suggests that this procedure reduces the incidence of shunt-dependent hydrocephalus and restores the cerebellum and brainstem to a more normal configuration.[39] However clinical results of fetal surgery for myelomeningocele are based on comparisons with historical controls, examine only efficacy not safety, and lack long-term follow-up.

The NIH has funded a multicenter randomized clinical trial (Management of Myelomeningocele Study [MOMS]) of 200 patients that will be conducted at three fetal surgery units: the University of California, San Francisco; the Children's Hospital of Philadelphia; and Vanderbilt University Medical Center, along with an independent data and study coordinating center, the George Washington University Biostatistics Center. Since the inception of the trial Vanderbilt has dropped out as a surgical site.

Primary objectives of this randomized trial are (1) to determine if intrauterine repair of fetal myelomeningocele at 19 to 26 weeks' gestation using a standard multilayer closure improves outcome, as measured by death or the need for ventricular decompressive shunting by 1 year of life, compared with standard postnatal care and (2) to determine if intrauterine repair of myelomeningocele can improve motor function as well as cognitive function as measured by the Bayley Scales of Infant Development mental development index at 30 months' corrected age.[82] The study was closed to new patient enrollment on December 7, 2010, after 183 patients had been randomized because of the efficacy of prenatal repair. Specifically, prenatal repair of spina bifida reduced the need for ventricular shunting to treat hydrocephalus and improved motor outcomes including the ability to walk at 30 months of age.[98] Prenatal repair of MMC was also associated with significant maternal and neonatal risks, including premature birth and uterine scar issues.

SACROCOCCYGEAL TERATOMA

Most neonates with sacrococcygeal teratoma survive and malignant invasion is unusual. However the prognosis of patients with sacrococcygeal teratoma diagnosed prenatally (by ultrasonography or elevated AFP levels) is less favorable. There is a subset of fetuses (fewer than 20%) with large tumors in whom hydrops develops from high-output failure secondary to extremely high blood flow through the tumor. Because hydrops progresses rapidly to fetal death, frequent ultrasonographic follow-up is mandatory. Excision of the tumor reverses the pathophysiology if it is performed before the mirror syndrome (maternal eclampsia) develops in the mother.[1,83] Attempts to interrupt the vascular steal by ablating blood flow to the tumor by alcohol injection or embolization have not been successful. Ultrasonographically guided radiofrequency ablation of the vascular pedicle has worked but with unacceptable damage to adjacent structures.

Gastroschisis

Patients born with gastroschisis require immediate surgical intervention after birth with either primary or staged closure of the abdominal wall. Despite closure of the abdominal wall defect, many infants face prolonged difficulty with nutrient absorption and intestinal motility. At birth, the intestines of these patients are frequently thickened and covered by a fibrinous "peel." Mesenteric shortening and intestinal atresia may also be present. The bowel damage may be due to constriction of the mesentery (like a napkin ring), causing poor lymphatic and venous drainage from the bowel, or to an inflammatory reaction to various substances in the amniotic fluid bathing the bowel.[84]

With advances in neonatal care, survival for gastroschisis is now more than 90% in most series.[84–86] Serial amniotic fluid exchange has been used to dilute putative inflammatory mediators and thus prevent bowel damage.[87] However our ability to select fetuses with damaged bowels is limited, and the volume of exchange may be inadequate to alter outcome.

Despite high survival rates the complications of gastroschisis remain severe. Gastroschisis is one of the leading causes of short-bowel syndrome and one of the leading indications for small bowel transplantation. The main challenge in fetal treatment of gastroschisis has been identifying biomarkers to distinguish the small subset of fetuses who will have poor outcomes for both counseling and potential treatment. Unfortunately most attempts at predicting outcome by prenatal markers have been unsuccessful. The only prenatal marker that has been reproducible has been multiple intra-abdominal dilated loops of intestine on prenatal US.[88,89]

INTESTINAL ABNORMALITIES

Nearly all abnormalities of fetal intestines are best managed postnatally. However pregnant women are frequently referred to pediatric surgeons for consultation. A common ultrasonographic finding is that of echogenic bowel, seen in up to 1.4% of all second-trimester ultrasonograms.[90] The vast majority of fetuses with echogenic bowel as an isolated anomaly have no clinical sequelae. However the presence of echogenic bowel does increase the risk of aneuploidy. Further, echogenic bowel can herald the presence of bowel injury from a variety of causes. The workup for echogenic bowel may include a detailed ultrasonogram of the fetus and an amniocentesis for karyotype for evidence of cytomegalovirus, toxoplasmosis, and parvovirus. Cystic fibrosis (CF) carrier testing for both parents and maternal serologic testing for recent cytomegalovirus and toxoplasmosis may also be performed. Follow-up with serial growth scans is recommended because these fetuses are potentially at risk for poor growth.

Evidence of frank bowel perforation is suggested by prenatal ultrasonographic findings of ascites, abdominal calcifications, pseudocysts, dilated loops of intestine, or polyhydramnios. The causes of bowel perforation in utero are similar to postnatal causes and are familiar to pediatric surgeons. They include intestinal atresias, meconium ileus, midgut volvulus, and intestinal ischemia. The majority of fetuses with evidence of bowel perforation usually require no surgery postnatally. However fetuses with pseudocysts or diffuse ascites are at higher risk for postnatal surgery and the possibility of long-term intestinal complications.[91]

Dilatation of intestine as an isolated finding usually indicates jejunal-ileal atresia. Without evidence of perforation, volvulus, or other complications, postnatal management results in excellent outcome.[92]

ANOMALIES OF MONOCHORIONIC TWINS

Identical twins may have separate placentas (dichorionic) or share a placenta (monochorionic). Monochorionic twins may have unequal blood flow or unequal shares of the placenta and are at risk for discordant growth or more severe anomalies such as TTTS and TRAP sequence, two of the anomalies of monochorionic twinning that frequently require fetal surgery. Consultation for complications in monochorionic twins represents the most frequent consultation to fetal diagnosis and treatment centers. Further, the laser treatment for TTTS described later on is the most common fetal surgery performed both in the United States and worldwide.

TWIN-TWIN TRANSFUSION SYNDROME

Branches of umbilical arteries and veins from one twin connect with branches of umbilical arteries and veins from the other twin on the surface of the placenta in all monochorionic twin pregnancies. In normal monochorionic twin pregnancies, the flow of blood is relatively balanced from one twin to the other.

TTTS is a complication of monochorionic multiple gestations resulting from an imbalance in blood flow through these vascular communications, or chorioangiopagus. This net imbalance in flow results in one twin (the "recipient") getting too much blood and becoming at risk for high-output cardiac failure and the other twin (the "donor) getting too little blood flow and becoming at risk for hypovolemia and hypoperfusion. Further, vascular mediators such as endothelin may exacerbate cardiac dysfunction in the recipient twin and cause progressive cardiac failure.[93]

It is the most common serious complication of monochorionic twin gestations, affecting between 4% and 35% of monochorionic twin pregnancies, or approximately 0.1 to 0.9 per 1000 births each year in the United States. Yet despite the relatively low incidence, TTTS disproportionately accounts for 17% of all perinatal mortality associated with twin gestations. Previously, standard therapy was limited to serial amnioreduction, which appears to improve the overall outcome but has little impact on the more severe end of the spectrum in TTTS. In addition survivors of TTTS treated by serial amnioreduction have an 18% to 26% incidence of significant neurologic and cardiac morbidity. Selective fetoscopic laser photocoagulation of chorioangiopagus has emerged as the gold standard for treatment of TTTS as demonstrated in a randomized trial in Europe.[22] This prospective randomized controlled trial compared fetoscopic laser coagulation of intertwin vessels to amnioreduction for severe TTTS, with the main outcome variable being survival of at least one twin. Survival of at least one twin was higher in the laser group compared with the amnioreduction group (76% versus 56%), with a decreased incidence of neurologic complications in the laser group. The authors concluded that laser coagulation for severe TTTS was superior to amnioreduction.[22]

TWIN REVERSED ARTERIAL PERFUSION SEQUENCE

Acardiac/acephalic twinning is a rare anomaly in which a normal "pump" twin perfuses an acardiac twin, resulting in TRAP sequence. TRAP sequence in acardiac monochorionic twin gestations compromises the viability of the morphologically normal pump twin. Selective reduction and obliteration of blood flow in the acardiac twin has been accomplished by a variety of techniques, including fetectomy; ligation, division, and cauterization of the umbilical cord; and obliteration of the circulation in the anomalous twin by alcohol injection, electrocautery, or radiofrequency ablation.[25,26] We have pioneered a technique using radiofrequency technology with ultrasonographic guidance. We have used a 14-gauge or 17-gauge radiofrequency ablation (RFA) probe placed percutaneously into the body of the acardiac twin with real-time ultrasonographic guidance, which effectively obliterates the blood supply of the acardiac fetus and protects the pump twin.[26,94] Using this technique survival in monochorionic diamniotic TRAP pregnancies was 92%, with a mean gestational age of 36 weeks. The natural history of TRAP sequence has been reported at greater than 50% mortality.[95] Recently the North American Fetal Therapy Network presented a national registry of 98 pregnant women with TRAP sequence treated by RFA and found an 80% overall survival from 12 centers.[96]

INHERITED DEFECTS CORRECTABLE BY FETAL STEM CELL TRANSPLANTATION

Various inherited defects that are potentially curable by hematopoietic stem cell (HSC) transplantation (e.g., immunodeficiencies, hemoglobinopathies, and storage diseases) can now be detected early in gestation. Postnatal bone marrow transplantation is limited by donor availability, graft rejection, graft-versus-host disease, and patient deterioration before transplantation, which often begins in utero. Transplantation of fetal HSCs early in gestation may circumvent these difficulties.[36,40,41]

The rationale for in utero rather than postnatal transplantation is that the preimmune fetus (<15 weeks) should not reject the transplanted cells, and the fetal bone marrow is primed to receive HSCs that migrate from the fetal liver. Thus myeloablation and immunosuppression may not be necessary. In addition in utero transplantation allows treatment before fetal health is compromised by the underlying disease. The disadvantage of treatment in utero is that the fetus is difficult to access for diagnosis and treatment. Definitive diagnosis using molecular genetic techniques requires fetal tissue obtained by transvaginal or transabdominal chorionic villus sampling, amniocentesis, or fetal blood sampling. Delivering even a small volume (<1 mL) of cells to an early-gestation fetus by intra-abdominal or intravenous injection requires skill and carries significant risks. The greatest potential problem with in utero transplantation of HSCs is that the degree of engraftment or chimerism may not be sufficient to cure or palliate some diseases. In diseases such as chronic granulomatous disease and severe combined immunodeficiency, relatively few normal donor cells can provide sufficient enzyme activity to alleviate symptoms. However a significantly higher degree of donor cell engraftment and expression in the periphery might be necessary to change the course of diseases such as ß-thalassemia or sickle cell disease. For diseases that require a high percentage of donor cells, a promising strategy is to induce tolerance in utero for subsequent postnatal booster injections from a living relative. The optimal source of donor HSCs for in utero transplantation is not known. Donor cells can be obtained from adult bone marrow or peripheral blood, from neonatal umbilical cord blood, or from the liver of an aborted fetus.

Clinical experience with fetal HSC transplantation is limited. Although engraftment has been successful in cases of severe combined immunodeficiency syndrome, for most other diseases low levels of engraftment after injection have limited clinical efficacy.[31,40,41]

PAST AND FUTURE OF FETAL INTERVENTION

Although only a few fetal defects are currently amenable to surgical treatment, the enterprise of fetal surgery has produced some unexpected spin-offs that have interest beyond this narrow therapeutic field. For pediatricians, neonatologists, and dysmorphologists, the natural history and pathophysiologic features of many previously mysterious conditions of newborns have been clarified by following the development of the disease in utero. For obstetricians, perinatologists, and fetologists, techniques developed during experiments in lambs and monkeys will prove useful in managing other high-risk pregnancies. For example an absorbable stapling device developed for fetal surgery has been applied to cesarean sections; radiotelemetric monitoring has applications outside fetal surgery; and videoendoscopic techniques have allowed fetal manipulation without hysterotomy. These techniques will greatly extend the indications for fetal intervention. Finally, the intensive effort to solve the vexing problem of preterm labor after hysterotomy for fetal surgery has yielded new insight into the role of nitric oxide in myometrial contractions and has spawned interest in treating spontaneous preterm labor with nitric oxide donors.

Fetal surgical research has yielded advances in fetal biology with implications beyond fetal therapy. The serendipitous observation that fetal incisions heal without scarring has provided new insights into the biological characteristics of wound healing and has stimulated efforts to mimic the fetal process postnatally. Fetal tissue seems biologically and immunologically superior for transplantation and gene therapy, and fetal immunologic tolerance may allow a wide variety of inherited nonsurgical diseases to be cured by fetal HSC transplantation.

The great promise of fetal therapy is that for some diseases the earliest possible intervention (before birth) produces the best possible outcome (the best quality of life for the resources expended). However the promise of cost-effective preventive fetal therapy can be subverted by misguided clinical applications—for example, a complex in utero procedure that only half saves an otherwise-doomed fetus for a life of intensive (and expensive) care. Enthusiasm for fetal interventions must be tempered by reverence for the interests of the mother and her family, by careful study of the disease in experimental fetal animals and untreated human fetuses, and by a willingness to abandon therapy that does not prove both therapeutically effective and cost-effective in properly controlled trials. Advances must be achieved in a thoughtful manner that balances the potential benefits with the attendant risks, including those to the most important patient, the pregnant woman.

The complete reference list is available online at www. expertconsult.com.

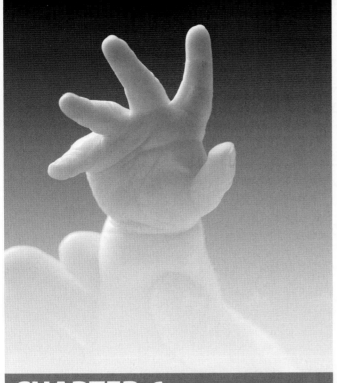

CHAPTER 6

Neonatal Physiology and Metabolic Considerations

Agostino Pierro, Paolo De Coppi, and Simon Eaton

Advances in neonatal intensive care and surgery have significantly improved the survival of neonates with congenital or acquired abnormalities. This has been matched by an improvement in our understanding of the physiology of infants undergoing surgery and their metabolic response to starvation, anesthesia, operative stress, and systemic inflammation.[1] Newborn infants who undergo surgery are not just small adults; their physiology in terms of thermoregulation and fluid and caloric needs can be very different, particularly if the neonate is premature or has intrauterine growth retardation (IUGR). This chapter focuses on the physiology and metabolism of newborn infants undergoing surgery, with particular emphasis on the characteristics of preterm neonates. In this chapter we discuss fluid and electrolyte balance, neonatal energy metabolism and thermoregulation, and the metabolism of carbohydrate, fat, and protein. In addition, we present the current knowledge on the neonatal response to operative trauma and sepsis, which represent two of the major factors that alter their physiology.

Premature, Small for Gestational Age, and Neonates with Intrauterine Growth Retardation

The greatest growth rate occurs during fetal life. In fact the passage from one fertilized cell to a 3.5-kg neonate encompasses an increase in length of 5000-fold, an increase in surface area of 61×10^6, and an increase in weight of 6×10^{12}. The greatest postnatal growth rate occurs just after birth. It is not unusual in neonates undergoing surgery to notice a period of slow or arrested growth during critical illness or soon after surgery.

Neonates can be classified as premature, term, or postmature according to gestational age. Any infant born before 37 weeks of gestation is defined as premature, term infants are those born between 37 and 42 weeks of gestation, and post-term neonates are born after 42 weeks of gestation. Previously any infant weighing less than 2500 g was termed premature. This definition is inappropriate because many neonates weighing less than 2500 g are mature or postmature but are small for gestational age (SGA); they have different appearance and different problems than do premature infants. The gestational age can be estimated antenatally or in the first days after birth using the Ballard score (Fig. 6-1).[2] By plotting body weight versus gestational age (Fig. 6-2),[3] newborn infants can be classified as small, appropriate, or large for gestational age. Head circumference and length are also plotted against gestational age to estimate intrauterine growth (Fig. 6-3).[3] Any infant whose weight is below the 10th percentile for gestational age is defined as SGA. Large for gestational age infants are those whose weight is above the 90th percentile for gestational age (see Fig. 6-2).[3] In general preterm infants weigh less than 2500 g, have a crown-heel length less than 47 cm, a head circumference less than 33 cm, and a thoracic circumference less than 30 cm. The preterm infant has physiologic handicaps due to functional and anatomic immaturity of various organs. Body temperature is difficult to maintain, there are commonly respiratory difficulties, renal function is immature, the ability to combat infection is inadequate, the conjugation and excretion of bilirubin is impaired, and hemorrhagic diathesis is more common.

Premature infants are usually further assigned to subgroups on the basis of birth weight as follows:

1. Moderately low birth weight (birth weight between 1501 and 2500 g): This group represents 82% of all premature infants. The mortality rate in this group is 40 times that in term infants.
2. Very low birth weight (birth weight between 1001 and 1500 g): This group represents 12% of premature infants. The mortality rate in this group is 200 times that in full-term newborns.
3. Extremely low birth weight (birth weight less than 1000 g): These neonates represent 6% of premature births but account for a disproportionate number of newborn deaths. The mortality rate is 600 times that in term infants.

The definition of IUGR is often confused and unclear in the medical literature. IUGR is usually defined as a documented decrease in intrauterine growth noted by fetal ultrasonography. IUGR can be temporary, leading to a normal-sized neonate at birth. There are two types of IUGR: symmetric and

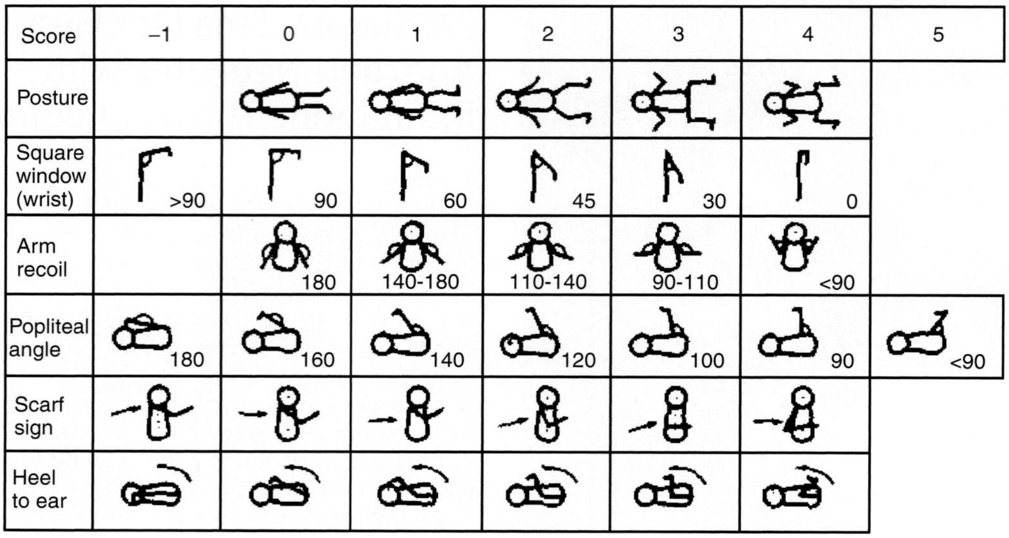

Score	−1	0	1	2	3	4	5
Posture		(image)	(image)	(image)	(image)	(image)	
Square window (wrist)	>90	90	60	45	30	0	
Arm recoil		180	140-180	110-140	90-110	<90	
Popliteal angle	180	160	140	120	100	90	<90
Scarf sign	(image)	(image)	(image)	(image)	(image)	(image)	
Heel to ear	(image)	(image)	(image)	(image)	(image)	(image)	

Physical Maturity

							Maturity Rating
Skin	Sticky, friable, transparent	Gelatinous, red, translucent	Smooth, pink, visible veins	Superficial peeling and/or rash; few veins	Cracking, pale areas; rare veins	Parchment, deep cracking; no vessels	Leathery, cracked, wrinkled
Lanugo	None	Sparse	Abundant	Thinning	Bald areas	Mostly bald	
Plantar surface	Heel-toe 40-50 mm: −1 <40 mm: −2	>50 mm, no crease	Faint red marks	Anterior transverse crease only	Creases anterior $^2/_3$	Creases over entire sole	
Breast	Imperceptible	Barely perceptible	Flat areola, no bud	Stippled areola, 1–2 mm bud	Raised areola, 3–4 mm bud	Full areola, 5–10 mm bud	
Eye/ear	Lids fused loosely: −1 lightly: −2	Lids open; pinna flat; stays folded	Slightly curved pinna; soft; slow recoil	Well-curved pinna; soft but ready recoil	Formed and firm, instant recoil	Thick cartilage, ear stiff	
Genitals (male)	Scrotum flat, smooth	Scrotum empty, faint rugae	Testes in upper canal, rare rugae	Testes descending, few rugae	Testes down, good rugae	Testes pendulous, deep rugae	
Genitals (female)	Clitoris prominent, labia flat	Clitoris prominent, small labia minora	Clitoris prominent, enlarging minora	Majora and minora equally prominent	Majora large, minora small	Majora cover clitoris and minora	

Maturity Rating

Score	Weeks
−10	20
−5	22
0	24
5	26
10	28
15	30
20	32
25	34
30	36
35	38
40	40
45	42
50	44

FIGURE 6-1   Ballard score for gestational age. (From Ballard JL, Khoury JC, Wedig K, et al: New Ballard score, expanded to include extremely premature infants. J Pediatr 1991;119:417–423.)

asymmetric. Symmetric IUGR denotes normal body proportions (small head and small body) and is considered a more severe form of IUGR.[4] Asymmetric IUGR denotes small abdominal circumference, decreased subcutaneous and abdominal fat, reduced skeletal muscle mass, and head circumference in the normal range. Infants with asymmetric IUGR show catch-up growth more frequently than do infants with symmetric IUGR, although 10% to 30% of all infants with IUGR remain short as children and adults. Premature infants are expected to have catch-up growth by 2 years of age. Those born after 29 weeks of gestation usually exhibit catch-up growth, whereas those born before 29 weeks of gestation are more likely to have a decreased rate of length and weight gain, which may be noted in the first week after birth and last up to 2 years.[5–7]

Predicting Neonatal Mortality

Various factors contribute to the mortality of neonates. The most common factors are listed in Table 6-1. Although neonatal mortality decreased markedly as a result of improvements in care, it appears to have reached a plateau[8] at which small improvements in neonatal care may be offset by other secular trends such as increases in premature birth. Birth weight and gestational age are strong indicators of mortality, but ethnicity is also a factor (Fig. 6-4).[9] The survival of neonates of 500 g and 22 weeks' gestational age approaches 0%. With increasing gestational age, survival rates increase to approximately 15% at 23 weeks, 56% at 24 weeks, and 79% at 25 weeks of gestation. Scoring systems to predict mortality would be particularly useful in neonatal surgery to plan treatment, to counsel parents, and to compare outcomes between different centers.

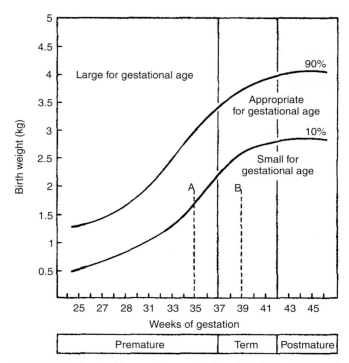

FIGURE 6-2 Level of intrauterine growth based on birth weight and gestational age of live-born, single white infants. (From Disturbances in newborns and infants. In Beers MF, Berkow R [eds]: The Merck Manual of Diagnosis and Therapy, 17th ed. White House Station, NJ, Merck Research Laboratories, 1999, pp 2127–2145.)

TABLE 6-1	
Major Causes of Mortality in Neonates Undergoing Surgery	
Preterm Neonates	*Term Neonates*
Necrotizing enterocolitis	Congenital anomalies
Congenital anomalies	Infection
Severe immaturity	Persistent pulmonary hypertension
Respiratory distress syndrome	Meconium aspiration
Intraventricular hemorrhage	Birth asphyxia, trauma
Infection	
Bronchopulmonary dysplasia	

or clinical parameters such as gestational age, birth weight, anomalies, acidosis, and fraction of inspired oxygen (FIO_2) (Clinical Risk Index for Babies [CRIB]).[10,11] CRIB includes 6 parameters collected in the first 12 hours after birth, and SNAP has 26 variables collected during the first 24 hours, and there have been various modifications to these scoring systems (e.g., CRIB-II, SNAP-II).[12] The authors have recently used[13] a modified organ failure score (Table 6-2) based on the Sepsis-related Organ Failure Assessment (SOFA) in use in adults and children to monitor the clinical status of neonates with acute abdominal emergencies who require surgery. Combining the surgeon's judgment and an objective score may produce an accurate assessment of the clinical progress of critically ill neonates and estimate their risk of mortality.

Fluid and Electrolyte Balance

BODY WATER COMPOSITION

The content and distribution of intracellular and extracellular water in the human body is defined as total body water (TBW) and it changes with age. TBW also varies with body fat content. Fat cells contain very little water; therefore children with more body fat have a lower proportion of body water than

However these scoring systems have not been developed and validated in neonatal surgery. Generic scoring systems for neonates are available but these do not take into consideration the anatomic abnormality requiring surgery. They are based on physiologic abnormalities such as hypotension-hypertension, acidosis, hypoxia, hypercapnia, anemia, and neutropenia (Score for Neonatal Acute Physiology [SNAP])

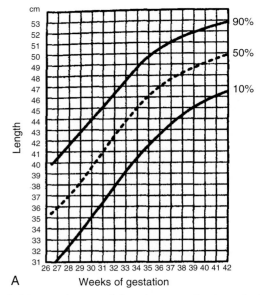

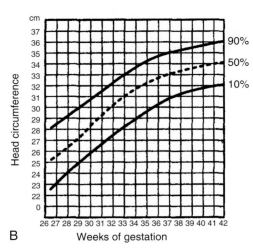

FIGURE 6-3 Level of intrauterine growth based on gestational age, body length (**A**), and head circumference (**B**) at birth. (From Disturbances in newborns and infants. In Beers MF, Berkow R [eds]: The Merck Manual of Diagnosis and Therapy, 17th ed. White House Station, NJ, Merck Research Laboratories, 1999, pp 2127–2145.)

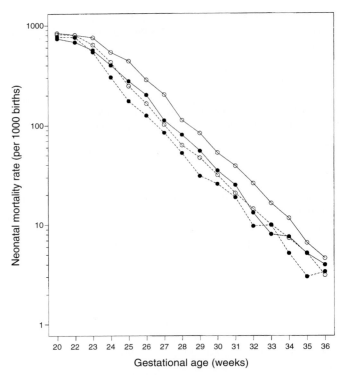

FIGURE 6-4 Neonatal mortality, by gestational age, for black (•) and white (○) infants in the United States. Solid lines denote data for 1989; dashed lines are for 1997. Data shown are for less than 37 weeks' gestation only. (From Demissie K, Rhoads GG, Ananth CV, et al: Trends in preterm birth and neonatal mortality among blacks and whites in the United States from 1989 to 1997. Am J Epidemiol 2001;154:307-315.)

fat, 90% of body mass is TBW, with 65% of body mass made up of extracellular fluid.[14] However these ratios alter throughout gestation as the amount of body protein and fat increases. TBW as a proportion of body mass declines and is approximately 70% to 80% by term.[15] TBW continues to decline during the first year of life reaching 60% of total body mass, which is consistent with adult age. This is accompanied by a decrease in the extracellular compartment fluid (ECF)/intracellular compartment fluid (ICF) ratio. The ECF is 60% of total body mass at 20 weeks' gestation, declining to 40% at term, whereas ICF increases from 25% at 20 weeks' gestation to 35% of body mass at term and then to 43% at 2 months of age. Because extracellular fluid is more easily lost from the body than intracellular fluid and infants have a larger surface area/body mass ratio, they are more at risk of dehydration than are older children and adults.

Among preterm infants, those who are SGA have a significantly higher body water content (approximately 90%) than appropriate for full-term infants (approximately 80%).[16] Blood volume can be estimated as 106 mL/kg in preterm infants, 90 mL/kg in neonates, 80 mL/kg in infants and children and about 65 mL/kg in adults.[17,18] Adequate systemic perfusion depends on adequate intravascular volume, as well as many other factors. However infants and children can compensate for relatively large losses in circulating volume, and signs and symptoms of shock may be difficult to detect if a child has lost less than 25% of the circulating volume. The movement of fluid between the vascular space and the tissues depends on osmotic pressure, oncotic pressure, hydrostatic pressure, and changes in capillary permeability. Understanding these factors is important when trying to anticipate changes in the child's intravascular volume.[19]

NEONATAL FLUID BALANCE

Before labor, pulmonary fluid production decreases while existing fluid is reabsorbed, and efflux through the trachea increases and accelerates during labor, thereby drying out the lungs. During labor, arterial pressure increases and causes shifts in plasma from the vascular compartment and a slight rise in hematocrit values. Placental transfusion can occur if

children with less fat. The water in body tissues includes the intracellular fluid, which represents the water contained within the cells, and extracellular fluid. Extracellular fluid is further subdivided into intravascular fluid (plasma), interstitial fluid (fluid surrounding tissue cells), and transcellular fluid (e.g., cerebrospinal, synovial, pleural, peritoneal fluid). During the first trimester, when only 1% of body mass is

TABLE 6-2

Modified Organ Failure Score*

To calculate the aggregate score, the worst value of each parameter in each time interval will be recorded. MAP = Mean Arterial Pressure

	Score				
Organ System	*0*	*1*	*2*	*3*	*4*
Respiratory Pao₂/Fio₂	>400	≤400	≤300	≤200 with respiratory support	≤100 with respiratory support
Renal (urine output)			<1 mL/kg /hr for 6 hours	<0.5 mL/kg /hr for 6 hours	Anuria
Hepatic (serum bilirubin in μmol/L and [in mg/dL])		20-32 [1.17-1.9]	33-101 [2.0-5.9]	102-204 [6.0-12.0]	>204 [> 12.0]
Cardiovascular (hypotension)	No hypotension	MAP < gestational age + age (weeks) mmHg	Dopamine ≤5 or dobutamine any dose	Dopamine >5 or epinephrine ≤0.1 or norepinephrine ≤0.1	Dopamine >15 or epinephrine >0.1 or norepinephrine >0.1
Coagulation (platelet count)	>150	≤150	≤100	≤50	≤20 or platelet transfusion

*P < .05 vs. preoperative sample.
From Hall NJ, Eaton S, Peters MJ, et al: Mild controlled hypothermia in preterm neonates with advanced necrotizing enterocolitis. Pediatrics 2010;125:e300-e308.

there is delayed clamping of the cord and the neonate is placed at or below the level of the placenta, resulting in up to 50% increase in red blood cells and blood volume. This polycythemia may have severe consequences such as neurologic impairment, thrombus formation, and tissue ischemia.[20] One day postpartum the neonate is oliguric. Over the following 1 to 2 days, dramatic shifts in fluid from the intracellular to extracellular compartment result in a diuresis and natriuresis that contributes to weight loss during the first days of life. This is approximately 5% to 10% in the term neonate and 10% to 20% in the premature newborn. The proportion of contributions from ECF and ICF to fluid loss is controversial and the mechanism is yet to be determined. This diuresis occurs regardless of fluid intake or insensible losses and may be related to a postnatal surge in atrial natriuretic peptide.[21] Limitations in the methodology of measuring ECF and ICF have limited our understanding of the processes. It has been demonstrated however that large increases in water and calorie intake are required to reduce the weight loss. Higher caloric intake alone reduces weight loss but the ECF still decreases. Subsequent weight gain appears to be the result of increases in tissue mass and ICF per kilogram of body weight but not ECF per kilogram of body weight. By the fifth day postpartum, urinary excretion begins to reflect the fluid status of the infant.

RENAL FUNCTION

The kidneys in neonates have small immature glomeruli and for this reason the glomerular filtration rate (GFR) is reduced (about 30 mL/min/1.73m^2 at birth to 100 mL/min/1.73m^2 at 9 months). Eventually renovascular resistance decreases, resulting in a rapid rise in GFR over the first 3 months of life followed by a slower rise to adult levels by 12 to 24 months of age. Premature and low-birth-weight infants may have a lower GFR than term infants, and the initial rapid rise in GFR is absent.

Urine osmolality is controlled by two mechanisms. Urine is concentrated in the loop of Henle using a countercurrent system dependent on the osmolality of the medullary interstitium. In neonates, the low osmolality in the renal medulla means the countercurrent system is less effective and urine concentration capacity is between 50 and 700 mOsm/kg compared with 1200 mOsm/kg in the adult kidney; therefore there is less tolerance for fluid imbalance.

COMMON FLUID AND ELECTROLYTE DISTURBANCES AND THEIR TREATMENT

Sodium

Serum sodium is the major determinant of serum osmolality and therefore extracellular fluid volume. Urinary sodium excretion is dependent on the GFR and therefore is low in neonates when compared with adults. Normal neonatal serum sodium levels are 135 to 140 mmol/L, controlled by moderating renal excretion. During the period of oliguria on the first day of life, sodium supplementation is not normally required. The normal maintenance sodium requirement after normal diuresis is 2 to 4 mmol/kg/day.

Hyponatremia Hyponatremia is defined when serum sodium concentrations are less than 135 mmol/L. Treatment depends on the fluid status of the patient and in case of hypovolemia or hypervolemia, fluid status should be corrected first. When normovolemic, serum sodium levels should be gradually corrected with NaCl infusion, but at a rate not exceeding 0.8 mEq/kg/hr. Symptoms are not reliable for clinical management because they are not often apparent until serum sodium levels fall to less than 120 mmol/L, and their severity is directly related to the rapidity of onset and magnitude of hyponatremia. If not promptly recognized, hyponatremia may manifest as the effects of cerebral edema: apathy, nausea, vomiting, headache, fits, and coma. Urine sodium concentrations can be useful to help determine the underlying cause of hyponatremia because the kidneys respond to a fall in serum sodium levels by excreting more dilute urine, but the secretion of antidiuretic hormone (ADH)/vasopressin in response to hypovolemia affects this. Urine sodium concentrations less than 10 mmol/L indicates an appropriate renal response to euvolemic hyponatremia. However if the urinary sodium concentration is greater than 20 mmol/L this can indicate either sodium leakage from damaged renal tubules or hypervolemia.

Hypernatremia Hypernatremia (serum sodium concentrations >145 mmol/L) may be due to hemoconcentration/excessive fluid losses (e.g., diarrhea). Symptoms and clinical signs include dry mucous membranes, loss of skin turgidity, drowsiness, irritability, hypertonicity, fits, and coma. Treatment is again by correction of fluid status with appropriate electrolyte-containing solutions. Other causes of hypernatremia are renal or respiratory insufficiency, or it can be related to drug administration.

Potassium

In the 24 to 72 hours postpartum, a large shift of potassium from intracellular to extracellular compartments occurs, resulting in a rise in plasma potassium levels. This is followed by an increase of potassium excretion until the normal serum concentration of 3.5 to 5.8 mmol/L is achieved. Therefore supplementation is not required on the first day of life, but after neonatal diuresis a maintenance intake of 1 to 3 mmol/kg/day is required.

Hypokalemia Hypokalemia is commonly iatrogenic, either due to inadequate potassium intake or use of diuretics but can also be caused by vomiting, diarrhea, alkalosis (which drives potassium intracellularly) or polyuric renal failure. As a consequence, the normal ion gradient is disrupted and predisposes to muscle current conduction abnormalities (e.g., cardiac arrhythmias, paralytic ileus, urinary retention, and respiratory muscle paralysis). Treatment employs the use of KCl.

Hyperkalemia Hyperkalemia can be iatrogenic or due to renal problems but can also be caused by cell lysis syndrome (e.g., from trauma), adrenal insufficiency, insulin-dependent diabetes mellitus, or severe hemolysis or malignant hyperthermia. As in hypokalemia, hyperkalemia alters the electrical gradient of cell membranes and patients are vulnerable to cardiac arrhythmias, including asystole. Treatment is with insulin (plus glucose to avoid hypoglycemia) or with salbutamol.

Calcium

Calcium plays important roles in enzyme activity, muscle contraction and relaxation, the blood coagulation cascade, bone metabolism, and nerve conduction. Calcium is maintained at a total serum concentration of 1.8 to 2.1 mmol/L in neonates and 2 to 2.5 mmol/L in term infants and is divided into three fractions. Thirty percent to 50% is protein bound and 5% to 15% is complexed with citrate, lactate, bicarbonate, and inorganic ions. The remaining free calcium ions are metabolically active and concentrations fluctuate with serum albumin levels. Hydrogen ions compete reversibly with calcium for albumin-binding sites and therefore free calcium concentrations increase in acidosis. Calcium metabolism is under the control of many hormones but primarily 1,25-dihydroxycholecalciferol (gastrointestinal absorption of calcium, bone resorption, increased renal calcium reabsorption), parathyroid hormone (bone resorption, decreased urinary excretion), and calcitonin (bone formation and increased urinary excretion). Calcium is actively transported from maternal to fetal circulation against the concentration gradient, resulting in peripartum hypercalcemia. There is a transient fall in calcium postpartum to 1.8 to 2.1 mmol/L and a gradual rise to normal infant levels over 24 to 48 hours.

Hypocalcemia   In addition to the physiologic hypocalcemia of neonates which is usually asymptomatic, other causes of hypocalcemia are hypoparathyroidism, including DiGeorge syndrome, and parathyroid hormone insensitivity in infants of diabetic mothers, which may also be related to hypomagnesemia. Clinical manifestations are tremor, seizures, and a prolonged QT interval on electrocardiography.

Hypercalcemia   This is less common than hypocalcemia but can result from inborn errors of metabolism such as familial hypercalcemic hypocalcuria or primary hyperparathyroidism. Iatrogenic causes are vitamin A overdose or deficient dietary phosphate intake. Less common causes in children are tertiary hyperparathyroidism, paraneoplastic syndromes, and metastatic bone disease.

Magnesium

As an important enzyme cofactor, magnesium affects adenosine triphosphate (ATP) metabolism and glycolysis. Only 20% of total body magnesium is exchangeable with the biologically active free ion form. The remainder is bound in bone or to intracellular protein, RNA, or ATP, mostly in muscle and liver. Gastrointestinal absorption of magnesium is controlled by vitamin D, parathyroid hormone, and sodium reabsorption. As previously stated, hypomagnesemia is often related to hypocalcemia and should be considered.

Acid-Base Balance

Acidosis (pH <7.35) and alkalosis (pH >7.45) can be generated by respiratory or metabolic causes. When the cause is respiratory—Pa_{CO_2} >45 mm Hg (acidosis) or <35 mm Hg (alkalosis)—treatment is with appropriate respiratory support. In case of metabolic causes—bicarbonate <21 mmol/L (acidosis) or >26 mmol/L (alkalosis)—it is useful to check the anion gap [$Na^+ - (Cl^- + HCO_3^-)$, which is normally 12 ± 2 mEq/L] to understand the underlying cause. Treatment should be directed toward any underlying cause, for example, metabolic acidosis caused by dehydration or sepsis. The slow infusion of buffers such as sodium bicarbonate or tris-hydroxymethylaminomethane (THAM, a sodium-free buffer) should be used as

therapeutic adjuncts. The amount of sodium bicarbonate required can be calculated using the following equation:

$$NaHCO_3 \text{ (mmol)} = \text{base excess} \times \text{body weight (kg)}$$

Acid-base balance is maintained by a complex system achieved by intracellular and extracellular buffer systems, respiration, and renal function. Intracellular systems consist of conjugate acid-base pairs in equilibrium as shown by the following equation (A = acid, H = proton):

$$HA \leftrightarrow H^+ A^-$$

The pH can be derived from the Henderson-Hasselbalch equation:

$$pH = \frac{pK + \log[A^-]}{[HA]}$$

where pK is the dissociation constant of the weak acid, [A^-] is the concentration of the dissociated acid, and [HA] is the concentration of the acid. The most important of these systems is the carbonic anhydrase system:

$$CO_2 + H_2O \leftrightarrow H^+ + HCO_3^-$$

Extracellular buffer systems are similar but the proton is loosely associated with proteins, hemoglobin, or phosphates and take several hours to equilibrate.

Respiratory compensation occurs through the carbonic anhydrase system, ridding the body of carbon dioxide and thereby shifting equilibrium to the left of the reaction and reducing the number of protons. The extent of the shift is influenced by the active transport of bicarbonate across the blood-brain barrier, thereby triggering central respiratory drive.

Normal extracellular pH is maintained at 7.35 to 7.45. Normal metabolic processes produce carbonic acid, lactic acid, ketoacids, phosphoric acid, and sulfuric acid, all of which are either excreted or controlled by a number of buffer systems.

In the neonate, loss of the contribution of the fetomaternal circulation and maternal respiratory and renal compensation mechanisms force adaptation and maturation. There is a suggestion that increased sensitivity of the respiratory centers to fluctuations in pH changes allow the neonate to control acid-base balance more. Increases in the intracellular protein mass allow greater intracellular buffering. The extracellular buffer systems are already functional.

Respiratory compensation becomes active as respiration is established. It relies on pulmonary function and lung maturity, and therefore neonates with lung disease may have impaired respiratory compensation. Carbon dioxide passes freely across the blood-brain barrier, allowing almost immediate response to respiratory acidosis from respiratory drive centers. The response to metabolic acidosis is delayed because interstitial bicarbonate requires a few hours to equilibrate with the cerebral bicarbonate.

Renal compensation is the most important mechanism available to the neonate for acid-base balance. Adjustments in urine acidity have been seen as soon as a few hours postpartum but it takes 2 to 3 days for it to fully mature. Consequent to the changes in renal function and perfusion described previously, the ability of the neonate to handle acid-base balance is limited in the first few days of life. Proximal tubules are responsible for the reabsorption of 85% to 90% of filtered bicarbonate but function less efficiently in the premature neonate. Reabsorption can also be affected by some drugs used in neonates. Dopamine inhibits sodium/proton pump activity in the proximal tubules and therefore decreases the amount of bicarbonate that is reabsorbed. The remaining bicarbonate reabsorption takes place in the distal tubules, but they differ from the proximal tubules in their absence of carbonic anhydrase. Aldosterone is the most important hormone affecting distal tubular function and stimulates proton excretion in the distal tubules. However the distal nephrons of the premature infant are developmentally insensitive to aldosterone. Protons are excreted in the urine as phosphate, sulfate, and ammonium salts. This increases with age and gestation. However the introduction of phosphate-containing drugs increases phosphate delivery to the distal tubules and therefore can increase the capacity to excrete H^+. Dopamine decreases the reabsorption of protons in the distal tubules thereby increasing proton excretion.

Intravenous Fluid Administration

Fluid Maintenance Fluid administration varies with age as a consequence of the variation of TBW composition and the different compensatory mechanisms. Newborns can have a very wide range of maintenance requirements, depending on clinical conditions. In addition, especially in preterm infants, fluid administration should also allow for physiologic weight loss over the first 7 to 10 days of life (up to a maximum of 10% of birth weight), always maintaining a urine output of greater than or equal to 0.5 mL/kg/hr (Table 6-3).

Not only the amount of fluids but also the type of fluid administered varies according to age. In newborns, 10%

dextrose solution is recommended. Sodium supplementation is not usually required in the first 24 hours (low urine output), and after that time can be given at 2 to 4 mmol/kg/day (adjusted primarily based on serum sodium values and changes in weight). Potassium (1 to 3 mmol/kg/day) and calcium (1 mmol/kg/day) are usually added after the first 2 days of life. In infancy and childhood various intravenous solutions are used (Table 6-4); probably the most common is 5% dextrose with one-half normal saline. Potassium is not usually necessary, except if intravenous fluid is given for a longer time. Fluids can be administered intravenously with peripherally or centrally placed catheters. In newborns, or in other situations in which dextrose is administered at more than 10%, peripheral administration is not recommended because of complications due to hyperosmolar solutions.

Energy Metabolism

Energy provides the ability to do work and is essential to all life processes. The unit of energy is the calorie or joule (J). One calorie = 4.184 J. One calorie equals the energy required to raise 1 g of water from 15° to 16° centigrade. The most widely used medical unit of energy is the kilocalorie (kcal), which is equal to 1000 calories. One joule equals the energy required to move 1 kilocalorie the distance of 1 meter with 1 newton of force. The first law of thermodynamics states that energy cannot be created or destroyed. Thus:

$$Energy\ in = Energy\ out + Energy\ stored$$

In the case of a neonate this can be expressed as:[22]

$$\begin{aligned} Energy\ intake = {}& Energy\ losses\ in\ excreta + Energy\ stored \\ & + Energy\ of\ tissue\ synthesis \\ & + Energy\ expended\ on\ activity \\ & + Basal\ metabolic\ rate \end{aligned}$$

ENERGY INTAKE

The principal foodstuffs are carbohydrates, fats, and proteins (see later). The potential energy that can be derived from these foods is energy that is released when the food is completely absorbed and oxidized. The metabolizable energy is somewhat less than the energy intake, since energy is lost in the feces in the form of indigestible elements and in the urine in the form of incompletely metabolized compounds such as urea from amino acids or ketone bodies from fats.

TABLE 6-3

Normal Maintenance Fluid Requirements

Premature infant	1st day of life	60-150 mL/kg/day
	2nd day of life	70-150 mL/kg/day
	3rd day of life	90-180 mL/kg/day
	>3rd day of life	Up to 200 mL/kg/day
Term infant	1st day of life	60-80 mL/kg/day
	2nd day of life	80-100 mL/kg/day
	3rd day of life	100-140 mL/kg/day
	>3rd day of life	Up to 160 mL/kg/day
Child > 4 weeks of age, up to 10 kg		100 mL/kg/day
Child from 10-20 kg		1000 mL + 50 mL/kg/day for each kg over 10
Child >20 kg		1500 mL + 20 mL/kg/day for each kg over 20

TABLE 6-4

Common Intravenous Fluids

Intravenous fluid	Glucose (g/100 mL)	Na$^+$ (mEq/L)	K$^+$ (mEq/L)	Cl$^-$ (mEq/L)	Osmolality (mOsm/L)
5% dextrose	5	—	—	—	252/277
10% dextrose	10	—	—	—	505/556
Normal saline (0.9% NaCl)	—	154	—	154	308
½ Normal saline (0.45% NaCl)	—	77	—	77	154
5% dextrose with ½ normal saline	5	77	—	77	406
5% dextrose with ¼ normal saline	5	34	—	34	329
Lactated Ringer solution	0	130	4	109	273
Hartmann's solution	0	131	5	111	278

Thus metabolizable energy can be calculated as the following equation:

Metabolizable energy = Energy intake −

Energy losses in urine and stool

The foodstuffs are metabolized through a variety of complex metabolic pathways. Complete metabolism of a food requires that it be oxidized to carbon dioxide, water, and in the case of proteins urea and ammonia. This metabolism takes place according to predictable stoichiometric equations.[23] The energy liberated by oxidation is not used directly but is used to create high-energy intermediates, from which the energy can be released where and when it is required. The main intermediates are ATP (all cell types) and creatine phosphate (muscle and brain) but there are others.

These intermediates store the energy in the form of a high-energy phosphate bond. The energy is released when the bond is hydrolyzed. Formation of these high-energy intermediates may result directly from a step in a metabolic pathway. More often however they are created indirectly as the result of oxidative phosphorylation in mitochondria, the process by which a compound is oxidized by the sequential removal of hydrogen ions, which are then transferred through a variety of flavoproteins and cytochromes until they are combined with oxygen to produce water. This process releases large amounts of energy, which is used to form the high-energy phosphate bonds in the intermediates. Thus the energy in food is used to produce high-energy intermediates, the form of energy that is used for all processes of life. This process is the main oxygen-consuming process in the body, and the continual requirement for ATP for all energy requiring processes explains why oxygen delivery to the mitochondria of every cell is crucial for survival of these cells and ultimately the body as a whole.

Respiratory quotient is calculated as carbon dioxide production divided by oxygen consumption and varies with the substrate that is being oxidized. It has a numeric value of 1.0 for glucose oxidation and 0.70 to 0.72 for fat oxidation, depending on the chain length of fat oxidized. Thus the respiratory quotient, measured by indirect calorimetry, reflects the balance of substrate use. This situation is complicated however by partial oxidation of, for example, fats to ketone bodies or carbohydrate conversion to lipids, which will give a respiratory quotient greater than 1. Tables of precise respiratory quotient values for individual carbohydrates, fats, and amino acids are available.[23]

Birth represents a transition from the fetal state, in which carbohydrate is the principal energy substrate (approximately 80% of energy expended) to the infant state, in which both carbohydrate and fat are used to provide energy.[24] This transition is evidenced by the change in respiratory quotient, which declines from 0.97 at birth to 0.8 by 3 hours of age,[25,26] such that fat provides around 60% to 70% of energy expenditure. This is probably due to the fact that newborns have some initial difficulty in obtaining enough exogenous energy to meet their energy needs and are thus more dependent on their endogenous energy stores. Thereafter the respiratory quotient has been shown to increase slightly during the first week of life,[26–28] which suggests that newborns may preferentially metabolize fat in the first instance. Low-birth-weight infants have a respiratory quotient higher than 0.9 because of their limited fat stores and dependence on exogenous glucose.[29]

ENERGY STORAGE

Although glucose is an essential source of energy, the circulation only contains approximately 200 mg glucose at birth in a term infant, which is only enough to support whole-body requirements for 15 minutes. The body does not store glucose directly because of osmotic problems, but glucose can be indirectly stored in the liver, kidneys, and muscles (and to a lesser degree in other cells) as glycogen. Muscle glycogen can only be used in situ, but liver and kidney glycogen can be used to produce glucose for metabolism in other sites. Glycogen stores in a term infant approximate 35 g (~140 kcal), enough to sustain energy requirements for between 12 and 24 hours. Energy is stored mainly as fat, which has two advantages. First, there is more energy stored per gram of fat (9 kcal/g) than glycogen (4 kcal/g). Second, although fat is stored as globules in adipose tissue and requires little hydration (~15% of its own mass in water), glycogen is stored as a hydrated polymer and so requires four times its own mass in water. Taking both these factors into consideration, 9.4 times as much glycogen mass (with its associated water) would need to be stored as the equivalent caloric amount of fat. A term infant has about 460 g of fat, which is capable of yielding 4140 kcal of energy on oxidation, enough energy for a 21-day fast. Protein largely performs functions other than energy storage, although some of the 525 g of protein (~60% intracellular; ~40% extracellular) in a term infant can be used as a source of energy during severe fasting, yielding 4 kcal/g. The serious consequences of oxidizing protein include wasting, reduced wound healing, edema, failure of growth/neurologic development, and reduced resistance to infection. The relative amounts of fat and carbohydrate stored as a proportion of body mass alter in the last trimester of gestation as the relative hydration decreases, so preterm infants have much lower caloric reserves than do term infants (Fig. 6-5).

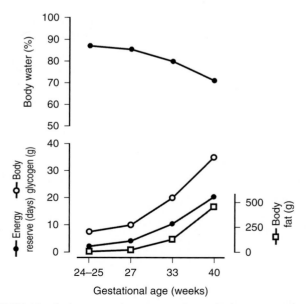

FIGURE 6-5 Body water and energy stores according to gestational age.

ENERGY OF GROWTH AND TISSUE SYNTHESIS

In stable mature adults little energy is needed for growth. However in neonates the energy requirements for growth are considerable. In infants up to 50% of the energy intake can be used for growth.[22,30] The energy required to lay down tissue stores includes two components: (1) the energy stored within the tissue itself (i.e., 9 kcal/g of fat, 4 kcal/g of carbohydrate or protein) and (2) the energy investment needed to convert the food into storable and usable substrates. Studies have shown this additional investment to be on the order of 5% to 30% of the energy value of the tissue.[31] The rate of growth of premature infants is on the order of 17 to 19 g/kg/day,[32] whereas that of full-term infants is 4 to 8 g/kg/day.[33] In addition, in rapidly growing premature infants more of the weight gain is as protein. Although protein has a lower energy value per unit weight than does fat, it requires a greater energy investment. Thus the energy cost of growth is much greater in the premature infant largely due to the rate of protein accretion.[34–37] In rapidly growing premature infants, this metabolic cost of growth has been estimated to be 1.2 kcal/g of weight gained, which represents about 30% of total energy expenditure.[34,37]

ENERGY LOSSES

Infants lose energy in the excreta. Because of the immaturity of the gut and kidney and potentially inadequate supply of bile acids, stool and urine losses may be proportionally higher than in adults. This is especially true for infants undergoing surgery or those with gastroenterologic problems. Conversely parenterally fed infants have low or absent energy losses in stools, although there may be urinary losses.

ENERGY USED IN ACTIVITY

Studies have shown that energy expenditure varies considerably with changes in the activity of the infant. Vigorous activity such as crying may double energy expenditure,[36] but because most of the time is spent sleeping,[36] the energy expended on activity is less than 5% of the total daily energy expenditure.[22] Studies have shown that daily energy expenditure is related to both the duration and level of activity.[27,35]

BASAL METABOLIC RATE AND RESTING ENERGY EXPENDITURE

Basic metabolic rate represents the amount of energy used by the body for homeostasis: maintaining ion gradients, neurologic activity, cell maintenance, synthesis of extracellular proteins such as albumin, and so on. Because of ethical considerations, it is not possible to completely starve a newborn for the 14 hours required for a measurement of basal metabolic rate. As a result resting energy expenditure (REE) is much more commonly used as the basis of metabolic studies. REE is influenced by a number of factors, including age, body composition, size of vital organs, and energy intake.

Age

The REE of a full-term, appropriate-for-gestational-age infant increases from 33 kcal/kg/day at birth, to 48 kcal/kg/day by the end of the first week of life.[38,39] It then remains constant for 1 month before declining. REE is higher in premature and SGA infants than in full-term and appropriate-for-gestational age infants.[40] The differences discussed probably reflect changes in body composition,[38] although it has been suggested that the increase in basal metabolism during the first week of life may represent increased enzyme activity in functioning organs.[41]

Body Composition

During the first weeks of life infants lose body water. This is accompanied by a well-recognized loss of body weight.[25] Immediately before birth, a term infant is approximately 75% water, but by 1 month of age the water content has reduced to 45%.[42,43] Thus the increase in REE observed during the first weeks of life may reflect the relative increase in body tissue and the relative decrease in body water. These differences in body composition also result in an alteration in the ratio of basal metabolic rate/nonprotein energy reserve (Fig. 6-6).

Size of Vital Organs

The brain, liver, heart, and kidneys account for up to 66% of basal metabolic rate in adults yet make up only 7% of total body weight. In infants these organs, particularly the brain, account for a greater proportion of body weight. It is believed that the brain alone may account for 60% to 65% of basal metabolic rate during the first month of life. In premature and SGA infants, the vital organs are less affected by intrauterine and extrauterine malnutrition than are other organs.[38,40] Thus their contribution to basal metabolism is even greater.[32] The brain alone may account for up to 70% of basal metabolism.[44] Premature and SGA infants also tend to have a greater proportion of metabolically active brown adipose tissue than relatively inactive white adipose tissue.[36] By contrast full-term appropriate-for-gestational age infants may have only 40 g of brown adipose tissue yet have 520 g of white adipose tissue.[38]

Dietary Intake

REE of infants is related to caloric intake and weight gain. A significant linear correlation of increasing REE with increasing energy intake has been demonstrated.[30] REE increased by 8.5 kcal/kg/day after a meal, which was equivalent to 5.7% of the gross energy intake, which correlates well with the energy cost of growth.[30] Salomon and colleagues[45]

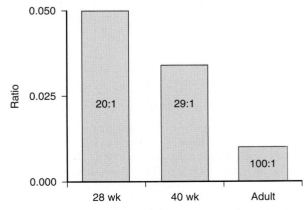

FIGURE 6-6   Ratio of basal metabolic rate/nonprotein energy reserve.

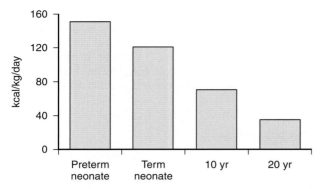

FIGURE 6-7   Energy requirements from the neonatal period to adulthood.

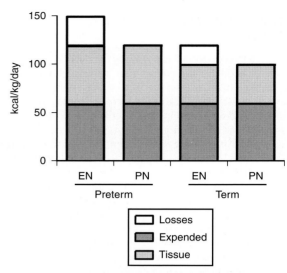

Losses
Expended
Tissue

FIGURE 6-8   Partition of energy metabolism in preterm and term infants receiving enteral nutrition (EN) or parenteral nutrition (PN). *Expended* includes basal metabolic rate, activity, the energy expended in laying down new tissue, and thermoregulation, *tissue* is the amount of energy actually stored in new tissue, *losses* include losses in stool and so on. Data from references 22, 36, 48, 49 and 52.

measured the diet-induced thermogenesis of each dietary constituent in infants. They found that amino acids increased REE by 11% (4.4% of caloric intake), fat increased REE by 8% (3% of caloric intake), and glucose did not increase REE at all. This study is somewhat at odds with the results of other studies that have shown that REE increases considerably after a glucose load, particularly at high doses.[46,47]

The energy metabolism of neonates is different from that of adults and children and this reflects the special physiologic status of the neonate. Newborns have a significantly higher metabolic rate and energy requirement per unit body weight than do children and adults: the total energy requirement for an extremely low-birth-weight (i.e., <1000 g) preterm infant fed enterally is 130 to 150 kcal/kg/day[48] and that of a term infant is 100 to 120 kcal/kg/day compared to 60 to 80 kcal/kg/day for a 10-year old child and 30 to 40 kcal/kg/day for a 20-year old individual (Fig. 6-7).[49–51] The partition of this energy is also different from that of adults. Of the 100 to 120 kcal/kg/day required by the term infant, approximately 40 to 70 kcal/kg/day is needed for maintenance metabolism, 50 to 70 kcal/kg/day for growth (tissue synthesis and energy stored), and up to 20 kcal/kg/day to cover energy losses in excreta.[22,35,36] Newborns receiving total parenteral nutrition require fewer calories (110 to 120 kcal/kg/day for a preterm infant and 90 to 100 kcal/kg/day for a term infant[52]) because of the absence of energy losses in excreta and the fact that energy is not required for thermoregulation when the infant is in an incubator. These data are summarized in Fig. 6-8.

Several equations have been published to predict energy expenditure in adults.[53] In stable neonates undergoing surgery, REE can be predicted from parameters such as weight, heart rate, and age using the following equation:[54]

Resting energy expenditure (cal/min)
$$= -74.436 + (34.661 \times \text{body weight in kilograms})$$
$$+ (0.496 \times \text{heart rate in beats/minute})$$
$$+ (0.178 \times \text{age in days})$$

$$(r = 0.92; F = 230.07; \text{significance } F < 0.00001).$$

The major predictor of REE in the preceding equation is body weight, which is also the strongest individual predictor of REE and represents the total mass of living tissue. The other predictors are heart rate, which provides an indirect measure of the hemodynamic and metabolic status of the infant, and postnatal age, which has been shown to influence REE in the first few weeks of life.

Thermoregulation

After delivery the relatively low ambient temperature and evaporation of the residual amniotic fluid from the skin further increase the heat loss from the newborn. Neonates are homeotherms. They are far more susceptible to changes in environmental temperature than are adults[28] because they have a small mass and relatively large surface area, they possess relatively little insulating tissue such as fat and hair, they are unable to make significant behavioral alterations such as increasing the central heating or putting on extra clothing, and they have limited energy reserves. The thermoneutral zone is of critical importance to infants[38] and is higher (32 to 34° centigrade for full-term appropriate-for-gestational age infants) than it is for adults.[55] There are a number of published tables giving the optimum environmental temperature for infants of different weights and ages.[55] Numerous studies have shown that the morbidity and mortality of infants nursed outside the thermoneutral zone, is significantly increased. There are however indications such as hypoxic ischemic encephalopathy in which therapeutic moderate hypothermia is used,[56] and the difference between iatrogenic hypothermia (potentially with rapid uncontrolled rewarming) and therapeutic controlled hypothermia (with slow controlled rewarming) should be emphasized.

RESPONSE TO COLD

Heat is lost through radiation/conduction/convection (70%), evaporation (25%), raising the temperature of feedings (3%), and with the excreta (2%).[38] The response of the infant to cooling depends on the maturation of hypothalamic regulatory centers and the availability of substrates for thermogenesis.[38] The initial response, which is mediated through the sympathetic nervous system, is to reduce heat losses by vasoconstriction[28] and to increase heat production by shivering and nonshivering thermogenesis. The most important site of nonshivering thermogenesis is the brown adipose tissue. This is well established by 22 weeks of gestation and makes up 90% of the total body fat by 29 weeks of gestation.[57] Other sites include the brain, liver, and kidneys. Studies have shown that the preferred fuels for nonshivering thermogenesis are free fatty acids.[58] The energy cost of thermoregulation in a cold environment is considerable. Even within the thermoneutral zone, thermoregulation can account for up to 8% of total energy expenditure.[59] The REE can double when full nonshivering thermogenesis is taking place.

Neonates undergoing major operations under general anesthesia frequently become hypothermic.[60,61] Compared with adults newborns experience greater difficulties in the maintenance of physiologic body temperature in the presence of a cold environmental challenge.[62] Hypothermia may increase the incidence of postoperative complications such as acidosis, impaired immune function, and delayed wound healing.[63] Newborns are not able to respond to cold exposure by shivering but have a highly specialized tissue, brown fat, capable of generating heat without the presence of shivering (nonshivering thermogenesis). As environmental temperature decreases, an increased blood flow to brown fat stores is observed and heat is produced in brown fat mitochondria. During an operation the neonate is exposed not only to a cool environment but also to a wide variety of anesthetic and paralytic agents that may have detrimental effects on heat production (energy expenditure) and core temperature.[64,65] Nonshivering thermogenesis is inhibited by anesthetic agents in experimental animals.[62,66] Albanese and associates[62] have shown that termination of general anesthesia during cold exposure causes a rapid and profound increase in nonshivering thermogenesis in rabbits. This may explain the sudden and rapid increase in energy expenditure observed in young infants at the end of an operation.[64,67]

It has long been known that brown adipose tissue is responsible for heat production, containing a protein (uncoupling protein 1) that dissipates the proton gradient formed across the mitochondrial inner membrane during substrate oxidation.[58] However it is only in recent years that a contribution of the proton leak to thermogenesis in liver has been postulated.[68] The magnitude of the proton leak may be a major determinant of metabolic rate.[69] Oxidative breakdown of nutrients releases energy, which is converted to usable chemical fuel (ATP) in the mitochondria of cells by oxidative phosphorylation. This is used to drive energy-consuming processes in the body. During oxidative phosphorylation, protons are pumped from the mitochondrial matrix to the intermembrane space. Proton pumping is directly proportional to the rate of oxygen consumption and generates and maintains a difference in electrochemical potential of protons across the inner membrane. Protons return to the matrix by one of two routes: the "phosphorylation pathway," which generates ATP, or by the "leak pathway," which is nonproductive and releases energy as heat. A significant proportion (20% to 30%) of oxygen consumed by resting hepatocytes in adult rats is used to drive the heat-producing proton leak.[70] This leak pathway in liver and other organs is a significant contributor to the reactions that compose the standard REE and therefore results in significant resting heat production.[71,72] The proton permeability of the inner mitochondrial membrane that is present in rat liver mitochondria is high in fetuses and is significantly reduced during early neonatal life and reaches the lowest maintained level in adults.[73] These authors suggest that this could provide a physiologic protective mechanism for thermal adaptation of newborn rats during the perinatal period before the establishment of brown adipose tissue thermogenesis.[73] It is conceivable that human newborns are "preprogrammed" with similar protective mechanisms that allow them to survive the stresses of birth (cold adaptation), surgery (cord division), and starvation (transient hypoglycemia).

Carbohydrate, Fat, and Protein Metabolism of the Neonate

The profound physiologic changes that take place in the perinatal period are reflected by equally dramatic changes in nutrition and metabolism. The fetus exists within a thermostable environment in which nutrition is continually supplied "intravenously" and waste products are equally efficiently removed. At birth, this continual nutrient supply ceases abruptly, resulting in a brief period of starvation. At the end of this period of starvation, nutrition also changes from the placental supply of glucose to milk, which is high in fat and low in carbohydrate. In addition the kidney and lung of the neonate have to become much more active metabolically and the neonate must maintain its own body temperature by activating both metabolic and physiologic mechanisms of thermogenesis and heat conservation, as described previously. The successful adaptation of the neonate to extrauterine life requires carefully regulated changes in glucose and fat metabolism, together with the use of stored protein reserves, until adequate nutritional supply of protein or amino acids, or both, is established. Toward the end of the neonatal period nutrition again changes as the infant is weaned onto a diet that is higher in carbohydrate and lower in fat than the milk diet of the neonatal period. Hence a healthy neonate is in a state of metabolic flux, and these changes must be carefully regulated in order to maintain growth and brain development in this "critical epoch." It is now known that nutrition and growth during the neonatal period are important later determinants of cardiovascular disease[74] and neurodevelopment.[75] Additional physiologic stresses caused by prematurity, infection, gastrointestinal dysfunction, anesthesia, and surgical stress present a considerable challenge to the neonate to maintain metabolic homeostasis. Careful management of nutrition and metabolism by surgeons and physicians is necessary to avoid additional morbidity and mortality caused by malnutrition and the neurologic sequelae of hypoglycemia or hyperglycemia.[76] The long-term metabolic, neurologic, and cardiovascular sequelae of surgery, parenteral nutrition, or sepsis during the neonatal period are unknown, but given the importance of this period on subsequent development, nutritional management of the neonate undergoing surgery is also likely to play a role in adult health.

NEONATAL GLUCOSE METABOLISM

Most of the energy supply (approximately 70% of total calories as carbohydrate, <10% as fat[24]) of the fetus comes from maternally supplied glucose. At birth the switch from a high-carbohydrate diet to a diet that is high in lipid and lower in carbohydrate (approximately 40% of calories as carbohydrate, 50% as fat[24]) means that the neonate must not only adapt to a difference in timing and magnitude of carbohydrate supply but also must regulate its own level of glycemia by insulin/glucagons, gluconeogenesis, and the other mechanisms of glucose homeostasis. The brain can use only glucose or ketone bodies; it is not able to oxidize lipids directly, so maintenance of euglycemia during the neonatal period is particularly important for favorable neurologic outcomes. Despite the greater supply of fats as a fuel source in neonates than in adults, glucose turnover is greater in neonates (3 to 5 mg/kg/min) than in adults (2 to 3 mg kg/min) partly due to the relatively increased brain/body mass ratio. Premature infants have an even greater glucose turnover rate (5 to 6 mg/kg/min).[77] In the premature and term infant, 90% of glucose is used by the brain, whereas this decreases to about 40% in adults.[78] The term infant has two important means of glucose production to maintain euglycemia: glycogenolysis and gluconeogenesis. Glucose production in term neonates originates from glycogenolysis (approximately 40%) and gluconeogenesis from glycerol (20%), alanine and other amino acids (10%), and lactate (30%).[79]

Glucagon/Insulin Axis in the Perinatal Period

Although the fetus is capable of synthesizing and releasing glucagon and insulin, the function of insulin during pregnancy is probably its promotion of anabolism and enhancing growth rather than regulating circulating glucose.[77] Glucagon is important for the induction of gluconeogenic enzymes during pregnancy, and the surge in glucagon at birth, which results from cord clamping, is probably responsible for the rapid postnatal increase in gluconeogenic capacity.[80] Islet cell function is relatively unresponsive for the first 2 weeks of neonatal life so that increases in insulin secretion and decreases in glucagon secretion are relatively slow in response to increased glucose concentration.[77] There is a similarly slow response to hypoglycemia in the neonate so that if a neonate starts to become hypoglycemic, it may be some time before insulin secretion is decreased and glucagon secretion is increased to stimulate gluconeogenesis. In addition insulin sensitivity is lower in end organs of neonates than in those of adults so that plasma insulin is less closely linked with blood glucose, whereas plasma glucagon is more closely linked to glycemia.[81,82] The maturation of the response to glucose is even slower in preterm infants than in term neonates.[83]

Glycogen and Glycogenolysis in the Perinatal Period

During the third trimester of pregnancy, storage of maternal glucose as glycogen takes place. Most fetal storage is in the liver, although some glycogen is stored in fetal skeletal muscle, kidney, and intestine, and only to a small degree in brain. Hepatic and renal glycogen is mobilized at and immediately after birth to maintain circulating glucose concentration; however the hepatic glycogen stores are exhausted within 24 hours of birth, or even sooner in premature neonates (who have had an abbreviated or no third trimester), SGA neonates, or neonates who have experienced extensive perinatal stress and have therefore had early catecholamine-stimulated mobilization of hepatic glycogen. Other tissues such as heart, skeletal muscle, and lung can metabolize stored glycogen intracellularly but cannot mobilize it to the circulation

because of a lack of the enzyme glucose-6-phosphatase. Mobilization and use of glycogen stores takes place in response to the perinatal surge in glucagon or catecholamine, or both.

Gluconeogenesis in the Neonate

Key enzymes of gluconeogenesis are present in the fetus from early in gestation and increase throughout gestation and during the neonatal period. However in vivo fetal gluconeogenesis has not been demonstrated and it is not known whether cytosolic phosphoenolpyruvate carboxykinase (necessary for gluconeogenesis from amino acids or lactate) or glucose-6-phosphatase (necessary for gluconeogenesis from all substrates and for glucose export after glycogenolysis) is expressed adequately to support gluconeogenesis by fetal liver. Glucose-6-phosphatase expression is low in the fetus but increases in activity within a few days of birth in term neonates.[84] Studies measuring gluconeogenesis from glycerol in preterm infants have suggested that some gluconeogenesis from glycerol can occur[85] but can only partly compensate a decrease in exogenous glucose supply in preterm infants, probably because of limitation at the level of glucose-6-phosphatase.[86] Parenteral glycerol[87] supports enhanced rates of gluconeogenesis in preterm infants, whereas no increase in gluconeogenesis was observed by provision of mixed amino acids[88] or alanine[89] to preterm neonates, supporting the hypothesis that gluconeogenesis from amino acids or lactate is limited by lack of phosphoenolpyruvate carboxykinase activity in preterm infants. Parenteral lipids stimulate gluconeogenesis in preterm infants,[88] probably by providing both carbon substrate (glycerol) and fatty acids. Fatty acid oxidation is indispensable for gluconeogenesis; although fatty acid carbon cannot be used for glucose, fat oxidation provides both an energy source (ATP) to support gluconeogenesis and acetyl coenzyme A (acetyl-CoA) to activate pyruvate carboxylase. In experimental animals the increase in the glucagon/insulin ratio at birth stimulates maturation of the enzymes of gluconeogenesis, particularly phosphoenolpyruvate carboxykinase, although little is known about the induction of gluconeogenesis in human neonates. Gluconeogenesis is evident within 4 to 6 hours after birth in term neonates.[90,91]

Neonatal Hypoglycemia

Blood glucose levels fall immediately after birth but rise either spontaneously from glycogenolysis/gluconeogenesis or as a result of feeding. This period of hypoglycemia is not considered of clinical significance, but the appearance of hypoglycemia subsequent to this should be avoided. However there is considerable controversy as to which blood glucose level should be considered the cutoff below which infants are considered hypoglycemic. It is also debated what the duration of hypoglycemia should be before preventive or investigational measures, or both, are instigated,[92] particularly as glucose concentrations fluctuate significantly during this period of massive metabolic, physiologic, and nutritional change. In addition the symptoms of neonatal hypoglycemia are nonspecific and may include the signs and symptoms shown in Table 6-5, many of which are subjective. Current recommendations for operational thresholds of circulating glucose levels are less than 45 mg/dL (2.5 mmol/L) for the term neonate with abnormal clinical signs, persistently less than 36 mg/dL (2.0 mmol/L) for the term neonate with risk factors for compromised metabolic adaptation, 47 mg/dL

TABLE 6-5

Signs and Symptoms of Neonatal Hypoglycemia

Jitteriness	Abnormal cry
Tremors	Cardiac arrest
Apnea	Hypothermia
Cyanosis	Tachypnea
Limpness/apathy/lethargy	Seizures

(2.6 mmol/L) for preterm neonates (although data is limited), and maintenance of blood glucose greater than 45 mg/dL (2.5 mmol/L) at all times in parenterally fed infants because of the likelihood of increased insulin (and therefore suppressed lipolysis and ketogenesis) in these neonates.[93] Causes of hypoglycemia in the neonatal period are shown in Table 6-6. Glucose metabolism is particularly important for the brain during this critical growth period, and hypoglycemia less than 2.6 mmol/L has been found to be associated with short-term neurophysiologic changes[94] and poor neurodevelopmental outcome.[95,96] However in these studies it is difficult to reliably delineate hypoglycemia as a risk factor independent from those of comorbidities and causes of hypoglycemia—such as prematurity, congenital hyperinsulinism,[97] SGA status,[96] or a diabetic mother[98]—and there is uncertainty concerning the frequency, degree, and duration

TABLE 6-6

Causes of Hypoglycemia in the Neonate

Associated with Changes in Maternal Metabolism

Intrapartum administration of glucose

Drug treatment
   Terbutaline, ritodrine, propranolol
   Oral hypoglycemic agents

Diabetes in pregnancy/infant of diabetic mother

Severe Rh incompatibility

Associated with Neonatal Problems

Idiopathic condition or failure to adapt

Perinatal hypoxia-ischemia

Infection/sepsis

Hypothermia

Hyperviscosity

Erythroblastosis fetalis, fetal hydrops

Exchange transfusion

Other
   Iatrogenic causes
   Congenital cardiac malformations

Intrauterine Growth Restriction

Endocrinology and Metabolism

Hyperinsulinism (e.g., congenital hyperinsulinism, Beckwith-Weidemann syndrome)

Other endocrine disorders
   Panhypopituitarism
   Isolated growth hormone deficiency
   Cortisol deficiency

Inborn errors of metabolism
   Glycogen storage diseases types 1a and 1b
   Fructose 1,6-diphosphatase deficiency
   Pyruvate carboxylase deficiency
   Fatty acid oxidation disorders

of hypoglycemia that may cause neurologic problems.[99] Recent advances in neonatal cerebral imaging modalities have suggested a wide spectrum of features that may result from neonatal hypoglycemia.[100] However there is remarkably little strong evidence regarding which blood glucose levels are the thresholds below which adverse neurodevelopmental sequelae are likely to result, and many normal healthy infants experience glucose levels below these thresholds without adverse effects.[101,102] It is likely that duration of hypoglycemia and other metabolic factors such as ketone body levels (see later) are important as determinants of outcome. Treatment of hypoglycemia in the neonate depends on the feeding route and whether risk factors have been identified. Frequent monitoring of blood glucose levels is necessary and treatment/investigation algorithms combine increased enteral feeds with intravenous administration of glucose if clinical signs of hypoglycemia are present.[92]

Neonatal Hyperglycemia

Neonatal hyperglycemia can also occur and has been recognized as representing several distinct clinical entities. Diabetes mellitus can present in the neonatal period, although the condition is rare, representing approximately 1 in 400,000 to 1 in 500,000 live births.[103,104] Both permanent and transient neonatal diabetes occurs. Transient neonatal diabetes mellitus, which usually resolves within 3 to 6 months but may lead to the development of permanent diabetes in childhood or adolescence, represents about 50% of cases and permanent neonatal diabetes mellitus represents the other 50%. Transient neonatal diabetes mellitus is due to paternal imprinting[105,106] and one of the molecular causes of the permanent form has been elucidated.[107] However most hyperglycemia in neonates is self-limiting, resolves spontaneously, and has few features in common with diabetes. Its frequency appears to be increasing in parallel with increased survival of extremely low-birth-weight infants who are fed parenterally and receive corticosteroids. The etiology of neonatal hyperglycemia is not well understood, but possible causes[92] include inability to suppress gluconeogenesis in response to glucose infusion, excessive glucose infusion rates, end-organ insulin resistance, low plasma insulin levels in combination with high catecholamine levels (e.g., due to corticosteroid administration), infection, or response to pain or surgery (see later). The management of hyperglycemia in the neonate is to manage the cause, for example, treat infection or pain or decrease excessive glucose infusion rates. There is still controversy regarding insulin administration:[108] on the one hand insulin infusion allows maintenance of high glucose infusion rates (and may therefore increase weight gain), whereas on the other hand there are reports of adverse effects. Neither the acute nor the long-term sequelae of hyperglycemia in the neonate are well understood. Ketosis or metabolic acidosis does not occur as a result of hyperglycemia, but osmotic diuresis and glycosuria may lead to dehydration. Hyperglycemia has been found to be associated with increased mortality in premature infants.[109–111] Hyperglycemia has also been associated with increased morbidity and mortality in neonates with necrotizing enterocolitis.[112] However, except for a study linking hyperglycemia with white matter injury in premature infants,[109] evidence for a cerebral pathologic cause and adverse neurodevelopmental outcome as a result of neonatal hyperglycemia is scant, although there is a risk of increased cerebral bleeds from osmotic shifts. There has been a great deal of interest in the tight control of blood glucose in patients in adult intensive care units after the study of Van Den Berghe and colleagues.[113] In very-low-birth-weight infants, insulin therapy to maintain normoglycemia was not found to improve outcomes,[114] whereas a recent study (including some neonates) in glucose control in a pediatric intensive care unit suggested that intensive insulin therapy improved short-term outcomes.[115] Hence it remains uncertain whether tight control of blood glucose concentration is beneficial in neonates or in specific subgroups of neonates.

NEONATAL LIPID AND FAT METABOLISM

Fat is the main energy source of the neonate, providing 40% to 50% of calories in milk or formula. As discussed earlier, fat oxidation becomes a major fuel used within 3 hours after birth.[25,26] In addition fat is the main store of energy within the body. Although most chain lengths of fatty acids can be used for energy, fatty acids, in the form of phospholipids and other fat-derived lipids, are extremely important structural components of cell membranes, and the function of these membranes is critically dependent on the availability of the correct chain length and degree of unsaturation of fatty acids. Thus throughout the period of growth of the neonate, an array of different fatty acids, either supplied by the diet or metabolized by the body, is essential to support growth, particularly that of the brain, which is rich in complex lipids.

Fatty Acid Oxidation and Ketogenesis in Neonates

Fatty acid beta oxidation is the major process by which fatty acids are oxidized, by sequential removal of two-carbon units from the acyl chain, providing a major source of ATP for heart and skeletal muscle. Hepatic beta oxidation serves a different role by providing ketone bodies (acetoacetate and β-hydroxybutyrate) to the peripheral circulation and supporting hepatic gluconeogenesis by providing ATP and acetyl-CoA to activate pyruvate carboxylase activity. In addition kidney,[116] small intestine,[117] white adipose tissue,[118] and brain astrocytes[119] may be ketogenic under some conditions. Ketone bodies are another significant fuel for extrahepatic organs, especially the brain, when blood glucose levels are low. Consequently, ketogenesis is extremely important to provide an alternative fuel for the brain when glucose levels may be fluctuating because of alterations in feeding pattern and adaptation of physiologic and metabolic homeostasis. For oxidation of the acyl groups of stored, ingested, or infused triacylglycerol to take place, nonesterified fatty acids must be released. This can take place distant from the site of use by the action of hormone-sensitive lipase (HSL) in the adipocyte or locally by the action of endothelial lipoprotein lipase (LPL).[120,121] Nonesterified fatty acids (NEFA) bound to albumin provide the main substrate that is taken up and oxidized by tissues. In addition intracellular triacylglycerol stores can also provide a significant source of acyl moieties for beta oxidation in the heart and skeletal muscle, again through the action of HSL. HSL and LPL are under control of the hormonal and nutritional milieu so that fatty acid oxidation is partly controlled by the supply of NEFA to the tissue.[122] In the immediate postnatal period the plasma levels of NEFA increase rapidly in response to the glucagon/catecholamine surge that stimulates lipolysis and the fall in insulin that occurs as a result of birth and cord division.[123,124] This lipolysis also results in the release of glycerol, which can be used as a gluconeogenic precursor (see previous discussion).[123,124] Ketone bodies are formed fairly soon after birth,[24,125–129] reaching 0.2 to 0.5 mmol/L in the first 1 postnatal day, and 0.7 to 1.0 mmol/L between 5 and 10 days,[125] although this may be impaired in premature or SGA infants.[126,128,130] During hypoglycemia, ketone body concentrations can raise to 1.5 to 5 mmol/L.[125] The enzymes of fatty acid oxidation and ketogenesis all increase in activity postnatally in experimental animals, accounting for this increase in capacity for fatty acid oxidation and ketogenesis,[24] although little is known about the induction of fatty acid oxidation enzymes in humans. Hydroxymethylglutaryl-CoA synthase is thought to be particularly important in the control of ketogenesis and is subject to short-term activation by glucagon, which may account for the rapid surge in ketogenesis at birth.[131]

Ketone Body Use

Little is known about the ontogeny of the enzymes of ketone body use in human tissues. Heart, muscle, kidney, and brain are all capable of ketone body use and the enzymes required have been shown in human tissue.[132–134] In rats the activities of the ketone body use enzymes are very active in neonatal brain and decrease at weaning, whereas they are lower than adult levels in neonatal muscle and kidney, suggesting preferential use by the brain.[24]

Neonatal Protein and Amino Acid Metabolism

In contrast to healthy adults who exist in a state of neutral nitrogen balance, infants need to be in positive nitrogen balance in order to achieve satisfactory growth and development. Infants are efficient at retaining nitrogen and can retain up to 80% of the metabolizable protein intake on both oral and intravenous diets.[34,135,136] Protein metabolism is dependent on both protein and energy intake. The influence of dietary protein is well established. An increased protein intake has been shown to enhance protein synthesis,[137,138] reduce endogenous protein breakdown,[139] and thus enhance net protein retention.[139,140] The influence of nonprotein energy intake on protein metabolism is more controversial. Protein retention can be enhanced by giving carbohydrate or fat,[141–146] which are thus said to be protein sparing. Although some studies have suggested that the protein-sparing effect of carbohydrate is greater than that of fat,[142,143,146] others have suggested that the protein-sparing effect of fat may be either equivalent to or greater than that of carbohydrate.[141,144,145] The addition of fat calories to the intravenous diet of newborns undergoing surgery reduces protein oxidation and protein contribution to the energy expenditure and increases protein retention.[144] In order to further investigate this positive effect on protein metabolism we studied the various components of whole protein metabolism by the combined technique of indirect calorimetry and stable isotope (^{13}C-leucine) tracer technique. Two groups of neonates receiving isonitrogenous and isocaloric total parenteral nutrition were studied: one group received a high-fat diet and the other a high-carbohydrate diet.[65] There was no significant difference between the two groups with regard to any of the components of whole-body protein metabolism: protein synthesis, protein breakdown, protein oxidation/excretion, and total protein flux. This study confirms previous observations that infants have high rates of protein turnover, synthesis, and breakdown, which may be up to eight times greater than those reported in adults. In newborn infants receiving parenteral nutrition, synthesis and breakdown of endogenous body protein far exceed intake and oxidation of exogenous protein. Infants are avid retainers of nitrogen, and carbohydrate and fat have an equivalent effect on protein metabolism. This supports the use of intravenous fat in the intravenous diet of newborns undergoing surgery.

The protein requirements of newborns are between 2.5 and 3.0 g/kg/day. Amino acids, the building blocks of protein, can be widely interconverted so that several are described as dispensable (or nonessential). These are alanine, aspartate, asparagine, glutamate, and serine. Others are described as indispensable (or essential): histidine, isoleucine, leucine, lysine, methionine, phenylalanine, threonine, tryptophan, and valine. There are yet other amino acids (arginine, cysteine, glycine, glutamine, proline, and tyrosine) that are not usually essential but can become limiting during metabolic stress such as sepsis. Sulfur amino acids (i.e., cysteine, methionine) and tyrosine, in particular, are abundant in acute-phase proteins, so their supply becomes particularly important during acute-phase responses. Human milk provides amino acids in the form of protein and as free amino acids. However milk proteins are not just important for their nutritive value but also possess other important properties such as antiinfective activity (IgA, IgM, IgG, lactoferrin, lysozyme).[147] Platelet-activating factor acetylhydrolase, a minor component of human milk, has been suggested to be responsible for some of the protective effects of breast milk against necrotizing enterocolitis.[148] The amino acid glutamine is of particular interest in premature neonates and neonates undergoing surgery.

The nitrogen source of total parenteral nutrition is usually provided as a mixture of crystalline amino acids. The solutions commercially available contain the eight known essential amino acids plus histidine, which is known to be essential in children.[140] Complications like azotemia, hyperammonemia, and metabolic acidosis have been described in patients receiving high levels of intravenous amino acids.[149] These complications are rarely seen with amino acid intake of 2 to 3 g/kg/day.[150] In patients with severe malnutrition or with additional losses (i.e., in those who have undergone jejunostomy or ileostomy) the protein requirements are higher.[140] The ideal quantitative composition of amino acid solutions is still controversial. Cysteine, taurine, and tyrosine seem to be essential amino acids in newborns. However the addition of cysteine in the parenteral nutrition of neonates does not cause any difference in the growth rate and nitrogen retention.[136] The essentiality of these amino acids could be related to the synthesis of neurotransmitters, bile salts, and hormones. The consequences of failure to supply these amino acids may be poor long-term neurologic or gastrointestinal function.[151] The incidence of abnormalities of plasma aminograms during parenteral nutrition is low. There are no convincing data at the moment to support the selection of one crystalline amino acid solution over another in newborns. Glutamine is a nonessential amino acid that has many important biologic functions, such as being a preferential fuel for the immune system and the gut. Various authors have postulated that glutamine may become "conditionally essential" during sepsis and that addition of glutamine to parenteral feedings of premature neonates or those undergoing surgery may help to preserve mucosal structure, prevent bacterial translocation, and hence reduce the number of infections and the time before full enteral feeding can be established.

Metabolic Response to Stress

The body has developed a system of responses to deal with various noxious stimuli that threaten survival. In some respects these responses are stereotypical and lead to the so-called stress response. Stress can be defined as "factors that cause disequilibrium to an organism and therefore threaten homeostasis."[152] Initiators of the stress response in newborns include operative trauma and sepsis. In this section we discuss the response to operative trauma. The physiologic changes due to sepsis are discussed in another chapter.

OPERATIVE TRAUMA

The stress response that follows operative procedures is initiated and coordinated by several messengers and affects whole body systems. The insult of operative trauma can be considered a form of "controlled" injury.

After surgery there are alterations in metabolic, inflammatory, endocrine, and immune system responses. These responses have evolved to enhance survival to trauma and infection in the absence of iatrogenic intervention. They limit patient activity in the area of injury to prevent secondary damage and start the healing process through the inflammatory signals produced. Changes in metabolism increase the availability of substrates needed by regenerating and healing tissue. The immune stimulation allows for the swift eradication of any causal or secondary opportunistic microbial invasion, whereas the subsequent immune paresis may allow for a dampening of this immune stimulation to allow for healing to ensue.

In contrast to adults the energy requirement of infants and children undergoing major operations seems to be modified minimally by the operative trauma per se. In adults trauma or surgery causes a brief "ebb" period of a depressed metabolic rate followed by a "flow phase" characterized by an increase in oxygen consumption to support the massive exchanges of substrate between organs (Fig. 6-9).[153] In newborns major abdominal surgery causes a moderate (15%) and immediate (peak at 4 hours) elevation of oxygen consumption and REE and a rapid return to baseline 12 to 24 hours postoperatively (see Fig. 6-9).[64] There is no further increase in energy expenditure in the first 5 to 7 days after an operation.[64,154] The timing of these changes corresponds with the postoperative increase in catecholamine levels described by Anand and associates.[155] The maximum endocrine and biochemical changes are observed immediately after the operation and gradually return to normal over the next 24 hours. It is of interest that infants who have a major operation after the second day of life have a significantly greater increase in REE than infants who undergo surgery within the first 48 hours of life. A possible explanation for this may be the secretion of endogenous opioids by the newborn. It has been suggested that nociceptive stimuli during the operation are responsible for the endocrine and metabolic stress response and that these stimuli may be inhibited by opioids.[155,156] This is supported by studies showing that moderate doses of opioids blunt the endocrine and metabolic responses to operative stress in infancy.[155,156] The levels of endogenous opioids in the cord blood of newborn infants are five times higher than plasma levels in resting adults.[157] Thus, it is possible that

ADULTS

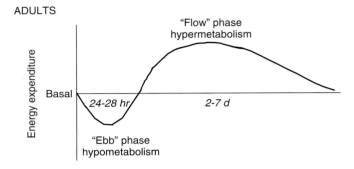

INFANTS

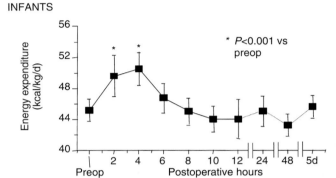

FIGURE 6-9 Postoperative variations in energy expenditure in adults and neonates undergoing major operations. Data for infants are expressed as mean ± SEM. (Adapted from Jones MO, Pierro A, Hammond P, et al: The metabolic response to operative stress in infants. J Pediatr Surg 1993;28:1258-1262; and Pierro A: J Pediatr Surg 2002;37:811-822.)

the reduced metabolic stress response observed in neonates less than 48 hours old is related to higher circulating levels of endogenous opioids. This may constitute a protective mechanism blunting the response to stress in the perinatal period. Chwals and colleagues[158] demonstrated that the postoperative increase in energy expenditure can result from severe underlying acute illness, which frequently necessitates surgery (i.e., sepsis or intense inflammation). REE is directly proportional to growth rate in healthy infants, and growth is retarded during acute metabolic stress. These authors suggest that energy is used for growth recovery after the resolution of the acute injury response in neonates undergoing surgery. The authors indicate that serial measurement of postoperative REE can be used to stratify injury severity and may be an effective parameter to monitor the return of normal growth metabolism in neonates undergoing surgery.

Operative trauma initiates a constellation of inflammatory pathways that regulate a whole-body response to operative stress, which is similar to that seen after injury. The responses can be initiated and controlled by both chemical/hormonal signals and afferent nervous signals. Some of the chemical signals responsible for the responses originate in the operative wound in response to cellular injury.

Cytokines

One of the key chemical messenger systems in the control and the coordination of the response to injury are cytokines. Cytokines are a group of low-molecular-weight polypeptides or glycoproteins, which act to regulate the local and systemic immune function and modulation of the inflammatory

response. They are active at very low concentrations, found usually at the picogram level, and their production is usually transient. Cytokines bring about their action by altering gene expression in target cells. They act in a paracrine and autocrine manner at concentrations in the picomolar to nanomolar range, but can have systemic effects if there is spill over into the circulation.

Cytokines generally have a wide range of actions in the body. Cytokines are not usually stored intracellularly and must therefore be synthesized de novo and released into the tissues on appropriate stimulation and gene transcription. One of the crucial controllers of cytokine gene regulation is nuclear factor kappa B (NFκB),[159,160] a protein transcription factor that enhances the transaction of a variety of cytokine genes. Lymphocytes are activated at the site of injury. The first cells to be recruited to the site of inflammation are monocytes and neutrophils, where they produce cytokines in the first few hours after the onset of a surgical or traumatic wound.[161] These cytokines are chemoattractant to other white cells.

Cytokines are divided into proinflammatory and antiinflammatory types on the basis of whether they stimulate the immune system or decrease or dampen the immune response. Although most cytokines have a clear proinflammatory or antiinflammatory response, a few have dual properties. Some cytokines may exhibit a proinflammatory action in a particular cell or certain conditions but an antiinflammatory response in a different cell or under different conditions.[162] The presence of antiinflammatory cytokines is of importance in abating the immune response to prevent excessive tissue destruction and death. The presence of naturally occurring inhibitors helps abate the otherwise catastrophic positive feedback loop that could lead to widespread tissue destruction from excessive inflammation. The cytokines that are commonly released after trauma include the proinflammatory interleukins (ILs) IL-1 and IL-6 and tumor necrosis factor-α (TNF-α) and the antiinflammatory IL-1ra and IL-10.

Both proinflammatory and antiinflammatory cytokines are produced in response to operative stress. The actual cytokine cascade is heterogeneous and is determined by various factors, which include the type and magnitude of the operation. The cytokine cascade in response to operations in adults has been well characterized.[163] There have been limited studies in neonates. Cytokines bond to specific membrane receptors of target organs. Their actions in the acute stress response include (1) changes in gene expression and proliferation, thereby affecting wound healing and immunocompetence; (2) release of counterregulatory hormones; and (3) facilitation of cell-to-cell communication.[164] Substrate use is also affected by cytokine release. Glucose transport is increased by TNF, hepatic gluconeogenesis is stimulated by IL-1, and hepatic lipogenesis is stimulated by IL-1, IL-6, and TNF. IL-1 and TNF also appear to promote muscle proteolysis. In neonates IL-6 increases maximally 12 hours after major surgery and the increase is proportional to the degree of operative trauma,[165] indicating that this cytokine is a marker of stress response in neonates. IL-1 and TNF may have a synergistic effect in producing the metabolic manifestations seen after injury and infection.[153] However systemic cytokine release cannot account for all the metabolic changes seen after injury because cytokines are not consistently found in the bloodstream of injured patients and systemic cytokine administration does not produce all the metabolic effects observed in injured adult individuals.

Other mediators of the response to tissue injury include *histamine*, a well-known chemical mediator in acute inflammation that causes vascular dilatation and the immediate transient phase of increased vascular permeability; *5-hydroxytryptamine (serotonin)*, a potent vasoconstrictor; *lysosomal compounds* released from activated neutrophils, monocytes, and macrophages; *lymphokines,* chemicals involved in the inflammatory cascade with vasoactive or chemotactic properties; the *complement system*, and the *kinin system*. These mediators cause vasodilation, increased vascular permeability, and emigration and stimulation of white blood cells. The postoperative changes that occur also affect the immune system. There is a period of immune stimulation that is often followed by a period of immune paresis. There is a proinflammatory response that is balanced by an antiinflammatory response. The balance often determines and predicts the development of complications and outcome in terms of morbidity and mortality.

Other responses may be initiated by peripheral and central nervous system stimulation. Peripheral efferent from pain receptors, for instance, can feed back to the central nervous system and produce some of the clinical signs of inflammation and the responses seen after operative stress. Indeed blockage of this afferent stimulus is associated with dampening of the stress response.[155] Fentanyl and morphine are commonly used in pediatric anesthesia for pain relief. Studies in preterm infants and neonates have shown that fentanyl blunts the metabolic response to operative stress.[155,156,166]

Endocrine Response

Various studies have characterized the endocrine response to surgery in infants and children.[167–169] These studies have revealed that the response lasts between 24 and 48 hours postoperatively. The response differs in some respects to that of adults, which usually lasts longer.[170,171] Compared with values seen after an overnight fast, there is an increase in insulin levels in the early postoperative period. However this increase in insulin levels is not proportional to the increase in glucose. There is a change in the insulin/glucose ratio in the postoperative period,[167,172] which lasts more than 24 hours postoperatively. Anand and colleagues[167] found that neonates exhibited an initial decrease in the insulin/glucose ratio in the immediate postoperative period that was restored by 6 hours. Ward-Platt and associates[172] found an instantaneous and continuous rise in the ratio in older infants and children.

Cortisol is significantly elevated and remains elevated for the first 24 hours postoperatively and is accompanied by a rise in catecholamines.[173,174] Both the hormones have antiinsulin effects. The rise in cortisol and catecholamines partially drives the postoperative hyperglycemic response and may be responsible for the relative insulin insensitivity in the postoperative period. Anand and colleagues found a very significant correlation between glucose and adrenaline levels in neonates at the end of abdominal surgery.[167] There is an increase in lactate levels in the postoperative period in both adults and infants/children.[156,175,176] The increase in lactate in the postoperative period is related to the alteration in glucose metabolism[167] and more acutely the presence of tissue hypoperfusion related to surgery.[176] The increase in lactate may represent a means of discriminating the magnitude of operative stress. Altogether the changes in hormone levels

are related to the magnitude of the operative stress and have been shown in some but not all procedures to be lessened by laparoscopic surgery.

Effect of Surgery on Glucose Metabolism in Neonates

Surgery in adults is well known to cause hyperglycemia, and a hyperglycemia response to surgery has also been well documented in neonates,[155,156,166,167,177–181] with the degree of hyperglycemia being negatively correlated with age.[181] In contrast to adults, however, in whom blood glucose concentration may remain high for several days postoperatively, the rise in glucose levels in neonates is short-lived, lasting only up to 12 hours. In an elegant study, Anand and Aynsley-Green showed a strong correlation between the degree of surgical stress and the increase in glucose levels.[168] In the same study stress scores were also strongly positively correlated with plasma levels of adrenalin, noradrenalin, glucagon, insulin, and less strongly with cortisol.[168] The hyperglycemic response to surgery is probably multifactorial, including increased glycogenolysis and gluconeogenesis in response to increases in plasma catecholamine and subsequently glucagon. In addition the insulin response to hyperglycemia may be inappropriately low, especially in preterm neonates undergoing surgery,[167] and tissues may become relatively refractory to insulin. Support for the hypothesis that these effects are driven by catecholamine release are provided by Anand's group, who in a series of studies showed that blunting of the catecholamine response to surgery by modulation of the anesthetic regimen led to a blunting of the hyperglycemic/endocrine response to surgery.[155,156,166] The timing of the adrenaline, noradrenaline, and glucose response to neonatal surgery is shown in Figure 6-10.

Carbohydrate conversion to fat (lipogenesis) occurs when glucose intake exceeds metabolic needs. The risks associated with this process are twofold: accumulation of the newly synthesized fat in the liver[182] and aggravation of respiratory acidosis resulting from increased carbon dioxide production, particularly in patients with compromised pulmonary function.[183] Jones and coworkers[184] have shown that there is a negative linear relationship between glucose intake (grams per kilogram per day) and fat use (oxidation and conversion to fat) expressed in grams per kilogram per day ($y = 4.547 - 0.254x; r = -0.937; P = <0001$) in infants undergoing surgery who receive parenteral nutrition. From this equation it was calculated that "net fat synthesis from glucose" exceeds "net fat oxidation" when the glucose intake is greater than 18 g/kg/day. Jones and colleagues[184] also found a significant relationship between glucose intake and carbon dioxide production (milliliters per kilogram per minute) ($y = 3.849 + 0.183x; r = 0.825; P = <0001$). The slope of this relationship was steeper when glucose intake exceeded 18 g/kg/day ($y = 2.62 + 0.244x; r = 0.746; P = <05$) than when glucose intake was less than 18 g/kg/day ($y = 5.30 + 0.069x; r = 0.264; P = .461$). Thus the conversion of glucose to fat results in a significantly increased production of carbon dioxide. Glucose intake exceeding 18 g/kg/day is also associated with a significant increase in respiratory rate and plasma triglyceride levels. In summary:

1. Glucose intake is the principal determinant of carbohydrate and fat use.
2. The maximal oxidative capacity for glucose in infants undergoing surgery is 18 g/kg/day, which is equivalent to the energy expenditure of the infant.

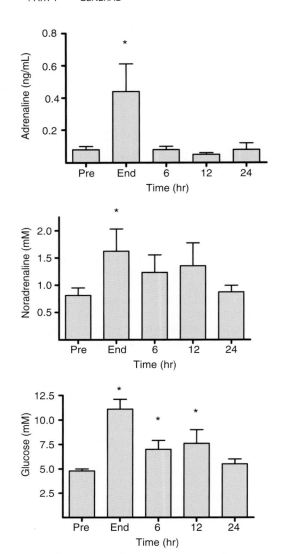

FIGURE 6-10 Response of adrenaline, noradrenaline, and glucose to surgery in neonates. (Data from Anand KJS, Brown MJ, Causon RC, et al: Can the human neonate mount an endocrine and metabolic response to surgery? J Pediatr Surg 1985;20:41-48.)

3. If glucose is given in excess of maximal oxidative capacity: (a) net fat oxidation ceases; (b) net fat synthesis begins; (c) the thermogenic effect of glucose increases and the efficiency with which glucose is metabolized decreases; (d) carbon dioxide production and respiratory rate increase; (e) plasma triglyceride levels increase.

It is advisable therefore in stable newborns undergoing surgery and requiring parenteral nutrition not to exceed 18 g/kg/day of intravenous glucose intake.[184,185]

Effect of Surgery on Fat Metabolism in Neonates

Surgery in neonates causes an increase in NEFA and ketone body levels,[156,166,167,180] which can be decreased by modulating the catecholamine release,[156,166] suggesting that catecholamine stimulation of lipolysis is responsible for this increase. Pierro and colleagues have studied intravenous fat use by performing an "Intralipid use test."[185] This consisted of infusing for 4 hours Intralipid 10% in isocaloric and isovolemic amounts to the previously given mixture of glucose and amino acids. Gas exchange was measured by indirect calorimetry to calculate the patient's oxygen consumption and carbon dioxide production, and net fat use. The study showed that (1) infants undergoing surgery adapt rapidly (within 2 hours) to the intravenous infusion of fat; (2) more than 80% of the exogenous fat can be oxidized; and (3) carbon dioxide production is reduced during fat infusion as a consequence of the cessation of carbohydrate conversion to fat.[185] This study did not measure the rate of fat use during a mixed intravenous diet including carbohydrate, amino acids, and fat. More recent studies on stable newborns undergoing surgery receiving fixed amounts of carbohydrate and amino acids and variable amounts of intravenous long-chain triglycerides (LCTs) fat emulsion have shown that at a carbohydrate intake of 15 g/kg/day (56.3 kcal/kg/day) the proportion of energy metabolism derived from fat oxidation does not exceed 20% even with a fat intake as high as 6 g/kg/day. At a carbohydrate intake of 10 g/kg/day this proportion can be as high as 50%.[186] This study seems to indicate that during parenteral nutrition in neonates undergoing surgery the majority of the intravenous fat infused is not oxidized but deposited. Net fat oxidation seems to be significantly influenced by the carbohydrate intake and by the REE of the neonate. When the intake of glucose calories exceeds the REE of the infant, net fat oxidation is minimal regardless of fat intake.[186] In order to use intravenous fat as an energy source (i.e., oxidation to carbon dioxide and water), it is therefore necessary to maintain carbohydrate intake at less than basal energy requirements.

Commonly used fat emulsions for parenteral nutrition in pediatrics are based on LCTs. The rate of intravenous fat oxidation during total parenteral nutrition can theoretically be enhanced by the addition of L-carnitine or medium-chain triglycerides (MCTS), or both, to the intravenous diet. Important differences have been observed between MCTS and LCTS with respect to physical and metabolic properties. MCTs are cleared from the bloodstream at a faster rate and are oxidized more completely for energy production than are LCTs. Therefore they seem to serve as a preferential energy source for the body. We have investigated the effects of MCTs on intravenous fat use during total parenteral nutrition in stable newborns undergoing surgery.[187] Two groups of neonates undergoing surgery and receiving total parenteral nutrition were studied: one group received LCT-based (100% LCTs) fat emulsion and the other group received an isocaloric amount of MCT-based (50% MCTs + 50% LCTs) fat emulsion. In newborns receiving carbohydrate calories in excess of measured REE (56 kcal/kg/day), net fat oxidation was not enhanced by the administration of MCT-based fat emulsion. Conversely in infants receiving carbohydrate calories less than REE (41 kcal/kg/day), the administration of MCT fat emulsion increased net fat oxidation from 0.6 ± 0.2 to 1.7 ± 0.2 g/kg/day. The administration of MCT-based fat emulsion did not increase the metabolic rate of the infants. Fats that are not used can become the substrates for free-lipid peroxidation and free-radical production. Peroxidation has been specifically linked with lipids in parenteral nutrition[188,189] and has been shown to be dependent on the amount of carbohydrate given: If net fat oxidation is not taking place because carbohydrate intake is high, more lipid is present to be peroxidized.[190]

Effect of Surgery on Protein and Amino Acid Metabolism in Neonates

Major operative stress in adults results in a negative nitrogen balance due to muscle protein catabolism. The neonate is already in a more precarious position regarding nitrogen balance, so if major protein catabolism were to take place in the neonate who undergoes surgery, growth and other important functions would be impaired. Nitrogen losses are increased after surgery in neonates,[191-194] and muscle protein breakdown has also been demonstrated by increased 3-methylhistidine excretion in these neonates.[155,166] However these changes are relatively short-lived and can be overcome by provision of additional dietary nitrogen or calories, or both. Powis and associates[195] investigated protein metabolism kinetics in infants and young children who had undergone major operations. Patients were studied for 4 hours preoperatively and for the first 6 hours after surgery. There were no significant differences in the rates of whole-body protein flux, protein synthesis, amino acid oxidation, and protein degradation between the preoperative and postoperative times, indicating that infants and children do not increase their whole-body protein turnover after major operations. It is possible that infants and children are able to convert energy expended on growth to energy directed to wound repair and healing, thereby avoiding the overall increase in energy expenditure and catabolism seen in the adult.[195] However little is known about the components of protein turnover in neonates who have surgery. The only available study, in six neonates with necrotizing enterocolitis, showed no differences in protein turnover between acute and recovery phases of the disease.[196]

The complete reference list is available online at www. expertconsult.com.

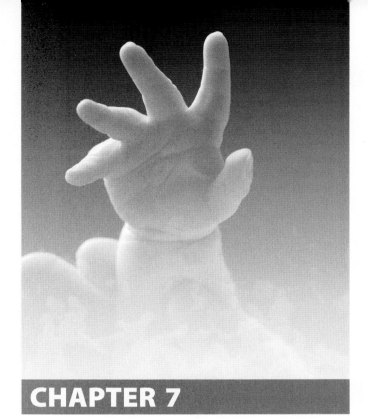

CHAPTER 7

Respiratory Physiology and Care

Jay M. Wilson and John W. DiFiore

"The body is but a pair of pincers set over a bellows and a stewpan and the whole fixed upon stilts."[1] This chapter discusses the bellows. In doing so we examine normal lung development, pulmonary physiology, devices (invasive and noninvasive) for patient monitoring, and devices designed to provide ventilatory support. Finally we discuss how to apply this information to the management of infants and children with respiratory failure in the modern intensive care unit.

The primary function of the respiratory system is the continuous absorption of oxygen and the excretion of carbon dioxide. This is achieved by bringing into close proximity massive amounts of air and blood while simultaneously humidifying inspired gas and filtering out contaminants. Ordinarily this process requires a minimal amount of work, but stressful conditions and disease can ultimately overwhelm the system. Since a reasonable understanding of the normal anatomy and physiology of the respiratory system is essential to the understanding and management of pulmonary diseases, we briefly review it here.

Lung Development

Lung development is divided into five phases: embryonic, pseudoglandular, canalicular, saccular, and alveolar. The boundaries between these phases are not sharp; they blend into one another with considerable overlap at any given time between areas within the lung, and they vary from person to person.[2]

EMBRYONIC PHASE

The human fetal lung originates in the 3-week-old embryo as a ventral diverticulum that arises from the caudal end of the laryngotracheal groove of the foregut.[3] This diverticulum grows caudally to form the primitive trachea. By 4 weeks the end of the diverticulum divides, forming the two primary lung buds. The lung buds develop lobar buds, which correspond to the mature lung lobes (three on the right side and two on the left side). By the sixth week of gestation the lobar buds have further subdivided to form the bronchopulmonary segments. During this time the vascular components of the respiratory system also begin their development. The pulmonary arteries form as a branch off the sixth aortic arch and the pulmonary veins emerge from the developing heart.

The primitive lung bud is lined by an epithelium derived from endoderm; it differentiates into both the respiratory epithelium that lines the airways[4] and the specialized epithelium that lines the alveoli and permits gas exchange.[5] The lung bud grows into a mass of mesodermal cells from which blood vessels, smooth muscle, cartilage, and other connective tissues that form the framework of the lung will differentiate.[6] Ectoderm contributes to the innervation of the lung (Fig. 7-1, A).[7]

PSEUDOGLANDULAR PHASE

From the seventh to sixteenth weeks of gestation, conducting airways and the associated pulmonary vasculature are formed by repeated dichotomous branching, resulting in 16 to 25 generations of primitive airways.[3] During this phase the lung has a distinctly glandular appearance (hence the term *pseudoglandular*) created by small epithelium-lined tubules surrounded by abundant mesenchyma (Fig. 7-1, B).[6] By the sixteenth week of gestation all the bronchial airways have been formed.[8-10] After this time further growth occurs only by elongation and widening of existing airways and not by further branching. During this period the respiratory epithelium begins to differentiate, cilia appear in proximal airways, and cartilage begins to develop from the surrounding mesoderm to support airway structures. The amount of cartilage supporting the airway decreases, moving distally from the trachea as smooth muscle cells increase. Alterations in the development of smooth muscle, cartilage, and vascular structures are responsible for many pulmonary disorders.

CANALICULAR PHASE

The canalicular phase takes place from the sixteenth to twenty-fourth weeks of gestation. During this time the basic structure of the gas-exchanging portion of the lung is formed and vascularized.

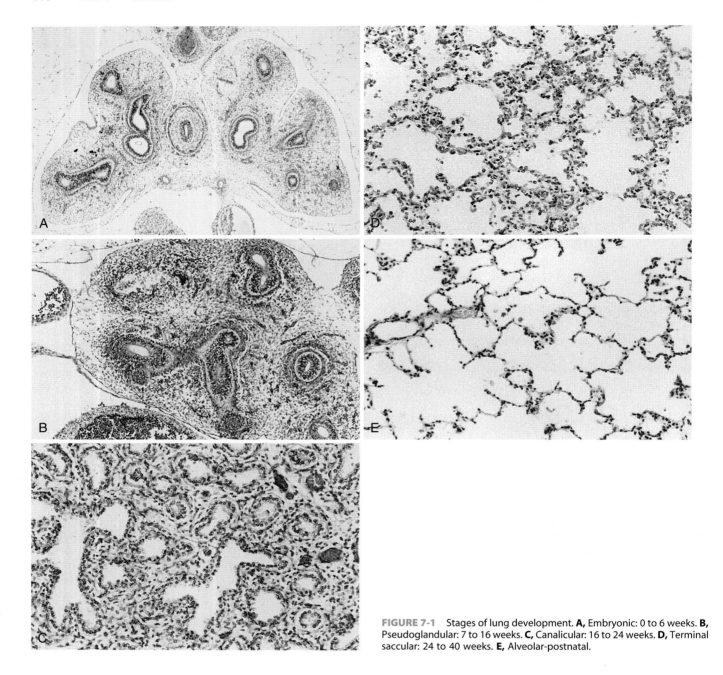

FIGURE 7-1 Stages of lung development. **A,** Embryonic: 0 to 6 weeks. **B,** Pseudoglandular: 7 to 16 weeks. **C,** Canalicular: 16 to 24 weeks. **D,** Terminal saccular: 24 to 40 weeks. **E,** Alveolar-postnatal.

Early in the canalicular period the lungs have a simple airspace configuration. Potential gas-exchanging structures are smooth-walled blind-ending channels that are lined by cuboidal epithelium and supported by abundant loose interstitium and scattered small blood vessels. As the canalicular period progresses interstitial tissue decreases, capillary growth increases, and these "channels" assume a more complex irregular pattern (Fig. 7-1, *C*).

At approximately 20 weeks' gestation differentiation of the primitive epithelial cells begins. The first morphologic evidence of this phase of differentiation is the growth of capillaries beneath the epithelial cells that line the primitive gas-exchanging channels. In one population of overlying epithelial cells, capillary ingrowth results in thinning of the cytoplasm, narrowing of the air-blood interface, and differentiation into type I pneumocytes—the cells ultimately responsible for gas exchange. In other overlying epithelial cells, the lamellar bodies that are associated with surfactant synthesis begin to appear; these bodies identify the type II cells that will ultimately produce surfactant. Although some investigators have concluded that the progenitor of type I cells is an undifferentiated epithelial cell, a more convincing body of evidence suggests that type I cells develop from differentiated type II cells.[11-15] By the end of the canalicular period, structural development of the lung has progressed to the point that gas exchange is possible.

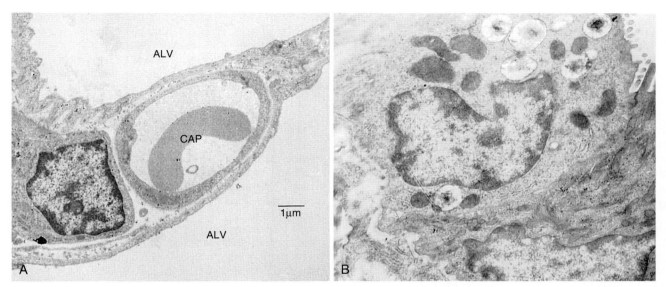

FIGURE 7-2 **A,** Electrophotomicrograph of a type I pneumocyte. Note the thin alveolar-arterial interface. **B,** Electrophotomicrograph of a type II pneumocyte. Note the lamellar bodies filled with surfactant. ALV, alveolar; CAP, capillary.

TERMINAL SACCULAR PHASE

The terminal saccular phase of lung development takes place from 24 weeks' gestation until term and is associated with remarkable changes in the appearance of the lung. Interstitial tissue becomes less prominent and airspace walls demonstrate marked thinning. Tissue projections into the distal airspace regions divide the distal airspaces into saccules, where capillaries are generally exposed to only one respiratory surface (Fig. 7-1, *D*). Later in the mature alveolus, each capillary is simultaneously exposed to at least two alveoli.[16]

The cells that line the terminal saccules of the human fetal lung at this stage of development are recognizable type I and type II pneumocytes. Morphologically they are indistinguishable from the corresponding cells described in neonatal or adult human lung tissue. However the surfactant produced by the early fetal lung differs biochemically from that produced later in gestation. Although no apparent morphologic differences in the lamellar bodies exists, immature lungs produce surfactant that is rich in phosphatidylinositol, whereas the surfactant produced by lungs late in gestation is rich in phosphatidylglycerol.[17]

ALVEOLAR PHASE

An alveolus is defined as an open outpouching of an alveolar duct lined almost exclusively by the thin processes of type I pneumocytes. Its interstitial capillaries are simultaneously exposed to at least two alveoli, and because the nuclei of all cells are located away from the gas-exchange surface, the barrier to gas exchange is usually only a few nanometers thick.[18] The barrier between the gas in the alveoli and the blood in the capillaries is composed of three layers: the thin processes of the type I cells, a basement membrane that appears to be common to the endothelial and alveolar cells, and the thin extensions of the endothelial cells (Fig. 7-2, *A*). The type I cell is responsible for gas exchange and the type II cell synthesizes and secretes surfactant.

At birth the lung has no mature alveoli but instead contains approximately 20 million primitive terminal sacs.[19-22] These sacs are lined by mature alveolar epithelium; they resemble large shallow cups.[9,19-22] At approximately 5 weeks after birth, these 20 million primitive terminal sacs begin to develop into the 300 million alveoli that will be present by 8 years of age, with the fastest multiplication occurring before 4 years of age (Fig. 7-1, *E*).[21-23] After age 8 years, increases in lung volume result from increases in alveolar size but not number.[21]

ARTERIAL GROWTH

The pattern of growth of pulmonary arteries differs depending on the location of the artery relative to the acinus. The preacinar region refers to the conducting airways and includes the trachea, major bronchi, and bronchial branches to the level of the terminal bronchiolus. The acinus refers to the functional respiratory unit of the lung and includes structures that are distal to the terminal bronchiolus (specifically the respiratory bronchioli, alveolar ducts, and alveoli). In the preacinar region the pulmonary artery gives off a branch to accompany each airway branch—a "conventional" artery that ultimately provides terminal branches to the acini. Many additional branches arise from the conventional arteries and pass directly into adjacent respiratory tissue to supply the peribronchial parenchyma; these are called *supernumerary* arteries.[8,24]

Mirroring the branching of bronchial airways, the development of all preacinar conventional and supernumerary arteries is complete by 16 weeks' gestation.[24,25] Subsequent changes in the preacinar arteries involve only size not number. In the intra-acinar region terminal branches of the conventional pulmonary arterioles supply the capillary bed. Concurrent with alveolar development these small vessels of the lung multiply rapidly after birth to keep pace with alveolar multiplication.

In adults complete muscularization of pulmonary arteries is found throughout the acinus, even in the walls of alveoli immediately under the pleura. In the fetus, however, complete muscularization of the arteries occurs only proximal to or at the level of the terminal bronchioli. Consequently only partially muscular or nonmuscular arteries are found within the acinus itself. New alveoli appear during early childhood simultaneously with the accompanying intra-acinar arteries. However muscularization of these arteries is a slow process.[9]

MEDIATORS OF FETAL LUNG DEVELOPMENT

Although a complete discussion of the genetics of lung development is beyond the scope of this chapter, some of the basic pathways are becoming better understood and are thus worthy of mention. Early lung bud development and airway branching involves the genes GATA6, HNF-3, FGF-10, SHH, and TGF-b. Alveolar development involves *platelet-derived growth factor, tropoelastin,* and glucocorticoids. Pulmonary vascular development involves TGF-b, VEGF-A, FOX, and integrin.[26] So far not enough is known about the genetics of lung development for it to be exploited clinically, but that day is probably not far off.

The distribution of fetal lung fluid has been exploited clinically. There is a large body of evidence supporting the role of lung liquid in normal and experimental fetal lung growth. Fetal lung fluid is a combination of plasma ultrafiltrate from the fetal pulmonary circulation, components of pulmonary surfactant, and other fluids from pulmonary epithelial cells. This fluid is produced constantly to keep the fetal lung inflated and at slightly positive pressure, which is essential to stimulate normal lung development. Naturally occurring airway occlusions in humans have resulted in large fluid-filled lungs that histologically have either normal or slightly distended alveoli.[27–31] In other instances intrauterine airway occlusion results in large lungs despite the presence of other anatomic abnormalities, such as Potter syndrome or congenital diaphragmatic hernia, that would normally lead to pulmonary hypoplasia.[32–34]

Experimental studies of normal fetal lambs have confirmed that retention of lung liquid leads to pulmonary hyperplasia, whereas drainage of liquid leads to hypoplasia. Fetal tracheal occlusion has also been shown to prevent pulmonary hypoplasia associated with fetal diaphragmatic hernia.[35–38] Since these initial studies, multiple experimental animal models of fetal tracheal occlusion have shown dramatic increases in lung growth. Subsequently several clinical trials of tracheal occlusion in association with congenital diaphragmatic hernia have shown some progress in alleviating the associated pulmonary hypoplasia, but preterm labor has continued to limit its application.[39,40] Postnatal intrapulmonary distention with perfluorocarbon liquid has also been shown to accelerate neonatal lung growth, but randomized clinical trials have been thwarted by regulatory issues.[26]

Although increased intrapulmonary pressure has been cited as the primary stimulus for lung growth in tracheal occlusion models, it is likely only a trigger for more complex downstream regulatory changes. Tracheal occlusion has been associated with increased expression or production of multiple growth factors, including keratinocyte growth factor, vascular endothelial growth factor, transforming growth factor-β2, insulin-like growth factor I, and many others, all of which may participate in a complex regulatory pathway for lung development enhanced by tracheal occlusion.[41–44]

Pulmonary Physiology

Shortly before birth epithelial cells cease production of lung fluid and begin to actively absorb it back into the fetal circulation. This process is facilitated by active sodium transport and is stimulated by thyroid hormone, glucocorticoids, and epinephrine.

At birth as the lung expands with the first few breaths, pulmonary arterial P_{O_2} increases and P_{CO_2} decreases. This results in pulmonary vasodilation, lowered pulmonary vascular resistance, and constriction of the ductus arteriosus. The loss of maternal prostaglandins further stimulates ductus arteriosus closure. Cessation of umbilical blood flow results in closure of the ductus venosus and a rise in the systemic vascular resistance, which in turn results in an increase in left-sided heart pressures above the pressure in the right side of the heart, resulting in closure of the foramen ovale. With this final right-to-left shunt closure, the transition from fetal to postnatal circulation is complete. Failure of any of these events can lead to persistence or recurrence of fetal circulation and respiratory failure.

The process of breathing is complex and involves contraction of the inspiratory muscles to generate negative pressure in the trachea to bring fresh air into the lungs. In the lungs the process of oxygen uptake and carbon dioxide elimination occurs by means of diffusion across the ultrathin alveolar capillary membrane. This process is critical not only to fuel the cells of the body with oxygen for metabolism but also to maintain appropriate acid-base status by careful regulation of carbon dioxide. Dysfunction in any part of this process can lead to respiratory failure and the need for mechanical ventilatory support.

LUNG VOLUMES

To understand the process of respiration, it is necessary to understand the terminology associated with the assessment of pulmonary function. The total volume of the lung is divided into subcomponents, defined as follows (Fig. 7-3):
- Functional residual capacity (FRC): The volume of gas in the lung that is present at the end of a normal expiration when airflow is zero and alveolar pressure equals ambient pressure
- Expiratory reserve volume: The additional gas that can be exhaled beyond FRC to reach residual volume
- Residual volume: The minimum lung volume possible; this is the gas that remains in the lung after all exhalable gas has been removed
- Total lung capacity: The total volume present in the lung
- Inspiratory capacity: The difference in inhaled volume between FRC and total lung capacity
- Vital capacity: The amount of gas inhaled from FRC to total lung capacity

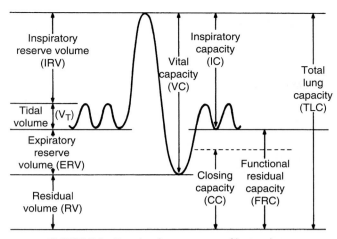

FIGURE 7-3   Functional components of lung volume.

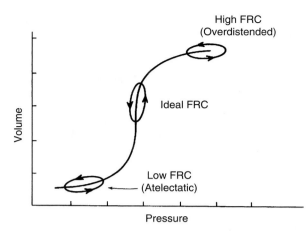

FIGURE 7-4   Static compliance curve with superimposed dynamic flow-volume loops for high, low, and ideal functional residual capacities (FRCs).

- Inspiratory reserve volume: The amount of gas inhaled from peak normal inspiratory volume to total lung capacity
- Tidal volume: The volume of a normal inspiration

Tidal volume, vital capacity, inspiratory capacity, inspiratory reserve volume, and expiratory reserve volume can be measured directly by spirometry. Conversely total lung volume, FRC, and residual volume cannot be measured by spirometry, and one of the following techniques must be used: (1) the nitrogen washout test, in which the nitrogen eliminated from the lungs while breathing pure oxygen is measured; (2) the helium dilution test, which measures the equilibration of helium into the lung; or (3) total-body plethysmography, which measures changes in body volume and pressure to calculate FRC using Boyle's law.[45]

CLOSING CAPACITY

Inspiratory pressure within the airway decreases as gas travels in a distal direction. Eventually the intraluminal pressure stenting the airway open equals the surrounding parenchymal pressure; this is called the *equal pressure point*.[46] Downstream of the equal pressure point, intraluminal pressure drops to less than surrounding parenchymal pressure, and airway closure occurs leading to unventilated alveoli and a physiologic shunt. In normal lungs little or no unventilated area exists at FRC. However any reduction in FRC (which frequently occurs in diseased lungs) will cause more areas of the lung to reach closing volume and become atelectatic and increase the shunt.[47] Conversely an increase in FRC (achieved by positive-pressure ventilation) may open some areas that were closed, thereby reducing the physiologic shunt.

PULMONARY COMPLIANCE

Pulmonary compliance is defined as the change in lung volume per unit change in pressure.[48] Dynamic compliance is the volume change divided by the peak inspiratory transthoracic pressure. Static compliance is the volume change divided by the plateau inspiratory pressure.[49] With the initiation of an inspiratory breath the transthoracic pressure gradient increases to a peak value. This increase is a function of elastic resistance of the lung and chest wall as well as airway resistance. The pressure then falls to a plateau level as the gas redistributes in alveoli. Consequently dynamic compliance is always lower than static compliance. Figure 7-4 demonstrates a standard static compliance curve.[50] Ventilation normally occurs in the steep portion of the curve, whereas large changes in volume occur in response to small changes in pressure. However at low and high volumes, large changes in pressure result in minimal changes in volume. In diseased lungs in which compliance has dropped into the flat portion of the curve, the goal of mechanical ventilation is to return it to the steep portion. Excessive pressure applied by the ventilator results in ventilation at the top of the curve where the process once again becomes inefficient.[51]

Changes in lung volume and pleural pressure during a normal breathing cycle, which reflect the elastic and flow-resistant properties of the lung, are displayed as a pressure-volume loop in Figure 7-5. The slope of the line that connects the end-expiratory and end-inspiratory points in the figure provides a measure of the dynamic compliance of the lung. The area that falls between this line and the curved lines to the right and left represents the additional work required to overcome flow resistance during inspiration and expiration, respectively.

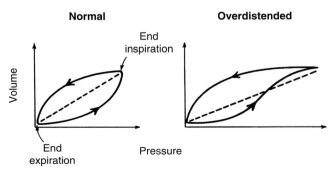

FIGURE 7-5   Dynamic pressure-volume loop demonstrating an idealized ventilatory cycle and overdistention during positive-pressure ventilation.

AIRWAY RESISTANCE

Resistance to gas flow is a function of the physical property of the gas (molecules interact with one another and with airway walls) as well as the length of the tube through which the gas travels. Most important, resistance is a function of the internal diameter of the tube. Because the airways in small children are narrow, a slight change in diameter secondary to airway swelling can result in a dramatic increase in resistance. Because airways are smaller at the base of the lung, resistance is greater there than in the apical region.[52] In addition the velocity of flow affects resistance because below critical velocity gas flow is laminar. However above critical velocity there is turbulent flow and resistance increases.

TIME CONSTANTS

The time constant is a product of the compliance and resistance of the lung and calculates how quickly exhalation can occur. Consequently increases in compliance or resistance of individual alveolar units or areas of the lung increase the time constant. One time constant is defined as the time required to complete 63% of tidal volume expiration (two, three, and four time constants = 87%, 95%, and 99%, respectively).[53] Because the resistance of the airways leading to individual alveoli varies depending on alveolar location, and because the compliance of individual alveoli also varies, the measured time constant is actually an average of many different time constants throughout the lung. The importance of understanding time constants becomes apparent when assisted mechanical ventilation is contemplated. In a lung with high compliance or high resistance the time constant is prolonged. Mechanical ventilator settings would consequently need to be adjusted to allow for near-complete expiration (three time constants, or 95% expiration) to avoid breath stacking and overdistention. Conversely in lungs with low compliance or low resistance, the time constant is less; under these circumstances an increase in minute ventilation should be accomplished with increases in respiratory rate rather than increases in tidal volume. Because of low compliance, tidal volume would be more likely to lead to high pressure and barotrauma.

PULMONARY CIRCULATION

Mixed venous blood from the systemic circulation collects in the right atrium, passes into the right ventricle, and then travels into the pulmonary capillary bed where gas exchange occurs. Blood subsequently drains into the left atrium where it is pumped into the left ventricle and ultimately into the systemic circulation. Desaturated blood that originates from systemic sources through the bronchial and pleural circulation represents 1% to 3% of the total volume of blood that exits the left atrium. In pathologic situations this anatomic right-to-left shunting can approach 10%.[54] In addition under any circumstance in which pressure in the right atrium exceeds that of the left atrium, the foramen ovale (which is anatomically patent in all neonates and in 20% to 30% of older children) becomes another major area for extrapulmonary right-to-left shunting.

Because blood is a fluid and is affected by gravity, in an upright individual blood pressure and thus blood flow in the pulmonary capillary bed are lowest at the apex of the lung and greatest at the base. Under normal circumstances pulmonary artery pressure is adequate to deliver some blood to the apex of the lung; however in pathologic situations such as hemorrhage or shock, blood flow to the apex can fall to zero, resulting in an area that is ventilated but not perfused; such areas are referred to as dead space. The lung can be divided into four regions designated progressively in a caudal direction from apex to base. In zone 1 (the apex) the alveolar pressure exceeds pulmonary artery pressure and little or no flow occurs. In zone 2 the arterial pressure exceeds alveolar pressure, but alveolar pressure exceeds venous pressure. In this region flow is determined by arterial-alveolar pressure differences. In zone 3 the pulmonary venous pressure exceeds alveolar pressure and flow is determined by the arterial-venous pressure differences. In zone 4 (the base) pulmonary interstitial pressure exceeds both pulmonary venous and alveolar pressure and flow in this region is determined by arterial interstitial pressure differences.[55]

Because oxygen is a pulmonary vasodilator, hypoxemia is a potent stimulus for vasoconstriction in the pulmonary vascular bed. In addition because acidosis is a pulmonary vasoconstrictor and alkalosis is a vasodilator, the partial pressure of carbon dioxide (Pco_2) indirectly affects the capillary bed because of its effect on pH.

PULMONARY GAS EXCHANGE

Diffusion

Oxygen and carbon dioxide pass between the alveolus and the pulmonary capillary bed by passive diffusion from higher to lower concentration.[56] Because diffusion in a gaseous environment is a function of molecular weight, oxygen diffuses more rapidly through air than carbon dioxide does. However because diffusion across the capillary alveolar membrane involves a shift from the gaseous phase to the liquid phase, solubility of the gas in liquid becomes rate limiting, so carbon dioxide (being far more soluble than oxygen) diffuses 20 times more rapidly.[57]

Diffusion is driven not only by differences in solubility but also by differences in partial pressure of the gases across the capillary alveolar membrane. Gas exchange is consequently most rapid at the beginning of the capillary where the differences in the partial pressure of oxygen (Po_2) and Pco_2 between the alveoli and the capillaries are greatest; gas exchange is virtually complete one third of the way across the pulmonary capillary bed.[58] Consequently in normal individuals the principal limiting factor for oxygen uptake at rest or during exercise is pulmonary blood flow.[59] Although the rate of diffusion is not rate limiting in the healthy state, when the alveolar capillary membrane is thickened, diffusion may become sufficiently impaired to prevent complete saturation of available hemoglobin. Carbon monoxide, which has diffusion characteristics similar to those of oxygen, is used to measure diffusion capacity.

Dead Space

Minute ventilation, which is defined as the total volume of air inspired each minute, is calculated as the product of the tidal volume and the respiratory rate. However the entire volume of gas does not participate in gas exchange; the portion of each tidal breath that ventilates only the oropharynx, larynx, trachea, and major conducting bronchi (the anatomic dead space) does not participate in gas exchange.[60] In addition to the anatomic dead space, a certain volume of gas ventilates unperfused alveoli and consequently does not participate in gas exchange. This is known as alveolar dead space and is minimal in the absence of disease. The combination of anatomic and alveolar dead space, known as physiologic dead space, is equal to approximately one third of the normal tidal volume; dead space that exceeds this amount is considered pathologic.[61]

Ventilation-Perfusion Matching

For optimal gas exchange, the ventilation (V) and perfusion (Q) to a given segment of the lung should be matched.[62] The V/Q ratios of different lung units are not identical,[58] but the averaged ratio of alveolar ventilation/blood flow in the lung is approximately 0.8. At the apex of the lung the V/Q ratio is higher; at the base of the lung the ratio is lower. Under normal circumstances V/Q mismatching is minimal and inconsequential. However in disease states mismatching can contribute significantly to the impairment of gas exchange. When blood flows through regions of the lung with no ventilation, a right-to-left shunt that can significantly decrease the arterial oxygen saturation is created.

Oxygen Transport

Oxygen is transported through the bloodstream in one of two ways. It may be transported in aqueous solution in the plasma or in chemical combination within hemoglobin in erythrocytes. The amount of oxygen transported in solution is negligible. Thus most oxygen is carried bound to hemoglobin in erythrocytes. At full saturation, 1 g of hemoglobin is capable of carrying 1.34 mL of oxygen. However the actual amount of oxygen carried by hemoglobin varies and is defined by a sigmoid-shaped curve referred to as the oxyhemoglobin dissociation curve (Fig. 7-6). Under normal circumstances hemoglobin is 100% saturated with oxygen; however the sigmoid

shape of this curve ensures that the oxygen carrying capacity of hemoglobin remains relatively high, even at a Po_2 as low as 60. As a result mild pulmonary disorders do not interfere with oxygen delivery. At the same time the steep area of the dissociation curve ensures that a large quantity of oxygen can be unloaded into the peripheral tissues as Po_2 drops. The oxyhemoglobin dissociation curve can be shifted to the left or right by changes in the affinity of hemoglobin for oxygen. A shift to the left results in a higher affinity of hemoglobin for oxygen and is caused by alkalosis,[63] hypothermia, decreased erythrocyte 2,3-diphosphoglycerate[64] (which often occurs in old banked blood),[65] or fetal hemoglobin.[66] In this situation, at a given Po_2, the hemoglobin is more saturated than normal and tissue perfusion should therefore be increased to deliver the same amount of oxygen for metabolic needs. A shift to the right is the result of a lowered affinity of hemoglobin for oxygen and is caused by acidosis,[63] hyperthermia, and an increased red blood cell 2,3-diphosphoglycerate content.[64] This rightward shift results in hemoglobin that is less saturated at a given Po_2 thereby allowing the unloading of more oxygen at lower rates of flow to the peripheral tissues.

Carbon Dioxide Equilibrium and Acid-Base Regulation

Because carbon dioxide is produced as an end product of metabolism, its rate of production is a function of metabolic rate. Under normal circumstances the amount of carbon dioxide produced is slightly less than the amount of oxygen consumed. This is defined by the respiratory quotient (R):

$$R = \frac{\text{Rate of } CO_2 \text{ output}}{\text{Rate of } O_2 \text{ uptake}}$$

Under normal circumstances, the respiratory quotient is 0.8, but it can vary from 1.0 to 0.7, depending on whether carbohydrate or fat is used as the principal source of nutrition. The lungs are primarily responsible for the elimination of carbon dioxide, and the rate of elimination depends on pulmonary blood flow and alveolar ventilation. Carbon dioxide is carried in the bloodstream in several forms. In aqueous solution it exists in a state of equilibrium as dissolved carbon dioxide and carbonic acid ($CO_2 + H_2O \rightleftharpoons H_2CO_3$). This equation normally is shifted markedly to the left. In erythrocytes, however, the enzyme carbonic anhydrase catalyzes the reaction, which shifts the equation to the right.[67,68] The ability of carbonic acid to dissociate and reassociate ($H_2C_3 \rightleftharpoons H^+ + HCO_5$) is an important factor in buffering plasma to maintain a physiologic pH. The relationship is defined using the Henderson-Hasselbalch equation. A small amount of carbon dioxide is also carried combined with hemoglobin in the form of carbaminohemoglobins.[67]

Monitoring

Because the condition of acutely ill infants and children can deteriorate rapidly, continuous surveillance of their physiologic status is necessary to provide ideal care. Many options for physiologic monitoring are available to the clinician in the modern intensive care unit; the most useful are discussed in this section.

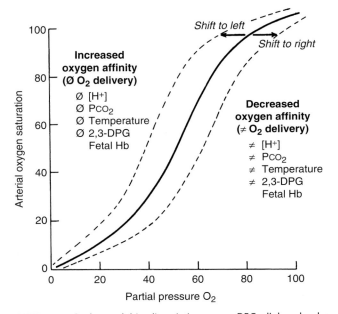

FIGURE 7-6 Oxyhemoglobin dissociation curve. DPG, diphosphoglycerate; Hb, hemoglobin.

NONINVASIVE MONITORING

Pulse Oximetry

Pulse oximetry provides continuous noninvasive monitoring of hemoglobin saturation. The principle of pulse oximetry is based on spectrophotometry and relies on the fact that oxygenated and deoxygenated hemoglobin transmits light at different frequencies. Oxygenated hemoglobin selectively absorbs infrared light (940 nm) and transmits red light (660 nm), whereas deoxyhemoglobin absorbs red light and transmits infrared light. The pulse oximeter probe contains two light-emitting diodes that pass light at the wavelengths noted through a perfused area of tissue to a photodetector on the other side. The photodiode compares the amounts of infrared, red, and ambient light that reach it to calculate the oxygen saturation in arterial blood (SaO_2).[69,70]

The advantages of pulse oximetry are that it is noninvasive and has a rapid response time, making changes in clinical status immediately apparent. Disadvantages of oximetry are that it is insensitive to large changes in arterial PO_2 at the upper end of the oxygenated hemoglobin dissociation curve. In addition at an oxygen saturation less than 70%, the true SaO_2 is significantly underestimated by most oximeters. When SaO_2 measurements are routinely less than 85%, determination of its correlation with actual partial pressure of oxygen in arterial blood (PaO_2) through the use of indwelling arterial catheters is necessary. Errors can also occur when other forms of hemoglobin exist.[71] The presence of carboxyhemoglobin and methemoglobin results in falsely elevated SaO_2 readings.[65] Conversely certain dyes such as methylene blue result in a marked decrease in measured SaO_2.[72] The presence of fetal hemoglobin, which has an absorption spectrum similar to that of adult hemoglobin, has no impact on the accuracy of SaO_2 measurements. Physical factors—including poor peripheral perfusion, abnormally thick or edematous tissue at the site of sensor placement, the presence of nail polish, and excessive ambient light—also lead to inaccurate readings.[73–75]

Capnometry

Capnometry is a noninvasive method that measures the end-tidal partial pressure of carbon dioxide in the expired gas.[76] As with pulse oximetry capnometry is based on the principle that carbon dioxide absorbs infrared light. Exhaled gas passes through a sampling chamber that has an infrared light source on one side and a photodetector on the other side. Based on the amount of infrared light that reaches the photodetector, the amount of carbon dioxide present in the gas can be calculated. Depending on the equipment, data can be reported as the maximum concentration of carbon dioxide (end-tidal carbon dioxide) or it can provide a display of the entire exhaled carbon dioxide waveform; this display is known as a capnogram.[77]

Two categories of carbon dioxide monitors exist: mainstream monitors and sidestream monitors.[78] Mainstream monitors, in which the sampling cell is connected to the airway between the ventilator and the endotracheal tube, respond faster to changes in carbon dioxide but must be heated to prevent water condensation. These chambers are consequently heavy and hot and must be supported to avoid contact with the patient. Sidestream monitors draw a continuous sample of gas from the respiratory circuit into the measuring cell. This system is lightweight and can theoretically be used in nonintubated patients[79]; however because of the longer transit time to the sampling chamber, this unit is slow in responding to changes in carbon dioxide.

Because the carbon dioxide that is measured in expired gases is a product of metabolic rate, pulmonary circulation, and alveolar ventilation, these variables must all be considered when interpreting changes in end-tidal carbon dioxide measurements.

Transcutaneous Measurement of Gas Tension

Measurement of PO_2 and PCO_2 at the skin surface is possible by means of transcutaneous monitoring.[80] The principle of this device is based on the fact that PO_2 and PCO_2 approximate arterial values in areas where blood flow exceeds the metabolic requirements of the tissue. To increase blood flow the devices used to measure transcutaneous PO_2 and PCO_2 contain a sampling electrode and a warming device to increase local blood flow.[81] The advantage of transcutaneous monitoring is that it may reduce the number of (but not eliminate the need for) arterial blood gas determinations required in a sick individual. One limitation of the device is that the measured transcutaneous PO_2 and PCO_2 are not equal to arterial blood gas tensions and can frequently be 5 to 10 mm Hg higher or lower than the arterial counterpart. Changes in peripheral perfusion caused by shock or vasopressors can make these values even more inaccurate.[82] Another disadvantage is that burns or blisters may occur at the electrode site because of the warming component. This requires frequent changing of the monitoring site, at which time recalibration is necessary.

INVASIVE MONITORING

Mixed Venous Oxygen Monitoring

Measurement of mixed venous oxygen saturation (SvO_2) may be the single most useful measurement in determining critical impairment in oxygen delivery to the tissues (usually interpreted as an SvO_2 <60%). Because the SvO_2 is a function of arterial saturation, cardiac output, and hemoglobin concentration, any deviation in these values is detected in the SvO_2.

Although a lowered SvO_2 does not identify the cause of the impairment, it provides several hints to solving the problem. Increasing the fractional concentration of oxygen in inspired gas (FIO_2) to elevate SaO_2, using pressors or volume expansion to increase the cardiac output, or increasing the hemoglobin concentration with transfusions can all be used to correct a critically low SvO_2. The SvO_2 can be monitored by intermittent measurement of blood withdrawn from a pulmonary artery catheter or by continuous monitoring using a pulmonary artery catheter equipped with a fiberoptic bundle.[83]

Arterial Catheterization

Indwelling arterial catheterization provides access for continuous monitoring of arterial blood pressure and intermittent arterial blood gas sampling. This method is indicated for patients who require frequent blood gas sampling or who are hemodynamically unstable.

In children the most common locations for arterial catheter placement are the radial, posterior tibial, or dorsalis pedis arteries. When placing a radial artery catheter, it is imperative to ascertain the patency of the ulnar artery by assessing blood flow to the hand and fingers while the radial artery is compressed (Allen test).[84] Otherwise ischemic necrosis of the hand may occur.[85] In newborn infants the umbilicus provides two additional arteries for access. The catheter tip is generally placed at one of two positions. The high position (T6 through T8) places the tip below the ductus arteriosus but above the major abdominal tributaries. The low position (L3 through L4) places the catheter tip between the renal arteries and inferior mesenteric arteries. These positions have the advantage of minimizing the potential complications of thrombus or embolus into the tributary vessels.

The advantage of direct arterial catheterization is that it provides the most accurate continuous measurement of blood pressure as well as the most accurate assessment of PaO_2 and $PaCO_2$. The disadvantage is that the technique is invasive and therefore involves a risk of infection,[2,86] embolization,[87] and thrombosis[88]; this risk increases with time.[89] Another complication is the potential for anemia because the presence of indwelling arterial lines has been associated with excessive blood testing.[90] Consequently daily assessment of the necessity of direct arterial monitoring is essential and catheters should be removed as soon as the patient can be managed without them.

In infants the right radial artery is unique in that it provides peripheral arterial access to preductal blood (i.e., blood ejected from the left ventricle before being mixed in the aorta with blood from a patent ductus arteriosus). When pulmonary hypertension exists (e.g., congenital diaphragmatic hernia), significant differences in preductal and postductal arterial saturation may occur and monitoring of both sites is often useful in guiding therapy.

Pulmonary Artery Catheterization

The pulmonary artery catheter enables the direct measurement of right atrial pressure, right ventricular end-diastolic pressure, pulmonary artery pressure, and SvO_2.[91-96] In addition calculation of cardiac output and left ventricular filling pressures can be calculated indirectly. Complications include cardiac arrhythmias in up to 50% of critically ill patients, conduction defects (6%), pulmonary infarction (<1%), pulmonary artery rupture (0.2%), catheter knotting, balloon rupture (5%), and infection.[97-102] Because of these safety concerns and the evolution of less invasive methods such as echocardiography, use of pulmonary artery catheters in noncardiac pediatric patients is now rare.

Mechanical Ventilators

A basic knowledge of mechanical ventilators is important for pediatric surgeons because many surgical procedures result in transient respiratory failure, and respiratory failure is the most frequent diagnosis requiring admission to neonatal and pediatric intensive care units.[103] The goals of mechanical ventilation are to achieve adequate excretion of carbon dioxide by maintaining alveolar ventilation, maintain adequate arterial oxygenation, expand areas of atelectasis by increasing lung volume, and reduce the mechanical work of breathing. While achieving these goals, mechanical ventilation must also avoid inflicting further injury from barotrauma or oxygen toxicity, or both.[104]

The first-generation ventilator developed by O'Dwyer in 1968 was powered by a foot pump and was not significantly improved on until 1970, when Siemens introduced the 900A. Since then ventilators have evolved from simple devices delivering bulk volumes of air based on cycling pressure and time to more advanced devices. Microprocessor-driven models provide new functions such as pressure support ventilation (PSV), mandatory minute ventilation, airway pressure release ventilation, and more recently proportional assist ventilation and volume-assured PSV.

CYCLING MECHANISMS

Mechanical Breath Phases

All ventilators deliver mechanical breaths that cycle through four distinct phases: inspiration, cycling, expiration, and triggering. Inspiration is the point at which expiratory valves close and fresh gas is introduced under pressure into the lungs. Cycling is the point at which inspiration changes to expiration and can occur in response to elapsed time, delivered volume, or pressure met. At this point inflow of gas stops and expiratory valves open to allow passive release of gas from the lungs. Triggering is the changeover from expiration to inspiration and can occur in response to elapsed time (control mode) or in response to a patient-initiated event (assist mode), such as changes in airway pressure or gas flow. Most of the recent refinements in ventilator design are aimed at decreasing the mechanical lag time between patient effort and ventilator response, thereby increasing patient comfort and reducing the work of breathing.[105,106]

VENTILATOR TYPES

Ventilators can be broadly classified into two groups: volume controlled and pressure controlled, based on the specific parameter by which the ventilator cycles are controlled.

Pressure-Controlled Ventilation

Pressure-controlled ventilation uses pressure as the main parameter to define inspiration. With pressure control the inspiratory phase ceases when a preset peak inspiratory pressure (PIP) is reached. Some ventilators, known as time-cycled ventilators, use a preset inspiratory time to determine inspiration but are pressure limited and thus classified as pressure ventilators. A variation of this, intermittent positive pressure ventilation using a time-cycled pressure limited continuous-flow ventilator, is currently the most common form of ventilation used in infants. The major advantage of pressure ventilation is that it allows careful control of PIP and mean airway pressure thereby avoiding barotrauma. The disadvantage is that tidal volume is a function of not only the difference between PIP and PEEP but also the inspiratory time and compliance. Consequently as lung compliance changes during the course of an illness, tidal volumes may change dramatically. Therefore use of pressure-cycled ventilators requires careful attention to the tidal volume being delivered at a given setting to avoid underventilation as compliance worsens or overdistention and barotrauma as compliance improves (see Fig. 7-5).

Volume-Controlled Ventilation

Volume-controlled ventilation uses a preset tidal volume to define inspiration. The major advantage of this type of ventilator is that a consistent tidal volume is delivered. However in reality, what is actually controlled is the volume of gas injected into the ventilator circuit not the volume of gas delivered into the patient's lungs. Humidification, compression of gas, distention of the compliant circuit, and the variable leak around an uncuffed endotracheal tube contribute to inaccurate control of delivered tidal volume. Frequently as the pathologic process progresses, adjustments in tidal volume and rate are necessary to maintain the desired minute ventilation and avoid high pressures and barotrauma. To avoid dangerously high PIPs most volume-cycled ventilators have a pressure-limit valve that prematurely interrupts inspiration when the preset limit is reached. Because this can lead to significant alveolar hyperventilation, a pressure-limit alarm sounds to alert the clinician that this is occurring. Volume-cycled ventilation is more commonly used in older children but can be used in infants.[104]

MODES OF VENTILATION

Modes of mechanical ventilation are classified on the basis of three factors: How is each breath initiated? How is gas flow controlled during breath delivery? How it is the breath ended? The mode indicates how the ventilator interfaces with the patient's own breathing efforts. Most pressure- and volume-cycled ventilators are capable of providing several modes, which vary from total control of ventilation to simple maintenance of PEEP without ventilatory assistance.

Control Mode

Total control is used when it is necessary to maintain complete control of the patient's ventilation.[79] Because the mechanisms for patient-triggered assist modes are disabled, it is generally necessary to paralyze and sedate the patient to eliminate asynchrony with the ventilator. The control mode is generally used when extremes of ventilation are necessary, such as very high minute ventilation requiring rapid respiratory rates.

Assist-Control Mode

Assist-control mode is similar to the control mode in that the variables of volume pressure and inspiratory time are preset. However the patient is allowed to override the preset respiratory rate with patient-triggered breaths, which are then completely supported by the ventilator. In the assist-control mode, each breath, whether the patient or the ventilator triggers it, is fully supported by the ventilator. This method may be advantageous if the goal is to reduce the work of breathing or disadvantageous in situations such as weaning, when exercise of the patient's respiratory muscles is desirable.[91] Another disadvantage is that in small infants with high respiratory rates, hyperventilation and asynchrony with the ventilator are common.

Intermittent Mandatory Ventilation

Intermittent mandatory ventilation (IMV) differs from the control and assist-control methods in that the ventilator controls are preset for mandatory inflations, but spontaneous unsupported ventilation is also allowed. The advantage of this method is that it allows exercise of the respiratory muscles. IMV is also an excellent weaning technique, and in infants with high respiratory rates it can avoid the hyperventilation seen with control modes. One disadvantage is the potential for asynchrony with the ventilator because a machine-driven inspiration may be stacked on top of a patient's spontaneous exhalation. This increases the work of breathing and may result in hypoventilation or even pneumothorax.[107]

Synchronized Intermittent Mandatory Ventilation

Synchronized IMV allows the mandatory ventilator-delivered breaths to be synchronized with the patient's spontaneous efforts. The obvious advantage of this mode is synchronization of breaths, which should reduce the work of breathing.[108] However spontaneous breaths in excess of the set rate are not supported, which results in uneven tidal volumes and a higher work of breathing during weaning. Other disadvantages relate to the sensitivity of the synchronizing mechanisms because a spontaneous inspiratory effort (usually identified by a change in airway pressure) that is not immediately responded to with a synchronous breath can actually increase the work of breathing.[91]

Pressure Support Ventilation

Pressure support ventilation (PSV) is a spontaneous mode of ventilation in which each breath is initiated by the patient but is supported by constant pressure inflation. This method has been shown to increase the efficiency of inspiration and decrease the work of breathing.[109,110] Like IMV, PSV is useful for weaning patients from mechanical ventilation. Unlike IMV, in which weaning involves decreasing the number of mandatory breaths with maintenance of inspiratory pressures, PSV involves steady decreases in the level of pressure support because the rate is controlled by the patient.

Continuous Positive Airway Pressure and Positive End-Expiratory Pressure

With continuous positive airway pressure (CPAP), a predetermined positive airway pressure is administered to the patient throughout the respiratory cycle.[111] The patient however is responsible for generating the tidal volume. This method increases the FRC and usually improves oxygenation by preventing atelectasis.[112] However this technique can increase the work of breathing.

Positive end-expiratory pressure (PEEP) provides continuous positive pressure throughout the ventilatory cycle, which can prevent atelectasis, increase FRC, and improve oxygenation. PEEP is commonly administered in the range of 2 to 10 cm/H_2O in neonates and 5 to 20 cm/H_2O in older children, although most ventilators can provide PEEP at significantly higher levels.

Inverse Ratio Ventilation

With inverse ratio ventilation, the inspiratory/expiratory time ratio is greater than 1 as opposed to the typical ratio of 1:2 to 1:5. It has been advocated for use in severe acute respiratory distress syndrome (ARDS) or acute lung injury to improve oxygenation while minimizing volutrauma or barotrauma.[1] This is because inverse ratio ventilation allows for increases in mean airway pressure without increases in tidal volume or PIP. Its use remains controversial; several small studies support its use but others report higher complication rates than with more conventional modes of ventilation.[113–117] However it should be considered when traditional modes of ventilation have failed to reverse hypoxemia despite high airway pressures.[118]

High-Frequency Ventilation

High-frequency ventilation (HFV) is defined as mechanical ventilation that uses a tidal volume less than or equal to dead space delivered at superphysiologic rates (>150 breaths per minute).[119] The potential advantages of HFV include smaller volume and pressure changes during the respiratory cycle, gas exchange at significantly lower pressures, and less depression of endogenous surfactant production. A large body of animal data suggests that ventilator-induced lung injury results from changes in pulmonary volume rather than from changes in pressure.[120] Large cyclic volume changes during conventional ventilation have been shown to disrupt the alveolar capillary interface, resulting in increased microvascular permeability and pulmonary interstitial edema.[121] This combination of fluid and protein in the interstitial and alveolar spaces results in surfactant inhibition, further reducing lung compliance. Conversely it has been shown that maintaining high lung volume with minimal changes in alveolar pressure or volume does not result in significant pulmonary injury.[122]

Several techniques of HFV exist. High-frequency positive-pressure ventilation is a modification of conventional pressure-limited ventilators, providing rates up to 150 breaths per minute.[123] High-frequency flow interrupters deliver high-pressure, short-duration breaths, with passive expiration.[40] High-frequency jet ventilators deliver short jet breaths at the distal end of the endotracheal tube; expiration is passive.[124] High-frequency oscillatory ventilation (HFOV) uses extremely small tidal volumes delivered at very high rates.[125,126] Unlike the other forms of HFV, the expiratory phase of oscillating ventilators is active.

The mechanism of gas exchange is poorly understood in HFV. With a tidal volume less than dead space volume, alveolar ventilation should equal zero, and the technique should not work. However the probable mechanisms are bulk axial flow, interregional gas mixing (pendelluft), and molecular diffusion.

Oxygenation is improved by recruiting or maintaining lung volume. Unlike conventional ventilation, which requires elevated peak pressure, mean lung volumes can be maintained with ventilation occurring around a relatively fixed intrapulmonary pressure.[127] Elimination of carbon dioxide is much more sensitive to changes in tidal volume than changes in rate.[128] Consequently when a lower P_{CO_2} is desired, it can be accomplished by reducing breathing frequency because the benefit of the increased volume output per stroke exceeds the detriment of decreasing the rate.

Currently there are two strategies for applying HFV. The high-volume strategy is designed for patients with atelectasis-prone lungs. The mean airway pressure is steadily increased in small increments while oxygenation is monitored. Risks of this approach include using inadequate pressure, thereby worsening atelectasis, or using excessive pressure, leading to injury and air leak.[129] The low-volume strategy is for patients with pneumothorax or air trapping.[130] A higher F_{IO_2} is frequently necessary with this strategy, and a higher Pa_{CO_2} (50 to 60 mm Hg) is frequently tolerated.

The initial clinical experience with HFOV (the most widely used HFV at present) was in premature infants with hyaline membrane disease.[131] That initial study did not show a particular benefit of HFV over conventional ventilation, but its methods have been criticized and its conclusions have not been corroborated by subsequent studies. Later studies of HFOV in neonates demonstrated a significant reduction in the incidence of chronic lung disease,[126] improvement in oxygenation, and reduction in the incidence of air-leak syndrome.[125] Several other studies have shown HFOV to be a reasonable alternative to extracorporeal membrane oxygenation (ECMO) for infants who meet ECMO criteria.[132,133]

Clinical data in older children are sparse; however, a series from Children's Hospital in Boston demonstrated that HFOV has some efficacy as a rescue therapy for pediatric patients who meet ECMO criteria.[134] In this study the high-volume strategy was used to rapidly attain and maintain optimal lung volume. A multicenter prospective randomized trial has since been completed, comparing HFOV with conventional mechanical ventilation in pediatric patients with diffuse alveolar disease or air-leak syndrome.[135] Those data showed that HFOV offered rapid and sustained improvements in oxygenation, and despite the use of higher mean airway pressures, a lower incidence of barotrauma was seen with HFOV than with conventional mechanical ventilation. However a 2009 Cochrane database analysis reported that although early observational studies and randomized studies did not show benefit of HFOV, important other changes in the practice of medicine including surfactant and inhaled nitric oxide (INO) might affect that and therefore recommended new prospective randomized controlled trials.

Extreme Modes of Gas Exchange

Extracorporeal Life Support Extracorporeal life support (ECLS) sits at the extreme end of the gas exchange spectrum. It supports or temporarily replaces the function of the heart or the lungs, or both, with an extracorporeal mechanical device. Further details and indications for its use are discussed in Chapter 8.

Intravascular Oxygenation Intravascular oxygenation involves an intracorporeal gas exchange device inserted into the inferior vena cava that functions similarly to the ECLS circuit. Space constraints in the inferior vena cava limit its use to a supportive role. This is discussed in greater detail in Chapter 8.

Extracorporeal Carbon Dioxide Removal Extracorporeal removal of carbon dioxide is similar to that in ECLS, but it is used when carbon dioxide elimination is the principal problem. This is discussed further in Chapter 8.

Liquid Ventilation Although the ability to provide gas exchange by means of a liquid medium was first demonstrated in the laboratory almost 30 years ago, liquid ventilation did not become a reality until 1990 when the first clinical evaluations were performed in moribund premature newborn infants with respiratory distress syndrome.[136] That study was the first to demonstrate that gas exchange could be supported clinically using a liquid medium. Since then additional clinical studies have been performed to assess the safety and efficacy of liquid ventilation in adults and children.[137–140]

To date the clinical trials of liquid ventilation have used perfluorocarbons as the liquid vehicle. Perfluorocarbons are clear, colorless, odorless fluids that have low surface tension and carry a large amount of oxygen and carbon dioxide. There are currently two methods of liquid ventilation: total liquid ventilation (TLV) and partial liquid ventilation (PLV). In TLV the lungs are completely filled with perfluorocarbon to FRC. Subsequently tidal volumes of additional perfluorocarbon are administered using a device similar to the ECMO circuit. The tidal volume of perfluorocarbon must pass through an external membrane oxygenator (where gas exchange occurs) before reentering the lungs. Because of the complexity of this process, to date TLV has been performed only in laboratory investigations. PLV in contrast is quite easy to perform and very similar to standard mechanical ventilation. In PLV the lungs are filled with the perfluorocarbon liquid to FRC. Tidal volume however is provided by a standard ventilator that uses gas.[138,141] The mixing of the liquid and the gas in the conducting airways of the lung allows the transfer of gases between the two mediums. Because of its ease of use, PLV has been used exclusively for all clinical trials to date.

The mechanism by which liquid ventilation improves gas exchange is probably a combination of a direct surfactant effect of the perfluorocarbon, resulting from its low surface tension, and a lavage effect that removes exudates in the peripheral airways. These two effects result in recruitment of atelectatic lung regions and better ventilation-perfusion matching.

After the initial clinical evaluation of perfluorocarbon liquid in newborns with respiratory distress, several other uncontrolled clinical studies were done in adults and children; these studies generally demonstrated improvement in pulmonary function with liquid ventilation.[137–139]

The only prospective randomized controlled trial of PLV in children was stopped prematurely; at the termination of the study the 28-day mortality rate was not significantly different between the control group and the PLV group.[142]

Investigational Adjuncts to Mechanical Ventilation

PRONE POSITIONING

Placing patients with ARDS in the prone position is purported to improve oxygenation by redistributing gravity-dependent blood flow into nonatelectic areas of nondependent lung by placing them in a dependent position. Several small series have demonstrated at least transient improvements in oxygenation,[39] whereas another failed to show significant improvements in ventilator-free days or survival. In addition this latter study noted significant complications with this technique.[143] Most recently a Cochrane database review determined that compared with the supine position, the prone position improved oxygenation, including desaturation episodes, when used for short periods or when patients were stable and in the process of weaning.[144] The value of this adjunct continues to be investigated.

INHALED NITRIC OXIDE

Nitric oxide is a potent short-acting pulmonary vasodilator that has been in clinical trial since the early 2000s. In neonates with primary pulmonary hypertension, it has been shown to improve oxygenation and decrease the use of ECLS. However despite a transient improvement in oxygenation, it has failed to improve ventilator weaning or survival in three large trials of patients with ARDS.[145,146]

In 2010 a Cochrane database report determined that there was insufficient evidence to support the use of INO in any category of ARDS in either adult or pediatric patients.[147] Despite these findings INO continues to be used widely in the pediatric and neonatal intensive care unit.

Pharmacologic Adjuncts in Acute Respiratory Distress Syndrome

Several pharmacologic adjuncts have been proposed for patients with ARDS, including prostaglandin E, acetylcysteine, high-dose corticosteroids, surfactant, and a variety of antioxidants. Unfortunately despite encouraging results from several small series, a recent meta-analysis of all published trials demonstrated no effect on early mortality and a greater number of adverse events in the active therapy arm in the prostaglandin, surfactant, and steroid trials.[148] Consequently none of these agents can be routinely recommended as adjunctive measures in the treatment of respiratory failure or ARDS at this time. Investigation continues.

Management of Respiratory Failure

The management of respiratory failure and infants and children is the subject of entire textbooks. Presented here will be the briefest of overviews. Respiratory failure is defined as inadequate oxygenation leading to hypoxemia or inadequate ventilation leading to hypercarbia. The first step in treating respiratory failure is to establish an adequate airway. Usually this is accomplished using an endotracheal tube, which can be placed either orally or nasally. However recent interest in noninvasive methods of respiratory support such as continuous positive airway pressure and bilevel positive airway pressure (BiPAP) occasionally allow mild respiratory distress or failure to be treated without intubation. If appropriate these methods can be evaluated first. The approximate internal diameter of the endotracheal tube can be estimated in children older than 2 years using the following formula:

$$\frac{16 + \text{age of child}}{4}$$

Traditionally in children older than 8 years, uncuffed tubes are often used, in which case there should be an air leak present when positive pressure between 20 and 30 cm H_2O is achieved. If properly cared for, these uncuffed tubes can be left in place for several weeks without fear of tracheal injury. Recently however softer cuffed tubes have become available and are used almost exclusively even in neonates in some units.

The goal of mechanical ventilation is to restore alveolar ventilation and oxygenation toward normal without causing injury from barotrauma or oxygen toxicity. In general this correlates to maintaining Pao_2 between 50 and 80 mm Hg, $Paco_2$ between 40 and 60 mm Hg, pH between 7.35 and 7.45, and mixed venous oxygen saturation at less than 70%.

Initial ventilator settings on pressure-cycled ventilators should be $FiO_2 = 100\%$, rate = 20 to 30 breaths per minute, PIP = 20 to 30 mm Hg, PEEP = 3 to 5 mm Hg, and inspiratory-expiratory ratio = 1:2. The aim is to provide an initial tidal volume of 6 to 8 mL/kg. PEEP should be used in cases of diffuse lung injury to support oxygenation. Support should be started at 2.0 cm H_2O and adjusted in increments of 1 to 2 cm H_2O. PEEP greater than 10.0 cm H_2O in infants and 15.0 cm H_2O in older children is rarely indicated. Sedation often enhances the response to mechanical support by allowing better synchrony between patient and machine. After the patient has been stabilized for a brief period, the ventilatory management must be individualized depending on the underlying physiologic condition.

MANIPULATING THE VENTILATOR SETTINGS

Various parameters can be preset on most ventilators, including the respiratory rate, PIP, PEEP, inspiratory time, and gas flow rate. When adjusting these parameters it is necessary to consider the pathologic condition present in the lung. Infants with primary pulmonary hypertension have very compliant lungs that are easily overdistended. In these patients adequate minute ventilation may be achieved with low PIP and PEEP, a short inspiratory time, and a moderate respiratory rate. Conversely a child with ARDS has noncompliant lungs and may require a relatively high PIP and PEEP, a short inspiratory time, and a high respiratory rate to achieve adequate alveolar ventilation. Obstructive disorders such as meconium aspiration syndrome and asthma have a longer time constant and require ventilation at a slower rate. After determining the initial settings, however, the patient's response must be evaluated and adjustments must be made to stay abreast of dynamic changes in pulmonary compliance and resistance that occur over time.

ADJUSTING THE PARTIAL PRESSURE OF CARBON DIOXIDE

The $Paco_2$ is directly related to alveolar ventilation and consequently to minute ventilation (tidal volume × respiratory rate). An increase in minute ventilation can be achieved by adjusting either tidal volume or more frequently respiratory rate. However at high rates or in lungs with prolonged time constants, increases in respiratory rate can lead to breath stacking, overdistention, reduced alveolar ventilation, and a subsequent rise in Pco_2.

ADJUSTING THE PARTIAL PRESSURE OF OXYGEN

In most conditions requiring mechanical ventilation, patchy atelectasis, caused by a drop in FRC toward closing capacity, results in a significant intrapulmonary shunt that is relatively insensitive to increases in FiO_2. Recruitment of the atelectatic areas by increasing the mean airway pressure is far more likely to be effective in increasing Pao_2. This can be achieved by increasing PIP, PEEP, or the inspiratory-expiratory ratio. High PIP has been shown to cause barotrauma, most likely as a result of overdistention of the more compliant (i.e., healthier) portions of the lung.[50] Consequently increases in PIP should be used sparingly. An increased PEEP is generally preferable to an increased PIP because the PEEP can recruit collapsed alveoli (by increasing FRC) thereby decreasing the intrapulmonary shunt without significant risk of barotrauma. However if a pressure-cycled ventilator is used, increases in PEEP without changes in PIP will result in a lower tidal volume and require adjustments in respiratory rate to maintain minute ventilation. Monitoring compliance also ensures that breaths are provided at the most compliant part of the ventilation curve.

WEANING

Weaning is the process during which mechanical ventilation is slowly withdrawn, allowing the patient to assume an increasing amount of the work of breathing. The specific technique of weaning depends on which form of ventilation is being used. Weaning from mechanical ventilation should be attempted only when the patient is hemodynamically stable on acceptable ventilator settings and is able to spontaneously maintain an acceptable $Paco_2$. In general this translates into an FiO_2 less than 0.4, PIP less than 30, PEEP less than 5, and ventilator-assisted breaths less than 15 per minute. The child should also have adequate nutrition and a ratio of dead space gas/tidal volume of less than 0.6 (normal = 0.3).

Weaning from IMV support involves a gradual decrease in the frequency of ventilator-delivered breaths. The rate of weaning depends on the patient's clinical condition and response. Monitoring the patient's spontaneous respiratory efforts and blood gas parameters can assist in this process. In older patients the IMV rate can be reduced to as low as 2 to 4 breaths per minute before the patient is extubated. Because of higher airway resistance in the smaller endotracheal tubes used in younger patients, extubation is generally attempted when the rate is reduced to 8 to 10 breaths per minute.

Weaning from PSV involves a slow decrease in the level of pressure support while monitoring the quality and quantity of the patient's spontaneous respiratory effort. In general this type of ventilation is withdrawn by reducing the pressure in increments of 1 to 2 cm H_2O.

WEANING FAILURE

Despite multiple indicators that predict successful weaning, 10% of patients will fail extubation. In most cases this failure is due to excessive respiratory load. This is manifested clinically as the development of rapid shallow breathing, worsening of lung mechanics, and increase in respiratory muscle load.[149,150] Factors that contribute to this are increased ratio of dead space gas/tidal volume, which accompanies the onset of rapid, shallow breathing; excessive carbon dioxide production caused by increased work of breathing; and, sometimes, excessive carbohydrate calories. Respiratory muscle fatigue due to increased respiratory load can cause prolonged (>24 hours) impairment in diaphragmatic and respiratory muscle function.[151] Consequently time must be allowed for recovery before attempting to wean again. Metabolic abnormalities such as acute respiratory acidosis decrease the contractility and endurance of the diaphragm.[152] Imbalances in phosphate, calcium, potassium, and magnesium also impair respiratory muscle function[153–155] as does hypothyroidism.[156] Correction of these variables toward normal ensures that the patient's best effort is being evaluated.

Complications of Mechanical Ventilation

Barotrauma is the principal complication of mechanical ventilation. It is caused by overdistention of alveoli by inappropriately high PIP or PEEP or excessive tidal volumes. The consequences of barotrauma include pneumothorax, pneumomediastinum, and pulmonary interstitial emphysema.[157] In addition, because barotrauma seems to be more closely related to volume changes than to pressure changes, the incidence and severity of barotrauma can potentially be lowered by the use of lower tidal volumes (5 to 7 mL/kg) and by accepting a lower pH and a higher P_{CO_2}—a ventilatory technique known as permissive hypercapnea.[158]

Oxygen toxicity is another complication of mechanical ventilation. The mechanism of injury is purported to be damage to the capillary endothelium, as well as type I and type II pneumocytes, from oxygen free radicals.[159] Every attempt should be made to maintain the F_IO_2 at less than 0.6 by adjusting mean airway pressure to improve intrapulmonary shunting and by accepting marginal levels of P_{O_2} (50 to 60 mm Hg) as long as S_{VO_2} remains adequate.

Bronchopulmonary dysplasia is a progressive chronic condition that may occur in 15% of infants who require mechanical ventilation. It is unclear whether the cause of this dysplasia is related to barotrauma or oxygen toxicity, or both. Consequently bronchopulmonary dysplasia can best be avoided by paying careful attention to providing adequate ventilatory support at the lowest possible pressures and oxygen concentration.

These complications are all a direct consequence of positive-pressure inflation of an organ designed to function in a negative-pressure environment. Consequently it is unlikely that any current or future variation of positive-pressure ventilation will ever be completely safe.

Other common complications not directly related to the mechanics of ventilation itself include nosocomial pneumonia acquired because of the ubiquitous nature of pathogens in the intensive care unit and breach of upper airway defenses by the endotracheal tube. Deep vein thrombosis and pulmonary emboli are not uncommon in older pediatric patients, and these patients should receive prophylaxis. Laryngeal trauma during intubation, tracheal stenosis caused by ill-fitting tubes and prolonged intubation, and sinusitis principally associated with nasal intubation round out the list of the more common complications. Most can be avoided or treated by careful attention to detail.

The complete reference list is available online at www.expertconsult.com.

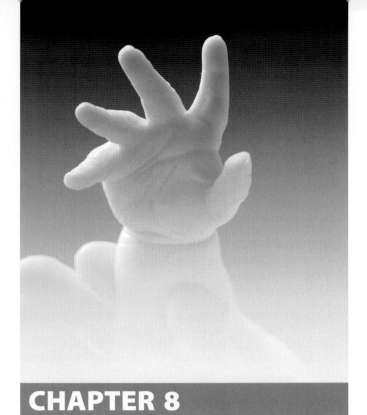

CHAPTER 8

Extracorporeal Life Support for Cardiopulmonary Failure

Ronald B. Hirschl and Robert H. Bartlett

Extracorporeal life support (ECLS) or extracorporeal membrane oxygenation (ECMO) denotes the use of prolonged extracorporeal cardiopulmonary bypass, usually through extrathoracic cannulation, in patients with acute reversible cardiac or respiratory failure who are unresponsive to conventional medical or pharmacologic management.[1,2] It is important to recognize that ECLS is not a therapeutic intervention; it simply provides cardiopulmonary support so that the patient is spared the deleterious effects of high airway pressure, high oxygen fraction in inspired air (FIO_2), vasoactive drugs, and perfusion impairment while reversible pathophysiologic processes are allowed to resolve either spontaneously or by medical or surgical intervention. The technology of ECLS is similar for all applications, but the indications, management, and results are best considered separately for adults, children, and neonates with either respiratory or cardiac failure. This chapter is limited to neonates and children with respiratory or cardiac failure.

In 1989 the active ECLS centers formed the Extracorporeal Life Support Organization (ELSO), which standardized many aspects of ECLS. ELSO maintains a registry of all cases treated by the member centers. Much of the information provided here is based on reports from the ELSO Registry.[3] As of January 2011 the ELSO Registry database reported 44,824 adult, pediatric, and newborn patients with cardiorespiratory failure who were supported with ECLS, with an overall 62% survival rate.[3,4]

Background

ECLS was first successfully applied in a newborn with respiratory failure in 1975.[5] By 1982 it had been used in 45 premature and full-term newborns with respiratory failure, demonstrating a survival of 55% and short-term normal growth and development in 80% of the survivors.[5-7] Three prospective, randomized trials compared the effectiveness of ECLS with that of conventional mechanical ventilation in full-term newborns with severe respiratory insufficiency. In 1985 our group used an adaptive design known as "play-the-winner," which weighted randomization toward the successful and away from the unsuccessful intervention.[8] The randomization scheme resulted in 11 patients who received ECLS and survived and 1 control patient who died. Although statistically significant in view of the 80% to 90% predicted mortality among the enrolled patients, this study was highly controversial and was not well accepted by the medical community. In 1989 O'Rourke and colleagues[9] conducted a randomized trial using a similar adaptive design. Survival in the control group was 6 of 10 patients (60%) and in the ECLS group 28 of 29 (97%) patients survived. A traditional randomized prospective study was performed in the United Kingdom that demonstrated a significant difference in survival between full-term newborns managed with ECLS (72%) and those managed by conventional means (41%).[10] Based on these studies ECLS is considered to be indicated in neonatal respiratory failure whenever the risk of mortality is high.[11] As of the beginning of 2011, 24,344 newborns had been managed with ECLS with a 75% survival rate.[3,12] Interestingly, the rate of use of ECLS in neonates has markedly decreased over the past two decades as newer ventilatory strategies have been developed and applied.

Timmons and associates[13] conducted a multicenter data collection study of pediatric respiratory failure in 1991. The only treatment variable that correlated with improved outcome was ECLS. This large database was further evaluated by Green and colleagues.[14] They did a matched-pair study of patients who were managed with ECLS (74% survival) compared with those managed by conventional means (53% survival). As of January 2011 there were 4771 cases of respiratory failure in children more than 30 days old in the registry, with an overall survival of 56%.

ECLS has been used successfully for pediatric cardiac failure since 1972. Intraoperative or postoperative cardiac failure is the most common indication, although preoperative use of ECLS is effective as a bridge to surgical palliation or anatomic repair.[15] In the past ECLS was the only mechanical support system available to support cardiac failure in children, but now ventricular assist devices such as the Berlin Heart (Berlin Heart AG, Berlin, Germany) are available, increasing in use, and may be associated with enhanced outcome.[16-18] The ELSO Registry documents 9453 cases of cardiac failure in newborns and children with an overall survival of 44%.

Indications

ECLS is indicated for acute severe respiratory or cardiac failure when recovery can be expected within 2 to 4 weeks. Severe cardiac or respiratory failure can be defined as any acute failure in which the mortality risk is greater than 50%; survival ranges from 50% to 90% in different categories of patients. In some cases the risk is easy to identify (e.g., cardiac arrest or inability to be removed from cardiopulmonary bypass in the operating room). In other cases it is more difficult to quantitate (e.g., a neonate with borderline oxygenation receiving 80% oxygen on moderate ventilatory settings with nitric oxide). Some scoring systems have been devised in these categories of patients to try to define high mortality risk:

1. Mortality risk in neonatal respiratory failure can be measured by an oxygen index (OI) that is based on arterial oxygenation (Pa_{O_2}) and mean airway pressure (MAP) despite and after all appropriate treatment. It is computed according to the following formula:

$$OI = (MAP \times F_{I}O_2 \times 100)/Pa_{O_2}$$

2. In the early ECLS studies an OI greater than 40 in three of five postductal arterial blood gas measurements (each drawn 30 to 60 minutes apart) was predictive of a mortality rate greater than 80%.[19,20] A randomized controlled study performed by our group suggested that "early" initiation of ECLS based on an OI greater than 25, which is predictive of a 50% mortality rate, is associated with a trend toward higher mental developmental scores and a lower incidence of morbidity at 1 year of age when compared with a control group of patients in whom ECLS was initiated at an OI greater than 40.[21] We currently consider institution of ECLS when a series of postductal arterial blood gas measurements demonstrates an OI greater than 25, with mandatory application of ECLS when the OI is greater than 40.

3. Criteria for high mortality risk among older children with respiratory failure are based on the OI or alveolar-arterial oxygen ($Pa_{O_2} - Pa_{O_2}$) gradient. Rivera and associates[22] suggest that a ventilation index (respiratory rate $\times$ Pa_{CO_2} $\times$ peak inspiratory pressure/1000) greater than 40 and an OI greater than 40 are associated with a mortality rate of 77%, and a combination of peak inspiratory pressure of 40 cm H_2O or greater and an $AaDO_2$ greater than 580 mm Hg are associated with a mortality of 81%. We consider $Pa_{O_2} - Pa_{O_2}$ greater than 600 on $F_{I}O_2$ 1.0—despite and after optimal treatment—an indication of high mortality risk in children.

4. Criteria for the initiation of ECLS in pediatric patients with cardiac failure include clinical signs of decreased peripheral perfusion, including oliguria (urine output <0.5 mL/kg per hour), metabolic acidosis, and hypotension despite the administration of inotropic agents and volume resuscitation.[23,24] ECLS is applied in pediatric cardiac patients in the setting of cardiogenic shock (20%), cardiac arrest (20%), and acute deterioration (10%); an additional 20% of patients are placed on ECLS directly in the operating room because of an inability to be weaned from heart-lung bypass.

Current relative contraindications for ECLS are as follows:

1. Prematurity. The lower limit for newborns is 1.5 kg and 30 weeks' gestational age because of a higher incidence of intracranial bleeding in smaller, younger infants.[25,26]

2. Pre-ECMO intracranial hemorrhage higher than grade 2.[27]

3. Prolonged mechanical ventilation. Mechanical ventilation for longer than 7 days in newborn and pediatric patients has been considered a contraindication to ECLS because of the high incidence of bronchopulmonary dysplasia and irreversible fibroproliferative pulmonary disease. However reviews of the ELSO Registry data suggest that the survival rate remains at approximately 50% to 60% after 14 days of pre-ECLS mechanical ventilation in neonatal and pediatric patients with respiratory failure.[28] We currently consider ECLS in any patient who has received mechanical ventilation for up to 14 days, keeping in mind that morbidity and mortality increase with time on the ventilator.

4. Cardiac arrest that requires cardiopulmonary resuscitation in the pre-ECLS period. This has been considered a contraindication to the institution of extracorporeal support. However survival rates of up to 60% have been observed among neonates who suffer cardiac arrest before or during cannulation.[12,29] Of those who survive at least 60% have a reasonable neurologic outcome. Similar survival rates (64%) without long-term sequelae were noted among pediatric patients with cardiac failure who endured cardiac arrest for 65 ± 9 minutes before the institution of ECLS.[30] Based on these data many centers now consider patients who sustain pre-ECLS cardiac arrest to be candidates for extracorporeal support.

5. Congenital diaphragmatic hernia (CDH) with severe pulmonary hypoplasia. Although CDH with severe pulmonary hypoplasia was originally a contraindication to ECLS,[31,32] it was subsequently demonstrated that a number of patients who met this exclusion criteria survived. Thus most centers now consider any patient with CDH a candidate for ECLS.[33–35] Other centers suggest that failure to generate a best preductal Pa_{O_2} greater than 100 mm Hg and a Pa_{CO_2} less than 50 mm Hg accurately identifies nonsalvageable newborns with CDH who should be excluded from ECLS.

6. Profound neurologic impairment, multiple congenital anomalies, or other conditions not compatible with meaningful life.

Additional relative contraindications for older children include the following:

1. Multiorgan system failure: In general organ system failure other than cardiac, pulmonary, and renal failure, which can be effectively supported with ECLS, are considered contraindications.

2. Major burns: Although thermal injury was previously considered a contraindication, ECLS has been applied in pediatric burn patients (mean of 46% of total body surface area burned), with survival in three of five patients.[36,37]

3. Immunodeficiency: Conditions associated with compromise of the immune system in the past have been considered contraindications to ECLS. Data from the ELSO Registry suggest however that survival is 31% with ECLS in pediatric patients with a diagnosis associated with immunocompromise although specific diagnoses such as bone marrow transplantation carry a poor outcome.[38]

4. Active bleeding.

5. An incurable disease process.

Methods of Extracorporeal Support

The goal of ECLS is to perfuse warmed arterialized blood into the patient.[1] To achieve this goal the extracorporeal blood flow is used most commonly in venoarterial (VA) mode for cardiac support and venovenous (VV) mode for respiratory support. VA mode provides complete support, but there are significant disadvantages: (1) a major artery must be cannulated and at least temporarily sacrificed, (2) the risk of dissemination of particulate or gaseous emboli into the systemic circulation is substantial, (3) pulmonary perfusion may be markedly reduced, (4) left ventricular output may be compromised owing to the presence of increased ECLS circuit-induced afterload resistance, and (5) the coronary arteries are perfused predominantly by the relatively hypoxic left ventricular blood.[37] VV access, either by two vessels or by a single vessel through a double-lumen catheter, supports gas exchange without the disadvantages of VA support. VV or double-lumen VV ECLS is now the preferred method for patients of all age groups who do not require cardiac support (Fig. 8-1).[39] Data from the ELSO Registry and a nonrandomized multicenter study suggest that bypass performed with the double-lumen VV configuration may increase the survival rate and reduce the incidence of intracranial hemorrhage in neonates.[40] However a matched-pairs analysis that corrected for pre-ECLS severity of cardiopulmonary dysfunction revealed no difference in either parameter between patients undergoing bypass with a double-lumen VV or a VA configuration.[32] Femoral and jugular cannulation is used for most children, although recent availability of the Avalon double-lumen cannulas (Avalon Laboratories, LLC, Rancho Dominguez, Calif.) from 13 to 31 French has broadened the use of double-lumen VV ECLS.

Arteriovenous support, typically through cannulation of the femoral artery and vein, is being applied for arteriovenous carbon dioxide removal (AVCO2R). This technique has been shown to be reduce $Paco_2$ and ventilatory requirements in adults with acute respiratory distress syndrome (ARDS) and children with asthma.[41,42]

Extracorporeal Life Support Circuit

The ECLS circuit comprises a pump, a membrane lung, and a heat exchanger (Fig. 8-2), as well as other devices associated with safety and monitoring functions. A full description of the technology, including device function and malfunction, is published in the ELSO's textbook.[43] Right atrial blood is drained by gravity siphon by a cannula placed through the right internal jugular or right femoral vein. Roller pumps are the most common perfusion devices used and require continuous servoregulation and monitoring to prevent the application of high levels of negative pressure to the drainage circuit and high levels of positive pressure, with a risk of circuit disruption, to the infusion limb of the circuit if occlusion occurs.[44] Application of high negative pressures to the drainage circuit (e.g., with a centrifugal

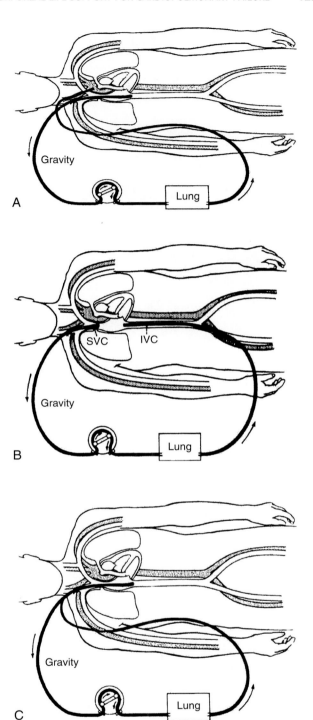

FIGURE 8-1 Three most common extracorporeal bypass configurations. **A,** Venoarterial configuration with drainage from the internal jugular vein and reinfusion into the carotid artery. **B,** Venovenous configuration with drainage from the internal jugular vein and reinfusion into the femoral vein. **C,** Venovenous configuration with a double-lumen cannula placed into the internal jugular vein. IVC, inferior vena cava; SVC, superior vena cava.

pump) results in hemolysis, damage to the endothelium of the right atrium or vena cava, and cavitation as air is drawn out of solution.

The artificial lung most commonly used is the Kolobow spiral coil (Medtronic, Minneapolis, Minn.) solid silicone

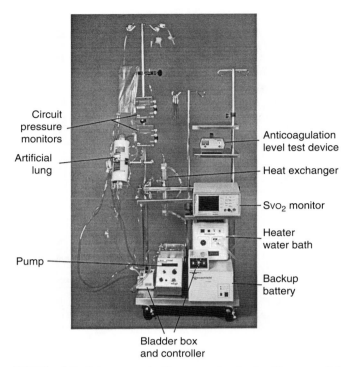

Circuit pressure monitors

Artificial lung

Pump

Anticoagulation level test device

Heat exchanger

Svo$_2$ monitor

Heater water bath

Backup battery

Bladder box and controller

FIGURE 8-2 Extracorporeal life support circuit. The essential components include the roller pump, the membrane lung, and the heat exchanger. The remainder of the devices shown perform monitoring and safety functions.

rubber membrane lung.[45] The size of the various ECLS components required as a function of patient weight is shown in Table 8-1. Hollow-fiber artificial lungs made of microporous materials are highly efficient with regard to gas exchange, have low resistance to blood flow, and are easy to prime. The disadvantage of the microporous membrane is the increased rate of condensation of water in the gas phase and the frequent need for replacement owing to the development of plasma leak.[46] Phospholipid adsorption onto the blood surface of the hollow fiber at the site of 5-μm pores is the mechanism by which the plasma leak occurs.[46] Artificial

lungs with hollow fibers that do not have pores resolve this problem and are preferred for ECLS. These devices have been used in Europe and Japan but are not available in the United States. Plasma leak is retarded in artificial lungs that use polymethylpentene fibers; such artificial lungs are being used more frequently in the United States and other parts of the world.[44]

The volume of the neonatal circuit is approximately 400 to 500 mL, which is one to two times the newborn blood volume. The circuit must therefore be primed carefully to perfuse the neonate at the onset of bypass with blood containing the appropriate pH, hematocrit, calcium, clotting factors, and electrolytes and at the appropriate temperature. However, as shown in Table 8-1, ECLS may be instituted in patients weighing more than 35 kg without the addition of blood to the priming solution.

Patient Management

Patient management is described in detail in the ELSO textbook.[43] The size of the venous cannula is the factor that determines the blood flow rate and therefore the level of extracorporeal support. The largest possible venous access cannula should be used; it should be of sufficient size to provide adequate blood flow (~100 mL/kg per minute) with the assistance of 100-cm H$_2$O gravity siphon pressure. The flow-pressure characteristics of a given cannula are determined by a number of geometric factors, including length, internal diameter, and side hole placement. The M number provides a standardized means for describing the flow-pressure relationships in a variety of vascular access devices.[47,48]

The first choice for venous access is the internal jugular vein because it is large and provides easy access to the right atrium through a short cannula. The femoral vein is the second choice for venous drainage access during ECLS and the first choice for drainage during VV support. In children younger than 5 years, the femoral vein is too small to function as the primary drainage site, and VV access is used in a jugular-to-femoral fashion or using a double-lumen VV cannula in young children. A proximal venous drainage cannula can be placed in the proximal internal jugular vein to enhance venous

TABLE 8-1

Circuit Components and Prime for Patients of Different Sizes Receiving Venovenous Support

	Weight (kg)					
	2-4	**4-15**	**15-20**	**20-30**	**30-50**	**50+**
Drainage tubing (in)	¼	¼	⅜	⅜	½	½
Raceway (in)	¼	¼	⅜-½	½	½	½
Oxygenator (m^2)	0.8-1.5	0.8-1.5	2.5-3.5	3.5-4.5	4.5	4.5 × 2
Cannulas* (French)	12-15	13-20	Inf: 16-19	Inf: 17-21	Inf: 21	Inf: 21
	DLVV†	DLVV†	Dr: 14-19	Dr: 17-21	Dr: 19-23‡	Dr: 21-23‡
Prime	RBC: 1-2 U	RBC: 1-2 U	RBC: 3 U	RBC: 4 U	RBC: 4 U§	RBC: 5 U§
	FFP: 50-100 mL	FFP: 50-100 mL	FFP: ½ U	FFP: 1 U	FFP:1 U	FFP: 1 U

*All cannulas are the shortest Biomedicus cannula available in the specified size. These are only guidelines, and individual patient variables must be considered.
†12 and 15 Fr DLVV cannulas are manufactured by Jostra. The 14 Fr DLVV cannula is manufactured by Kendall. Cannulas 13 to 31 Fr are manufactured by Avalon.
‡The M-number (2.4) of the 23 Fr Biomedicus (38 cm) custom cannula is nearly the same as that of the 29 Fr Biomedicus (50 cm) cannula.
§Normosol (3 L) with 12.5 g albumin and 1 g CaCl is usually used.
DLVV, double-lumen venovenous; Dr, drainage; ECLS, extracorporeal life support; FFP, fresh frozen plasma; Inf, infusion; NA, not applicable; RBC, red blood cells; U, units.

drainage to the extracorporeal circuit.[49] One study demonstrated a reduction in intracranial hemorrhage after initiation of the use of such a cannula when compared with historical controls.[50] An ELSO Registry study however failed to demonstrate an effect on intracranial hemorrhage or survival during routine use of a proximal venous drainage cannula. (F. L. Fazzalari, R. B. Hirschl, T. Delosh, R. H. Bartlett, oral communication, 1994).

The size of the reinfusion cannula is less critical than that of the venous drainage cannula, although it must be large enough to tolerate the predicted blood flow rate at levels of total support without generating a pressure greater than 350 mm Hg proximal to the membrane lung. When only respiratory support is required, the reinfusion cannula may be placed into the femoral vein to provide VV support. Rich and associates[52] demonstrated advantages in terms of reduced blood recirculation and overall oxygenation when the femoral cannula was used for drainage and the internal jugular cannula was used for reinfusion. When cardiovascular support is required, the first choice for placement of a cannula into the arterial circulation is the carotid artery in all age groups because it provides easy access to the aortic arch. Few complications have been associated with carotid artery cannulation and ligation in newborns and children.[53,54] The second choice for arterial access is the femoral artery. Distal perfusion of the lower extremity arterial circulation may be required when the femoral artery is cannulated and may be achieved through antegrade perfusion of the common femoral artery or retrograde perfusion of the posterior tibial artery.[55] However arch perfusion and oxygenation, and therefore heart and brain circulation, are poorly achieved with femoral artery reinfusion. This may be overcome and carotid artery cannulation-ligation avoided using the technique of venoarterial-venous (VAV) ECLS in which a drainage cannula is placed into the femoral vein and reinfusion cannulas into the femoral artery and internal jugular vein. Reinfusion into the femoral artery is limited to that required to maintain blood pressure, thus allowing a substantial portion of arterialized blood to reinfuse through the internal jugular vein, providing oxygenation of the blood perfusing the aortic arch.

The cannulation procedure is usually performed by direct cutdown using local anesthesia (Fig. 8-3). The tips of the arterial and venous cannulas (see Table 8-1 for sizes) are optimally located at the opening of the right brachiocephalic artery and the inferior aspect of the right atrium, respectively. The double-lumen VV cannula must be placed so that the tip is in the midright atrium, with the reinfusion ports oriented toward the tricuspid valve to minimize recirculation of reinfused blood. Percutaneous access to the internal jugular and femoral veins is the routine and preferred approach to cannulation in adults and children older than 3 years. Sequentially larger dilators are placed over a wire, and a Seldinger technique allows final access of the cannula itself into these large veins. A 12 or 15 French double-lumen VV cannula is amenable to percutaneous introduction into the internal jugular vein in neonates. The Avalon cannula can be placed by a percutaneous approach in patients of all ages. This cannula has distal and proximal drainage ports with a midcannula reinfusion lumen. As such the cannula design is intended for placement of the distal tip into the inferior vena cava with the reinfusion lumen opening positioned at the level of the tricuspid valve.

The cannulas are connected to the ECLS circuit and cardiopulmonary bypass is initiated. Flow is increased over

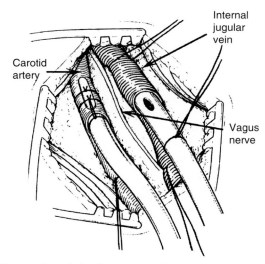

FIGURE 8-3 Cannulation for venoarterial extracorporeal support. The transverse right supraclavicular incision is shown. In neonates the cannulas are placed 2.5 cm into the artery and 6.0 cm into the vein. They are secured using two circumferential 2-0 silk ligatures with a small piece of plastic vessel loop placed underneath to protect the vessels from injury during decannulation. One of the ends of the marking ligature is tied to the most distal circumferential suture for extra security.

the ensuing 10 to 15 minutes to levels of approximately 100 mL/kg. Once a patient is receiving extracorporeal support there is typically rapid cardiopulmonary stabilization. All paralyzing agents, vasoactive drugs, and other infusions are discontinued during VA support; some pressor or inotropic support may be necessary when VV bypass is used.[39] Ventilator settings are adjusted to minimal levels (peak inspiratory pressure <25 and FiO_2 <0.4) to allow the lung to rest and any air leaks secondary to barotrauma to seal.[1] Application of positive end-expiratory pressure in the range of 12 to 14 cm H_2O during the course on extracorporeal support has been demonstrated to decrease the duration of ECLS from 132 ± 55 hours to 97 ± 36 hours.[56] Because only partial bypass is used, oxygenation and carbon dioxide elimination are determined by a combination of native pulmonary function and extracorporeal flow. The mixed venous oxygen saturation (SvO_2) is conveniently monitored by a fiberoptic Oximetrix catheter placed in the venous limb of the circuit, which allows one to determine the adequacy of oxygen delivery in relation to oxygen consumption, especially during VA ECLS. Pump flow is adjusted to maintain oxygen delivery so that the SvO_2 is greater than 70% during VA support and, because of the effects of reinfusion into the venous system, greater than 85% during VV support. The $PaCO_2$ is inversely proportional to the flow rate of gas ventilating the membrane lung.

Cannulation for Cardiac Support

Deterioration in myocardial function is observed in approximately 7% of neonates after initiation of ECLS.[57-59] This "myocardial stun" usually occurs in patients with exaggerated levels of hypoxia, with more frequent episodes of cardiac arrest, and who required more frequent epinephrine pressor support before ECLS. It typically resolves over the first 24 to 48 hours after initiation of ECLS.

If the left ventricle does not eject (no arterial pulse contour), the left ventricle and atrium will distend and cause pulmonary edema. If this occurs balloon or blade atrial septostomy may be required to decompress the left oximetry and allow the resolution of pulmonary edema and eventual improvement in cardiac function.[60]

Heparin is titrated to prevent thrombus formation throughout the course of ECLS. The level of anticoagulation is monitored hourly by the whole-blood activated clotting time (ACT).[1,2] The ACT is maintained at 50% to 60% above normal (180–220 seconds for the Hemochron device [ITC, Edison, NJ]).[61] Transfusion of red blood cells to maintain the hematocrit at greater than 45% and fresh frozen plasma to maintain the fibrinogen levels at greater than 200 mg/dL are frequently required. Platelets are transfused to maintain the platelet count at greater than 100,000/mm^3, although the decrease in platelet function and count associated with extracorporeal support appears to be only transiently corrected by platelet administration.[62] Stallion and colleagues[63] suggested that maintaining the platelet count at greater than 200,000/mm^3 appears to be associated with a decrease in bleeding complications. We continue to maintain the platelet count at greater than 100,000/mm^3, except in patients who are at high risk for or have ongoing hemorrhage, in which case the platelet count is maintained at greater than 150,000/mm^3.

Diuresis or hemofiltration is titrated to normal "dry" weight. Renal function may be transiently impaired during ECLS; therefore use of a hemofilter placed in the circuit to supplement urine output may be necessary in some patients.[64,65] Routine use of a hemofilter may reduce time on ECLS and mechanical ventilation.[66] Renal insufficiency that develops before or during ECLS can also be easily managed by a hemofilter or continuous renal replacement therapy placed in the extracorporeal circuit as necessary.[67] Nutrition remains a high priority in a critically ill patient requiring ECLS.

Most operative procedures performed during ECLS are carried out in the intensive care unit, although as comfort with ECMO transport increases, travel to the operating or cardiac catheterization suite is becoming more routine.[68] Either isoflurane gas anesthesia administered through the oxygenator of the ECLS circuit or intravenous anesthesia with fentanyl or sufentanil and vecuronium may be used. Nagaraj and associates[69] described 44 procedures performed in 37 neonates receiving ECLS. These procedures consisted of recannulation or repositioning of cannulas (14), tube thoracostomy (11), cardiac surgery (6), cardiac catheterization (4), repair of CDH (5), and thoracotomy (4). Hemorrhagic complications, which occurred in 46% to 55% of patients, were associated with a higher mortality. Therefore one should strongly consider whether the procedure is necessary (e.g., placement of thoracostomy tubes for small pneumothoraces) or whether the operation can be delayed until ECLS is discontinued. During procedures performed while the patient is receiving ECLS, electrocautery should be used generously, the ACT reduced to a maximum of 160 to 180 seconds, and the platelet count maintained at greater than 150,000/mm^3. One should also consider perioperative administration of aminocaproic acid (Amicar).[70]

Repair of CDH can be done before, during, or after ECLS. Practice changed when we realized that pulmonary dysfunction is caused by hypoplasia and vasospasm and not the

hernia. Connors and colleagues[71] first described the repair of CDH in six newborns at a mean of 25 hours after initiation of ECLS, with four survivors. Lally and coworkers[72] reported a 43% survival rate among 42 newborns undergoing diaphragmatic hernia repair while receiving extracorporeal support. Vazquez and Cheu[73] reported that up to 48% of patients with CDH who require ECLS undergo repair while receiving extracorporeal support. Other studies suggest that operative repair in a newborn with CDH can be performed after discontinuation of ECLS, continued resolution of pulmonary hypertension, and ventilator weaning. Based on data from the ELSO Registry, Vazquez and Cheu[73] demonstrated that surgical hemorrhage requiring transfusion occurred in 38% of CDH repaired while the patient was receiving ECLS versus 18% and 6% of those repaired before and after, respectively. Wilson and coworkers[70,74] observed a reduction in blood loss and transfusion requirement in a group of 22 patients receiving ECLS in whom repair was performed electively before decannulation. In these patients the ACT was maintained at the 180- to 200-second level, and aminocaproic acid was administered continuously for 72 hours postoperatively or until decannulation in all patients. Reexploration for hemorrhage was not required.[75] Bryner and associates[75] suggested that survival is enhanced when repair is performed following discontinuation of ECLS. In general our current practice is to repair the hernia after weaning the patient from ECLS, although there is a trend across the United States toward early repair while the patient is receiving ECLS.

When pulmonary function improves, ECLS flow is decreased, leading to a "trial off" (without ECLS). During VV bypass, the gas phase of the membrane lung can simply be capped indefinitely so that the patient remains on extracorporeal blood flow but without the artificial lung's contribution to gas exchange. Patients receiving VA bypass are tested by clamping the lines (no flow). Such trials are performed on a daily basis when cardiopulmonary physiology suggests improvement with optimal pressor support and are frequently accompanied by echocardiographic evaluation in patients with cardiopulmonary compromise.

Once it has been determined that ECLS can be discontinued, the cannulation site incisions are opened and the right carotid artery or internal jugular vein, or both, are ligated. The carotid artery can be repaired after a course of VA extracorporeal support, although there is no proven benefit and there is the potential risk of distal embolism, late stenosis or thrombosis, and development of atherosclerosis.[14,49,76,77] The internal jugular vein can be repaired as well, especially in patients with congenital heart disease who will require future percutaneous access.[78] A central line or Broviac catheter may be placed into the vein during decannulation with a surprisingly low risk of infection.[79] Percutaneously placed cannulas can simply be removed and pressure applied without concern about the patient's anticoagulation status. The femoral artery, if used, is repaired and the femoral vein is ligated.

The duration of ECLS (mean ± standard deviation) is 170 ± 126 hours for neonates with respiratory failure, 260 ± 224 hours for children with respiratory failure, and 151 ± 140 hours for patients with heart failure. Reasons to discontinue extracorporeal support other than when indicated by improvement of cardiopulmonary function include the presence of irreversible brain damage, other lethal organ failure, and uncontrollable bleeding. Neonates with CDH or pneumonia and pediatric patients with cardiac or pulmonary failure may require substantially longer periods on ECLS before resolution of the cardiopulmonary process is observed. On occasion a second course of ECLS is required and results in survival rates of 44% in children.[80]

Complications

In general the complications associated with ECLS fall into one of three major categories: (1) bleeding associated with heparinization, (2) technical failure, and (3) neurologic sequelae, a majority of which are secondary to the hypoxia and hemodynamic instability that occur before the onset of extracorporeal support.

The average number of patient complications per ECLS case is 2.1.[81] Because of systemic heparinization, bleeding complications are the most common and devastating.[82] Intracranial hemorrhage occurs in approximately 13% of neonates, 5% of pediatric patients, and 4% of cardiac patients. It is the most frequent cause of death in newborns managed with ECLS.[83] Because of the associated heparinization, intracranial hemorrhage may be unusual in terms of both extent and location.[84,85] The mechanism by which it occurs in newborns receiving ECLS is multifactorial. In addition to heparin administration, platelet function and number are decreased for up to 48 hours after discontinuation of ECLS, as are coagulation factor levels.[86] Wilson and colleagues[77] noted a reduction in the incidence of intracranial hemorrhage, compared with historical controls, among a cohort of 42 newborns considered to be at high risk for bleeding complications who received 100 mg/kg of aminocaproic acid just before or after cannulation, followed by a continuous infusion of 30 mg/kg per hour until decannulation. The incidence of intracranial hemorrhage is clearly increased in patients who are premature, especially those less than 37 weeks' gestational age. Although carotid ligation and institution of ECLS in normal animals do not affect carotid artery or cerebral blood flow, initiation of ECLS in the setting of hypoxia results in augmentation of carotid artery and cerebral blood flow and loss of cerebral autoregulation.[87] In addition, decreases in Pa_{CO_2} result in marked decreases in cerebral blood flow.[88] Therefore carotid artery and internal jugular vein ligation along with rapid institution of ECLS in the setting of hypoxia or hypercarbia may result in alterations in cerebral blood flow and cerebral autoregulation, with the potential induction of intracranial hemorrhage in a patient who has undergone anticoagulation.

Bleeding at extracranial sites is observed in 21% of neonatal patients, 44% of pediatric respiratory patients, and 40% of neonatal and pediatric cardiac patients. These sites of bleeding include gastrointestinal hemorrhage (2% to 5%), cannulation site bleeding (up to 6%), bleeding at another surgical site (neonatal respiratory patients, 6%; pediatric respiratory patients, 24%, neonatal and pediatric cardiac patients, 28%), and a miscellaneous group of bleeding sites, including pericardial, intrathoracic, and retroperitoneal (7% to 15%). Bleeding during ECLS is managed by maintaining the platelet count at greater than 150,000/mm³ and decreasing the ACT to a maximum of 160 to 180 seconds. Occasionally discontinuation of heparin or, if tolerated, temporary discontinuation of

bypass with normalization of the coagulation status may be necessary to achieve resolution of the bleeding.[89] If hemorrhage persists, aggressive surgical intervention is indicated. Administration of recombinant factor seven may be effective when nonsurgical bleeding is present, although thrombotic complications, including development of ECLS circuit or systemic arterial clots, is a concern.[90–94] We have found that intra-abdominal or intrathoracic packing with planned daily reexploration allows control of hemorrhage in most situations. Only in extreme circumstances should permanent discontinuation of bypass be considered in a patient with persistent cardiopulmonary failure. Heparin-induced thrombocytopenia occurs occasionally and argatroban or lepirudin may be used to provide systemic anticoagulation.[95,96]

Neurologic injury induced either before or after the onset of ECLS is a constant concern. Many neonates must endure the insult of hypoxia or ischemia before the institution of bypass and it has been suggested that ligation of the carotid artery in the minutes before the onset of ECLS, at a time when hypoxemia and hemodynamic instability are maximized, results in a further decrease in cerebral tissue oxygenation, which in turn might exacerbate the neurologic injury.[97] However Streletz and colleagues[98] noted no increase in the electroencephalographic abnormalities present before and during ECLS among 145 neonates. In addition Walsh-Sukys and associates[99] in a prospective evaluation of 26 neonates managed with conventional mechanical ventilation and 43 neonates managed with ECLS, noted a similar 25% rate of neurodevelopmental impairment in both groups at 8 to 20 months of age. The incidence of any neurodevelopmental impairment at 1 year of age was 28% among survivors of both groups in the United Kingdom neonatal randomized study.[10]

Seizures have been noted in 10% to 13% of patients undergoing ECLS.[100] The presence of seizures in newborns during ECLS portends a poor prognosis: 50% to 65% with electrographic seizures during ECLS either died or were developmentally delayed at 1 to 2 years of age.

Hemolysis (serum hemoglobin >100 mg/dL) occurs in 6% to 12% of patients. This complication is likely due to red blood cell trauma during extracorporeal support, which is often related to clot formation within the circuit or overocclusion of the roller pump. Centrifugal pumps have been associated in the past with development of hemolysis over time, likely caused by heat generation.[101] Newer generation magnetically levitated centrifugal pumps, which are magnetically suspended and therefore associated with minimal friction, can be used without major concerns about hemolysis generation. Hyperbilirubinemia is noted in 8% of patients and renal insufficiency in 10%. Pneumothorax (occurring in 4% to 14%) and pericardial tamponade are life-threatening intrathoracic complications that manifest with increasing Pa_{O_2} and decreasing peripheral perfusion and Sv_{O_2}, followed by decreasing ECLS flow and progressive deterioration. Initial emergent placement of a pleural or pericardial drainage catheter, followed by thoracotomy for definitive treatment of a pericardial tamponade, may be lifesaving.

Technical complications occurred in 15% of the neonatal and pediatric cases reported to the ELSO Registry.[102] The average number of mechanical complications per ECLS case was 0.71.[102] The most notable technical complications include the presence of thrombus in the circuit (26%), cannula problems (10%), oxygenator failure (9%), pump malfunction

TABLE 8-2

Extracorporeal Life Support Organization Registry: Summary Data on Neonatal Respiratory Failure Cases Managed with Extracorporeal Life Support (as of January 2011)

Primary Diagnosis	Number of Patients	Number Survived	Percent Survived
Congenital diaphragmatic hernia	6147	3139	51
Meconium aspiration syndrome	7743	7255	94
Persistent pulmonary hypertension of the newborn/persistent fetal circulation	4043	3134	78
Respiratory distress syndrome/hyaline membrane disease	1496	1263	84
Sepsis	2635	1967	75
Other	2606	1639	75
Total	24,670	18,397	75

TABLE 8-3

Pediatric Respiratory Failure Cases Managed with Extracorporeal Life Support at the University of Michigan between November 1982 and January 2011

Primary Diagnosis	Number of Patients	Number Survived	Percent Survived
Viral pneumonia	56	47	84
Bacterial pneumonia or sepsis	29	21	72
Aspiration	14	11	79
Trauma	7	7	100
Acute respiratory failure	57	34	60
ARDS	23	19	83
Other	76	59	78
Total	255	191	75

(2%%), and presence of air in the circuit (4%). The effect of technical complications on survival was not substantial, although there was a significant decrease among neonatal patients, from 84% without technical complications to 80% with them.

Results and Follow-Up

A total of 44,824 cases have been reported to the ELSO Registry since 1975.[3,103] Of these, there have been 24,344 cases of neonatal respiratory failure, 4771 cases of pediatric respiratory failure, and 4232 cases of newborn cardiac failure, and 5221 of pediatric cardiac failure. The number and diagnosis of neonatal respiratory failure survivors are given in Table 8-2. Overall survival is 75%, with the best survival noted among neonatal patients with the diagnoses of meconium aspiration syndrome (94% survival), respiratory distress syndrome (84%), and persistent pulmonary hypertension of the newborn (78%). Patients with CDH continue to have the poorest survival among those who receive ECLS, likely because of the "irreversible" pulmonary hypoplasia associated with that condition. In fact the survival rate in patients with CDH who require ECLS has fallen from a high of 71% in 1987 to the current rate of 51%. The total number of neonatal respiratory ECLS cases peaked in 1992 with 1516 cases. There was a trend downward in the total number of neonatal cases to a low of 707 in 2009 owing to improved results with neonatal respiratory management, including the use of nitric oxide and high-frequency oscillatory ventilation.[3]

The experience with pediatric patients with respiratory failure who were managed with ECLS at the University of Michigan is shown in Table 8-3 and demonstrates an overall survival rate of 75% since 1982.[3,104] Patients in the younger age groups demonstrate greater survival rates, including 100% survival in infants younger than 1 year of age. The ELSO Registry demonstrates that pediatric respiratory cases are accumulating at a rate of 200 to 300 per year, with an overall survival rate of 56% (Table 8-4).[3] One of the most frequent diagnoses is viral pneumonia, which is dominated by respiratory syncytial virus, an entity associated with 49% to 58% survival.[23,105]

TABLE 8-4

Extracorporeal Life Support Organization Registry: Summary Data on Pediatric Respiratory Failure Cases Managed with Extracorporeal Life Support (as of January 2011)

Primary Diagnosis	Number of Patients	Number Survived	Percent Survived
Bacterial pneumonia	533	303	57
Viral pneumonia	989	623	63
Aspiration	205	136	66
Pneumocystis	30	15	50
Acute respiratory failure	817	417	51
ARDS	523	286	55
Other	1761	912	52
Total	4858	2692	55

ARDS, acute respiratory distress syndrome.

Other studies from individual centers also suggest that the survival rate of pediatric patients with respiratory failure managed with ECLS is 41% to 53%.[74,106] An approximately 50% survival rate is noted in pediatric patients with multiorgan system failure and in those with overwhelming septic shock who are managed with ECLS.[107] Green and colleagues,[108] analyzing data from the ELSO Registry, demonstrated that the survival rate in pediatric patients with respiratory failure who receive ECLS for longer than 2 weeks was similar to the survival rate of patients supported for shorter periods. However judgment must be used regarding the reversible nature of the respiratory dysfunction, the presence of associated organ system failure, and the development of complications associated with ECLS in determining whether continuation is warranted after prolonged periods on ECLS.

The ELSO Registry results for cardiac support cases are summarized in Table 8-5.[3] The number of pediatric cardiac cases reported to the registry is increasing steadily and currently is approximately 600 to 750 cases each year, the vast majority of which are pediatric cardiac surgical cases.[3]

TABLE 8-5

Extracorporeal Life Support Organization Registry: Summary Data on Cardiac Failure Cases (Children Aged 1 Day to 16 Years) Managed with Extracorporeal Life Support (as of January 2011)

Primary Diagnosis	Number of ECLS Runs	Number Survived	Percent Survived
Congenital defect	7243	2959	41
Cardiac arrest	221	82	37
Myocarditis	306	199	65
Cardiomyopathy	628	375	60
Cardiogenic shock	178	77	43
Other	1273	602	47
Total	9849	4294	44

The overall survival is 41%. Almost all patients are managed with VA bypass. The survival rate has been thought to be poor (0% to 25%) in patients with an anomaly that consists of a single ventricle, but Allan and colleagues[109,110] demonstrated a survival to discharge of 48% in patients with shunted single-ventricle physiology and 81% in patients who underwent cannulation for hypoxemia as opposed to hypotension-cardiovascular collapse. Although Ziomek and coworkers[111] demonstrated a 47% survival among 17 patients in whom ECLS was initiated in the operating room, other studies suggest a poor outcome when ECLS is initiated in the operating room, at a point more than 50 hours after operation, or when continued for more than 6 to 9 days.[111] Data from numerous centers demonstrate a survival rate ranging from 46% to 53%,[112,113] with Klein and colleagues[114] observing a survival rate of 61% among 39 infants and children. The cause of death was lack of improvement in cardiovascular function in 37% of patients and major central nervous system damage in 15%, suggesting that earlier intervention with ECLS could improve outcome.[113] In a large series from Children's Hospital of Philadelphia, ECLS was used for 3.4% of children undergoing cardiac operations; the overall survival was 39%.[115] Survival among patients in whom ECLS was a bridge to heart transplantation was 40% to 60%.[116] Using ECLS in pediatric patients with cardiac failure following cardiac transplantation is associated with a long-term survival of 46%.[117]

ECLS has been effective in other clinical situations such as blunt trauma in children and adults, with survival rates of approximately 65%.[118,119] ECLS has also been successfully applied to patients with tracheal anomalies requiring repair, those with alveolar proteinosis who require pulmonary lavage, and those with pulmonary hypoplasia due to in utero renal insufficiency, asthma, sickle cell disease, and pulmonary failure after lung transplantation.[120-127] ECLS has been successfully applied to the management of pediatric and adult patients with H1N1 pneumonia.[128] Another application of ECLS has been in the form of extracorporeal cardiopulmonary resuscitation in pediatric patients with cardiogenic shock, post-traumatic hypotension, hypothermia, arrhythmias, and cardiac arrest, with the ELSO Registry and the literature overall demonstrating an approximately 40% survival.[129-131] Patients with mediastinal malignancies and airway compromise may be stabilized on ECLS during operative biopsy in order to avoid the risk of cardiopulmonary collapse associated with general anesthesia.[132] Those with hypothermia due to cold water drowning or winter mishaps may also be successfully warmed using this technology.[133,134] Donation after cardiac death is a new approach in which patients in whom support is being withdrawn or those with irreversible cardiac arrest are placed on ECMO support after death is declared thus allowing organ support until harvest can be performed.[135] This management strategy has the promise of enhancing available organs for transplantation.

Multiple studies have involved the long-term follow-up of newborn and pediatric patients after a course of ECLS. Most documented normal neurologic function in 70% to 80% of patients, although at least two studies document that approximately 50% of school-aged patients undergoing ECMO have abnormalities on careful neurologic assessment.[136-141] Such studies demonstrate that neurologic morbidity is no different in ECLS-managed newborns than in those managed by conventional mechanical ventilation. Pulmonary function tests at 8 years of age after neonatal courses on ECMO document measurable pulmonary sequelae in approximately half of the patients, with newborns with CDH being most affected.[142]

Patients with CDH who are managed with ECLS demonstrate a high incidence of morbidity, including gastroesophageal reflux in up to 81%, the need for tube feeding in up to 69%, the development of chronic pulmonary disease in up to 62%, the development of extra-axial fluid collections or enlarged ventricles in 30%, and growth delay in 40% to 50%.[143-145] These problems tend to resolve with time. The neurodevelopmental outcome among newborns with CDH was not dissimilar to that of other ECLS-treated children. Although most patients with cardiac and pediatric respiratory failure demonstrate few sequelae at follow-up, long-term studies in these groups have been less complete.

Four studies have evaluated the relative cost of treating newborn patients with ECLS compared with more conventional means.[20] Pearson and Short[146] found that the average daily charge for neonates receiving ECLS was twice that for patients receiving conventional mechanical ventilation, but the mean hospital stay was decreased by 50% in the ECLS group. Hospital charges were 43% lower in the ECLS group compared with the conventionally treated group when only the survivors were considered. The most recent randomized controlled trial comparing the outcome and costs of ECLS and standard management in newborn respiratory failure revealed average total costs of £73,979 or the ECLS group when compared with £33,435 or those managed by conventional means (UK prices, 2005).[147]

Maintaining a patient on extracorporeal support for days or weeks requires a prepared, organized, well-trained, and highly skilled team of physicians, respiratory therapists, nurses, and ECLS technicians. It is not a technique to be undertaken in a haphazard fashion on the spur of the moment without prior preparation and organization. The current recommendations by the American Academy of Pediatrics Committee on the Fetus and Newborn suggest that neonatal ECLS centers be established only at recognized level III regional centers with appropriate educational programs, ongoing research activity, and infant follow-up programs.[148]

Future of Extracorporeal Life Support

Although current devices allow safe and effective prolonged extracorporeal support, the future of ECLS depends on improvements in component technology, accompanied by circuit simplification and autoregulation. Safe nonocclusive pumps; leak-free low-resistance artificial lungs; circuit coatings that obviate the need for systemic anticoagulation, and simplified percutaneous single-cannulation systems are now either available or on the horizon. Once a compact servoregulated device is developed with the ability to provide extracorporeal support without anticoagulation, ECLS will be a simple technique rather than a complex labor-intensive intervention.[149] At that point the indications for extracorporeal support will broaden as the technique is applied to a wider population of patients with less severe cardiopulmonary insufficiency.

One of the major benefits of the ECLS experience may be the ability to explore the pathophysiology of cardiac and respiratory failure. Improved understanding of pulmonary and cardiac organ failure may lead to new preventive measures and improved treatment modalities that eventually eliminate the need for ECLS in patients with cardiorespiratory failure.

The complete reference list is available online at www.expertconsult.com.

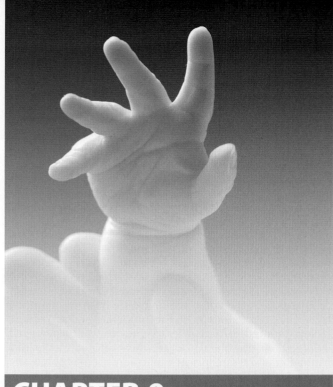

CHAPTER 9

Neonatal Cardiovascular Physiology and Care

Albert P. Rocchini

To appropriately manage the cardiovascular needs of your patient, it is important to understand normal cardiovascular physiology. This chapter summarizes normal fetal and neonatal cardiovascular physiology and describes principles that are necessary for the medical management of common cardiovascular problems in neonates.

Cardiovascular Physiology

Regardless of age, the major variables that affect cardiovascular function are preload (end-diastolic volume), heart rate, arterial pressure (afterload), and contractility (inotropic state of the heart).[1-3] At all ages, increasing myocardial muscle length, heart rate, and other factors that alter the inotropic state of the heart have a positive effect on cardiac function, whereas increasing afterload has a negative effect. However, in the intact animal or human, it is almost impossible to change one of these factors without also affecting another. The net

physiologic response is the combined effect of the intervention. For example, in an isolated muscle preparation, increasing rate of stimulation of the muscle will always result in an increase in the force of contraction.[2] However, in animals and children, pacing the heart at a faster rate will cause a decrease in stroke volume and no change or even a slight decrease in cardiac output. These opposite effects result from the difficulty in controlling the interaction of venous return, end-diastolic volume, inotropic state, heart rate, and afterload.

In addition, the subject's age can affect cardiovascular function. For example, in the fetus, increases in systemic afterload have a much greater effect on fetal right ventricular function (decreasing it) than left ventricular function, whereas, in the infant, increases in systemic afterload have a much greater effect on left ventricular function (decreasing it) than on right ventricular function.[4] The following sections focus individually on heart rate, preload, afterload, and contractility in the fetus and neonate.

HEART RATE

Changes in heart rate have the same effect on ventricular output in both the immature and the adult heart.[5] Increases in heart rate induced by atrial pacing also can result in a decrease of ventricular performance. Stroke volume falls with an increase in heart rate, a consequence of decreasing end-diastolic filling time and end-diastolic volume; however, because the decrease in stroke volume is usually proportional to the increase in heart rate, the net effect is either no change or a slight fall in cardiac output. In comparison with the adult, the fetus and neonatal infant have a relatively high resting heart rate. Because of the high basal heart rate, a neonate's cardiac output can rarely be increased by increasing heart rate. Similarly, in the neonate or fetus, decreases in heart rate to near adult levels, 60 beats/minute, are usually associated with marked decreases in cardiac output. Unlike pacing, a spontaneous increase in heart rate is usually associated with an increase in cardiac output. A spontaneous heart rate change differs from a similar change in heart rate resulting from atrial pacing, because the underlying stimuli that cause the spontaneous rate change also will affect inotropy, venous return, and/or afterload. For example, an increase in venous return that maintains end-diastolic volume, despite a rate-induced shortening of diastolic filling, can result in an increase in stroke volume. Similarly, if the stimulus to increase heart rate is associated with an increase in contractility, even though venous return may not increase, the increase in heart rate will still result in an increase in cardiac output. Exceptions to the positive effect of a spontaneous increase in heart rate on cardiac output can usually be explained by an increase in arterial pressure.[3] The negative effect of afterload on ventricular function results in a fall in stroke volume and cardiac output.

PRELOAD

At all ages, ventricular output depends on end-diastolic volume. An increase in stroke volume or cardiac output occurs when end-diastolic volume is increased (the Frank-Starling relation).[1,6] This relation depends on both the number of cross-bridge attachments that can be made at a given sarcomere length, and the sarcomere length depends on myofilament sensitivity to calcium.[7] Although this relationship exists in

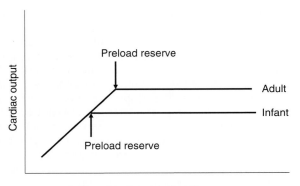

FIGURE 9-1   The Frank-Starling relation between cardiac output and left ventricular end-diastolic pressure. The point at which further increases in end-diastolic volume result in no further increase in cardiac output is referred to as preload reserve *(arrow)*. Since the neonatal myocardium is stiffer and less compliant, the preload reserve occurs at lower pressure than in the mature adult heart.

both the newborn and the adult, the magnitude of the relationship is frequently diminished in the newborn. It is well known that when left ventricular end-diastolic pressure is high, only small increments in end-diastolic volume and stroke volume follow from a further increase in filling pressure. As can be seen in Figure 9-1, the end-diastolic pressure at which further increases result in little change in cardiac output is called preload reserve. In the newborn, because the myocardium is immature and has greater stiffness (reduced compliance), the preload reserve occurs at a lower pressure than in the adult.[8]

AFTERLOAD

The cardiovascular function of both the immature and adult heart is negatively affected by an increase in afterload.[3,9,10] There is a maturational difference in the effect of afterload on myocardial function. The immature ventricle cannot eject against arterial pressures well-tolerated by the adult heart. This quantitative difference in response to afterload results from the weaker contraction of the immature myocardium (corrected for muscle cross-sectional area) and the thinner ventricular wall of the immature heart. Afterload also has a quantitatively different effect on right and left ventricular function. In both the neonate and the adult, increases in arterial pressure have a much greater negative effect on stroke volume of the right ventricle than that of the left. In the fetus and neonate with a widely patent ductus arteriosus, this difference is a consequence of the relatively larger right ventricular stroke volume, end-diastolic volume, and free wall curvature in the presence of similar right and left ventricular free wall thicknesses.[10] Because of Laplace's law, systolic wall stress of the right ventricle is greater than that of the left ventricle in the face of similar arterial pressures. This increase in right ventricular systolic wall stress causes the right ventricular ejection to be more negatively affected by an increase in arterial pressure.

CONTRACTILITY

An intervention that does not alter preload or afterload yet increases the force of contraction or increases cardiac output is said to have a positive inotropic effect. This positive effect

usually arises from either an increase in the sensitivity of the myofilaments to calcium or an increase in the cytosolic calcium transient. The immature heart responds to positive inotropic agents with an increase in left ventricular output; however, in comparison with the adult heart, this response is reduced. In cardiac muscle, the movement of calcium through the dihydropyridine-sensitive calcium channel is essential for calcium-induced calcium release from the sarcoplasmic reticulum.[11-15] Calcium-induced calcium release amplifies the effect of the calcium current on cytosolic calcium concentration.[15,16] In the absence of calcium-induced calcium release, trans-sarcolemmal calcium flow results in a contraction whose peak force is only a fraction of that achieved in the presence of the amplification system. Both the dihydropyridine-sensitive calcium channels and the sarcoplasmic reticulum calcium release channels (ryanodine receptors) are necessary for calcium-induced calcium release. Compared with the adult, the immature heart has a greater dependence on extracellular calcium, since it has reduced calcium-induced calcium release. The reduced dependence of the adult myocardium on extracellular calcium results from maturation of the sarcoplasmic reticulum. Both absolute and relative sarcoplasmic reticulum volume increases with age as does sarcoplasmic reticulum calcium release. For example, ryanodine has little effect on the force of contraction of the newborn myocardium. The immaturity of the sarcoplasmic reticulum and the greater dependence of the newborn heart on extracellular calcium concentrations are two explanations for why calcium channel blockers, such as verapamil, are poorly tolerated in the newborn.

Fetal Circulation

In addition to understanding how preload, afterload, heart rate, and contractility effect neonatal cardiovascular function, it is important to understand how birth affects the cardiovascular system. The fetal circulation differs from the adult circulation in a number of ways. The adult circulation is characterized as blood flow in series, that is, blood returns to the heart from the venous system to the right atrium and ventricle and is then injected into the lungs for oxygenation. Oxygenated blood then returns through the pulmonary veins to the left atrium and ventricle and is then ejected into the arterial system. The right ventricle works against the low afterload of the pulmonary circulation, whereas the left ventricle works against the high afterload of the systemic circulation. In the fetus, oxygenation and carbon dioxide elimination take place in the placenta. Oxygenated blood flows to the fetus through the umbilical veins, which connect to the inferior vena cava through the ductus venous.[17-19] The oxygenated umbilical blood flow mixes with the poorly oxygenated portal blood from the gastrointestinal tract. Because of the eustachian valve in the right atrium, the higher saturated umbilical venous blood preferentially streams across the foramen ovale into the left atrium,[20,21] whereas the lower saturated blood from the distal inferior vena cava and from the superior vena cava enters the tricuspid valve and is directed to the right ventricle. Although there are preferential patterns of flow, some of the blood from the placenta does enter the tricuspid valve, and some of the blood from the distal inferior vena cava and superior vena cava enters the foramen ovale. Both right and left ventricles pump to the systemic circulation. The right ventricular output is directed through the ductus arteriosus to the descending thoracic aorta, and the left ventricular output is directed although the aortic valve to the ascending aorta. Because of the preferential streaming of umbilical venous return, most oxygenated blood goes to the left ventricle and is distributed to the heart and cerebral circulations, whereas the lower oxygenated blood goes to the right ventricle and is distributed to the pulmonary arteries, abdominal organs, and placental arteries.[19]

Because of this unique fetal circulation, many types of congenital heart disease that are not compatible with life after birth are well tolerated in utero. For example, infants with hypoplastic or atretic left or right ventricular outflow tracts develop normally in utero, whereas after birth these lesions are fatal unless surgery is performed. With birth there is a rapid transformation from the fetal circulation to the adult circulation. This transformation involves elimination of the umbilical–placental circulation, establishment of an adequate pulmonary circulation, and separation of the left and right sides of the heart by closure of the ductus arteriosis and foramen ovale. Figure 9-2 depicts the fetal, immediate postbirth, and a few days postbirth hemodynamics.[22] Persistence of the fetal circulation after birth means that adequate pulmonary circulation is not achieved and fetal channels have not been closed. For example, infants with congenital diaphragmatic hernia have persistence of the fetal circulation because of high pulmonary resistance resulting from poor oxygenation and persistent patency of the foramen ovale and ductus arteriosus.

Neonatal Management of Common Cardiovascular Problems

CONGESTIVE HEART FAILURE

The common causes of heart failure in the neonate include rhythm disturbances and congenital cardiovascular malformations. Table 9-1 lists common congenital heart lesions and the age at which congestive heart failure is likely to occur. In the infant with cyanotic congenital heart disease, congestive heart failure usually occurs with lesions that have large amounts of pulmonary blood flow or regurgitant atrioventricular (AV) valves. The ultimate management of heart failure is to treat the underlying congenital malformation; however, medical management is essential to stabilize the infant and enable surgical correction to be performed with a reduced risk. The standard medical management includes the principles of rate control, preload control, afterload control, and improvement in contractility. Because of the high resting heart rate of the neonate, one cannot use increasing heart rate to increase cardiac output in the neonate. In fact, chronic supraventricular tachycardia, frequently the result of an atrial ectopic focus, is a cause of congestive cardiomyopathy.

Preload control is the mainstay of symptomatic therapy for heart failure. This is accomplished with the use of diuretics. The most common diuretic used to treat heart failure in the infant is furosemide (Lasix). Table 9-2 lists many of the commonly used diuretics and current dose recommendations.

One diuretic that may have more benefit than just symptomatic therapy is spironolactone (Aldactone).[23,24] Recent evidence suggests that in addition to causing fluid retention aldosterone can cause myocardial fibrosis. There are now a number of clinical trials in adults that suggest that chronic blockade of mineralocorticoid receptors results in improved cardiac remodeling.[24] It is important when considering the use of diuretics to avoid too much diuresis. If the child's preload is reduced below their preload reserve, cardiac output will decrease (see Fig. 9-1).

Afterload agents work by decreasing ventricular loading, predominately by reducing systemic vascular resistance. The pharmacologic agents that are most useful in altering afterload are vasodilators (see Table 9-2). These agents are important therapeutic agents in the treatment of infants with heart failure secondary to a large left to right shunt, severe atrioventricular and semilunar valve regurgitation, dilated cardiomyopathy, and postoperative low-output states.[25–29] Angiotensin-converting enzyme inhibitors are the most commonly used class of afterload reducing agents.[30–33] In addition to reducing ventricular afterload, in adults with congestive cardiomyopathy, they have been shown to also improve cardiovascular remodeling.[24] Another means of afterload control is low-dose beta-receptor blockade. Low-dose beta-blockade has been used successfully in the treatment of congestive cardiomyopathy. This agent works by interfering with the deleterious effects of increased sympathetic activity.[34,35]

With gram-negative septic shock or anaphylactic shock, it may be necessary to increase systemic afterload. In this situation, although systemic blood flow is high, because of severe vasodilation, the cardiac output is not high enough to maintain arterial pressure. The pharmacologic agents that are used in this situation are epinephrine, norepinephrine, and vasopressin.[36,37]

The final group of agents used to treat congestive heart failure in infants and young children are agents that increase the inotropy of the heart (see Table 9-2). The oldest agent in this class is digitalis. Digoxin is still the most commonly used chronic inotropic agent. It increases contractility by inhibiting the sodium-potassium-ATPase pump, resulting in an increase in intracellular sodium, which, in turn, stimulates calcium entry into the cell by the sodium-calcium exchanger; the increased intracellular calcium leads to increased contractility. Recent studies have suggested that digitalis also helps heart failure by inhibiting sympathetic nerve traffic and thus decreasing cardiac metabolic demands.[38] In addition to digoxin, there are other intravenous inotropic agents, the majority of which stimulate the beta-adrenergic receptor in the heart, which, in turn, increases production of adenyl cyclase activity and ultimately contractility. These agents are especially useful in managing severe acute congestive heart failure and cardiogenic shock. Depending on the individual agent, blood pressure can be either increased or slightly decreased. For example, dopamine can cause alpha-receptor stimulation with some degree of vasoconstriction,[39] whereas dobutamine tends to produce more systemic vasodilatation and either slightly decreases or has no effect on systemic pressure.[38,40] Milrinone is another intravenous inotrope that is frequently used in the infant. Milrinone is a phosphodiesterase inhibitor and increases contractility by inhibiting the breakdown of cyclic $3'5'$-adenosine monophosphate (c-AMP). Besides being a positive inotropic agent, it reduces afterload as well. Thus

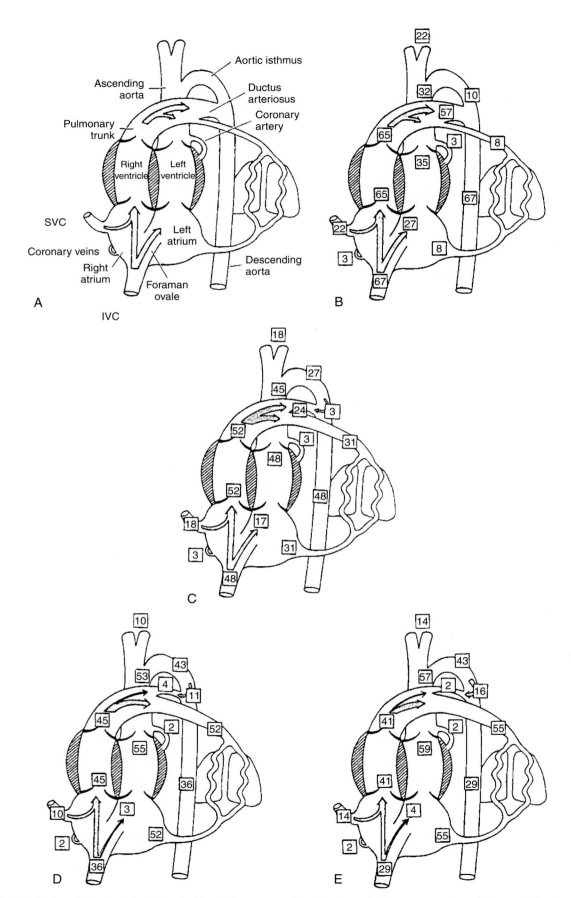

FIGURE 9-2 Distribution of the circulation in the fetal lamb. Percentages of combined ventricular output are shown in boxes. **A,** Anatomy of the fetal circulation. **B,** Undisturbed state. **C,** After ventilation with 3% oxygen, so as not to alter fetal blood gases. **D,** After ventilation with oxygen. **E,** After ventilation with oxygen and umbilical cord occlusion. IVC, inferior vena cava; SVC, superior vena cava. (From Rudolph AM: The fetal circulation and its adjustments after birth. In Moller JH, Hoffman JIE [eds]: Pediatric Cardiovascular Medicine. Philadelphia, Churchill Livingstone, 2000, p 62.)

TABLE 9-1
Causes of Congestive Heart Failure at Various Ages

Fetus to Day 1 of Life	First Week to 6 Weeks of Life	6 Weeks to 3 Months of Life	Greater Than 6 Months of Life
Tachyarrhythmias	Critical aortic stenosis	Ventricular septal defects	Myopericarditis
Anemia and/or hemolytic disease	Co-arctation of the aorta (simple or complex)	Patent ductus arteriosus	Endocarditis
Atrioventricular valve regurgitation	Hypoplastic left heart syndrome	Atrioventricular septal defects	Primary pulmonary hypertension*
Heart block	Interrupted aortic arch	Atrial septal defects*	Rheumatic heart disease
Cardiac or pericardial tumors*	Critical pulmonary stenosis	Tachyarrhythmias	Kawasaki disease
Arteriovenous malformations (usually brain or liver)*	Common mixing lesions (truncus, single ventricle, etc.)	Anomalous left coronary artery form the pulmonary artery	Postoperative congenital heart disease
Birth asphyxia	Tachyarrhythmias	Myocarditis or cardiomyopathy	Neuromuscular disease
Fetal–maternal or fetal–fetal transfusions	Obstructed or nonobstructed total anomalous pulmonary venous return	Nonobstructive total anomalous pulmonary venous return	Cardiomyopathies (restrictive, hypertrophic, and dilated)
Myocarditis	Myocarditis or cardiomyopathy		Systemic hypertension
Hyperviscosity	Systemic hypertension*		Collagen vascular disease*
Premature closure of the foramen ovale or patent ductus*	Endocrine disorders: thyroid disease, adrenal insufficiency, parathyroid disease*		Drugs: anthracycline, ipecac, cocaine, heavy metal, etc.
Semilunar valve insufficiency (i.e., absent pulmonary valve, aortic to LV tunnel)*	Persistent pulmonary hypertension		Anemia: sickle cell, thalassemia, hemolytic anemias, etc.*
	Patent ductus arteriosus (especially premature infants)		
	Infant of diabetic mother		

*Rare causes of heart failure.
LV, left ventricle.

TABLE 9-2
Medications Used to Treat Congestive Heart Failure

Class	Drug	Dose	Dosing Interval	Comments
Diuretic	Hydrochlorothiazide	2.0-3.0 mg/kg up to 50 mg/day	bid	Will increase uric acid level
	Furosemide	0.5-2.0 mg/kg up to 6 mg/kg/day	qd or bid	
	Spironolactone	1.0-3.3 mg/kg	bid	Potassium-sparing, used with causing with CEI
	Metolazone	0.2-0.4 mg/kg	qd	
ACE	Benazepril	0.2 mg/kg up to 10 mg/day	qd	Contraindicated in pregnancy, check serum potassium, creatinine. Cough and angioedema are side effects
	Captopril	0.3-0.5 mg/kg up to 6 mg/kg	tid	
	Enalapril	0.08 mg/kg up to 5 mg/day	qd-bid	
	Lisinopril	0.07 mg/kg up to 40 mg/day	qd	
ARB	Irbesartan	6-12 years: 75-150 mg/day	qd	Contraindicated in pregnancy, check serum potassium, creatinine
	Losartan	0.7 mg/kg/day up to 50 mg/day	qd	
Beta-blocker	Metoprolol	1.0-2.0 mg/day up to 6.0 mg/kg/day	qd	
Vasodilator	Hydralazine	0.75 mg/kg up to 7.5 mg/kg	qid	Tachycardia, fluid retention, lupus-like syndrome
	Prazosin	0.05-0.1 mg/kg up to 0.5 mg/kg	tid	
Inotrope	Digoxin	Digitalizing dose 20-40 µg/kg depending on age Maintenance dose 5-10 µg/kg	bid	
	Dobutamine	2.0-20 µg/kg/min IV		
	Dopamine	2.0-20 µg/kg/min IV		
	Milrinone	Loading dose 0.05-1 mg/kg then 0.5-0.75 µg/kg/min		
	Epinephrine	0.05-2 µg/kg/min IV		

ACE, angiotensin-converting enzyme inhibitor; ARB, angiotensin receptor blocker; CEI, converting enzyme inhibitor.

milrinone is likely to lower blood pressure slightly. It is also useful in producing some degree of pulmonary artery vasodilation and is therefore an ideal agent for the infant with severe congestive heart failure and pulmonary artery hypertension.[20]

If pharmacologic therapy is not enough to maintain adequate cardiac output, mechanical devices can be used to support the circulation. The most commonly used mechanical support device is extracorporeal membrane oxygenation. More recently ventricular assist devices have been used in infants with end-stage cardiomyopathy as a bridge to cardiac transplantation.[22,41,42]

ABNORMALITIES IN CARDIAC RHYTHM

Heart Block

Both slow and fast heart rates can severely compromise the cardiovascular circulation of an infant. Complete heart block may be either congenital or acquired and occurs in 1 per 20,000 live births.[43–45] There is a strong association between maternal connective tissue disease and congenital complete heart block. A mother with systemic lupus erythematosus has a 1 in 20 risk of having a child with complete heart block if she is anti-Ro positive.[46] Maternal immunoglobulin G antibodies to soluble ribonucleoprotein antigens (anti-Ro and anti-La) cross the placenta after the 12th to 16th week of gestation. This transfer of antibodies results in an inflammatory response in the fetal heart, particularly the conduction system, with destruction of the atrioventricular node.[45–51] Complete heart block in the neonate may or may not need treatment. The decision of whether to place a pacemaker in an infant with heart block depends on the presence of in utero heart failure (hydrops) or the development of postnatal congestive heart failure. Heart rate alone is usually not an indication for pacemaker placement; however, if the infant's heart rate remains at less than 50 beats/minute, a pacemaker is frequently required. Some forms of congenital heart disease also have a high incidence of heart block. These lesions include the Ebstein anomaly of the tricuspid valve and corrected transposition of the great arteries.

Tachyarrhythmias

Tachyarrhythmias can also occur in the infant and young child and cause heart failure. The most common type of tachyarrhythmia is supraventricular tachycardia. The incidence of paroxysmal supraventricular tachycardia is 1 in 250 to 1000 children.[4] It occurs most commonly in males younger than 4 months of age and frequently is even present in the fetus. The pathologic mechanism underlying the tachycardia is usually either the result of Wolff-Parkinson-White (WPW) syndrome (an accessory pathway between the atria and ventricles) or atrioventricular nodal reentry (dual conduction pathways within the atrioventricular node). If the supraventricular tachycardia is sustained, heart failure will likely occur within 24 to 48 hours. The treatment for supraventricular tachycardia, regardless of cause, is similar. If the infant becomes acidotic or hypotensive, immediate synchronized direct-current cardioversion should be performed at a dosage of 1 to 2 watt-second/kg.[52] If the infant is stable and relatively asymptomatic, then in most situations any intervention that increases AV node refractoriness is likely to work. In the infant, application of ice or an ice-water bag directly to the center of the infant's face recruits the diving reflex and stops the tachycardia. A rapid intravenous infusion of adenosine is also very effective in terminating supraventricular tachycardia.[53] The usual dose is a 100 μg/kg bolus, increasing by 100 μg-increments to a maximum of 400 μg/kg. A few serious side effects associated with adenosine administration included atrial fibrillation, ventricular tachycardia, asystole, apnea, and bronchospasm. Because of these potential side effects, adenosine should be administered in an area where cardioversion and cardiopulmonary resuscitation can be performed.

Children with supraventricular tachycardia and mild to moderate congestive heart failure may be initially treated with adenosine; however, other pharmacologic agents, such as digoxin, amiodarone, and procainamide may be helpful if adenosine fails to convert the tachycardia. Table 9-3 lists many of the commonly used antiarrhythmic agents and current dose recommendations. In infants, the intravenous route is the preferred method for administration of digoxin. The digitalizing dose interval may be given as frequently as every 2 to 4 hours. If tachycardia persists after three doses, one more dose equivalent to one fourth of the total digitalizing dose may be given. If the tachycardia has still not converted vagal stimulation or adenosine may be effective in terminating the tachycardia after digitalization. The maintenance dose of digoxin should be determined according to the total digitalizing dose required to terminate the tachycardia and is one eighth of the total digitalizing dose twice daily. Digoxin should be avoided in patients with a wide QRS tachycardia and when WPW syndrome is considered as a possible cause. Digoxin in the presence of WPW with atrial fibrillation can result in an acceleration of the ventricular response and resultant ventricular fibrillation.

Esmolol or propranolol, which may further depress cardiac function, should be used with caution in the critically ill infant with congestive heart failure. Once the tachycardia has been terminated and the congestive heart failure controlled, beta blockers can be used as effective long-term antiarrhythmic therapy in infants with supraventricular tachycardia.

Amiodarone is now being used with increasing frequency for the emergency treatment of supraventricular tachycardia, especially in the postoperative patient. Intravenous administration of amiodarone has been reported to terminate the tachycardia within 2 hours of the initial bolus in more than 40% of patients.[54,55] The major side effects of amiodarone include hypotension, decreased ventricular function, and bradycardia.

Intravenous procainamide can be very effective in patients with refractory supraventricular tachycardia. The combination of procainamide and a beta blocker is especially effective in treating refractory atrial flutter in the neonate.

Verapamil, although an effective agent to treat supraventricular tachycardia in the adult, is contraindicated in the infant with congestive heart failure. Use of verapamil in infants has resulted in cardiovascular collapse and death.[56,57]

In our institution, we frequently use esophageal overdrive pacing to convert supraventricular tachycardia in the infant. Esophageal pacing has the advantage of not only treating the arrhythmia but also helping to make a definitive diagnosis of the tachycardia. Overdrive pacing involves pacing the atrium via the esophagus at a rate slightly higher than the rate of the tachycardia. With cessation of pacing, sinus rhythm will usually return. Esophageal pacing is effective in most forms of supraventricular tachycardia, including atrial flutter.[58,59]

TABLE 9-3

Commonly Used Pharmacologic Agents to Treat Tachyarrhythmias

Drug	Dosage	Onset of Action	Potential Adverse Effects	Drug Interactions	Cardiovascular Contraindications	Comments
Adenosine	100-150 µg/kg given rapid IV; double dose sequentially to maximum of 300 µg/kg	< 5 sec	Dyspnea, bronchospasm, headache, chest pains, AV block/asystole, PVCs, atrial fibrillation, torsades de pointes, hypotension	Theophylline-adenosine is less effective Digoxin: increases risk of VT Diazepam-potentiated effects of adenosine	Prolonged QT interval Second- or third-degree AV block, except in the presence of pacemaker Sick sinus syndrome	Have defibrillator available when administering, in the event of ventricular rate acceleration, torsade de pointes, or VF
Amiodarone	Bolus: 5 mg/kg during 10 min Infusion of 10-15 µg/kg/day	Within 5 min of initial bolus	Hypotension, sinus arrest, or bradycardia, AV block	Digoxin: increases digoxin levels Procainamide: causes increased levels of amiodarone Warfarin: increases INR	Sick sinus syndrome or AV block, except if pacemaker present Cardiogenic shock	Closely monitor blood pressure, heart rate and rhythm Hypotension can be treated with volume and calcium
Esmolol	Load: 500 µg/kg during 1-2 min Maintenance: 50-200 µg/kg/min	Within 1-2 min	Hypotension, dizziness, headache, nausea, bronchospasm, decreased cardiac output	Digoxin: increases level Morphine: causes increased esmolol level	Sinus bradycardia, second- or third-degree heart block, cardiogenic shock, overt heart failure	Use with caution in patients with decreased renal function, diabetes, or asthma
Procainamide	Load: infants 7-10 mg/kg during 45 min, older children 12 mg/kg Infusion 40-50 µg/kg/min, occasionally may need up to 100 µg/kg/min	Within 30 min	Hypotension, increased ventricular response with atrial flutter, bradycardia, asystole, depressed ventricular function, fever myalgia, AV block, confusion, dizziness and headache	Amiodarone: causes increased concentration of procainamide Digoxin: causes increased digoxin levels	Second- and third-degree AV block without pacemaker Congestive heart failure Prolonged QT interval	Continuous ECG and BP monitoring Monitor potassium levels; if potassium decreases arrhythmias may increase

AV, atrioventricular; BP, blood pressure; ECG, electrocardiogram; INR, international normalization ratio; PVCs, premature ventricular contractions; VF, ventricular fibrillation; VT, ventricular tachycardia.

Ventricular tachycardia is extremely unusual in the newborn. It is most commonly seen in infants with intracardiac tumors, such as rhabdomyomas and in infants with long QT syndrome.

MANAGEMENT OF SELECTIVE TYPES OF CONGENITAL HEART DISEASE

Certain types of congenital heart disease are frequently associated with other congenital lesions that require general surgical procedures to be performed in the newborn period. For example, tetralogy of Fallot and ventricular septal defects are common in infants with tracheoesophageal fistulas, anal atresia, and other lesions common to the VATER complex (vertebral defects, imperforate anus, tracheoesophageal fistula, and radial and renal dysplasia). Interrupted aortic arch, truncus arteriosus, and tetralogy of Fallot are frequently present in infants with the DiGeorge syndrome. Hypoplastic left heart syndrome has been reported to occur in infants with congenital diaphragmatic hernia. More than 60% of infants with Down syndrome have congenital heart disease (patent ductus arteriosus, ventricular septal defects, atrioventricular septal defects, and tetralogy of Fallot). Because of the strong association of congenital heart disease with other congenital anomalies that require general

surgery in the newborn period, a cardiology consultation and echocardiogram are frequently necessary prior to the surgical procedure. The exact management of the infant depends on the type of congenital heart disease.

In infants with restricted pulmonary blood flow, such as seen with tetralogy of Fallot and/or pulmonary atresia, ductal patency is necessary in order to maintain adequate oxygenation. If a ductus was present in fetal life, it can usually be maintained patent with the administration of prostaglandin E_1, at a starting dose of 0.1 to 0.05 µg/kg/minute. If the ductus is patent, I use low-dose prostaglandin (0.02 to 0.03 µg/kg/minute) to maintain its patency; if the ductus is virtually closed, I start with a higher dose of prostaglandin until patency is achieved and then cut back to low-dose therapy. Side effects associated with prostaglandin administration include apnea, seizures, fevers, hypotension, and flushing. Once the infant has been stabilized, then more definitive therapy can be contemplated. At our institution, whenever possible, we choose complete repair of these lesions rather than palliation, with a systemic to pulmonary artery shunt.

In infants with hypoplastic left heart syndrome initial management requires that an atrial septal defect be present and that ductal patency be maintained. In these infants, systemic blood flow is directly related to pulmonary artery resistance, and oxygen saturation is inversely related to pulmonary vascular resistance (i.e., as pulmonary resistance decreases, pulmonary blood flow increases, resulting in higher oxygen saturation and lower systemic blood flow). The ideal systemic oxygen saturation in an infant with hypoplastic left heart syndrome is about 80%. When oxygen saturations are in the high 80s to low 90s, the ratio of pulmonary to systemic blood flow is usually greater than 4:1, and systemic hypoperfusion is usually present; when oxygen saturation is in the high 70s to low 80s, the pulmonary to systemic flow ratio is nearly balanced. Ideally, I like to let these infants maintain spontaneous respirations, and I withhold supplemental oxygen. In some cases, it may be necessary to cause pulmonary vasoconstriction, which can be accomplished by placing the infant in a mixture of room air and nitrogen. The lower inspired oxygen concentration will cause pulmonary artery vasoconstriction, which will result in a reduction in pulmonary blood flow and maintenance of adequate systemic perfusion. Once the infant has been stabilized, it is my policy to perform Norwood palliation. In some selected cases, cardiac transplantation may be the best surgical option for the infant.

Infants with ventricular septal defects or atrioventricular septal defects usually have no symptoms from their heart disease during the first month of life. Congestive heart failure from a ventricular septal defect is usually the result of excess pulmonary blood flow. The two major determinants of left to right shunt flow across a ventricular septal defect are the size of the defect and the ratio of pulmonary arteriolar to systemic arteriolar resistance. In a term infant, it usually takes from 4 to 6 weeks for the pulmonary resistance to drop to normal levels; thus infants with large septal defects do not usually develop heart failure until the second month of life. Causes of early heart failure in an infant with a ventricular septal defect include prematurity and other associated cardiac lesions. The two lesions most often associated with the early development of congestive heart failure are the presence of a co-arctation of the aorta and, in the case of atrioventricular septal defect, the presence of significant atrioventricular valvular regurgitation.

The complete reference list is available online at www. expertconsult.com.

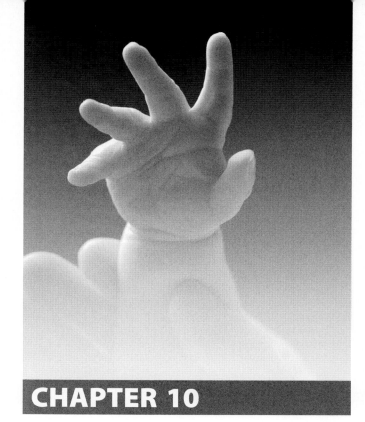

CHAPTER 10

Sepsis and Related Considerations

Allison L. Speer, Tracy C. Grikscheit, Jeffrey S. Upperman, and Henri R. Ford

Despite advances in neonatology and pediatric critical care, sepsis remains a challenging problem for the health care provider. Sepsis is a leading cause of morbidity and mortality in infants and children, and, unfortunately, its incidence continues to rise.[1,2] In their most recent reports, the Centers for Disease Control and Prevention and the National Center for Health Statistics cited septicemia as the tenth leading cause of death and bacterial sepsis of the newborn as the eighth leading cause of infant death in the United States.[3] In addition, sepsis-related health care costs represent a significant economic burden to society, with almost $17 billion spent annually in the United States alone.[4]

There are only a handful of epidemiologic studies of sepsis and even fewer regarding pediatric sepsis. One of the challenges to the study of sepsis has been the lack of standardized terminology. Consistent definitions may be crucial for early diagnosis and goal-directed therapies to improve mortality from sepsis. Furthermore, they may enhance the design and evaluation of future trials. The first part of this chapter outlines the evolution of sepsis terminology as well as its epidemiology. Emerging therapies for sepsis are typically aimed at enhancing or modulating the immune system or destroying the invading microbe. Therefore it is important to fully understand host

defense mechanisms as well as microbial virulence. The second section covers the pathogenesis of sepsis, with a focus on the determinants of infection: host defense mechanisms and bacterial virulence. The third part of this chapter examines the diagnosis of sepsis, with a focus on the Goldstein consensus criteria[5] and the PIRO system (Predisposing conditions, the nature and extent of the Insult or Infection, the magnitude of the host Response, and the degree of concomitant Organ dysfunction).[6] The fourth and final part discusses principles of management, with concentration on the Surviving Sepsis Campaign (SSC)[7,8] and the American College of Critical Care Medicine (ACCM)[9]/Pediatric Advanced Life Support (PALS)[10] guidelines for the management of pediatric and neonatal sepsis.

Sepsis Terminology and Epidemiology

TERMINOLOGY

Historically, confusing terminology and a lack of standardized definitions had obscured diagnosis and treatment as well as interpretation of clinical research trials on sepsis and its related syndromes. The American College of Chest Physicians/ Society of Critical Care Medicine (ACCP/SCCM) 1991 Consensus Conference established the current definitions of sepsis and its related syndromes with the goal of improving early diagnosis and thereby facilitating early therapeutic intervention.[11] They also reasoned that the ACCP/SCCM 1992 consensus criteria, or the Bone criteria, would help to standardize research protocols, which would enable improved application of information derived from clinical studies.

Sepsis is defined as the development of the systemic inflammatory response syndrome (SIRS) resulting from a confirmed infection. According to the Bone criteria, SIRS is characterized by the presence of two or more of the following: (1) temperature greater than 38° C or less than 36° C, (2) heart rate greater than 90 beats per minute, (3) respiratory rate greater than 20 breaths per minute or $Paco_2$ less than 32 mm Hg, or (4) an alteration in the white blood cell count, such as greater than 12,000/mm³, less than 4,000/mm³, or greater than 10% immature neutrophils (bands). When sepsis is associated with acute organ dysfunction, it is referred to as severe sepsis.[11] Septic shock, by contrast, is defined as sepsis-induced hypotension (<90 mm Hg or reduction by 40 mm Hg or more from baseline in the absence of other causes) persisting despite adequate fluid resuscitation, along with signs of organ hypoperfusion, such as lactic acidosis, oliguria, or acute alteration in mental status. However, SIRS may also occur in the absence of infection as a result of trauma, burns, pancreatitis, or other triggers (Fig. 10-1). Septicemia and septic syndrome are confusing and ambiguous terms that should no longer be used.

According to Bone and colleagues,[11] detection of altered organ function in an acutely ill patient constitutes a syndrome that is termed multiple organ dysfunction syndrome (MODS). In contrast to organ failure, organ dysfunction is a dynamic process and a continuum of physiologic derangements that evolve with time. They argue that terms such as *sequential organ failure*[12] or *multiple systems organ failure*[13] are inadequate and should

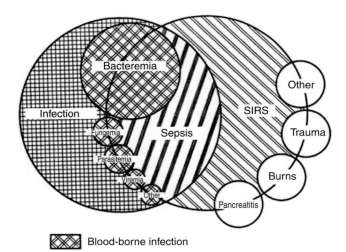

FIGURE 10-1 The interrelationship between systemic inflammatory response syndrome (SIRS), sepsis, and infection. (Used with permission from Bone RC, Balk RA, Cerra FB, et al: Definitions for sepsis and organ failure and guidelines for the use of innovative therapies in sepsis. Chest 1992;101:1644-1655.)

be eliminated from use. MODS develops by two relatively distinct, but not mutually exclusive, pathways that may be described as either primary or secondary. Primary MODS is the direct result of a well-defined insult in which organ dysfunction occurs early and can be directly attributed to the insult itself. Secondary MODS develops as a consequence of the host response (SIRS) in organs remote from the initial insult, typically after a latent period following the inciting injury.

The Bone criteria have been widely adopted in both clinical practice and research trials.[14–17] A MEDLINE search dated January 1992 to May 2010 yielded more than 50,000 publications using SIRS as a keyword. Despite this proliferation of articles, analysis of a recent physician attitudinal survey revealed that only 22% (114 of 529) of intensivists and 5% (26 of 529) of other physicians defined sepsis according to the ACCP/SCCM 1992 consensus criteria.[18] The failure to adopt these criteria and the concurrent growth of clinical trial data provided the impetus for a review of the 1992 definitions of sepsis and its related conditions. The 2001 International Sepsis Definitions Conference, sponsored by the SCCM, European Society of Intensive Care Medicine, ACCP, American Thoracic Society, and the Surgical Infection Society, undertook this task. These experts and opinion leaders ultimately upheld the ACCP/SCCM 1992 consensus criteria and expanded the list of signs and symptoms of sepsis to reflect clinical bedside experience (Table 10-1).[6]

EPIDEMIOLOGY

The ACCP/SCCM 1992 consensus criteria have been applied in several epidemiologic surveys of sepsis during the last 15 years.[2,4,14,19–22] Although standardized terminology is now used, information on the incidence of sepsis and patient outcomes continues to be limited, and published results are conflicting. Two European studies reported the incidence of sepsis in adult intensive care units (ICUs) and drew some interesting conclusions regarding prognosis. Brun-Buisson and colleagues reported the incidence of severe sepsis in adult ICUs in French public hospitals to be 6.3%,[19] while Alberti and

TABLE 10-1
Diagnostic Criteria for Sepsis

Infection* documented or suspected, and some of the following[†]:

General variables
  Fever (core temperature greater than 38.3° C)
  Hypothermia (core temperature < 36° C)
  Heart rate > 90 bpm or > 2 SD above the normal value for age
  Tachypnea
  Altered mental status
  Significant edema or positive fluid balance (>20 mL/kg over 24 hours)
  Hyperglycemia (plasma glucose > 120 mg/dL or 7.7 mmol/L) in the absence of diabetes

Inflammatory variables
  Leukocytosis (WBC count > 12,000 μL^{-1})
  Leukopenia (WBC count < 4000 μL^{-1})
  Normal WBC count with > 10% immature forms
  Plasma CRP > 2 SD above the normal value
  Plasma procalcitonin > 2 SD above the normal value

Hemodynamic variables
  Arterial hypotension (SBP < 90 mm Hg, MAP < 70, or an SBP decrease > 40 mm Hg in adults or < 2 SD below normal for age)
  Svo_2[†] > 70%[†]
  Cardiac index[†,‡] > 3.5 L × min^{-1} × M^{-23}

Organ dysfunction variables
  Arterial hypoxemia (Pao_2/Fio_2 < 300)
  Acute oliguria (urine output < 0.5 mL/kg/hr or 45 mmol/L for at least 2 hours)
  Creatinine increase > 0.5 mg/dL
  Coagulation abnormalities (INR > 1.5 or aPTT > 60 seconds)
  Ileus (absent bowel sounds)
  Thrombocytopenia (platelet count < 100,000 μL^{-1})
  Hyperbilirubinemia (plasma total bilirubin > 4 mg/dL or 70 mmol/L)

Tissue perfusion variables
  Hyperlactatemia (>1 mmol/L)
  Decreased capillary refill or mottling

Modified and used with permission from Levy MM, Fink MP, Marshall JC, et al: 2001 SCCM/ESICM/ACCP/ATS/SIS International Sepsis Definitions Conference. Crit Care Med 2003;31:1250-1256.
*Infection is defined as a pathologic process induced by a microorganism.
[†]Svo_2 saturation > 70% is normal in children (normally, 75% to 80%), and CI 3.5 to 5.5 is normal in children; therefore NEITHER should be used as signs of sepsis in newborns or children.
[‡]Diagnostic criteria for sepsis in the pediatric population are signs and symptoms of inflammation plus infection with hyperthermia or hypothermia (rectal temperature > 38.5° C or < 35° C), tachycardia (may be absent in hypothermic patients), and at least one of the following indications of altered organ function: altered mental status, hypoxemia, increased serum lactate level, or bounding pulses.
aPTT, activated partial thromboplastin time; BPM, beats per minute; CRP, C-reactive protein; INR, international normalized ratio; MAP, mean arterial blood pressure; SBP, systolic blood pressure; SD, standard deviation(s); Svo_2, mixed venous oxygen saturation; WBC, white blood cell.

colleagues found a higher adult ICU-specific incidence of infection in Europe (21.1%). They stratified the data into the following categories: infection without SIRS (17.9%), sepsis (28.3%), severe sepsis (23.9%), and septic shock (29.9%), according to the ACCP/SCCM 1992 consensus criteria.[20] Alberti and colleagues identified the majority of infections to be gram-negative bacilli, followed by gram-positive cocci. However, even though the incidence of community-acquired (11.9%) versus hospital-acquired (9.2%) infection was similar, nosocomially infected patients had poorer outcomes.[20] Interestingly, Brun-Buisson and colleagues demonstrated that patients with culture-negative, clinically suspected severe sepsis had the same 28-day mortality (60%) as patients with documented infection (56%).[19]

Before 2000, only two epidemiologic studies had been conducted in the United States that used the ACCP/SCCM 1992 consensus criteria.[21,22] Neither study provided accurate information on population incidence (including children) or the costs of care. In 1995, Rangel-Frausto and colleagues published a prospective epidemiologic study of the sequential progression of SIRS to sepsis, severe sepsis, and, finally, septic shock in a single institutional cohort.[21] They demonstrated a stepwise increase in positive blood cultures (17%, 25%, 69%, respectively) and in mortality rates along the hierarchy from SIRS (7%), to sepsis (16%), severe sepsis (20%), and septic shock (46%).[21] Interestingly, Rangel-Frausto and colleagues confirmed the findings of Brun-Buisson and colleagues that culture-negative patients had similar morbidity and mortality rates as culture-positive patients.[21] Another U.S. study by Sands and colleagues, however, reported very different results from the European epidemiologic studies. Their prospective, multi-institutional, observational study involving eight academic tertiary care centers, published in 1997, estimated the hospital-wide incidence of sepsis at 2.0%, with ICU patients accounting for 59%.[22] Bacteremia was documented in only 28% of the study population, with gram-positive organisms as the most frequent isolates. The 28-day mortality was 34%.[22] The lower incidence of sepsis, bacteremia, and the improved mortality rates compared with the European studies are likely due to the fact that this study enrolled patients hospital-wide, including healthier non-ICU patients in addition to sicker ICU patients. The differences in types of bacteria responsible for sepsis in the U.S. study by Sand and colleagues versus the European study by Alberti and colleagues may reflect geographic as well as institutional differences.

In an effort to better define the incidence, costs, and outcomes of sepsis in the United States, two important studies using the ACCP/SCCM 1992 consensus criteria were published in 2001[4] and 2003.[2] Angus and colleagues conducted a large observational cohort study to determine incidence, costs, and outcomes of severe sepsis.[4] Using 1995 state hospital discharge records from seven large states, they estimated 3.0 cases per 1,000 population, 2.26 cases per 100 hospital discharges (51.1% from the ICU),[4] and a national incidence of 751,000 cases per year. Major differences were identified between children and adults. The incidence of severe sepsis increased greater than100-fold with age (0.2/1000 in children to 26.2/1,000 in patients > 85 years old). The annual total cost nationally was $16.7 billion, with an average cost per case of $22,100.[4] Costs were higher in infants, nonsurvivors, ICU patients, surgical patients, and those with more organ failure.[4] The mortality of severe sepsis also increased with age (10% in children to 38.4% in patients > 85 years old, and 28.6% overall).[4]

Martin and colleagues published an epidemiologic study in the *New England Journal of Medicine* in 2003 that analyzed sepsis from 1979 to 2000 using a nationally representative sample of all nonfederal acute care hospitals in the United States.[2] They suggested that Angus and colleagues may have overestimated the incidence of severe sepsis by a factor of 2 to 4, because the estimated number of deaths exceeded the combined numbers of deaths reported in association with nosocomial bloodstream infections and septic shock. Martin and colleagues identified more than 10 million cases of sepsis occurring during approximately 750 million hospitalizations over the 22-year study period. The incidence of sepsis increased from 82.7 cases per 100,000 population to 240.4 cases per 100,000 population, for an increase of 8.7% per year. Martin and colleagues suggested that possible reasons for a true increase in the incidence of sepsis included increasing microbial resistance, the epidemic of human immunodeficiency virus (HIV) infection, and the increased use of invasive procedures, immunosuppressive drugs, chemotherapy, and transplantation.

Martin and colleagues[2] identified several other important changes that occurred during the 22-year study period. Gram-negative infections predominated until 1987, when gram-positive bacteria became more prevalent, increasing by an average of 26.3% per year. In 2000, gram-positive bacteria accounted for 52.1% of sepsis cases, whereas gram-negative bacteria were responsible for 37.6%. Of note, fungal organisms increased by 207% during the study period. Despite a decline in mortality rates from sepsis from 1979 to 2000, the increased incidence of sepsis resulted in a significant increase in the number of in-hospital deaths resulting from sepsis, increasing from 43,579 (21.9 per 100,000 population) to 120,491 (43.9 per 100,000 population). Racial disparities were also striking, with nonwhites having almost twice the risk of sepsis as whites. The highest risk was among African-American men, in whom sepsis occurred at the youngest age and resulted in the most deaths. Martin and colleagues did not focus on the pediatric population. The significant differences between pediatric and adult patients observed in the study by Angus and colleagues[4] and the scarce data on the epidemiology of sepsis in children became the incentive for a follow-up study by the University of Pittsburgh research group.

Using the same 1995 hospital discharge and population database that Angus and colleagues had studied, Watson and colleagues estimated 42,364 cases of pediatric severe sepsis per year nationally (0.56 cases per 1,000 population per year).[14] The incidence was 15% higher in boys than in girls and highest in infants (5.16/1000) compared with older children (0.20/1000 in those 10 to 14 years of age).[14] Half of all children had underlying comorbidity.[14] The majority of infectious causes were either respiratory (37.2%) or primary bacteremia (25.0%), although this varied by age, with bacteremia being more common in neonates and respiratory infections predominating in older children.[14] The mean length of stay (LOS) was 31 days with very-low-birth-weight (VLBW) newborns, weighing less than 1500 g at birth, accounting for 40% of the total hospital days.[14] Estimated annual total costs were $1.97 billion nationally, with a mean cost of $47,050, which is significantly more than the $22,100 cost per case for adults and children combined quoted by Angus and colleagues.[14] Thirty-one percent of the costs were incurred by VLBW newborns.[14]

Watson and colleagues demonstrated that hospital mortality was 10.3% (4,383 deaths nationally or 6.2 per 100,000 population), and more than one fifth were low-birth-weight newborns weighing less than 2500 g at birth.[14] Not surprisingly, hospital mortality was higher in children with neoplasms, HIV infection, and those undergoing surgical procedures.[14] The risk of death increased with increasing number of dysfunctional organs (7.0% with single-organ failure to 53.1% for patients with greater than or equal to four-organ systems failing).[14] Although sepsis-associated mortality in children has fallen from 97% in 1966[23] to 10.3% in 1995[14] and remains lower than adult sepsis-associated mortality, without a doubt, sepsis is still a significant health problem in infants and children.

Pathogenesis

The pathogenesis of sepsis is summarized in Figure 10-2. Bacterial invasion secondary to barrier failure leads to the local release of lipopolysaccharide (LPS), with consequent formation of an LPS–lipopolysaccharide binding protein (LBP)–CD14–Toll-like receptor-4 (TLR-4) complex on neutrophils, macrophages, and endothelial cells. Signaling via

this complex results in activation of the complement system, clotting cascade, as well as various inflammatory cells. This process leads to the release of inflammatory mediators, which up-regulate adhesion molecules and promote chemotaxis of neutrophils and macrophages. The activated cells release microbicidal agents typically designed for bacterial killing but which may promote distant organ injury and SIRS if the inflammatory process is "uncontrolled." Predictably, immuno-compromised infants and children, as well as preterm and term neonates who classically have significant host defense impairment, are particularly vulnerable to infections. Such infections may elicit an inflammatory response, which may be exaggerated at times and result in significant host tissue destruction. Failure to control either the infection itself or the host inflammatory response may follow a predictable course along the sepsis continuum: SIRS, sepsis, severe sepsis, septic shock, MODS, and, ultimately, death.[21]

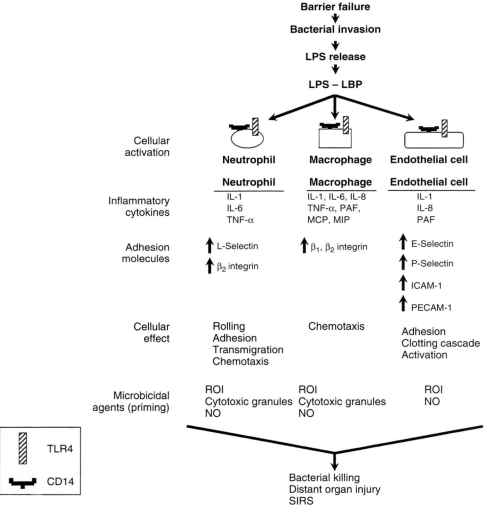

FIGURE 10-2   Pathogenesis of systemic inflammatory response syndrome (SIRS). Bacterial invasion secondary to barrier failure leads to the local release of lipopolysaccharide (LPS), with consequent formation of an LPS–lipopolysaccharide binding protein (LBP)–CD14–Toll-like receptor 4 (TLR-4) complex on neutrophils, macrophages, and endothelial cells, resulting in cellular activation. Inflammatory cytokines are released, up-regulate adhesion molecules, and promote chemotaxis of neutrophils and macrophages. (The complement system, clotting cascade, and lymphocyte population may also be activated, but this is not shown in the diagram.) The activated cells release microbicidal agents typically designed for bacterial killing, but they may be injurious and promote distant organ injury and SIRS if the inflammatory process is uncontrolled. ICAM, intercellular adhesion molecule; IL, interleukin; MCP, monocyte chemotactic protein; MIP, macrophage inflammatory protein; NO, nitric oxide; PAF, platelet-activating factor; PECAM, platelet-endothelial cell adhesion molecule; ROI, reactive oxygen intermediate (or species); TNF, tumor necrosis factor.

This section on pathogenesis examines the determinants of infection: host defense mechanisms and bacterial virulence. Host defense mechanisms include barriers to infection and host immunity. The host immune system classically mounts a well-orchestrated response aimed at destroying the invading microbe. Both cellular immunity (neutrophils, monocyte-macrophages, and lymphocytes) and humoral factors (immunoglobulins, complement, and cytokines) will be discussed, because they represent the final common pathway for the development of SIRS. Bacterial virulence is then examined in detail. Impairment or failure of the intrinsic host defense mechanisms and significant virulence of invading microbes increase the likelihood of successful establishment of infection and development of sepsis. This section ends with a separate discussion of impaired neonatal host defense mechanisms.

HOST DEFENSE MECHANISMS

Barriers to Infection

Host defense mechanisms begin with anatomic barriers to infection: the presence of indigenous microbial flora on the skin, oropharynx, respiratory, gastrointestinal, and genitourinary tracts. These ubiquitous host bacteria prevent colonization by foreign or pathogenic microbes by blocking adherence to the epithelial barrier or by competing for nutrients. Each organ system has additional local protective mechanisms as well. The largest organ in the body, the skin, limits bacterial replication by maintaining a relatively acidic environment as well as undergoing regular desquamation, which severely hinders bacterial adherence. Gastric acidity impedes bacterial replication and colonization. Intestinal mucus and peristalsis as well as the cilia of the respiratory epithelium prevent bacterial adherence. Immunoglobulin A (IgA)-rich secretions in the oropharynx, nasopharynx, and tracheobronchial tree also impair bacterial adherence to the mucosa. For infection to occur, there must be either a breach in the integrity of the normal protective barrier or a sufficiently virulent microbe must penetrate the barrier (Fig. 10-3). Barrier failure may be caused by trauma or direct tissue injury, surgery, malnutrition, burns, immunosuppression, shock, and reperfusion injury following ischemia.[24] For example, during ischemia, consumption of adenosine triphosphate results in the accumulation of adenosine diphosphate, adenosine monophosphate, inosine, and hypoxanthine. Xanthine oxidase activity is also increased, but its effect is initially blunted because oxygen is required to oxidize hypoxanthine to xanthine. However, during reperfusion, oxygen is supplied, hypoxanthine is oxidized,

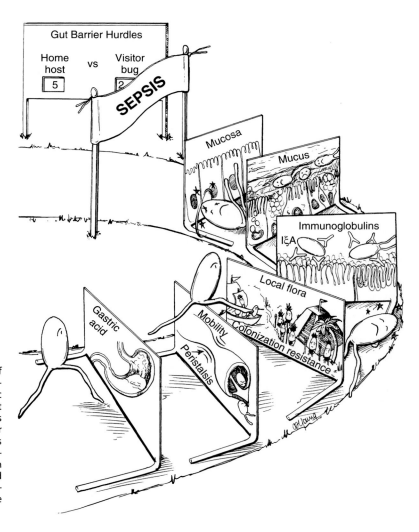

FIGURE 10-3 The gut barrier is envisioned as a series of hurdles that bacteria must overcome to penetrate the epithelial layer and disseminate systemically. First hurdle: Gastric acid lowers intragastric pH, promoting a hostile environment for bacterial growth. Second hurdle: Coordinated peristalsis continually sweeps bacteria downstream, thus limiting their attachment to the mucosal surface. Third hurdle: Indigenous microbial flora (aerobes and anaerobes) prevent the overgrowth of pathogenic Gram-negative aerobic bacteria. Fourth hurdle: IgA, a nonbactericidal immunoglobulin, coats and aggregates bacteria, preventing their attachment to the mucosal surface. Fifth hurdle: Intestinal mucus forms a weblike barrier to prevent bacterial attachment to the enterocyte.

and toxic reactive oxygen intermediates (ROIs), or species such as superoxide (O_2^-) and hydrogen peroxide (H_2O_2), are formed. These ROIs can mediate direct tissue injury and thus result in gut barrier failure.[25–28] This results in adherence of bacteria, with subsequent penetrance and internalization. The development of clinical infection (bacterial survival and replication within the host) is dependent on the virulence of the microbe and its ability to evade both the local cellular and humoral host defense mechanisms.

Cell-Mediated Immunity

Neutrophils Neutrophils constitute the first line of defense in response to infection, tissue injury, or other triggers of inflammation. Egress from the circulation into the tissues is a highly regulated process that involves complex interactions between receptors on the phagocytes and the vascular endothelial cells. These interactions are partially governed by cytokines or other inflammatory mediators. The sequence of events occurs as follows: (1) neutrophil adherence to the endothelium, (2) migration of the neutrophil through the endothelium to the site of injury or inflammation (diapedesis), and (3) stimulation or priming of the neutrophil for killing.

Neutrophil adherence is regulated by adhesion molecules on both the neutrophil and the endothelial cell. There are three classes: selectins, integrins, and the immunoglobulin superfamily. Selectins direct the first step in the adhesion cascade, which involves the rolling of the neutrophil along the vascular endothelium. Specifically, leukocyte (L)-selectin binds endothelial (E)-selectin and platelet (P)-selectin, which are both present on activated endothelial cells.[29]

Migration of the neutrophil to the site of inflammation requires the formation of a firm adhesion between the neutrophil and endothelial cell. This step is governed by the β_2 integrin CD11b/CD18 on the neutrophil and the intercellular adhesion molecule-1 (ICAM-1) on the endothelial cell.[30] Interestingly, patients with leukocyte adhesion deficiency are susceptible to recurrent bacterial infections, because they lack the β_2 integrin receptor CD11b/CD18. Their neutrophils fail to adhere to the endothelium and therefore diapedesis cannot occur.[31]

Lipopolysaccharide released by bacteria enhances neutrophil–endothelial interactions directly and indirectly. LPS stimulates the release of inflammatory mediators, such as tumor necrosis factor-α (TNF-α), interleukin-1 (IL-1), and interferon-γ (IFN-γ), which upregulate E-selectin and ICAM-1 expression on endothelial cells.[29,32] In addition, LPS forms a complex with LBP, which then binds to the CD14 molecule and TLR-4 on the neutrophil (and monocyte) and leads to up-regulation of the β_2 integrin CD11b/CD18. Thus LPS plays an important role in neutrophil adhesion and migration.[33,34]

After the firm adhesion step, neutrophil diapedesis is regulated by platelet-endothelial cell adhesion molecule-1 (PECAM-1), which normally maintains the vascular permeability barrier and modulates transendothelial migration of neutrophils and monocytes.[35–38] Antibodies to PECAM-1 lead to leaky barriers and inhibit neutrophil transmigration.[39] In addition to PECAM-1, neutrophil egress requires the presence of a chemotactic gradient through the extracellular matrix. A wide variety of chemotaxins abound at sites of inflammation, such as small bacterial peptides, monocyte chemotactic protein-1 (MCP-1), platelet-activating factor (PAF), and leukotriene B_4. Probably the two most important chemotaxins for neutrophil diapedesis are IL-8 and C5a. Interaction between specific receptors on the neutrophil and the chemotaxin evokes a cascade of secondary intracellular signaling events: translocation of protein kinase C from the cytoplasm to the cell membrane, protein kinase C–dependent phosphorylation, and an increase in free calcium in the cytosol. This results in conformational changes in the cytoskeleton of the neutrophil that allow its transendothelial egress and rapid movement toward the chemotactic gradient.[40] As one would expect, specific monoclonal antibodies against adhesion molecules disrupt the neutrophil–endothelial cell interaction and inhibit neutrophil chemotaxis, thus potentially impairing the ability to fight bacterial infection.[41]

The final step in the neutrophil response to infection is the phagocytosis of the microbe with subsequent intracellular killing. Phagocytosis is greatly enhanced by prior opsonization of the bacteria with specific immunoglobulins. This results in complement activation, the deposition of additional ligands or receptors on the bacterial surface, and the facilitation of neutrophil adherence to the microbe. This interaction results in the complete internalization of the microbe into endosomal compartments known as phagosomes. Prior stimulation or priming of the neutrophil by inflammatory cytokines or chemotaxins activates it for more efficient killing. Bacteria are then killed by the fusion of lysosomes containing potent microbicidal agents with the phagosome. In the phagolysosome, both oxygen-dependent and oxygen-independent pathways facilitate microbial killing.

The major oxygen-dependent mechanisms involve the formation of ROIs by the enzyme nicotinamide adenine dinucleotide phosphate oxidase. The active form of the enzyme is assembled in the cell membrane and catalyzes the reduction of molecular oxygen (O_2) to superoxide (O_2^-), the so-called respiratory burst. Superoxide is converted to hydrogen peroxide (H_2O_2) by superoxide dismutase. H_2O_2, in turn, can react with superoxide in the presence of iron or other metals to give the potent ROI hydroxyl radical ($^\circ OH$). Alternatively, H_2O_2 can react with chloride (Cl^-) in the presence of myeloperoxidase, an enzyme found in the cytoplasmic granules, to give the highly reactive hypochlorous acid (HOCl). HOCl, in turn, reacts with endogenous nitrogen-containing compounds to form the powerful oxidizing agents chloramines, which account for much of the neutrophil's cytotoxicity.[42,43]

The principal oxygen-independent microbicidal pathway is affected mainly by a number of peptides contained in specific cytoplasmic granules, including lysozyme, elastase, lactoferrin, cathepsin, and defensins. Many of these peptides act synergistically to promote microbial killing. For instance, defensins and elastase increase bacterial membrane permeability, allowing penetration by other microbicidal peptides or ROIs.

Monocytes-Macrophages The monocyte-macrophage shares many similarities with the neutrophil in host defense mechanisms because it arises from the same stem cell as the granulocyte. The stem cell gives rise to the monoblast, which differentiates into a promonocyte, and then the monocyte. Once released into the bloodstream, monocytes migrate to various tissues and organs, where they terminally differentiate into macrophages. These mature macrophages are characterized by the acquisition of specific granules containing enzymes as well as receptors for growth factors and complement.[44–46]

Macrophages play an important role in the host defense against intracellular pathogens. Like neutrophils, they migrate to sites of inflammation in response to various chemotaxins, such as C5a, bacterial peptides, foreign antigens, and cytokines (IL-1, TNF-α, and MCP-1). They also express adhesion molecules, such as L-selectin as well as β_2 and β_1 integrins. The latter is an important distinction from the neutrophil, because it allows the macrophage to migrate to sites of inflammation in patients lacking the β_2 integrin receptor (i.e., leukocyte adhesion deficiency). Macrophages can phagocytose and kill many common bacteria, though less efficiently than the neutrophil. The macrophage's mechanisms of intracellular killing closely resemble those of the neutrophil, with both oxygen-dependent and oxygen-independent pathways. However, in addition to the production of ROIs, macrophages make a substantial amount of the potent molecule nitric oxide (NO), which is also microbicidal.

NO is the product of the conversion of arginine to citrulline by nitric oxide synthase (NOS). There are three isoforms of NOS: NOS-1 (neuronal NOS) and NOS-3 (endothelial NOS) are calcium dependent and are expressed constitutively at low levels. NOS-2 (inducible NOS or iNOS) is usually absent except when induced in response to inflammatory mediators (e.g., LPS, cytokines) and is the principal isoform found in macrophages.[47,48] NO has been shown to have both cytotoxic and cytostatic activity against a wide range of microorganisms in vitro and in vivo; these include bacteria, viruses, fungi, mycobacteria, parasites, and *Chlamydia*.[49] However, there is no clear evidence that human phagocytes produce sufficient amounts of NO to account for its antimicrobial activity.[48] In fact, data suggest that NO must react with ROIs to exert cytotoxicity.[50] The precise nature of this reaction is not completely understood. Under certain conditions NO may be cytostatic or cytotoxic, while under others, it may be cytoprotective.[48,51,52]

Following the phagocytosis of bacteria and intracellular killing, antigenic fragments derived from these microbes are processed by the macrophage and then presented to T lymphocytes in the context of major histocompatibility complex (MHC) class II molecules. This interaction elicits specific immune responses that amplify the cytokine (and cellular) response to further enhance microbicidal activity. This highly specialized function is one of the key distinguishing features of the macrophage in the host defense against microbes.

Lymphocytes Although neutrophils and monocytes-macrophages represent the major effectors of the host defense against microbes, certain microorganisms are able to evade their cytotoxic arsenal. These organisms must be eliminated through different means. The lymphocytes, and, to a lesser extent, the natural killer (NK) cells form the secondary line of defense against invading microbes.

Lymphocytes arise from a hematopoietic stem cell in the bone marrow. Early in the differentiation pathway, the lymphoid progenitor cell undergoes maturation in one of two distinct compartments, where it acquires its phenotypic and functional characteristics. Certain cells leave the bone marrow to undergo a process of "education" or maturation in the thymus. These mature T cells migrate from the thymus to reside in peripheral lymphoid organs, such as the spleen, lymph nodes, and intestinal Peyer patches. Other cells undergo maturation either in the bone marrow or fetal liver,

where they become committed to immunoglobulin synthesis (B cells).

Both B cells and T cells play an important role in the elimination of microbes. B cells, in particular, produce opsonizing antibodies that facilitate phagocytosis of encapsulated organisms. They also secrete other immunoglobulins, such as IgA, that play a central role in mucosal immunity by preventing bacterial adherence and invasion. In addition, B cells participate in antibody-dependent cell-mediated cytotoxicity. T lymphocytes, in contrast, are the principal effectors of cell-mediated immunity against intracellular pathogens. T-cell–mediated killing requires: (1) recognition of the inciting antigen or microbe, (2) cellular activation, (3) clonal expansion, and (4) targeted killing.

Antigen presentation and recognition are governed in part by a family of normally occurring cell surface proteins known as major histocompatibility proteins. There are two classes of MHC proteins: class I, which is expressed in virtually all nucleated cells, and class II, which is expressed primarily in antigen-presenting cells (APCs), such as macrophages, dendritic cells, and B lymphocytes. These cells phagocytose bacteria, processing or breaking down the organism into smaller fragments or peptides that are then bound to the MHC class II proteins and inserted into the cell membrane of the APCs. T cells bearing the same MHC molecules are then able to recognize this MHC-peptide complex on the APC. Interaction between this complex and specific ligands on T helper (TH) cells (CD4+) leads to cytokine production, recruitment of additional phagocytic cells, and proliferation of different classes of lymphocytes: B cells, TH cells, and CD8+ cytotoxic T lymphocytes (CTLs). Ultimately, microbial killing is promoted primarily by the CTLs. Infected cells that cannot process antigen in the context of an MHC class II protein form a complex between MHC class I molecules in the cell and antigenic peptides derived from the invading pathogen. This complex is readily recognized and targeted for destruction by the CTLs. Thus although only APCs can process antigen in the context of MHC class II molecules and elicit a TH response, all cells infected by an intracellular pathogen can present foreign antigen in association with MHC class I molecules, which serve as the target for the CTLs.

T-cell activation is dependent on two important events: stimulation by the T-cell receptor signal-transducing protein complex CD3 and simultaneous cross-linking of the CD4 or CD8 ligand to the appropriate MHC peptide complex on an APC or infected cell (CD4–MHC class II–APC and CD8–MHC class I–infected cell). T-cell activation initiates a cascade of events leading to calcium mobilization, activation of protein kinases, and transcription/translation of specific genes encoding proteins that will help to eliminate the pathogen. These proteins include perforins and serine proteases in CTLs and various cytokines in TH cells. Activated CTLs bind to cells expressing the MHC peptide complex and release cytotoxic granules, such as perforin, which can "perforate" the cell membrane creating a hole that leads to osmotic lysis. Alternatively, CTLs may release serine proteases that induce apoptosis in the infected cell without affecting the effector cell.[53–55] Similar to the CTL, NK cells, which are a variant of the lymphocyte family, can also use granule exocytosis to kill infected target cells. In addition, these cells possess Fc receptors for immunoglobulin and therefore can participate in antibody-dependent cell-mediated cytotoxicity. Two classes of TH cells have been described based on their cytokine profile: TH1 cells produce IL-2 and IFN-γ, while TH2 cells produce IL-4, IL-5, IL-10, and IL-13. Other cytokines, such as IL-3 and granulocyte-macrophage colony-stimulating factor, are produced by both TH1 and TH2 cells. TH1 cells evoke primarily a T-cell–mediated response characterized in part by recruitment of macrophages to the site of infection, followed by macrophage activation by IFN-γ.[56,57] In contrast, TH2 cytokines shift the balance toward a humoral (B-cell) response.

Humoral Factors

Thus far, we have emphasized the importance of cell-mediated immunity in the host defense against microbes. However, this cellular response is a highly complex phenomenon that is often initiated and optimized by diverse humoral factors, including immunoglobulins, complement activation, and cytokines, which is discussed in this section.

Immunoglobulins Immunoglobulins or antibodies represent a class of proteins that are synthesized by mature B lymphocytes or plasma cells, mainly as a result of cognate interaction between a TH cell and an antigen-presenting cell bearing an MHC-plus-peptide complex. This interaction may lead to cytokine synthesis and B-cell proliferation and maturation, with production of distinct classes of immunoglobulin. The primary role of antibodies in the host defense against microbes is to prevent bacterial adherence to, and subsequent invasion of, susceptible host cells. The mechanisms involved in this process include opsonization of the microbe to facilitate phagocytosis and complement activation with deposition of complement fragments on bacterial membranes to further enhance phagocytosis and subsequent bacterial killing. Neutralization of intrinsic microbial toxins or virulence factors to impede bacterial attachment to cell surfaces also occurs. There are five major classes of immunoglobulins: IgA, IgG, IgM, IgD, and IgE. Among these groups, IgG, IgM, and IgA are the predominant antibodies that mediate the host defense against microbes.

IgM is the largest of the immunoglobulins. It is the main component of the initial response to infection or antigenic stimulus. As such, it has a half-life of only 5 to 6 days, and its level declines steadily as IgG levels increase. Because of its size, IgM is found exclusively in the intravascular space, serving as an efficient bacterial agglutinin and as a potent activator of the complement system.

IgG is perhaps the most abundant antibody, constituting nearly 85% of serum immunoglobulins. It is found in both intravascular and extravascular (tissue) spaces. It is the only immunoglobulin that crosses the placenta from the mother to the fetus. IgG is the predominant class of antibody directed against bacteria and viruses. The biological potency of the molecule resides in its ability to opsonize bacteria by binding the antigen with its Fab component, while simultaneously binding the Fc receptor on the neutrophil, monocyte, or macrophage with its own Fc component. Moreover, IgG aggregates can activate the complement system.

Antibodies of the IgA isotype play a critical role in local mucosal immunity. They are synthesized by plasma cells within lymphoid tissue situated subjacent to the epithelial surfaces where they are secreted. IgA is released as a dimer and acquires a secretory component as it passes through the epithelial cell to exit at the mucosal surface in the form of secretory IgA. The latter serves as an antiseptic paint that binds pathogenic microbes and thus prevents their attachment, colonization, and subsequent invasion of tissue. Note, however, that IgG, IgM, and, to a lesser extent, IgE can also play a role in local mucosal immunity, especially in patients with congenital IgA deficiency.

Complement System Although antibodies are effective at recognizing antigenic determinants on microbial pathogens, they are unable to independently kill the microorganisms. Following opsonization, they must rely on phagocytes to ingest the microbe and on complement activation to further enhance or augment their opsonic ability to neutralize and ultimately kill the ingested pathogen. There are two distinct pathways for complement activation: classical and alternative. Antigen-antibody complexes are the predominant initiators of the classical pathway. In contrast, bacterial cell wall fragments, endotoxin (or LPS), cell surfaces, burned and injured tissue, and complex polysaccharides are capable of activating the alternative (properdin) pathway. Stimulation through either pathway initiates a cascade of events that can lead to marked complement activation as a result of an elaborate amplification process. The most critical point in this cascade occurs at C3, where both pathways converge to form C3a and C3b. C3a is both a vasodilator and a chemotaxin for phagocytes. The C3b molecule, in contrast, is the most critical component of the complement cascade, because this enzyme permits dramatic amplification of the system by facilitating further cleavage of C3 to C3a and C3b, as well as enhanced C3b production by the alternative pathway. Moreover, C3b is the most potent biologic opsonin, with cell surface receptors present on most phagocytes. Deposition of C3b on the surface of bacteria can promote its lysis by activating the distal components of the complement cascade (C8 and C9), which insert into and damage the cell membrane, resulting in osmotic lysis. In the process, another even more potent chemotaxin, C5a, is released, a molecule that is also capable of inducing a respiratory burst in the phagocyte and thus facilitates bacterial killing.

Cytokines The mediators that regulate the complex interactions among the various cellular effectors in the cytotoxic arsenal against microbes are generally known as cytokines. They represent a heterogeneous class of glycoproteins that are secreted by a variety of cells, including neutrophils, monocytes-macrophages, B and T lymphocytes, NK cells, endothelial cells, and fibroblasts. In general, there is extensive pleiotropy and redundancy in cytokine function. Some cytokines serve to amplify the inflammatory response, while others function to limit its extent.

Proinflammatory cytokines, such as TNF-α, IL-1, IL-6, IL-8, IL-11, and IL-18 share a number of similar properties; other cytokines that confer more specific immunity against certain pathogens, such as IL-2, IL-4, IL-12, and IL-13, also exhibit a number of similarities. Anti-inflammatory cytokines, such as IL-10 and transforming growth factor-β, neutralize the biological activities of the proximal mediators of inflammation——the monocytes-macrophages and their secretory products.

Tumor necrosis factor-α is one of the earliest inflammatory mediators released in response to infection. The predominant source of TNF-α is the monocyte-macrophage, although NK cells, mast cells, and some activated T cells also produce it, but to a lesser extent. TNF-α exerts a number of important functions in the inflammatory response. At low levels, it may (1) enhance endothelial cell adhesiveness for leukocytes; (2) promote neutrophil chemotaxis or recruitment to sites of inflammation; (3) stimulate the production of other proinflammatory cytokines that mimic TNF function, such as IL-1, IL-6, and IL-8; (4) prime neutrophils and monocytes-macrophages for microbial killing; and (5) up-regulate the expression of MHC class I molecules on target cells to facilitate killing. However, excess or uncontrolled TNF production, as occurs in overwhelming sepsis, may contribute to profound hemodynamic instability because of cardiovascular collapse, depressed myocardial contractility, and disseminated intravascular coagulation.

Interleukin-1 is released relatively early during the inflammatory response to infection or injury. It is produced by monocytes-macrophages and by epithelial, endothelial, and dendritic cells in response to endotoxin challenge or TNF stimulation. There are two biologically active forms of the molecule: IL-1α, which may be membrane associated, and IL-1β, which is active in soluble form. They share similar properties with TNF-α, including induction of other cytokines, such as IL-2, IL-6, and IL-8. However, unlike TNF-α, they exert little or no effect on MHC class I expression, nor do they play a role in hemodynamic collapse.

Interleukin-6 is the most important regulator of hepatic production of acute phase reactants, such as C-reactive protein. It is produced by a variety of cells, including mononuclear phagocytes, TH2 cells, and fibroblasts, in response to tissue injury, infection, TNF, and IL-1. It stimulates B-cell differentiation and enhances CTL maturation. IL-6 acts through a membrane-bound receptor that can shed and continue to regulate IL-6 activity away from the site of production.[58]

Interleukin-8 is secreted by monocytes-macrophages, T cells, endothelial cells, and platelets in response to inflammation, IL-1, and TNF. It is one of the most potent chemotactic and activating factors for neutrophils. IL-8 belongs to a family of chemoattractants that includes other chemokines, such as MCP-1, MCP-2, and MCP-3; macrophage inflammatory protein (MIP-1a, MIP-1b); and RANTES (regulated on activation, normal T expressed and secreted). These mediators are released early in inflammation, mainly by monocytes-macrophages but also by neutrophils and platelets. MIP-1a and MCP-1 may act in an autocrine fashion to recruit additional mononuclear phagocytes to sites of inflammation, thus potentially amplifying the inflammatory response. Another proinflammatory macrophage product, migration inhibitory factor, appears to be induced by TNF at sites of inflammation and serves to trap macrophages at those sites and elicit further TNF-α production by them.[59] RANTES is a lymphocyte-derived chemoattractant that promotes macrophage chemotaxis, up-regulates adhesion molecules, and enhances the release of inflammatory mediators.[59] Other chemoattractants include PAF, which is secreted by endothelial cells and macrophages, and leukotriene B4. In addition to serving as a chemoattractant for neutrophils, PAF up-regulates CD11b/CD18 (β$_2$ integrin) on the neutrophil.[60] In general, the chemoattractants not only recruit phagocytes to sites of inflammation but also appear to prime these cells for subsequent cytotoxic effector function.[61–63]

Other cytokines that play an important role in the elimination of invading microbial pathogens include products of TH1 cells, such as IL-2 and IFN-γ, as well as products of TH2 cells, such as IL-4 and IL-13. In general, TH1 cytokines are produced in response to bacterial, viral, or protozoan infections, and TH2 cytokines are secreted mostly in response to metazoa or allergens.[64,65] IL-2, the prototypical T-cell growth factor, directly amplifies the immune response by inducing cellular proliferation. It also augments killing by activating NK cells.

Interferon-γ is perhaps one of the most important macrophage activating factors. It stimulates the macrophage to express MHC class II molecules, which is necessary for antigen processing and for amplification of the immune response. In addition, it induces NOS activity (NOS-2), which is critical for intracellular killing of invading pathogens.[49,66] IFN-γ may enhance microbial killing by inducing TNF-α production and TNF-α receptor expression by macrophages and by activating NK cells. IFN-γ is also produced by activated CTLs in response to IL-2 and antigen expressed in the context of MHC class I molecules and by NK cells in response to IL-12.

Interleukin-12, primarily a macrophage product, is the most potent inducer of IFN-γ production by NK cells. In addition, it influences the uncommitted TH cell to differentiate into the TH1 phenotype, secreting IL-2 and IFN-γ.[60] IL-12 can support most of the functions performed by IL-2, except perhaps its proliferative effect. Therefore IL-12 plays an important role in the elimination of intracellular organisms.

The role of TH2 cytokines, such as IL-4 and IL-13, is less clear. Although they partly promote monocyte differentiation and may induce the expression of adhesion molecules in the endothelium, they are mostly responsible for immunoglobulin isotype switching in B cells, leading predominantly to IgG4 and IgE production.

Cytokine production and signaling are central to the sepsis response. Yet, under similar clinical and demographic circumstances, individuals may exhibit distinct responses to an identical stimulus. One possible explanation is differential protein expression between the two patients. For example, whereas a traumatic insult in one patient may lead to overwhelming sepsis and result in admission to the intensive care unit, another individual may exhibit a more attenuated response characterized by fever and tachycardia for a couple of hours, followed by resolution of the symptoms. Proteins may be expressed differently for a number of reasons, but one significant factor may be the genetic makeup of the individual. Gene polymorphisms or single nucleotide polymorphisms are differences in nucleic acid base pairs that occur every 100 bases. The change in base pairs that occurs in the promoter region of the gene may lead to overproduction or underproduction of a gene product. Recent evidence suggests that the presence of one gene polymorphism may serve as a marker for additional protective gene polymorphisms.[67] Cytokine gene polymorphisms may explain differences in the inflammatory response among individuals.[68]

Bacterial Virulence

Microbial pathogens possess unique biochemical properties known as virulence factors, which permit the successful establishment of infection within the host. If these virulence factors escape the host immune system, the net result will be sufficient multiplication or persistence of the microorganism within the host to cause significant damage to local tissue or allow transmission of the microorganism to other susceptible hosts.

The first and perhaps the most critical step in the process of microbial infection is adherence of the pathogenic microorganism to the cell surface. Some organisms multiply at the site of attachment, while others use this attachment as a prerequisite for microbial invasion. Elimination of this first step may completely abrogate colonization and invasion by microbial pathogens.

The process of microbial adherence requires specific interaction between specific molecules on the surface of the bacteria, known as adhesins, and specialized receptors on the host cell. Bacterial fimbriae or pili are perhaps the best studied adhesins that have been shown to promote bacterial adherence to mucosal surfaces. Members of the Enterobacteriaceae family exhibit prominent, morphologically similar pili—type I fimbriae—that permit their attachment to the d-mannose receptor sites on epithelial cells.[69,70] Further, certain bacteria, such as *Escherichia coli,* can simultaneously express different types of adhesins—type I, X, and P fimbriae—a property that clearly enhances the microbe's ability to attach to host surfaces.[71] Other adhesins include invasins, proteins that not only mediate bacterial attachment but also facilitate entry into the host, and hemagglutinin, which is expressed on pathogens such as *Bordetella pertussis, Salmonella typhimurium,* and influenza virus.[71] The host also secretes proteins that indirectly facilitate bacterial adherence; these include proteins of the extracellular matrix, namely, fibronectin, laminin, collagen, and vitronectin. These proteins share a common peptide sequence, Arg-Gly-Asp (RGD), which is also found on many microbial pathogens that bind to mammalian cells.[72] For instance, *Staphylococcus aureus* and *Streptococcus pyogenes* are known to bind fibronectin on epithelial surfaces.[71] Fortunately, bacterial binding to extracellular matrix proteins is usually of low affinity and rarely leads to microbial invasion.

Bacterial adherence allows microorganisms to penetrate the intact epithelial barrier of the host and eventually replicate. However, the mere adherence of the bacteria may not be sufficient for subsequent entry into the host cell. Bacterial internalization requires a high-affinity interaction between adhesins and specific receptors on the cell surface. The integrin receptors appear to be the primary targets on the cell surface for these interactions, because they can bind bacterial adhesins as well as extracellular matrix proteins, such as fibronectin, laminin, collagen, and vitronectin. It is the affinity of this interaction that determines whether the microbe becomes internalized or remains adherent to the host cell surface.[72]

Other bacterial virulence factors may also facilitate internalization. For instance, the cell surface protein invasin, found on *Yersinia* species, serves a dual purpose as an adhesin and an enhancer of bacterial invasion. It binds to β_1 integrins on the cell surface, resulting in internalization of *Yersinia*. Transfer of the invasin gene to nonpathogenic *E. coli* renders the organism capable of internalization and host tissue invasion.[72,73] Another variant of the invasin gene, termed the attachment invasion locus, has been identified in *Yersinia* species that cause clinical disease but not in those species that do not cause clinical infection. This molecule may serve as a potential marker of bacterial virulence.

Once bacterial internalization has occurred, the microbe is now located in an endosomal compartment, known as a phagosome, and must escape the intracellular host defense mechanisms to multiply. For internalized bacteria to survive, (1) fusion of the host cell lysosome with the phagosome to form a phagolysosome must be avoided, (2) acidification of the phagolysosome must be prevented, or (3) the antibacterial activity of the phagolysosome must be neutralized. Successful avoidance of these host defense mechanisms permits the establishment and multiplication of the organisms within the host. Bacterial toxins may play an important role in this process either by causing direct damage to host cells or by interfering with host defense mechanisms. For instance, diphtheria toxin creates a layer of dead cells that serves as a medium for bacterial growth. *Clostridium difficile* secretes both an enterotoxin (toxin A) and a cytotoxin (toxin B) that can damage the mucosal epithelium. *Clostridium perfringens* secretes numerous exotoxins with well-defined roles in the microbe's virulence. These toxins are enzymes with specific targets; they include hyaluronidase, collagenase, proteinase, deoxyribonuclease, and lecithinase. Several organisms, such as *Haemophilus influenzae, Streptococcus pneumoniae, Neisseria meningitidis,* and other bacteria that infect the oral cavity produce proteases that are capable of neutralizing local host defense mechanisms.[74] *S. aureus* is able to neutralize ROIs, such as hydrogen peroxide, through the production of catalase.

Likewise, bacterial endotoxins have potent biological properties. LPS consists of three regions: an O-specific side chain, a core polysaccharide, and an inner lipid A region. Most of the biological properties of LPS (also known as endotoxin) are attributed to the lipid A region. In fact, lipid A is believed to be the principal mediator of septic shock. LPS (especially the lipid A component) triggers an inflammatory cascade, leading to the release of various inflammatory mediators, including arachidonic acid derivatives, leukotrienes, and proinflammatory cytokines, and complement activation. Endotoxin interacts with inflammatory cells by binding to a complex consisting of soluble and membrane-bound receptors; this leads to a cascade of signaling events that result in increased expression of proinflammatory cytokines. These inflammatory mediators are responsible for the hemodynamic and metabolic events that characterize SIRS.

Another method of evading the host defense mechanisms is for the bacteria to avoid phagocytosis or engulfment by the professional phagocytes, such as the neutrophils and macrophages. Streptococci secrete a streptolysin that inhibits neutrophil migration or chemotaxis and impairs phagocyte cytotoxicity. Encapsulated organisms cannot be eliminated unless specific opsonizing antibodies that bind to the surface of the bacteria and facilitate their attachment to the Fc receptors on the neutrophil are present. These organisms are virulent pathogens in splenectomized patients, especially those younger than 4 years, with 50% mortality for overwhelming postsplenectomy sepsis found in some studies. Finally, certain microbial pathogens may avoid phagocytosis by binding the Fc receptor of IgG with the bacterial cell wall protein A, which is found in many bacteria, including virulent strains of staphylococci. This interaction prevents binding of the Fc receptor of the IgG antibody to the Fc receptor of the neutrophil.

Neonatal Host Defense

In general, neonates, especially premature infants, show increased vulnerability to bacterial infections and sepsis. This predisposition is closely linked to intrinsic deficiencies in the neonatal host defense apparatus. For term neonates, production of neutrophils is near the maximal level. Neutrophils constitute approximately 60% of circulating leukocytes; 15% of these neutrophils are immature (bands). These percentages are substantially lower in premature infants. Perhaps one of the most important factors in neonates' increased propensity for bacterial infections is their relative inability to significantly increase the levels of circulating neutrophils in response to stress or infection, resulting primarily from a limited neutrophil storage pool (20% to 30% that of adults) and, to a lesser extent, to increased margination of neutrophils.[75,76] Therefore systemic infections in neonates often lead to severe neutropenia. In fact, the relative degree of depletion of the neutrophil storage pool is a predictor of fatal outcome in neonatal sepsis.[75]

In addition to an already diminished storage pool, neonatal neutrophils show decreased adhesion to activated endothelium.[77,78] This process may be due to decreased L-selectin expression on the surface of neonatal neutrophils and an inability to up-regulate cell surface β_2 integrin.[69,70] Consequently, the neutrophils are unable to form the high-affinity adhesion to the endothelium that is necessary to effectively respond to a chemotactic gradient and migrate into tissues at sites of inflammation. In fact, several studies have shown that chemotaxis of neonatal neutrophils is substantially less than that of adult neutrophils.[79,80] Further, accumulating evidence suggests that abnormal signal transduction following the binding of chemotactic receptors to membrane receptors on neonatal neutrophils may also contribute to impaired chemotaxis.

Under normal conditions, neonatal neutrophils bind, ingest, and kill bacteria as effectively as adult neutrophils do. However, in the presence of a suboptimal concentration of opsonins, neonatal neutrophils are less efficient at phagocytosis,[81] an important consideration, because neonatal serum is deficient in opsonins. Neonatal neutrophils show normal production of superoxide but a relative decrease in the amount of hydroxyl radical and in the number of specific granules (defensins).[82] Therefore they may exhibit decreased oxygen-dependent and oxygen-independent microbial killing.[82] However, the deficiencies in microbicidal activity appear to be less critical than the substantial reduction in the neonatal neutrophil storage pool and the impairment in neutrophil chemotaxis, except perhaps in the presence of a high bacterial load, when efficient microbial killing becomes crucial.

Although the neonatal neutrophil storage pool may be diminished, the number of monocytes per blood volume in term infants appears to be equal to or greater than that of adults.[83] However, migration of these monocytes to sites of inflammation is significantly delayed compared with adults. Possible explanations for this relative delay in migration include decreased generation of chemoattractant factors for monocytes, impaired monocyte chemotaxis (as has been shown for neutrophils), and inability to up-regulate adhesion molecules on the surface of neonatal monocytes. Yet numerous studies have shown that neonatal monocytes have normal chemotaxis; others suggest that they may have normal migratory capacity but fail to properly orient toward the chemotactic gradient. Similarly, there are several conflicting reports regarding the expression of adhesion molecules on the surface of neonatal monocytes. Some studies show increased expression of β_2 integrins, while others suggest that these molecules are down-regulated in activated and resting neonatal monocytes. Nevertheless, once they reach the site of active inflammation,

neonatal monocytes phagocytose and kill bacteria as effectively as adult monocytes do. They probably use microbicidal mechanisms similar to adult monocytes because they can generate comparable levels of ROIs. However, data on NO production by neonatal monocytes relative to adult monocytes are scant. Activated neonatal monocytes and macrophages produce substantially less IL-6 and TNF-α than their adult counterparts. IL-1 production, in contrast, is equivalent.

Term neonates have a substantially greater number of circulating T lymphocytes than adults do. They also have a greater proportion of CD4+ versus CD8+ T cells compared with adults. These T cells express predominantly a virgin phenotype secondary to their relative lack of exposure to foreign antigens. However, they proliferate effectively in response to mitogenic stimuli. Stimulated neonatal T cells produce large quantities of IL-2. In contrast, production of other cytokines, such as TNF-α, IFN-γ, IL-3, IL-4, IL-5, and IL-10, is either moderately or significantly suppressed.[84–86] Neonates show decreased T-cell–mediated (CTL) cytotoxicity; this phenomenon may be due in part to the relative lack of prior antigenic exposure and the deficiency in cytokine production. Alternatively, the relative decrease in T-cell function may be the result of impaired monocyte-macrophage chemotaxis, resulting in diminished MHC-restricted cognate interactions between antigen-presenting cells and TH cells. Thus cytokine production is significantly reduced, and the inflammatory response is not amplified.

Term neonates also show relative immaturity of B-cell function and development. Although neonatal B cells can differentiate into IgM-secreting plasma cells, they do not differentiate into IgG- or IgA-secreting plasma cells until much later. IgM is more abundant in neonatal than in adult secretions. In contrast, virtually all circulating neonatal serum IgG is derived from maternal placental transfer. In fact, it is not until the third or fourth month of life that neonatal IgG production begins to account for a greater proportion of circulating IgG. As a result, the fetus is protected against most infectious agents for which the mother has adequate levels of circulating IgG antibodies, but not against those microbes that elicit a different immunoglobulin isotype, such as E. coli and Salmonella. Premature neonates are particularly vulnerable to such infections, because they do not receive sufficient maternal IgG. IgM and secretory IgA, which is detected in neonatal secretions within the first week of life and is abundant in breast milk, may provide compensatory protection against bacterial infection.

In term neonates, the percentage of NK cells, which play an important role against intracellular pathogens by promoting target cell lysis in a non–MHC-restricted fashion, is similar to that of the adult. However, they are functionally and phenotypically immature (CD56−).[87,88] At birth, their lytic potential is only 50% of that of adult NK cells, and they do not reach mature levels until late in infancy. This phenomenon may be partly due to decreased cytokine production (especially IFN-γ) in neonates, as previously discussed.

In general, because of their reduced levels of immunoglobulins, neonates rely primarily on the alternative (antibody-independent) pathway of complement activation. However, a substantial proportion of term and preterm neonates exhibit a significant reduction in components of both the classic and the alternative pathways of complement activation. The level of C9, a terminal component of the complement system that is critical for killing gram-negative organisms, is diminished, especially in preterm infants. The relative opsonic capacity of both term and preterm neonates is also impaired. This observation may be the result of inefficient cross-linking of the opsonin C3b after it has been deposited on the microorganism. Alternatively, it may reflect diminished levels of fibronectin, which plays an important role in cell adhesion and facilitates the binding of certain bacteria to phagocytes. Neonates also show decreased production of the potent chemotactic factor C5a. These defects further predispose term and preterm neonates to bacterial infections, because in addition to their already reduced neutrophil storage pool and their depressed levels of immunoglobulin, they cannot effectively use the most potent biologic opsonin, C3b, which is also responsible for amplification of the complement pathway. In addition, they have a decreased influx of phagocytes and impaired killing at the sites of infection owing to the decrease in C5a and in C9.

Diagnosis

GOLDSTEIN CRITERIA

Although definitions of the sepsis continuum have been published for adults,[6,11] no such work had been done for the pediatric population until 2002, when an international panel of 20 experts in sepsis convened to modify the published adult consensus definitions for children.[5] Physiologic and laboratory variables used to define SIRS, sepsis, severe sepsis, and MODS required modification for the different developmental stages in children. In addition, comparing pediatric sepsis studies had been very difficult because of the disparity in inclusion criteria and the myriad of pediatric definitions for the sepsis continuum in the literature before 2004. Therefore establishment of age group specific consensus definitions of the pediatric sepsis continuum should facilitate the interpretation and comparison of pediatric clinical trials. The following definitions and guidelines published by Goldstein and colleagues provide a uniform basis for diagnosing sepsis in children (Tables 10-2 to 10-4).

Age Group–Specific Definitions for Abnormal Vital Signs and Leukocyte Count

Specific definitions for abnormal vital signs and leukocyte count were established in six clinically and physiologically meaningful age groups (see Table 10-2). Premature infants were excluded, because their care occurs primarily in neonatal intensive care units; diagnosis in this group of unique patients will be discussed later. Age groups were defined as newborn (0 days to 1 week), neonate (1 week to 1 month), infant (1 month to 1 year), toddler and preschool (2 to 5 years), school-age child (6 to 12 years), and adolescent and young adult (13 to <18 years).

Definitions of the Pediatric Sepsis Continuum

Definitions of the pediatric sepsis continuum were established (see Table 10-3). There are several key differences in the terminology of sepsis and its related syndromes between adults and children. The major distinction is that the diagnosis of pediatric SIRS requires that a temperature or leukocyte abnormality be present. This requirement reflects the fact that tachycardia and tachypnea are common presenting symptoms of many pediatric disease processes and are not specific to SIRS or sepsis. A core temperature measured by rectal, bladder, oral, or central catheter probe is required. Temperatures taken through the tympanic, toe, or axillary route are not sufficiently accurate. Notably, bradycardia may be a sign of SIRS in the newborn age group. Although a positive culture confirms the presence of infection, the definition of infection in children also includes specific clinical examination findings, such as petechiae and purpura in the setting of hemodynamic instability; fever, cough, and hypoxemia in the setting of leukocytosis and pulmonary infiltrates; or a distended tympanitic abdomen with fever and leukocytosis associated with perforated bowel.

Pediatric Organ Dysfunction Criteria

The definition of pediatric septic shock remains problematic, because children typically maintain their blood pressure until they are gravely ill. Thus, unlike adults, there is no requirement for systemic hypotension to make the diagnosis of septic shock, because shock may occur long before hypotension is present in children. Pediatric septic shock is defined as sepsis and cardiovascular organ dysfunction, as noted in Table 10-4. Although adult organ dysfunction criteria have been applied to various pediatric populations, they may be inappropriate for children. Thus the consensus conference established pediatric organ dysfunction criteria (see Table 10-4) based on those used in the Pediatric Logistic Organ Dysfunction, Pediatric-MODS, and Multiple Organ System Failure scores as well as the criteria used in the open-label recombinant human activated protein C study.[5]

TABLE 10-2				
Age Group Specific Definitions for Abnormal Vital Signs and Leukocyte Count				
Age Group	*HR (Beats/Minute)*	*RR (Breaths/Minute)*	*SBP (mm Hg)*	*WBC count (WBCs $\times$ 10³/mm)*
Newborn (0 day-1 week)	>180 or <100	>50	<65	>34
Neonate (1 week-1 month)	>180 or <100	>40	<75	>19.5 or <5
Infant (1 month-1 year)	>180 or <90	>34	<100	>17.5 or <5
Toddler/preschool (2-5 years)	>140	>22	<94	>15.5 or <6
School-age child (6-12 years)	>130	>18	<105	>13.5 or <4.5
Adolescent/young adult (13 to <18 years)	>110	>14	<117	>11 or <4.5

Modified and used with permission from Goldstein B, Giroir B, Randolph A, et al: International pediatric sepsis consensus conference: Definitions for sepsis and organ dysfunction in pediatrics. Pediatr Crit Care Med 2005;6:2-8.
HR, heart rate; RR, respiratory rate; SBP, systolic blood pressure; WBC, white blood cell.

TABLE 10-3

Definitions of the Pediatric Sepsis Continuum

Systemic Inflammatory Response Syndrome (SIRS)*

The presence of at least two of the following four criteria, **one of which must be abnormal temperature or leukocyte count:**

1. Core[†] temperature of $> 38.5°$ C or $< 36°$ C.
2. Tachycardia, defined as a mean heart rate > 2 SD above normal for age in the absence of external stimulus, chronic drugs, or painful stimuli; or otherwise unexplained persistent elevation over a 0.5- to 4-hour time period **OR for children < 1 year old: bradycardia, defined as a mean heart rate < 10th percentile for age in the absence of external vagal stimulus, beta-blocker drugs, or congenital heart disease; or otherwise unexplained persistent depression over a 0.5-hour time period.**
3. Mean respiratory rate > 2 SD above normal for age or mechanical ventilation for an acute process not related to underlying neuromuscular disease or the receipt of general anesthesia.
4. Leukocyte count elevated or depressed for age (not secondary to chemotherapy-induced leukopenia) or $> 10\%$ immature neutrophils.

Infection

A suspected or proven (by positive culture, tissue stain, or polymerase chain reaction test) infection caused by any pathogen OR a clinical syndrome associated with a high probability of infection. Evidence of infection includes positive findings on clinical exam, imaging, or laboratory tests (e.g., white blood cells in a normally sterile body fluid, perforated viscus, chest radiograph consistent with pneumonia, petechial or purpuric rash, or purpura fulminans)

Sepsis

SIRS in the presence of or as a result of suspected or proven infection.

Severe Sepsis

Sepsis plus one of the following: cardiovascular organ dysfunction OR acute respiratory distress syndrome OR two or more other organ dysfunctions. Organ dysfunctions are defined in Table 10-4.

Septic Shock

Sepsis and cardiovascular organ dysfunction as defined in Table 10-4.

Modified and used with permission from Goldstein B, Giroir B, Randolph A, et al: International pediatric sepsis consensus conference: Definitions for sepsis and organ dysfunction in pediatrics. Pediatr Crit Care Med 2005;6:2-8.
*See Table 10-2 for age group specific definitions for abnormal vital signs and leukocyte count.
[†]Core temperature must be measured by rectal, bladder, oral, or central catheter probe.
Modifications from the adult definitions are in **boldface**; SD, standard deviation(s).

DIAGNOSIS OF NEONATAL SEPSIS

The diagnosis of neonatal sepsis, particularly in premature newborns and VLBW infants, remains a challenge. As previously discussed, the neonate's host defense mechanism is markedly impaired, and this problem is even more pronounced in the preterm neonate. These infants may not manifest the same clinical signs as older patients. Sepsis should be suspected in any newborn with temperature instability, apnea, respiratory distress or tachypnea, cardiovascular instability (including tachycardia, bradycardia, and hypotension), reduced perfusion or poor color, feeding intolerance or diarrhea, and poor tone or lethargy, particularly in the presence of a maternal history of premature onset of labor, prolonged (>24 hours) rupture of membranes, clinically proven chorioamnionitis, colonization of the genital tract with pathogenic bacteria (e.g., group B *Streptococcus* or *E. coli*), urinary tract infection, or sexual intercourse near the time of delivery, because these are all independent risk factors for the development of neonatal infection. In fact, these risk factors increase the rate of systemic infection more than 10-fold.[89]

TABLE 10-4

Pediatric Organ Dysfunction Criteria

Cardiovascular Dysfunction

Despite administration of isotonic intravenous fluid bolus ≥ 40 mL/kg in 1 hour:

Decrease in BP (hypotension) < 5th percentile for age or systolic BP < 2 SD below normal for age*

OR

Need for vasoactive drug to maintain BP in normal range (dopamine > 5 µg/kg/min or dobutamine, epinephrine, or norepinephrine at any dose)

OR

Two of the following:

  Unexplained metabolic acidosis: base deficit > 5.0 mEq/L
  Increased arterial lactate > 2 times upper limit of normal
  Oliguria: urine output < 0.5 mL/kg/hr
  Prolonged capillary refill: >5 seconds
  Core to peripheral temperature gap $> 3°$ C

Respiratory[†]

$Pao_2/Fio_2 < 300$ in absence of cyanotic heart disease or preexisting lung disease

OR

$Paco_2 > 65$ torr or 20 mm Hg over baseline $Paco_2$

OR

Proven need[‡] or $>50\%$ Fio_2 to maintain saturation $\geq 92\%$

OR

Need for nonelective invasive or noninvasive mechanical ventilation[§]

Neurologic

Glasgow Coma Score ≤ 11

OR

Acute change in mental status with a decrease in Glasgow Coma Score ≥ 3 points from abnormal baseline

Hematologic

Platelet count $< 80,000$/mm³ or a decline of 50% in platelet count from highest value recorded during the past 3 days (for chronic hematology/oncology patients)

OR

International normalized ratio > 2

Renal

Serum creatinine ≥ 2 times upper limit of normal for age or twofold increase in baseline creatinine

Hepatic

Total bilirubin ≥ 4 mg/dL (not applicable for newborn)

OR

ALT 2 times upper limit of normal for age

Modified and used with permission from Goldstein B, Giroir B, Randolph A, et al: International pediatric sepsis consensus conference: Definitions for sepsis and organ dysfunction in pediatrics. Pediatr Crit Care Med 2005;6:2-8.
*See Table 10-3.
[†]Acute respiratory distress syndrome must include a Pao_2/Fio_2 ratio ≤ 200 mm Hg, bilateral infiltrates, acute onset, and no evidence of left heart failure. Acute lung injury is defined identically, except the Pao_2/Fio_2 ratio must be ≤ 300 mm Hg.
[‡]Proven need assumes oxygen requirement was tested by decreasing flow with subsequent increase in flow if required.
[§]In postoperative patients, this requirement can be met if the patient has developed an acute inflammatory or infectious process in the lungs that prevents him or her from being extubated.
ALT, alanine transaminase; BP, blood pressure; SD, standard deviation(s).

BIOCHEMICAL MARKERS

Although the Goldstein consensus criteria establish important and useful definitions for the sepsis continuum in children, these are largely based on clinical and some laboratory findings.

Current research targets to improve the diagnosis of pediatric sepsis include various biochemical inflammatory markers. These may prove to be objective criteria and perhaps more reliable than some physiologic variables. Investigators have reported elevated sedimentation rate, C-reactive protein, base deficit, IL-6, procalcitonin level, adrenomedullin, soluble CD14, soluble endothelial cell/leukocyte adhesion molecule 1, MIP, and extracellular phospholipase A_2 as potential biochemical markers of SIRS.[90–104] Although some of these markers are sensitive, most lack specificity, and none of them is sufficiently robust to add to the consensus definition of SIRS at this time. However, in the future, it may be possible to incorporate biochemical and immunologic markers in the diagnostic criteria for pediatric SIRS.

PIRO SYSTEM

An emerging concept in sepsis research is the PIRO system, which stratifies patients on the basis of their *P*redisposing conditions, the nature and extent of the *I*nsult or *I*nfection, the magnitude of the host *R*esponse, and the degree of concomitant *O*rgan dysfunction.[6] The PIRO system is analogous to the tumor-node-metastasis (TNM) system for oncology in that it can be used to assess risk and predict outcome in septic patients, assist with enrollment of patients into clinical trials, and determine the likely patient response to specific therapies. Specifically, the PIRO system should be able to discriminate morbidity arising from infection and morbidity arising from the response to infection based on a patient's I and R scores and their outcomes. Thus the PIRO system has the potential to help researchers develop and clinicians choose the most appropriate treatments for septic patients, because therapeutics that modulate the host response may adversely affect the body's ability to contain an infection.

A recent retrospective analysis of two large global databases of patients with severe sepsis (PROWESS-840 patients and PROGRESS-10,610 patients) was undertaken to generate and validate the PIRO system. In PROWESS, the correlation between the PIRO total score and in-hospital mortality rates was 0.974 ($P < 0.0001$), and in PROGRESS it was 0.998 ($P < 0.0001$). The investigators concluded that the PIRO system appears to accurately predict mortality, can develop into an effective model for staging severe sepsis, and may prove useful in future sepsis research.[105] Brilli and colleagues suggest that a modified PIRO system for pediatric sepsis should be developed and applied to future clinical pediatric sepsis trials, assuming the adult PIRO system is proven to be successful and adds a useful new dimension to clinical trials.[106,107]

Management

PREVENTION

Given the rising incidence of sepsis and growing health care burden, management of pediatric sepsis should begin with prevention. In neonates, early onset sepsis can potentially be prevented or reduced with appropriate prenatal and peripartum management, especially in complicated pregnancy.

Active management of early postpartum newborns based on their risk profile with antibiotic prophylaxis is also important. Prevention of neonatal late onset sepsis and sepsis in older children is dependent on infection control practices that reduce hospital-acquired infection, such as frequent handwashing, contact precautions, invasive device care, sterilization of equipment, and epidemic control methods. Although good outcome studies of individual interventions are difficult because of power restrictions, intervention bundle studies indicate that combined implementation of infection control techniques reduces the risk of nosocomial infection.[108,109] One pediatric study by Costello and colleagues found that an intervention bundle in their pediatric cardiac ICU reduced the central-line–associated bloodstream infection rate from 7.8 infections per 1000 catheter-days to 2.3 infections per 1000 catheter-days.[110] Furthermore, Brilli and colleagues were the first to demonstrate a significant, sustained reduction in pediatric ventilator-associated pneumonia (VAP) rates following the use of an intervention bundle. After implementation of their VAP prevention bundle, VAP rates decreased from 7.8 cases per 1,000 ventilator days in fiscal year 2005 to 0.5 cases per 1,000 ventilator days in 2007.[111]

EARLY GOAL-DIRECTED THERAPY

Surviving Sepsis Campaign

After prevention, the cornerstone of treatment is early diagnosis and goal-directed therapeutic interventions. In 2002, the European Society of Intensive Care Medicine, International Sepsis Forum, and SCCM launched the surviving sepsis campaign (SSC) in an effort to improve sepsis outcomes by establishing evidence-based guidelines to standardize care. These internationally accepted guidelines (endorsed by 11 professional societies) were published in 2004 and updated in 2008.[7,8] Previous studies have found that the development and publication of guidelines are infrequently integrated into bedside practice in a timely fashion and may not change clinical behavior.[112–117] Recognizing that guideline implementation is a significant challenge, Levy and colleagues conducted the SSC performance improvement initiative at 165 sites internationally to assess the impact of guideline compliance on the hospital mortality of 15,022 patients. Compliance increased linearly over the 2-year study period and unadjusted hospital mortality decreased from 37% to 30.8% in the same period. The adjusted odds ratio for mortality improved the longer a site participated in the campaign. The authors commented that the campaign was associated with a sustained, continuous quality improvement in sepsis care and a reduction in reported hospital mortality rates, although these findings do not necessarily reflect cause and effect.[118] Although the SSC guidelines primarily pertain to the adult population, both the 2004 and 2008 publications address pediatric considerations in sepsis.

American College of Critical Care Medicine/ Pediatric Advanced Life Support Guidelines

The same year the SSC was launched, the ACCM published their clinical practice parameters for hemodynamic support of pediatric and neonatal patients in septic shock.[9] Multiple studies have reported that these guidelines are useful, effective, and improve outcomes in infants and children with sepsis.[10] For instance, Han and colleagues demonstrated that although resuscitation practice among community physicians was consistent with the ACCM/PALS guidelines in only 30% of patients, when practice was in agreement with guideline recommendations, a lower mortality was observed (8% vs. 38%). Notably, every hour that went by with persistent shock was associated with a greater than twofold increase in odds of mortality.[119] In a retrospective study of the 2003 Kids' Inpatient Database, including nearly 3 million pediatric discharge records, overall hospital mortality from severe sepsis was estimated to be 4.2%, 2.3% in previously healthy children, and 7.8% in children with comorbidities.[120] This lower mortality rate is distinct from the previous estimate of 10.3% by Watson and colleagues, using 1995 hospital discharge and population data. Survival from severe sepsis in 2003 may have improved, in part, as a result of guideline implementation.[14] In a randomized controlled trial, de Oliveira and colleagues reported that treatment adhering to the ACCM/PALS guidelines with central venous oxygen saturation ($Scvo_2$) goal-directed therapy resulted in reduced 28-day mortality for severe sepsis and septic shock (11.8% vs. 39.2%, $P = 0.002$).[121] These studies support the implementation of the early, goal-directed therapy recommended by the ACCM/PALS guidelines.

The ACCM/PALS guidelines were updated in 2007 with continued emphasis on (1) first-hour fluid resuscitation and inotrope drug therapy directed to restore threshold heart rate (HR), normal blood pressure (BP), and capillary refill less than or equal to 2 seconds and (2) subsequent intensive care unit hemodynamic support directed to achieving $Scvo_2$ greater than 70% and cardiac index (CI) of 3.3 to 6.0 L/minute/m². The changes recommended were few but include the following: (1) the use of peripheral inotropes (not vasopressors) until central access is attained is recommended, because mortality increased with delay in establishing central access and subsequent inotrope use. (2) Etomidate is not recommended for children with septic shock unless it is used in a randomized controlled trial; atropine and ketamine may be used for invasive procedures in children with septic shock, but no recommendation is made for sedative/analgesic use in newborns with septic shock. (3) Cardiac output (CO) may be measured not only with a pulmonary artery catheter, but also with Doppler echocardiography, a pulse index contour CO catheter, or a femoral artery thermodilution catheter. Therapy should be directed to maintain a CI 3.3 to 6.0 L/min/m² or superior vena cava (SVC) flow greater than 40 mL/min/kg in VLBW infants. (4) Several new potential rescue therapies, including enoximone, levosimendan, inhaled prostacyclin, and intravenous (IV) adenosine, should be further evaluated in the appropriate patient settings. (5) Fluid removal is recommended using diuretics, peritoneal dialysis, or continuous renal replacement therapy in adequately fluid resuscitated patients who cannot maintain fluid balance by native urine output, which can be identified by the development of new-onset hepatomegaly, rales, or greater or equal to 10% body-weight fluid overload.

SURVIVING SEPSIS CAMPAIGN AND AMERICAN COLLEGE OF CRITICAL CARE MEDICINE/PEDIATRIC ADVANCED LIFE SUPPORT RECOMMENDATIONS AND MANAGEMENT ALGORITHMS

The recommendations of both the updated SSC and ACCM/PALS guidelines for the management of pediatric and neonatal sepsis are summarized in two algorithms: the time-sensitive, goal-directed stepwise management of hemodynamic support for infants and children (Fig. 10-4) and for newborns (Fig. 10-5) in septic shock. These recommendations and management algorithms are discussed in detail below.

Initial Resuscitation

Once the diagnosis of sepsis is made, aggressive early intervention should ensue. The principal objective is to restore oxygen delivery to the tissues in view of the decreased peripheral oxygen utilization and the increased oxygen demand. This goal can be achieved by ensuring that the patient is adequately resuscitated. Evidence suggests that children who present with sepsis are often grossly underresuscitated.[119,122] Contrary to adult septic shock, low CO, not low systemic vascular resistance (SVR), is associated with mortality in pediatric septic shock.[123–132] Therefore children frequently respond well to aggressive volume resuscitation, with attainment of the therapeutic goal of a CI 3.3 to 6.0 L/minute/m².[124,132] Ceneviva and colleagues demonstrated that outcome can be significantly improved when aggressive fluid resuscitation is used for fluid-refractory, dopamine-resistant septic shock.[124,132] Additionally, they make an important point: Unlike adults, children with fluid-refractory shock are frequently hypodynamic and respond to inotrope and vasodilator therapy; because hemodynamic states are heterogeneous and change with time, an incorrect cardiovascular therapeutic regimen should be suspected in any child with persistent shock.[132]

Airway, Breathing, and Circulation During the first 15 minutes of the initial resuscitation, the airway, breathing, and circulation, or ABCs, should be maintained or restored. The airway must first be secured followed by establishment of oxygenation and ventilation. Finally, assessment of perfusion and blood pressure should be performed. Hypoglycemia and hypocalcemia should also be corrected during these first 15 minutes.[10] Missed hypoglycemia can result in neurologic devastation. It is crucial to rapidly diagnose and promptly treat hypoglycemia with appropriate glucose infusion in the septic patient.[10] A 10% dextrose-containing isotonic intravenous (IV) solution can be run at maintenance rate and titrated as needed to provide age appropriate glucose delivery to prevent hypoglycemia. The target plasma glucose concentration is greater than or equal to 80 mg/dL. Hypocalcemia is a frequent, reversible cause of cardiac dysfunction.[133,134] Calcium replacement therapy should be aimed at normalizing ionized calcium concentration, because serum calcium is often bound to albumin and may appear falsely low in malnourished patients.[10]

Crystalloid Versus Colloid Fluid infusion is best begun with boluses of 20 mL/kg isotonic saline or colloid, and initial volume resuscitation commonly requires 40 to 60 mL/kg but

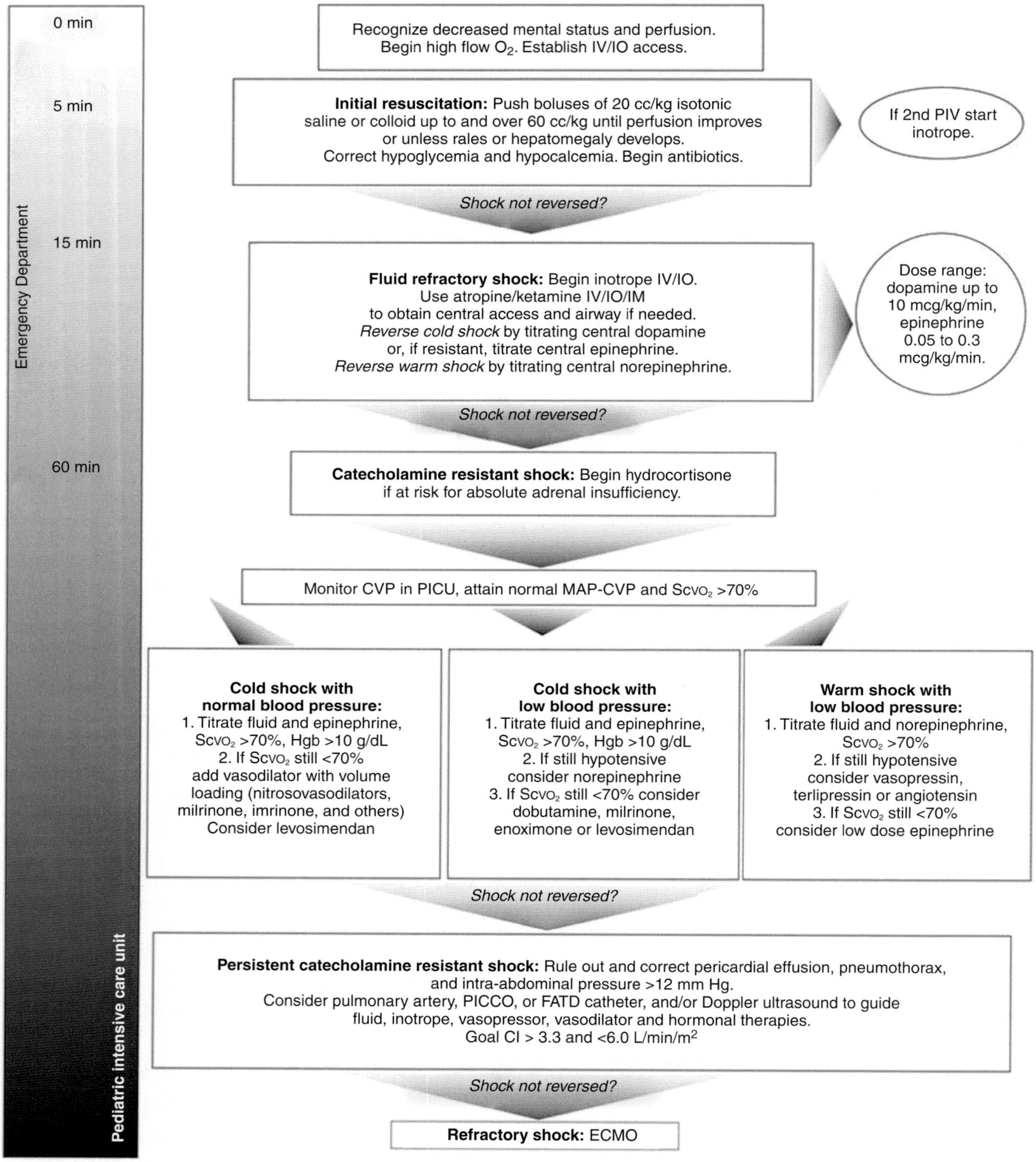

0 min

Recognize decreased mental status and perfusion.
Begin high flow O_2. Establish IV/IO access.

5 min

Initial resuscitation: Push boluses of 20 cc/kg isotonic
saline or colloid up to and over 60 cc/kg until perfusion improves
or unless rales or hepatomegaly develops.
Correct hypoglycemia and hypocalcemia. Begin antibiotics.

If 2nd PIV start
inotrope.

Shock not reversed?

15 min

Fluid refractory shock: Begin inotrope IV/IO.
Use atropine/ketamine IV/IO/IM
to obtain central access and airway if needed.
Reverse cold shock by titrating central dopamine
or, if resistant, titrate central epinephrine.
Reverse warm shock by titrating central norepinephrine.

Dose range:
dopamine up to
10 mcg/kg/min,
epinephrine
0.05 to 0.3
mcg/kg/min.

Shock not reversed?

60 min

Catecholamine resistant shock: Begin hydrocortisone
if at risk for absolute adrenal insufficiency.

Monitor CVP in PICU, attain normal MAP-CVP and $ScvO_2$ >70%

Cold shock with normal blood pressure:	**Cold shock with low blood pressure:**	**Warm shock with low blood pressure:**
1. Titrate fluid and epinephrine, $ScvO_2$ >70%, Hgb >10 g/dL 2. If $ScvO_2$ still <70% add vasodilator with volume loading (nitrosovasodilators, milrinone, imrinone, and others) Consider levosimendan	1. Titrate fluid and epinephrine, $ScvO_2$ >70%, Hgb >10 g/dL 2. If still hypotensive consider norepinephrine 3. If $ScvO_2$ still <70% consider dobutamine, milrinone, enoximone or levosimendan	1. Titrate fluid and norepinephrine, $ScvO_2$ >70% 2. If still hypotensive consider vasopressin, terlipressin or angiotensin 3. If $ScvO_2$ still <70% consider low dose epinephrine

Shock not reversed?

Persistent catecholamine resistant shock: Rule out and correct pericardial effusion, pneumothorax,
and intra-abdominal pressure >12 mm Hg.
Consider pulmonary artery, PICCO, or FATD catheter, and/or Doppler ultrasound to guide
fluid, inotrope, vasopressor, vasodilator and hormonal therapies.
Goal CI > 3.3 and <6.0 L/min/m^2

Shock not reversed?

Refractory shock: ECMO

Emergency Department

Pediatric intensive care unit

FIGURE 10-4 Algorithm for time-sensitive, goal-directed stepwise management of hemodynamic support in infants and children. CI, cardiac index; CVP, central venous pressure; FATD, femoral artery thermodilution; Hgb, hemoglobin; IM, intramuscular; IO, intraosseous; IV, intravenous; MAP, mean arterial pressure; PICCO, pulse index contour cardiac output; PICU, pediatric intensive care unit; PIV, peripheral intravenous (line); $ScvO_2$, central venous oxygen saturation. (Used with permission from Brierley J, Carcillo JA, Choong K, et al: Clinical practice parameters for hemodynamic support of pediatric and neonatal septic shock: 2007 update from the American College of Critical Care Medicine. Crit Care Med 2009;37:666-688.)

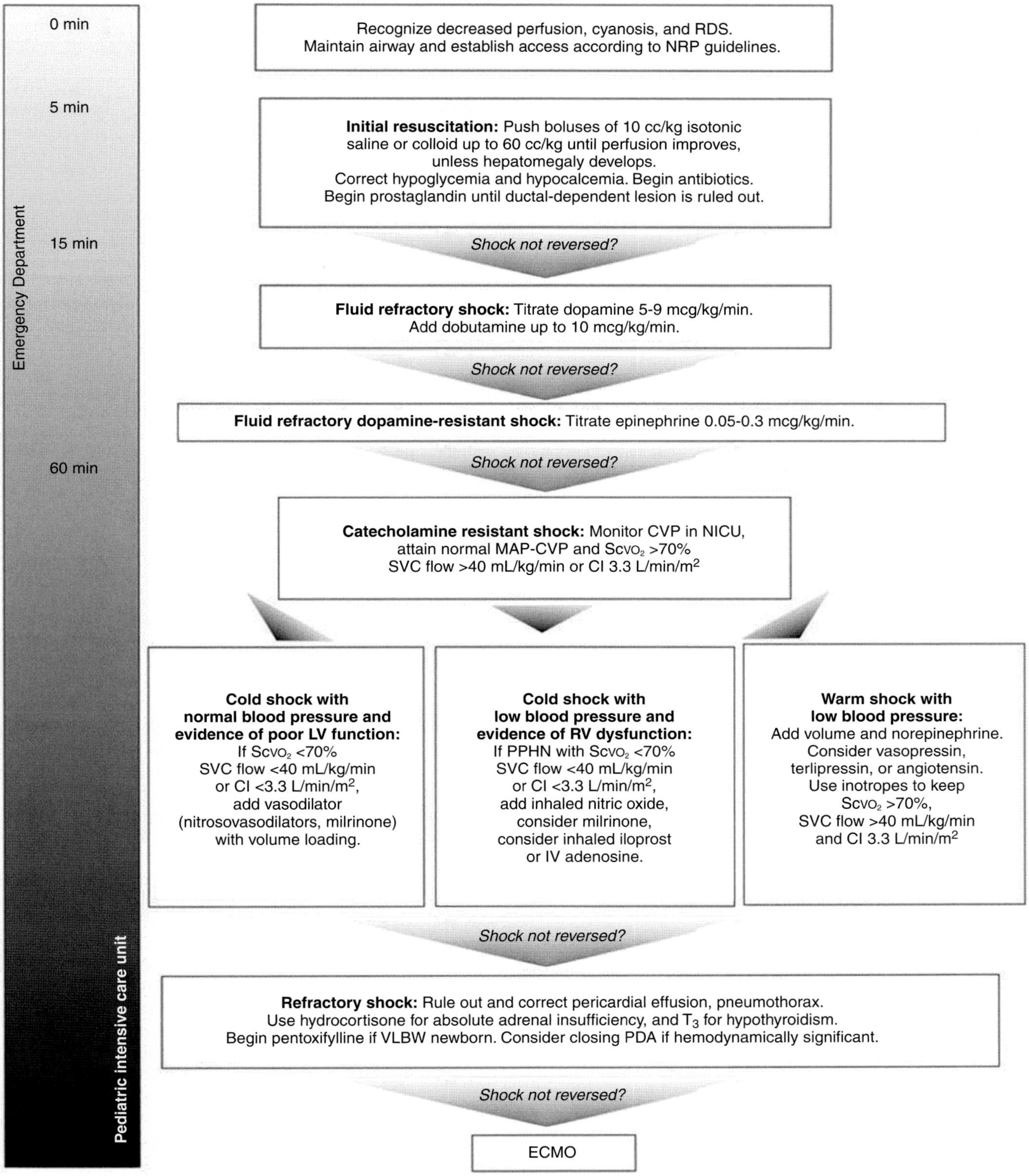

FIGURE 10-5 Algorithm for time-sensitive, goal-directed stepwise management of hemodynamic support in newborns. CI, cardiac index; ECMO, extracorporeal membrane oxygenation; LV, left ventricular; MAP, mean arterial pressure; NICU, neonatal intensive care unit; NRP, Neonatal Resuscitation Program; PDA, patent ductus arteriosus; PPHN, persistent pulmonary hypertension; RDS, respiratory distress syndrome; RV, right ventricular; Scvo$_2$, central venous oxygen saturation; SVC, superior vena cava; T$_3$, triiodothyronine; VLBW, very low birth weight. (Used with permission from Brierley J, Carcillo JA, Choong K, et al: Clinical practice parameters for hemodynamic support of pediatric and neonatal septic shock: 2007 update from the American College of Critical Care Medicine. Crit Care Med 2009;37:666-688.)

can be as much as 200 mL/kg.[119,122,131,135–145] Of note, large volumes of fluid for resuscitation in children have not been shown to increase the incidence of acute respiratory distress syndrome[122,146] or cerebral edema.[122,147] The use of either crystalloid or colloid is acceptable, because three randomized controlled trials have compared the use of colloid versus crystalloid resuscitation in children with dengue shock and found no difference in mortality.[144,145,148]

Blood Products The use of blood transfusion during resuscitation is less well defined. Two small pediatric observational studies have looked at the use of blood to restore intravascular volume; however, no recommendations were made by the investigators.[149,150] A recent randomized controlled trial by Lacroix and colleagues found that a lower transfusion threshold can decrease transfusion requirements without increasing adverse outcomes in stable critically ill children. They demonstrated similar outcomes in 637 pediatric patients managed with a transfusion threshold of hemoglobin (Hb) 7 g/dL versus 9.5 g/dL (38 vs. 39 patients developed new or progressive MODS, and 14 vs. 14 patients died within 28 days).[151] However, these results should be interpreted with caution. Their study population was stable critically ill children defined by mean arterial pressure (MAP) not less than 2 standard deviations (SD) below normal mean for age and no escalation of cardiovascular treatment for at least 2 hours prior to enrollment. Therefore these results may not be applicable to unstable children in septic shock with severe hypoxemia, hemodynamic instability, active blood loss, or cyanotic heart disease.[152] Children in septic shock may benefit from early blood transfusion to restore preload and achieve minimum Scvo$_2$. Although the task force members for the updated ACCM/PALS guidelines report the use of conservative goals for blood transfusion in routine clinical illness (consistent with the randomized controlled trial by Lacroix and colleagues[151]), they suggest that transfusion to a goal Hb greater than 10 g/dL to achieve an Scvo$_2$ greater than 70% is warranted in children with septic shock.[10] They base their recommendation on the previously mentioned report by de Oliveira and colleagues that the use of the 2002 ACCM/PALS guidelines and continuous Scvo$_2$ monitoring improved mortality (11.8% vs. 39.2%) and that the treatment group received more blood transfusions directed toward improving Scvo$_2$ to greater than 70% (45.1% vs. 15.7%).[121]

Fresh frozen plasma (FFP) may be used to correct abnormal prothrombin time and partial thromboplastin time, but should be infused, not pushed as a bolus, because it may produce acute hypotensive effects resulting from vasoactive kinins and high citrate concentration.[10] FFP has been proposed as an adjunctive therapy for septic neonates, especially premature neonates who are deficient in IgG, IgM, IgA, and complement. However, no benefit was found when FFP was administered prophylactically to infants with suspected infection.[153]

Antibiotics Broad-spectrum antibiotics should be administered after appropriate cultures have been obtained during the initial resuscitation period.[8,10] The SSC guidelines recommend that at least two blood cultures be obtained before antibiotics are begun, with at least one drawn percutaneously and one drawn through each vascular access device unless it was inserted recently (<48 hours).[8,154] Cultures of other sites, preferably quantitative, such as urine, cerebrospinal fluid, respiratory secretions, wounds, or other body fluids should also be obtained before antibiotic therapy if not associated with a significant delay in antibiotic administration. Acquiring appropriate cultures prior to antibiotic administration is essential to confirm infection and the responsible pathogens, which will later allow de-escalation of antibiotic therapy after receipt of the susceptibility profile. However, it should not prevent prompt administration of antimicrobial therapy.[8] In the presence of septic shock, each delay of an hour in administering effective antibiotics is associated with a measurable increase in mortality of 7.6%.[155] The SSC guidelines recommend starting IV antibiotics as early as possible, certainly within the first hour of recognition of septic shock and severe sepsis.[8]

It is also imperative that the initial empirical antimicrobial therapy be broad enough to cover all likely pathogens and penetrate in adequate concentrations into the presumed source of sepsis. Failure to initiate appropriate antibiotics against the pathogen that is subsequently identified as the causative organism correlates with increased morbidity and mortality.[156–159] Equally important is the subsequent tailoring of the antibiotic regimen once the causative pathogen and its susceptibilities are identified. This helps to reduce the development of antimicrobial resistance and the likelihood of superinfection with resistant organisms such as *Candida* species, *Clostridium difficile*, or vancomycin-resistant *Enterococcus faecium*.[8]

Selection of appropriate antibiotic therapy is challenging because dynamic epidemiology, multidrug-resistant bacteria, and opportunistic infection make optimal broad-spectrum antimicrobial coverage a moving target. In term and preterm neonates, group B streptococcus and *Escherichia coli* account for most of the bacterial isolates.[160] Although the incidence of coagulase-negative *Staphylococcus aureus* and *Candida* species infections in neonates is rising,[161] historically, the most common organisms identified in adults and older children include *E. coli, Pseudomonas aeruginosa, Klebsiella*, and *Bacteroides* species. However, the epidemiology is constantly changing, now with an increase in gram-positive isolates.[2,162] It is diffcult to define the epidemiology of infective organisms because it changes with time, is unique to each hospital, and varies by patient age.

The RESOLVE trial, a randomized controlled trial that found a lack of proof of efficacy and an increased risk of bleeding of recombinant human activated protein C in pediatric sepsis, may have inadvertently provided some current data on the global bacteriology of pediatric sepsis.[162] The study enrolled 477 patients, aged between 38 weeks corrected gestational age and 17 years, from 104 study sites in 18 countries between November 2002 and April 2005. The most common site of infection was the lung in approximately 37%, followed by the blood in just less than one third of patients. Pure gram-positive infections were more common than pure gram-negative infections, consistent with the data of Martin and colleagues on the rising incidence of gram-positive infections beginning in 1987.[2] The most frequent isolates in lung infections were *Staphylococcus aureus,* followed by *Pseudomonas aeruginosa* and *Candida albicans. Neisseria meningitides* and coagulase-negative *Staphylococcus* were the most common cause of bacteremia.

The SSC guidelines recommend empiric antimicrobial therapy for not more than 3 to 5 days, with reduction to the most appropriate single therapy as soon as the susceptibility profile is known. The duration of antibiotics should

TABLE 10-5

Threshold Heart Rates and Perfusion Pressure for Age Groups

Age Group	HR (BPM)	Perfusion Pressure* (mm Hg)
Term newborn	120-180	55
<1 year	120-180	60
<2 years	120-160	65
<7 years	100-140	65
<15 years	90-140	65

Modified and used with permission from Brierley J, Carcillo JA, Choong K, et al: Clinical practice parameters for hemodynamic support of pediatric and neonatal septic shock: 2007 update from the American College of Critical Care Medicine. Crit Care Med 2009;37:666-688.

*Perfusion pressure is defined as [mean arterial pressure – central venous pressure] or [mean arterial pressure – intra-abdominal pressure].

BPM, beats per minute; HR, heart rate.

TABLE 10-6

The American College of Critical Care Medicine Hemodynamic Definitions of Shock

Shock
Decreased perfusion manifested by altered decreased mental status
Decreased urine output < 1 mL/kg/hr

Cold Shock
Shock plus the following:
Capillary refill > 2 seconds
Diminished peripheral pulses
Mottled cool extremities
Low CI with either high SVR and normal BP or low SVR and low BP

Warm Shock
Shock plus the following:
Flash capillary refill
Bounding peripheral pulses
High CI with low SVR and low BP

Fluid-Refractory Shock
Shock persists despite ≥ 60 mL/kg fluid resuscitation (when appropriate)

Catecholamine-Resistant Shock
Shock persists despite use of catecholamines
    Dopamine up to 10 µg/kg/min
    Epinephrine 0.05-0.3 µg/kg/min
    Norepinephrine

Refractory Shock
Shock persists despite goal-directed use of inotropic agents, vasopressors, vasodilators, and maintenance of metabolic (glucose and calcium) and hormonal (thyroid, hydrocortisone, insulin) homeostasis

Modified and used with permission from Brierley J, Carcillo JA, Choong K, et al: Clinical practice parameters for hemodynamic support of pediatric and neonatal septic shock: 2007 update from the American College of Critical Care Medicine. Crit Care Med 2009;37:666-688.

BP, blood pressure; CI, cardiac index; SVR, systemic vascular resistance.

typically be 7 to 10 days unless the patient has an undrainable focus of infection, immunologic deficiency, or a slow clinical response.

Source Control In addition to early broad-spectrum antimicrobial therapy, obtaining emergent source control immediately following initial resuscitation is crucial.[163] Source control includes drainage of abscesses, debridement of infected necrotic tissue, and removal of a potentially infected device after other vascular access has been established.[164] Of course, the selection of optimal source control methods must weigh the benefits and risks of the specific intervention, because it may cause further complications, such as bleeding, fistulas, and inadvertent organ injury. Ideally, source control should be accomplished with the least amount of physiologic disturbance possible.[165]

Resuscitation Goals During resuscitation, several clinical signs and hemodynamic variables can be used to direct treatment to the goal of normal perfusion. Initial fluid resuscitation and inotrope drug therapy are directed toward maintaining threshold HR and perfusion pressure appropriate for age (Table 10-5) and capillary refill less than or equal to 2 seconds. Perfusion pressure is defined as MAP minus central venous pressure (CVP) or MAP minus intra-abdominal pressure (IAP). Subsequent intensive care unit hemodynamic support is directed to goals of $ScvO_2$ greater than 70% and CI 3.3 to 6.0 L/min/m^2.[10] Goal urine output is greater than 1 mL/kg/hour in children and greater than 2 mL/kg/hour in neonates. Of note, in VLBW newborns, a MAP of 30 mm Hg is considered the absolute minimum tolerable blood pressure, because a MAP less than 30 mm Hg is associated with poor neurologic outcome and survival in this population.[166] Because blood pressure does not necessarily reflect CO, it is recommended that normal CO and/or SVC flow, measured by Doppler echocardiography, be a primary goal in these extremely premature infants.[167–177]

Fluid-Refractory Shock If shock is not reversed with fluid alone, the algorithm (see Figs. 10-4 and 10-5) proceeds to the treatment of fluid-refractory shock (see Table 10-6 for hemodynamic definitions of shock). Fluid boluses should be continued unless new onset hepatomegaly or rales develop, which suggest fluid overload. Diuretics, peritoneal dialysis, or continuous renal replacement therapy are indicated for patients who have been adequately fluid resuscitated but cannot maintain subsequent fluid balance by native urine output. No large randomized controlled trial has been performed comparing continuous renal replacement therapy with intermittent dialysis. A retrospective study of 113 critically ill children reported that patients with less fluid overload before continuous venovenous hemofiltration had better survival.[178] Therefore the SSC guidelines recommend instituting continuous venovenous hemofiltration before significant fluid overload occurs. The updated 2007 ACCM/PALS guidelines are consistent with the SSC guidelines and recommend intervention for 10% body-weight fluid overload. Fluid-refractory shock mandates the addition of an inotrope to fluid resuscitation through a second peripheral IV line or through intraosseous (IO) access until central access is obtained. In the case of peripheral infiltration with any catecholamine, its adverse effects may be antagonized by local subcutaneous infiltration of phentolamine (1 to 5 mg diluted in 5 mL of normal saline).[10]

First-line inotrope support in children includes: mid-dose dopamine (5 to 9 µg/kg/minute), dobutamine, or epinephrine (0.05 to 0.3 µg/kg/minute). Dobutamine is preferred when there is low CO with adequate or increased SVR.[132,179–192] This is in contrast to the first-line agent in adults, norepinephrine, which is used in fluid-refractory vasodilated, and often hypotensive, septic shock.[193–196] Again, the majority of adults with fluid-refractory, dopamine-resistant shock have high CO and low SVR, while children with this condition predominantly have low CO.[10] Dobutamine or mid-dosage dopamine can be used to increase cardiac contractility in patients with impaired contractility on echocardiogram with normal blood pressure.[10] Dobutamine- or dopamine-refractory low CO shock may be reversed with epinephrine infusion.[132,197–200] Epinephrine is more commonly used in children than in adults.

The next step in fluid-refractory shock is the establishment of a definitive airway, if needed, and central vascular access for subsequent inotrope and vasopressor infusion. The work of breathing uses up to 40% of CO. Therefore intubation and mechanical ventilation can help to reverse shock in the pediatric population.[10] The updated 2007 ACCM/PALS guidelines recommend volume loading and peripheral or central, inotropic/vasoactive drug support before and during intubation if there is hypovolemia and cardiac dysfunction. Etomidate is not recommended. The sedative/induction regimen of choice is ketamine, with atropine pretreatment and benzodiazepine postintubation. A short-acting neuromuscular blocker can be used to facilitate intubation as long as airway patency can be maintained.[10] Once the airway and central vascular access are obtained, vasopressors should be initiated. Cold shock (see Table 10-6) is treated with central dopamine, or, if resistant, central epinephrine. Although dopamine remains the first-line vasopressor for fluid-refractory hypotensive shock in the setting of low SVR, it may not work as well in patients less than 6 months old. Dopamine causes vasoconstriction by releasing norepinephrine from sympathetic vesicles as well as acting directly on alpha-adrenergic receptors. Because infants less than 6 months old have immature sympathetic innervation, their releasable stores of norepinephrine are reduced. However, dopamine-resistant shock usually responds to high-dose epinephrine or norepinephrine.[132,201–203] Warm shock (see Table 10-6) is reversed by infusing central norepinephrine. Some committee members who updated the 2007 ACCM/PALS guidelines advocate the use of low-dose norepinephrine as a first-line agent for fluid-refractory hypotensive, hyperdynamic shock. Although the use of norepinephrine as a first-line agent for fluid-refractory shock is more common in adults than in children, there is no level I evidence to recommend one catecholamine versus another.[8] However, most guidelines recommend dopamine and norepinephrine as first-line agents, followed by epinephrine, phenylephrine, or vasopressin.[8]

Stabilization and Continued Resuscitation

Catecholamine-Resistant Shock If shock is not reversed with fluid and catecholamines, the algorithm (see Figs. 10-4 and 10-5) then proceeds to the treatment of catecholamine-resistant shock (see Table 10-6 for hemodynamic definitions of shock). Care is now directed within the pediatric intensive care unit (PICU) or neonatal intensive care unit (NICU). For those patients at risk for absolute adrenal insufficiency, steroids should be initiated at this time. Management of catecholamine-resistant shock then depends on whether a patient has cold or warm shock and what are his or her specific hemodynamics.

Steroids Unlike adults, children are at higher risk for absolute adrenal insufficiency.[10] If a child is at risk of absolute adrenal insufficiency or adrenal pituitary axis failure and remains in shock despite epinephrine or norepinephrine infusion, then hydrocortisone can be administered. High-risk pediatric patients include those with purpura fulminans and Waterhouse-Friederichsen syndrome, congenital adrenal hyperplasia, prior recent steroid use for chronic illness, and children with pituitary or adrenal abnormalities. Hydrocortisone should ideally be administered after obtaining a blood sample for subsequent determination of baseline cortisol concentration. Absolute adrenal insufficiency in children is defined by basal cortisol of less than 18 µg/dL and a peak adrenocorticotropic hormone (ACTH)-stimulated cortisol concentration of less than 18 µg/dL.[10]

There is a lack of data on steroids for septic shock in the pediatric literature. The few studies that have been published demonstrate variable results. In a randomized controlled trial of 98 children with dengue shock, hydrocortisone therapy resulted in improved mortality (18.75% vs. 44%).[204] A second randomized controlled trial of 97 pediatric patients with dengue shock syndrome reported that response to a single IV dose of hydrocortisone (50 mg/kg) as measured by mortality, duration of shock, and amount of replacement fluids required was virtually identical between the two groups.[205] It was concluded that hydrocortisone was of no value in the treatment of dengue shock syndrome. Of note, both studies were underpowered, did not measure cortisol levels in these children, but did match the two cohorts for age, sex, and illness severity. Thus it is difficult to conclude if steroids truly provide a survival benefit. In fact, some investigators have reported that steroid therapy may be harmful for children with sepsis. In a recent retrospective cohort study using the Pediatric Health Information System database, investigators reported that the use of any corticosteroids in children with severe sepsis was associated with increased mortality (30% vs. 18%, odds ratio 1.9, 95% confidence interval 1.7 to 2.2).[206] An important limitation of this study is the lack of illness severity data. Although steroids may have been given preferentially to more severely ill children with a presumed higher probability of mortality, steroid use was an independent predictor of mortality in multivariate analysis.[206] Taking these studies and several case series under consideration, the updated 2007 ACCM/PALS guidelines continue to recommend hydrocortisone only for pediatric patients with absolute adrenal insufficiency, as defined by peak cortisol concentration of less than 18 µg/dL following corticotropin stimulation, or adrenal-pituitary axis failure and catecholamine-resistant shock.[10]

The steroid dose continues to be controversial, but the current recommendation is between 2 mg/kg/day (stress dose) and 50 mg/kg/day (shock dose) of IV hydrocortisone as a continuous infusion or as intermittent boluses, with a plan to wean off as tolerated to minimize potential long-term toxicities such as developmental delay.[10] Although the SSC guidelines now recommend IV hydrocortisone for adult septic shock patients if BP is inadequate with appropriate fluid resuscitation and vasopressor therapy and without cortisol testing, whether this approach should be adopted in pediatric and/or neonatal sepsis without classical adrenal or hypophyseal pituitary axis insufficiency depends on the results of pending prospective randomized clinical trials.[8,10]

Cold Versus Warm Shock Management of catecholamine-resistant shock can be divided into three groups: (1) cold shock with low CI, high SVR, and normal BP; (2) cold shock with low CI, low SVR, and low BP; and (3) warm shock with high CI, low SVR, and low BP. The goals for the treatment of catecholamine-resistant shock are the same as mentioned previously: attainment of a normal perfusion pressure (MAP minus CVP) for age, as well as maintenance of $ScvO_2$ greater than 70% and CI 3.3 to 6.0 L/min/m^2.

Cold shock with low CI, high SVR, and normal BP is first treated with fluids and epinephrine. Normotensive pediatric patients with a low CO and high SVR require afterload reduction to improve blood flow by increasing ventricular emptying. If $ScvO_2$ remains less than 70%, a short-acting vasodilator should be initiated with volume loading. Sodium nitroprusside or nitroglycerin are first-line vasodilators in patients with epinephrine-resistant septic shock and normal BP, and it may reduce ventricular afterload and result in an improved CO.[207-212] If there is continued low CO, or toxicity develops (e.g., cyanide, isothiocyanate, or methemoglobin toxicity), then a type III phosphodiesterase inhibitor should be used next. Type III phosphodiesterase inhibitors are rarely used in adults with septic shock, because catecholamine-refractory low CO and high SVR is uncommon; however, this hemodynamic state is present in a majority of children with fluid-refractory, dopamine-resistant shock. Therefore use of type III phosphodiesterase inhibitors, such as milrinone and inamrinone (formerly amrinone), is an alternative approach to improve CO and lower SVR in the pediatric population.[213-219] Their mechanism of action is to increase intracellular cyclic adenosine monophosphate (cAMP) by blocking its hydrolysis. This ultimately has the same effect as beta-adrenergic agonists, because they increase intracellular cAMP by stimulating its production. One limitation of type III phosphodiesterase inhibitors is their long half-lives, requiring loading doses with fluid boluses to reach steady state as well as the possibility of slowly reversible toxicities, such as hypotension, tachyarrhythmias, or both, particularly in the setting of abnormal renal (milrinone clearance) or liver (inamrinone clearance) function.[8]

Other vasodilators that have been used in children include prostacyclin, pentoxifylline, dopexamine, and fenoldopam.[220-225] Pentoxifylline, in particular, has been shown to decrease production of TNF and increase survival in murine endotoxin shock,[226] and a randomized controlled trial reported improved outcome with the use of daily 6-hour pentoxifylline infusions in very premature infants with sepsis.[227,228] A Cochrane analysis concurs that this vasodilator and anti-inflammatory agent is a promising therapy deserving evaluation in a multicenter trial.[229] Finally, levosimendan should be considered as a rescue therapy for recalcitrant low CO catecholamine-resistant shock. Levosimendan increases calcium/actin/tropomyosin complex binding sensitivity and has some type III phosphodiesterase inhibitor and adenosine triphosphate-sensitive potassium channel activity. This drug therefore allows improved contractility at a fundamental level, because one of the pathogenic mechanisms of endotoxin-induced heart dysfunction is desensitization of calcium/actin/tropomyosin complex binding.[230-235]

Cold shock with low CI, low SVR, and low BP is also first treated with fluids and epinephrine, but if hypotension persists, norepinephrine should be considered to increase SVR.

If $ScvO_2$ is still less than 70%, dobutamine or milrinone should be considered to increase $ScvO_2$ by improving cardiac contractility. Finally, enoximone or levosimendan should be considered as well. Enoximone is a type III phosphodiesterase inhibitor with 10 times more β_1 than β_2 cAMP hydrolysis inhibition. Therefore it can increase cardiac contractility with a lower risk of undesired hypotension than milrinone or inamrinone.[236-238] Levosimendan, in the setting of cold shock with low CI, low SVR, and low BP, when added to norepinephrine, will improve CO and $ScvO_2$ as well.

Warm shock with high CI, low SVR, and low BP is treated first with fluids and norepinephrine. Again, some committee members for the updated 2007 ACCM/PALS guidelines advocate the use of low-dose norepinephrine as a first-line agent for fluid-refractory hypotensive (low SVR) hyperdynamic (high CO) shock.[10] If the patient remains hypotensive, the use of vasopressin, terlipressin, or angiotensin can help to restore BP. In patients with vasodilatory septic shock and hyporesponsiveness to catecholamines, vasopressin has been shown to increase MAP, SVR, and urine output.[239-249] Terlipressin, a long-acting form of vasopressin, has demonstrated similar effects with reversal of vasodilated shock as well.[247,250] Angiotensin has been reported to increase BP in patients refractory to norepinephrine, although its clinical role remains to be defined.[251] If $ScvO_2$ remains less than 70%, low-dose epinephrine should be considered to improve cardiac performance as the above potent vasoconstrictors can reduce CO.

Persistent Catecholamine-Resistant Shock If shock is not reversed with fluid, catecholamines, steroids, and other adjunctive therapies the algorithm (see Figs. 10-4 and 10-5) then proceeds to the treatment of persistent catecholamine-resistant shock (see Table 10-6 for hemodynamic definitions of shock). It is important at this point to rule out and correct several potential occult conditions: (1) pericardial effusion requiring pericardiocentesis, (2) pneumothorax requiring thoracentesis or tube thoracostomy, (3) hypothyroidism requiring thyroid hormone replacement therapy, (4) ongoing blood loss requiring hemostasis and/or transfusion, (5) increased intra-abdominal pressure requiring diuretics and/or peritoneal drainage for IAP greater than 12 mm Hg and surgical decompression for greater than 30 mm Hg, (6) necrotic tissue requiring debridement, or (7) excessive immunosuppression or immune compromise mandating a wean of immunosuppressants and restoration of immune function. In addition, therapy can be guided to the goal of CI 3.3 to 6.0 L/min/m^2 by the use of pulmonary artery, pulse contour cardiac output, or femoral arterial thermodilution catheters and/or Doppler ultrasonography. Once these feasibly reversible causes are addressed and monitoring has been optimized, if shock persists, the algorithm (see Figs. 10-4 and 10-5) advances to refractory shock and extracorporeal membrane oxygenation (ECMO) as an alternative to consider.[10]

Refractory Shock Extracorporeal membrane oxygenation is a viable therapy for refractory pediatric and neonatal septic shock, although its long-term impact is not known.[8,10] Most centers use refractory shock or PaO_2 less than 40 mm Hg after maximal therapy as an indication for ECMO support.[10] Persistent hypotension and/or shock with venovenous ECMO should be treated with dopamine/dobutamine or epinephrine.

Inotrope requirements will usually diminish after venoarterial ECMO. Neonates (80%) and children (50%) have similar survival whether or not the indication for ECMO is refractory respiratory failure or refractory shock from sepsis.[10] Although ECMO survival is similar in pediatric patients with and without sepsis, thrombotic complications can be more common in sepsis.[10]

One U.S. study analyzed 655 patients from a national registry to examine the influence of sepsis on survival from ECMO.[252] The study found that systemic sepsis does not independently influence survival in pediatric ECMO and concluded that although neurologic complications occur more frequently in septic patients on ECMO, this therapy should not be withheld solely because of sepsis. Another study examined the use of ECMO in 12 patients from the United Kingdom and Australia with refractory cardiorespiratory failure resulting from meningococcal disease.[253] The pediatric risk of mortality score ranged from 13 to 40 (median 29, median predicted risk of mortality 72%), and overall, 8 of the 12 patients survived, with six leading functionally normal lives at a median of 1 year (4 months to 4 years) of follow-up. There is a role for ECMO therapy in pediatric and neonatal patients with refractory septic shock, although it remains to be better defined.

OTHER CONSIDERATIONS

Intravenous Immunoglobulin

A promising adjuvant therapy in the treatment of sepsis is the administration of polyclonal intravenous immunoglobulin (IV Ig). A recent randomized controlled trial of polyclonal IV Ig in 100 pediatric sepsis syndrome patients aged 1 to 24 months demonstrated a significant reduction in mortality, LOS, and progression to complications such as disseminated intravascular coagulation.[254] The SSC guidelines therefore recommend consideration of IV Ig in pediatric severe sepsis, although more studies may be needed to validate this therapy.

Recombinant Human Activated Protein C

Recombinant human activated protein C (rhAPC), also known at drotrecogin alfa (activated), or Xigris, is indicated for the reduction of mortality in adult patients with severe sepsis who have a high risk of death (Acute Physiology and Chronic Health Evaluation, or APACHE, II score ≥ 25) or MODS and no contraindications. rhAPC is contraindicated in clinical situations where bleeding could lead to significant morbidity or death, such as active internal bleeding, recent (<3 months) hemorrhagic stroke, recent (<2 months) intracranial/intraspinal surgery or severe head trauma, trauma with an increased risk of life-threatening bleeding, presence of an epidural catheter, or intracranial neoplasm or mass lesion.[8] The evidence that rhAPC reduces mortality in adult patients with a high risk of death and does not benefit patients at a lower risk of death, but rather increases risk of serious bleeding, is based on the PROWESS[6] (stopped early for efficacy) and ADDRESS[255] (stopped early for futility) randomized clinical trials. An open-label study (EVAO) in children with severe sepsis demonstrated that pharmacokinetics and pharmacodynamics of rhAPC are similar to that in adults.[256] Before EVAO was completed, a global open-label trial in adults and children with severe sepsis (ENHANCE) was initiated to gather additional data for mortality and safety.[257] In the ENHANCE study, the 28-day mortality rate for children was 13.4%, and 5.9% had serious bleeding events during rhAPC infusion, such as central nervous system (CNS) bleed in 2.7% of children.[258] This was followed by the only randomized placebo-controlled trial of rhAPC in children, the RESOLVE (REsearching severe Sepsis and Organ dysfunction in children: a gLobal perspectiVE) trial, which was stopped early for futility.[162] Because of the low mortality rate of children with sepsis, the primary end point for efficacy in the RESOLVE trial was a reduction in the composite Time to Complete Organ Failure Resolution (CTCOFR) score. The RESOLVE trial showed no significant difference between groups in CTCOFR score or in 28-day mortality. This is quite different from the adult data in the PROWESS trial, which demonstrated a statistically significant reduction in 28-day mortality. It is also important to point out that although there was no difference in the incidence of serious bleeding events between the RESOLVE study groups, more rhAPC patients had CNS bleeding than placebo patients. Furthermore, four of the five patients in the rhAPC group with a CNS bleed were younger than 60 days and weighed less than 4 kg. The SSC guidelines therefore recommend against the use of rhAPC in children because of lack of proof of efficacy and increased risk of bleeding.[8]

NEONATAL SEPTIC SHOCK

Although the algorithms for time-sensitive, goal-directed stepwise management of hemodynamic support are similar for pediatric patients (see Fig. 10-4) and newborns (see Fig. 10-5) with septic shock, there are several important differences between children and neonates that the clinician should consider.

During the initial resuscitation period, it is crucial to distinguish septic shock from cardiogenic shock resulting from closure of a patent ductus arteriosus in newborns with ductal-dependent complex congenital heart disease. These patients should be started on prostaglandin infusion until an echocardiogram is performed to rule out complex congenital heart disease.

Neonatal septic shock is also complicated by the physiologic transition from fetal to neonatal circulation. In utero, 85% of fetal circulation bypasses the lungs via the ductus arteriosus and foramen ovale. Suprasystemic pulmonary vascular resistance maintains this flow pattern in the antenatal period. However, at birth, inhalation of oxygen results in reduced pulmonary vascular resistance, which allows blood flow through the pulmonary circulation. Closure of the ductus arteriosus and foramen ovale complete this transition.

During sepsis of the newborn, both acidosis and hypoxia can increase pulmonary vascular resistance and arterial pressures, leading to persistent pulmonary hypertension (PPHN). The patency of the ductus arteriosus is maintained, ultimately resulting in persistent fetal circulation. Right ventricular work is increased and can lead to right ventricular failure with right to left shunting at the atrial/ductal levels, manifested by tricuspid regurgitation, hepatomegaly, and cyanosis. Therefore treatment of PPHN requires reduction of pulmonary artery pressures aimed at reversing right ventricular failure. After fluid resuscitation and initiation of catecholamines, if right ventricular dysfunction is present, treatment of PPHN should begin. The patient should be hyperoxygenated with 100% oxygen, and inhaled NO should be administered as the first treatment when available. Historically, metabolic alkalization (up to pH 7.50) with $NaHCO_3$ or tromethamine was instituted until inhaled NO was available, but this is no longer a common practice. Inhaled NO's greatest effect is typically seen at 20 ppm. Refractory PPHN may be treated with inhaled prostacyclin and/or IV adenosine with variable response.[10]

Key differences in fluid resuscitation between children and neonates include the type of fluid used as well as the rate of infusion. Although crystalloid or colloid can be used to resuscitate children with septic shock and the use of blood transfusion is suggested for Hb less than 10 g/dL to achieve $Scvo_2$ greater than 70% because this is associated with increased survival, the recommendation for neonates is crystalloid for Hb greater than 12 g/dL and packed red blood cells for Hb less than 12 g/dL. Ideally, all packed red blood cells should come from one donor, to limit transfusion reaction risks. Indications for diuretics and complete renal replacement therapy are the same. Furthermore, standard volume resuscitation and vasopressor therapy practices for preterm infants in septic shock use a more cautious, graded approach. This is likely because of anecdotal reports of hemorrhage after rapid shifts in blood pressure in preterm infants at risk for intraventricular hemorrhage (<30 weeks' gestation). Finally, rapid fluid administration can further increase left to right shunting, with ensuing pulmonary edema in the case of VLBW infants who are unable to close their ductus arteriosus because of immature muscle constriction. The majority of these infants are treated medically with indomethacin and the minority with surgical ligation.

Other considerations in neonates include external warming, because their mechanisms of thermogenesis are immature. Also, newborns are at increased risk of hypoglycemia because of reduced glycogen stores and muscle mass for gluconeogenesis; therefore appropriate dextrose infusion should be initiated to maintain serum glucose concentration with frequent monitoring.[10]

Management of pediatric and neonatal sepsis is challenging. It is clear that early diagnosis and time-sensitive, goal-directed therapies are associated with decreased morbidity and mortality in children with sepsis. Emerging novel therapies and improved understanding of existing treatments through both experimental studies and clinical trials will continue to improve current management in an effort to maximize patient survival.

The complete reference list is available online at www. expertconsult.com.

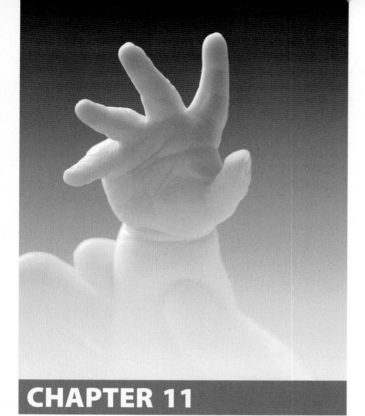

CHAPTER 11

Surgical Implications of Hematologic Disease

Kelly Walkovich and Raymond J. Hutchinson

Hematologists and pediatric surgeons frequently interact with each other in the comprehensive management of pediatric surgical patients. The evaluation and management of anemia, thrombocytopenia, platelet dysfunction, clotting factor deficiencies, and thrombosis are the common meeting grounds; in addition, maintenance of indwelling central venous lines and the judicious use of transfusion therapy often raise questions of interest to both groups of physicians. The most important considerations in each of these areas are discussed here.

Anemia

An inadequate mass of red blood cells (RBCs), resulting in insufficient delivery of oxygen to the tissues, can occur for three major pathophysiologic reasons:[1] inadequate production or maturation of RBCs in the bone marrow (e.g., Diamond-Blackfan anemia, transient erythroblastopenia of childhood), loss of red cell mass as a result of bleeding (e.g., gastrointestinal blood loss from Meckel diverticulum) or splenic sequestration (as seen in sickle cell diseases), or (3) RBC destruction (hemolytic disorders).[1] Clearly, a thorough history and physical examination provide invaluable data when planning the workup for a pale child or for the evaluation of a low hematocrit or hemoglobin concentration noted on a complete blood cell count (CBC). In pediatric medicine and surgery, individual and family histories are particularly relevant because of the frequency of congenital and genetic anemias.

In taking the medical history, items of importance include evidence of intrauterine bleeding in the mother or neonatal hemolysis (e.g., from placental abruption or erythroblastosis fetalis, respectively), history of neonatal jaundice or neonatal bleeding, the rate of development of pallor, the presence of scleral icterus, and a history of rectal bleeding. The family history is relevant for identifying other family members with history of anemia or treatment for anemia, splenectomy, or cholecystectomy. A complete physical examination includes assessment for jaundice and degree of pallor, documentation of the size of the spleen and lymph nodes, evaluation for signs of bleeding (including testing the stool for blood), and assessment of cardiovascular stability.

The CBC yields much information regarding the causes of anemia. It provides information regarding two lineages in addition to the red cell lineage: the white cell (myeloid) and the platelet (megakaryocytic). Involvement of more than one hematopoietic lineage often indicates a production problem occurring in the bone marrow; hence, bone marrow aspiration and biopsy are typically done early in the workup of children with multiple cytopenias. The mean corpuscular volume (MCV) allows the classification of anemias into microcytic, normocytic, and macrocytic categories; this can be a useful diagnostic clue and can facilitate a directed workup. Similarly, a mean corpuscular hemoglobin concentration that exceeds 36 is highly suggestive of the presence of a large number of spherocytes, as seen in hereditary spherocytosis.[2] The RBC distribution width index provides information about the size distribution of circulating red cells, allowing the physician to categorize the red cell population as homogeneously small or large or as heterogeneous. This information, when coupled with the MCV, allows a more cost-effective workup. Figure 11-1 provides an algorithm for the workup of a patient with anemia.

NONHEMOLYTIC ANEMIAS

Underproduction of RBCs because of marrow failure or as a result of deficiency of an essential nutrient, such as iron, is a common mechanism that can lead to severe degrees of anemia. Such severe anemia may present a dilemma when evaluating a patient for a surgical procedure.

Marrow Failure

One major clue to the existence of bone marrow failure is the presence of multilineage cytopenias. The concomitant existence of anemia with neutropenia or thrombocytopenia suggests (1) the existence of primary marrow failure resulting from constitutional aplastic anemia (Fanconi anemia) or acquired aplastic anemia or (2) failure of the bone marrow as a result of infiltrative disease, which occurs in cases of acute

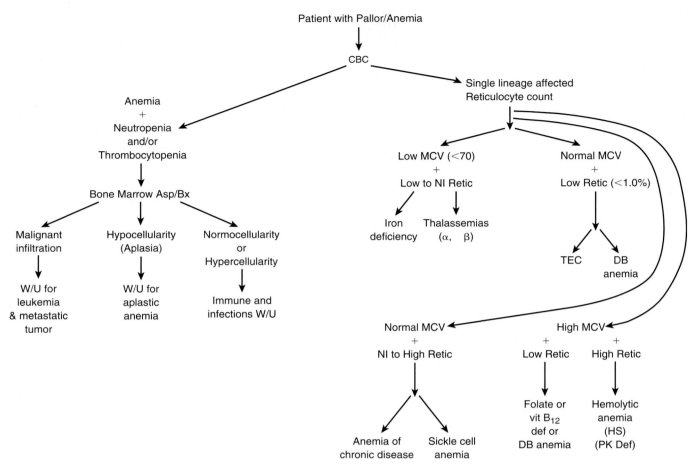

FIGURE 11-1   Algorithm for the workup of a patient with anemia. Asp/Bx, aspirate/biopsy; CBC, complete blood count; DB, Diamond-Blackfan; Def, deficiency; HS, hereditary spherocytosis, MCV, mean corpuscular volume; Nl, normal; PK def, pyruvate kinase deficiency; Retic, reticulocyte; TEC, transient erythroblastopenia of childhood; W/U, workup.

leukemia or metastatic neuroblastoma. Bone marrow aspiration and biopsy can often quickly resolve uncertainty regarding the diagnosis.

Fanconi anemia is transmitted in an autosomal recessive pattern but affects boys slightly more often than girls (1.2:1).[3] The hematologic presentation is variable, with a single cell lineage often affected early, followed by evolution to multilineage aplastic anemia. The age at presentation ranges from birth to 55 years (median, 6.5 years).[3] Patients affected by Fanconi anemia often exhibit congenital malformations (e.g., cutaneous hyperpigmentation, anomalies of the thumb and radial side of the forearm, microsomy, mental retardation).[4] They are predisposed to malignancies (e.g., leukemia and liver tumors) as a consequence of the associated chromosomal breakage.[5–7] Additional genetic cytopenic syndromes that can progress to multilineage involvement, and thus bear consideration when discussing aplasia, are congenital (CAMT) amegakaryocytic thrombocytopenia, Shwachman-Diamond neutropenia, and dyskeratosis congenita.[3]

Acquired aplastic anemia is idiopathic in at least 50% of cases; commonly observed associations include occurrence after hepatitis B or after the use of drugs such as chloramphenicol, sulfonamides, phenothiazines, and anticonvulsants.[8] Although administration of anabolic steroids (oxymetholone) can lead to improvement in the blood counts of patients with

Fanconi anemia,[3] their use is now largely restricted to patients who are not candidates for stem cell transplantation because of concern regarding a negative impact on the outcome of transplantation.[9] Multiagent immunosuppressive therapy with cyclosporine and intravenous antithymocyte globulin, with or without corticosteroids, produces durable responses in approximately 75% of patients with severe acquired aplastic anemia.[10,11] For children with Fanconi anemia or severe acquired aplastic anemia, allogeneic hematopoietic stem cell transplantation offers a potentially curative treatment option.[9,11] Granulocyte colony-stimulating factor (G-CSF) is used in neutropenic patients with Fanconi anemia with benefit,[3] whereas its use in patients with severe acquired aplastic anemia is of uncertain benefit.[12]

Anemia associated with single-lineage erythroid hypoplasia is characterized by normal white blood cell and platelet counts, a low reticulocyte count (<1.0%), and the absence of erythroid precursors on marrow aspirate smears. Two conditions should come to mind when confronted with this clinical picture: Diamond-Blackfan anemia (congenital hypoplastic anemia) and transient erythroblastopenia of childhood (TEC). The former condition is characterized by elements of persistent fetal erythropoiesis, such as a high fetal hemoglobin percentage on hemoglobin electrophoresis, increased erythrocyte adenosine deaminase activity, retained expression of fetal red cell antigen i, and high MCV of red cells.[13] Patients with TEC usually do not exhibit these features.[14] TEC resolves within 2 to 8 weeks, which is consistent with suppression due to a presumed viral cause.[15–17] Corticosteroids are the mainstay of therapy for Diamond-Blackfan anemia; prednisone 2 mg/kg per day is used initially, followed by tapering to alternate-day dosing or less frequently as the patient's condition allows.[13] Patients with Diamond-Blackfan anemia occasionally become transfusion dependent; in rare cases, patients require allogeneic bone marrow transplantation.[18–20] Although RBC transfusions are occasionally required for patients with TEC, most do not require therapy because recovery is sufficiently rapid.

Blood Loss

Anemia is an important manifestation of acute and chronic hemorrhage. Significant acute hemorrhage is usually accompanied by signs of cardiovascular stress, consisting of peripheral vasoconstriction, hypotension, tachycardia, and oliguria.[21] If the patient loses more than 30% of the total blood volume, hypovolemic shock often occurs. After acute hemorrhage, it may take several hours before the full effect on the hemoglobin and hematocrit levels can be assessed; a precipitous drop in these values within 1 to 2 hours of the hemorrhage usually indicates blood loss in excess of 20% of the total volume.[22]

Conversely, chronic blood loss resulting from low-grade, slow, or intermittent bleeding is usually not associated with the symptoms of cardiovascular stress. Patients with chronic anemia often exhibit a compensated picture that may not require intervention with transfusion. When transfusion is unavoidable, a judicious approach should be taken because multiple transfusions carry notable risks, including transmission of viral infection[23] and transfusion hemosiderosis.[24]

Sequestration of blood in the spleen is another mechanism of significant blood loss that can lead to anemia.[25] Splenomegaly caused by hemolytic anemias, portal vascular anomalies, or primary pathologic conditions of the liver can lead to sequestration of blood in dilated splenic sinusoids.

The therapeutic approach to the management of patients with anemia resulting from blood loss varies according to the rate at which the anemia developed. To restore blood volume and oxygen carrying capacity to a patient who has lost a large amount of blood, it may be necessary to transfuse a unit of blood quickly. This can usually be accomplished safely, even in young children, over a 15- to 30-minute period, as long as the volume and rate of delivery are adjusted to the child's size and estimated blood loss. Excessive volume expansion can usually be prevented through careful monitoring of the heart rate, arterial blood pressure, venous pressure, and core and peripheral temperatures.[21] Patients with chronic anemia that has gradually reached a level that compromises cardiopulmonary status should receive transfusions of RBCs in amounts that are appropriate to restore cardiopulmonary function to a compensated level. Overtransfusion should be avoided; this is particularly relevant for children with chronic anemia requiring repeated transfusions. For such children, frequent transfusions may result in transfusion hemosiderosis; the greater the number of RBC units transfused, the greater the iron load transfused. After the serum ferritin level exceeds 1000 μg/L, transferrin becomes saturated, and patients are at risk for cardiac and hepatic iron deposition[24]; these patients

should be considered for chelation therapy with intravenous or subcutaneous deferoxamine[24] or oral deferasirox (Exjade).[26] Patients in whom moderate anemia develops from blood loss or aggressive hemolysis should undergo slow transfusion back to the baseline level in aliquots of 5 to 10 mL/kg over 2 hours each, with time allowed between aliquots for reequilibration and reassessment of the patient's cardiac status.

Nutritional Anemias

Iron-deficiency anemia results from inadequate intake of dietary iron, poor absorption, misutilization as a result of defective transport, loss of iron through bleeding, or sequestration of iron in an atypical location (e.g., the lungs in cases of pulmonary hemosiderosis). The age of the patient influences whether he or she will become iron deficient. In infants, who experience rapid expansion of blood volume during growth, 30% of the iron required for hemoglobin production must come from the diet. In adult men, only 5% is derived from the diet,[27] and the remainder is generated by RBC degradation.

The American Academy of Pediatrics[28] recommends dietary iron intake of 1.0 mg/kg per day to a maximum of 15 mg/day for full-term infants, starting by age 3 months. Preterm infants weighing between 1500 and 2500 g require 2 mg/kg per day from dietary and supplemental sources to a maximum of 15 mg/day, starting no later than 2 months of age. Recommendations for very-low-birth-weight infants are even higher: 4 mg/kg per day for those weighing less than 1500 g at birth. In older children and adults, dietary iron requirements vary, depending on growth and gender:

4 to 10 years: 10 mg/day
11 to 16 years: 18 mg/day
Adult men: 10 mg/day
Adult women: 18 mg/day

The peak age range for the development of nutritional iron deficiency is 6 months to 2 years. During this period, children make the transition from being dependent on breast milk or iron-fortified formula to a mixed diet of milk (often cow's milk) and solid foods. Depending on which foods constitute most of the child's diet, dietary iron may be adequate or inadequate. Children who depend heavily on cow's milk, at the expense of solid foods, are especially prone to iron-deficiency anemia. The typical presentation for such children is the gradual development of pallor, a hemoglobin concentration of 3.0 to 6.0 g/dL, and an MCV of 45 to 60 fL. Older individuals are much less likely to experience iron-deficiency anemia, especially from an inadequate diet, unless they participate in fad diets.

Consumption of unprocessed cow's milk by infants, intestinal parasitic infestations, and preexistent iron deficiency may lead to intestinal blood loss. The use of aspirin or aspirin-containing medications may increase intestinal blood loss sufficiently to cause anemia. Other anatomic sources of blood loss and iron deficiency include the following: (1) in the perinatal period—fetal-maternal hemorrhage, placental injury at delivery, and twin-to-twin transfusion through placental communications; (2) in older children—Meckel diverticulum, intestinal duplication, hemorrhagic telangiectasia, and, rarely, bleeding ulcers or gastroesophageal reflux.

The diagnosis of iron deficiency is made by confirming the existence of microcytic, hypochromic anemia in the context of a clinical situation that suggests a possible cause of the deficiency. The low MCV and mean corpuscular hemoglobin concentration should be corroborated with a careful review of the blood smear. Serum iron studies that measure the serum iron level, total iron-binding capacity, and serum ferritin level finalize the diagnosis. The typical pattern consists of a low serum iron level, high total iron-binding capacity, and low serum ferritin level, consistent with low total-body iron stores. Finally a therapeutic trial of iron should result in an increasing reticulocyte count within 1 week, and the hemoglobin and hematocrit levels should rise soon thereafter.

Treatment consists of the administration of oral iron (ferrous sulfate) at a dose of 6 mg/kg per day of elemental iron. Because ferrous sulfate is only 20% elemental iron, this fact must be taken into consideration when calculating the dose (e.g., a 325-mg tablet of ferrous sulfate contains 65 mg of elemental iron). The iron must be continued for 3 to 4 months. Correction of the anemia, correction of microcytosis, and elevation of the free erythrocyte protoporphyrin level usually occur within that period.[29]

HEMOLYTIC ANEMIAS

The sickle cell diseases, β-thalassemia, hereditary spherocytosis, and glucose-6-phosphate dehydrogenase and pyruvate kinase deficiencies all have potential ramifications for pediatric surgeons.

Sickle Cell Diseases

The sickle hemoglobinopathies present early in life with episodes of painful crisis, acute chest syndrome, bacteremia, and splenic sequestration.[30] In a report of the Cooperative Study of Sickle Cell Disease, patients with homozygous sickle cell anemia and those with sickle cell–hemoglobin C disease demonstrated significant incidence rates of painful crisis, acute chest syndrome, and bacteremia; however, all 20 deaths in a cohort of 694 infants followed for 10 years occurred among the patients with homozygous sickle cell anemia.[30] It was also clear from this study that most hand-foot syndromes occurred among the homozygous sickle cell anemia patients in the first 3 years of life.

Several sequelae of the sickle cell disorders are of interest to pediatric surgeons. Painful vasoocclusive crises occasionally masquerade as acute abdominal events that typically require surgical intervention (e.g., appendicitis). Because painful crises are usually accompanied by an elevated leukocyte count, this parameter is not useful in distinguishing appendicitis from a painful crisis. Serial examinations and collaborative evaluation with a hematologist who is skilled in the evaluation of patients with sickle cell diseases reduce the frequency of unnecessary and potentially harmful surgical interventions during painful crises.

Acute chest syndrome can represent a life-threatening situation. Correction of this process requires rapid transfusion to raise the oxygen carrying capacity of the blood and lower the percentage of hemoglobin S to reverse the sickling process; often this is accomplished by exchange transfusion.

For patients with repeated episodes of splenic sequestration, the surgeon may be called on to remove the spleen to reduce the risk of subsequent sequestration, which is characterized by rapid drops in hemoglobin concentration, hematocrit value, and platelet count. At times, progressive sequestration may lead to hypovolemic shock and have life-threatening implications. Historically, splenectomy was justified only after two episodes of sequestration because of

concern for splenectomy in young patients (younger than 4 years).[25] However, recent work suggests that splenectomy can safely be performed after one major episode of sequestration.[31] Similarly, the development of symptomatic cholelithiasis usually dictates that cholecystectomy be performed.[32] Patients with sickle cell anemia have a high incidence of perioperative morbidity.[33] Complications that occur at an increased rate in patients with sickle cell disease undergoing surgery include painful crises, acute chest syndromes, and transfusion reactions due to erythrocyte alloimmunization.

Another consideration for pediatric surgeons managing patients with sickle cell diseases is related to the percentage of sickle hemoglobin and the safety of general anesthesia. In the past, RBC transfusion to lower the percentage of sickle hemoglobin to less than 30% was the preferred approach. However, data suggest that patients do just as well with a more conservative approach that aims at achieving a preoperative hemoglobin level of 10 g/dL but does not attempt to lower the hemoglobin S level below an arbitrary cutoff point.[34] Care should be taken to ensure adequate blood oxygenation during a surgical procedure, but excessive transfusion should be avoided.

Further, reducing preoperative transfusions reduces the risk of alloimmunization and transfusion reactions. The development of non-ABO erythrocyte antibodies occurs in 8% to 50% of patients with sickle cell disease, varying with the number of RBC transfusions administered.[35] Clearly, the development of these antibodies adds complexity to surgical procedures and increases the risk of reactions with subsequent transfusions. RBC phenotyping with matching for E, C, and Kell group antigens is recommended because it reduces the risk of alloimmunization.[36,37] Several published studies have questioned the benefit of aggressive preoperative transfusion, suggesting that young patients undergoing low-risk surgery do not require transfusion.[34,38] For others, a conservative transfusion regimen designed to increase the plasma hemoglobin concentration to 10 g/dL offers as much benefit as an aggressive regimen aimed at decreasing the hemoglobin S concentration, with a lower risk of complications.[34]

Postoperative complications of surgery vary, depending on the type of surgical procedure performed, the age of the patient, the status of disease activity and disease-related organ dysfunction, the presence of infection, evidence of chronic lung disease, pregnancy in female patients, and the genetic form of sickle cell disease.[33] Preoperative assessment of lung function with a chest radiograph, oxygen saturation determination, and pulmonary function tests, and of renal function with serum blood urea nitrogen and creatinine measurements, blood pressure measurement, and screening for urinary infection and proteinuria, offer useful strategies for decreasing intraoperative risks.

β-Thalassemia

β-Thalassemia is characterized by the inability to synthesize normal amounts of β-chain hemoglobin polypeptide,[39] resulting in ineffective erythropoiesis. Patients with homozygous β-thalassemia become dependent on RBC transfusions early in life. As a consequence of extramedullary hematopoiesis, splenomegaly is a frequent finding. Splenic sequestration of RBCs often leads to an enhanced transfusion requirement. When the RBC transfusion requirement exceeds 250 mL/kg per year, splenectomy should be considered because it often reduces the transfusion requirement.[40]

Hereditary Spherocytosis and Erythrocyte Enzyme Deficiencies

Hereditary spherocytosis and RBC enzyme deficiencies, such as glucose-6-phosphate dehydrogenase and pyruvate kinase deficiencies, result in hemolytic anemia, often associated with gallstone formation. When cholelithiasis is symptomatic, cholecystectomy is necessary. In the case of hereditary spherocytosis, when patients maintain a relatively high reticulocyte count (>10%) in the presence of moderate to severe anemia, splenectomy should be considered when patients reach the age of 5 to 6 years.[41] Splenectomy reduces the risk of the development of gallstones, and it minimizes the chance of a precipitous drop in the hemoglobin concentration when a patient with hereditary spherocytosis experiences a viral infection. Partial splenectomy may offer an alternative in the future, with the definitive risks and benefits yet to be determined, possibly in a randomized clinical trial.[42] The therapeutic value of splenectomy also needs to be considered in patients with other types of hemolytic anemia, such as pyruvate kinase deficiency and refractory autoimmune hemolytic anemia.

Thrombocytopenia and Disorders of Platelet Function

Bleeding manifestations attributable to platelets can either be the result of quantitatively too few platelets, (i.e. thrombocytopenia), or qualitatively abnormal platelets (i.e. dysfunctional platelets).

Thrombocytopenia is defined as a platelet count less than 150,000/μL, although clinically significant manifestations are generally apparent only at platelet counts less than 100,000/μL. Thrombocytopenia can have either a genetic or an acquired origin.

GENETIC THROMBOCYTOPENIA

Although rare, several genetic conditions should be considered when thrombocytopenia is diagnosed early in life. Both thrombocytopenia with absent radii (TAR) and CAMT present in the newborn period and are inherited in an autosomal recessive fashion with normal platelet size. As the name implies, TAR is a clinical diagnosis based on variable thrombocytopenia, ranging from 10,000 to 100,000/μL in association with limb abnormalities, most commonly bilateral radius aplasia.[43] No underlying molecular mechanism for TAR has been identified. The thrombocytopenia generally improves over the first year of life, requiring only supportive care with platelet transfusions, and progression to bone marrow failure is rare. Although the thrombocytopenia is expected to resolve within the first year, it should be noted that in the original case series of TAR patients published in 1969, 35% mortality was observed due to intracranial and gastrointestinal bleeds, with the majority of deaths occurring before age 1 year.[44] In addition, many other skeletal abnormalities as well as nonskeletal abnormalities—macrocephaly, short stature, facial dysmorphism, renal malformations, cardiac defects, and capillary hemangiomas—are common in patients with TAR and often require subspecialist care. In contrast, CAMT often presents within the first year of life with more severe thrombocytopenia

and elevated serum thrombopoietin levels, and a distinct lack of megakaryocytes in the bone marrow in the absence of other congenital malformations.[43,45] Most patients with CAMT experience bone marrow failure within the first few years of life; patients are also at an increased risk of myelodysplasia and acute leukemia. Bone marrow transplant, preferably with a matched sibling donor, is the only definitive treatment for CAMT. Other bone marrow failure syndromes, in particular Fanconi anemia, can present as isolated thrombocytopenia in infancy before progression to a complete aplastic state. However, the classic physical stigmas of Fanconi anemia (i.e., anomalies of the forearm and thumb, as well as chromosomal breakage analysis with diepoxybutane or mitogen C testing) typically permits distinction between the diagnoses.[3]

In addition, familial thrombocytopenias, including conditions with reduced or increased platelet size, can be appreciated in early childhood. Wiskott-Aldrich syndrome is an X-linked familial microthrombocytopenia due to a defect in the WAS protein, which manifests as thrombocytopenia with small-volume platelets, eczema, and frequent infections due to T-lymphocyte abnormalities and immunoglobulin M deficiency.[46,47] Autoimmune conditions and malignancies, particularly B-cell dyscrasias, are common in patients with Wiskott-Aldrich syndrome.[48] The more rare macrothrombocytopenias can either be related to other disease entities (e.g., velocardiofacial syndrome or pseudo–von Willebrand's disease) or to isolated *MYH-9* macrothrombocytopenia with leukocyte inclusions, hearing loss, or nephritis, or a combination of these conditions.[49]

ACQUIRED THROMBOCYTOPENIA

Acquired thrombocytopenia can arise from a number of sources, for example, intrauterine exposure to maternal antibodies with antiplatelet surface antigen specificity arising from exposure to certain therapeutic drugs, various viral infections, or the existence of a maternal autoimmune state. Likewise, certain classes of drugs are more likely to induce thrombocytopenia, including antibacterial drugs (e.g., trimethoprim-sulfamethoxazole), anticonvulsant drugs (e.g., phenytoin, carbamazepine), and antipsychotic drugs (e.g., chlorpromazine). Three disorders merit special mention: neonatal alloimmune thrombocytopenia, immune thrombocytopenic purpura, and heparin-induced thrombocytopenia (HIT).

Neonatal alloimmune thrombocytopenia (NAIT) is the most common cause of severe thrombocytopenia in fetuses and newborns.[50] NAIT occurs when an infant's mother becomes sensitized to a foreign paternal platelet antigen inherited by the infant and expressed on platelets during gestation. The mother develops an antiplatelet IgG titer when the maternal-fetal blood barrier breaks down, allowing the infant's platelets to enter the maternal circulation; IgG antibody then crosses back through the placenta to the infant. Platelet counts less than 50,000/μL should prompt consideration for screening for NAIT. The platelet antigen most frequently responsible for this sensitization is PLA1, an antigen for which 98% of the population is positive. Random platelet transfusions generally do not provide a sustained rise in the infant's platelet count, especially when a common antigen, such as PLA1, has led to sensitization; such transfused platelets are rapidly destroyed. Despite their rapid destruction, random donor platelets may be useful if other treatments are not readily available, especially if the bleeding is life-threatening. As such they are generally the first line of treatment in suspected cases of NAIT. Conversely, the use of maternal platelets (i.e., PLA1 or other specific antigen-negative platelet) typically leads to a sustained rise in the infant's platelet count; when the mother's postpartum condition allows platelet pheresis, this can be a lifesaving intervention. Platelet transfusion is recommended in well, term infants with a platelet count less than 30,000/μL and for premature infants with a platelet count less than 50,000/μL. In infants with intracranial hemorrhage, a platelet count greater than 100,000/μL is the goal. Besides platelet transfusions, intravenous immunoglobulin (IVIG) 1 g/kg per day for 1 to 3 days depending on response, plus/minus intravenous (IV) methylprednisolone 1 mg/kg (maximum 30 mg) every 8 hours, can be administered for marked thrombocytopenia.[51] NAIT usually resolves in 2 to 4 weeks. It should be noted that unlike Rh disease, NAIT can occur with the mother's first pregnancy, and no preventive measures similar to Rh immune globulin (Rhogam) exist. Like Rh disease, however, NAIT is anticipated to be worse with each subsequent pregnancy.[51]

Immune thrombocytopenic purpura occurs in children and adolescents of all ages, but the majority of patients are between 2 and 10 years of age. It often occurs after a viral infection and is believed to be caused by a misdirected antiviral immune response, with antibodies cross-reacting with platelets and leading to splenic consumption.[52] It is a clinical diagnosis based on the acute onset of isolated thrombocytopenia that is frequently concurrent with the abrupt onset of petechiae, bruising, or mucous membrane bleeding, or a combination of these conditions, in an otherwise healthy child. Unlike adults, the majority of children will have spontaneous remission, with at least two thirds of patients having a normal platelet count within 6 months.[53] However, because of the severity of the thrombocytopenia (often <10,000/μL platelets) and the small, less than 1%, associated risk of intracranial hemorrhage,[54] many children are treated with IVIG 0.8 to 1 g/kg IV, anti-D immunoglobulin 75 μg/kg, or oral prednisone.[55] All three treatments can provide a temporary increase in platelet counts. One should note that anti-D immunoglobulin has been reported to cause brisk hemolysis leading to rare renal failure or death, so care should be taken to provide adequate hydration and to monitor for hemoglobinuria.[56] Before prednisone is used, consideration should be given to performing a bone marrow aspiration to rule out leukemia, because leukemia may be partially, but inadequately, treated by prednisone. Platelet transfusions are only clinically indicated in life-threatening bleeding situations and should be used concurrently with IVIG 0.8 to 1 g/kg IV and methylprednisolone 30 mg/kg (maximum 1 g) IV. In children with refractory, symptomatic immune thrombocytopenic purpura, splenectomy or rituximab can be considered.

HIT is an immune-mediated side effect of heparin therapy characterized by thrombocytopenia and paradoxical increased risk for thrombosis. Although previously considered rare in neonates and children, HIT is now recognized to occur in up to 1% to 2% of certain pediatric patient populations, particularly those receiving cardiac surgery or intensive care unit (ICU) care, or both.[57] The thrombocytopenia usually begins 5 to 10 days after the heparin is initiated, although it can occur within the first 48 hours if the patient has previously received heparin.[58] Unlike most other drug-induced thrombocytopenias, which classically lower the platelet count to less than 10,000/μL, HIT typically drops the platelet count by at least 50%, with a resultant platelet count ranging from 20,000 to 150,000/μL, with a median platelet count of 50,000/μL.[59] It should be noted that 10% of patients with HIT have platelet nadirs in the normal range[60]; thus, a normal platelet count does not nullify a diagnosis of HIT. Thrombosis can also precede thrombocytopenia.[60] The risk for HIT is greater with therapeutic rather than prophylactic doses of heparin, for bovine- than for porcine-derived heparin, and for unfractionated as opposed to low-molecular-weight heparin (LMWH).[61]

To make a diagnosis of HIT, both clinical and laboratory features must be present: a triggering agent (i.e., a form of heparin), a significant fall in platelet count with the typical timing, and the identification of heparin-dependent antibodies. A clinical score to assess the pretest probability of HIT has been proposed[62] and is frequently used despite not being validated in a pediatric population. Treatment of HIT requires immediate discontinuation of heparin once HIT is suspected. In addition, because of the risk of significant thrombosis, transition to an alternative anticoagulant is recommended. Warfarin should not be used as a substitute for heparin during an acute HIT episode because it can result in an abrupt decrease in protein C levels, placing the patient at greater risk for thrombotic complications.[63] LMWH to replace unfractionated heparin should also be avoided because of the appreciable cross-reactivity between the two agents. Instead, the alternative agents danaparoid,[64] lepirudin,[57] argatroban[65] or fondaparinux[66] should be considered.

DISORDERS OF PLATELET FUNCTION

Cutaneous or mucous membrane bleeding despite a normal platelet count suggests the presence of a disorder of platelet function, which may be either acquired or inherited.

Medications are a common cause of acquired platelet function defects. Aspirin, although rarely used in children because of the risk of Reye syndrome, is well documented to inhibit platelet cyclooxygenase irreversibly, resulting in deficiency of thromboxane A_2 and inhibition of platelet aggregation.[67] Since platelets are unable to synthesize new proteins, the action of aspirin is permanent and lasts the life of the platelet. Unlike aspirin, ibuprofen is a reversible cyclooxygenase inhibitor, and although data is limited there is some evidence to suggest that platelet function may normalize within 24 hours of cessation of regular ibuprofen use.[68]

Of the inherited platelet dysfunction disorders, von Willebrand disease is the most prevalent.[69] This disorder is characterized by mucosal bleeding caused by abnormal platelet adhesion and aggregation that arises from subnormal levels of factor VIII activity and von Willebrand factor. A number of variants of von Willebrand disease are known to exist; most are transmitted in an autosomal dominant fashion. Recombinant factor VIII/von Willebrand factor concentrate is the treatment of choice to normalize hemostasis. Desmopressin (DDAVP), a synthetic analog of the antidiuretic hormone vasopressin, which transiently increases levels of factor VIII and von Willebrand factor by releasing them from storage pools in the blood can also be used to minimize bleeding. Care should be taken with desmopressin use because patients are at risk for the development of hypo-natremia and seizures. Particular attention should be given to the amount of perioperative fluid the patient receives, and serum sodium levels should be measured during the perioperative period. If factor VIII/von Willebrand factor concentrate is not available, cryoprecipitate can be used. Each unit of cryoprecipitate contains 80 to 100 U of factor VIII and 80 U of von Willebrand factor. A dose of cryoprecipitate providing 10 U of factor VIII/kg of body weight is generally sufficient to achieve adequate hemostasis for surgery. It should be noted that cryoprecipitate is a second-line agent, since during the processing of cryoprecipitate there is no viral inactivation. Failure to correct von Willebrand disease deficiencies before a patient undergoes surgery increases the risk for mucosal bleeding or surface bleeding, or both.

Two other rare inherited platelet dysfunction disorders are Bernard-Soulier syndrome and Glanzmann thrombasthenia.[69] Both conditions are due to a defect in platelet adhesion and can result in severe bleeding. In Bernard-Soulier syndrome the defect is in the GPIb-IX-V platelet surface complex, whereas in Glanzmann thrombasthenia the defect is in the platelet membrane complex GPIIb-IIIa. The two diagnoses can be differentiated by platelet aggregation testing, as Bernard-Soulier syndrome classically demonstrates no agglutination in response to ristocetin but shows otherwise normal agglutination, but Glanzmann thrombasthenia shows a normal ristocetin response despite an absent response to other agents. For bleeding episodes, platelet concentrate transfusion is the appropriate corrective measure. However, patients quickly become resistant to platelet transfusions because of the high risk of alloimmunization.

Disorders of Coagulation

In evaluating children for bleeding tendencies, the physician should begin with a review of items relevant to a bleeding history. Specifically, this includes inquiring about the occurrence of frequent, large (greater than quarter-sized) bruises in unusual places or after minor trauma, oozing or frank bleeding from the umbilical stump, gum bleeding, epistaxis, hemarthroses, menorrhagia, hematuria, gastrointestinal bleeding, or intracranial bleeding. Moreover, bleeding symptoms from procedures (such as a hematoma with intramuscular injections) and history of bleeding with circumcision, dental extractions, or other surgical procedures should be ascertained. A history of anticoagulation use (i.e., aspirin, heparin, enoxaparin [Lovenox], warfarin) should be obtained. Finally, taking a family history of bleeding tendencies is essential, and that history can either enhance or reduce the probability of diagnosing a bleeding disorder in the patient being evaluated.

The physical examination also provides important information. Bleeding in the skin or mucous membranes (gingival bleeding, petechiae, ecchymoses), soft tissues (hematomas), joints, or on funduscopic examination should be noted.

A good initial laboratory screening panel includes a CBC, prothrombin time (PT), and activated partial thromboplastin time (aPTT) (Table 11-1). Historically, a bleeding time has also proved useful. However, since the bleeding time is subject to considerable variation related to the experience of the person performing the test, the patient's skin temperature, and the length and depth of the incision, the bleeding time is now

rarely used. If it is used, the normal range for the bleeding time is 3.5 to 11.5 minutes. Times in the 12- to 15-minute range should be viewed circumspectly, whereas values in excess of 15 minutes are prolonged and abnormal. The CBC is useful to determine the presence of an adequate number of platelets. The PT detects deficiencies of factor VII and factors in the common pathway (Fig. 11-2). The normal range for the PT is 11 to 12 seconds. The most sensitive of the global screening tests is the aPTT. The aPTT detects deficient clotting factors in the intrinsic and common pathways. However, mild deficiencies of factors VIII and IX will not be recognized, and deficiencies of factor VII and factor XIII will not be detected at all by the aPTT.

Specific assays to determine the presence of a single factor deficiency are available. If a satisfactory determination cannot be achieved despite attempts to identify one or more factor deficiencies, a search for a plasma inhibitor should be initiated. This can be accomplished by performing mixing studies with the aPTT or PT, depending on which result is more abnormal. For these studies, normal plasma is mixed with the deficient (patient) plasma in a range of ratios (1:3, 1:1, 3:1). Failure to correct the test completely at the 3:1 (normal patient) mix ratio suggests the presence of an inhibitor. In contrast, factor deficiencies should be totally corrected at the 1:3 mixture and certainly at the 1:1 mixture.

COAGULATION FACTOR DEFICIENCIES

The most common inherited factor deficiencies include hemophilia A (factor VIII deficiency) and hemophilia B (factor IX deficiency). Hemophilia occurs in approximately 1 in 5000 boys, with hemophilia A accounting for 80% to 85% of the patients and hemophilia B accounting for the remaining 15% to 20%; there are no ethnic predilections.[70] These disorders are inherited as X-linked recessive traits and as such almost exclusively affect boys. Although the majority of patients will have a family history of hemophilia or a bleeding history suggestive of hemophilia, it should be noted that in a third of patients, the diagnosis of hemophilia is the result of a new mutation.[71]

Both factors VIII and IX are critical for thrombin development; thus, deficiency of either leads to bleeding manifestations characterized by oozing or delayed hemorrhage because, although the initial platelet plug is capable of forming, thrombin clot formation is delayed and not robust. Usual bleeding symptoms include bleeding with circumcision, oral bleeding (particularly in infancy from a torn frenulum), easy bruising, hemarthroses, and intramuscular hemorrhage. The frequency and severity of bleeding strongly correlate with the level of active factor. For hemophilia A and B, factor levels of less than 3% are associated with spontaneous hemorrhage into joints and soft tissues. In general factor levels greater than 30% have essentially normal hemostasis. For joint bleeding and bleeding emergencies, such as central nervous system (CNS) bleeding or hemorrhage into the psoas muscle, specific factor recombinant products should be administered rapidly to achieve 100% factor replacement.

The diagnosis of factor VIII deficiency can be made at birth with a prolonged aPTT and a confirmatory low factor VIII level. In the evaluation of factor IX deficiency, however, the physician must consider the physiologic delay in achieving normal levels of the vitamin K–dependent factors (factors II,

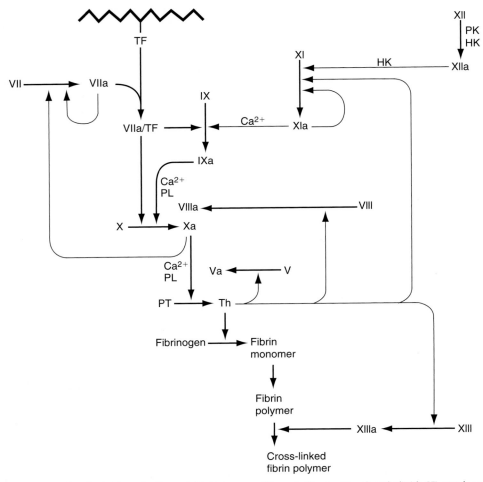

FIGURE 11-2 Coagulation cascade. HK, high-molecular-weight kininogen; PK, prekallikrein; PL, phospholipid; PT, prothrombin; TF, tissue factor; Th, thrombin. (From Schafer AI: Coagulation cascade: An overview. In Loscalzo J, Schafer AI [eds]: Thrombosis and Hemorrhage. Boston, Blackwell Scientific, 1994.)

VII, IX, and X) in infants. Although confounding the interpretation of the factor IX level in infants, the physiologic delay does not lead to misinterpretation of the near-complete deficiency seen in severe to moderate hemophilia B. A prolonged aPTT with a subsequent factor IX level of less than 10% is consistent with a diagnosis of hemophilia B. Infants with levels in the 10% to 50% range should be retested at 3 to 6 months of age or earlier if clinically significant bleeding occurs. All newborn infants suspected of having hemophilia should have a head ultrasonogram to evaluate for intracranial hemorrhage because 1% to 2% of infants with hemophilia have been reported to have CNS bleeding.[72,73]

Once a diagnosis of hemophilia is made, patients requiring surgery should have a careful presurgical evaluation, including laboratory evaluation for the development of an inhibitor. Specific factor concentrate should be administered before surgery to achieve a level of 100 to 150 U/dL for factor VIII and 80 to 100 U/dL for factor IX, and factor levels should be maintained at 50 to 60 U/dL for 7 to 14 days postoperatively.[70] In trauma scenarios swift action should be taken to provide 100% factor correction before imaging. This is particularly true for head trauma cases because patients with hemophilia experience intracranial hemorrhage 20 to 50 times more frequently than does the general population.[74]

OTHER FACTOR DEFICIENCIES

Besides the more common factor VIII and IX deficiencies, other factor deficiencies do occur, such as abnormalities in fibrinogen, the soluble precursor of fibrin that is mainly produced in the liver. Dysfibrinogenemias are disorders of fibrinogen function caused by structural defects in the protein; more than 300 abnormal fibrinogens have been described. In contrast, afibrinogenemia is due to a complete absence of fibrinogen.

Afibrinogenemia usually manifests in the neonatal period, with 85% of patients presenting with umbilical cord bleeding,[75] although later age at onset is not unusual. Patients with afibrinogenemia often have mucosal and other bleeding (e.g., bleeding from skin, gastrointestinal tract, and CNS), with intracranial hemorrhage reported as the main cause of death.[76] Hemarthrosis, however, is notably infrequent (particularly compared with patients with severe hemophilia), with joint bleeding observed in 25% of patients.[77] The diagnosis of afibrinogenemia is confirmed by the absence of immunoreactive fibrinogen. The partial thromboplastin time (PTT), PT, and thrombin time (TT) will all be infinitely prolonged because all these tests rely on the formation of fibrin as an end point. Generally fibrinogen levels greater than 50 mg/dL are sufficient

TABLE 11-1

Tests to Detect Bleeding Disorders

Test	Parameters Measured
Platelet count	Platelet number
Bleeding time	Systemic primary hemostasis Defect of platelet number or function Defect in platelet-vessel wall interaction Primary vascular disorder
Prothrombin time (PT)	Extrinsic and common pathways: factors VII, X, V; prothrombin; fibrinogen
Activated partial thromboplastin time (APTT)	Intrinsic and common pathways: factors XII, IX, XI, VIII, X, V; prothrombin; fibrinogen; prekallikrein; high-molecular-weight kininogen
Thrombin time	Fibrinogen
Fibrinogen quantitation	Level of fibrinogen in plasma (mg/dL)
Fibrin degradation products	Breakdown products of fibrinogen or fibrin-elevated with increased fibrinolysis or disseminated intravascular coagulation
D-dimer assay	Fibrin-specific degradation product; indicator of both thrombin and plasmin generation
Euglobulin lysis time	Screening test of fibrinolytic activity
Mixing study (using PT or APTT)	Presence of a circulating anticoagulant
Antithrombin III (ATIII) activity	Level of the antithrombotic ATIII
Protein C, protein S antigen activity	Levels of the antithrombotic proteins C and S
Activated protein C resistance assay	Presence of mutant, functionally deficient factor V Leiden (predisposing to thrombosis)

Data from Schafer AI: Approach to bleeding. In Loscalzo J, Schafer AI (eds): Thrombosis and Hemorrhage. Boston, Blackwell Scientific, 1994; Comp PC: Approach to thrombosis. In Loscalzo J, Schafer AI (eds): Thrombosis and Hemorrhage. Boston, Blackwell Scientific, 1994; and Santoro SA: Laboratory evaluation of hemostatic disorders. In Hoffman R, et al (eds): Hematology: Basic Principles and Practice. New York, Churchill Livingstone, 1991.

TABLE 11-2

Clotting Factor Deficiencies

Deficient Factor	Clinical Relevance
I	Risk of hemorrhage at levels <50 mg/dL
II	Mild bleeding tendency after injuries, dental extractions, surgery
V	Mild bleeding tendency (menorrhagia, significant bleeding after injury or surgery)
VII	Variable bleeding tendency (intracranial hemorrhage in newborns, menorrhagia)
VIII	Moderate to severe bleeding tendency at levels <5%
IX	Moderate to severe bleeding tendency at levels <5%
X	Variable bleeding tendency (neonatal hemorrhage, bleeding after trauma, menorrhagia)
XI	Mild bleeding tendency (menorrhagia, epistaxis, postoperative bleeding)
XII	Generally asymptomatic
Prekallikrein	Asymptomatic
High-molecular-weight kininogen	Asymptomatic

for hemostasis; fibrinogen concentrates, cryoprecipitate, or fresh frozen plasma, or all of these, can be used for fibrinogen replacement as needed.

Unlike afibrinogenemia, which is often diagnosed in childhood, dysfibrinogenemia is often recognized only in adulthood in patients with menorrhagia, prolonged bleeding from trauma or surgery, or abnormal screening laboratory values. The diagnosis of dysfibrinogenemia depends on assays that demonstrate that the functional contribution of fibrinogen to coagulation is abnormal. Most patients with dysfibrinogenemia do not require treatment, but fibrinogen concentrates, cryoprecipitate or fresh frozen plasma, or all of these, can be used for patients with significant bleeding.

Other recognized clotting factor deficiencies and their propensity for associated clinical bleeding are listed in Table 11-2. Deficiencies of prothrombin (factor II), factor V, and factor XI predispose to mild bleeding tendencies, whereas deficiencies of factors VII and X result in variable bleeding tendencies, with some patients demonstrating significant hemorrhagic events. Of note, deficiencies of the contact-activated factors—factor XII (Hageman factor), prekallikrein, and high-molecular-weight kininogen—are not associated with bleeding, and identification of a deficiency should not preclude required surgery.

ACQUIRED DEFECTS OF COAGULATION

The most common causes of acquired hemorrhagic defects include drug-induced bleeding, disseminated intravascular coagulation (DIC), liver disease, vitamin K deficiency, massive transfusion, and acquired inhibitors to coagulation proteins.[78]

Many drugs have been associated with bleeding, the most obvious of which are the therapeutic anticoagulant medications (i.e., warfarin, heparin, low-molecular-weight heparin) and antiplatelet agents (e.g., aspirin, clopidogrel). Other medication classes, namely β-lactam antibiotics,[79] tricyclic[80] and selective serotonin reuptake inhibitor[81] antidepressants, H2-receptor antagonists,[82] and calcium channel blockers,[83] among others, have been identified as interfering with platelet function, but they rarely result in clinical bleeding. Of note, however, valproic acid, an anticonvulsant agent commonly used to treat pediatric generalized tonic-clonic and absence seizures, has been identified as having several effects on coagulation[84,85] (bone marrow suppression,[86,87] development of antiplatelet antibodies,[88] fibrinogen depletion,[89,90] and induction of factor XIII deficiency[91,92]), and has occasionally been reported to have significant bleeding complications associated with its use.

In patients with clinical bleeding due to drug-induced hemorrhagic defects, the suspected offending agent should be discontinued. Vitamin K and fresh frozen plasma should be considered to reverse warfarin coagulopathy. In addition, platelet transfusions should be used for significant or persistent bleeding, or both.

DIC is an acquired systemic disorder caused by in vivo activation of the coagulation mechanism, resulting in the transformation of fibrinogen to fibrin, which generates thrombi in the microcirculation, with secondary fibrinolysis.[78] The vast majority of DIC cases are due to sepsis from infectious causes, although leukemia and other malignancies, cavernous hemangiomas, acute anaphylaxis, snake bites, abruptio placentae, and trauma can all be the precipitating cause. The diagnosis of DIC is facilitated by reviewing the peripheral blood smear and identifying schistocytes and thrombocytopenia. Other supporting laboratory tests include prolonged PT/aPTT and decreased fibrinogen with increased D-dimer and fibrin degradation products. A decrease in protein C, protein S, and antithrombin III (ATIII) may also be seen.

Treatment of DIC centers on the correction of the underlying cause and supportive care. Further therapy should be determined by the patient's general condition and the hemorrhagic or thrombotic manifestations. Heparin may be indicated in children with purpura fulminans and signs of thrombosis; however, routine use of heparin, particularly in less severe forms of DIC, is questionable. In the presence of decreased ATIII levels, heparin may not be effective. ATIII concentrate or fresh frozen plasma can be used as supplements. The patient's platelet count and fibrinogen level can be monitored as indices of response to therapy. For patients with primarily hemorrhagic manifestations and little, if any, thrombosis, the administration of platelets and fresh frozen plasma is indicated if bleeding is moderately severe and associated with a decreasing platelet count and prolonged PT/aPTT.

Severe liver disease is often associated with significant clotting factor deficiency. The healthy liver is the site of synthesis of most coagulation factors, including fibrinogen; prothrombin; factors V, VII, IX, X, XI, XII and XIII; prekallikrein; and high-molecular-weight kininogen.[78] In addition, the liver is the source of the natural anticoagulants antithrombin III, protein C, and protein S, as well as inhibitors of fibrinolysis, antiplasmin and alpha-1 antitrypsin. Because the liver is also involved in the clearance of activated clotting factors, liver failure can lead to DIC. However, severe hepatic injury or failure is more typically associated with a hemorrhagic tendency due to the insufficient production of clotting factors. Increased fibrinolysis resulting from decreased hepatic synthesis of inhibitors may also contribute to the hemorrhagic tendency. Measuring factor VIII and factor V levels in a patient can serve as markers of liver function. High factor VIII levels (indicating a lack of liver clearance) and low factor V levels (indicating a lack of liver production) correlate with poor liver function. Treatment of the underlying liver condition and supportive care with fresh frozen plasma or specific factor concentrates, or both, is most useful.

Vitamin K stores are deficient in most normal newborns; this deficiency has the potential to result in a severe bleeding diathesis. Without early supplementation, infants may bruise, have cephalohematomas, and experience gastrointestinal or umbilical hemorrhage, and oozing from puncture sites. Platelet and fibrinogen levels are normal in these infants, but marked prolongation of the PT and aPTT is noted because of the deficiency of vitamin K, thus interfering with the development of essential calcium-binding sites on the vitamin K–dependent coagulation factors,[93] including factors II, VII, IX, and X. Administration of parenteral vitamin K leads to quick cessation of bleeding and correction of the clotting test results. Breast-feeding accentuates the vitamin K deficiency because breast milk contains far less vitamin K (2 to 15 μg/L) than does cow's milk (60 μg/L).[94] Hemorrhagic disease in newborns can be prevented by intramuscular administration of vitamin K shortly after birth. A dose of 0.5 to 1.0 mg of vitamin K1 oxide is recommended; this dose far exceeds the requirement of 25 μg.[78,95]

Although newborns rely on exogenous sources of vitamin K, older infants absorb vitamin K from the colon, and synthesis by bacteria is the primary source. In older children and adults, vitamin K is absorbed from the ileum. The daily requirement of 1 μg/kg is supplied by green leafy vegetables in the diet and is stored in the liver.[96] Thus, malabsorption resulting from cystic fibrosis, biliary atresia, chronic hemolytic anemia with secondary cholelithiasis, and obstructive jaundice, as well as other disorders leading to dysfunction of the upper small intestine, can result in vitamin K deficiency. In addition exogenous medications, namely warfarin, can lead to vitamin K deficiency. Administration of vitamin K intravenously at a dose of 5 to 10 mg leads to clinical improvement within a few hours and correction of the prolonged PT and aPTT within 24 hours.[78]

Massive transfusion therapy, defined as replacing at least one blood volume in 24 hours, can result in significant bleeding resulting from hypothermia, dilutional coagulopathy, platelet dysfunction, fibrinolysis, or hypofibrinogenemia.[97] Agents such as aprotinin, a serine protease inhibitor that modulates the systemic inflammatory response, have been used as effective hemorrhage prophylaxis in cardiac[98] and orthopedic surgeries.[99] In addition activated factor VII has been used as a rescue therapy for life-threatening bleeding.

Several acquired inhibitors to coagulation proteins are known, namely, inhibitors to factors VIII and IX, inhibitors associated with acquired Willebrand syndrome, and lupus anticoagulants (LA). The LAs are the most commonly identified in children and are often recognized after a prolonged aPTT is noted during a routine presurgical evaluation or in association with an infection.[100] The LAs are a group of antibodies against proteins bound to phospholipids; they can be identified by a noncorrecting mixing study. Generally LAs resolve spontaneously within days to weeks and do not require a change in the operative plan.[78]

THROMBOTIC DISORDERS

The naturally occurring anticoagulants ATIII, protein C, and protein S work to contain excessive in vivo blood coagulation. Thrombosis often results when the activity of one or more of these anticoagulants is deficient.

ATIII is a physiologic inhibitor of thrombin and activated factor V. In addition ATIII is a heparin cofactor that is essential to heparin therapy and is a major inhibitor of blood clotting. This cofactor, which is synthesized in the liver, has a biologic half-life of 2 to 5 days. Congenital ATIII deficiency occurs at a frequency of 1 per 2000 to 5000 individuals.[101] Thrombotic events are often first noted in the second and third decades of life. Surgery, trauma, infection, and pregnancy predispose to thrombotic events. Large amounts of heparin may be required for effective anticoagulation in patients with ATIII deficiency because ATIII is necessary for full heparin activity. Diagnosis is made through a specific assay for ATIII. Oral anticoagulation with warfarin has been the mainstay of therapy. However, purified concentrates of ATIII are available and can be used at a dose of 50 IU/kg for the short term to prevent thrombosis in high-risk situations, such as acute thrombosis, during surgery, or during the third trimester of pregnancy.[102]

Both protein C and protein S are vitamin K–dependent plasma proteins that act in concert to inactivate procoagulants, thereby reducing the risk for thrombosis. Protein C functions by inactivating factors V and VIII; in its active form, protein C also indirectly facilitates clot lysis.[103] Deficiency of protein C is inherited as an autosomal dominant trait. The homozygous state in infants is characterized by purpura fulminans, retinal thrombotic events with retinal detachment and loss of vision, and other thrombotic events.[104] Heterozygous deficiency of protein C is often asymptomatic during childhood but causes venous thrombosis in adolescents and young adults. Heterozygotes generally have levels of approximately 50%, but these individuals are still at risk for other thrombotic events. Diagnosis is made with a specific assay for protein C. Although it has a role in preventing thrombosis in homozygous individuals who are essentially deficient of protein C, warfarin should be used cautiously, if at all, in heterozygous individuals because their thrombotic tendency can be exacerbated by a further reduction in vitamin K–dependent protein C. In fact, heterozygotes often experience purpuric, thrombotic cutaneous lesions while receiving warfarin, which is a contraindication to its use. Further lowering of the protein C level presumably causes these side effects. Heparin should be used to treat acute venous thrombosis, and protein C concentrates are available to facilitate the management of acute thrombosis in protein C–deficient patients.

Protein S acts as a cofactor for protein C. Deficiency of protein S is associated with recurrent venous thrombosis. Heterozygotes with 35% to 50% of the normal levels of the protein experience recurrent thromboses in adolescence and early adulthood.[105] The same guidelines for use of heparin in treating venous thrombosis apply to patients who are deficient in protein S (as well as those deficient in ATIII and protein C). Caution should be exercised when warfarin is used in protein S–deficient patients.

Besides deficiencies in ATIII, protein C, and protein S, genetic mutations such as factor V Leiden or prothrombin 20210 are associated with an increased risk of venous thromboembolism. Other acquired states, such as increased factor VIII levels with significant infection or inflammatory states, anticoagulation protein deficiencies due to consumption in processes like DIC, and production of parainfectious antiphospholipid antibodies, can all contribute to a prothrombotic state.

One of the largest acquired risk factors for venous thrombosis is the presence of a central venous catheter. More than 50% of deep venous thromboses in children and greater than 80% in neonates are related to indwelling central venous catheters.[105,106] The signs and symptoms of a venous thromboembolism are dependent on the location and chronicity of the clot. For example, acute extremity deep venous thrombosis presents with unilateral limb swelling, whereas acute superior vena cava thrombosis may result in swelling of the face and neck. However, chronic venous thromboembolism may have no signs or symptoms or may have appreciable dilated superficial collateral veins or evidence of venous stasis. Venography is the gold standard for diagnosis of a clot; however, because of the invasive nature of venography, compression ultrasonography with Doppler, computed tomography, and echocardiography are used routinely to diagnosis and follow thrombi. Once a diagnosis of acute venous thromboembolism is identified, initial anticoagulant therapy most frequently relies on unfractionated heparin or LMWH. The latter has become increasingly favored because of its subcutaneous dosing, decreased need for frequent blood monitoring, and decreased risk for the development of HIT. The starting dose of LMWH in nonneonates commonly begins at 1 mg/kg with no bolus given. In full-term infants, the LMWH dose generally is increased to 1.5 mg/kg.[107] The LMWH dose should be titrated to achieve a therapeutic anti-Xa level of 0.5 to 1.0.[78] Unfractionated heparin, however, may be preferred in patients with an increased risk of bleeding or labile clinical status. Nonneonates commonly are loaded with a 50- to 75-U/kg dose of unfractionated heparin, followed by an infusion of 15 to 25 U/kg per hour. Full-term neonates generally require increased doses. The therapeutic anti-Xa range for unfractionated heparin is 0.3 to 0.7.[78] Patients with a known, resolved risk factor generally require treatment for 3 to 6 months; patients with no known clinical risk factor require 6 to 12 months of treatment; and patients with a chronic risk factor or congenital thrombophilia may require indefinite treatment.[78]

Transfusion Therapy

Greater accessibility to improved blood products has increased the survival of critically ill patients who need enhanced oxygen delivery, intravascular volume expansion, and improved coagulability. The estimated blood volume for infants and young children weighing 10 to 30 kg is approximately 75.4 mL/kg,[108] whereas that for older children and adolescents is 55 to 75 mL/kg.[109] RBC transfusions should be used to correct pathophysiologic events that cause inadequate oxygen delivery and resultant tissue hypoxia. The decision to transfuse RBCs should be based on several factors: signs of tissue hypoxia (tachycardia, tachypnea), extent of blood loss, rate at which anemia has developed, age of the patient, and concomitant or subsequent physiologic stress that the patient may be forced to undergo (e.g., infection, pulmonary compromise, surgery). Transfused RBCs survive for a relatively long time; less than 1% of the number transfused is destroyed daily.[110]

Typically, the number of transfused cells in the recipient's circulation decreases steadily over 110 to 120 days.

Historically, whole blood was the preferred product for transfusion in patients with severe acute blood loss. However, with the increased use of blood fractionation to produce several products from each unit of blood, greater emphasis is now placed on the use of packed RBCs in conjunction with a plasma substitute, if necessary. For hemorrhage of moderate severity, packed RBCs are as effective as citrated whole blood.[108] For severe hemorrhage, plasma substitutes are required when packed RBCs are transfused to prevent an unacceptable increase in hematocrit levels.[110]

To restore blood volume and oxygen carrying capacity to a patient who has lost a large amount of blood, it may be necessary to transfuse a unit of blood quickly. This can usually be accomplished in the same way as discussed previously in the section on blood loss resulting from anemia. When replacement is less urgent, 10 to 15 mL/kg is transfused over 1 to 2 hours. Massive transfusions that involve replacing an amount of blood equal to the patient's blood volume in 24 hours carry the risk of citrate toxicity, electrolyte imbalance, decreased release of oxygen to tissues resulting from diminished RBC 2,3-bisphosphoglycerate content, pulmonary microembolism, decreased core temperature (if massive amounts of cold blood have been transfused), and thrombocytopenia or DIC. Prevention and successful treatment of the side effects of massive transfusion require careful reassessment of the patient during and after transfusion.

Various plasma substitutes, such as dextran, modified fluid gelatin, and hydroxyethyl starch, have been used to expand plasma volume in hypovolemic patients. However, the possibility of allergic reactions and abnormal bleeding has tempered enthusiasm for their use. Perfluorocarbon compounds, in which oxygen is highly soluble, have been shown to act as effective blood substitutes for oxygen delivery in animals.[111] However, side effects, including lowered platelet count,[112] diminished macrophage function,[113] and activation of complement with resultant pulmonary changes,[114] have severely hampered the use of these compounds; they have undergone evaluation in clinical trials and are currently not recommended for clinical use.[115]

TRANSFUSION IN PATIENTS WITH CANCER OR IMMUNODEFICIENCIES

The basic principle of transfusing to correct altered hemodynamics and insufficient delivery of oxygen applies when treating immunodeficient patients and those with cancer. No absolute value of peripheral blood hemoglobin concentration or hematocrit below which transfusion is mandated exists. In fact, absolute threshold criteria for transfusion therapy are being abandoned in many centers as a result of concerns about transfusion risks, the high cost of transfusion therapy, and the growing perception that many patients can tolerate lower hemoglobin values than previously believed without adverse physiologic effects. Clearly, the age of the patient, the rate at which hemoglobin or hematocrit values are falling, and concomitant problems influence the decision to transfuse. Children younger than 10 years tolerate hemoglobin values as low as 6 to 7 g/dL without adverse effects. Nevertheless, a rapid decline to this level usually requires RBC transfusion. Similarly, concomitant infection, space-occupying pulmonary disease, pleural effusion, cardiomyopathy, CNS insult, or injury to any major organ may mandate earlier transfusion. The immune state of the patient often warrants special consideration with respect to the type of RBC product chosen and the handling of that product. Many patients with primary immunodeficiency and those with immunodeficiency secondary to therapy should receive blood products that have been irradiated at a level of 2500 to 3000 cGy to prevent graft-versus-host disease.[116] In addition, severely immunocompromised patients, such as bone marrow transplant recipients, who are serologically cytomegalovirus (CMV) negative at the time of transfusion should receive CMV-negative or CMV-safe (leukocyte-reduced) blood products. In fact, many blood banks are releasing only leukocyte-reduced cellular products for all transfusion recipients.

CHOICE OF RED BLOOD CELL PRODUCT

Fresh whole blood is a suitable choice for use in exchange transfusions when the whole blood being removed from the patient is being replaced (milliliter for milliliter) and when patients with massive blood loss resulting from acute hemorrhage are being treated. For patients in whom excessive increases in intravascular volume may cause problems, other RBC products are preferred.

Packed RBCs are the product of choice for patients with moderate acute blood loss or chronic anemia resulting from underproduction of RBCs or hemolysis. Advantages of packed RBCs include removal of the anticoagulant citrate and 60% to 70% of the plasma.[117] This consideration is particularly important for patients with volume overload or poor cardiac function, or both.

One advantage of washed RBCs is that 85% to 90% of the leukocytes and more than 95% of the plasma have been removed[117]; however, additional expense is incurred for the preparation of this product. Washed RBCs can be used to transfuse patients with a history of nonhemolytic transfusion reactions.

More than 90% of the white blood cells have been removed from frozen deglycerolized RBCs, with retention of minimal plasma (≈0.5% of original plasma).[117] This product is often chosen for patients who require chronic transfusions.

Leukocyte-reduced RBCs are relatively free of leukocytes (≈70% removed)[117] and may be less likely to transmit CMV and other viruses. This product is advantageous for patients with a history of transfusion reactions and for immunodeficient patients at risk for CMV disease.

Each of the products mentioned has a place in transfusion therapy. However, physicians who use these products should bear in mind the appropriate indications for each and the increased cost associated with additional processing of RBCs (e.g., washing, freezing, thawing).

TRANSFUSION REACTIONS, TOXICITY, AND OTHER COMPLICATIONS

Citrate toxicity resulting from transfusion of the plasma anticoagulant citrate, which binds calcium, may manifest as symptomatic hypocalcemia. Development of this toxicity is the major drawback for using whole blood for rapid RBC and volume replacement.

Transfusion reactions take several forms and usually occur because of patient exposure to proteins from plasma, RBCs, white blood cells, or platelets to which the individual has a natural or an acquired sensitivity. Reactions occur in 2% to 3% of transfusions; of these, 41% are febrile and nonhemolytic, 58% are urticarial, and 1% are delayed hemolytic.[118] For patients with repeated urticaria, the use of washed or frozen RBCs in conjunction with pretreatment of the recipient with an antihistamine or corticosteroid may reduce the incidence of recurrence. Febrile nonhemolytic reactions are usually caused by acquired antibodies to plasma protein or leukocyte alloantigens and occur exclusively in patients with a history of previous transfusion or pregnancy. Pretreatment of the patient with antipyretic agents, antihistamines, or corticosteroids may alleviate symptoms. Because of the sophisticated quality control measures currently in place in modern blood banks, hemolytic reactions are rare. Fever, chills, pain in the abdomen and lower back, tachycardia, hypotension, hemoglobinuria, renal failure, and shock may be manifestations of a hemolytic reaction caused by major blood group incompatibility. When these symptoms are associated with transfusion, the infusion should be stopped, and a sample of the patient's blood should be sent to the blood bank along with the remainder of the aborted RBC unit. Delayed transfusion reactions occur 3 to 10 days after transfusion, are caused by minor blood group sensitization from previous transfusion, and are usually less severe than reactions due to major blood group incompatibility.

The risk of transfusing infectious agents in blood products has been reemphasized by the acquired immunodeficiency syndrome (AIDS) epidemic. Although less than 5% of AIDS cases have been caused by blood transfusion, fear of acquiring the human immunodeficiency virus (HIV) from transfused blood products remains high because of the associated risk of mortality. Preferential collection of blood products from volunteer donors and HIV screening have reduced the risk for HIV transmission to 1 in 2.3 million units of blood product transfused.[119]

The risk of transmitting certain hepatitis viruses, CMV, and Epstein-Barr virus must also be considered when ordering transfusions. Screening for hepatitis B and hepatitis C has had a positive effect on reducing the risk of acquiring these viruses from transfusions; hepatitis A is not considered to be a risk of transfusion. With the use of volunteer donors and screening for the hepatitis B antigen, the incidence of transfusion-acquired hepatitis B has fallen to 1 in 280,000 transfusions.[120] The use of hepatitis B vaccine for patients who are likely to receive multiple transfusions is a recommended practice. A screening test is now used to detect the hepatitis C virus in the blood of potential donors, and the use of this test has resulted in a risk of 1 in 1.8 million for acquiring this infection through transfusion.[119] CMV is carried in transfused lymphocytes, and infusion of such lymphocytes in immunodeficient individuals can cause serious infection. Use of frozen or washed RBCs, blood products from CMV-negative donors, or leukocyte-reduced RBCs reduces the risk of acquiring CMV-related illness for immunodeficient individuals.[121,122]

Graft-versus-host disease is a potential transfusion-related problem for immunodeficient individuals. This disorder, which is well documented to occur after allogeneic bone marrow transplantation, has been recognized in an increasing number of immunodeficient patients receiving transfusions and in other patients who happen to share an HLA haplotype with the donor. Transfusion-associated graft-versus-host disease (TA-GVHD) has been reported from many countries and centers.[123,124] High fever, scaly maculopapular erythematous rash, diarrhea, hepatocellular damage with morbid elevation of liver enzyme levels, and pancytopenia characterize TA-GVHD. The disorder typically occurs in adults 8 to 12 days after transfusion, whereas in newborns TA-GVHD typically presents as fever on day 28 after transfusion.[123] Overall mortality remains greater than 90%, with most deaths occurring within 1 month of onset.[123,124] Steroids, antithymocyte globulin, cyclophosphamide, and anti–T-cell monoclonal antibodies have been disappointing in the treatment of this disease. TA-GVHD is readily avoided by irradiation of all cellular blood products to be transfused to immunodeficient patients and others at risk of TA-GVHD. Irradiation of cellular products with doses of 2500 to 3000 cGy lethally damages lymphocytes without adversely affecting the function of RBCs, platelets, and neutrophils.[123] The treated blood product is not radioactive and can be handled by hospital personnel in the usual fashion. TA-GVHD has not been demonstrated

definitively to occur after transfusion of fresh frozen plasma or frozen RBCs.[124]

Transfusion-related acute lung injury (TRALI) is now the leading cause of transfusion-related morbidity and mortality worldwide,[125,126] given the reductions achieved in infectious risk and hemolytic transfusion reactions. The pathophysiology relates to transfusions of biologically active substances in the blood product; these include donor antibodies that cross-react with leukocyte antigens in the host and lipids and other biologic response modifiers that accumulate in blood during storage.[125] In 2004, the National Heart, Lung, and Blood Institute convened a working group to develop a consensus definition of TRALI.[127] The criteria include

- Satisfying the criteria for acute lung injury (ALI)[128]:
  - Hypoxemia
  - Bilateral infiltrates on chest radiograph
  - Pulmonary artery occlusion pressure less than 18 mm Hg or no clinical evidence of left atrial hypertension
- Onset of signs and symptoms less than 6 hours after transfusion
- No ALI may have been present before transfusion

The patient's clinical course should determine whether the ALI is related to the transfusion. Critically ill patients are those most at risk for TRALI, with the risk factors including septic shock, pulmonary sepsis, aspiration, multiple transfusions, drug overdose in the ICU, long-bone fracture, pulmonary contusion, cardiopulmonary bypass, and burn.[125] Further, there is an independent, dose-dependent relationship between transfusion and the subsequent development of ALI. Mortality rates range from 6% to 15%, with the rate rising to 41% for patients in the ICU.[125,126] The differential diagnosis includes transfusion-associated circulatory overload, an anaphylactoid transfusion reaction, and transfusion of contaminated blood products.[125] Signs and symptoms include severe dyspnea, tachypnea, worsening or new hypoxemia, fever, occasional hypotension, and cyanosis temporarily related to receiving a transfusion.[126] Treatment centers on ventilatory support, fluid management, and reduction in transfusions.[125] If transfusions are necessary, consideration should be given to using washed RBCs and possibly the use of male-only plasma-containing blood products.[125,126] The differentiation of TRALI from transfusion-associated circulatory overload and circulatory overload is accomplished by careful evaluation of clinical signs and symptoms.[129,130]

Platelet Transfusion

The normal platelet count in children and adults ranges from 150,000/μL to 450,000/μL[131]; levels in newborns are occasionally as low as 100,000/μL.[132] Once released into the bloodstream, platelets circulate for approximately 8 to 10 days. Patients with platelet counts less than 10,000/μL are clearly at risk for hemorrhage,[133,134] whereas individuals with platelet counts less than 50,000/μL carry a risk for bleeding during surgical intervention.[135] Replacing circulating platelets with a transfusion of platelet concentrate reduces the risks for spontaneous bleeding in patients with platelet counts less than 10,000/μL and of intraoperative and postoperative bleeding in individuals with platelet counts less than 50,000/μL.[136]

Random donor concentrates are obtained from whole blood collections through a two-step centrifugation procedure.[137,138] An initial soft spin brings down the RBCs and leaves the platelets suspended in the supernatant plasma. The platelet-rich plasma is then centrifuged at high speeds to pellet the platelets, resulting in a platelet button that is resuspended in 50 mL of plasma. The platelet concentrate is then stored at 20°C to 24°C for up to 5 days. The pH of the concentrate should be maintained at 6.0 or higher.

Single-donor platelets are collected by apheresis techniques; approximately 3×10^{11} platelets, which is equal to four to six individual concentrates, are contained in 200 to 3600 mL of plasma.[139] These platelets can be stored for up to 5 days. Single-donor collections are useful for transfusion in patients who have become alloimmunized to random donor concentrates. Identification of compatible single donors through trial and error or by HLA matching prospective donors often results in greater augmentation of the platelet count after transfusion for patients with alloantibodies to platelets. The use of 1-hour posttransfusion platelet counts in patients who are apparently alloimmunized to random donor platelet concentrates is of value in determining the need for single-donor or HLA-matched platelets.[140] If the patient is not septic or sequestering platelets in the spleen, failure to demonstrate an increase in the circulating platelet count 1 hour after transfusion of random donor concentrates usually indicates the existence of platelet alloantibodies. Platelet concentrates are usually used for patients with thrombocytopenia and concomitant bleeding or thrombocytopenia of sufficient magnitude to impart a significant threat of bleeding during surgery or other invasive procedures. When surgery or invasive procedures are required, administration of prophylactic transfusions to thrombocytopenic patients is reasonable for platelet counts less than 50,000/μL.[135] The same threshold for platelet transfusion is reasonable for patients with head trauma and thrombocytopenia. Many oncology centers transfuse patients with cancer in a prophylactic manner, with the threshold for transfusion ranging from 10,000 to 30,000/μL.[134,141,142] Data suggest that minimal risk for bleeding exists when the platelet count is greater than 10,000/μL provided that the patient is afebrile and uninfected. Finally, it is important to consider that platelet concentrates can be used to stop bleeding resulting from impaired platelet function (e.g., Glanzmann thrombasthenia, Bernard-Soulier syndrome) or in acquired platelet functional defects (e.g., aspirin ingestion).

To stop bleeding in a patient with thrombocytopenia, an increase in the platelet count of about 40,000/μL is thought to be necessary.[143] For children, 0.1 U of concentrate per kilogram of body weight usually produces an increment of 40,000 to 50,000/μL; similarly, 4 U/m^2 of body surface area accomplishes the same result.[143] In clinical practice, a minimum of 2 U of platelet concentrate is administered, even to infants. This algorithm can be applied to meet the needs of patients with thrombocytopenia undergoing surgery. A platelet count obtained 1 hour after the platelet transfusion usually provides an accurate assessment of the increment achieved; in bleeding patients, cessation of bleeding is the ultimate index. The half-life of transfused platelets averages approximately 4 days; concomitant fever, infection, or conditions favoring platelet consumption decrease platelet survival.[144] The use of ABO-compatible platelets may lengthen survival, although this is controversial.[144,145] Use of single-donor platelets or HLA-matched platelets often lengthens platelet survival in an allosensitized recipient. When a patient demonstrates increments of less than 10,000/μL on two or three successive administrations of random donor platelets, consideration should be given to using single-donor or HLA-matched platelets. However, if a patient with thrombocytopenia is a candidate for bone marrow transplantation from a related donor, use of matched platelets from family members should be avoided to prevent sensitization to minor antigens, because this might increase the potential for graft rejection.

Platelet concentrates are administered through blood filters. The standard 170-μm screen filters remove blood clots and are commonly used to administer platelet concentrates.[146,148] Contemporary microaggregate blood filters remove lymphocytes while allowing platelets to pass through. These filters may reduce the risk for febrile transfusion reactions and may prevent sensitization to HLA antigens through the removal of lymphocytes.[146] However, filters used to prepare leukocyte-reduced RBCs should not be used to transfuse platelet concentrates because they also remove most of the platelets.[147] Irradiation of platelet units to 2500 cGy is appropriate to lower the risk for GVHD in high-risk patients. Platelet function measured by in vitro assays is not altered by this dose of radiation.[148,149]

Small amounts of Rh-positive RBCs in platelet concentrates may be sufficient to stimulate the production of anti-D in Rh-negative individuals.[143,150] Administration of Rh immune globulin may prevent this sensitization in Rh-negative female recipients of platelet concentrates. Transfusion reactions caused by leukoagglutinins that combine with leukocytes and platelets may occur during or shortly after a platelet transfusion.[139,143] Fever and rigor are often associated with reactions to platelet transfusions. Decreasing the rate of infusion may reduce the risk of a febrile reaction. Acetaminophen, intravenous corticosteroids, and parenteral meperidine can be used to ameliorate this type of reaction. Allergic transfusion reactions are characterized by hives and occasional hypotension or bronchospasm.[139,143] Antihistamines and occasionally epinephrine are useful to treat allergic reactions.

A small risk for the transmission of viral infection is associated with the transfusion of platelet concentrate. In addition, because platelets are stored at room temperature, the possibility of bacterial contamination must be considered when patients who have undergone transfusion experience fever, chills, hypotension, or DIC.

The complete reference list is available online at www.expertconsult.com.

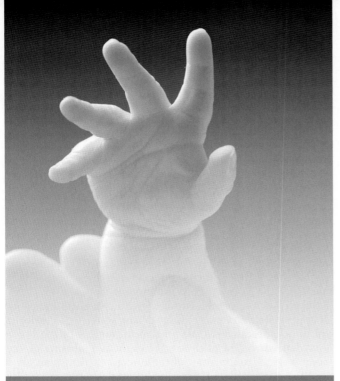

CHAPTER 12

Nutritional Support in the Pediatric Surgical Patient

Daniel H. Teitelbaum, Imad F. Btaiche, and Arnold G. Coran

The development of modern nutritional support is the result of numerous investigators' contributions during the past 350 years. The first known person to attempt to deliver intravenous nutrition was Sir Christopher Wren, the architect of St. Paul's Cathedral in London, in 1658. Wren used hollow goose quills to infuse wine into dogs. In the 18th century, Claude Bernard, the first modern physiologist, infused numerous substrates into animals. He discovered that intravenously administered sugars could be effectively metabolized only if they were predigested by gastric juices. Thus it was then that the first understanding of the digestion of carbohydrates took hold.[1] In the 1930s, Elman[2] delivered the first successful infusion of protein, as hydrolysates of casein, into patients. In 1949, Rhoads and Vars[3] developed an apparatus for a continuous infusion of intravenous substances into dogs. It was used to definitively show that weight gain could be achieved in puppies by means of intravenous nutrition. Critical refinements in the intravenous solutions, filtration of the infusate, and the use of a central venous catheter allowed Dudrick to infuse concentrated solutions of glucose and amino acids into patients.[4–6] This technique rapidly changed the ability to parenterally nourish adult and pediatric patients. One of the most dramatic cases of the use of parenteral nutrition (PN) was in a newborn with jejunoileal atresia; the infant was maintained by this route for more than 22 months and had weight gain and increased head circumference.[6] Application of this technique in other infants led to dramatic improvements in survival of patients who previously would have died after surgical correction of their congenital anomaly. The past 50 years has led to dramatic developments in both specialized enteral and parenteral products for infants and children.

Normal Pediatric Growth

Growth and development are unique features to pediatric patients that greatly affect the goals and objectives of nutritional support. The term newborn infant grows at a rate of 25 to 30 g per day during the first 6 months of life, leading to a doubling of the birth weight by 5 months of age.[7] The average infant triples the birth weight by 12 months. By 3 years of age, the weight is 4 times the birth weight, and by completion of the first decade, the weight increases 20-fold. Body length increases by 50% by the end of the first year of life and increases threefold at the end of the first decade of life. The preterm infant's growth pattern is quite distinct from term infants. Most nutrients are accumulated by the fetus in the third trimester of pregnancy. Thus fat accounts for only 1% to 2% of body weight in a 1-kg infant compared with 16% in a term (3.5-kg) infant. An anticipated loss of 15% of a preterm infant's birth weight is usual in the first 7 to 10 days of life, compared with a 7% to 10% weight loss for a term infant, both of which comprise a shedding of excess body water. After this initial period of weight loss, a preterm infant of less than 27 weeks' gestation gains weight at a slower rate of approximately 10 to 20 g per day, because he/she has not yet entered the accelerated weight gain of the third trimester.[8]

Nutritional Assessment

Nutritional assessment is a critical aspect of the initial evaluation of all surgical patients.[9] The incidence of malnutrition in surgical patients has been well documented in several reviews, and this group comprises 35% to 45% of inpatients.[10] Classical work by Cooper and colleagues[11] showed that 18% to 40% of pediatric surgical patients have malnutrition. This rate of malnutrition has also been shown in other pediatric patients.[12] Aside from surgery, other patients at risk for malnutrition include those with large open wounds with concomitant loss of protein and increased metabolic needs, extensive burns, blunt trauma, and sepsis. An important question is how long the gastrointestinal tract will be dysfunctional after major surgery; this information must be integrated into the nutritional support delivered in the perioperative period. Nutritional assessment can be divided into subjective and objective components. Two basic tools are available: the Mini Nutrition Assessment[13] and the Subjective Global Assessment (SGA). The SGA is performed during the history and physical examination. This should include an evaluation of weight loss

(5% for mild to 10% for moderate to severe malnutrition), anorexia, vomiting, and physical evidence of muscle wasting (indicative of severe malnutrition), and modifications of this have been made for pediatrics, though not as well validated as for adults.[14] SGA has been shown to be an accurate mode of assessing malnutrition for both inpatients as well as non-hospitalized patients. Additionally, although not fully substantiated in young children, both of these nutrition tools have been directly correlated with Acute Physiology and Chronic Health Evaluation (APACHE) II scores and hospital mortality in surgical patients[15,16] The objective portion of the assessment begins with the basic anthropometric measurements of height, weight, and head circumference. Measurements are placed on a standardized growth curve, such as that of the National Center for Health Statistics. From these growth charts, the expected weight for height index can be calculated. As length and head circumference are less affected by excess fat or postoperative fluid fluctuations, length is an excellent indicator of long-term body growth. Acute changes in nutritional status will have a more immediate effect on body weight than length and will decrease the child's weight for height index. Chronic undernutrition, however, will result in a lag in both height and weight. These changes in growth are probably best expressed using a Z-score for weight for length ratios as well as weight, length, and head circumference for age. A number of automated and free software programs are available for such evaluations, such as from the World Health Organization (WHO Anthro [version 3.1, June 2010]). Once patients are more than 2 years of age, this can best be reflected by the child's body mass index (BMI); however, expression of BMI as a Z-score can often add a very useful perspective. Special growth charts are also available for monitoring the growth of children with special health-care needs (e.g., Down syndrome, Prader-Willi syndrome, myelomeningocele, achondroplasia, cerebral palsy). Use of these can give a very important perspective about where a child's growth should lie.[17] An increasingly important group of patients to assess nutrition on are those children with obesity.[18] Assessment of such children requires a high index of suspicion. Although BMI measures weight rather than adiposity, it is still regarded as one of the best tools to perform this assessment, and it is a fairly strong predictive of adult obesity and associated medical complications resulting from an obese state.[19]

BIOCHEMICAL MEASUREMENTS OF NUTRITIONAL STATUS

Serum albumin level has been used as an indication of chronic nutritional status. However, albumin turnover is slow ($t_{1/2}$ of 20 days). Therefore other plasma proteins, such as prealbumin binding protein ($t_{1/2}$ of 2 days) and retinol-binding protein ($t_{1/2}$ of 12 hours) are indications of a more current nutritional status. There are no established norms for prealbumin or retinol-binding protein in infants and young children.[20] Further, visceral proteins lack specificity under stress and inflammatory conditions, and they are affected by non-nutritional factors. Therefore their levels should be interpreted in the context of nutritional history, underlying diseases, and medication therapy. Ideally, a baseline level is obtained, and then subsequent levels may be used to establish the effects of disease and/or nutritional supplementation.

Other parameters that can be useful for measuring nutritional status include bone age and dental status. Malnutrition is a common cause of delayed bone maturation.[21]

DIRECT MEASUREMENT OF BODY COMPOSITION

Various methods have been created during the past 25 years to more directly measure the body composition of adults and children. Although many of these methods are not readily accessible to most clinicians and, rather, are used for experimental purposes, some, are becoming more commonly used in pediatric clinical settings. Measurement of body water has been done for several years using isotope dilution techniques. This is based on the principle that fat is anhydrous so that most of the isotope is directed into the water compartments of the body.[22] This assumption is not always true; however, such measurements can give an excellent indication of approximate amounts of body fat and water.[23,24] Bioelectrical impedance analysis uses the measurement of the body's impedance to a flow of electrical current as a measure of total body water. Extrapolation of these measurements can allow for the determination of other body compartments, including total body adipose tissue. More recently, dual photon absorptiometry and dual energy x-ray absorptiometry have been used to measure bone mineral content and amounts of fat and body water.[25,26] The accuracy of the instruments is excellent, and because of the low amounts of radiation exposure, dual energy x-ray absorptiometry is becoming the method of choice for measuring pediatric body composition. Standards have only been established down to approximately 6 to 8 years of age[27]; therefore further work is required to understand the use of these measures in small children and infants.

Nutritional Requirements

ENERGY REQUIREMENTS

The energy needs of infants and children are unique. Estimates of premature infants show that a 1-kg infant has only a 4-day nutritional reserve, and a full-term infant may live for no more than 1 month without nutrition.[28,29] In children, energy is required for maintenance of body metabolism and growth. A gross estimate of calorie expenditure can be obtained by using the Dietary Reference Intakes (DRIs) for energy requirements, based on the child's age, weight, height, and physical activity, and also based on the Food and Nutrition Board, Institute of Medicine, and National Academy of Sciences guidelines (Dietary Reference Intakes: Recommended Intakes for Individuals in 2006) (http://www.iom.edu/Reports.aspx). Predictive equations (e.g., from the World Health Organization, Schofield equations, and so forth) provide an estimate of the resting energy expenditure (REE), but none are extremely accurate. Other estimates use the amount of calories per length or height for children with chronic health conditions and special health-care needs (e.g., Down syndrome, Prader-Willi syndrome, myelomeningocele, and cerebral palsy; see Table 12-13).

Energy requirements vary depending on age as well as the physiologic status of the child (Table 12-1). Periods of active growth and extreme physical activity will increase energy requirements. The average distribution of kilocalories in

TABLE 12-1

Energy Requirements

Daily Energy Requirements (Total kcal/kg) for Pediatric Patients	
Preterm neonate	90-120
<6 months	85-105
6-12 months	80-100
1-7 years	75-90
7-12 years	50-75
>12-18 years	30-50

Mirtallo J, Canada T, Johnson D: Task Force for the Revision of Safe Practices for Parenteral Nutrition. Safe practices for parenteral nutrition. JPEN J Parenter Enteral Nutr 2004;28:S39-S70.

TABLE 12-2

Daily Fluid Requirements for Pediatric Patients

Body Weight	Amount
<1500 g	130-150 mL/kg
1500-2000 g	110-130 mL/kg
2-10 kg	100 mL/kg
>10-20 kg	1000 mL for 10 kg + 50 mL/kg for each kg >10
>20 kg	1500 mL for 20 kg + 20 mL/kg for each kg >20

Mirtallo J, Canada T, Johnson D: Task Force for the Revision of Safe Practices for Parenteral Nutrition. Safe practices for parenteral nutrition. JPEN J Parenter Enteral Nutr 2004;28:S39-S70.

a well-balanced diet is as follows: protein, 15%; fat, 35%; and carbohydrate, 50%. Although careful clinical examination is important in making a determination of the child's status, Baker and colleagues[30] showed that the depleted state could not be reliably detected on the basis of the weight-to-height ratio, triceps skinfold, mid–upper arm circumference, hand strength, albumin concentration, total protein level, or creatinine-to-height ratio. Actual measurement or estimation of metabolic rate and energy needs is the best method of following the nutritional status. Commonly used nomograms may significantly underestimate or overestimate energy expenditure.[31–33] One of the most accurate methods of measuring energy expenditure is indirect calorimetry.[34] In indirect calorimetry, carbon dioxide (CO_2) production and O_2 consumption are measured using a metabolic cart. The sample is best measured in intubated infants, yielding a resting energy expenditure. The energy expenditure or metabolic rate, as measured in cubic centimeters of oxygen per minute, can be converted to calories per hour or per day, if the substrates are known. All measurements are only approximations of caloric needs, for which the surgeon must further adjust according to the clinical course of the patient. Such measurements give an excellent way to monitor patients, particularly those children who are in an intensive care unit setting.[35] In contrast to adults, the rise in REE postsurgery is much less. Mitchell and colleagues[33] found that the REE of postoperative cardiac patients fell to values less than those of normal healthy children who had not undergone surgery. This finding was also confirmed in the study by Letton and colleagues,[36] who examined energy expenditure in young infants in the postoperative period. These studies suggested that reliance on recommended daily allowance (RDA) values may result in overfeeding postoperative children (see the section on complications from overfeeding later). Measurements are critical, because those infants starting with poor nutritional status, or more aggressive surgery (e.g., cardiopulmonary bypass), may have significantly greater energy needs.[37] Indirect calorimetry, however, may be difficult in young infants with uncuffed endotracheal tubes, where an air leak may lead to significant inaccuracies in results. Typically, parenteral energy requirements are lower than enteral or oral requirements because of less thermogenesis with the parenteral route and absence of energy loss in stools.

WATER

The water content of infants is higher than that of adults (75% of body weight versus 65%) and is proportional to muscle mass. Fluids provide the principal source of water; however, some water is derived by the oxidation of food and body tissues. Requirements for water are related to caloric consumption; so, infants must consume much larger amounts of water per unit of body weight than adults. In general, calorie requirements (kcal/kg/day) are matched to the amount of fluid needs mL/kg/day). The daily consumption of fluid by healthy infants is equivalent to 10% to 15% of their body weight, in contrast to only 2% to 4% by adults. In addition, the normal-content food for infants and children is much higher in water content than that of adults; the fruit and vegetables consumed by infants and children contain about 90% water. Only 0.5% to 3% of fluid intake is retained by infants and children. About 50% is excreted through the kidneys, 3% to 10% is lost through the gastrointestinal tract, and 40% to 50% is insensible loss. Estimation of daily maintenance fluid requirements in infants and children are shown in (Table 12-2).[38]

PROTEIN

The requirement for protein in infants is based on the combined needs of growth and maintenance (Table 12-3). Two percent of the infant's body weight, compared with 3% of the adult's body weight, consists of nitrogen. The average intake of protein should comprise approximately 15% of total calories administered. Two percent of an infant's body weight, compared with 3% of an adult's body weight, consists of nitrogen. Most of the increase in body nitrogen occurs during the first year of life. The nutritional value of protein is based not only on the amount of nitrogen available but also on the amino acid composition of the protein.[39] Protein provides 4 kcal/g of energy and should be included in estimates of energy (caloric) delivery. Twenty amino acids have been identified, of which eight amino acids (phenylalanine, valine, threonine, tryptophan, isoleucine, methionine, leucine, lysine) are generally considered essential for humans, with an additional four amino acids (cysteine, tyrosine, arginine, histidine)

TABLE 12-3

Daily Protein Requirements (g/kg) for Pediatric Patients*

Preterm neonates	3-4
Infants (1-12 months)	2-3
Children (>10 kg or 1-10 years)	1-2
Adolescents (11-17 years)	0.8-1.5

Mirtallo J, Canada T, Johnson D: Task Force for the Revision of Safe Practices for Parenteral Nutrition. Safe practices for parenteral nutrition. JPEN J Parenter Enteral Nutr 2004;28:S39-S70.
*Assumes normal age-related organ function.

considered conditionally essential in infants. New tissue cannot be formed unless all of the essential amino acids are present in the diet simultaneously; the absence of only one essential amino acid will result in a negative nitrogen and protein balance. Further, the use of taurine supplementation has been shown to decrease the severity of PN-associated cholestasis.[40] It has also been suggested that proline is essential in preterm infants, although this has yet to be confirmed.[41]

Protein requirements are typically based on age and adjusted based on nutritional status, stress level, severity and type of injury, kidney and liver functions, and other clinical conditions. In general, estimated protein requirements for children based on age are: 0 to 2 years, 2 to 3 g/kg/day; 2 to 13 years, 1.5 to 2 g/kg/day; and 13 to 18 years, 1.5 g/kg/day.[42] Protein requirements are markedly higher in term neonates and infants ranging from 2 to 3 g/kg/day. This estimate is based on several sources. Extrapolation of data on fetal absorption across the placenta during the last trimester indicates protein needs to be 2.2 g/kg/day.[43,44] Delivery of greater amounts of protein to neonates has generally been associated with elevated blood urea nitrogen levels. Protein requirements in premature infants are higher than term infants and range from 3 to 3.5 g/kg/day.[44,45] Such delivery is critical to provide optimal growth and neurodevelopment in infants. In very-low-birth-weight infants, this requirement may approach 3.85 g/kg/day.[46] Such added protein loads must be balanced against the immaturity of the renal system, and the development of uremia should be monitored.[47,48] In particular, taurine is essential for normal neural and retinal development.[49]

Two amino acids that may have significant benefit to the integrity of the gastrointestinal mucosa and the immune status of patients are glutamine and arginine. Although these amino acids are not truly essential, the organism may require additional usage of these during periods of stress. Glutamine has been shown to prevent PN-associated atrophy of the intestine in animals, however, and possibly in humans.[50,51] The efficacy of glutamine in bowel adaptation has been called into question.[52–54] However, a recent meta-analysis of all clinical studies using glutamine showed that glutamine dipeptide significantly reduced the length of hospital stay, and decreased risk of infectious complications rates in surgical patients.[55] Arginine has also been shown to improve nitrogen retention, wound healing, and the immune status.[56,57] However, at least in animal models, early administration of arginine has been shown to worsen the prognosis of animals, because of the activation of nitric oxide within the gastrointestinal tract.[58]

CARBOHYDRATES

Carbohydrates provide a major and most immediate source of energy through parenteral and enteral routes. Carbohydrates can be provided in one of three ways: monosaccharides (glucose and fructose), disaccharides (lactose, sucrose, and maltose), and complex carbohydrates (starches). Because the body is capable of forming sugars from amino acids, no essential amount of carbohydrate has been defined. However, the addition of small amounts of carbohydrates prevents breakdown of somatic protein sources and thus acts as a protein-sparing substrate.[59] This effect leads to suppression of endogenous glucose production as well as to endogenous glucose oxidation, thereby preventing the oxidation of amino acids that have been derived from skeletal muscles. The body

has a limited ability to store glucose, although the substrate is essential and almost continuously needed by the central nervous system. Dextrose is the most common source of carbohydrate, and it yields 3.4 kcal/g. Glucose metabolism may occur aerobically through the tricarboxylic acid cycle, theoretically yielding a maximum of 38 moles of adenosine triphosphatase (ATP)/mole of glucose. Anaerobically, glucose metabolism through the glycolytic cycle yields 2 moles of ATP/mole of glucose, with lactic acid as an end product. Glucose is formed in the liver by means of gluconeogenesis (formation of glucose from noncarbohydrates precursors), which uses alanine and other amino acids from skeletal muscle and lactic acid from the breakdown of glycogen in skeletal muscle through the Cori cycle. Immediately after a meal, glucose absorption contributes to the bulk of circulating glucose. As soon as 4 hours after the meal, these sources are rapidly depleted, and glycogen from the liver becomes a major source of energy for the next 8 to 12 hours. Newborn infants have relatively limited glycogen reserves (34 g), most of which reside in the liver. Thus relatively short periods of fasting can lead to a hypoglycemic state.

The primary enteral carbohydrate delivered to neonates and young infants is lactose.[3] Lactose is broken down into glucose and galactose in the intestines by disaccharidases (e.g., lactase), which are located along the intestinal epithelial border. Because lactose is the predominant carbohydrate of small children, lactase levels remain sufficiently high in most infants until they are at least 2 or 3 years of age. Nonlactose formulas that are soy-based and contain sucrose or corn syrup may provide adequate amounts of carbohydrates (see Enteral Nutrition later). Preterm infants may be unable to digest certain carbohydrates, particularly lactose, because lactase activity in the intestines is inadequate. Thus for premature infants, formulas that have a 50/50 mixture of lactose and glucose polymers are ideal.

Supplementation with inadequate amounts of carbohydrates may lead to a ketotic state, whereby fat and muscles are broken down for gluconeogenesis. Stable infants should receive approximately 40% to 45% of their total caloric intake as carbohydrates. Glucose intolerance does occur and is not only manifested by hyperglycemia but also commonly by hypertriglyceridemia (see the section on hyperglycemia later). Delivery of carbohydrates in amounts greater than the body can use will result in hyperglycemia and lipogenesis (see the section on complications from enteral feeding later).

FAT

Intravenous lipids have the highest caloric density of the three major nutrients (9 kcal/g). In general, intravenous lipids should comprise between 30% to 50% of all non-nitrogen calories. Lipids have the advantage of being an excellent source of energy and essential fatty acids (EFAs). Linoleic acid is essential for neonates, older children, and adults. Deficiencies of linoleic acid may occur rapidly in neonates. Withholding lipids from the PN of a neonate for as few as 2 to 3 days may lead a biochemical deficiency of fatty acids.[60,61] A deficiency of fatty acids in infants may result when less than 1% of the caloric intake is linoleic acid; in general, 2% to 4% of dietary energy should come from essential fatty acids. Manifestations of fatty acid deficiency include scaly skin, hair loss, diarrhea, thrombocytopenia, and impaired wound healing.[62] Absence of trace amounts of linolenic acid may also be the cause of visual and behavioral disorders. Fatty acids are an excellent source of energy to all tissues of the body except erythrocytes and the brain. With time, however, the brain can also use fatty acids as an energy source once they are converted to ketones. Fatty acids are carried into the mitochondria for β-oxidation by the carnitine transferase system (see later).

Essentially, two types of fatty acids exist: saturated and unsaturated. Saturated fatty acids lack double carbon bonds and are generally derived from animals. Unsaturated fatty acids have at least one double bond, the position of which is designated by a prefix omega (ω). The two major polyunsaturated fatty acids are linoleic acid, which is an ω-6 fatty acid, and α-linolenic acid, which is an ω-3 fatty acid. Omega-6 fatty acids are usually derived from plants, and ω-3 fatty acids are usually derived from fish oils. Both of these polyunsaturated fats are essential for the development of cell membranes and the central nervous system (CNS), as well as for the synthesis of arachidonic acid and related prostaglandins. Thromboxanes derived from ω-6 fatty acids are potential mediators of platelet aggregation, whereas thromboxanes, derived from ω-3 fatty acids, are potent anticoagulants, as well as docosahexaenoic acid (DHA), which has important roles for CNS development and modulation of inflammatory conditions. Further, ω-6 fatty acids, which form arachidonic acid, also contribute to the formation of prostaglandin (PG) E_2, a known immunosuppressant, whereas ω-3 fatty acids contribute to the formation of PGE_1 and PGE_3, which do not have an immunosuppressive effect. A 1:1 ratio of ω-6 to ω-3 fatty acids seems to be ideal, based on experimental data from animals that survived burns.[63] No data are available on the ideal ratio in neonates or children.

Essential fatty acid deficiency shows an elevated triene-to-tetraene ratio of greater than 0.2, where trienes consist of 5,8,11-eicosatrienoic acid and tetraenes consist of linoleic and arachidonic acids and an eicosatrienoic/arachidonic acid, and low plasma levels of one or more of the essential fatty acids. Overall, any infant not receiving the full amount of lipids should be monitored at least once a month for essential fatty acid deficiency. Absolute values of linoleic and 1-linolenic acid can be ordered, and actually may yield a better perspective for the clinical development of EFA deficiency.

MINERALS, TRACE ELEMENTS, AND VITAMINS

The normal daily requirement of vitamins has been recently revised by the Food and Drug Administration.[64] Vitamins are essential components or cofactors of various metabolic reactions. Most commercial infant formulas contain adequate amounts of vitamins to meet known daily requirements. Such requirements were established by the American Medical Association (AMA) in the 1970s.[65] Infants who receive other types of formula or human milk may require additional vitamin supplementation.

Fat-Soluble Vitamins

Vitamin A Vitamin A is principally stored in the liver and is involved in formation of retinoic acid for vision and the coordination of cell cycles. Deficiencies of vitamin A may lead to night blindness, xerophthalmia, poor growth, and impaired resistance to infection. It is also clear, however, that low levels of vitamin A predispose infants to long-term pulmonary disease, and vitamin A levels are low in such infants.[66] In a recent Cochrane review, eight studies were reviewed, and it was found that vitamin A supplementation was associated with a prevention in the development of bronchopulmonary dysplasia (BPD).[67] Neurodevelopment at 18 to 22 months of age was not different between those treated with and without vitamin A. Excessive amounts of vitamin A can be quite deleterious to infants. As little as 6000 µg of retinol daily can produce anorexia, desquamation of the skin, and increased intracranial pressure.[68]

Vitamin D Vitamin D is essential for bone formation and mineral homeostasis. A deficiency may occur with fat malabsorption; however, overuse of vitamin D may lead to hypercalcemia.[69] Most formulas contain adequate amounts of vitamin D (approximately 60 IU/100 kcal). No evidence to support the supplementation of vitamin D to infants for better bone growth beyond that provided by standard formulas exists. During the past decade, a greater appreciation of the link between deficient immune status and low vitamin D levels has been examined in pediatric children. In fact, this association may account for an increased risk of pediatric asthma and food allergies.[70]

Vitamin E Vitamin E seems to have significant antioxidant affects. Vitamin E may prevent the neuropathy seen in infants with biliary atresia as well as muscle weakness in children with cystic fibrosis.[71] The dose of vitamin E required for full-term infants is approximately 0.7 IU/100 kcal of energy intake. Because of its antioxidant action, vitamin E has been used to decrease lung injury in neonates with bronchopulmonary dysplasia. It does appear that usage of vitamin E is beneficial in this regard.[72] It also appears that vitamin E is beneficial in the prevention of retinopathy in premature infants[73]; and it may have a benefit in reducing the incidence of intraventricular hemorrhage.[74]

Vitamin K Vitamin K is required at birth to prevent coagulopathy in newborns and should be administered soon after delivery.[75] Vitamin K is included in most formulas; however, larger amounts may be needed in infants with prolonged episodes of diarrhea. Assessment of deficiencies is most readily done by attaining a prothrombin time.

Water-Soluble Vitamins

Deficiencies of water-soluble vitamins are rare in formula-fed and breast-fed babies. B vitamins are needed for carbohydrate, protein, and fat metabolism as well as oxidation and reduction reactions. Deficiencies may be seen with short-bowel syndrome and manifest as chelosis and lethargy. Abnormal levels of vitamin B_1 (thiamine) are generally the first signs of vitamin B deficiency and can be detected with an erythrocyte transketolase enzyme assay. Vitamin C is required for optimizing several enzyme reactions and has direct antioxidant effects. Excessive amounts of vitamin C may lead to nephrolithiasis and interference with vitamin B_{12} absorption.

TABLE 12-4

Daily Parenteral Trace Element Requirements and Supplementation in Parenteral Nutrition According to the ASPEN Guidelines

Age Group	Zinc	Copper	Manganese	Chromium	Selenium
Adults (mg/day)	2.5-5	0.3-0.5	0.06-0.1	0.01-0.015	0.02-0.06
Adolescents > 40 kg (mg/day)	2-5	0.2-0.5	0.04-0.1	0.005- 0.015	0.04-0.06
Preterm infant < 3 kg (µ/kg/day)	400	20	1	0.05-0.3	1.5-2
Term infant 3-10 kg (µ/kg/day)	50-250	20	1	0.2	2
Children 10-40 kg (µ/kg/day)	50-125	5-20	1	0.14-0.2	1-2

Mirtallo J, Canada T, Johnson D: Task Force for the Revision of Safe Practices for Parenteral Nutrition. Safe practices for parenteral nutrition. JPEN J Parenter Enteral Nutr 2004;28:S39-S70.

ASPEN, American Society for Parenteral and Enteral Nutrition.

Trace Elements

Trace elements comprise less than 0.01% of the total body weight in humans.[76] They often function as metalloenzymes, which maximize enzymatic reactions, but may also act as soluble ionic cofactors or nonprotein organic molecules. Without supplementation, specific deficiencies of many of these factors have been manifested clinically in patients maintained on long-term PN as well as those with short-bowel syndrome or malabsorptive conditions. Table 12-4 lists the recommended doses of trace elements.

Zinc Zinc has several biochemical functions, including formation of metalloenzymes, ribonucleic acid (RNA) conformation, and membrane stabilization.[77] In addition, zinc seems to play a critical role in the maintenance of a normal immunologic system. Deficiencies in zinc can arise from various sources that are common in pediatric surgical patients; such sources include the short-bowel syndrome, thermal burns, peritoneal dialysis, inflammatory bowel disease, and other causes of diarrhea. Clinical manifestations of zinc deficiency include growth retardation, alopecia, skin lesions (acrodermatitis enteropathica), impaired lymphocyte function, impaired wound healing, and zinc deficiency can actually lead to diarrhea.[78] Supplementation in infants should be a minimum of 400 µg/kg/day. Because gastrointestinal losses can be higher during episodes of diarrhea and sepsis, higher doses are indicated in these instances. In addition, zinc deficiency may impair recovery of the intestines after massive resection.[79]

Copper Copper is a critical trace element for metalloenzyme function. The main site of copper storage, distribution, and excretion is the liver. Copper deficiency has been reported in patients receiving PN formulas that are not supplemented with copper.[80] Manifestations of copper deficiency include microcytic, hypochromic anemia; neutropenia; hypothermia; mental status changes; and, in children, growth retardation and skeletal demineralization. Removal of copper from infants and children may lead to an aplastic anemic condition, which can be fatal.[81]

Selenium During the past decade, selenium has been acknowledged as an essential trace element. Selenium is a component of a selenoenzyme that helps catalyze glutathione peroxidase, an enzyme system that is necessary to reduce free radicals. The most practical way of measuring selenium levels is by assaying glutathione peroxidase activity in erythrocytes. Selenium levels dramatically decline after as few as 6 weeks of PN.[82] Without the addition of selenium, deficiencies are generally manifested by cardiomyopathy as well as by peripheral myositis with associated muscle tenderness.

Manganese, Chromium, and Molybdenum Although no clear-cut cases of manganese deficiency have been documented in the literature, manganese is an essential element for many organisms and is believed to also be essential for humans. Animals that are deficient in manganese show growth retardation and ataxia in the newborn period.[83] Excess deposition of manganese has been shown to occur in both the liver and brain of infants on prolonged PN, and clinicians should have a very low threshold of eliminating Mn from the trace element package of infants who have developed PN-associated liver disease (PNALD).[84] Chromium seems to have its predominant action as a potentiator of insulin action. Deficiencies of chromium can lead to poor glucose tolerance.[85] Molybdenum is important in the oxidative metabolism of purines and sulfur-containing compounds[86] but is not typically supplemented in PN. Deficiencies of molybdenum are associated with increases in serum uric acid levels.

Enteral Nutrition

Enteral nutrition (EN) includes oral nutritional supplementation and tube feedings. EN should be the primary source of nutrients if the gastrointestinal tract is functional. Even when full feedings are not tolerated enterally, the provision of small volumes of "trophic" feedings may prevent further deterioration of intestinal function.

INDICATIONS

Infants in a state of good health before surgery or trauma can sustain 5 to 7 days without significant energy intake and without serious systemic consequences, provided that adequate nutritional support is initiated thereafter. Premature infants less than 32 to 34 weeks' gestation do not generally have a maturely coordinated suck and swallow. Feedings must therefore be provided enterally either by bolus every 2 to 3 hours or by continuous feedings. The overall growth patterns are exceedingly poor for premature infants. In addition, the younger an infant's gestational age, the greater the percentage who are discharged with growth restriction. In fact, almost 100% of infants born at 24 weeks' gestational age will be discharged with a diagnosis of growth restriction. Therefore aggressive feeding even within the first 24 hours of life is generally considered advisable. Enteral feedings are begun after the resolution of the postoperative ileus. There are many high-calorie formulas available to address variable needs (Tables 12-5 (infant) and 12-6 (pediatric). Children who have specific

TABLE 12-5

Infant Formulas

Formula	kcal/ mL	Protein (g/L)	Protein (% kcal)	Protein Source	Carbohydrate Source	Carbohydrate (% kcal)	Fat Source	Fat (% kcal)	Indications
Similac Special Care (Ross)	0.81	24	12	Nonfat milk, whey	Lactose, corn syrup solids	41	MCT oil, soy oil, coconut oil	47	Prematurity
Neosure (Ross)	0.73	21	11	Nonfat milk, whey	Lactose, corn syrup solids	42	MCT oil, soy oil, coconut oil	48	Prematurity, discharge formula
Enfamil (Mead Johnson)	0.67	14	8.5	Whey, nonfat milk	Lactose	43.5	Palm olein, soy oil, coconut oil, sunflower oil	48	Standard
Similac (Ross)	0.67	14	8	Nonfat milk, whey	Lactose	43	Soy oil, coconut oil, safflower oil	49	Standard
	0.81	17	8	Nonfat milk, whey	Lactose	43	Soy oil, coconut oil, safflower oil	49	
Prosobee (Mead Johnson)	0.67	17	10	Soy isolate, methionine	Corn syrup solids	42	Palm olein, soy oil, coconut oil, sun oil	48	Lactose intolerance, galactosemia
Isomil (Ross)	0.67	17	10	Soy isolate, methionine	Corn syrup, sucrose	41	Soy oil, coconut oil, safflower oil	49	Lactose, malabsorption, galactosemia
Nutramigen (Mead Johnson)	0.67	19	11	Casein hydrolysate, cystine, tyrosine, tryptophan	Corn syrup solids, modified cornstarch	41	Palm olein, soy oil, coconut oil, sun oil	48	Protein intolerance
Pregestimil (Mead Johnson)	0.67	19	11	Casein hydrolysate, cystine, tyrosine, tryptophan	Corn syrup solids, modified cornstarch, dextrose	41	MCT oil, Corn oil, Soy oil, safflower oil	48	Protein intolerance, cystic fibrosis, neonatal cholestasis, short-bowel syndrome
Alimentum (Ross)	0.67	19	11	Casein hydrolysate, cystine, tyrosine, tryptophan	Sucrose, modified tapioca, starch	41	MCT oil, safflower oil, soy oil	48	Protein intolerance, neonatal cholestasis
Neocate (Scientific Hospital Supplies)	0.67	21	12	Free amino acids	Corn syrup solids	47	MCT oil, safflower oil, corn oil, soy oil, sun oil	41	Food allergy, protein intolerance, short-bowel syndrome
Enfaport Lipil (Mead Johnson)	1	35	14	Calcium caseinate, Sodium caseinate	Corn syrup solids	41	MCT oil (84%), soy oil	45	Chylothorax, LCHAD deficiency

LCHAD, long-chain hydroxyacyl-CoA dehydrogenase deficiency; MCT; medium-chain triglyceride.

Composition of infant and pediatric formulas is summarized in Tables 12-5 and 12-6, respectively. Enfamil (Mead Johnson) and Similac (Ross, Columbus, Ohio) both have milk-based proteins and contain lactose as the carbohydrate source. There are only limited reasons to use soy formulas. The soy-based products include Prosobee (Mead Johnson) and Isomil (Ross). Both contain corn syrup solids as a carbohydrate source. Isomil also contains sucrose. Soy formulas are indicated to manage galactosemia and primary or secondary lactase deficiency. Soy formulas should not be used in patients with a documented allergy or intolerance to milk protein, because one third of infants who have an allergen-induced reaction to cow's milk are also intolerant of soy. Therefore a protein hydrolysate or elemental formula is recommended in infants who have milk-protein intolerance. Protein hydrolysates include Nutramigen (Mead Johnson), Alimentum (Ross), and Pregestimil (Mead Johnson). Alimentum and Pregestamil also provide 50% to 55% of fat as medium-chain triglycerides (MCT). If infants have continued symptoms of protein intolerance when ingesting a protein hydrolysate, then an amino acid–based formula may be provided. For the infant population, Neocate (Scientific Hospital Supplies, Gaithersburg, Md.) is the only amino acid–based formula available. Children older than 12 months of age who continue to be intolerant of milk protein may respond well to Peptamen, Jr (Clintec, Chicago, Ill.), which is a whey protein hydrolysate. If an amino acid–based formula is needed in children older than 12 months of age, options include Neocate 1+ (Scientific Hospital Supplies), L-emental (Gala/Gen/Nutrition Medical, Arden Hills, Minn.), and Elecare (Ross). Neocate 1+ and Elecare both have long-chain triglycerides. Sixty-eight percent of the fat in L-emental is derived from MCT. The authors thank Megan Perkowski, RD, for her contribution and editing of this table.

TABLE 12-6

Pediatric Formulas

Formula	kcal/ mL	Protein (g/L)	Protein (% kcal)	Protein Source	Carbohydrate Source	Carbohydrate (% kcal)	Fat Source	Fat (% kcal)	Indications
Pediasure (Ross)	1.0	30	12	Milk protein concentrate, whey protein, soy isolate	Corn maltodextrin, sucrose	53	Safflower oil, soy oil, MCT oil	35	Standard, oral feeds, tube feeds
Boost (Mead Johnson)	1	42	17	Milk	Corn syrup, sucrose	68	Canola oil, corn oil, sunflower oil	15	Standard, oral feeds, tube feeds
Peptamen, Jr (Clintec)	1.0	30	12	Hydrolyzed whey	Maltodextrin	55	MCT, soy oil, canola oil	33	Short-bowel syndrome, cholestasis, pancreatitis
L-emental (GalaGen/ Nutrition Medical)	0.8	40	16	L-Amino acids	Maltodextrin, modified starch	82	Safflower oil	2	Short-bowel syndrome, IBD, pancreatitis
Elecare (Ross)	0.67	21	15	L-Amino acids	Corn syrup solids	43	MCT, safflower oil, soy oil	42	Malabsorption, food allergies
Suplena (Ross)	1.8	45	10	Sodium caseinate, milk protein isolate	Corn maltodextrin, sucrose	51	Safflower oil, soy oil, canola oil	48	Renal failure

IBD, inflammatory bowel disease; MCT, medium-chain triglyceride.
The authors thank Megan Perkowski, RD, for her contribution and editing of this table.

underlying diseases associated with malabsorption may benefit from specialized formulas. Once oral feeds are clinically possible they should begin. Delay in initiating oral nutrient swallowing will result in long-term oral aversion.

DELIVERY MODALITIES

Aside from oral intake, a number of modalities are available for enteral delivery. These include nasogastric and nasojejunal feedings. Children receiving gastric feedings tolerate a higher osmolarity and volume than those being fed into the small bowel. Furthermore, gastric acid may benefit digestion, has a bactericidal effect, and is associated with less-frequent gastrointestinal complications.[7] Auscultation of air insufflated into the tube is inadequate. Confirmation must be obtained by aspiration of gastrointestinal contents or radiographic confirmation.[87] For patients requiring feedings for more than 8 weeks, a more permanent feeding access (e.g., gastrostomy tube) should be considered. The preoperative assessment usually consists of an upper gastrointestinal series followed by a 24-hour pH probe study if the results of the upper gastrointestinal study are abnormal. If either of these studies reveals reflux, a fundoplication should be done at the time the gastrostomy tube is placed. Assessment of gastric emptying should also be done before surgery, with a nuclear gastric-emptying study.[88,89] The most common procedure for gastrostomy placement is a percutaneous endoscopic gastrostomy (PEG) tube.[90] An improvement in gastrostomy tubes is the gastrostomy "button." The button is made of nonreactive Silastic components. It has a valve placed into a low-profile device that lies almost flush with the abdominal wall, and it can be capped between uses.[91] These buttons may now be placed at the same time as the percutaneous endoscopic procedure.[92] It has been reported that the incidence of complications is less with a PEG technique compared with other approaches; however, several complications have been described, including improper placement (i.e., close to the pylorus), inadvertent placement through an adjacent loop of bowel, necrosis of the tract of the gastrostomy tube, and technical failures that require laparotomy.[93]

Use of jejunal tubes is plagued with problems, including involuntary dislodgement of transpylorically placed tubes and catheter obstruction because of inspissation of feedings or instillation of medications. Short-term complications of surgically-placed J-tubes include intra-abdominal abscess and volvulus with bowel infarction. Long-term complications include intestinal obstruction and peritonitis. When using tubes passed distal to the pylorus, continuous drip feedings are recommended to prevent the development of diarrhea and other symptoms of dumping. Verification of the location of the tube is mandatory before beginning enteral tube feedings. This requires either aspiration of enteric contents or radiologic confirmation.

ENTERAL FORMULAS

The choice of formula depends on the age of the patient and the condition of the gastrointestinal tract. In general, term infants should be maintained on human milk (see later) or a standard 20 kcal/oz formula (see Tables 12-5 and 12-6). Cow milk–based formulas for term infants contain nutrients that closely approximate the nutritional profile of human milk. Some formulas have added arachidonic acid (ARA) and docosahexaenoic acid (DHA), the two fatty acids that are found in human milk and believed to be essential for brain and eye development; however, no strong evidence-based literature supports the need for this. A lactose-based formula is generally the first choice, because it is the most physiologically

TABLE 12-7

Enteral Nutrition Administration to Preterm Infants

Birth Weight (g)	≤1000	>1000 to <1250	1250 to 1500	>1500 to 2000	>2000 to 2500
Volume of first feeding Schedule of feeding	10-20 mL/kg/day	10-20 mL/kg/day	20 mL/kg/day	20 mL/kg/day	5 mL every 3 hours
Volume rate of feeding advances	10-20 mL/kg/day	10-20 mL/kg/day	20 mL/kg/day	20 mL/kg/day, may advance as tolerated	5 mL every other feed as tolerated

Btaiche I, Khalidi N, Kovacevich D (eds): The Parenteral and Enteral Nutrition Manual, ed 9. Ann Arbor, Mich, 2010, University of Michigan, University of Michigan Hospitals and Health Centers.

similar to human milk and is the least expensive. Soy formulas are indicated to manage galactosemia and primary or secondary lactase deficiency. Soy formulas should not be used in patients with a documented allergy or intolerance to milk protein, because one third of infants who have an allergen-induced reaction to cow's milk are also intolerant of soy. Therefore a protein hydrolysate or elemental formula is recommended in infants who have milk-protein intolerance. Further, soy formulas are not recommended for premature infants, because of their high aluminum content, which may contribute to osteopenia.

Calories from enteral nutrition can be added by increasing the volume delivered, increasing the concentration of the formula, or by supplementing the feedings. Formula concentrations may be increased to 30 kcal/oz; however, highly concentrated formulas may be difficult for some infants to digest, because they have a higher renal solute load and it may take time for them to build up tolerance. Higher concentrations have also been associated with a necrotizing enterocolitis–type process.[94] Formula supplementation can be done by the addition of a glucose polymer or fats (as medium-chain triglycerides or vegetable oil). Each 0.5 g of glucose polymer added to an ounce of standard formula increases calories by 0.06 kcal/mL, therefore creating a total caloric delivery of 0.73 kcal/mL. The addition of 0.5 g of oil to formula increases calories by 0.13 kcal/mL or a total of 0.8 kcal/mL. Caution must be taken when supplementing calories in this fashion, because it may compromise the ability of the infant to consume sufficient amounts of protein or minerals if the amount of formula is limited. However, up to 2 g of glucose polymer or 1 g of oil per ounce of formula can be added safely.

Standard premature infant formulas are milk-based formulas that provide 22 to 24 calories/ounce, and are optimized for required vitamins, minerals, and trace element needs. A portion of fat is provided as medium-chain triglycerides (MCT) to compensate for the limited bile salt pool in young infants. MCTs can be absorbed directly through the basolateral surface of the epithelial cell without the need for bile salts. MCTs, however, cannot be used to prevent essential fatty acid deficiency (all of which are long-chain triglycerides). The carbohydrate is composed of glucose polymers, as well as lactose, to optimize carbohydrate absorption in the presence of limited lactase activity. Premature infants are at increased risk for necrotizing enterocolitis. This risk is not increased with gastrointestinal (GI) priming feeds; however, excessive advancements in the rates of these feedings have been shown to put neonates at increased risk. In general, feeding advancements should not exceed 20 mL/kg/day.[61] Whether feedings are given through a bolus or continuous methods does not appear to influence hospital outcomes or days to reach full feeding.[95,96]

Administration of Enteral Nutrition

For preterm infants, a feeding protocol is typically followed to maintain consistency of practice and reduce the incidence of necrotizing enterocolitis, and these guidelines are now well established.[97,98] For term infants, intermittent enteral feeding can be initiated at 2 to 5 mL/kg every 3 to 4 hours. Feeding is advanced in increments of 2 to 5 mL/kg every two feedings to a goal rate as tolerated. Guidelines have been revamped for safe delivery of enteral nutrition, and are given in Table 12-7 for term and premature infants. Feeding residuals are checked before each intermittent feeding, and enteral nutrition is held if the residual volume is greater than twice the administered volume.

HUMAN MILK

Human milk has a variety of advantages compared with commercial formulas. The American Academy of Pediatrics advocates nursing until 1 year of age; yet, the majority of mothers in the United States stop nursing by the infant's second month of life.[99] Breast-feeding provides both nutrition as well as passive immunologic protection to the neonate. Breast milk contains 87% water and provides 0.64 to 0.67 kcal/mL. The fat content of breast milk is fairly high, at 3.4 g/dL. The protein content of human milk (0.9%) is lower than that of bovine milk or commercial formulas but appears much better absorbed because of the higher amounts of whey content. Casein, which predominates in bovine milk, is a complex of protein and calcium. The whey fraction contains primarily lactalbumin and, as well, lactoferrin, an iron-binding protein that is bacteriostatic to *Staphylococcus aureus* and *Escherichia coli* by restricting iron availability.[100] Additionally, ingestion of human milk allows for the acquisition of passive immunity by the transfer of both immunoglobulins and lymphocytes from the mother.[101] Breast milk also contains elevated levels of cysteine, which is potentially essential for a neonate, and taurine, which is needed for bile salt excretion and neurologic and retinal development. Despite similar amounts of trace elements, human milk allows for a more efficient absorption of these elements compared with commercial formulas. The immunologic advantages of breast milk include the transmission of both humoral as well as cellular factors to the neonate.[101] Although human milk has many advantages, high demands for calcium, phosphorus, electrolytes, vitamins, and trace elements cannot be achieved with human milk alone. Because of this, human milk fortifiers (one pack per ounce) should be added to breast milk fed to preterm infants. Supplementation should continue until the child achieves the weight of a term infant. When human milk fortifier is added to human milk, the hang time of the final reconstituted formula is 2 hours. Because of reports of vitamin D deficiency and rickets in breast-fed infants, the American Academy of Pediatrics recommends beginning, within the first few days of life, a daily supplementation of vitamin D 400 IU to all breast-fed and non–breast-fed infants who do not receive at least 1000 mL of daily vitamin D-fortified formula or milk.[102]

COMPLICATIONS OF ENTERAL FEEDING

The gastrointestinal tract generally tolerates feedings quite well once the postoperative ileus has resolved. Not uncommonly, the critically ill child will sustain a loss of a significant portion of the absorptive function, often because of a lactase deficiency. Symptoms are generally manifested by cramping, diarrhea, or emesis. Symptoms will often improve with the initiation of a lactose-free diet. Enteral nutrition is the preferred route of feeding when oral nutrition is not possible or adequate. In the critically ill child, frequent interruptions of enteral feeding for procedures, feeding intolerances, fluid restriction, or gastrointestinal dysmotility result in suboptimal enteral nutrition delivery.[103,104] The gastrointestinal tract generally tolerates increased volume more readily than increased osmolarity. Therefore in situations of gastrointestinal dysfunction, such adverse symptoms can be avoided by initiating ¼-strength formula and slowly advancing the formula concentration. Second, administration of formula by continuous drip may be better tolerated than bolus feedings. The risk of gastroesophageal reflux and dumping symptoms are thereby greatly reduced. Aspiration is a major risk of enteral feedings. Rapid-bolus nasogastric feedings may lead to a high incidence of reflux. Complications can be decreased with the use of a slow, continuous infusion or, preferably, with jejunal feedings.[105] However, this latter method has become controversial. Although patients with delayed gastric emptying (e.g., infants with sepsis, recent trauma, electrolyte imbalance, or receipt of opiates) or those who are comatose may be at risk for aspiration; in stable patients, a continuous infusion through a nasogastric tube is associated with no higher incidence of aspiration than is infusion through a nasoduodenal tube.[106] When the patient's clinical condition allows, raising the backrest or the head of the bed to 30 to 45 degrees during continuous feeding decreases the risk of aspiration.[107] Third, care must be taken to ensure that the enteral formula does not become contaminated, either during preparation or at the bedside. Expiration times should be observed. Finally, pectin, Metamucil, Lomotil, paregoric, or Imodium may be required for those who have lost a significant amount of their bowel length (see Short-Bowel Syndrome section). Assessment of adequate absorption can be carried out most readily by the testing of the stool for the absorption of carbohydrates, by measuring stool pH, and detecting for reducing substances. The presence of a stool pH less than 5.5 or a reducing substance of greater than one-half percent indicates the passage of unabsorbed carbohydrates into the stool, and once detected, should lead to a decrease in the formula concentration of carbohydrate.

Parenteral Nutrition

Parenteral nutrition (PN) is the intravenous administration of balanced and complete nutrition to support anabolism, prevent weight loss, or promote weight gain. Because acute illness causes mobilization of energy and protein stores, appropriate and timely nutrition should be provided to prevent malnutrition and promote speedy recovery.[108] PN is indicated when oral or enteral feeding is not possible, or as a supplemental nutrition when enteral feeding fails to meet nutritional needs. PN should be used for the shortest time possible, and oral or enteral feeding should be initiated as soon as clinically feasible. Although enteral feeding can prevent gut atrophy and reduce the risk of PN-associated hepatobiliary complications,[109–111] a recent meta-analysis showed that the incidence of complications resulting from enteral and parenteral nutrition are essentially the same.[112]

INDICATIONS FOR PARENTERAL NUTRITION

Parenteral nutrition is ideal for maintaining nutrition in infants and children who are unable to tolerate enteral feedings. Clinical conditions in children likely requiring PN include gastrointestinal disorders (short-bowel syndrome, malabsorption, intractable diarrhea, bowel obstruction, protracted vomiting, inflammatory bowel disease, enterocutaneous fistulas), congenital anomalies (gastroschisis, bowel atresia, volvulus, meconium ileus), radiation therapy to the gastrointestinal tract, chemotherapy resulting in gastrointestinal dysfunction, and severe respiratory distress syndrome in premature infants. Very-low-birth-weight infants are generally intolerant of enteral feeding and require PN during the first 24 hours following birth. Signs of starvation may be seen in underfed premature infants in as soon as 1 to 2 days. Although older children and adults generally do not require PN unless periods of starvation extend beyond 7 to 10 days, young infants require PN if periods of starvation extend beyond 4 to 5 days.

Protein and calories are essential for growth but must be provided in appropriate proportions for their optimal utilization. Very-low-birth-weight infants are born with limited nutritional reserves, loose protein in desquamated epidermal cells and urine, and quickly use their somatic protein reserves for energy if inadequate nutrition is provided early after birth. Providing early nutrition within 24 hours after birth is essential for the transition from fetal to extrauterine life to prevent growth failure and neurodevelopmental delays. Therefore prompt initiation of PN within a few hours after birth is essential. Further, because very-low-birth-weight infants have shown decreased plasma amino acid levels following birth, protein intake at about 3.8 to 4.0 g/kg/day improves nitrogen retention and stimulates weight gain.[113,114]

VENOUS ACCESS

The type of venous access varies depending on the nutritional needs of the patient. Although peripheral PN may be used for a limited number of days, the high risk of using peripheral veins is extravasation of the solution with a subsequent inflammatory response and potential skin necrosis. Since the mid-1990s, a percutaneous intravenous catheter (or PIC-line) has been used. These catheters are relatively small in diameter (2-Fr or 22-gauge). They are placed through the child's peripheral veins, in the upper or lower limbs, and passed into the central venous system. These catheters are extremely well tolerated in adults and children; they can often be maintained for several weeks with reasonably low infection rates.[115,116] Unlike the placement of a Broviac-type catheter, which requires local or general anesthesia, PIC-lines can generally be placed in the neonatal intensive care unit (NICU) with minimal sedation. Another advantage of these catheters is avoidance of pneumothorax, because access is through the extremities rather than the chest. The cost of the peripheral access devices is considerably less than that of Broviac-type catheters; however, PIC-lines have similar or higher incidences of venous thrombosis, and comparable rates of infection and complications.[117]

For infants and children who require longer durations of infusion, central venous PN may be administered through a tunneled Silastic catheter (e.g., Broviac, 2.7- or 4.0-Fr). Such a catheter often has a woven Dacron cuff. Although the tunneling of the catheter and cuff has not been shown to reduce catheter sepsis, the use of a cuff can prevent accidental dislodgement.[118] The catheter may be placed into the superior or inferior vena cava. The ideal position for the tip of the catheter is the junction of the right atrium and the superior vena cava. The child's facial, external jugular, subclavian, or saphenous veins are ideal locations for access. In children who weigh less than 750 g, the internal jugular or femoral vein may need to be used because of the small caliber of other vessels.

PARENTERAL NUTRITION: COMPOSITION AND REQUIREMENTS

Parenteral nutrition is a source of macronutrients (amino acids, dextrose, lipid emulsions), micronutrients (multivitamins, trace minerals), fluids, and electrolytes.

Amino Acids

Pediatric parenteral crystalline amino acid formulas provide essential and nonessential amino acids specifically balanced to meet the needs of the developing child. Neonatal-specific amino acid formulas are formulated to closely reproduce the plasma amino acid profile of breast-fed infants. These formulas have led to greater weight gain and improved nitrogen balance in infants compared with standard amino acid formulas.[119] Some amino acids, such as cysteine, tyrosine, glycine, and taurine, are considered conditionally essential for the child. Taurine supplementation for premature infants is essential to promote bile acid conjugation and to improve bile flow[120] and has been shown to decrease the degree of PN-associated cholestasis.[40] Premature infants are at risk for taurine deficiency as a result of elevated renal taurine losses and their low capacity for taurine synthesis resulting from low cystathionase enzyme activity.[49,121] Amino acids are a source of energy (4 kcal/g) and nitrogen for protein synthesis. Parenteral amino acids should provide approximately 10% to 15% of total calories. Amino acids are started at 1 g/kg/day and advanced to goal over 2 to 3 days. To simulate intrauterine protein accretion rates, low-birth-weight infants may need up to 3.85 g/kg/day of amino acids.[46,122] Amino acid requirements are 2.5 to 3 g/kg/day in term infants, 1.5 to 2 g/kg/day in older children, and 1 to 1.5 g/kg/day in adolescents. Amino acid doses should be adjusted based on the patient's clinical condition and nutritional status. For example, higher amino acid doses are required for wound healing. Patients with liver failure and hyperammonemia require lower amino acid doses. Higher amino acid doses are required in patients

treated with dialysis or continuous renal replacement therapies to make up for losses through the dialysis membrane and filter.[123,124]

Dextrose

Hydrous dextrose is the major source of energy and provides carbon skeletons for tissue accretion. Dextrose also acts as a protein-sparing substrate by preventing breakdown of somatic protein stores by suppression of gluconeogenesis.[125] In most children and adolescents receiving PN, parenteral dextrose usually provides 50% to 60% of total calories. The caloric value of hydrous dextrose is 3.4 kcal/g. In infants, PN should be initiated at a dextrose infusion rate of 4 to 8 mg/kg/min to maintain adequate serum glucose concentrations. Lower amounts of glucose in a young neonate will lead to hypoglycemia because of inadequate hepatic production of glucose. Dextrose infusion is thereafter advanced at a daily rate of 2 mg/kg/min until the nutritional goal is achieved. The maximum dextrose infusion rate should not exceed 10 to 14 mg/kg/min, which can usually be achieved when PN is administered through a central venous catheter.[126,127] Premature infants with hypoglycemia or failure to thrive may require higher dextrose infusion rates up to 20 mg/kg/min to maintain euglycemia and promote adequate growth.

Lipid Emulsions

Intravenous lipid emulsions are a condensed source of energy and essential fatty acids, providing 9 kcal/g of energy. The caloric value of lipid emulsions varies with the lipid emulsion concentration. Lipid emulsions at 10%, 20%, and 30% concentrations yield 1.1 kcal/mL, 2 kcal/mL, and 3 kcal/mL, respectively. Currently marketed intravenous lipid emulsions in the United States are made of long-chain triglycerides (LCT). Lipids usually provide 30% to 50% of the non-nitrogen caloric needs or about 20% to 30% of total calories. Typically, lipid emulsions in infants and children are initiated at a dose of 1 g/kg/day and advanced by 1 g/kg/day to a maximum of 3 g/kg/day. Gradually increasing the daily lipid intake (0.5 or 1 g/kg/day) does not seem to improve lipid clearance. However, the lipid emulsion is cleared better[128,129] and lipid utilization is improved[130] when lipid is infused continuously over 24 hours rather than intermittently or for part of the day. Keeping the intravenous lipid infusion rate below 0.12 g/kg/hour improves lipid clearance.

There are also differences between the clearances of lipid emulsions. The 20% lipid emulsion is favored rather than the 10% emulsion because of its better clearance as a result of its lower phospholipid content.[131,132] Because lipid emulsions are derived from vegetable oils, they are also a natural source of variable amounts of vitamin K[133] and vitamin E isomers.[134,135]

Multivitamins

Pediatric parenteral multivitamins contain a combination of water-soluble and fat-soluble vitamins that are added to the daily PN (Table 12-8). Several pediatric multivitamin formulas are available in the United States. No parenteral multivitamin products are currently available to specifically meet the needs of premature infants. Pediatric parenteral multivitamins provide low vitamin A and high water-soluble vitamins to premature infants. Higher vitamin A intake may be essential in

TABLE 12-8

Pediatric Intravenous Multivitamin Formulation and Requirements for Infants and Children Up to 11 Years of Age

Vitamin	Composition (per 5 mL)
Fat-Soluble Vitamins	
Vitamin A	2300 IU
Vitamin D	400 IU
Vitamin E	7 IU
Vitamin K	200 μ
Water-Soluble Vitamins	
Thiamine (B_1)	1.2 mg
Riboflavin (B_2)	1.4 mg
Niacin (B_3)	17 mg
Pantothenic acid (B_5)	5 mg
Pyridoxine (B_6)	1 mg
Cyanocobalamin (B_{12})	1 μ
Biotin (H)	20 μ
Folate	140 μ
Ascorbic acid (C)	80 mg
Dose	<1 kg: 1.5 mL/day; 1 to <3 kg: 3.25 mL/day; >3 kg: 5 mL/day

Mirtallo J, Canada T, Johnson D: Task Force for the Revision of Safe Practices for Parenteral Nutrition. Safe practices for parenteral nutrition. JPEN J Parenter Enteral Nutr 2004;28:S39-S70.

TABLE 12-9

Daily Electrolyte and Mineral Requirements for Pediatric Patients*

Electrolyte	Preterm Neonates	Infants/ Children	Adolescents and Children >50 kg
Sodium	2-5 mEq/kg	2-5 mEq/kg	1-2 mEq/kg
Potassium	2-4 mEq/kg	2-4 mEq/kg	1-2 mEq/kg
Calcium	2-4 mEq/kg	0.5-4 mEq/kg	10-20 mEq
Phosphorus	1-2 mmol/kg	0.5-2 mmol/kg	10-40 mmol
Magnesium	0.3-0.5 mEq/kg	0.3-0.5 mEq/kg	10-30 mEq
Acetate	As needed to maintain acid-base balance		
Chloride	As needed to maintain acid-base balance		

*Assumes normal age-related organ function and normal losses.
Mirtallo J, Canada T, Johnson D: Task Force for the Revision of Safe Practices for Parenteral Nutrition. Safe practices for parenteral nutrition. JPEN J Parenter Enteral Nutr 2004;28:S39-S70.

low-birth-weight infants who are at increased risk for lung disease.[136] Depletion of water-soluble vitamins occurs rapidly under stressful conditions. Thiamine is a cofactor for normal dextrose metabolism. Dextrose is normally metabolized to pyruvate, which is then converted to acetyl coenzyme A, which undergoes oxidation through the citric acid cycle. If thiamine deficiency occurs, pyruvate is instead converted to lactate, which can result in lactic acidosis.[137] Lactic acidosis has been reported in patients who received dextrose infusions without thiamine supplementation,[138,139] and fatalities from lactic acidosis resulting from thiamine deficiency were also reported during periodic multivitamin shortages in the United States.

Trace Elements

Standard pediatric trace mineral formulas contain zinc, copper, manganese, and chromium, and some formulas have added selenium. Trace element formulas are designed to meet the recommendations of the American Gastroenterological Association (AGA)-AMA and the Society of Clinical Nutrition for daily intravenous supplements of trace minerals in the absence of deficiencies.[65] The Safe Practice Guidelines by the American Society for Parenteral and Enteral Nutrition (ASPEN) recently issued different guidelines with lower daily parenteral trace element requirements and supplementation (see Table 12-4).[140] Trace element status varies with the patient's underlying clinical conditions, and are mentioned in a preceding section of this chapter. Whenever trace elements are restricted or supplemental doses are given, blood trace element concentrations should be periodically measured to avoid deficiencies or toxicities.

Fluids and Electrolytes

A parenteral nutrition solution should be not be used to manage acute fluid and electrolyte losses. Instead, patients should receive a separate intravenous solution for fluid and electrolyte supplementation (Table 12-9). In the home setting, fluid and electrolyte requirements are incorporated into the PN admixture for convenience of administration. Maintenance fluid and electrolyte requirements in children are shown in the respective chapters. Electrolyte adjustments in PN are based on serum electrolyte concentrations. Adjustments should account for all electrolyte sources and losses, acid-base status, clinical conditions, and medications that affect electrolyte balance.

Sodium   Sodium can be provided in PN solutions in the form of chloride, acetate, or phosphate salts. Neonates and especially premature infants develop a natruresis during the first 1 to 2 weeks following birth, resulting from their immature kidney function. Because adequate sodium intake is essential for protein synthesis and tissue development, adequate sodium supplementation is necessary and is guided by serum and urine sodium levels.[141] Premature infants may require as much as 8 mEq/kg/day of sodium, and this decreases with age such that in older children needs range from 1 to 2 mEq/kg/day. Maximum sodium concentration in PN solutions should not exceed normal saline solution equivalent (154 mEq of sodium/L).

Potassium   Potassium can be provided in PN solutions in the form of chloride, acetate, or phosphate salts. Higher potassium requirements are needed during anabolism[142] and to correct any gastrointestinal or renal potassium losses. Potassium concentrations in the PN solution should not exceed 120 mEq/L, and potassium infusion rates in infants and children should not exceed 0.5 mEq/kg/hour[143]; in adolescents dosage should be at 0.7 mEq/kg/hour. With higher potassium infusion rates, the patient should be placed in the intensive care unit on a cardiac monitor.

Chloride and Acetate   The chloride to acetate ratio in the PN solution can be adjusted based on the patient's acid-base status. Acetate is converted in vivo to bicarbonate at a 1:1 molar ratio. A high acetate-to-low chloride ratio is indicated to help correct the metabolic acidosis, such as resulting from lower intestinal bicarbonate losses. High acetate may also be used to help a child compensate for a respiratory acidosis. Premature infants are especially at risk for acid-base changes because of their inadequate response resulting from inefficient hydrogen ion excretion and bicarbonate reabsorption by the kidneys.[141,144] A low acetate-to-high chloride ratio minimizes the bicarbonate load in patients with metabolic alkalosis such as resulting from excessive gastric fluid and electrolyte losses. Great caution should be used when adjusting the chloride-to-acetate ratio because dramatic acid-base changes may rapidly occur.

Calcium and Phosphate   Calcium and phosphate requirements in infants and children are greater compared with adults because of increased demands for growth. Corticosteroids and loop diuretics that are commonly used in neonatal and pediatric intensive care patients can further increase calcium requirements by increasing calcium losses. Following birth, hypophosphatemia is commonly observed in premature infants, resulting from high urinary phosphate excretion.[145] Because phosphates dissociate into monobasic and dibasic forms, depending on solution pH, they should be dosed in millimoles (mmol) instead of mEq to avoid dosing errors. Calcium and phosphate should be provided in adequate ratio and amounts to optimize bone mineralization and prevent metabolic bone disease.[146] Bone mineralization is optimized at an intake ratio of 2.6 mEq of calcium:1 mmol of phosphorus (1.7 mg calcium:1 mg phosphorus).[147] Inadequate calcium and phosphorus supplementation is problematic because of a solubility limitation. As such, enteral calcium and phosphorus supplementation may be required. Also, cysteine hydrochloride, an acidic compound that can be added to the PN solution, can be used to lower the solution pH and allow higher calcium and phosphate amounts in PN. An acidic medium favors the formation of monovalent phosphates instead of the divalent phosphates that otherwise would bind to calcium. Cysteine hydrochloride is added to the neonatal PN solution at a dose of 40 mg/g of amino acids.[148] Calcium and phosphorus can safely be added to PN when the concentrations provided satisfy the following equation:

$$\text{Calcium (mEq)} + \text{Phosphorus (mmol)}$$
$$< 30 \text{ (per 1000 mL of PN)}$$

Because of these solubility issues, the full needs for optimal tissue and bone growth may not be met unless calcium and phosphorus are also provided enterally.

ADDITIVES TO PARENTERAL NUTRITION

Heparin

The addition of heparin to the PN solution at a concentration of 0.5 to 1 units/mL[149] maintains the patency of the venous catheter,[150] and reduces vein irritation.[151] Further, heparin is a cofactor of lipoprotein lipase, an enzyme released from the vascular endothelium, which enhances the clearance of lipid particles and thus enhances lipid clearance.[152] Heparin should not be used in patients with bleeding or at risk for bleeding, or in patients with thrombocytopenia.

Histamine-2 Receptor Antagonists

Histamine-2 receptor antagonists, such as ranitidine, famotidine, and cimetidine, are compatible with PN and may be added to the PN solution for stress ulcer prophylaxis or to decrease gastric secretions.

Regular Insulin

Regular insulin is compatible with the PN solution. However, insulin therapy is difficult to regulate in infants, and intravenous insulin should be administered as a separate intravenous infusion to allow safe titration of the insulin dose.

Iron Dextran

Iron deficiency anemia may occur in PN-dependent patients. Iron is not routinely added to PN. Iron dextran is the most common parenteral iron available for use when oral iron absorption is unreliable or results in gastrointestinal intolerance and is the only parenteral iron formulation that can be added to PN solutions. Because iron can be used as a substrate for bacterial proliferation, iron dextran should be avoided in infected patients. Because severe anaphylactic side effects may occur with iron dextran, an intravenous test dose must be first administered before the total dose is given. Although not recommend by manufacturers, its use during the first 4 months of life has been safely done by many qualified groups. Daily iron dextran doses up to 1 mg/kg have been added to neonatal PN to prevent iron deficiency anemia. Iron replacement calculations can be found in Table 12-10. The estimated total iron dextran dose can be equally divided into incremental doses and added to the daily supply of non–lipid-containing PN solution until the total replacement dosage is given. Iron dextran at therapeutic doses is incompatible with lipid emulsions.[153] Other potentially safer intravenous iron preparations are iron sucrose and sodium ferric gluconate; however, a test dose of these other iron preparations must also be given to determine the potential for an adverse reaction. Their use has been predominately in renal failure patients but also appears effective in children.[154]

Carnitine

Carnitine is a quaternary amine required for the transport of long-chain fatty acids into the mitochondria, where they undergo oxidation.[155] Premature infants are at risk for carnitine deficiency because of their limited carnitine reserves and reduced ability for carnitine synthesis.[156] Reduced fatty acid oxidation and elevated serum triglyceride concentrations have been correlated with low plasma carnitine concentrations.[157] Although many enteral formulations contain carnitine, PN solutions are carnitine-free. Supplementation of L-carnitine to PN normalized plasma carnitine concentrations[158] and improved fatty acid oxidation. Premature infants who develop

TABLE 12-10
Intravenous Iron Replacement Therapy
Calculation for Total Iron Replacement Dose
mL of iron dextran = 0.0476 × weight (kg) × (Hb$_n$ − Hb$_o$) + 1 mL per 5 kg of body weight (up to a maximum of 14 mL)
1 mL of iron dextran = 50 mg of elemental iron
Hb$_n$ = desired hemoglobin (g/dL). The desired hemoglobin is 12 if patient weighs < 15 kg or 14.8 if patient weighs > 15 kg.
Hb$_o$ = measured hemoglobin (g/dL)
Maximal Daily Iron Replacement Dose
Infants weighing < 5 kg: 25 mg
Children weighing 5-10 kg: 50 mg
Children > 10 kg: 100 mg

unexplained hypertriglyceridemia during lipid infusion may benefit from L-carnitine supplementation at a dose of about 10 mg/kg/day.[159] In neonates, L-carnitine 20 mg/kg/day for 8 weeks resulted in higher-than-normal plasma total carnitine concentrations. Doses of L-carnitine exceeding 20 mg/kg/day in infants are unlikely of clinical benefit. Larger oral L-carnitine doses have caused seizures, diarrhea, nausea, abdominal cramps, and may negatively affect growth by possibly increasing the infant's metabolic rate. Parenteral L-carnitine doses of 48 mg/kg/day in low-birth-weight infants increased protein oxidation, decreased nitrogen balance, and increased the time to regain birth weight.[160]

COMPLICATIONS OF PARENTERAL NUTRITION

Despite more than 40 years of experience with PN, complications continue to be a major obstacle in the care of pediatric patients. Complications of PN can be classified into metabolic, respiratory, hepatobiliary, and infectious.

Metabolic Complications

Hyperglycemia Hyperglycemia in patients receiving PN is primarily the result of excessive dextrose infusion. Factors that exacerbate glucose intolerance include sepsis, surgery, diabetes, pancreatitis, prematurity, and corticosteroid therapy. Elevated blood glucose may coincide with PN initiation, but endogenous insulin secretion usually adjusts within 48 to 72 hours. Untreated hyperglycemia causes osmotic diuresis that can lead to hyperosmolar, hyperglycemic, nonketotic dehydration with electrolyte disturbances,[127] impaired phagocytosis,[161] and liver steatosis.[162] Intensive insulin therapy to maintain tight glucose control in critically ill patients has variably affected patient outcomes and was associated with increased incidence of hypoglycemia. Although an earlier study in critically ill surgical adult patients showed decreased patient morbidity and mortality with continuous insulin infusion to maintain blood glucose levels between 80 to 110 mg/dL,[163] a recent large multicenter study reported that a more permissive glycemic target range of 140 to 180 mg/dL is desirable, because tight glycemic control was associated with increased patient mortality.[164] Data in pediatric intensive care unit patients showed that intensive insulin therapy targeting age-adjusted blood glucose levels was associated with decreased inflammatory response, reduced secondary infections, a shorter length of intensive care unit stay, and increased incidence of hypoglycemia.[165] Although uncontrolled hyperglycemia is unacceptable, there is disparity in practice of glycemic control in pediatric intensive care units, and the long-term outcomes and optimal blood glucose targets in these children remain unknown.[166]

The first attempt in managing hyperglycemia is to decrease the dextrose load or reduce the infusion rate. However, this may compromise nutritional intake, because dextrose is the major source of calories in PN. If reducing dextrose does not improve hyperglycemia, insulin therapy is then indicated. Because infants have a variable response to insulin therapy,[167] adding insulin to the PN solution should be avoided. Instead, a regular insulin drip should be initiated and titrated based on serial glucose checks.

Hypoglycemia Hypoglycemia with PN is usually the result of a sudden reduction of the PN infusion rate. In patients who receive PN during a portion of the day ("cycled"), hypoglycemia may be avoided by gradually reducing the rate during the 1 to 2 hours prior to discontinuation. Capillary glucose levels (chemsticks) should be monitored 15 to 60 minutes (typically 30 minutes) after PN is discontinued to check for any reactive hypoglycemia. Premature infants are at very increased risk for hypoglycemia because of their underdeveloped metabolic response[168]; cycling of PN in this group of patients is typically not safely performed until the child is more mature. If PN is unavoidably to be discontinued, intravenous administration of 10% dextrose in water, following PN discontinuation, will prevent symptomatic hypoglycemia.[9] Iatrogenic hypoglycemia can result from insulin therapy. If insulin is added in PN, adjustments to the insulin dose, guided by regular capillary glucose level checks, are necessary when metabolic stress decreases, pancreatitis resolves, or when corticosteroid therapy is tapered or discontinued.

Hypertriglyceridemia High dextrose infusion is the primary cause of hypertriglyceridemia in PN patients. Excessive carbohydrate intake enhances hepatic and adipose tissue lipogenesis.[169] Other factors that predispose to hypertriglyceridemia in pediatric patients receiving PN include prematurity,[170] lipid overfeeding,[171,172] critical illness, and sepsis.[173] Although the tendency would be to reduce lipid infusion, a reduction in dextrose would be far more effective. However, the dextrose infusion rate should not be decreased to less than 4 mg/kg/minute in infants, a minimum rate required for protein-sparing effect. If hypertriglyceridemia persists despite reducing glucose intake, the lipid emulsion dose and rate should be decreased to keep triglyceride levels less than 275 mg/dL. A lipid dose of 0.5 to 1 g/kg/day in children would prevent essential fatty acid deficiency. If the 10% lipid emulsion is used, switching to the 20% lipid emulsion is recommended because of its better clearance.[174] Carnitine deficiency should be ruled out, especially in premature infants and those with renal insufficiency, because it may also be a cause of hypertriglyceridemia (see previous).

Metabolic Acidosis Metabolic acidosis may result from excessive chloride (hyperchloremic acidosis may occur with serum chloride levels >130 mEq/L) or high amino acid load in PN. The addition of cysteine hydrochloride to the PN solution to improve calcium and phosphate solubility may also cause acidemia,[48] which may also lead to just the opposite effect—a leaching of calcium from the infant's bones. Premature infants and patients with liver or renal disease are at increased risk for metabolic acidosis and should be closely monitored for acid-base changes.

Electrolyte Disturbances Hypokalemia, hypomagnesemia, and hypophosphatemia may result from increased requirements during anabolism and protein synthesis (refeeding syndrome), which is particularly common in the severely malnourished patient. Slow advancement of feeding with electrolyte repletion is recommended.[142] Phosphate is required intracellularly for generation of high-energy phosphate bonds and bone formation, and intracellular shift of phosphate occurs with carbohydrate infusion.[175] Severe hypophosphatemia may lead to hypoventilation, neurologic and cardiac disturbances, and coma.[176] Apparent hypocalcemia in malnourished patients is often secondary to a reduced serum albumin concentration with proportionally low total serum calcium. Hyperkalemia, hypermagnesemia, and hyperphosphatemia may result from increased intake in combination with decreased renal function and hypercatabolism.

Metabolic Bone Disease   Metabolic bone disease, including osteopenia, osteomalacia, and rickets, is a complication in PN-dependent patients. Diagnosis is often difficult and may not be evident until a pathologic fracture is observed. Biochemical markers may reveal elevated serum alkaline phosphatase concentrations, hypercalciuria, low to normal plasma parathyroid hormone (PTH), and low 1,25 dihydroxyvitamin D.[177,178] Several factors predispose to PN-associated metabolic bone disease, including calcium and phosphorus deficiency, excessive losses of calcium resulting from diuretics, excessive vitamin D intake,[179] and aluminum toxicity.[180] Maximizing calcium and phosphorus intake is most important to improve bone mineralization. Calcium deficit is the result of limitations on the amount of calcium supplementation and the resultant hypercalciuria from amino acids,[181] with secondary metabolic acidosis.[182] Aluminum, a contaminant of the PN solution, is another possible cause of metabolic bone disease. Aluminum causes bone remodeling by impairing calcium fixation in bones,[183] impairing PTH secretion, or reducing the formation of active vitamin D.[184] Premature infants and patients with renal failure are at highest risk for aluminum toxicity resulting from their reduced ability for aluminum elimination. Additional vitamin D administration may actually be dangerous, because vitamin D may also play a role in the pathogenesis of metabolic bone disease; however, the exact mechanism is unknown. Withdrawing vitamin D from these patients leads to improvement in bone demineralization, resolution of bone pain, positive calcium balance,[179] and normalization of plasma active vitamin D and PTH concentrations.[185]

Hepatobiliary Complications

Hepatobiliary complications associated with PN include cholestasis, steatosis, and cholelithiasis. Multiple factors may predispose to PN-associated hepatobiliary complications, including prematurity, overfeeding, PN dependence, absence of enteral stimulation for gall bladder contraction, short-bowel syndrome, and recurrent sepsis.[186,187] Cholestasis is the most common hepatobiliary complication in children receiving PN. Jaundice may occur as early as 2 to 3 weeks after PN initiation. A serum conjugated bilirubin concentration greater than or equal to 2 mg/dL is commonly used as a biochemical marker of cholestasis.[187] A rapid rise in direct bilirubin is a strong predictor of impending hepatic failure. Use of a taurine-supplemented PN solution has been shown to decrease the degree of cholestasis in premature infants and those with necrotizing enterocolitis.[40] In infants with short-bowel syndrome, a direct bilirubin greater than 2.5 mg/dL for more than 4 months was associated with an 80% mortality[189] and suggests a potential criteria for referring patients for transplant evaluation.[190] Strategies to prevent or reduce PN-associated liver disease (PNALD) include initiation of enteral feeding, weaning PN, avoiding overfeeding,[191] balancing calories,[192] "cycling" PN,[193,194] and avoiding and promptly treating sepsis.[192] Pharmacologic interventions include improving bile flow with the administration of bile acids or use of cholecystokinin, both have been studied in controlled

prospective trials without any proven benefit.[195,196] Oral antibiotics, such as oral gentamicin and metronidazole have been used to decrease intestinal bacterial overgrowth and reduce bacterial translocation.[197] During the past decade, it has become apparent that soybean-based intravenous fat emulsions are a causative agent of PNALD. Strategies to either reduce the amount of these fats[198] or replace them with a fish-oil–based intravenous fat[199–201] have proven successful in reversing PNALD, thus making soybean fats a potential contributing factor to this disease process.

Infectious Complications

Sepsis is one of the most frequent and serious complications of centrally infused PN in infants and children.[202] Fever and sudden glucose intolerance are suggestive of sepsis. Persistent hyperglycemia has been shown to increase infection rates, and intensive control is recommended.[203] Microbial culturing of PN should be performed if PN is suspected as a source of microbial contamination, though this is a rare occurrence with the use of strict sterile compounding techniques. Catheter-related infections remain the main cause of sepsis in patients receiving PN. Although not specific for children, guidelines for the diagnosis and treatment of central venous access infections have recently been established by the Infectious Disease Society of America[204] and the European Society of Parenteral and Enteral Nutrition.[205] Microorganisms may enter the bloodstream (1) along the catheter tract, starting at the skin exit site; (2) through a contaminated intravenous solution; (3) by breaks in sterility at the catheter hub–blood drawing or cleaning intravenous tubing; or (4) from a distant septic site or the GI tract. The catheter in this case, acts as a foreign body focus for bacterial growth. The most important factors in reducing the incidence of septic complications are placement of catheters under strict aseptic conditions and meticulous care of the catheter sites. Factors that correlate with catheter-related infections include prolonged catheterization, use of the catheter for multiple purposes, manipulation of the catheter hub, and chronic PN therapy. Most series report an incidence of 0.5 to 2.0 infections per 1000 catheters-days for a nonimmunosuppressed patient with a central venous catheter.[206,207] For immunosuppressed patients (e.g., hematology or oncology patients), a rate of 2 to 3 infections per 1000 catheter-days is generally reported.[208,209] A considerably higher rate of infection is found in children with the short-bowel syndrome; this rate ranges from 7 to 9 infections per 1000 catheter-days.[210–213] Several measures have proven effective in preventing catheter-related infections, including the use of sterile barriers and topical disinfectants during catheter insertion, use of antimicrobial-coated catheters, and regular catheter flushing. Although some individual studies have shown benefit with chlorhexidine-impregnated catheters, a recent review found no benefit but did suggest beneficial reduction of infections when catheters were either heparin-coated or antibiotic-impregnated.[214] Use of chlorhexidine-impregnated dressings has been shown to reduce pediatric catheter infections.[215] Guidelines for the prevention and management of catheter-related infections have been published elsewhere.[216,217] In general, nonpermanent polyvinyl chloride lines should be removed with catheter sepsis; however, more than 80% of patients with a Silastic catheter (e.g., Broviac or Hickman) will be able to have the infection cleared with intravenous antibiotics. Another technique to treat such infections is the antibiotic-lock technique. This technique allows delivery of markedly higher doses of antibiotics into the catheter with allowance of the antibiotic to remain in the lumen while it is not in use.[218,219] This allows use of antibiotics that would normally have such high minimal inhibitory concentrations (MIC) that systemic use would result in renal failure (e.g., nafcillin for a staphylococcal line infection). Antibiotic lock methods are used routinely in some centers but are probably most useful in patients who may not tolerate an aminoglycoside or vancomycin. Because of this problem, as well as the risk of developing resistant organisms in the patient, ethanol-lock therapy has become commonly used to both treat as well as prevent the development of pediatric central venous-line infections.[220–222] Overall, the use of ethanol lock can reduce infections by almost 10-fold. However, complications may occur because of the risk of precipitation of heparin or citrate with ethanol, which requires that these two agents *not* be used when patients are receiving ethanol lock.[221] Additionally, ethanol may weaken plastics in the catheter and should *not* be used if the device is composed of polyurethane.[223] Because of the high failure rate of antibiotics, most patients with a *track* infection should have the line removed. Most children with fungal infections should also have the catheter removed, because of reports of fatalities and high failure rates with attempts at trying to salvage the line with antifungal therapy.[224] Attempting to maintain a catheter with a *Candida* infection is associated with a mortality of up to 25% and the low chance of clearing the infection with the line in place (13%).[225] Only a relatively short course of antifungal agents needs to be given after the catheter is removed (7 to 14 days); however, the results of blood cultures must be negative.[226] For unusual cases in which central venous access has been lost because of previous placement of several catheters, a trial of antifungal agents with the line in place may be attempted. An uncommon fungal organism associated with PN is *Malassezia furfur*. This organism thrives in a lipid-rich environment, but as long as lipids are withheld, it generally responds to antifungal treatment without catheter removal.

Complications from Overfeeding

Overfeeding can lead to a number of adverse consequences. The administration of excessive dextrose may lead to osmotic diuresis and subsequent dehydration resulting from serum glucose levels exceeding renal tubular reabsorption threshold. Immunologic suppression has also been associated with overfeeding and is believed to be due to an inactivation of the complement system, as well as a depression of natural killer activation (see previous section on hyperglycemia). Overfeeding may also adversely affect the liver, because excessive glucose, which is not oxidized, is converted into fat (lipogenesis). These changes may lead to elevated serum triglyceride levels and hepatic steatosis that may be injurious to the liver. Additionally, overfeeding from carbohydrates associated with lipogenesis will lead to high carbon dioxide production, as reflected by an elevated respiratory quotient (RQ).[227] A RQ value exceeding 1 may represent overfeeding, and this high level may exacerbate ventilatory impairment in a critically ill child, because it represents excessive carbon dioxide production. Overfeeding should be avoided and caloric needs are best assessed in the critically ill child using indirect calorimetry. Overfeeding critically ill patients may also lead to fluid retention that may further compromise respiratory function.

Technical Complications

In recent years, the incidence of technical complications caused by the placement of central venous lines in infants and children has been greatly reduced by careful attention to technique and by radiologic confirmation of catheter position. The incidence of cardiac arrhythmias caused by catheter irritation has been greatly reduced by placing the tip of the catheter at the junction of the superior vena cava and right atrium. Another important point is to ensure that a subclavian catheter is not inserted too medially, because this could lead to a pinching of the catheter between the first rib and clavicle, with the potential shearing off of the distal catheter into the heart.[228] Even with the proper positioning of a silicone catheter, thrombosis of the vein in which the catheter resides can occur, especially in the critically ill patient with sepsis and reduced circulation. Thrombosis of the great vessels will require anticoagulation and catheter removal. Pulmonary embolism and infection of these thrombi have been reported in infants and small children.[229] Thrombolytic therapy has proven effective in clearing the catheter of clots and avoiding the need for catheter replacement.[230] This procedure may be repeated at least twice to ensure removal of thrombus. Patients with long-term indwelling lines may have occlusion from either lipids or calcium deposits. These patients should also receive a trial of ethanol and dilute hydrochloric acid.[231] Since 1996, use of percutaneous intravenous central catheters (PICCs) has become the dominant mode of PN delivery in the United States.[232] This mode of insertion has the advantage of avoiding many of the complications associated with central venous catheters and can be often easily inserted on the floor with little or no sedation[233,234]; however, thrombotic events are more frequent than with centrally placed catheters. A reduction in these thrombotic events is seen if the catheters are placed in a central position, rather than in the juncture of the periphery and central venous system.

ADMINISTRATION OF PARENTERAL NUTRITION

Neonates are generally started on PN within the first 12 hours after birth; and many centers now stock a pre-made 10% dextrose (D10%) solution for such use in their units. Neonates tend to be somewhat intolerant of large amounts of dextrose or amino acids for the first 2 to 3 days of life. Dextrose solution concentrations are generally initiated at 10% to 12.5%, and the concentration is slowly increased on a daily basis to between 20% and 25%. Monitoring of the patient's glucose levels and electrolyte balance and checking for glucosuria will confirm whether the child can tolerate this level of dextrose administration. PN may be administered through a peripheral or central venous catheter. The risk of developing phlebitis in peripheral veins is greater when the PN solution osmolarity exceeds 600 to 900 mOsm/L.[235] Intravenous solutions with higher osmolarities must be infused through a central vein. The maximum dextrose concentration in peripherally infused solutions in infants and children is 12.5%. Because lipid emulsions are isotonic solutions, coinfusion of lipids with peripheral PN protects the veins and prolongs the viability of peripheral intravenous catheters.[236] Because calcium phosphate precipitates are potentially life threatening in PN solutions, the Food and Drug Administration has recommended that PN solutions be infused through an inline filter. A 0.22-μ filter is used for non–lipid-containing PN solutions, whereas a 1.2-μ filter is used for total nutrient admixtures to allow lipid particles (0.5μ in diameter) to pass through the filter. PN should be initiated as a continuous infusion spanning 24 hours. For patients receiving long-term PN, delivery may be given spanning a shortened period of time (e.g., 16 hours).

Importantly, to avoid hypoglycemia or hyperglycemia, the rate of infusion needs to be reduced by half for 1 to 2 hours before terminating or starting up infusion each day. Additionally, neonates, particularly premature infants, have limited glycogen reserves and generally do not tolerate cycling of PN. A suggested guideline for writing orders for neonatal PN is given in Figure 12-1. Adequate maintenance of catheters and

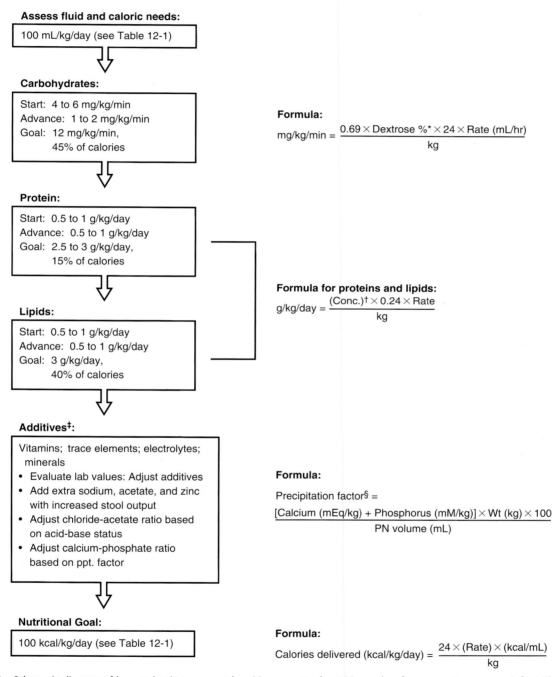

Assess fluid and caloric needs:

100 mL/kg/day (see Table 12-1)

Carbohydrates:

Start: 4 to 6 mg/kg/min
Advance: 1 to 2 mg/kg/min
Goal: 12 mg/kg/min,
45% of calories

Formula:

$$mg/kg/min = \frac{0.69 \times Dextrose\ \%^* \times 24 \times Rate\ (mL/hr)}{kg}$$

Protein:

Start: 0.5 to 1 g/kg/day
Advance: 0.5 to 1 g/kg/day
Goal: 2.5 to 3 g/kg/day,
15% of calories

Formula for proteins and lipids:

$$g/kg/day = \frac{(Conc.)^\dagger \times 0.24 \times Rate}{kg}$$

Lipids:

Start: 0.5 to 1 g/kg/day
Advance: 0.5 to 1 g/kg/day
Goal: 3 g/kg/day,
40% of calories

Additives‡:

Vitamins; trace elements; electrolytes; minerals
• Evaluate lab values: Adjust additives
• Add extra sodium, acetate, and zinc with increased stool output
• Adjust chloride-acetate ratio based on acid-base status
• Adjust calcium-phosphate ratio based on ppt. factor

Formula:

Precipitation factor§ =

$$\frac{[Calcium\ (mEq/kg) + Phosphorus\ (mM/kg)] \times Wt\ (kg) \times 100}{PN\ volume\ (mL)}$$

Nutritional Goal:

100 kcal/kg/day (see Table 12-1)

Formula:

$$Calories\ delivered\ (kcal/kg/day) = \frac{24 \times (Rate) \times (kcal/mL)}{kg}$$

FIGURE 12-1 Schematic diagram of how to begin to approach writing parenteral nutrition orders for a neonate or young infant. Fluids should be adjusted based on the infant's gestation age and body weight.
*Dextrose concentration should be used as the percent number (i.e., 20 for 20%). Conc, concentration; PN, parenteral nutrition; ppt, precipitation.
†The concentration in this formula should be written as the percent number (i.e., 4.25 for 4.25%).
‡See relevant tables for each of these additives.
§If the amino acid concentration is greater than 1.5%, the precipitation factor should be less than 3. If the final amino acid concentration is greater than 1% and less than 1.5%, a precipitation factor should be less than 2. Also, for an amino acid concentration less than 1%, calcium and phosphate should not be added. Adjustments to this formulation need to be done if additives (e.g., cysteine) are placed in the parenteral nutrition.

prevention of infection demands meticulous care, because catheters are a common source of sepsis in neonates.[211] Maintenance of all of these catheters requires that the skin site be cleansed with an antiseptic solution and dressed in a dry fashion every other day.[237] Tubing and infusion bags are changed every 72 hours, along with a new inline filter. Tubing used to deliver lipids must be changed every 24 hours.

Monitoring of Laboratory Values

Monitoring of laboratory values is essential, because aberrations in these values are common in pediatric patients, particularly at the initiation of PN. Table 12-11 gives a suggested guide for such monitoring. A complete blood count, glucose, blood urea nitrogen, creatinine, and electrolytes (sodium, potassium, chloride, carbon dioxide) levels should be measured at initiation and on a biweekly basis. Liver function tests (alanine aminotransferase, aspartate aminotransferase, lactate dehydrogenase, alkaline phosphatase, and total direct bilirubin) should be done, and magnesium, albumin, calcium, and phosphorus levels should be checked at initiation and weekly. Triglyceride levels should be maintained until the desired level of fat intake is reached.

TABLE 12-11

Guidelines for Blood Laboratory Monitoring of Nutrition Support in Parenteral Nutrition–Dependent Pediatric Patients

	Initial	Daily	2 to 3 Times/ Week	Weekly	As Indicated
Glucose	X	X	X		
BUN, creatinine	X	X	X		
Sodium, potassium, chloride, carbon dioxide	X	X	X		
AST, ALT, LDH, alkaline phosphatase, total and direct bilirubin, GGTP	X			X	
Magnesium, calcium, phosphorus	X			X	
Albumin, total protein	X			X	
Triglycerides	X*			X	
Hb, Hct, CBC, platelets, PT	X				X
Copper, zinc, selenium, chromium, manganese, iron					X
TIBC, ferritin					X
Vitamin concentrations					X
Chemsticks					X
Ammonia					X
Blood cultures					X

*Measured once goal lipid infusion reached.
ALT, alanine transaminase; AST, aspartate transaminase; BUN, blood urea nitrogen; CBC, complete blood count; GGTP, gamma-glutamyl transpeptidase; Hb, hemoglobin; Hct, hematocrit; LDH, lactate dehydrogenase; PT, prothrombin time; TIBC, total iron-binding capacity.

Special Problems in the Nutritional Support of the Pediatric Surgical Patient

NUTRITION IN THE PEDIATRIC SURGICAL PATIENT

The surgical patient responds to the stress of surgery quite differently than older children or adults.[238] The metabolism of children is markedly affected by operative stress. The time period of increased energy expenditure, however, is much shorter than in adults.[239] Induction of anesthesia has profound effects on body metabolism, with agents such as fentanyl having a beneficial effect in reducing the catabolic effect.[240] Moreover, protein turnover and catabolism seems not to be affected by major operative procedures in neonates. PN, however, in surgical neonates is associated with increased production of oxygen-free radicals, and this may contribute to suppression of the immune status. Thus utilization must be tempered with any potential benefit. A discussion of the use of nutrition support both preoperatively and postoperatively follows.

INDICATIONS FOR PREOPERATIVE NUTRITION

In malnourished adults, provision of enteral feedings preoperatively for 2 to 3 weeks may reduce postoperative wound infections, anastomotic leakage, hepatic and renal failure, and length of hospital stay.[241,242] Data for PN support are less clear. A meta-analysis demonstrated only a marginal benefit of preoperative PN. Little benefit, and possible increase in complications, was noted in mildly or moderately malnourished patients.[243] The most significant benefit has been documented in severely malnourished patients who have developed fewer noninfectious complications if receiving perioperative PN (PN presurgery for 7 to 15 days, and postsurgery for 3 days).[244] However, PN patients were noted to have an increased infection rate that could not totally be explained by the use of central venous catheters. This suggests that the use of PN may actually predispose patients to increased infectious complications. Thus unless there are clear indications of severe malnutrition (see Subjective Global Assessment in the previous section on nutritional assessment), a delay in operative management in order to provide preoperative PN is *not* indicated.[9] An extrapolation of these findings to neonatal patients is difficult because of their limited nutritional stores. However, because of similarities in the metabolic response to surgery, it seems reasonable to apply these same conclusions to the pediatric population.

INDICATIONS FOR POSTOPERATIVE NUTRITION

Use of aggressive postoperative nutritional support is even more controversial. In critically ill adult patients, early enteral nutrition within 24 to 48 hours of admission to the intensive care unit has been shown to reduce infectious complications.[245,246] However, gastrointestinal complications and feeding intolerance can be a considerable limitation to the adequate delivery of enteral nutrition.[247] These data suggest that, when used, postoperative nutrition should be started early, using a combination of PN and EN until the gastrointestinal tract fully recovers. A recent controlled study examining the effect of postoperative PN in children demonstrated a positive effect on nitrogen balance and levels of insulin growth factor-1 (IGF-I); however, no clinical benefit was noted.[248] The effect of PN on postoperative healing has been negligible. In the postoperative period, there are higher infection rates in patients on PN. Meta-analysis studies show that there is an actual adverse effect to postoperative PN.[243] Although prolonged starvation postoperatively places patients at adverse risk,[249] postoperative PN should be restricted to infants who will not tolerate even a short period of starvation or to older children who will probably not start enteral nutrition for at least 5 to 7 days. In well-nourished adolescents, this period of time should increase to 7 to 10 days.[9]

NUTRITIONAL SUPPORT IN THE CRITICALLY ILL SURGICAL PATIENT

Nutritional care of the critically ill or septic postoperative patient represents a much greater challenge. Clinically, a critically ill child manifests poor enteral feeding, anorexia, and often a paralytic ileus. Insulin resistance results in hyperglycemia and hypertriglyceridemia. Control of this hyperglycemia has been shown to have a significantly beneficial effect in preventing sepsis.[203] Visceral protein stores become progressively reduced with time. Although measurements of albumin may change slowly because of its long half-life ($t_{1/2} > 18$ days), other measures of visceral protein status, such as prealbumin levels ($t_{1/2} = 2$ days), will better reflect these metabolic derangements. Estimates of energy needs during this time are important. Energy needs of postoperative or septic critically ill infants have not uncommonly been overestimated. Almost one third of an infant's energy needs is provided to support growth (30 to 35 kcal/kg/day). Because a cessation of growth occurs during periods of sepsis and critical illness, a marked decrease in energy needs may ensue. In a study of critically ill, postoperative infants, the mean measured basal energy expenditure was only 43 kcal/kg/day.[36] However, results are extraordinarily variable, further emphasizing the utility of performing indirect calorimetry. The use of indirect calorimetry can also yield information on the respiratory quotient (see previous) and aid in the prevention of overfeeding. Combined enteral and PN feedings in critically ill adult patients on ventilator support is controversial and may not be recommended.[250] Although not as well studied in neonates, data from meta-analyses in adult patients suggest that PN has little proven benefit to most critically ill surgical patients, and thus supplementation should be used sparingly in the initial few days of support until it is determined that the length of starvation will exceed 5 to 7 days.[251]

BILIARY ATRESIA

The infant with biliary atresia, even after a clinically successful hepatic portoenterostomy, will typically have lower than normal amounts of bile flow into the intestine. This subsequently leads to a profound defect in fat digestion and absorption. Such a deficit may leave the infant with an essential fatty acid deficiency and inadequate absorption of fat-soluble vitamins.[252] Consequently, this will lead to a lack of bone mineralization as well as failure to thrive. The essential goals for such

an infant are to provide adequate calories using a formula that maximizes fat intake. A commonly used formula in these patients is Pregestimil (Mead Johnson & Company, Evansville, Ind.). This formula has a large amount of medium-chain triglycerides and sufficient linoleic acid to prevent fatty acid deficiency in the face of decreased absorption. Use of this formula has been shown to increase growth in such patients.[253] Portagen (Mead Johnson & Company) should not be used in cholestatic infants, because it does not provide sufficient essential fatty acids to prevent deficiency. When PN is needed, a standard crystalline amino acid solution should be used; there is no proven benefit to hepatic formulas. Breast-feeding, although generally ideal in infancy, should be used cautiously in patients with biliary atresia. Breast milk has a much higher fat content than commercially available formulas and may not be well tolerated in these children. Vitamin supplementation is critical in patients with biliary atresia (Table 12-12). Unfortunately, supplemental vitamins are rarely covered by medical insurance payers despite the fact that they are medically necessary. Frequent monitoring of vitamin levels is essential to ensure sufficient supplementation is being achieved. The addition of water-soluble vitamins to levels greater than those provided in standard infant formulas should be carried out by the administration of a multivitamin preparation. Iron, zinc, and calcium deficiencies should be ruled out. From a practical perspective, it may be difficult and expensive to administer so many vitamins to a small infant. Many have used a combination form of fat-soluble vitamins (vitamins A, D, E, and K [ADEK] 0.5 mL/kg); however, vitamin K may be inadequate in this formulation, and additional supplementation (2.5 mg/day) should be given. Vitamin levels should be followed and deficiencies corrected with individual vitamins. Protein metabolism is impaired in children with biliary atresia, increasing from 4% to 9% of energy expenditure in healthy infants to 17% in patients with biliary atresia.[254] Pierro and colleagues[255] have shown that resting energy expenditure was about 29% higher than expected in infants with biliary atresia and that only 35% of the metabolizable energy intake was retained for growth in these children. Optimal growth and nutrition in infants with biliary atresia has recently been associated with improved outcomes and should be a major goal for pediatric surgeons.[256]

TABLE 12-12

Vitamin Therapy in Cholestasis

Name	Dose	Supplied As
Vitamin A	10,000-15,000 IU/day	3-mg tablets
(Aquasol A; Centeon)	(50,000 IU = 15 mg)	3-mg, 7.5-mg, or 15-mg capsules
		50,000 IU/mL drops
Vitamin D: 1,25(OH)$_2$D$_3$	0.01-0.05 μg/kg/day	0.25 and 0.5 μg capsules
(Rolcaltrol; Roche Laboratories)		0.1 μg/mL/liquid
Vitamin E TPGS (Liqui-E; Twinlab)	25 IU/kg/day	26.7 IU/mL liquid
Vitamin K	2.5-5 mg/day	5-mg tablets

SHORT-BOWEL SYNDROME

The nutritional support of a child with the short-bowel syndrome (SBS) is complex and requires a multidisciplinary approach with the pediatric surgeon, pediatric gastroenterologist, pharmacist, and dietitian working together. Although initially the child's main or sole caloric source will be through PN, enteral feedings should be initiated as soon as possible after the onset of the short-bowel syndrome. Enteral feedings will both stimulate small-bowel adaptation and prevent the development of PN-associated cholestasis. The ideal enteral solution should be isotonic. The protein source should be predominately elemental. Dipeptides and tripeptides have often been advocated, because this source of protein is most easily and efficiently absorbed.[257] Although data are limited, others have found better feeding tolerance with the use of an elemental (pure amino acid) enteral nutrition formula.[258] The formula should have at least 50% of medium-chain triglycerides because this type of fat is well absorbed through the basolateral wall of the intestinal enterocytes and into the portal venous circulation. However, medium-chain triglycerides contain no essential fatty acids; thus these fats cannot be the sole source of lipids in these patients, and supplemental long-chain triglycerides should be provided to prevent essential fatty acid deficiency. Tables 12-5 and 12-6 give recommended formulas for children of different ages. Despite the use of these elemental formulas early in the initiation of feedings, more complex diets, particularly human milk, appear to have the greatest benefit in achieving intestinal adaptation, and a modified regular diet should eventually be initiated.[259]

High stool output is associated with excessive losses of zinc, magnesium, sodium, bicarbonate, and potassium.[260] These losses must be monitored. Total-body sodium depletion has been shown to be associated with failure to thrive, despite the administration of adequate amounts of calories.[261] A simple way to detect such a deficit is to measure a spot urine sodium. A urine sodium of less than 10 mEq/L may well indicate total-body sodium depletion, and supplementation (sodium chloride or sodium bicarbonate, as indicated) by the oral route should be given on a daily basis.[262] A major obstacle to feeding advances may be high stool output. The etiology of this high output may include infections, malabsorption, rapid transit, as well as bile acid irritation of the colonic epithelium.[263] The child's stool should intermittently be assessed for infections. Additionally, measurement of stool pH, reducing substances, and qualitative fecal fats should be checked. Stool pH less than 5.5 and an elevated reducing substance level (greater than 0.5%) indicate carbohydrate malabsorption. Formulas with sucrose as the carbohydrate will not yield a positive reducing substance test despite carbohydrate malabsorption. Elevation in fecal fats will suggest fat malabsorption, which may require modification of the child's enteral diet (i.e., increase the percentage of medium-chain triglycerides). An increase in stool alpha-1 antitrypsin would indicate a protein malabsorption, although much less commonly encountered. Use of a resin binder (e.g., cholestyramine) will markedly reduce bile acid irritation and has proven extremely effective in many infants who have their small bowel in continuity with a portion of the colon. However, excessive use of bile acid binders, such as cholestyramine, may result in depletion of the circulating bile acid pool and thereby further limit fatty acid absorption. Because many infants with short-bowel syndrome have dysmotility, it is only after all other etiologies have been eliminated (i.e., infectious, bacterial overgrowth, bile acid irritation, and potentially correctable malabsorption) that an agent to reduce motility (e.g., Imodium) should be considered.

OBESITY

Obesity has become a worldwide issue, with a striking increase in obesity rates being reported in North America as well as Europe and Asia.[264,265] Rates in the United States demonstrate a greater than threefold increase in obesity during the past 30 years. The implications of this rise in obesity are dramatic. First, more than 50% of children who are diagnosed with obesity will carry this excess weight into adulthood. Second, a number of secondary complications have been manifested in these children, including the prediabetic condition of syndrome X, type 2 diabetes mellitus, coronary artery disease, and obstructive sleep apnea.[266,267] Additional problems include bone and joint disease and cholelithiasis. The difficulty in the diagnosis of obesity has hampered the identification and treatment of many of these children. Although a National Institutes of Health (NIH) consensus has established a BMI of greater than 40 as morbid obesity,[268] BMIs change dramatically during adolescence and do not follow a linear curve. A more consistent diagnosis is based on the number of standard deviations from the mean using Centers for Disease Controls (CDC) standardized growth curves.[269] In this regard, at risk for overweight is defined as being at the 85th percentile, and overweight is defined as being at the 95th percentile.[264] Factors influencing the development of obesity are environmental as well as genetic.[270] The risk of obesity increases to 80% if one parent is also obese.[271]

Treatment of this condition is complex, and no ideal approach has been advanced. For the pediatric surgeon, use of surgery may be appropriate; however, it is essential that a team approach be applied to these children.[272] This approach includes pediatricians, nurses, nutritionists, psychiatric support, as well as the surgeon. The key issues when contemplating surgical intervention for obese adolescents include a careful patient evaluation and selection based on sufficient maturity to understand the implications of this lifelong decision, as well as the willingness to participate in follow-up for the rest of their lives. Vitamin and nutrient deficiencies are very common in such patients and require monitoring on an every-6-month basis.[273] Levels that are commonly deficient include protein, vitamin B_{12}, folate, iron, calcium, vitamin D, and thiamine.

FAILURE TO THRIVE

Malnutrition in childhood is associated with poor growth and development. The diagnosis of failure to thrive is based on a weight more than two standard deviations less than the mean weight percentile (Z score of 2.0) resulting in a child falling at 2.1%.[274] Failure to thrive is symmetric, in which height, length, and development of other body organs fall below the fifth percentile, or asymmetric, in which the weight is below the fifth percentile but length and head circumference are within normal limits. In general, patients with symmetric failure to thrive have more profound malnutrition and suffer from greater neurologic underdevelopment than those with asymmetric failure to thrive; the latter patients have relatively normal cognitive development. Recent investigations have shown that abnormal cognitive development in patients with failure to thrive probably results from a poor social environment and is often reversible.[275,276]

The approach to feeding a patient with failure to thrive should include a multidisciplinary assessment of medical, social, and psychological factors. A systematic evaluation to rule out neurologic pathology, swallowing disorders, feeding aversion, malabsorption, and metabolic disorders should be done. A trial of feeding the child in a hospital setting can often identify a problem with the child's home and social environment. Nutritional support for an infant should begin at approximately 50 kcal/kg/day and be increased by 20 to 25 kcal/kg/day as long as gastrointestinal tolerance to the feeding is adequate. Stool weight should be less than 150 g/day in young infants. Feedings may increase to 150 to 240 kcal/kg/day to achieve adequate catch-up growth,[277] but overshooting is not uncommon, and such high energy delivery states demands close clinical observation.

Supplementing the formula with additional potassium (up to 5 mEq/kg/day) may also be required during the first week of nutritional rehabilitation. Levels of potassium, magnesium, and phosphate need to be closely monitored, because they often drop rapidly after the initiation of feedings. One simple method to calculate caloric needs is that for each gram of weight gain desired per day, 5 additional calories should be provided.

CHILDREN WITH SPECIAL CARE NEEDS

Between 10% and 20% of children in the United States have special health care needs because of chronic illness and developmental disorders.[278] For several of these disorders, pediatric surgeons take an active part in the nutritional care of the patients. Some of the disorders include several neurologic impairments; developmental delay; cerebral palsy; and such genetic syndromes as trisomies 13, 18, and 21 and Cornelia de Lange and Rett syndromes. Pediatric surgeons are often responsible for providing nutritional access in many of these patients as well as for maintaining nutritional care before and after surgery. Potential factors that may contribute to poor nutrition in these patients include feeding disorders, uncoordinated tongue movements, poorly coordinated swallowing reflexes, gastroesophageal reflux with associated nutrient loss, and increased energy expenditure caused by muscle spasticity or athetosis (a mixed pattern of too much and too little muscle tone). Because measuring energy expenditure in these children may be impractical, estimates of energy needs can be

TABLE 12-13

Guidelines for Estimating Caloric Requirements Based on Height in Children with Developmental Disabilities

Condition	Caloric Recommendation
Ambulatory, ages 5 to 12 years	13.9 kcal/cm height
Nonambulatory, ages 5 to 12 years	11.1 kcal/cm height
Cerebral palsy with severely restricted activity	10 kcal/cm height
Cerebral palsy with mild to moderate activity	15 kcal/cm height
Athetoid cerebral palsy, adolescence	Up to 6000 kcal/day
Down syndrome, boys, ages 1 to 14 years	16.1 kcal/cm height
Down syndrome, girls, ages 1 to 14 years	14.3 kcal/cm height
Myelomeningocele	Approximately 50% of RDA for age after infancy; may need as little as 7 kcal/cm height to maintain normal weight
Prader-Willi syndrome	10-11 kcal/cm height (maintenance) 9 kcal/cm height (to promote weight loss)

RDA, recommended daily allowance.

From Nelson JK, Moxness KE, Jensen MD, Gastineau CF: *Mayo Clinic Diet Manual*, ed 7, St Louis, 1994, Mosby-Year Book. Used with permission.

based on previous studies of resting energy expenditure. Children with spastic-type (hypertonia) cerebral palsy may have lower energy needs than normal; adolescents require a total of approximately 1200 to 1300 kcal/day.[279,280] Children with athetosis may require a higher-than-normal calorie intake, sometimes more than twice the RDA. Children with myelomeningocele are far less active than their peers; for that reason, their energy needs are approximately only 50% to 60% that of normal children (Table 12-13).

If the child's body habitus is markedly abnormal, a more appropriate estimate of energy needs should be based on surface area rather than weight. Repeated assessments of the child's growth during nutritional supplementation are essential, because obesity in these children is common. Obesity can cause a considerable burden on the family and caregivers because of the increased difficulty in moving an overweight child.

The complete reference list is available online at www. expertconsult.com.

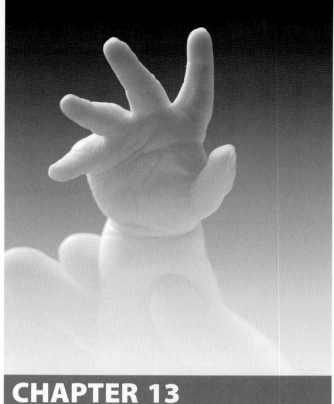

CHAPTER 13

Pediatric Anesthesia

Ira S. Landsman, Stephen R. Hays,
Christopher J. Karsanac, and Andrew Franklin

Dr. Marc Rowe, a leader in pediatric surgery, noted, "no matter how skilled and experienced the pediatric surgeon, safe conduct of the newborn patients through the perioperative period requires an equally competent pediatric anesthesiologist."[1] Anesthetic management of both neonates and older children must take into account the process of rapid growth and development. The child's variable anatomic, physiologic, pharmacologic, and psychological characteristics, as well as the magnitude of the surgical problem, influence anesthetic care. This chapter provides an overview of important issues in pediatric anesthesia and pain management that are directly related to clinical management.

Physiologic Considerations

During the first 3 months of life, circulatory and ventilatory adaptation is completed, thermoregulation processes change, the sizes of body fluid compartments shift toward adult values, skeletal muscle mass increases, and hepatic enzyme systems and renal function mature. Over the next 2 years, the child approaches adult physiologic but not psychological maturity. Between the ages of 18 months and 5 years, children

demonstrate sufficient awareness of their surroundings so that psychological aspects of care become an issue. Anxiolytic agents may be useful in the child's preoperative preparation. Healthy preschool-aged children (2 to 6 years) present relatively few technical problems to the anesthesiologist, but the child's fear, apprehension, and lack of cooperation are of concern. Anxiety treatment before surgery in school-aged children (6 to 18 years) may also be necessary.

Newborns can feel acute pain and process established pain (postoperative pain). At birth peripheral nociceptors function similarly to mature receptors.[2] However, the nerves responsible for transmitting the immediate chemical, thermal, and mechanical painful stimuli to the central nervous system (CNS) are not fully mature, nor are the inhibitory pathways from the CNS mature.[3] In the past, because of their inconsistent response to pain, neonates did not receive adequate analgesia for procedures known to cause pain in adults.[4-6] However, neonates of various gestational ages clearly respond to painful stimuli by measurable physiologic, metabolic, and clinical changes, and analgesia and anesthesia attenuate these changes.[7]

Neonates are sensitive to anesthetic agents and have inefficient mechanisms of drug metabolism and elimination.[8] Until infants are 1 month old, there is a marked interpatient difference in the volume of distribution, sensitivity of the CNS, and quality and quantity of transport proteins such as albumin and α_1-acid glycoprotein. These interpatient differences contribute to neonates' varied and often unpredictable responses to anesthetic agents.

After the first several weeks of life, drug metabolism gradually becomes so efficient that many of the opioid agents, such as fentanyl and morphine, have a shorter half-life in infants and young children than in older children and adults. The doses per body weight of intravenous (IV) anesthetic agents (e.g., thiopental and propofol) are higher in the first 6 months of life than during any other period (Fig. 13-1).[9] During the first year of life, the concentration of inhalation agent needed to maintain anesthesia is greater than during any other period (Table 13-1 and Fig. 13-2). However, the infant's heart is more sensitive to these higher concentrations.

Anesthetic Risk and Common Complications

Recent animal studies have stimulated debate and concern that anesthetic gases and drugs may be toxic to the immature developing brain.[10,11] Jevtovic-Todorovic and associates[10] began this recent controversy after publishing the results from a study in which 7-day-old rats were exposed to commonly used anesthetics for a total of 6 hours. The authors found that these rats exhibited learning/memory deficits, and histologic specimens of the brain revealed widespread apoptotic neurodegeneration and deficits in hippocampal synaptic function. The results of this study caused concern throughout the pediatric anesthesia community and was the subject of a Federal Drug Administration (FDA) advisory committee meeting.[12-15]

The FDA committee found that at present practice changes would be ill advised. On the one hand there is no doubt that animals varying from rats to primates have exhibited signs of neurotoxicity when exposed to higher levels of anesthetic

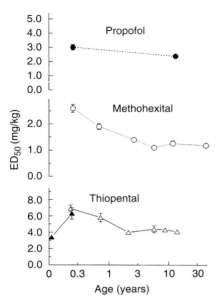

FIGURE 13-1 Estimated ED_{50} (dose of a drug that will induce anesthesia in 50% of patients) plus or minus the standard error in various age groups. Methohexital is indicated by open circles, thiopental by open or filled triangles, and propofol by filled circles. The vertical scales were adapted to yield the same height at ED_{50} for children 7 to 16 years of age. (From University and University Hospital of Lund: Intravenous Induction of Anesthesia in Infants and Children. Lund, Sweden, Studentlitteratur, 1991.)

TABLE 13-1

Age Versus Mean Minimum Alveolar Concentration of Inhaled Anesthetics in Children

Age (mo)	Halothane[*]	Isoflurane	Desflurane[‡]	Sevoflurane[§†]
1	0.87	1.6	9.16	3.2-3.3
2	1.08	1.9	9.4	3.2-3.3
14	0.97	1.8	8.72	2.5
44	0.91	1.6	8.54	2.5
480	0.76	1.2	7.5	2.5

*Data from Cook DR, Marcy JH: Pediatric anesthetic pharmacology. In Cook DR, Marcy JH (eds): Neonatal Anesthesia. Pasadena, CA, Appleton Davies, 1988.
†Data from Cameron CB, Robinson S, Gregory GA: The minimum anesthetic concentration of isoflurane in children. Anesth Analg 1984;63:418.
‡Data from Taylor RH, Lerman J: Minimum alveolar concentration of desflurane and hemodynamic responses in neonates, infants, and children. Anesthesiology 1991;75:975.
§Data from Lerman J, et al: The pharmacology of sevoflurane in infants and children. Anesthesiology 1994;80:814.

agent than is normally experienced by human infants and children. On the other hand 4 million children are exposed to anesthesia, and predictable patterns of brain injury have yet to be identified.[14] More animal studies are needed with doses and duration of exposure that reflect human exposure to these agents.[16] More important, clinical studies evaluating neurodevelopment in children exposed to anesthetic drugs are critical to better understand the effect of general anesthesia on neurologic development. Two multicenter clinical protocols for studying these issues have been developed and implemented.[11,13]

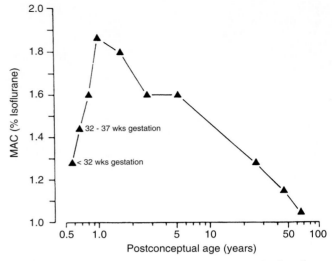

FIGURE 13-2 Minimum alveolar concentration (MAC) of isoflurane according to gestational age. (From LeDez KM, Lerman J: The minimum alveolar concentration [MAC] of isoflurane in premature neonates. Anesthesiology 1987;67:301.)

The American Society of Anesthesiologists (ASA) risk classification system is used by anesthesiologists to estimate the severity of their patients' medical conditions and to determine the relative risk for morbidity and mortality secondary to the anesthetic agent, not the surgery.[17,18] The ASA classification system does not predict surgical risk, because the type of operative procedure is not taken into consideration.[19] The ASA classification allows the anesthesiologist to tailor the plan for anesthesia based on the patient's underlying condition. The six ASA classes are as follows:

ASA 1: normal healthy patient
ASA 2: patient with mild systemic disease
ASA 3: patient with severe systemic disease
ASA 4: patient with severe systemic disease that is a constant threat to life
ASA 5: moribund patient who is not expected to survive without the operation
ASA 6: A declared brain-dead patient whose organs are removed for donor purposes
E: Any patient in whom an emergency operation is required

Because of their medical complexity, patients in ASA classifications 3 and 4 should have a consultation with an anesthesiologist before the day of surgery. The Vanderbilt Children's Hospital recommendations for preoperative visit are shown in Table 13-2.

Death caused by anesthesia alone is uncommon. Mortality related to anesthesia varies from 1 in several hundreds of thousands for healthy children undergoing routine procedures to greater than 1:10,000 in neonates and infants with congenital or neurologic diseases.[20,21] Keenan and colleagues suggested that the use of pediatric anesthesiologists for all infants younger than 1 year might decrease anesthetic morbidity in this group.[23] Auroy and associates observed that a minimum of 200 pediatric cases per year per pediatric anesthesiologist is necessary to reduce the incidence of complications and improve the safety in pediatric practice.[24]

TABLE 13-2

Summary of Fasting Recommendations to Reduce the Risk of Pulmonary Aspiration*

Ingested Material	Minimum Fasting Period (hr)[†]
Clear liquids[‡]	2
Breast milk	4
Infant formula	6
Nonhuman milk[§]	6
Light meal[¶]	6

*These recommendations apply to healthy patients who are undergoing elective procedures. They are not intended for women in labor. Following these guidelines does not guarantee that complete gastric emptying has occurred.

[†]Fasting periods apply to all ages.

[‡]Examples of clear liquids are water, fruit juices without pulp, carbonated beverages, clear tea, and black coffee.

[§]Because nonhuman milk is similar to solids in terms of gastric emptying time, the amount ingested must be considered when determining an appropriate fasting period.

[¶]A light meal typically consists of toast and clear liquids. Meals that include fried or fatty foods or meat may prolong gastric emptying time. Both the amount and the type of food ingested must be considered when determining an appropriate fasting period.

Data from ASA Practice Guidelines for Preoperative Fasting and the Use of Pharmacologic Agents to Reduce the Risk of Pulmonary Aspiration: Application to Healthy Patients Undergoing Elective Procedures, A Report by the American Society of Anesthesiologists. 1999.

The Pediatric Perioperative Cardiac Arrest Registry (POCA) was created in 1994 in an attempt to determine the clinical factors and outcomes associated with cardiac arrest in anesthetized children.[25] Through this registry, it was determined that anesthesia-related cardiac arrest occurred most often in patients younger than 1 year and in patients with severe underlying disease. Cardiac arrest during emergency surgery, especially in children with severe underlying disease, was associated with increased mortality. In this study, medication-related problems accounted for 37% of all cardiac arrests and 64% of arrests in ASA 1 and ASA 2 patients. A POCA update published in 2007 revealed that the decreased use of halothane (a potent cardiac depressant) in favor of sevoflurane decreased the number of cardiac arrests due to medications from 37% to 15%.[26] The most common causes of cardiac arrest in the POCA update were hypovolemia from blood loss and metabolic complications from blood transfusion.

LARYNGOSPASM

Laryngospasm is a common complication of inhalation anesthesia in children. Laryngospasm is defined as glottic closure caused by reflex constriction of the intrinsic laryngeal muscles.[27] If not treated quickly laryngospasm makes ventilation of a patient's lungs difficult and can lead to hypercarbia, hypoxia, cardiac collapse, and death. Although the majority of laryngospasm episodes are self-limited or responsive to conservative maneuvers, the anesthesiologist must be prepared to treat laryngospasm to restore normal ventilation.

The incidence of laryngospasm is higher in children than in adults. Olsson and Hallen studied the incidence of laryngospasm in 136,929 patients of all ages over an 11-year period (1967 to 1978) and found an incidence of 8.7 per 1000 patients.[28] They reported that the laryngospasm incidence during general anesthesia correlated inversely with age, with higher rates in children between birth and 9 years (17.4 per 1000 patients) and the highest incidence in infants between birth and 3 months (28.2 per 1000 patients). In adolescent patients, a significantly higher laryngospasm incidence was found in boys than in girls (12.1 versus 7.2 per 1000 patients). The study also showed that children with upper respiratory infections or bronchial asthma had a very high laryngospasm rate (95.8 per 1000 patients).

Treatment of incomplete airway obstruction includes removing the irritating surgical stimulus, removing debris from the larynx, and deepening anesthesia. Lung ventilation is facilitated by applying gentle continuous positive airway pressure as 100% oxygen is administered through a tight-fitting facemask. If airway maneuvers do not improve ventilation, a muscle relaxant is required. Intramuscular (IM) or IV succinylcholine will relax the vocal cords, allowing adequate lung ventilation.[29]

POSTOPERATIVE APNEA

Former preterm infants receiving general anesthesia are at risk for postoperative apnea. Regardless of whether they have a history of apnea, premature infants and full-term infants less than 44 weeks' postconceptual age may develop apnea in the postoperative period.[30-32] Postoperative apnea is defined as cessation of breathing or no detectable air flow for 15 seconds or longer, or less than 15 seconds with bradycardia. The cause of this phenomenon is unknown. Recovery from general anesthesia may unmask immature central respiratory regulation or decrease upper airway tone; both factors are believed to be responsible for postoperative apnea.[33] Although postoperative apnea usually develops in the first 2 hours after the anesthesia, it may present as long as 12 hours after anesthesia.

Several investigators have tried to establish a postconceptual age after which healthy premature infants with no history of neonatal apnea can be discharged on the day of surgery. Unfortunately, the recommendations vary from 44 weeks to 60 weeks.[32,34-36] The variance of recommendations are based in part on the sophistication of monitoring. The more sophisticated the monitoring, the higher the rate of identified apneic spells. Because considerable controversy exists, each hospital must develop its own policy. It is reasonable to monitor former premature infants for 24 hours if their postconceptual age is 55 weeks or less. Obviously, children with serious medical or neurologic problems or a history of significant and recurrent neonatal apnea are exceptions to this recommendation.

So far, anemia is the only independent risk factor identified that increases the likelihood of postoperative apnea in this at-risk population.[33,37] It has been recommended that anemic preterm infants with hematocrit values less than 30% have elective surgery delayed and receive iron supplementation until the hematocrit is greater than 30%. If surgery cannot be deferred, anemic infants must be observed and monitored very carefully for postoperative apnea.

OBSTRUCTIVE SLEEP APNEA SYNDROME

Obstructive sleep apnea syndrome (OSAS) is a disorder of breathing during sleep that is characterized by prolonged partial upper airway obstruction (obstructive hypopnea) or intermittent complete obstruction (obstructive sleep apnea, OSA) with or without snoring. OSAS is also associated with moderate to severe oxygen desaturation that disrupts normal sleep-time breathing and normal sleep patterns.[38] The most common cause of OSAS among children is upper airway narrowing with adenotonsillar hypertrophy. OSAS also occurs in infants and children with upper airway narrowing due to craniofacial anomalies and in those with neuromuscular diseases, including cerebral palsy and muscular dystrophy.[39,40]

In recent years, the epidemic increase in the prevalence of obesity during childhood seems to be contributing to substantial changes in the cross-sectional demographic and anthropometric characteristics of the children being referred for evaluation of OSAS. Although less than 15% of all symptomatic habitually snoring children were obese (i.e., >95% for age and gender) in the early 1990s, more than 50% fulfilled the criteria for obesity among all referrals to a Kentucky sleep center.[40,41]

Symptoms of OSAS include nocturnal snoring, breathing pauses, gasping, use of accessory muscles of respiration, enuresis, and excessive sweating.[42] In addition, children with OSAS have a host of sequelae, which are usually reversible after adenotonsillectomy but can lead to perioperative complications during and after surgery. Children with OSAS have a higher incidence of postoperative respiratory complications, including prolonged oxygen requirements, airway obstruction requiring a nasal airway, and major respiratory compromise requiring airway instrumentation.[43]

To date, the subpopulation of children with OSAS that must be monitored in the hospital is still unknown. Children who are most likely to experience postoperative respiratory complications and have a higher postoperative respiratory disturbance index on their postoperative polysomnogram include children younger than 3 years of age, children with severe OSAS diagnosed by preoperative polysomnography, and those with associated medical conditions such as hypotonia, morbid obesity, failure to thrive, or severe structural airway abnormalities.[44,45] These children are not candidates for outpatient surgery and should receive medical care in centers with pediatric inpatient facilities and pediatric intensive care unit support. High-risk patients should be monitored overnight with continuous pulse oximetry because standard apnea monitoring is unable to detect obstructive apnea and hypopnea. Patients can be discharged when significant oxygen desaturation during sleep has resolved.

Preanesthesia Evaluation and Preparation

The primary purpose of a preoperative visit is to obtain information about the surgical problem and medical history and to assess the child's ability to tolerate anesthesia. The preoperative evaluation permits the identification of abnormalities that should be corrected before administration of an anesthetic; these disorders include severe anemia, sickle cell abnormalities, acute systemic infections, and active lower respiratory processes such as asthma, bronchopulmonary dysplasia, and cystic fibrosis.

In addition, the preoperative visit should be used to address the child's and parent's anxiety about the scheduled surgery and anesthesia. Preoperative behavioral evaluation

programs are common in major pediatric hospitals. These preparation programs may provide narrative information, hospital tours, role rehearsal, and child life counseling.[46,47] Outpatient surgery programs may minimize a young child's separation anxiety. Ordinarily, a simple explanation of what the patient can expect before induction of anesthesia reduces the element of surprise and can be used to reinforce preoperative teaching materials. In older children, the preoperative visit allows the anesthesiologist to establish rapport, which fosters trust and may enhance cooperation. In some clinics, parents actively participate in the anesthesia induction process.[47,48] For some but not all parents and preschool-aged children, this joint experience minimizes fear and anxiety.

PREOPERATIVE FASTING

The patient's stomach must be empty to prevent aspiration of stomach contents into the lungs during anesthesia induction. However, the patient should also be optimally hydrated. These two goals are compatible and are not difficult to achieve. Patients who are fed at the usual mealtimes and sleep through the night present no particular problems if procedures are scheduled for the early morning hours.

Numerous studies have failed to document an increased pulmonary aspiration risk when fasting guidelines are relaxed.[49,50] The perioperative fasting guidelines developed by the ASA are listed in Table 13-2.[51] These guidelines allow children to ingest clear liquids up to 2 hours before scheduled surgery. Infants and toddlers can be fed breast milk up until 4 hours before surgery, and infants and young children can be fed formula up until 6 hours before surgery.

If these details are not clearly stated in an itemized fashion with specific times, fluids may inadvertently be withheld from some children, particularly infants, for excessively long periods. Procedures should be scheduled according to age, with the youngest patient being the first on the operating schedule. Both the surgeon and the anesthesiologist must be alert to delays and ensure that the infant's fluid restriction is revised accordingly.

PREANESTHESIA MEDICATIONS

Various drugs and routes of administration have been described as parts of premedication regimens. In the past, many anesthesiology departments created their own unique mixtures of sedative-hypnotic, narcotic, and antisialagogue medications, which were usually administered by the IM route. The goal of this premedication was to allay anxiety, provide analgesia, decrease autonomic (vagal) reflexes, decrease airway secretions, and reduce the volume and acidity of gastric fluid. The oral or nasal route is now preferred.

Premedication should provide a rapid level of short-term sedation that allows easy separation of the child from the parents and a smooth induction of anesthesia. Because children are usually not in pain before elective surgery, the use of opioids as part of standard premedication is not required. Antisialagogues were useful when diethyl ether and cyclopropane were the commonly used inhalation anesthetics. The newer inhalation agents do not significantly increase the quantity of oral secretions, thereby eliminating the need for anticholinergic premedication.

Midazolam is a popular, short-acting benzodiazepine that is now used frequently for preoperative sedation. It is an anxiolytic, hypnotic, and anticonvulsant agent, with antegrade but not retrograde amnestic properties.[52,53] At physiologic pH, midazolam becomes lipophilic, allowing quick absorption by the gastrointestinal tract and rapid entry into the CNS.[52] Sedative doses of IV midazolam can depress the hypoxic ventilatory drive and attenuate reflex cardiorespiratory responses to hypoxemia.[54] When combined with opioids, IV midazolam is likely to place unmonitored patients at significant risk for apnea and hypoxemia.[55]

In children, sedation with midazolam can be delivered by the intranasal, oral, rectal, IV, or IM route. The bioavailability of intranasal midazolam is 51% of the IV dose, and the speed of onset is 45% faster than with the rectal route.[56] Wilton and colleagues reported that intranasal midazolam given to children between 18 months and 5 years of age at a dose of 0.2 mg/kg calmed the patient within 5 to 10 minutes of administration.[57] Davis et al. found that intranasal midazolam at a dose of 0.2 to 0.3 mg/kg produced excellent sedation without prolonging recovery from anesthesia or time to hospital discharge in infants and small children undergoing very short ambulatory surgical procedures.[58] Cardiorespiratory depression has not been encountered when recommended doses of intranasal midazolam (0.2 to 0.3 mg/kg) or oral midazolam (0.5 to 0.75 mg/kg) are administered to otherwise healthy children for preoperative sedation.[57,59] Commercially prepared oral midazolam produces satisfactory sedation and anxiolysis within 10 to 20 minutes of consumption.[60] Oral midazolam prepared from the IV product has an onset time between 20 and 30 minutes.

Intranasal midazolam can cause mild, transient burning of the nasal mucosa, and amounts greater than 1 mL of a 0.5% solution (5 mg/mL) may produce choking and coughing. If more than 1 mL of 0.5% midazolam is necessary, the oral route is usually better tolerated. Oral midazolam prepared from the IV product should be flavored with sweetened clear liquids or syrup to mask the bitter taste. It has been demonstrated that commercially prepared oral midazolam has a more consistent bioavailability and pH characteristics. This stability allows doses as low as 0.25 mg/kg while still producing adequate sedation.[60]

Preoperative medication given to increase the pH of gastric fluid or to promote gastric emptying is not needed in healthy children, because pediatric pulmonary aspiration is rare.[61,62] Clear liquids administered to infants, children, and adults up to 2 hours before surgery do not alter residual gastric volume.[63] In fact, some children who have consumed liquids have a lower residual gastric volume and a higher gastric pH than controls who have had nothing by mouth (NPO).

Fluid Requirements

MAINTENANCE FLUID REQUIREMENTS

Various calculations involving body weight, surface area, and calorie expenditure have been used to determine fluid therapy for full-term infants and children.[64–66] Body weight and calorie expenditure, as well as estimates of insensible water loss, renal water requirement, stool water loss, and water needed for growth, determine the amount of fluid needed for maintenance. Calorie expenditure is related to size: infants weighing 1 to 10 kg require 100 calories/kg; small children weighing 10 to 20 kg require 1000 calories/day plus 50 calories/day for each kilogram greater than 10 kg; older children weighing more than 20 kg require 1500 calories/day plus 25 calories/day for each kilogram greater than 20 kg. For every 100 calories that the patient consumes, 67 mL of water is required for solute excretion; an additional 50 mL per 100 calories is associated with insensible loss, but 17 mL per 100 calories is produced by oxidation. Thus, infants and children need 100 mL of water for each 100 calories expended. Assuming that there are 25 hours in a day, a simple formula can be used to calculate the hourly maintenance fluid needed by healthy full-term infants and children. For children weighing 1 to 10 kg, the hourly maintenance fluid requirement (MFR) is 4 mL/kg per hour. For patients weighing 10 to 20 kg, the hourly MFR is 4 mL/kg per hour for the first 10 kg, plus 2 mL/kg per hour for each kilogram between 10 and 20 kg. For patients weighing more than 20 kg, the MFR is calculated as 4 mL/kg per hour for the first 10 kg, plus 2 mL/kg per hour for the next 10 kg, plus 1 mL/kg per hour for each additional kilogram greater than 20 kg. For example, a 28-kg child requires 68 mL of maintenance fluid per hour.

For every 100 mL of water given to an infant or child, 3 mEq Na^+, 2 mEq K^+, 2 mEq Cl^-, and 5 g glucose (to prevent ketosis) are required. It is more convenient to equalize the sodium and chloride requirements at 3 mEq. For routine IV fluid therapy, 5% dextrose in 0.25% normal saline meets these requirements. However, this is not an ideal fluid for intraoperative use, as noted later.

Premature or Critically Ill Infants

Many factors influence water and electrolyte balance in premature or critically ill infants. The infant's gestational age, postnatal age, weight, renal solute load, and maximum renal concentrating ability are variables. Tissue destruction and catabolism that result from disease, stress, infection, reduced bowel activity, phototherapy, and gastric or intestinal drainage affect fluid therapy. These issues are reviewed by Bell,[65] Rowe,[67] and Hammarlund.[68]

INTRAOPERATIVE FLUID REPLACEMENT

Intraoperative fluid replacement involves the initiation of fluid management or, alternatively, a continuation of ongoing therapy. Fluid replacement can simply consist of replacing the deficit from preoperative fasting and providing maintenance fluids. Fluid therapy can also be complex when preoperative deficits, translocated fluids, and variable blood loss are part of the equation.

Estimated Fluid Deficit

The fluid deficit incurred during fasting should be replaced during anesthesia. Assuming a child is healthy at the time of fasting, the fluid deficit is estimated by multiplying the hourly MFR by the number of hours the patient has had nothing by mouth. This deficit can be replaced during surgery and if necessary in the recovery room. Maintenance fluids should continue in conjunction with replacement fluids.

Role of Glucose

Surgery may cause the release of stress hormones that decrease insulin sensitivity, so serum glucose levels are usually elevated during surgery. If serum glucose concentrations become too high, glycosuria and osmotic diuresis ensue. Hyperglycemia may contribute to neurologic damage subsequent to episodes of severe ischemia and hypoxia.[69–71] Several studies have shown that healthy infants and children remain euglycemic for up to 17 hours after the start of a fast. These studies suggest that healthy infants and children do not require glucose-containing solutions during surgery.[72,73] Frequent monitoring of blood sugar should accompany fluid and glucose therapy in patients who are at high risk for hypoglycemia (e.g., premature infants and those who are small for gestational age, children on total parenteral nutrition, and patients with diabetes).

Choice of Intraoperative Fluid

For most patients, lactated Ringer solution can be used to provide maintenance and replacement fluids for intraoperative losses. The electrolyte composition of lactated Ringer is similar to that of serum. Hyponatremia with associated neurologic complications can occur if hypotonic solutions are used for fluid maintenance and replacement of third space fluid losses.

Surgical trauma is associated with isotonic transfer of fluids from the extracellular fluid compartment to the interstitial compartment.[74] This acute sequestration of edematous fluid to the interstitial compartment is called third-space loss. The greater the third-space volume losses, the greater the loss of intravascular volume. The magnitude of third-space loss varies with the surgical procedure and is usually highest in infants having intraabdominal surgery. In pediatric patients, estimated third-space loss is 6 to 10 mL/kg per hour during intraabdominal surgery, 4 to 7 mL/kg per hour during intrathoracic surgery, and 1 to 2 mL/kg per hour during superficial surgery or neurosurgery. Generally, lactated Ringer solution is used to restore third-space losses. In cases of massive volume replacement, some advocate using 5% albumin to restore one third to one fourth of the loss. The end point of third-space replacement therapy is maintenance of adequate blood pressure, tissue perfusion, and urine output.

BLOOD REPLACEMENT

Blood replacement depends on the patient's needs, and clear communication between the surgeon and the anesthesiologist is crucial. Accurately measuring blood loss and assessing the limit of safe blood loss in infants are vital parts of any replacement regimen. Weighing sponges and using calibrated miniaturized suction bottles and visual estimates define the magnitude of blood loss. Allowable blood loss is determined by calculating the starting blood volume and measuring the hemoglobin or hematocrit of the patient.[75,76] Other factors used to determine allowable blood loss include the patient's age, cardiopulmonary status, and general medical condition. These factors are also used to determine the risk versus benefit of blood transfusion.

Estimating Allowable Blood Loss

Several methods have been proposed for estimating allowable blood loss. The formulas range from simple to complex, but all involve an estimate of blood volume. Allowable blood loss can be calculated using the following equation:

$$ABL = Weight \ (kg) \times EBV \times [Ho - Hl]/H,$$

where ABL is allowable blood loss, EBV is estimated blood volume, Ho is the original hematocrit, Hl is the lowest acceptable hematocrit, and H is the average hematocrit ([Ho + Hl] / 2).

This equation assumes that blood loss and replacement are gradual and exponential. Estimated blood volume is approximately 90 mL/kg for neonates, 80 mL/kg for infants and children, and 65 to 78 mL/kg for adolescents. This equation has general applicability for all age groups.

The ideal fluid to replace blood loss until the lowest acceptable hematocrit value is reached is a matter of controversy.[77–79] Generally, lactated Ringer solution is given in an amount equal to 2 to 3 times the estimated amount of lost blood except in situations of massive transfusion when massive transfusion protocols are followed (see later).

Blood Products

Blood component therapy depends on the clinical setting and the availability of various blood products. Fresh whole blood (i.e., blood that was obtained less than 4 hours previously) has limited availability. Thus treatment with component therapy rather than fresh whole blood is the rule rather than the exception.[80,81] Packed red blood cells (RBCs) have a hematocrit value between 55% and 75% and are relatively hyperkalemic (K ± 15 to 20 mEq/L) and acidotic (pH <7.0). The estimated rise in hematocrit for every 10 mL/kg of packed RBCs (assuming a hematocrit of 70%) depends on the patient's age, size, and estimated blood volume (Table 13-3).

The need for platelets during surgery can be predicted from the preoperative platelet count. Platelets are mobilized from the spleen and bone marrow as bleeding occurs. An infant with a high preoperative platelet count (>250,000/mm³) may not need a platelet transfusion until two to three blood volumes are lost, whereas an infant who has a low count (<150,000/mm³) may need platelets after only one blood volume is lost. Two platelet packs/10 kg increases the platelet count by 50,000 to 100,000/mm³.

Fresh frozen plasma (FFP) is indicated for emergency reversal of warfarin, for correction of microvascular bleeding in the presence of elevated prothrombin time and partial thromboplastin time, and as part of a massive transfusion protocol.[81] Ten to 20 ml/kg of FFP usually raises the level of coagulation factors by 20%. FFP contains the highest concentration of citrate per unit volume of any blood product; thus rapid FFP

TABLE 13-3

Estimated Rise in Hematocrit with Increasing Blood Volume

	Blood Volume (mL/kg)	Estimated Rise Age in Hematocrit*
Premature Infants	100	6.30
Term infants	90	7.00
Preschool-aged children	80	7.7
School-aged children	75	8.2
Adults	65	9.3

*The estimated rise in hematocrit for every 10 mL/kg of packed red blood cells (RBCs) (assuming a hematocrit of 70%) depends on the patient's age, size, and estimated blood volume.

causes the greatest change in ionized calcium. Under most circumstances, mobilization of calcium and hepatic metabolism of citrate are sufficiently rapid to prevent precipitous decreases in ionized calcium. However, because infants' calcium stores are small, rapid infusion of FFP can acutely decrease ionized calcium and cause significant decreases in arterial blood pressure.[82] Treatment of acute hypocalcemia includes IV calcium chloride (10 mg/kg) or calcium gluconate (30 to 60 mg/kg), which effectively increases ionized calcium and ameliorates hemodynamic changes.

When blood loss approaches one blood volume many centers have established massive transfusion protocols.[83] These protocols help prevent the acidosis, hypothermia, and coagulopathy seen when only packed RBCs are infused during massive hemorrhage.[79] The goals of these protocols are to improve communication between the surgeon, anesthesiologist, and blood bank to expedite delivery of appropriate quantities of blood products to the patient care team. Although the transfusion and coagulation management in children experiencing severe hemorrhage is not well studied, it is prudent to develop a massive transfusion protocol. The goal of transfusion is to deliver blood products that resemble whole blood. Current data support the use of plasma-to-RBC-to-platelet at 1:1:1.[84,85]

Inhalation Anesthetic Agents

Several inhalation agents are available for induction and maintenance of anesthesia. The choice of agent depends on the age of the child and the disease process. Each agent has general and specific advantages and disadvantages (Table 13-4). None ensures hemodynamic stability. In patients with significant cardiac depression or hemodynamic instability, inhalation agents are generally avoided or used in markedly reduced concentrations. In healthy children, most inhalation agents can be used safely and successfully regardless of age.

To spare children an awake placement of an IV catheter, anesthesia is often induced by inhalation. However, inhalation anesthesia in children has some risk and is associated with an increased incidence of bradycardia, hypotension, and even cardiac arrest.[25,86] These risks have been reduced with the use of sevoflurane rather than halothane.[26] In premature or critically ill infants, the incidence of untoward effects from potent inhalation agents is attributed to age-related differences in uptake, anesthesia requirements, and cardiovascular system sensitivity. The uptake of inhalation anesthetics is more rapid in infants and small children than in adults because of major differences in blood-gas solubility coefficients,

TABLE 13-4

Inhalation Anesthetics

Agent	Advantages	Disadvantages and Precautions
Nitrous oxide	Inexpensive	Should be used as a supplement to other inhalation or intravenous anesthetics to provide complete general anesthesia
	Odorless	
	Rapid onset and recovery of clinical effects	In critically ill patients, can be a potent vasodilator
	When combined with potent inhalation anesthetics, side effects of potent agents are reduced	Expands gas-containing spaces, such as the intestines or middle ear; increases the expansion of pneumothorax and pneumocephalus
	Activates the sympathetic nervous system, which attenuates cardiac depression or vasodilatation caused by potent inhalation agents	Exposure to operating room atmosphere contamination may cause neuropathies
Halothane	Nonpungent odor	Causes cardiac depression manifested as bradycardia and decreased myocardial contractility
	Effective inhalation induction agent	
	Bronchodilator (like all potent inhalation agents)	Causes halothane-associated hepatitis (rare in children)
		Sensitizes the myocardium to the arrhythmogenic properties of epinephrine; however, infants and children require higher doses of epinephrine to stimulate ventricular arrhythmias than do adolescents and adults
Isoflurane	Maintains myocardial contractility and heart rate	Pungent odor
	Minimal sensitization of the myocardium to the arrhythmogenic properties of epinephrine	Not an effective inhalation induction agent
		Can cause bradycardia in neonates and young infants
		May cause hypotension by decreasing systemic vascular resistance
Sevoflurane	Nonpungent odor	More expensive than halothane
	Effective inhalation induction agent	Metabolized by liver, releasing free fluoride ions; theoretical risk for renal diabetes insipidus
	Low blood-gas coefficient	
	Maintains myocardial contractility and heart rate	Degradation in Baralyme and soda lime, forming potentially toxic metabolites
	Minimal sensitization of the myocardium to the arrhythmogenic properties of epinephrine	Increased incidence of postanesthesia delirium
Desflurane	Low blood-gas coefficient	Pungent odor
	Maintains myocardial contractility and heart rate	Poor inhalation induction agent
	Minimal sensitization of the myocardium to the arrhythmogenic properties of epinephrine	High incidence of laryngospasm
		Expensive
		Increased incidence of postanesthesia delirium

blood-tissue solubility coefficients, body composition, ratio of alveolar ventilation to functional residual capacity, and distribution of cardiac output.[87-89] Thus, early in the course of anesthesia induction, infants have higher tissue concentrations of the drug in the brain, heart, and muscle than do adults.

MINIMUM ALVEOLAR CONCENTRATION

The minimum alveolar concentration (MAC) is the minimum concentration of an inhaled anesthetic at 1 atm of pressure that prevents skeletal muscle movement in response to a surgical incision in 50% of patients. The MAC of a volatile anesthetic changes with the patient's age (see Table 13-1). LeDez and Lerman[91] showed that premature infants younger than 32 weeks' gestation have a lower MAC for isoflurane than do neonates of longer gestation. For all anesthetic agents, the MAC is highest at 6 to 12 months of age. The increased MAC requirement in conjunction with the rapid uptake of anesthetic makes infants and children very susceptible to anesthetic overdose.[92,93]

NITROUS OXIDE

Because nitrous oxide is a nonpotent inhalation agent with a MAC of 105%, it is usually used as an adjunct to the more potent inhalation agents. Nitrous oxide reduces the side effects of these agents by reducing the amount required for effective analgesia. During the induction phase of anesthesia, nitrous oxide hastens the uptake of potent inhalation agents. Eger and Saidman[93a] noted that nitrous oxide is more soluble than nitrogen in blood and thus distends any air-containing space, such as the intestines, to which it is carried. As a result, nitrous oxide is usually avoided in patients with closed pneumothorax, intestinal obstruction, or air in the cerebral ventricles. Nitrous oxide has been implicated in lymphocyte depression, testicular damage, birth defects, and miscarriages with chronic exposure, so it is important to adequately scavenge this gas in the operating suite.

HALOTHANE

Halothane was once the most commonly administered anesthetic agent in children because it was less likely than isoflurane and desflurane to cause airway irritability. However, halothane was not an ideal induction agent because of its potential to cause bradycardia, hypotension, and ventricular ectopy secondary to induced sensitivity to catecholamines. In the United States, sevoflurane (because of its cardiovascular safety profile) has replaced halothane as the induction agent of choice.[94]

ISOFLURANE

Isoflurane has a lower solubility coefficient than that of halothane, so induction and recovery with isoflurane is faster than with halothane. However, isoflurane causes moderate to severe airway irritability if used as an induction agent.

The cardiovascular effects of isoflurane in children are well documented. Unlike adults, unpremedicated infants 5 to 26 weeks of age who were anesthetized with isoflurane showed a decrease in heart rate similar to that seen with halothane and a decrease in blood pressure half that seen with halothane.[95] In

children older than 2 years who did not receive atropine, isoflurane preserved heart rate and cardiac function better than did halothane.[96] Halothane and isoflurane both reduced blood pressure. Isoflurane reduced peripheral vascular resistance but preserved cardiac output. Gallagher and colleagues[97] compared the anesthetic effects of halothane and isoflurane on cardiac function in 15 older children using pulsed Doppler echocardiography.[97] Cardiac output, heart rate, and myocardial contractility were preserved with isoflurane, but contractility was decreased with halothane. Kotrly and associates[98] found that isoflurane preserved the baroreceptor response in adults more than halothane did.

DESFLURANE

Desflurane is a potent inhalation agent. The blood-gas solubility is low and similar to nitrous oxide.[99] Because it is a pungent airway irritant, desflurane results in an unacceptably high incidence of laryngospasm, coughing, and hypoxia when used as an induction agent in children.[100-102] Patients anesthetized with desflurane have a faster emergence from general anesthesia.

The cardiovascular profile of desflurane is age dependent.[100] When desflurane was given at a MAC of 1 before incision, the arterial blood pressure decreased approximately 30% compared with awake values, and the heart rate decreased significantly or remained the same. Thus at a MAC of 1, desflurane, like isoflurane and halothane, seems to attenuate the baroreceptor response in children. Weiskopf and colleagues[103] also demonstrated that in adults, rapid increases in desflurane from a MAC of 0.55 to 1.66 can transiently increase arterial blood pressure and heart rate; this excitation is associated with an increase in sympathetic and renin-angiotensin system activity.

SEVOFLURANE

Sevoflurane is a potent inhalation agent with a low blood-gas solubility coefficient. It does not have a pungent odor and has replaced halothane as the inhalation anesthetic of choice for infants and children.[104,105] Clinical studies with sevoflurane inpediatric patients have found shorter times to emergence than with halothane.[94] This may be related to the low blood-gas solubility. Sevoflurane has fewer cardiovascular side effects than halothane.[94,108-112] Wodey and colleagues[111] compared cardiovascular changes at equipotent concentrations of sevoflurane and halothane in infants. They concluded that in infants, sevoflurane decreases cardiac output less than does halothane, and a minor decrease in contractibility is compensated by a greater decrease in systemic vascular resistance (SVR) without a change in heart rate.[111] Unlike halothane, sevoflurane does not increase the sensitivity of the myocardium to the arrhythmogenic effects of epinephrine.[113] Sevoflurane causes a significant decrease in respiratory resistance, and it is an effective bronchodilating agent.[114]

One theoretical concern surrounding the use of sevoflurane is that it is metabolized in the liver by the cytochrome system, with the subsequent release of fluoride and the potential for renal diabetes insipidus. However, renal concentrating ability and normal creatinine clearance have been demonstrated in adult volunteers subjected to prolonged sevoflurane exposure. In addition to in vivo metabolism, sevoflurane undergoes degradation by soda lime and barium hydroxide lime (Baralyme) to produce two potentially toxic olefins, compound A and compound B. Although human exposure to sevoflurane administered by circle absorption systems has not demonstrated toxicity, animal studies have yielded conflicting histologic evidence of chemical-induced toxicity.[97,115,116] Frink and associates[117] concluded that the concentrations of compound A measured in pediatric patients during sevoflurane anesthesia using a 2-L flow circle system were low, and there was no evidence of abnormal renal or hepatic function up to 24 hours after anesthesia.

Emergence Delirium

The advent of the use of volatile anesthetics in children brought with it the new entity of emergence delirium (ED). ED is a dissociated state of consciousness in which children are inconsolable, irritable, uncompromising, or uncooperative, or a combination of these behaviors.[118] It occurs in 2% to 80% of children, depending on the age of the patients, anesthetics used, and the type of surgery. It usually occurs within 30 minutes after the conclusion of the anesthesia procedure and is typically self-resolving within 30 minutes.[119] Children experiencing ED are disruptive to the postanesthesia care unit (PACU) and increase the risk of injury to themselves and others; ED is also associated with parent dissatisfaction with the hospital care. The current theories on the causes of ED involve the direct interaction of volatile agents on neurons. The two most prominent theories are an uneven susceptibility of neurons to volatile anesthetics or direct, low-level activation of excitatory neurons by volatile anesthetics.[120,121]

The main risk factors are age, perioperative anxiety, and the anesthetics used, with volatile agents causing the most ED.[119] Preventive measures include preoperative anxiolysis, avoidance of volatile anesthetics, and preemptive treatment. Multiple agents have been used for preemptive treatment, and most are given 10 minutes before the patient wakes up. They include fentanyl, propofol, ketamine, nalbuphine, and dexmedetomidine. Once a child is in ED, fentanyl, midazolam, propofol, or dexmedetomidine can be used for treatment.

Dexmedetomidine, a highly specific and selective α_2-adrenergic agonist, is becoming an important drug in the treatment of ED. It can be given either preoperatively as an anxiolytic agent, intraoperatively for ED avoidance, or postoperatively for the treatment of ED. Currently, there are six prospective clinical trials that have shown that dexmedetomidine significantly reduces the incidence of ED when given to children before recovery from volatile anesthetics.[122] Doses range from 0.15 to 1 µg/kg given either as a bolus or infusion before completion of surgery. Once a child is in ED, a single bolus dose of 0.5 µg/kg can be used as treatment. Side effects are minimal and usually consist of bradycardia with a concomitant decrease in blood pressure.

Neuromuscular Blocking Agents

Neuromuscular blocking agents (i.e., muscle relaxants) are used to facilitate endotracheal intubation, to provide surgical relaxation, and to facilitate controlled mechanical ventilation. This is accomplished through blockade of the nicotinic acetylcholine receptor site on the neuromuscular junction. The use of neuromuscular blocking agents reduces the need for potent inhaled anesthetics or IV sedative-hypnotics. Throughout infancy, the neuromuscular junction matures physically and biochemically. The contractile properties of skeletal muscle change, and the amount of muscle in proportion to body weight increases. As a result, the neuromuscular junction is variably sensitive to relaxants.[123] In addition, age-related changes in the volume of distribution of relaxants, their redistribution and clearance, and possibly their rate of metabolism occur. These factors influence the dose-response relationships of relaxants and the duration of neuromuscular blockade.[124–126]

When allowances are made for differences in the volume of distribution and for the type and concentration of anesthetic, infants seem to be relatively resistant to succinylcholine and relatively sensitive to nondepolarizing relaxants (Table 13-5). The degree of neuromuscular blockade should be monitored with a nerve stimulator during the course of the operation, and the patient should be treated with a dose of the selected agent sufficient to achieve the desired degree of block. The paralysis caused by nondepolarizing relaxants should be reversed at the end of each operation unless postoperative mechanical ventilation is planned. Anticholinesterase drugs, such as neostigmine and edrophonium, combined with anticholinergics are given to prevent muscarinic side effects. The effectiveness of reversal is judged by muscle strength, adequacy of ventilation, and response to nerve stimulation. Minimum criteria for withdrawing assisted ventilation should include good muscle tone, flexing of the arms and legs, and adequate respiratory effort.

Neuromuscular blocking agents have no sedative, hypnotic, or analgesic effects, but they may indirectly decrease metabolic demand, prevent shivering, decrease nonsynchronous ventilation, decrease intracranial pressure, and improve chest wall compliance. Major organ failure, up-regulation of acetylcholine receptors, malnutrition, electrolyte and acid-base abnormalities, drug interactions, and muscle atrophy can also have a profound influence on the kinetics and dynamics of relaxants. In addition, repeated doses of relaxants over relatively long periods without monitoring of neuromuscular transmission may lead to prolonged muscle weakness despite discontinuation of therapy. Knowledge of neuromuscular pharmacology and its modification by age, concurrent medications, and concurrent disease processes permits a more rational use of neuromuscular blocking agents in patients in intensive care.

COMPLICATING CONDITIONS OF DEPOLARIZING BLOCKING AGENTS

The use of succinylcholine for elective pediatric procedures has been abandoned secondary to multiple case reports of cardiac arrest from hyperkalemia due to undiagnosed muscular dystrophy. Life-threatening hyperkalemia can also be caused by succinylcholine in all of the following situations: burns on greater than 8% of the body, upper motor neuron lesions, lower motor neuron lesions, crush injuries, neuromuscular diseases, and chronic ongoing sepsis. It is also a known triggering agent of malignant hyperthermia (MH). The FDA issued the following "Black Box" warning in 1993 because of previous listed potential complications:

> Since there may be no signs or symptoms to alert the practitioner to which patients are at risk, it is recommended that the use of succinylcholine should be reserved for emergency intubation or

TABLE 13-5

Muscle Relaxants

Agent	Type	Dose	Metabolism and Excretion	Advantages	Disadvantages and Precautions
Succinylcholine	Short acting; depolarizing	IV: 1.0-2.0 mg/kg IM: younger than 6 mo, 4.0-5.0 mg/kg; older than 6 mo, 3.0-4.0 mg/kg	Pseudocholinesterase	Rapid onset; rapid recovery; may be delivered through intravascular or intramuscular routes	Masseter muscle spasm; trigger for malignant hyperthermia; bradycardia; hyperkalemia leading to life-threatening arrhythmias; myoglobinemia (muscle injury); muscle fasciculations; increased intraocular pressure; prolonged neuromuscular blockade with pseudocholinesterase deficiency Avoid in patients with muscular dystrophy; multiple trauma >24 hr; burns >24 hr; spinal cord injury >24 hr; malignant hyperthermia–susceptible
Mivacurium	Short acting; nondepolarizing	Intubation: 0.2 mg/kg Maintenance: 0.1 mg/kg	Plasma cholinesterase	Recovery time 10 min; infusion possible	Histamine release; unpredictable intubating conditions
Atracurium	Intermediate acting; nondepolarizing	Intubation: 0.5 mg/kg Maintenance: 0.15 mg/kg	Ester hydrolysis; Hoffman degradation	Recovery time 30 min regardless of age; can be used in renal and kidney disease; infusion possible	Histamine release; (metabolite of Hoffman degradation); epileptogenic in high doses
Cisatracurium	Intermediate acting; nondepolarizing	Intubation: 0.1 mg/kg Maintenance: 0.03 mg/kg or 1-2 mcg/kg/min continuous	Ester hydrolysis; Hoffman degradation	Recovery time 30 min; no cardiovascular effects; infusion possible	
Rocuronium	Intermediate acting; nondepolarizing	Intubation: 0.6 mg/kg (onset 50-80 sec) or 1.2 mg/kg (onset 30 sec) Maintenance: 0.1 mg/kg	Liver and renal	Recovery time 15-40 min (dose dependent); can be used for rapid-sequence intubation; infusion possible	Slight vagolytic effect
Vecuronium	Intermediate acting; nondepolarizing	Intubation: 0.1 mg/kg Maintenance: 0.02 mg/kg	Kidney and liver	Recovery time approx 30 min in children; no histamine release at up to 0.4 mg/kg; no effect on cardiovascular system	Long-acting muscle relaxant in infants; recovery time approx 70 min.
Pancuronium	Long acting; nondepolarizing	Intubation: 0.1 mg/kg Relaxation: 0.02 mg/kg	Kidney and liver	Recovery time approximately 50 min; inexpensive	Vagolytic effect; tachycardia; hypertension; histamine release

IV, intravenous.

in instances where immediate securing of the airway is necessary (e.g., laryngospasm, difficult airway, full stomach, or for IM route when a suitable vein is inaccessible).

Succinylcholine is broken down by plasma cholinesterase and is the reason for the short period of paralyzation (3 to 5 minutes). However, 1 in 3000 to 1 in 10,000 patients may be homozygous for an alternative version of the plasma cholinesterase enzyme. This enzyme has limited ability to bind and break down succinylcholine. In this patient population, muscle paralysis from succinylcholine can last up to 8 hours.[127]

Malignant Hyperthermia

MH is a life-threatening condition characterized by hyperthermia, hypermetabolism, and muscle injury that occurs in response to a triggering agent. Potent inhalation agents (not nitrous oxide) and the depolarizing muscle relaxant succinylcholine are two potent triggers in children. Triggers that stimulate MH cause excessive release of Ca^{2+} from the sarcoplasmic reticulum of skeletal muscle into the myoplasm, resulting in a chain of metabolic events that culminates in heat production, cell injury, hyperkalemia, and myoglobinemia.[128] The mortality rate for untreated MH is greater than 60%; rapid treatment with dantrolene reduces mortality to almost zero.

The incidence of fulminant MH is approximately 1 in 50,000 to 1 in 100,000 in adults and 1 in 3,000 to 1 in 15,000 in children. Most cases of MH occur in patients thought to be healthy. Predisposition to MH is a familial condition of multigenetic inheritance. First-degree relatives are at high risk; second-degree relatives have a lower but significant risk of MH developing in response to the appropriate triggering agents. Patients with Duchenne muscular dystrophy are thought to be at high risk for the development of MH. Other diseases associated with the development of MH are central core disease and King-Denborough syndrome.

The classic signs of MH include tachycardia, ventricular dysrhythmias, tachypnea, a rapid increase in temperature to greater than 39.5° C, rigidity of the jaw or generalized rigidity, metabolic and respiratory acidosis, and decreased mixed venous oxygen saturation. Associated laboratory values include hyperkalemia, hypercarbia, respiratory and metabolic acidosis, increased creatine phosphokinase and lactate levels, blood clotting abnormalities, and myoglobinuria.

The clinical diagnosis of MH should be considered before signs of hypermetabolism and elevated temperature reach extremes. The early signs of the disorder include tachypnea, tachycardia, increased end tidal carbon dioxide ($ETCO_2$), and ventricular dysrhythmias. These signs must be evaluated quickly because they can have many causes, such as iatrogenic hyperthermia, sepsis, pheochromocytoma, hyperthyroidism, ventilator valve malfunction with rebreathing of carbon dioxide, inadequate levels of anesthesia, and faulty temperature and $ETCO_2$ monitors.

Management of an acute episode of MH is outlined in Table 13-6. The cornerstone of treatment is IV dantrolene, which must be diluted with sterile, preservative-free, distilled water. The initial IV dose is 2.5 mg/kg, although much higher doses may be required. The usual dose limit of 10 mg/kg may be exceeded if necessary.[129] Dosing of dantrolene should be guided by clinical and laboratory signs and carried out every 5 minutes until metabolic acidosis has resolved. Dantrolene decreases the release of calcium from the sarcoplasmic reticulum by decreasing the mobility of calcium ions or the protein that transports calcium across membranes and is specific for skeletal muscle.[130,131] Dantrolene attenuates muscle hypermetabolism, reducing muscle rigidity and restoring normal muscle function. As skeletal muscle function normalizes, serum potassium levels decrease and abnormal lactic acid production slows.[132] Patients respond to dantrolene within 20 minutes. The $ETCO_2$ begins to decrease in 6 minutes, and arterial blood gas analysis demonstrates significant resolution of metabolic and respiratory acidosis within 20 minutes.[132] By 45 minutes, metabolic and respiratory acidosis and hyperthermia should be resolved. Dantrolene treatment at higher doses is necessary if metabolic dysfunction persists.[129]

Parents of an affected child may wish to have a muscle biopsy and contracture testing because negative findings mean that other relatives have no increased risk of MH.

In patients with a personal history or a strong family history of MH, surgery can be safely performed under regional or local anesthesia. General anesthesia with nontriggering agents can also be used. All nondepolarizing muscle relaxants and IV anesthetic agents are safe to use in patients who are susceptible to MH. Monitoring for the early signs of MH and initiating quick treatment are the most important aspects of caring for these patients.

Intravenous Anesthetic Agents

PROPOFOL

Propofol is a sedative-hypnotic, lipophilic IV agent used for induction and maintenance of anesthesia. It has become the IV agent of choice because of its favorable pharmacokinetic profile. The pharmacokinetics of propofol are characterized by rapid distribution, metabolism, and clearance. After termination of an infusion, redistribution to the peripheral tissues results in a prompt decrease in plasma concentration. Propofol is eliminated by hepatic conjugation to inactive metabolites, and excretion is by the renal route.[133]

Multiple studies have shown that the dose of propofol needed for induction is indirectly related to age. A typical induction dose is between 2.5 and 3.5 mg/kg.[134–137] Although the mechanisms that contribute to different dose requirements in younger children compared with older children have not been delineated, Westrin[137] hypothesized that because infants have a greater cardiac output in relation to body weight and a larger vessel-rich component, arterial peak concentration reaching the brain may be lower than that achieved in adults.

Propofol can induce hypotension, but the mechanism through which this occurs has not been clearly established.[135,138,139] Aun and associates[138] compared the hemodynamic responses to an induction dose of thiopental (5 mg/kg) or propofol (2.5 mg/kg) in 41 healthy children aged 8 months to 12 years. Heart rate, blood pressure, and velocity of flow were measured. The 28% to 31% reduction in mean arterial pressure after propofol administration was significantly greater than that after thiopental administration (14% and 21%, respectively). The 10% to 15% reduction in cardiac index was similar for both drugs. The children studied tolerated the hypotensive episodes without requiring pharmacologic intervention. Hannallah and associates[135] noted that like adults, children anesthetized with propofol have a slower heart rate than those given a volatile agent. Atropine may be useful to attenuate the bradycardia that can develop in young children when propofol and an IV opioid are used to maintain anesthesia. Keyl and colleagues[140] concluded that the vagally mediated heart rate response to cyclic peripheral baroreflex stimulation was markedly depressed during propofol anesthesia; there was also an impaired blood pressure response to cyclic baroreceptor stimulation.

TABLE 13-6

Management of Acute Episodes of Malignant Hyperthermia

Stop inhalation anesthetics immediately

Cancel or conclude surgery as soon as possible

Hyperventilate with high-flow 100% oxygen

Administer IV dantrolene (2.5 mg/kg) and repeat as needed

Give more dantrolene if signs of the condition reappear

Initiate cooling with hypothermia blanket, IV cold saline solution (15 mL/kg for 10 min), ice packs in the axillary region and groin, and lavage of body cavities with cold saline solution if core temperature is >37° C. Stop cooling when core temperature falls to 38° C

Correct metabolic acidosis with 1.0 to 2.0 mEq/kg sodium bicarbonate as an initial dose

Administer calcium (10 mg/kg calcium chloride) or insulin (0.2 U/kg) in 50% dextrose in water (1 mg/kg) to treat the effects of hyperkalemia

Administer lidocaine (1 mg/kg) to treat ventricular arrhythmias

Maintain urine output at 2 mL/kg/hr with furosemide (1 mg/kg) and additional mannitol if needed.

Insert arterial and central venous catheters

Repeat venous blood gas and electrolyte analysis every 15 min until signs of the disorder resolve and vital signs normalize

Pain at the site of injection occurs in up to 50% of patients receiving propofol through a vein in the dorsum of the hand.[141] Pain on injection of propofol can be attenuated or eliminated by injection through a large antecubital vein or by adding 0.1 mg/kg of lidocaine to every 2 to 3 mg/kg of propofol drawn into the syringe.[142]

Long-term sedation with propofol in the pediatric population is not recommended. Five deaths of infants and children (4 weeks to 6 years old) involving propofol infusions were reported in 1992.[143] These deaths involved lipemia, metabolic acidosis, hyperkalemia, and rhabdomyolysis. Further case reports have delineated what is now called propofol infusion syndrome (PIS). Risk factors for PIS include young age and propofol infusion rates of 70 μg/kg/min or greater for longer than 48 hours. However, there are reports of PIS in cases in which infusions were continued for less than 48 hours at lower levels.[144]

THIOPENTAL

Thiopental is a barbiturate induction agent that can be administered by the IV or rectal route. The dose required for IV induction varies with age. Several studies[145,146] confirmed previous findings by Cote and colleagues[147] and Brett and Fisher,[148] who showed that thiopental requirements are higher in children (Fig.13-3). Barbiturates decrease cerebral blood flow and intracranial pressure. The direct myocardial depression and venodilatation caused by thiopental are well tolerated by healthy children.[145] In patients who are hemodynamically compromised, however, these cardiovascular effects can result in significant hypotension. Thiopental should be avoided in children who are dehydrated, have heart failure, or have lost a significant amount of blood. Side effects seen with an induction dose of thiopental include hiccups, cough, and laryngospasm. Valtonen and associates[149] reported these side effects in 20% of children aged 1 to 6 years. Extravasation can cause tissue injury caused by thiopental's alkalinity. Barbiturates also cause histamine release, which is why they are often avoided in patients with a history of asthma.[150,151]

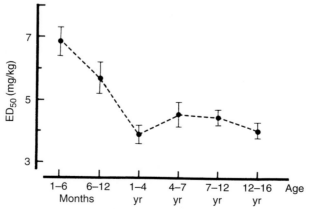

FIGURE 13-3 Estimated ED$_{50}$ (the dose of a drug that will induce anesthesia in 50% of patients) plus or minus the standard error for thiopental in various age groups. (From Jonmarker C, Westrin P, Larsson S, Werner O. Thiopental requirements for induction of anesthesia in children. Anesthesiology 1987;67:104.)

KETAMINE

Ketamine is a derivative of phencyclidine that antagonizes N-methyl-D-aspartate (NMDA) receptors. It causes a central dissociation of the cerebral cortex along with causing cerebral excitation. It is an excellent analgesic and amnestic, with recommended doses of 1 to 3 mg/kg IV, 5 to 10 mg/kg IM, or 5 to 10 mg/kg PO. The IV dose has a duration of 5 to 8 minutes. Glycopyrrolate or similar antisialagogue should be given for the copious secretions associated with ketamine use.

Ketamine increases heart rate, cardiac index, and systemic blood pressure. It also causes bronchodilation with minimal effects on respiration.[152,153] There is no direct effect on pediatric pulmonary artery pressure as long as ventilation is controlled. Its systemic effects are sympathetically mediated. However, ketamine will cause bradycardia and a decrease in systemic vascular resistance in patients who are depleted of catecholamine. Also, it is the only IV anesthetic to increase both intracranial pressure and intraocular pressure. Therefore, it is relatively contraindicated in patients in whom these increases could be detrimental.

ETOMIDATE

Etomidate is a steroid-based hypnotic that has minimal effects on the hemodynamics or cardiac function of a patient at clinical doses. It also has minimal effects on respiratory parameters. Therefore, it is useful in pediatric patients with known or anticipated hemodynamic instability. The main drawbacks to its routine use are pain with injection and adrenal suppression even after one dose. Typical dosages for induction are 0.2 to 0.3 mg/kg IV.

Monitoring

NONINVASIVE MONITORING

The ASA has established standards for basic anesthesia monitoring, which include continuous evaluation of the patient's oxygenation, ventilation, circulation, and temperature during the use of all anesthetics. Delivery of an adequate oxygen concentration is ensured by measuring the inspired concentration of oxygen in the patient's breathing system using an oxygen analyzer on the anesthesia machine. Blood oxygenation is measured by pulse oximetry. Ventilation is ensured by qualitative clinical signs such as chest excursion, observation of the reservoir breathing bag, and auscultation of breath sounds as well as continual monitoring for the presence of end-tidal carbon dioxide. When ventilation is controlled by a mechanical ventilator, a continuous device that is capable of detecting the disconnection of system components is used. Circulation is monitored by a continuously displayed electrocardiogram, arterial blood pressure reading, and heart rate, which is determined and evaluated at least every 5 minutes. In addition, adequate circulation is ensured by auscultation of heart sounds, palpation of a pulse, monitoring of a tracing of intraarterial pressure, ultrasonographic pulse monitoring, or pulse plethysmography or oximetry. Temperature monitoring is required to aid in the maintenance of appropriate body temperature during all anesthesia.[154]

Temperature Monitoring

The oral or nasal cavity is the most common site for temperature measurement in the pediatric population. Midesophageal or nasopharyngeal temperature better reflects core temperature compared with rectal or tympanic measurements. However, tympanic temperature theoretically provides ideal information because it most closely reflects the temperature of the brain. Rectal temperature is also a common site for temperature measurement, despite the following disadvantages: (1) potential for perforation of the bowel wall with a stiff thermistor probe wire, (2) potential dislodging of the probe, and (3) excessive warming of the thin tissues of the perianal and coccygeal area by the circulating warm water mattress. A more fundamental objection is that rectal temperatures, in general, do not promptly track rapid temperature changes, such as those that occur during deliberate hypothermia or rewarming.

Pulse Oximetry

Continuous, noninvasive monitoring of arterial oxygen saturation (Sao_2) can be accomplished by pulse oximetry. The oximeter is usually placed on a finger or toe, but any site is acceptable as long as a pulsating vascular bed can be interposed between the two elements. Two wavelengths of light chosen for their relative reflectance with oxygenated versus deoxygenated hemoglobin illuminate the tissue under the probe. Through expansion and relaxation, the pulsating vascular bed changes the length of the light path, thereby modifying the amount of light detected. The result is a characteristic plethysmographic waveform, and artifacts from blood, skin, connective tissue, or bone are eliminated. This technique is accurate with oxygen saturation values from 70% to 100%. Reduction in vascular pulsation—for example, with hypothermia, hypotension, or the use of vasoconstrictive drugs—diminishes the instrument's ability to calculate saturation. In addition to a continuous indication of Sao_2, the pulse oximeter usually provides a continuous readout of pulse rate and amplitude.

Capnography

The presence of end tidal CO_2 ($ETco_2$) is the gold standard in confirming proper endotracheal tube placement and measuring the adequacy of ventilation. Plotting $ETco_2$ versus time produces the classic time-capnograph curve. In Figure 13-4, *A*, the curve represents an ideal time-capnograph tracing during quiet respiration with no rebreathing of exhaled gas. The maximum value of $ETco_2$ at number 4 represents alveolar gas, which is in equilibrium with arterial CO_2 ($Paco_2$). In the absence of any ventilation-perfusion (V/Q) mismatch, the value at 4 should be within 2 to 4 mm Hg of $Paco_2$. Any discrepancy that is larger points to an increase in V/Q mismatch due to larger dead-space ventilation.

An ideal capnographic tracing cannot always be obtained, but the abnormal curve may be diagnostic or highly suggestive of certain types of problems involving the patient, the anesthesia circuit, or the ventilation technique. In Figure 13-4, *B*, several capnographic tracings are presented that represent changes or pathologic features in ventilation. In all of these, the maximum obtained $ETco_2$ is no longer indicative of $Paco_2$.

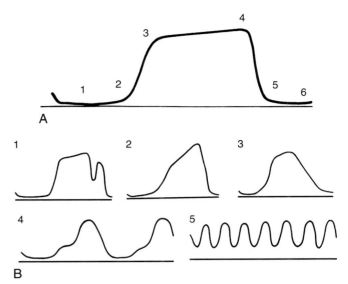

FIGURE 13-4   **A,** Ideal capnographic tracing. Exhalation begins *(1)*. Anatomic dead space is cleared *(1-2)*. Dead-space air mixes with alveolar gas *(2-3)*. Alveolar plateau *(3-4)*. End-tidal maximum value; inspiration begins *(4)*. Dead-space air is cleared *(4-5)*. Inspiratory gas is devoid of carbon dioxide *(5-6)*. **B,** Types of capnographic tracings: Efforts at spontaneous breathing with incomplete neuromuscular blockade *(1)*. Respiratory obstruction *(2)*. Lack of sustained pressure resulting from a large leak in the breathing system *(3)*. In the Mapleson D system, when large amounts of fresh gas flow at small tidal volumes, the expired carbon dioxide is diluted and achievement of a stable alveolar plateau is prevented *(4)*. The effect of partial rebreathing of carbon dioxide from the expiratory limb of the Mapleson D system, when fresh gas flows at small amounts, is excessively rapid ventilation and small tidal breaths *(5)*.

Monitoring Neuromuscular Function

The only satisfactory method of monitoring neuromuscular function is stimulation of an accessible peripheral motor nerve and observation or measurement of the response of the skeletal muscle supplied by this nerve. Various nerve stimulators are commercially available. Usually, the ulnar nerve is stimulated at the wrist with surface electrodes, and the response of the adductor pollicis brevis is noted. Supramaximal electrical stimuli are necessary to ensure full activation of the nerve. The evoked response to single repeated nerve stimuli at 0.1 Hz or train-of-four stimulation at a low frequency (2 Hz for 2 seconds) allows continuous monitoring of neuromuscular transmission after the administration of muscle relaxants. Tetanic rates of stimulation (50 Hz), train-of-four ratios, or double-burst stimulation allow the assessment of neurotransmission after reversal.

In adults clinical signs of adequate neuromuscular transmission include the ability to sustain a head lift for 5 seconds in conjunction with a vital capacity of at least 15 to 20 mL/kg or a negative inspiratory force of 30 cm H_2O. Because an infant cannot lift the head for 5 seconds, the ability to flex its arms or legs is a reliable sign of adequate neuromuscular transmission. Because vital capacity cannot easily be determined in infants, inspiratory force is measured instead. The ability to sustain tetany of 30 to 50 Hz for 5 seconds or a near-normal train-of-four ratio (>0.7) is also a reliable sign of adequate neuromuscular transmission.

INVASIVE MONITORING

The availability of sophisticated noninvasive monitoring devices has reduced the need for invasive monitoring. The need for invasive monitoring is driven more by patient condition than by surgical procedure.[155] Intraarterial and, to a lesser degree, central venous and pulmonary artery catheters are required for the continuous measurement of pulse, intravascular pressures, and serial arterial blood gas concentrations, blood chemistry values, and coagulation abnormalities intraoperatively and postoperatively for extended periods in critically ill patients.

The most desirable site for arterial sampling is the right radial artery, where the concentration of oxygen tension most closely resembles that of the carotid artery. Postductal arteries have lower oxygen tension in the presence of right-to-left shunting and may become occluded during procedures such as repair of coarctation of the aorta. When the radial artery is not available, the femoral, dorsalis pedis, or posterior tibial artery may be used. In infants, the brachial and axillary arteries are generally avoided because of the risk of loss of the limb. Femoral artery catheterization may be complicated by joint injury, and cannulation of the superficial temporal artery is associated with a risk of temporal lobe infarction resulting from retrograde perfusion of the vessel during flushing. Despite their accessibility during the first 10 days of life, umbilical arteries are a limited option because the incidence of infection is high. In addition, because of the risk for thrombosis and embolism, the catheter tip must be carefully positioned above the diaphragm or below the third or fourth lumbar vertebra away from the origins of the celiac, mesenteric, and renal arteries. Also, when blood is sampled from below a patent ductus arteriosus in a patient with right-to-left shunting, oxygen saturation in the umbilical arteries may be less than that of the carotid or right radial artery and thus lead to the administration of dangerously high oxygen concentrations.

The indications for central venous catheterization, and especially for flow-directed pulmonary artery (Swan-Ganz) catheters, are limited in infants and children. The procedure is probably indicated more often for patients in the intensive care unit than for those in the operating room. Central venous catheterization is indicated for patients having operations involving major blood loss, shock, and low-flow states. The preferred route of access for either catheter is the internal jugular vein, although the subclavian and femoral veins are alternatives. Placing the catheter and monitoring the pressure in a major vein returning blood to the heart allows proper maintenance or adjustment of the patient's circulating blood volume.[155] Possible complications include atrial or ventricular arrhythmias, thromboembolic phenomena, hemothorax, pneumothorax, and infection.

Pain Management

Children of all ages feel pain. Although progress remains to be made, recent interest in and awareness of pain in pediatric patients, along with philosophical shifts and technical advances, have markedly improved pain management for children.[156,157]

Appropriate care of pediatric surgical patients entails pain management tailored to each child's age, emotional and developmental maturity, and surgical procedure. Children's ability to both experience pain and to tolerate potent analgesia has been questioned.[158,159] Many pediatric patients undergo surgery without adequate pain management. Historically, up to 40% of children undergoing surgical procedures have reported moderate to severe pain on the first postoperative day.[160] Although many children continue to receive inadequate perioperative analgesia, the evolution of integrated, multidisciplinary approaches has dramatically improved treatment strategies for pediatric surgical patients.[161] Preoperative, intraoperative, and postoperative strategies for minimizing pain should be based on the planned surgical procedure, anticipated severity of postoperative pain, anesthesia technique, and expected course of recovery.[162] Children must be reassessed at frequent intervals, with analgesic regimens modified accordingly.

Acute pain is a physiologic response to actual or impending tissue damage and may provide helpful information regarding the location and nature of injury or illness. Accordingly, there is often reluctance to provide potent analgesia to patients who will potentially undergo surgical procedures before obtaining a definitive diagnosis. It is now increasingly recognized that this dramatically undertreats pain in such patients, particularly children.[163] Appropriately titrated analgesia not only relieves pain and reduces distress but also often allows a more thorough and accurate evaluation, particularly in frightened or uncooperative pediatric patients. IV morphine, for example, provides significant analgesia to children with acute abdominal pain without masking focal tenderness or impairing the clinical diagnosis of appendicitis.[164] The traditional teaching that potent analgesia must be withheld from patients, including children, who may potentially have diagnoses requiring surgery is invalid and should be abandoned.

PERIOPERATIVE PLANNING AND GENERAL APPROACH

The goal of perioperative pain management is to maximize patient comfort while minimizing side effects such as excessive sedation or respiratory depression. Multiple techniques are available and are chosen and titrated to effect based on each child's particular needs. Planning begins with the preoperative anesthesia evaluation and continues throughout the surgical procedure and postoperative period.

Nonpharmacologic techniques, such as distraction and guided imagery, may augment analgesia, enhance patient cooperation, and minimize pharmacologic therapy.[165] Nonopioid analgesics most commonly include acetaminophen, nonsteroidal antiinflammatory agents, and ketamine. Oral opioids are often adequate for the treatment of mild to moderate pain, whereas IV opioids are the mainstay of therapy for moderate to severe pain. Persistent requirement for IV opioids can be managed with continuous infusion or patient-controlled analgesia (PCA) modalities. Regional anesthesia may also be used as part of a comprehensive analgesia regimen. A useful paradigm that can be applied to pediatric pain management is the World Health Organization's analgesic ladder (Fig. 13-5).[166]

DEVELOPMENT AND PHYSIOLOGY

Children of all ages feel pain, but the type and intensity may vary dramatically. Although peripheral nociceptors are fully functional at birth,[167–170] central modulation and pain

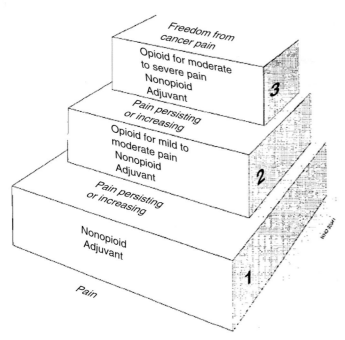

FIGURE 13-5 First proposed in 1986 as a protocol for managing cancer pain, the analgesic ladder has become a popular and effective model for pain management in a variety of settings and can be applied to pediatric surgical patients. (From World Health Organization: Cancer Pain Relief: With a Guide to Opioid Availability, ed 2. Geneva, World Health Organization, 1996, p 15.)

perception in children are not well understood. Further, many reflex pathways allowing the expression of nociception are structurally and functionally immature in neonates and young infants.[171] Thus, although peripheral nociceptors register painful stimuli, central processing of pain in these young patients is more variable, and their ability to indicate pain perception is more limited. The response of infants and young children to pain is therefore unpredictable, particularly in premature neonates,[170] which often leads to inadequate pain management.

HYPERSENSITIZATION AND PREEMPTIVE ANALGESIA

Acute pain is a physiologic response to actual or impending tissue damage. Untreated, persistent, or severe pain, however, may contribute to potentially detrimental pathophysiologic processes.[170,172] Tissue injury and inflammation enhance peripheral nociceptor activity, resulting in hypersensitivity to mechanical and chemical stimuli. In animal models, dorsal horn neurons respond to sustained afferent stimulation with neurophysiologic and morphologic changes consistent with increased excitability. The development of peripheral and central hypersensitization may alter normal sensory perception (dysesthesia), accentuate pain due to noxious stimuli (hyperalgesia), and produce pain in response to normally innocuous processes (allodynia), suggesting that hypersensitization at the cellular and neurophysiologic level correlates with clinical hypersensitivity to pain.

Preemptive analgesia before tissue injury may inhibit stimulation of nociceptive pathways, blunting the neuroendocrine stress response and preventing the development of peripheral and central hypersensitivity.[173] General anesthesia alone is ineffective for such purposes; nonsteroidal antiinflammatory drugs (NSAIDs), opioids, and a variety of local anesthesia techniques have been studied in animal models, with variable results.[173–175] Animal models generally suggest that preemptive analgesia, before noxious stimuli decreases dorsal horn neuron hyperexcitability, blunts observed pain behaviors and lowers clinical analgesic requirements. Human studies, however, have yielded conflicting and frequently negative results, particularly in children.[176–182] Subjective pain scores, objective assessments, and analgesic requirements are not dramatically affected in most patients by varying the timing of the analgesic technique before or after surgery. Preemptive analgesia as a strategy for blunting hypersensitization and reducing perioperative pain remains a subject of ongoing investigation and controversy.[183–187]

PAIN ASSESSMENT

Pain assessment in pediatric patients can be challenging. Preverbal or developmentally delayed children may be unable to convey the severity or even the presence of pain to caregivers. In patients of any age, it may be difficult to distinguish pain from agitation. Nonetheless, pain in children should be recognized, assessed, and treated promptly.

Numerous tools have been developed and prospectively validated to allow ongoing quantitative assessment of pain in children of all ages and developmental skills.[188,189] In preverbal, young, or developmentally delayed patients, numerous tools allow the quantitative assessment of pain intensity by generating a pain score derived from the objective assessment of various pain-associated behaviors. The recently developed neonatal pain, agitation, and sedation scale (N-PASS) is a useful tool to assess pain in neonates 0 to 100 days of age and may also be applied to intubated or extremely premature children.[190–192] The face, legs, activity, cry, and consolability (FLACC) scoring system is valid and reliable for pain assessment in patients 5 to 16 years of age. Analog scales, useful for school-aged patients, use drawings or photographs of faces in varying degrees of distress, with colors, arrows, lines, or numbers (usually 0 to 10) for patients to indicate their level of pain.[193] Subjective, self-reported analog pain scores and objective, behavioral assessment pain scores in children are often discordant,[194] likely reflecting difficulties in distinguishing pain, agitation, and other causes of distress. The particular pain assessment tool chosen is less important than application of the tool to the appropriate population and consistent use of the tool in each patient over time.

NONOPIOID ANALGESICS

Often overlooked, nonopioid analgesics are important adjunctive agents in pediatric pain management. They are often adequate for mild to moderate pain and may reduce opioid requirement in cases of moderate to severe pain.[195] Unlike opioids, nonopioid analgesics generally demonstrate a ceiling effect: exceeding recommended doses does not significantly improve analgesia but does increase the risk of side effects and toxicity.[196] Common nonopioid analgesics for children include acetaminophen, various NSAIDs, and in appropriate settings ketamine (Table 13-7).

TABLE 13-7

Common Nonopioid Analgesics for Children

Drug	Dose	Comments
Acetaminophen	20 mg/kg PO load (max 1000 mg), then	Good antipyretic
	15 mg/kg PO (max 1000 mg) q4h	Hepatic toxicity with overdose
	40 mg/kg PR load (max 1300 mg), then	
	20 mg/kg PR (max 1300 mg) q4h	
	Max 4 g/24 hr PO or PR	
Selected nonsteroidal anti-inflammatory drugs (NSAIDs)		
Choline magnesium trisalicylate	10 mg/kg PO or PR (max 1000 mg) q6h	Good antipyretic
	Max 4 g/24 hr	Only NSAID without platelet dysfunction
		No association with Reye syndrome
Ibuprofen	10 mg/kg PO or PR (max 800 mg) q6h	Good antipyretic
	Max 4 g/24 hr	
Ketorolac	0.5 mg/kg IM or IV (max 30 mg) q6h	Poor antipyretic
	Total duration must be <5 days	Potentially significant platelet dysfunction
Ketamine (requires appropriate personnel and monitoring)	4.0-10.0 mg/kg PO (adult dose, 300-500 mg)	Anticholinergic agent; reduces sialorrhea
	3.0-5.0 mg/kg IM (adult dose, 150-300 mg)	Benzodiazepine; may prevent agitation
	0.5-1.0 mg/kg IV (adult dose, 50-100 mg)	Increases intracranial pressure; may precipitate seizures

IM, intramuscular; PO, orally; IV, intravenous.

Acetaminophen

Acetaminophen remains popular for the management of mild to moderate pain in children and as an antipyretic. Acetaminophen is a potent inhibitor of cyclooxygenase but has virtually no antiinflammatory activity and therefore few gastrointestinal, renal, or hematologic complications. The primary toxicity of acetaminophen is hepatic injury, seen with acute and chronic overdose. Acetaminophen may provide complete analgesia for mild to moderate pain and reduces opioid requirements in the treatment of moderate to severe pain, particularly when given on a scheduled basis. Procedural and perioperative analgesia with acetaminophen is enhanced by NSAIDs.[197]

Acetaminophen is available in a variety of oral and rectal preparations in the United States (see Table 13-7); IV preparations are available in other countries. The total dose should not exceed 4 g/day.

Rectal absorption of acetaminophen is slower and bioavailability is more variable than with oral administration, requiring higher doses for equivalent analgesia.[198] Although rectal acetaminophen has been shown to reduce pain scores and lower opioid requirements after surgical procedures, including myringotomy tube placement and inguinal hernia repair,[199] at least 40 mg/kg must be given.[200]

Nonsteroidal Antiinflammatory Drugs

Like acetaminophen, NSAIDs may provide adequate analgesia for mild to moderate pain and are useful in conjunction with opioids in the management of moderate to severe pain.[202,201] NSAIDs are particularly effective for musculoskeletal pain. Unlike acetaminophen, NSAIDs have significant antiinflammatory activity. NSAIDs reduce mesenteric and renal perfusion and impair platelet function, potentially causing gastrointestinal ischemia, renal insufficiency, and bleeding. Risk is higher with elevated doses or prolonged administration.

Choline magnesium trisalicylate is the only NSAID that does not cause significant platelet dysfunction and may be useful in patients with coagulopathy or those who are at risk for bleeding during surgery. Pediatric aspirin use has declined dramatically since the described association with Reye syndrome in children with primary varicella.[196] Although choline magnesium trisalicylate is an aspirin derivative, it has no known association with Reye syndrome; nonetheless, it may be prudent to limit its use in children to patients who have previously had primary varicella or received varicella immunization. Choline magnesium trisalicylate is available in liquid and tablet preparations; the liquid preparation can be given rectally at the same dose to patients unwilling or unable to tolerate oral administration (see Table 13-7). The total dose should not exceed 4 g/day.

The most widely used oral NSAID in children in the United States is ibuprofen, available in a variety of liquid, tablet, and capsule preparations (see Table 13-7). An IV formulation is now available but is licensed only for medical closure of patent ductus arteriosus in infants. Ibuprofen is a moderate-potency analgesic and an excellent antipyretic with an impressive pediatric safety record, but it is still underused for procedural and perioperative pain management in children.[201] The liquid preparation can be given rectally at the same dose as choline magnesium trisalicylate. The total dose should not exceed 4 g/day.

Ketorolac is the only NSAID available for IV use as an analgesic (see Table 13-7). Indomethacin may be given IV but is approved only for medical closure of patent ductus arteriosus in infants. Ketorolac is a high-potency NSAID with an analgesic efficacy similar to that of many opioids and provides superior perioperative analgesia compared with other NSAIDs or acetaminophen.[203] Ketorolac may be particularly useful in patients who are intolerant of opioids, or in procedures that involve a high risk of postoperative nausea and emesis. Initially approved only for IM administration, ketorolac is safe and effective when given IV.[204] Oral ketorolac administration is approved for adults but not for children.

The volume of distribution and plasma clearance rate of ketorolac in children are roughly twice those in adults, but the overall elimination half-life is similar.[205] As the most potent NSAID, ketorolac also has the highest incidence of side effects; total duration of therapy must not exceed 5 days to avoid potentially serious gastrointestinal and renal complications. Given its ability to compromise mesenteric perfusion, ketorolac should probably be avoided in infants at risk for necrotizing enterocolitis.

Significant platelet dysfunction may develop after a single dose of ketorolac, and its use in patients at high risk for bleeding is controversial. Initial experience indicated greater intraoperative blood loss during tonsillectomy in children receiving perioperative ketorolac,[198] and retrospective studies reported higher rates of postoperative hemorrhage.[206,207] Other retrospective studies suggested otherwise,[208] and prospective, randomized trials have shown only statistically insignificant trends toward increased bleeding.[209] The product literature warns against using ketorolac in patients at high risk of bleeding; it is probably prudent to avoid administering ketorolac to such patients until more definitive information is available.

Ketamine

Ketamine can be used as an adjuvant analgesic in perioperative pain management. More recently, ketamine has been recommended for procedural analgesia and sedation in children in a variety of settings[210,211] and has become particularly popular in pediatric emergency departments, given its favorable safety profile.[212,213] Concomitant administration of anticholinergic agents to prevent sialorrhea, and benzodiazepines to decrease the likelihood of hallucinations and delirium, has traditionally been recommended. Recent data suggest these practices are of limited efficacy.[214] Adequate monitoring and immediate availability of appropriate resuscitation equipment and personnel are mandatory for children receiving Oketamine.[215]

OPIOID ANALGESICS

Reluctance to use opioids in children is a common excuse for inadequate pain management in the pediatric population. Opioids are the mainstay of pharmacologic therapy for moderate to severe pain, however, and have established roles in procedural and perioperative pain management for children.[216] Acting on various subtypes of opioid receptors throughout the CNS, opioids cause dose-dependent pain relief and respiratory depression; other side effects include somnolence, miosis, decreased gastrointestinal motility, nausea, and urinary retention. Many opioids induce histamine release, causing urticaria, pruritus, nausea, bronchospasm, and occasionally hypotension. Pruritus is more common, and typically more intense, with neuraxial administration, likely owing to the CNS opioid effect rather than histamine release. Opioid side effects can be managed with a variety of agents (Table 13-8).

The opioid receptor antagonist naloxone rapidly reverses opioid effects. Mild respiratory depression or somnolence can be treated with IV naloxone 1.0 µg/kg titrated every 1 to 2 minutes as needed; doses of 10 to 100 µg/kg should be reserved for apnea or coma secondary to opioid overdose. Higher or repeated doses may be necessary. Naloxone may precipitate withdrawal in opioid-dependent patients, and pulmonary edema has been reported with higher doses. A low-dose naloxone infusion (0.25 µg/kg/min) may reduce the incidence of unwanted opioid side effects without significantly affecting analgesia for patients on patient-controlled opioid analgesic regimens.[217] Opioid analgesics do not generally have maximum effective doses. Recommended doses are for initial administration in opioid-naive patients; titration to clinical effect is required, and higher doses may be necessary. Increased dosage requirements (tolerance, tachyphylaxis) are often observed with prolonged administration or persistent pain. Opioid therapy longer than 7 to 10 days may result

---

TABLE 13-8

Agents for Management of Opioid Side Effects

Side Effect	Agent	Dose	Comments
Apnea, coma	Naloxone	10-100 µg/kg IV or IM q1-2 min PRN Usual initial max: 400 µg Higher or repeated doses may be required	Resedation may occur Withdrawal in opioid-dependent patients Higher doses may cause pulmonary edema
Mild respiratory depression, mild sedation	Naloxone	1.0 µg/kg IV or IM q1-2 min PRN Usual initial max: 400 µg Higher or repeated doses may be required	Resedation may occur
Constipation	Docusate	5.0 mg/kg PO (max 100 mg) bid	Stool softener
Nausea	Metoclopramide	0.1 mg/kg IV (max 10 mg) q6h PRN	Extrapyramidal side effects
	Ondansetron	0.1 mg/kg IV (max 4.0 mg) q6h PRN	Expensive
	Promethazine	0.25-0.5 mg/kg PO, PR, or IV (max 25 mg) q6h PRN	May cause somnolence
Pruritus	Diphenhydramine	0.5-1.0 mg/kg PO or IV (max 50 mg) q6h PRN	May cause somnolence
	Hydroxyzine	0.5-1.0 mg/kg PO or IV (max 50 mg) q6h PRN	May cause somnolence
	Nalbuphine	0.05 µg/kg IV (max 5.0 mg) q4h PRN	For pruritus from neuraxial opioid
	Naloxone	1.0 µg/kg/hr IV infusion	For pruritus from neuraxial opioid

IM, intramuscular; IV, intravenous; PO, orally; PRN, as needed;

in physical dependence, requiring weaning before discontinuation to avoid withdrawal.[218] Tolerance and dependence may occur independently. Addiction, a psychopathologic condition of volitional drug-seeking behavior, rarely develops in children receiving appropriately dosed opioids for analgesia and is not a valid reason to withhold therapy.[216] Opioids are commonly administered in conjunction with sedative-hypnotic agents, particularly benzodiazepines, increasing the risk of respiratory depression and desaturation.[219–221] Careful titration of doses, appropriate monitoring, and full capability to manage complications, including respiratory depression and apnea, are essential. Appropriate reversal agents should be available.

Opioid use in neonates and young infants has been the subject of much investigation and controversy. Historical studies in rats and humans suggested increased permeability of the neonatal blood-brain barrier to opioids, particularly morphine, and greater clinical respiratory depression.[222,223] It has more recently and more accurately been realized that the pharmacologic properties and clinical effects of morphine,[224–228] fentanyl,[229] and indeed all opioids in human neonates are subject to great individual variability. In general, opioid clearance is decreased and elimination is more prolonged in neonates than in older children, with values approaching adult levels by several months of age. There is no intrinsic reason to withhold opioid therapy from children of any age provided that doses are individualized to each patient and titrated to clinical effect.

Oral Opioids

When pain needs allow and gastrointestinal function permits, oral opioids offer freedom from parenteral therapy. Onset of action is relatively slow, rendering oral opioid therapy unsuitable for the acute management of severe pain. Several lower-potency oral opioids are used commonly in children (Table 13-9), providing adequate analgesia for mild to moderate pain.

Codeine, available in liquid and tablet preparations, is commonly used in combination with acetaminophen. Codeine has a high rate of gastrointestinal upset. Hydrocodone, available in liquid and tablet preparations, is also usually used in combination with acetaminophen or an NSAID. Hydrocodone tends to cause less gastrointestinal upset than does codeine. Oxycodone is available in tablet preparations containing only oxycodone or in combination with acetaminophen or an NSAID; liquid preparations contain only oxycodone. This analgesic causes little gastrointestinal upset and is generally well tolerated. Sustained-release oxycodone is available for chronic therapy.

Although often given IV, higher-potency opioids may also be given orally (Table 13-10). The histamine release induced by morphine may cause urticaria, pruritus, bronchospasm, and even hypotension at higher doses, although these are less common with oral administration. Sustained-release oral morphine is available for chronic therapy. Hydromorphone causes less histamine release than does morphine. Methadone is particularly useful for chronic therapy in opioid-dependent patients.[230] Treatment of psychopathologic opioid addiction with methadone may be undertaken only in federally licensed facilities.

Oral transmucosal fentanyl citrate (OTFC) is a formulation of fentanyl in a lozenge attached to a stick. Oral transmucosal

TABLE 13-9

Lower-Potency Oral Opioids for Children

Drug	Dose	Comments
Codeine	1.0 mg/kg PO q4h (adult dose, 30-60 mg)	Tablet and liquid preparations
		Usually in combination products with acetaminophen
		High rate of GI side effects
Hydrocodone	0.2 mg/kg PO q4h (adult dose, 10-15 mg)	Tablet and liquid preparations
		Usually in combination products with acetaminophen or NSAID
		Moderate rate of GI side effects
Oxycodone	0.1 mg/kg PO q4h (adult dose, 5-10 mg)	Tablet preparations as oxycodone or in combination products with acetaminophen or NSAID
		Liquid preparation as oxycodone
		Low rate of GI side effects
		Sustained-release product available for chronic therapy

GI, gastrointestinal; NSAID, nonsteroidal anti-inflammatory drug; PO, orally.

fentanyl citrate may provide effective preanesthetic sedation in children,[231,232] as well as analgesia and sedation for painful procedures,[233] although nausea and emesis are common. Appropriate monitoring is required.

Intravenous Opioids

IV opioids are the mainstay of therapy for moderate to severe pain (see Table 13-10). Subcutaneous or IM administration, although pharmacologically reliable, causes additional pain and distress, particularly in children, and should be avoided.[234–236] Side effects are more common and potentially more serious with IV opioids, mandating appropriate monitoring and prompt management of complications. Neonates and young infants receiving IV opioids should be monitored particularly closely, and doses should be reduced by 25% to 50%. Equipotent doses of opioids entail a similar risk of side effects.[216]

Morphine is the traditional IV opioid analgesic but hydromorphone causes less histamine release. Although historically popular, meperidine offers no significant advantages over other opioids and causes no less hepatobiliary spasm at equipotent doses. Meperidine is useful at lower doses for the treatment of shivering but is no longer recommended as a primary analgesic.[216,218,237,238] A benefit of IV methadone is its longer duration of action with dosing regimens suggested at 6 to 12 hours. Pediatric surgical patients receiving intraoperative methadone require less subsequent analgesia than those receiving intraoperative morphine.[235] The risk of respiratory depression and other opioid side effects is also prolonged with methadone.

Fentanyl is commonly used for procedural and perioperative pain management in children because of its rapid onset and short duration of action. Fentanyl is highly lipophilic; high-dose, repeated, or sustained administration results in

TABLE 13-10

Higher-Potency Opioids for Children

Drug	Dose*	Comments
Fentanyl	5-15 μg/kg PO (adult dose, 400 μg)	Oral preparation for single-dose use
	0.5-1.0 μg/kg IV (adult dose, 50-100 μg) q1h	Rapid infusion may cause chest wall rigidity in infants
	Infusion: 0.5-1.0 μg/kg/hr (adult dose, 50-100 μg/hr)	Transdermal patch not for acute management
	Patch: 25 μg = 1 mg/hr IV morphine	
Hydromorphone	20-40 μg/kg PO (adult dose, 2.0-4.0 mg) q3h	Less histamine release than morphine
	10-20 μg/kg IM, IV, or SC (adult dose 1.0-2.0 mg) q3h	
	Infusion: 4 μg/kg/hr (adult dose, 0.2-0.3 mg/hr)	
Meperidine	1.0 mg/kg PO, IM, IV, or SC (adult dose, 50-100 mg) q3h	Neurotoxic metabolite may cause seizures; higher risk with renal disease
	Infusion: not recommended	No hepatobiliary advantages
Methadone	0.1 mg/kg PO (adult dose, 5-10 mg) q6-12h	Useful for long-term therapy, including palliative care
	0.05 mg/kg IV (adult dose, 2.5-5.0 mg) q6-12h	Treatment of opioid addiction must be in a federally licensed facility
	Infusion: not generally used	
Morphine	0.3 mg/kg PO (adult dose, 15-30 mg) q3h	Histamine release may cause urticaria, pruritus, bronchospasm, hypotension
	0.1 mg/kg IM, IV, or SC (adult dose, 5-10 mg) q3h	
	Infusion: 0.02 mg/kg/hr (adult dose, 1.0-1.5 mg/hr)	High dose and rapid administration increase histamine release
		Sustained-release oral preparation available for chronic therapy

*Recommended doses are for initial administration in opioid-naive patients; titration to clinical effect is required, and higher doses may be necessary. Doses should be reduced 25% to 50% in neonates and young infants.
IM, intramuscular; IV, intravenous; PO, orally; SC, subcutaneous.

significant tissue accumulation and a markedly prolonged duration of effect.[239] Fentanyl is also available as a transdermal patch that provides continuous transcutaneous absorption, mimicking IV infusion; one 25-μg fentanyl patch is roughly equivalent to 1.0 mg/hour IV morphine. Onset is slow, and absorption is somewhat variable. Although useful in some settings for the management of chronic pain, transdermal fentanyl is not indicated for acute pain management.[216,240]

Continuous infusion is an effective means of providing analgesia to infants and children requiring more than occasional doses of IV opioids. Respiratory depression is uncommon in healthy patients at suggested doses, which neither prevent spontaneous ventilation nor hamper weaning from mechanical ventilatory support.[241] Methadone infusion is generally neither necessary nor helpful in most children because of the drug's long half-life. Adequacy of analgesia, level of sedation, and degree of respiratory depression should be followed closely, and the infusion titrated as required. All patients receiving continuous opioid infusions should probably receive continuous pulse oximetry, with cardiorespiratory monitoring for neonates and young infants. Doses in opioid-naive neonates and young infants should generally be reduced by 25% to 50%.[242,243]

Patient-Controlled Analgesia

Historically, it has been all too common to provide opioids only after patients feel pain. This can lead to a vicious circle of symptomatic pain followed by frequently delayed administration of medication, with the resultant risk of persistent pain or excessive sedation (Fig. 13-6).[244] This pattern exposes patients to potentially significant opioid side effects while providing only intermittent analgesia. Optimally, opioid levels should be maintained above the threshold for analgesia but below that for obtundation or apnea, preserving a balance between desired efficacy and undesired toxicity (Fig. 13-7).[245] Intermittent bolus dosing of opioids at appropriate intervals

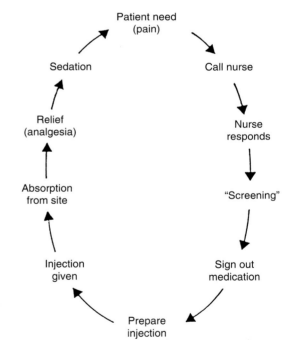

FIGURE 13-6 Vicious circle of conventional opioid therapy. (From Graves DA, Foster TS, Batenhorst RL, et al: Patient-controlled analgesia. Ann Intern Med 1983;99:360-366.)

before patients experience pain may maintain opioid levels within this analgesic window, but this is time-consuming for staff and entails the risk of drug accumulation. Continuous opioid infusion eventually establishes a pharmacologic steady state but lacks easy short-term adjustment. A safe, effective, and readily titratable modality for IV opioid administration in children is PCA.[200,244,246]

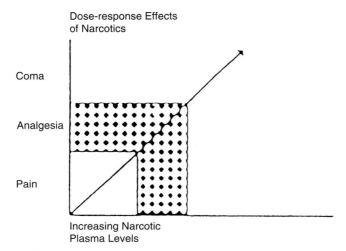

Dose-response Effects
of Narcotics

Coma

Analgesia

Pain

Increasing Narcotic
Plasma Levels

FIGURE 13-7 Analgesic window of opioid therapy. Idealized dose-response curve shows the continuum from pain to analgesia to coma associated with increasing plasma opioid levels. The shaded area depicts the analgesic window between inadequate pain relief and excessive sedation. (From Berde CB: Pediatric postoperative pain management. Pediatr Clin North Am 1989;36:921-940.)

TABLE 13-11

Patient-Controlled Analgesia Regimens for Children

Drug	Demand Dose*	Basal Infusion (if used)
Fentanyl	0.5-1.0 µg/kg IV (adult dose, 50-100 µg)	0.5-1.0 µg/kg/hr IV (adult dose, 50-100 µg/hr)
Hydromorphone	4 µg/kg IV (adult dose, 0.2-0.3 mg)	4 µg/kg/hr IV (adult dose, 0.2-0.3 mg/hr)
Meperidine	Not recommended	
Methadone	Not generally used	
Morphine	0.02 mg/kg IV (adult dose, 1.0-1.5 mg)	0.02 mg/kg/hr IV (adult dose, 1.0-1.5 mg/hr)

*Generally every 8-10 min for patient-controlled analgesia; every 15-60 min for nurse- or parent-controlled analgesia. Recommended opioid doses are for initial administration in opioid-naive patients; titration to clinical effect is required, and higher doses may be necessary. Doses should be reduced 25% to 50% in neonates and young infants.
IV, intravenous.

With PCA, opioid delivery is controlled by a device that allows administration of small doses of drug in response to patient request, usually by pressing a button; an appropriate lockout interval is programmed to prevent excessive administration. Analgesia is excellent, and with appropriate doses, serious complications are rare.[235] With proper instruction, most school-aged children can safely and effectively use PCA for opioid delivery.[235,247] Nurse- or parent-controlled analgesia can be used for children unable or unwilling to control their own pumps,[249,250] although the risk of respiratory depression increases if dosing intervals are not adequately adjusted, particularly in combination with basal infusions.[251] Overall risk of complications with so-called PCA by proxy in children is not elevated compared with the PCA, although risk of serious complications requiring intervention may be somewhat increased.[252] Morphine is the most common choice for PCA, but hydromorphone or fentanyl can be used (Table 13-11). Meperidine PCA is not recommended because

of the increased risk of toxicity with sustained administration. Methadone PCA has been described in pediatric cancer patients with significant opioid requirements and tolerance to other agents,[253] but it is neither necessary nor helpful in most children because of the drug's long half-life. Routine PCA regimens provide a specified dose every 8 to 10 minutes for patient-controlled administration or every 15 to 60 minutes for nurse- or parent-controlled administration. Longer dosing intervals may be safer in younger or more medically fragile patients. Concomitant basal infusion to ensure ongoing analgesia and sustain drug levels during sleep has been advocated[254] but has not been shown to improve analgesia significantly.[255,256] PCA basal infusions in adults have been shown to increase the risk of respiratory complications,[257,258] but this has not been observed in children. PCA basal infusions in pediatric patients, although safe, appear to offer little analgesic benefit except in the setting of significant opioid tolerance. Patients receiving PCA should be assessed frequently, and doses and intervals should be adjusted appropriately. Continuous pulse oximetry is recommended for children receiving any opioid infusion. Cardiorespiratory monitoring may be appropriate in very young or medically fragile patients. Instruction of patients, families, and caregivers regarding appropriate PCA use is essential.

Regional Anesthesia

Regional anesthesia with a local anesthetic can be provided by topical application or direct infiltration at desired sites or by myriad peripheral nerve, plexus, or neuraxial blocks. An advantage of regional anesthesia is that pain relief is often provided without reliance on opioids or other systemic agents, although these may be needed in some children despite apparently successful block.[259] Greater apprehension and variability in developmental and emotional maturity in pediatric patients may explain this unpredictable requirement for supplemental analgesia. Regional anesthesia in children entails a lower risk of adverse effects, including nausea, sedation, and respiratory depression, than does systemic opioid therapy.[245,259,260,261] Regional anesthesia may be particularly advantageous in patients with potentially increased sensitivity to opioids, including neonates and children with chronic respiratory disease. In some settings, regional anesthesia in children has been shown to improve surgical outcomes.[255] Topical anesthesia can be applied to children without sedation or anesthesia. Infiltration anesthesia can be accomplished in cooperative or older children, or it can be performed during surgical procedures. In contrast to adult practice, peripheral nerve, plexus, and neuraxial blocks in children are most commonly performed after induction of general anesthesia.[263,264] Theoretically, this prevents the detection of complications, including paresthesias, failed block, or injection into undesired sites or structures; fortunately, serious complications of regional techniques in anesthetized children are rare.[234,265,266] Performance of regional anesthesia after induction but before surgical incision offers the advantages of lighter intraoperative anesthesia and more rapid emergence and recovery.[267] The use of ultrasonographic imaging to visualize anatomic structures and facilitate placement of peripheral and neuraxial blocks has grown in popularity over the past few years.

TABLE 13-12

Maximum Recommended Doses of Local Anesthetics

	Maximum Recommended Dose Local Anesthetic (mg/kg)*
Bupivacaine	3.0
Levobupivacaine	3.0
Lidocaine	5.0
Prilocaine	7.0
Ropivacaine	4.0

*Addition of a vasoconstrictor such as epinephrine or phenylephrine to local anesthetic solutions may prolong absorption and modestly increase the maximum recommended dose, but this is not reliable.

TABLE 13-13

Topical Anesthetic Formulations

Product	Ingredients	Comments
ELA-Max	Liposomal lidocaine 4% or 5%	Apply for 30 min
		No dressing required
		Nonprescription
EMLA	Lidocaine 2.5% + prilocaine 2.5%	Apply for 1-4 hr
		Requires occlusive dressing
		Prilocaine may cause methemoglobinemia
Numby Stuff	Iontocaine (lidocaine 2% + epinephrine 1:100,000)	Apply for 10 min
		Requires specialized electrodes, generator
		Tingling sensation may frighten some children
TAC	Cocaine 4%-11.8% + tetracaine 0.5%-1% + epinephrine 1:2000-4000	Apply for 20 min
		Avoid mucous membranes
		Avoid terminally perfused areas
		Potential cocaine toxicity

Ultrasonographically guided blocks may decrease the overall local anesthetic requirement, and thereby toxicity, by providing real-time data regarding spread of the injected solution in proximity to the targeted structure. This imaging modality is also likely to decrease risk of complications such as inadvertent intrathecal, intravascular, intrapleural, or intraperitoneal injection. Although small-scale studies suggest improvement in outcome, larger-scale studies are currently under way regarding the improved safety and efficacy of ultrasonographic guidance over conventional methods of nerve blockade.[268-271] Lidocaine provides dense analgesia but has a relatively short duration of action and often induces motor block. In topical preparations, lidocaine is commonly combined with prilocaine, which may cause methemoglobinemia, particularly in large doses or in small patients. Bupivacaine is widely used in children because of its longer duration of action and relative selectivity for sensory over motor block. It is highly cardiotoxic, however, and thresholds for cardiac and neurologic toxicity are similar; dysrhythmias may occur before obtundation or seizures are noted. Ropivacaine has moderately greater selectivity for sensory over motor block than does bupivacaine, with a relatively higher threshold for cardiac toxicity, but widespread use is limited primarily by cost. Adherence to maximum recommended doses (Table 13-12) reduces the risk of toxicity.

TOPICAL ANESTHESIA

Numerous formulations of local anesthetics provide cutaneous analgesia without the need for injection (Table 13-13), potentially reducing or eliminating the need for systemic analgesia and sedation.

Eutectic mixture of local anesthetics (EMLA) cream is a combination of 2.5% lidocaine and 2.5% prilocaine. Applied in a thick layer and covered with an occlusive dressing for at least 60 minutes, EMLA provides effective cutaneous analgesia for minor procedures, including circumcision and even chest tube removal.[188,272-275] Analgesia increases with application up to 4 hours.[276] EMLA cream is easy to apply; patients and families can do so at home. Side effects include erythema, blanching, and rash. The prilocaine component has caused concern about the risk of methemoglobinemia, particularly with generous application or in infants, but this is rare when the product is used appropriately.

Several other preparations of topical anesthetics are available. ELA-Max is an over-the-counter preparation of 4% or 5% liposomal lidocaine.[277] Numby Stuff is a unique system of topical anesthesia using mild electrical current to promote rapid iontophoretic intradermal transport of a solution of 2% lidocaine and 1:100,000 epinephrine.[278,279] TAC (tetracaine, adrenaline, cocaine) is available in a variety of preparations and provides effective cutaneous analgesia for the repair of superficial lacerations in children.[280-283]

INFILTRATION ANESTHESIA

Infiltration with local anesthetic provides effective analgesia for minor procedures and can be performed in cooperative or older patients without sedation or anesthesia. Any appropriate solution may be used. The acid pH of many local anesthetic solutions enhances solubility and prolongs shelf life but is responsible for much of the pain associated with injection. Buffering pH helps reduce pain in awake patients and may increase efficacy. Addition of 1.0 mEq sodium bicarbonate to 10 mL local anesthetic significantly reduces pain during injection without precipitation of the solution.[284] The bicarbonate is added immediately before use. Infiltration anesthesia provides adequate analgesia after minor, but not major, surgical procedures.[285] The technique is straightforward, and the risk of local anesthetic toxicity is low if maximum recommended doses are not exceeded. Wound infiltration during inguinal hernia repair in children provides analgesia similar to that afforded by ilioinguinal-iliohypogastric nerve block[286,287] or caudal block[288] for 2 to 4 hours after the procedure. Longer-term analgesia is inferior, however.[289]

PERIPHERAL NERVE AND PLEXUS BLOCKS

Successful block of virtually any peripheral nerve or plexus is possible with appropriate equipment and sufficient practitioner interest.[289,290] Regional anesthesia has been advocated for potentially optimizing analgesia, minimizing opioid requirements, and improving pulmonary function.[291] Peripheral nerve blocks are readily performed in children; several are particularly applicable to pediatric surgical patients. Plexus blocks are performed less frequently in children than in adults, often secondary to practitioner inexperience but also because of logistic challenges in the application of adult techniques to pediatric practice. IV regional anesthesia of the extremity, or Bier block, has been described in children,[292] but its application may be limited by the risk of local anesthetic toxicity. Performance of peripheral nerve and plexus blocks before surgical incision offers the theoretical advantages of preemptive analgesia and lessened overall pain experience, but this has not been reliably demonstrated in clinical practice, particularly in children.[176,177,182] Timing appears to be less important than the regional block's performance.

RECTUS SHEATH BLOCK

Recent interest in umbilical surgery in children, particularly the application of laparoscopic techniques, has prompted research on the use of regional anesthesia for such procedures. Terminal cutaneous branches of the lower thoracic intercostal nerves supply the skin of the anterior abdominal midline. Although infiltration anesthesia is readily accomplished in this area, specific nerve block offers the advantage of prolonged analgesia. Rectus sheath block for repair of umbilical and paraumbilical hernias in children has been described[293] and with minor modifications has been described as paraumbilical block.[294] Injection is made halfway between the umbilicus and the lateral linea alba (Fig. 13-8).[294] A blunt-bevel needle is

introduced through the skin with slight medial angulation until a pronounced give or "pop" is felt as the needle pierces the external rectus sheath. After negative aspiration for blood and a negative test dose to reduce the likelihood of intravascular injection, 0.25 to 0.5 mL/kg of local anesthetic is deposited; little or no resistance should be felt. The needle may be withdrawn and a subcutaneous weal made toward the umbilicus for improved coverage of distal cutaneous braches. Injection is then repeated on the contralateral side. Rectus sheath block can be used at other dermatomal levels for the repair of midline ventral hernias above or below the umbilicus.[290]

ILIOINGUINAL-ILIOHYPOGASTRIC BLOCK

The ilioinguinal and iliohypogastric nerves are terminal cutaneous branches of the lumbar plexus. The ilioinguinal nerve arises from the first lumbar spinal nerve roots and supplies much of the external genitals and part of the proximal thigh; the iliohypogastric nerve arises from the 12th thoracic and 1st lumbar spinal nerve roots to innervate the skin of the anterior abdominal wall above the inguinal ligament. The two nerves are usually blocked in conjunction, providing analgesia for procedures on the ipsilateral groin, including inguinal hernia repair and orchiopexy.[295]

Injection is made 1 to 2 cm medial and 1 to 2 cm superior to the anterior superior iliac spine (Fig. 13-9).[267] A blunt-bevel needle is introduced perpendicular to the skin until a distinct give or "pop" is felt as the needle pierces the Scarpa fascia, adherent to the aponeurosis of the external oblique muscle. After negative aspiration for blood and a negative test

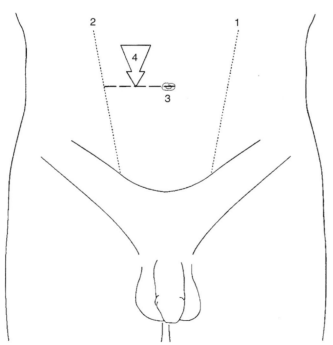

FIGURE 13-8   Landmarks for rectus block at the umbilicus. Injection is made halfway between the umbilicus and the lateral linea alba. Left and right lateral lineae albae (*1* and *2*). Umbilicus (*3*). Right-sided injection site (*4*). The left-sided injection site is symmetrically located. (From Courreges P, Poddevin F, Lecoutre D: Para-umbilical block: A new concept for regional anaesthesia in children. Paediatr Anaesth 1997;7:211-214.)

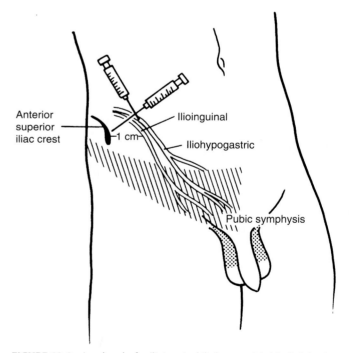

FIGURE 13-9   Landmarks for ilioinguinal-iliohypogastric block. Injection is made 1 to 2 cm medial and 1 to 2 cm superior to the anterior superior iliac spine. Cutaneous innervation of the ilioinguinal nerve includes much of the external genitals and part of the proximal thigh; cutaneous innervation of the iliohypogastric nerve includes the skin of the anterior abdominal wall above the inguinal ligament. (From Yaster M, Maxwell LG: Pediatric regional anesthesia. Anesthesiology 1989;70:324-338.)

dose to reduce the likelihood of intravascular injection, 0.5 to 1.0 mL/kg of local anesthetic is deposited. Total volume of local anesthetic required for adequate blockade may be reduced with ultrasonographic guidance.[296] The needle may be withdrawn and a subcutaneous weal made toward the umbilicus for improved coverage of distal cutaneous branches of the iliohypogastric nerve. Ilioinguinal-iliohypogastric block provides only cutaneous analgesia; supplemental anesthesia is required for visceral manipulation. Because of this lack of visceral coverage, ilioinguinal-iliohypogastric block is inferior to caudal block at blunting the neuroendocrine stress response to orchiopexy.[297] The ilioinguinal-iliohypogastric block may also be paired with a caudal block for superior analgesia.[298] Bilateral block can be performed, but application may be limited in small children by the dose of local anesthetic required.

FASCIA ILIACA BLOCK

The femur and anterior thigh receive innervation from the femoral nerve; the medial and lateral proximal thigh are supplied by the obturator and lateral femoral cutaneous nerves, respectively. Simultaneous block of all three nerves can be accomplished by various techniques, including fascia iliaca block, with resultant analgesia of the proximal leg, although sparing the posterior thigh. This block is appropriate for procedures involving the bony femur or soft tissues of the proximal thigh and may be particularly useful in children

undergoing quadriceps muscle biopsy for evaluation of myopathy, in whom volatile anesthetic agents are best avoided. Fascia iliaca block is increasingly common in pediatric practice[290,299] and ultrasonographic guidance appears to result in a technically superior block.[300] Injection is made 1 to 2 cm medial and 1 to 2 cm inferior to the anterior superior iliac spine, just inferior to the junction of the middle and lateral thirds of the inguinal ligament (Fig. 13-10).[289] A blunt-bevel needle is introduced with slight inferior and lateral angulation, perpendicular to the iliac wing, until two distinct gives or "pops" are felt as the needle pierces first the fascia lata and then the fascia iliaca; the former is usually more pronounced than the latter. Alternatively, the needle may be advanced until encountering the iliac wing and then withdrawn slightly. After negative aspiration for blood and a negative test dose to reduce the likelihood of intravascular injection, 0.5 to 1.0 mL/kg of local anesthetic is deposited; little or no resistance should be felt. Continuous fascia iliaca block in children has been described.[301] Bilateral block can be performed, but application may be limited in small children by the dose of local anesthetic required.

PENILE BLOCK

Penile block provides analgesia for circumcision and other distal penile procedures, including simple hypospadias repair; caudal block is preferred for more proximal procedures, such as repair of complex hypospadias.[302–305] In general, penile

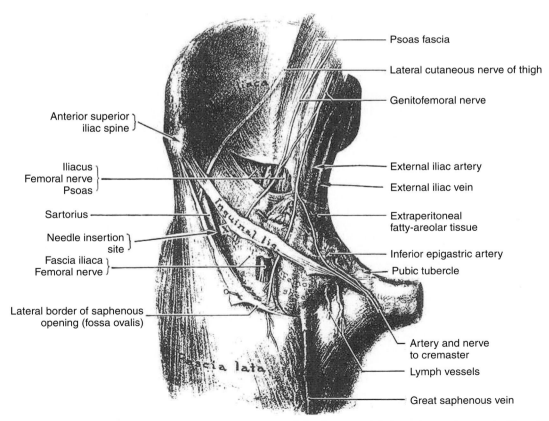

FIGURE 13-10   Landmarks for fascia iliaca block. Injection is made 1 to 2 cm medial and 1 to 2 cm inferior to the anterior superior iliac spine, just inferior to the junction of the middle and lateral thirds of the inguinal ligament. (From Sethna NF, Berde CB: Pediatric regional anesthesia. In Gregory GA [ed]: Pediatric Anesthesia, ed 3. New York, Churchill Livingstone, 1994, pp 281-318.)

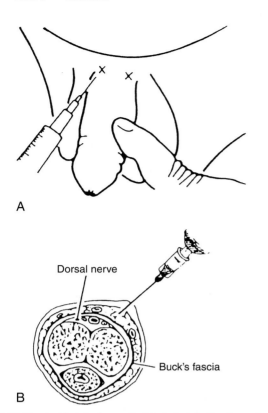

FIGURE 13-11   Landmarks for penile block. **A,** Injection is made at the base of the penis lateral to the midline at approximately the 10 and 2 o'clock positions. **B,** The dorsal vein, two dorsal arteries, two dorsal nerves, and three corpora of the penis lie beneath the Buck fascia. (**A** From Yaster M, Maxwell LG: Pediatric regional anesthesia. Anesthesiology 1989;70:324-338. **B** From Rice LJ, Hannallah RS: Local and regional anesthesia. In Motoyama EK, Davis PJ [eds]: Smith's Anesthesia for Infants and Children, 5th ed. St Louis, CV Mosby, 1990, pp 393-426.)

block has fewer complications than does caudal block, in particular a lower incidence of motor block, but caudal block has a higher success rate and provides more prolonged analgesia. Penile block is not free of risk; puncture of dorsal penile vessels may lead to hematoma,[306] and gangrene of the glans penis has been reported. Local anesthetic solutions for penile block should not contain epinephrine or other vasoconstrictors. Injection is made at the base of the penis lateral to the midline at approximately the 10 and 2 o'clock positions (Fig. 13-11).[267,309] Alternatively, a single injection can be made in the midline. A blunt-bevel needle is introduced perpendicular to the skin until a distinct give or "pop" is felt as the needle pierces the Buck fascia. After negative aspiration for blood and a negative test dose to reduce the likelihood of intravascular injection, 0.5 to 1.0 mL/kg of local anesthetic, up to 10 mL, is deposited; little or no resistance should be felt. The process is then repeated on the contralateral side. Ring block at the base of the penis superficial to the Buck fascia provides equivalent analgesia and may reduce the risk of hematoma.[306]

NEURAXIAL BLOCK

Neuraxial block involves either spinal or epidural techniques. Spinal block, with injection of anesthetic directly into the cerebrospinal fluid of the spinal subarachnoid space, is performed almost exclusively for procedures in infants at high risk of apnea after general anesthesia, although continuous spinal techniques are occasionally used for palliative analgesia. Epidural block, with injection of anesthetic into the potential space between the ligamentum flavum and the dura mater, is a far more common technique for procedural and perioperative pain management in children. Anesthetic can be administered as a single injection or by repeated injections or continuous infusion through an indwelling catheter. Contraindications to neuraxial block include patient or parent refusal, coagulopathy predisposing to neuraxial hematoma, local or systemic infection carrying the risk of neuraxial abscess or meningitis, increased intracranial pressure, and anatomic deformity. Most contraindications are relative; risks and benefits must be weighed in each patient.

CAUDAL BLOCK

The most common neuraxial block in children is caudal block,[267] in which the epidural space is accessed via the sacral hiatus created by the failure of fusion of the spinous process of the fifth sacral vertebra. The technique is relatively straightforward, the success rate is high, and the complication rate is low.[310,311]

Injection is made between and slightly inferior to the sacral cornua (Fig. 13-12).[267] A blunt-bevel needle is introduced with approximately 45 degrees of cephalad angulation until a distinct give or "pop" is felt as the needle pierces the sacrococcygeal ligament, the most inferior aspect of the ligamentum flavum. If bone is encountered, usually representing the posterior aspect of anterior sacral elements, the needle is withdrawn slightly and redirected more parallel to the skin. Correct positioning of the needle tip within the epidural space is confirmed by loss of resistance to injection. After negative aspiration for blood and a negative test dose to reduce the likelihood of intravascular injection, the full dose of anesthetic is injected. Serious complications associated with caudal block include intravascular or intraosseous injection, inadvertent dural puncture with resultant spinal anesthesia, injury to pelvic contents, and hematoma; these complications are rare.[312] Caudal block is most commonly performed as a single injection of anesthetic providing reliable analgesia below the umbilicus in patients weighing less than approximately 30 kg. Perhaps because of their lower overall sympathetic tone, infants and children do not generally demonstrate hemodynamic instability after neuraxial block. Caudal block in pediatric patients induces significant changes in regional

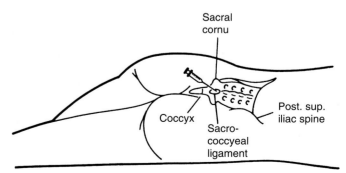

FIGURE 13-12   Landmarks for caudal block. Injection is made between and slightly inferior to the sacral cornua. (From Yaster M, Maxwell LG: Pediatric regional anesthesia. Anesthesiology 1989;70:324-338.)

blood flow but does not significantly alter heart rate or blood pressure.[313] The agents administered determine the duration of analgesia after caudal block. Local anesthetic may provide analgesia for several hours and does not cause urinary retention at usual doses.[314] Bupivacaine 0.0625% to 0.25% is used most commonly. The addition of an opioid prolongs analgesia but increases the risk of side effects, particularly respiratory depression. Duration of analgesia and risk of side effects are greater with increasing opioid hydrophilicity, which promotes uptake into the cerebrospinal fluid and enhances distal spread. Caudal fentanyl, a highly lipophilic opioid, can be used for outpatient and ambulatory surgery in children. Caudal morphine, a highly hydrophilic opioid, provides analgesia for more than 12 hours but entails a significant risk of side effects, including pruritus and respiratory depression, for up to 24 hours.[315,316] Neuraxial morphine should not be used for outpatient analgesia. Caudal hydromorphone provides more prolonged analgesia than does caudal fentanyl, with less risk of respiratory depression than does caudal morphine. Caudal administration of clonidine[317,318] and ketamine[319] has been described and may be particularly advantageous in patients with potentially increased sensitivity to opioids, including neonates and children with chronic respiratory disease.

CONTINUOUS TECHNIQUES

Single-injection caudal block works well for pain anticipated to last less than 24 hours; even caudal morphine does not provide reliable analgesia beyond this time frame. For pain of longer duration, continuous techniques are preferred. Excellent analgesia can be provided by repeated injection or continuous infusion of anesthetic through indwelling epidural catheters, which can be placed via caudal, lumbar, or thoracic approaches to the epidural space in children.[320–322] Cervical epidural catheters for palliative care in children have been reported,[323,324] and tunneled catheters for prolonged analgesia have been described.[325] Epidural catheters are commonly placed directly at the desired vertebral level in patients weighing more than 5 to 10 kg. Once the epidural space is reached, the epidural catheter is advanced through the needle. Threading more than 3 cm beyond the needle often causes catheter coiling at the level of insertion.[326] The risk of spinal cord damage when placing thoracic or lumbar epidural catheters is always a concern, especially in the anesthetized or heavily sedated patient; these fears are largely theoretical, although neurologic complications have been reported.[327] Inserting the epidural catheter in the low lumbar or caudal space (after termination of the spinal cord) and threading a styletted catheter cephalad to the desired level may decrease the risk of direct spinal cord injury with high rates of success, particularly in neonates and young infants in whom the epidural fat is more gelatinous and the epidural space is largely free of fibrous septa.[263] This technique is often paired with conventional radiography, fluoroscopy, nerve stimulation, or electrocardiographic guidance to confirm correct catheter placement.[328–331] Ultrasonographic imaging of the spine may allow calculation of the skin-to-epidural space distance, localization of important bony and soft tissue landmarks, and even direct visualization of the epidural catheter in certain cases.[332–334]

Skin preparation with chlorhexidine rather than iodine-containing solutions confers a lower risk of subsequent catheter colonization.[335] The agent selected for epidural infusion

TABLE 13-14	
Agents for Epidural Infusion in Children*	
Local Anesthetic[†]	*Opioid*[†,‡]
Bupivacaine 0.0625%-0.1% (max dose 0.4 mg/kg/hr)	Fentanyl 0.5-1.0 µg/kg/hr (adult dose, 50-100 µg/hr)
OR	OR
Levobupivacaine 0.0625%-0.1% (max dose 0.4 mg/kg/hr)	Hydromorphone 2.0-4.0 µg/kg/hr (adult dose, 150-300 µg/hr)
OR	OR
Lidocaine 0.1%-0.5% (max dose 3 mg/kg/hr)	Morphine 3.0-6.0 µg/kg/hr (adult dose, 250-500 µg/hr)
OR	AND/OR
Ropivacaine 0.1%-0.2% (max dose 0.5 mg/kg/hr)	Clonidine 0.25-0.5 µg/kg/hr (adult dose, 25-50 µg/hr)

*Thoracic catheters commonly deliver 0.2-0.3 mL/kg/hr (max 5-10 mL/hr); lumbar catheters, 0.3-0.4 mL/kg/hr (max 10-15 mL/hr); and caudal catheters, 0.4-0.5 mL/kg/hr (max 15-20 mL/hr).
[†]Recommended local anesthetic and opioid doses should be reduced 25% to 50% in neonates and young infants.
[‡]Recommended opioid doses are for initial administration in opioid-naive patients; titration to clinical effect is required, and higher doses may be necessary.

depends on the dermatomal position of the catheter tip relative to the site of pain as well as on the distribution and intensity of analgesia desired. Numerous combinations of local anesthetic and opioid are commonly used in the United States (Table 13-14); other agents are used in other countries.[336,337] Concomitant administration of local anesthetic and opioid is synergistic and enables dose reductions of both agents, minimizing motor block and decreasing the risk of opioid side effects.[245,338] If the epidural catheter tip has been appropriately positioned in close dermatomal proximity to the site of pain, diluted local anesthetic with a lipophilic opioid such as fentanyl may be sufficient. If the epidural catheter tip is at a dermatomal level distant from the painful area, or if this area covers multiple dermatomes, addition of an increasingly hydrophilic opioid such as hydromorphone or morphine may be necessary. Epidural opioids provide excellent analgesia but are associated with side effects, including pruritus, nausea, urinary retention, and respiratory depression; risk of side effects increases with increasing opioid hydrophilicity. Opioid side effects can be managed with a variety of agents (see Table 13-8). Clonidine can be used to reduce or eliminate opioids in an epidural infusion, providing similar analgesia but avoiding opioid side effects.[339,340] This may be particularly advantageous in patients with potentially increased sensitivity to opioids, including neonates and children with chronic respiratory disease.

Close observation of patients receiving epidural infusions is essential. Continuous pulse oximetry and cardiorespiratory monitoring have been recommended for any child receiving an epidural opioid.[338] Alternatively, all patients receiving epidural infusions may be provided continuous pulse oximetry, with cardiorespiratory monitoring reserved for patients at increased risk of respiratory depression. Neonates and young infants, children with neurologic or pulmonary disease, and patients receiving a hydrophilic opioid such as morphine may merit more intensive monitoring.[234] Level of consciousness, adequacy of analgesia, degree of motor and sensory block, and presence of side effects should be assessed regularly and frequently for all patients receiving epidural infusions. Continuous neuraxial techniques require significant caregiver diligence and expertise but provide superb analgesia for children with severe pain.

COMMENTS

Appropriate pain management in children requires an understanding of developmental and physiologic issues unique to pediatric patients. A coherent plan encompassing the entire perioperative course should be developed, providing analgesia in proportion to pain and preempting pain whenever possible. Numerous tools are available to perform ongoing quantitative assessment of pain in all children.

Nonpharmacologic techniques may reduce the need for pharmacologic agents, and nonopioid analgesics may reduce the need for opioids. Opioids, however, remain the mainstay of therapy for moderate to severe pain and in appropriate doses can be used in patients of any age. Regional anesthesia with local anesthetic optimizes analgesia and reduces the need for systemic agents. Topical and infiltration anesthesia may be provided or specific peripheral nerve, plexus, or neuraxial blocks may be performed. Pain management is individualized, pain relief is assessed regularly, and regimens are modified as needed to optimize analgesia, minimize side effects, and facilitate recovery.

The complete reference list is available online at www. expertconsult.com.

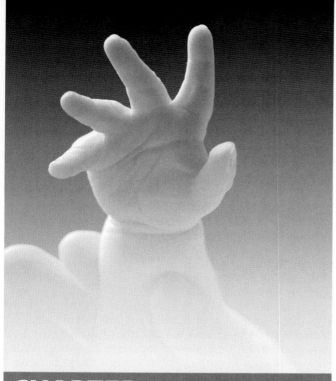

CHAPTER 14

Clinical Outcomes Evaluation and Quality Improvement

Tamara N. Fitzgerald and R. Lawrence Moss

Decades of increasing resources for medical research and the explosion of information technology have created an enormous increase in the body of information available to practicing surgeons. In pediatric surgery, as in all disciplines, clinicians strive to offer their patients the benefit of all available data to provide the best care. Evidence-based medicine (EBM) is the practice of identifying the best available scientific evidence and applying this evidence to the medical care of patients. Sackett defined EBM as "the integration of best research evidence with clinical expertise and patient values."[1] EBM exists in two forms: the application of data to the care of individual patients and the development of evidence-based guidelines to guide the care of groups of patients within an institution or health system.

Actual medical decision making is best accomplished through a process by which the physician and patient (or family in the case of children) come to a health care decision based on the best available evidence, thoughtful application of the evidence to the patient, and personal factors such as quality-of-life and social or religious preferences. The development of clinical guidelines is a collaborative process by which relevant and knowledgeable practitioners critically review existing data and develop a plan of care for a set of patients with a particular disease process.[2] Patients treated by these guidelines are then followed prospectively to ensure that the anticipated improved outcome is realized. Guidelines are continually modified in an iterative process so that they can be refined, updated, and improved.

Several sources provide an extensive review of the principles of EBM and can provide the pediatric surgeon with a more detailed description than space allows here.[1,3–5] In this chapter, we provide an overview of the concepts that we believe are essential to the practicing pediatric surgeon who wishes to use most effectively the ever-growing body of information to provide the most rational, scientifically based, and current care to his or her patients. The first section discusses the concepts of study design and the second section focuses on the interpretation of data from clinical studies. The third section reviews the concepts of quality and outcomes assessment of one's own practice or institution in comparison to a standard.

Study Design and Sources of Evidence

A basic understanding of the types of evidence that exist and the advantages and limitations of each study design is essential for the modern clinician. Varying levels of evidence are available for almost any imaginable clinical problem. The ability to understand which type of evidence a given study provides is critical to being able to determine the relevance of the study's findings to a particular patient or clinical situation. The spectrum ranges from personal anecdotal experience to large, multicenter clinical trials that examine specific questions in a rigorous but perhaps tangentially relevant manner. There is a hierarchy in study design, and the rating system used to evaluate diagnostic tests and therapies is described in Table 14-1. Studies are discussed in the following sections in order of increasing scientific rigor and reliability: case reports, case series, cross-sectional studies, case-control studies, retrospective cohort, prospective cohort, and randomized clinical trials.

CASE REPORTS

Often when a clinician encounters a rare or interesting problem, it becomes the topic for a case report. In surgery, case reports are often used to introduce a novel procedure or technique. They are anecdotal in nature and represent the experience of just one or a few cases. Although they provide very little objective data, they serve to identify new disease processes or unexpected responses to treatment. They may also provide information and motivation for more rigorous clinical investigation. Case reports are particularly useful in the field of pediatric surgery in which the clinician frequently encounters rare or "never seen before" anomalies and responses to treatment. They can help the clinician realize possibilities beyond those discussed in a standard text and can allow the field to learn more collectively about rare conditions than would ever

TABLE 14-1

Rating System Used to Evaluate Diagnostic Tests and Therapies

Evidence Rating in Support of a Diagnostic Test

Class I	Evidence obtained from a blinded prospective study Patient population represents a broad spectrum of persons with disease
Class II	Evidence provided by a blinded prospective study Patient population may be a narrow spectrum of persons with disease
Class III	Evidence provided by a retrospective study Patient population may be a narrow spectrum Test is applied in a blinded evaluation
Class IV	Any design in which test is not applied in blinded evaluation Evidence may be provided by expert opinion alone May be a descriptive case series (without controls)

Evidence Rating in Support of a Therapy

Class I	Prospective RCT
	Masked outcome assessment in a representative population
	Meets the following criteria:
	  a. Primary outcome is clearly defined
	  b. Exclusion/inclusion criteria are clearly defined
	  c. Adequate accounting for dropouts and crossovers
	  d. Relevant baseline characteristics are presented and equivalent

Class II	Prospective matched group cohort study with masked outcome assessment RCT that lacks one criteria listed in a-d above
Class III	Other controlled trials in which outcome assessment is independent of treatment
Class IV	Evidence from uncontrolled studies, case series, or case reports

RCT, randomized controlled trial.

be possible in a single practice or institution. However, the data in a case report are anecdotal and the application of any anecdotal data to one's own patient is quite limited.

CASE SERIES

A case series is the observational experience of a surgeon or group of surgeons and reports on a series of patients with a particular disease or treatment. As such, there is usually no comparison between groups or any information about the outcome of a different treatment. Furthermore, the patient population usually represents a select group that has been referred to that surgeon or center for a particular reason, and the surgeon has often selected patients who are thought to be likely to do well with the procedure. This phenomenon is often referred to as "cherry picking." Data on patients at the same center who did not receive the operation being studied or data comparing the institution's patients with the disease to broader populations of patients are usually not provided. This markedly limits the reader's ability to determine the relevance of the results to his or her patients.

In case series, it is difficult for the authors to maintain objectivity. Investigators are often introducing a procedure or treatment that they truly believe "works" and they are motivated to demonstrate their success. Therefore, adverse events may be underreported and outcomes exaggerated. This bias is usually introduced subconsciously even with the best of intentions. In comparing one case series to another case series, there may also be variations in disease severity, comorbid conditions, operative technique, and postoperative care that are not addressed. Therefore, one cannot reliably make decisions about which treatment is superior based on case series data. In pediatric surgery, case series compose the vast majority of the clinical evidence.[6]

Consider the treatment for necrotizing enterocolitis (NEC). For years there were multiple case series that presented conflicting data as to whether laparotomy or peritoneal drainage was superior in the management of intestinal perforation. Proponents of laparotomy claimed superior results, whereas those in favor of peritoneal drainage reported data supporting a less invasive approach. Not until clinical trials were performed was it determined that the type of operation performed does not influence survival or other clinically pertinent early outcomes.[7–9]

The limitations of case series can also be seen in the history of in utero tracheal occlusion for congenital diaphragmatic hernia (CDH). In animal models, tracheal occlusion was shown to induce lung growth and respiratory maturation. Case series data were then published that showed tracheal occlusion improved lung function.[10] However, when a prospective randomized trial was conducted, the outcomes for infants treated with in utero tracheal occlusion were no better than those treated with standard postnatal care. In this randomized trial, survival in the control group was much higher than anticipated. Tracheal occlusion did not improve survival or morbidity rates.[11,12]

CROSS-SECTIONAL STUDIES

Cross-sectional studies are useful for characterizing the prevalence of a condition or risk factor in a particular population. Measurements are made at a specified time in a population, one patient at a time. There is no longitudinal component of the investigation. For example, all children in the emergency room during a certain month may have their blood drawn once to determine the incidence of antibodies indicating prior exposure to a particular virus. These studies can be inexpensive and easy to conduct.

However, cross-sectional studies may not detect certain data depending on the timing and method of data collection. A good example is the hidden mortality of CDH. In Norway mortality from CDH was thought to be 30%, as reported from hospital records. However, on a more comprehensive survey of neonatal deaths it was found that many infants died soon after birth from CDH and never presented to a major referral center. The true incidence of CDH was at least 1 in every 5000 live births and the actual mortality from CDH was closer to 66%.

Cross-sectional studies have other limitations. Although they are useful for characterizing the prevalence of a condition or a risk factor in a study population, their inability to demonstrate a temporal relationship limits the ability to infer causation. However, these studies do provide preliminary data to justify further epidemiologic investigation.

CASE-CONTROL STUDY

The case-control study begins with choosing an outcome of interest, with a goal to evaluate for exposures that are associated with this outcome. By design, these studies are retrospective.

Patients with a particular diagnosis (cases) are compared with similar individuals who are otherwise healthy (controls). For example, an investigator wishes to determine what factors are associated with the development of NEC in the newborn intensive care unit (NICU). Newborns with NEC are identified and comprise the case group. A second set of newborns would then be chosen from the NICU who do not have NEC (controls), but are "similar" in every other way to the case group. "Similar" is subject to interpretation and choosing the two groups appropriately is the key to success in this study.

A case-control study compares the relative prevalence of factors that might be associated with the outcome in the case and control groups. Using the example of patients with NEC, one might find that the incidence of a particular type of feeding was twice as prevalent in the group of newborns with NEC (cases) than other babies (controls). The study identifies the association but tells the investigator nothing definitive about the cause of NEC. It is entirely possible that the mode of feeding had nothing to do with the cause of NEC. Perhaps newborns fed the particular type of feeding were more likely to be small for gestational age or perhaps they were likely to come from a particular socioeconomic group with a high incidence of NEC. The case-control study can provide interesting hypotheses for further study but is only able to identify the odds of an association between a risk factor and outcome and *not* the relative risk of the outcome given the risk factor. This is a nuanced but critical difference.

It is also important that case controls studies "match" for the prevalence of certain characteristics that are known to affect the outcome so that the characteristics are found at the same prevalence in each group (e.g., gestational age). Ideally this requires that the investigators know in advance what all the factors are. This is, of course, not possible. If this was known, the study would be unnecessary.

This study design is easy to perform with relatively little expense. It is an efficient means to study rare conditions and infrequent outcomes, and several exposure variables can be studied simultaneously. Therefore this study design lends itself well to logistic regression models, which help elucidate the manner in which one factor is associated with another and to clarify the relationship of each individual factor to the outcome.

Disadvantages of case-control design include the tendency for bias and the fact that identifying all important potential confounding factors is almost impossible. Recall bias and survivorship bias are two notable problems. Recall bias stems from the phenomenon that those affected by a disease are more likely to remember potential risk factors than those not affected. For example, in neonates born with birth defects, mothers may be more likely to remember potential teratogenic exposures compared with those mothers with healthy newborns. Survivorship bias occurs when data from survivors are included and data from deceased patients are either excluded or cannot be obtained. This type of bias may also result when patients with poor outcomes are lost to follow-up.

A recent study regarding perforated appendicitis provides a good example of case-control design.[13] In this multi-institutional study, children with perforated appendicitis in whom postoperative abscess developed made up the case group, whereas those who did not develop an abscess comprised the control group. Multivariate analysis with logistic regression was used to determine the factors that were independently associated with postoperative abscess development. A sample population consisting of 75% of the data was used to create the model, and then the model was tested on the remaining 25% of the data. The results showed that several factors were independently associated with abscess formation. Although this design was not able to show that these factors were causative of abscess formation, this information could be used to develop treatment guidelines that could then be evaluated prospectively.

RETROSPECTIVE COHORT

A retrospective cohort study is designed to compare the outcomes of two groups of patients after an exposure. In surgical studies, the exposure is typically the operation. The study is conceptualized and the hypothesis is created after the patients have been treated and the outcome has occurred. This creates important limitations. For example, suppose that an investigator wished to determine if laparoscopic fundoplication reduces the length of hospital stay. He or she must first define a set of criteria that determines the cohorts: for example patients younger than 15 years of age with reflux confirmed by pH probe who underwent fundoplication. Patients are then identified who meet these criteria and assigned to one of two cohorts based on whether their operation was open or laparoscopic.

Several limitations are immediately apparent. One could ask why some patients in the study underwent laparoscopic fundoplication while others had an open procedure. Certainly, there was no effort to have any similarity between the two study groups because the study was not conceived when the treatment was done. It is very likely that there are large differences in patient characteristics and in the characteristics of the surgeons performing the procedure. It is also likely that the criteria for operation versus medical therapy were different in the two cohorts. Although it is important for investigators to report on covariates (factors that may affect outcome, such as age, neurologic status, and length of medical treatment) it is impossible to ensure that they will be equal between the cohorts or to make appropriate statistical adjustments when they are not. Further, it is not even possible for the investigators to know what covariates might be important or to what degree. A further limitation is the subjectivity of the outcome variables. Outcomes like death are objective, but the timing of when a surgeon chooses to discharge a patient is subjective.

Data in a retrospective cohort study must be retrieved from the medical record. The record is frequently incomplete or inaccurate.[14] The record was created before the study was designed and solely to meet the clinical needs at the time. Therefore it is almost inconceivable that all or even most of what the investigator wishes to find will be present or available in a consistent manner.

A retrospective cohort study can use either concurrent or historical controls. Concurrent controls were treated during the same period as the study patients. Remember that just because they are treated during the same period does not mean that they have the same characteristics, but at least this design does not have the additional limitations seen in studies using historical controls.

Historical controls were treated during different periods. Factors that can change over time include but are not limited to referral patterns, operating surgeons, indications and contraindications for operation, availability and quality of nonoperative treatments, accuracy of tests to measure the disease or outcome, prevailing practice patterns, and even the natural history of disease. Returning to our example of laparoscopic versus open fundoplication, many of these factors have changed over the past decade.[15,16] Medical therapy for reflux has evolved considerably.[17] Our ability to define severity of reflux objectively through pH and impedance measurements has improved.[18] The subset of patients with reflux who are referred for operation has changed considerably over time.[19]

PROSPECTIVE COHORT

A prospective cohort study is designed to compare the outcomes of two groups of patients after an exposure. The study is planned and inclusion and exclusion criteria are created before the patients are enrolled and data collected. The resulting data are more complete than a retrospective study because the investigators can observe and record the appropriate findings as they occur. Various outcome measures can be prespecified and recorded, such as length of stay, disease recurrence, or side effects. Patients are followed until a set end point is reached. For example, intestinal failure has been studied in neonates with NEC. All neonates with suspected or confirmed NEC, as defined by preset entry criteria, were enrolled. Study end points were defined as the development of intestinal failure or the achievement of full enteral feeds. Risk factors such as birth weight, antibiotic use, requirement for mechanical ventilation, exposure to enteral feeding, and small-bowel resection at surgery were monitored and recorded.[20]

The strength of this study design is a predetermined set of criteria to assess outcomes. This protects against "data mining," a phenomenon in which one may find a statistically significant difference in outcomes between groups if multiple outcomes are investigated. For example, an investigator may perform a study to investigate whether birth weight, race, or sex are associated with the development of esophageal reflux. If the study is completed and none of the factors investigated was found to be related to reflux, the investigator may be disappointed and want to search other factors. He may then look back into the medical record for the presence of asthma, mechanical ventilation, or obesity. If the investigator continues to expand the number of outcomes investigated, he or she will eventually find an association, most likely based on chance and not a true relationship. Therefore predetermined outcomes in the prospective cohort study protect against "data mining."

Several limitations are inherent to this study design. Foremost, there is no randomization. To return to our previous example of neonates with NEC,[20] these babies may receive surgery or drain placement in the instance of a bowel perforation. However, the decision for operation was made by individual surgeon preference, not a randomization process. The choice of intervention (drain placement versus laparotomy) could influence the length of mechanical ventilation or time to enteral feeds. The extent of small-bowel resection was also determined at operation, and different surgeons are likely to have different thresholds for bowel that should be removed. However, the length of bowel remaining will certainly be a factor in how the infant will tolerate enteral feeds.

Although this study design is inferior to a randomized clinical trial, it is sometimes the only appropriate study that can be performed.[21] Prospective cohort studies can provide valuable information on outcomes and are less expensive to perform than are randomized trials. They can be used to generate data so that randomized trials can then be performed.

Prospective observational studies can raise ethical concerns. Ethicists and other members of the research community have questioned whether investigators have an obligation to address the underlying needs of special populations and not just exploit their condition for the purposes of research. This is of particular interest in disadvantaged communities and developing countries.[22]

The degree of study validity lies in the similarity and selection of groups and in the definition of the cohort. Statistical methods can be used to take into account inequalities in the cohort, but when possible, covariates that are likely to affect outcomes between groups must be matched. If highly selective inclusion criteria are used, this may limit the general applicability of the results. Because patients are not randomized, bias may select patients into treatment groups. Also, investigator bias may alter outcomes. For example, investigators have studied long-term pulmonary function after extracorporeal membrane oxygenation (ECMO).[23] Cohorts consisted of infants with meconium aspiration syndrome, CDH, sepsis, or persistent pulmonary hypertension. Because of the invasive nature of ECMO, it would have been unethical to subject patients with these diseases to ECMO if it was not necessary. However, these cohorts represent infants with very different disease processes, and the disparity of disease states may explain the difference in their lung function, which may or may not be related to ECMO. They were also compared with healthy infants who never received ECMO. Therefore bias is difficult to remove from this study design, and it is difficult to ascertain from this study the role that ECMO has in preserving lung function.

An additional challenge in the pediatric population is that disease states tend to be rare and a multicenter approach may be needed to gain enough patients. For this reason, these studies can often be expensive. However, they are useful to characterize the natural history of a disease and relative risks. Prospective cohort studies can also be used to develop multi-institutional prospective databases, which can be used to study multiple risk factors and outcomes simultaneously. One such example is the database generated by the National Institute of Child Health and Human Development Neonatal Research Network, a consortium of 16 tertiary neonatal centers within the United States. Among other studies, this database has been used to examine the incidence and morbidity of short-bowel syndrome.[24]

PROSPECTIVE RANDOMIZED CONTROLLED TRIAL

The randomized controlled trial (RCT) is the gold standard to compare treatment outcomes and acquire necessary data.[25] The first RCT in health care was reported in the 1940s.[26] To illustrate the importance of rigorous scientific inquiry, Sacks and associates compared RCT and historical control trials (HCT) by searching the literature for therapies studied by both methods. Seventy-nine percent of HCTs found the therapy better than the control regimen, but only 20% of RCTs agreed. Biases in patient selection may weight the outcome of HCTs in favor of new therapies.[27] Unfortunately, information gained from nonrandomized studies continues to guide many of our treatment decisions because of the lack of RCTs.[28] In 2001, there were only 134 RCTs in pediatric surgery, accounting for 0.17% of the articles published in 33 years.[29]

In RCTs the study population and the disease of interest are clearly defined, and patients are randomized into two treatment groups but are otherwise treated identically. It is essential that the only variable that differs between the two groups is the one that is being studied. Theoretically the randomized design ensures that any observed differences should be due to the treatment and not to other factors. By randomly assigning patients into two groups, there is a built-in control for unknown clinical parameters that may influence treatment response. Thus the randomization process should eliminate confounding covariates. The RCT is the gold standard of clinical evidence and is the most powerful study design. In addition to research benefits, patients may also benefit from participation in trials because participating centers may focus increased attention and resources on these patients and their disease processes. Participating patients have been shown to have improved outcomes regardless of assignment.[30]

The main weaknesses of the RCT are that they are time intensive and expensive to conduct. It is not unusual for a trial to cost upward of $5000 per patient.[31] Additional staff may be required to conduct surveys, obtain informed consent, record results, analyze data, and organize protocol requirements. For surgeons participating in the study, there is an increase in paperwork and administrative oversight.[32] As previously noted, pediatric disease states are rare and therefore an appropriately powered study will require the participation of several institutions and surgeons. This can significantly increase the complexity of data acquisition and maintenance of study uniformity.[33]

The RCT should include a broad patient population. If the inclusion criteria are too narrow, the results may not be applicable to a larger patient population.[34] For example, if an investigator wishes to study the routine use of a nasogastric tube after laparotomy in children, but then excludes all emergency cases and children with developmental delays, the results of the study are applicable only to elective cases in developmentally normal children. Likewise, if a trial is conducted in a geographic region that is racially homogeneous, the results of the study may not apply to children of other racial backgrounds.[35]

In addition, the ability of a randomized trial to control chance is limited by sample size. Therefore the RCT must be appropriately powered to yield accurate results. In many RCTs, the sample size calculation is not reported, is frequently incorrect, and is based on erroneous assumptions.[36] The CONSORT group is an international consortium that has issued guidelines for conducting and reporting results of RCTs.[37] It provides a minimum set of recommendations for reporting RCTs. In this way, authors can report trial findings in a complete and transparent fashion, thereby facilitating critical interpretation of the results. The CONSORT statement comprises a 25-item checklist.[38] According to this statement, calculation of sample size must be reported and justified. The CONSORT statement has been adopted by several journals, including the *Journal of Pediatric Surgery*.[39,40]

Conducting a surgical RCT poses several challenges. If the condition under investigation is rare, or if there is difficulty enrolling patients, the RCT may take years to conduct and there is a chance that the therapy may be obsolete before the trial has been completed. Surgical techniques may evolve over the course of the study. Skill level is variable between surgeons and therefore the outcome is operator dependant. It is difficult to standardize an operation, as surgeons have different techniques, operating facilities, and learning curves.[41] Most pediatric surgery RCTs require a multicenter study, which increases the variability in clinical care and makes consistency across patients difficult.

One such example is the Necrotizing Enterocolitis Trial (NET). This RCT has enrolled patients from neonatal surgical units in Europe, Asia, Australia, and Africa. In this study, infants were randomized to peritoneal drainage or laparotomy. The results indicated that peritoneal drainage does not immediately improve clinical status and that the evidence does not support using peritoneal drainage as a temporizing measure.[8] Similarly, a second study conducted in the United States and Canada showed that the choice of operation did not influence survival or other short-term clinical outcomes.[9] To accomplish statistical power in both of these trials, patients from a large geographic region were enrolled. These examples illustrate that enacting study protocols, standardizing the care of patients, and collecting data is more complex when multiple institutions must coordinate efforts.

True blinding of the investigators in a surgical RCT is difficult. In RCT involving medication, it is relatively simple to give one group of patients the therapeutic drug and the control group a placebo. However, if one group of patients receives laparoscopic surgery and the control group receives the traditional open procedure, both surgeon and patient will know which operation was performed. Some investigators have chosen to openly discuss the operation with patients and families and not attempt a blinded approach. This approach has been applied to open versus laparoscopic pyloromyotomy for pyloric stenosis. In the seminal study performed by St. Peter and colleagues, patients were randomly assigned to open or laparoscopic pyloromyotomy, but both the surgeon and the guardians knew the procedure to be performed. Postoperative pain management, feeding schedule, and discharge criteria were standardized for both groups. The laparoscopic technique was found to be superior to the open method in several outcomes.[42] However, one could argue that the surgeon's operating time or the perception of postoperative pain could be influenced by the knowledge of which technique was performed.

Investigators have attempted multiple blinding strategies in these situations. For example, while the patient is still under anesthesia, the surgeon may place identical wound dressings for both the laparoscopic and open operations.[43] When it is not possible to blind the investigators performing the procedures, it may be possible to blind the investigators evaluating the outcome. For example, a common scenario occurs in trials involving carotid endarterectomy versus stenting. In this situation, the patient and surgeon know the procedure performed, but a blinded practitioner such as a neurologist can assess for postoperative stroke symptoms and neurologic deficits.[44] When the outcome is soft (such as length of stay or pain), blinding is more difficult. Hard outcomes such as death or postoperative laboratory values are affected less by the blinding process.

In addition to study blinding, randomization may also pose a problem in surgical RCT. Patients may initially agree to be randomized but may change their minds after learning to which treatment group they have been randomized. For example, in a RCT comparing best medical therapy with surgery, patients may agree to be randomized, but after being placed in the best medical therapy group may decide that they would really like to receive surgical therapy or vice versa. In this scenario, investigators often address the problem with the "intention to treat" approach, whereby all patients are included in the analysis despite which treatment they did or did not receive. This analysis should be adequately performed and described in the data reporting.[45]

SUMMARIES OF EVIDENCE

To make evidence-based decisions for a particular patient or group of patients, data from multiple sources must be combined. No single data source, not even a well-conducted RCT, can provide all the evidence that a practitioner needs to choose the appropriate course of therapy for a patient. The medical literature is full of papers that combine evidence, and three examples are discussed here: review articles, meta-analysis, and systematic reviews.

Review Articles

Reading a review article on a disease process or treatment of interest can be an excellent first step toward familiarization with the current literature. It is a compilation of the existing literature and evidence deemed important or relevant by the author. However, the quality of the review is largely dependent on the author. The referenced articles are typically chosen by the author and the comments regarding the validity of these articles or their relevance to patient care are usually the author's opinion. In many cases the review may not be comprehensive because conflicting evidence is omitted.

For example, there may be an author who has written extensively about the repair of abdominal wall defects. This author is asked to write a review article on the topic by a respected journal. Imagine that this author is a long-standing advocate of early cesarean section and delivery. The author may be more likely to reference articles from institutions that share this view. He or she may be more familiar with the theoretical physiologic benefit of this approach and perhaps more likely to reference experimental studies with this perspective versus opposing views. Consider that the author is very experienced with this disorder and has a large referral base. She is likely to include excellent outcomes from her own institution in the review. These excellent outcomes could be due to myriad ways that her institution provides quality care that might have nothing to do with the fact that the treated babies were delivered by early cesarean section. The result is an article that provides important information on the topic but is decidedly slanted toward one viewpoint.

The author is probably a highly ethical and well-intentioned individual who truly believes in the superiority of her approach. Nevertheless, the structure of a review article and the lack of rigorous constraints on selection of articles and methods of review are likely to produce a result that strongly reflects the author's views. This is not necessarily negative, as viewpoints of experts can be of great value. However, it is crucial that the reader of a review article understand its

inherent limitations and is able to place its conclusions in the broader perspective of other types of evidence. We would go so far as to suggest that even this chapter on EBM reflects our own biases and viewpoints and should be considered in the context of other information written by those with a different outlook.

Meta-analysis

When there are data from several sources, a meta-analysis can be performed by combining the results of multiple clinical studies into aggregate data (Fig. 14-1). True meta-analysis is the analysis and compilation of data from randomized trials, but in the absence of RCTs, other data types are sometimes combined as well. It is assumed that the quality of studies is comparable and that the patient populations are equivalent. It also assumes that measurement techniques and factors examined are similar. The quality of the meta-analysis is therefore directly related to whether these assumptions are true and also to the quality of the original data.

In pediatric surgery, meta-analysis has been limited by the small number of RCTs and prospective cohort data. For example, meta-analysis was performed to evaluate laparoscopic versus open appendectomy in the pediatric population.[46] At the time of this analysis, only 30 studies had been performed over a 10-year period that matched the inclusion criteria. Of these studies, 12 were retrospective, 11 were prospective, and only 7 were randomized. Only 14 of the studies contained at least 50 patients in each group (laparoscopic or open). Therefore, meta-analysis is an important tool to gain a big-picture approach to a particular treatment and to incorporate data from multiple sources, but it is ultimately limited by the quality of the original data.

Systematic Reviews

Systematic reviews use algorithms to search, analyze, and combine the existing literature. Often both published and unpublished results are included in the search. The rigorous search algorithm minimizes bias, and these reviews provide a highly accessible source of quality information. Unfortunately in pediatric surgery, there are limited topics on which systematic reviews have been performed because of the lack of primary data.

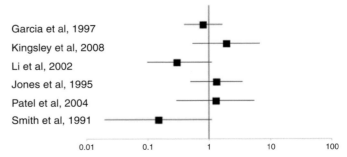

FIGURE 14-1 A forest plot illustrates the relative strength of treatment effects in multiple RCTs contributing to a meta-analysis. The relative risk of a treatment in a single RCT is represented by a square, and the CI is represented by the extent of the horizontal line. The area of each square is proportional to the study's weight in the meta-analysis. When multiple studies fall either to the left or the right of the central axis (relative risk = 1), this indicates a strong treatment effect. When studies are scattered to the left and right of the central axis, this indicates a weak treatment effect.

An excellent source of systematic reviews is the Cochrane Collaboration and Best Evidence. The Cochrane Collaboration is an international consortium of physicians, statisticians, and epidemiologists. It is the first, largest, and most successful group, and they have provided a model for consortiums that have followed. The mission of the group is to review the scope of the world's literature, primarily through RCTs. Only treatments are included. Usually, diagnostic tests or risk factors are not reviewed. The resulting reviews can be found in the Cochran Collaboration database[47] and PubMed.

Best Evidence is another review that is edited by experts in EBM and tends to be highly clinical in nature. Unlike the Cochran Collaboration, Best Evidence also includes analyses on therapy, diagnosis, cost effectiveness, and complications.

Application of Clinical Evidence

HYPOTHESIS TESTING

When reviewing a study, one must have a basic understanding of the statistical methods and pitfalls that can result in erroneous conclusions. The discipline of statistics is dependent on the notion of chance, that there is a random nature to all outcomes. When two groups are compared (treatment versus no treatment), the null hypothesis is that there is no difference between the groups. The P value is the probability that the observed difference is due to chance alone. Results are commonly considered statistically significant when $P < 0.05$ (there is less than a 5% chance that the difference observed was by chance). If multiple outcomes are examined, at $P = 0.05$, 1/20 of these outcomes will occur by chance alone. Therefore it is easy to see how multiple hypothesis testing can result in erroneous conclusions. This is often referred to as "data mining" or "sifting the data." The most simple statistical method to correct for multiple comparisons is to define significance as the desired P value (usually $P < 0.05$) divided by the number of comparisons. This is called the Bonferroni correction. The confidence interval (CI) is the probability that the same difference would occur if the study were repeated an infinite number of times. Therefore, a CI of 95% means that a difference would be seen in 95% of the repetitions of the study. There are many tests available to calculate P and CI. The correct test is dependent on the number of observations, number of groups compared, whether the data is continuous versus categorical, and if risk adjustment is required.

SUBJECTIVE VERSUS OBJECTIVE DATA AND RISK

Many kinds of outcomes can be studied, and data can be either objective (such as laboratory values or vital signs) or subjective (pain scales or physical examination). Objective data are more easily analyzed with statistical methods, and the results are often more straightforward to interpret. However, subjective data can be validated by using multiple observers. For example, if one outcome of a study is a radiographic finding, this type of data may vary depending on the radiologist examining the case. If multiple radiologists report their findings on the radiograph and are blinded to the opinions of their peers, a measurement of interobserver variability can be obtained. The measurement is known as the kappa value, for which a value of one indicates complete agreement between observers and a value of zero indicates no agreement.

Event rates and risk are important concepts to understand when deciding how a study result should impact the current standard of care. The event rate (ER) is the probability that an outcome will occur in a defined population. The control event rate is the probability that an outcome will occur with standard therapy, and the experimental event rate is the probability of the outcome with experimental therapy. Relative risk reduction and absolute risk reduction are the proportional and absolute risk values reduced by the experimental treatment, respectively. Number needed to treat (NNT) is the number of patients who need to be treated to prevent one adverse event. Therefore the impact of therapy depends on the event rate in the population, and the magnitude of risk reduction is greater for common events.

ERROR

All diagnostic tests and clinical studies contain errors. A type I error is rejecting the null hypothesis when it is true. This is also referred to as the false-alarm rate or the false-positive rate. In other words, a difference is observed when there is none. Alpha is the probability of a type I error, and when alpha is low, the specificity of a study is high.

The type II error is failing to reject the null hypothesis when it is false (the study does not find a difference when one exists). When the type II error is small, the sensitivity is high. Usually this type of error occurs because the sample size was too small. Beta is the probability of a type II error and can be minimized by performing power calculations during the planning of the study to ensure an adequate sample size. The study's statistical power should be stated in the results section of the manuscript. Unfortunately, no amount of statistical prowess can compensate for insufficient power. Therefore, for the results of a study to be reliable, type I and II errors must be minimized.

IDENTIFYING BIAS AND DETERMINING VALIDITY

Many types of bias exist and can be pervasive and difficult to recognize. Selection bias refers to an imperfection in the selection process. This can result in subjects who are not typical of the target population or subjects who are more likely to have the outcome of interest. For example, a study may conclude that laparoscopic colon resection is superior to the open technique. However, a bias may exist if patients who presented with nonemergent conditions were offered the laparoscopic procedure, whereas patients who presented with an acute abdominal process were treated with the open procedure.

Information bias can be introduced by the way data is obtained. Patients who are interviewed may recall different events than patients filling out a survey. However, patients completing an anonymous survey may be more likely to give truthful responses than those being interviewed. Recall bias refers to a selective memory of past events. For example, parents of children with digestive disorders or food allergies may be more likely to remember what the child ate in previous days than families with healthy children.

Before data from a study can be used in clinical decision making, the clinician must ask about the applicability and validity of the study. The characteristics of the patients in the study should be similar to the patient who will be treated. The clinician must ask, "Are the patients in the study similar to my patient?" and "Does the sensitivity analysis include values that my patient would use?" Also, the validity of the study must be examined. The evidence needs to meet minimum criteria and the conclusions must be logical and complete.[25] If there are "soft spots" in the evidence, these should be dealt with appropriately. If possible, the analysis should be validated in a prospective study.

GUIDELINES AND PATHWAYS

Once several valid studies have been performed and there exists a body of clinical evidence, guidelines and pathways can be constructed. Health care entities are increasingly relying on clinical guidelines, which typically focus on managing a particular type of patient. Guidelines are useful for cost savings, outcomes improvement, and error reduction. The difference between algorithms, guidelines, and pathways is an important distinction. An algorithm is a checklist or detailed list of instructions to carry out a specific task. A guideline is a standardized set of recommendations for a specific problem. A pathway combines several practice guidelines into a set of recommendations and may track a patient through diagnosis, management, rehabilitation, and follow-up.

Guidelines can be created to improve outcomes, to minimize variation in practice between physicians, or to contain excessive costs. To create a guideline, practitioners agree on a standard of care based on the available evidence. If the evidence is inadequate, that step is either decided on by consensus or left to the discretion of the physician. It is important that key members of the community "buy in" to the guidelines for implementation to run smoothly. Outcomes should be measured before and after implementation for validation purposes. However, it has been shown that implementing guidelines improves patient outcomes.[48] This is due in part to the observation that obtaining consistency may be more important than finding the "best" guideline.

Advantages of guidelines include reduction in errors of omission (forgetting an order) and reduction in errors of commission (e.g., drug dosage errors). There is an increase in efficiency and a potential cost savings, and guidelines often minimize confusion among staff. Hospital lengths of stay are decreased and patients have better outcomes. Potential disadvantages include loss of physician autonomy and potential dissonance if not all providers agree with the guidelines, as there is a recommended acceptance of the value judgments inherent in the guideline. It may become cumbersome if different entities (e.g., Medicare and the American Heart Association) promote different guidelines. If guidelines do not account for individual variation between patients, harm can result. There is a potential for legal liability if an undesirable outcome results despite proper adherence. For this reason, clinicians are ultimately responsible for deciding if a guideline is valid and whether or not it is applicable to their patient.

In summary, before applying current evidence to patient care, the clinician must carefully analyze the available data. This includes understanding the benefits and limitations of the study design, as well as the statistical analysis and significance of the data. The clinician must determine if a study result is applicable to a particular patient. Over time, applying this information to patient care can improve the quality of care. Introducing guidelines and pathways is one way to improve patient outcomes, and must be validated. Therefore clinicians should have a basic understanding of quality assessment.

Outcomes and Measuring Quality of Care

QUALITY OF CARE ASSESSMENT

There is growing recognition that there is great variation in surgical care between institutions and practitioners. Patients and families want to make informed decisions and are asking for more data regarding their health care choices. In addition, clinical leaders want to improve the quality of care. Therefore there is a need to assess performance and patient outcomes. A good performance measure will guide patients toward hospitals and clinicians with better results. Performance analysis can include structural, process, and outcome measures. Transparency of performance measures leads all institutions to take steps to improve results and elevates the overall level of medical care.

Specific Measurements

There are three widely used measures to determine healthcare "quality": structure, process, and outcome. Health care structure consists of elements that are fixed characteristics of the system that will not vary between individual providers. Examples of structural measures include nurse/patient ratios and whether or not there is a dedicated intensive care team. Measures of health care structure are expedient and inexpensive because the data are generally obtained from preexisting administrative records. Measures tend to be efficiently analyzed; a single measure may be compared to several outcomes. Unfortunately the number of measurements is limited and measures do not reflect individual performance, which many clinicians find unfair. An example of comparing structural measures would be evaluating the inpatient mortality rates of teaching versus nonteaching hospitals. One may find that mortality is higher in teaching facilities. Although the correlation may be strong, the analysis reveals little about the causative relationship between the variables. It is possible that quality of care is worse in teaching hospitals. It is also possible that teaching hospitals have more complex or high-risk cases. The ability to perform accurate risk adjustment is relevant here as it is to both process and outcome measures as well.

A second way to measure health care quality is to evaluate processes of care. These are services provided, medications prescribed, and other interventions applied to the care of patients. Process measures reflect care that patients actually receive and are directly actionable for quality improvement. An example of a process measure would be determining how many patients are asked to rate their level of pain as part of routine vital signs or whether patients receive the appropriate antibiotics before surgical incision. One benefit of process measures is that risk adjustment is often unnecessary. For example, it is well established that all patients receiving surgery should receive an antiseptic skin preparation before incision. Therefore it is unnecessary to collect data regarding illness severity for the purposes of risk adjustment. Process measures are designed to determine how closely the care actually delivered resembles the care that the facility intended to deliver.

Because process measures are easy to implement and enforce, they are often the focus of regulatory agencies. The Surgical Care Improvement Project (SCIP) is a national partnership that was formed to improve patient safety by decreasing postoperative complications.[49] SCIP focuses on antibiotic prophylaxis, perioperative glucose control, appropriate preoperative hair removal, postoperative normothermia, perioperative beta blockade, and venous thromboembolism prophylaxis. For example, the SCIP guidelines suggest that antibiotics should be received within 1 hour before surgical incision, should be appropriately selected for the procedure to be performed, and should be discontinued within 24 hours of surgery. Compliance with these types of guidelines can be easily monitored and publically reported.

Unfortunately, studies have shown that institutions that score high on process measures do not necessarily have better outcomes. For example, a recent study compared the rate at which facilities provided timely and appropriate preoperative antibiotics to actual wound infection rates. Many of the centers with the highest rate of compliance with antibiotic use unexpectedly had the highest rate of wound infections.[50] In addition, hospitals that scored high on performance measures for the treatment of heart failure did not show any difference in patient outcomes within 1 year of discharge.[51] An additional limitation is that there is currently a lack of reliable data infrastructure. Many databases contain information on outcomes, and lack information on process of care. Therefore, measures may be difficult to define with existing databases, and the link between the measure and important patient outcomes is variable.

The third type of measurement is outcome data, which is the measurement most familiar to clinicians. End points can include variables such as mortality, complications, length of hospital stay, patient satisfaction, and readmission. Direct outcome measurements are appealing because they have inherent face validity and directly address variables that are most clinically important. Outcome measures are easily accepted by clinicians and hospitals. For example, ability to compare morbidity and mortality between centers in the Veterans

Administration (VA) Hospitals through the National Surgical Quality Improvement Program (NSQIP) allowed improvements to be instituted that improved patient outcomes.[52] Collection of accurate outcome data requires a highly skilled data collection team and is time and resource intensive. Comparative outcome data between centers is of limited value without adequate risk adjustment. For example, hospitals and physicians who avoid high-risk patients or complicated procedures may appear to have better outcomes if a thorough risk adjustment is not performed. The most robust and accurate models for risk adjustment in surgical patients have been developed by the American College of Surgeons' NSQIP.[53,54]

Improving Performance

Several organizations use performance measures to make recommendations regarding guidelines and to focus efforts to improve outcomes. The National Quality Forum (NQF), Joint Commission of Accreditation of Healthcare Organizations (JCAHO), and the Center for Medicare and Medicaid Services (CMS) have focused mainly on process measures and hospital-based care. The LeapFrog Group is a consortium of employers and health care payers who developed an extensive set of quality measures for value-based purchasing assessment.[55]

Databases and Networks

Several collaborative efforts have been undertaken to create databases for quality improvement and outcomes research. The most well known is NSQIP, which was developed to improve the quality of surgical care on a national level. The American College of Surgeons (ACS) adopted this system after it was successfully implemented in the VA system. NSQIP provides reliable and risk-adjusted outcomes data. Because of the national scope of the project, surgical quality can be compared between hundreds of institutions. A rigorously trained clinical nurse reviewer collects information from the medical record. Data are collected prospectively and reported as the observed/expected ratio for mortality and numerous specific morbidities. Since the implementation of NSQIP in the VA system, 30-day mortality and morbidity were reduced by 45% and 27%, respectively (Fig. 14-2).[52] This translates to tens of thousands of lives saved.

The most important strength of NSQIP is that risk adjustment is done effectively and in a manner that is widely accepted as valid. Also, participating institutions can access

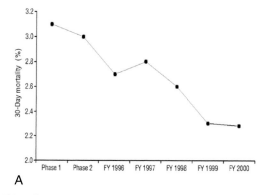

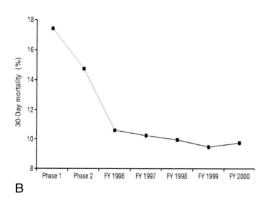

FIGURE 14-2 Thirty-day postoperative mortality **(A)** and morbidity **(B)** for all major operations performed in the Veterans Affairs hospitals throughout the NSQIP data collection process. A 27% and 45% decrease in mortality and morbidity, respectively, were observed.[60] FY = fiscal year.

their own outcomes and compare their results against others. The program is expensive to implement, as it requires an annual fee as well as the salary of a dedicated nurse. It is not yet designed for assessing procedure-specific performance. At this juncture NSQIP provides informative data regarding general and vascular surgery in adults. The program is evolving to provide procedure- and specialty-specific outcomes in many disciplines. A separate pediatric program is under development.[56]

The Children's Oncology Group provides a wonderful success story of how large cooperative trials and evidence-based practice were used to decrease mortality for children with cancer. Through modification of therapeutic regimens based on multicenter RCTs, this group was able to decrease mortality from acute lymphocytic leukemia by 70%, without the development of any new drugs.[57,58] More recently, the American Pediatric Surgical Association (APSA) Outcomes and Clinical Trials Center was established in 2000. The objective of the center is to promote evidence-based guidelines through research efforts and outcomes analysis. Capabilities of the center include project coordination, database management, and data analysis.[59] These research efforts will no doubt be instrumental in providing new outcomes data, which will then be used to determine clinical guidelines.

Conclusions

With the numerous sources of data available to surgeons, the application of EBM to patient care has become a complex and rewarding endeavor. Study design in many ways determines the strength of the data and to which patients the results can be applied. Therefore it is essential that pediatric surgeons understand the strengths and limitations of clinical studies and basic principles of statistics when evaluating clinical evidence. In addition, outcomes research and quality of care measurement is in a state of evolution and is already influencing the practice of surgery. Therefore clinicians should continue to carefully evaluate clinical evidence, as well as their own outcomes, so that we can constantly improve the health of our patients.

The complete reference list is available online at www. expertconsult.com.

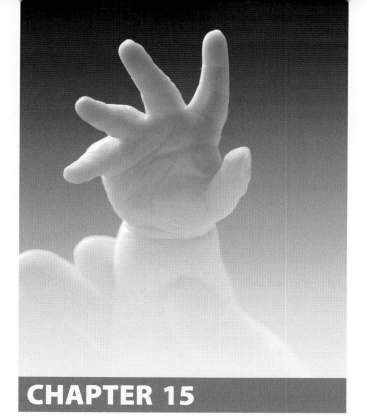

CHAPTER 15

Ethical Considerations

Benedict C. Nwomeh and Donna A. Caniano

Ethics is concerned with questions of right and wrong. Medical ethics, also known as bioethics, outlines the standards, principles, and rules of conduct that govern physician behavior, the practice of medicine, and the conduct of biomedical research and training. However, although the core principles of medical ethics are immutable, our notion of what constitutes ethical practice is constantly challenged by evolving cultural norms, particularly within the milieu of an increasingly multicultural society and the rapid pace of technologic advancement. Furthermore, there are significant overlaps between the distinct disciplines of law and medical ethics, such that evolving standards of one affects the other.[1] Thus a new statute or court ruling sets a standard of conduct that often compels adjustment in the rules of ethical conduct. Conversely, the pronouncement of new ethical guidelines by professional medical organizations frequently influences the work of legislatures and the courts. Ethics tells us what we ought to do but the law stipulates what we must do. Together, law and ethics define the rules of conduct within which medicine is practiced, but like medicine itself, both are dynamic disciplines that undergo constant adjustment.

Beauchamp and Childress have articulated certain *prima facie* principles that define the most fundamental foundations of medical ethics.[2] The tetrad of principles includes beneficence, nonmaleficence, autonomy, and justice. The first two of these principles, beneficence and nonmaleficence, are derived from the Hippocratic obligations to "act in the best interests of the patient" and to "do no harm." The other two principles, based on relatively recent concepts, are (1) autonomy, which respects the right of competent persons to give informed consent for medical treatment and to have control over their bodies and (2) justice, which involves the fair and equitable distribution of the benefits (and risks) of medical care to all persons.

Although principle-based and duty-based ethics tend to be given the most attention, some ethicists make a strong case for virtue-based ethics and contend that virtue is derivable from the nature of medicine as a human activity and is an irreducible element in medical ethics.[3] Ethical principles, per se, focus on the action or actions that give rise to dilemmas, such as withdrawing life-sustaining treatment from a terminally ill patient. In contrast, virtue ethics emphasizes the agents (physicians) and the recipients (patients) of principle-based actions and decisions. Pellegrino and Thomasma cite the relevance of virtues such as trust, compassion, prudence, justice, courage, phronesis or common sense, fortitude, integrity, honesty, and self-effacement in confronting practical problems such as care of the poor, research with human subjects, and the conduct of the healing relationship.[3] In practice, physicians' ethical behavior is shaped as much by the core ethical principles as by the special bond that sickness and the response to it creates between healer and patient. In addition, pediatric surgeons are challenged by issues that are distinctive to the profession of surgery and other factors that are unique to the care of infants and children.

In this chapter we review some of the basic ethical concepts and responsibilities pertinent to pediatric surgery and explore thorny issues related to the extremes of prenatal care and the end of life. We address common surgical and ethical dilemmas in operative management, such as in adolescent bariatric surgery. We also highlight new areas of ethical concerns such as surgical error, and aspects of professionalism in the relationships between physicians and industry. Finally, we discuss the ethical imperatives of multiculturalism and why the prevailing ethical landscape should not deter much needed research and innovation in pediatric surgery.

Resolution of Ethical Dilemmas

The essence of pediatric surgery was underscored by Potts in his classic monograph *The Surgeon and the Child*, in which he noted that "the satisfaction of correcting a deformity in a newborn infant lies in the fact that all his life lies before him. Parents hope for miracles, but are grateful for the best that can be given by a mere human being."[4]

This profound statement is applicable, whether the pediatric surgeon is repairing a major congenital anomaly, treating a devastating traumatic injury, or resecting a malignancy. However, in the course of providing the best possible care to children and their families, the pediatric surgeon will occasionally encounter ethical and moral issues.

A classic moral dilemma arises when two or more conflicting ethical principles support mutually inconsistent actions. A common situation is when there is a conflict between the principles of autonomy and beneficence—when parents desire a course of treatment for their child that does not align with the opinion of the pediatric surgeon. The pediatric surgeon may also encounter moral dilemmas in the form of moral uncertainty and moral distress when the prognosis is unclear for a given condition, when two or more equally valid treatment options are available, or when parents disagree with each other, or the surgical recommendations, or both. Therefore the need often arises to resolve the moral basis by which decisions should be made, who should make those decisions, and how decisions should be implemented.

Little[5] has identified five pillars that mark the moral domain of the surgeon-patient relationship: rescue, proximity, ordeal, aftermath, and presence. These factors may be present in other therapeutic relationships as well, but they have a special intensity in surgery. The term *rescue* acknowledges the elements of surrender and dependency that patients and their families experience when they have little control over the proposed surgical remedy. This situation can be mitigated if the pediatric surgeon confronts and negotiates the patient's (and family's) surrender and dependency within the context of the surgeon's power. *Proximity* refers to surgeons' acknowledgment of the close, intimate interactions they have with their patient, who must forgo their autonomy, acknowledge dependency, face risk, and yet place trust in the surgeon. *Presence* is both a virtue and a duty for surgeons, to be a visible and engaged presence throughout the entire surgical experience. In pediatric surgery, this professional obligation extends to the long-term follow-up of patients, often into young adulthood.

The foregoing ethical and moral principles and virtues are brought to bear in the ordinary course of a pediatric surgeon's daily work, in which ethical dilemmas are frequently encountered. Resolution of ethical problems in a given pediatric surgical patient requires a patient-centered approach that uses all members of the health care team working together in a manner that promotes respect for all parties and all views.

As we and others have noted, successful outcomes require that the team (1) develop common moral language for the discussion of moral issues, (2) have training in how to articulate their views about issues, (3) have common experiences on which to base recommendations, and (4) agree on a moral decision-making method for all to use in the course of their deliberations.

Bayliss and Caniano previously outlined the following set of guidelines to provide a framework for the effective resolution of difficult moral problems[6]:

1. Identify the decision makers. For most cases in pediatric surgery, the decision makers will be the parents, unless the patient is a mature minor.
2. Ascertain "value data" from the parents and other relevant family members. These may include their views on the sanctity of life, spirituality and religious beliefs, cultural norms, and community values.
3. Collect all relevant medical information, including the prognosis. Clarify the areas of uncertainty and identify whether additional diagnostic testing would be of value in the decision making process.
4. Define all treatment options, including their benefits, risks, and chances of achieving the desired outcomes.
5. Provide the parents with a professional recommendation for the best treatment option.
6. Seek a consensus resolution that can be accepted by all participants.

In order for the above paradigm to be successful, the health care team must accept that rational people of good will may hold divergent views that are irreconcilable, even after extended discussions. The goal of reaching a consensus decision should be viewed as a successful outcome for all participants.

Informed Consent and Assent

The doctrine of informed consent is based primarily on the ethical principle of respect for individual autonomy, but also on beneficence and justice. These three pillars, established in the Belmont Report[7] to guide human subjects' research, have become the basis for ethical and legal requirements for informed consent for research as well as clinical care. Respect for patients' *autonomy* recognizes the right of each person to make their own decisions. The principle of *beneficence* requires physicians to propose only those interventions intended to promote the well being of the patient, and *justice* requires that the patient be treated in the same manner as any other individual under similar circumstances.

In pediatric surgery, fulfillment of a child's autonomy typically requires surrogate decision makers (in most cases, the parents) to speak, understand, and consent on behalf of infants, children, and adolescents. In some cases, court-appointed guardians or other spokespersons may fulfill this role, depending on applicable laws. In some jurisdictions, and in certain specific circumstances, adolescent patients may be granted authority to make their own decisions about the health care they receive. This situation is particularly applicable to adolescents with chronic illnesses, such as sickle cell disease, cystic fibrosis, and advanced malignancies. However, when an adolescent's consent to or refusal of surgery is in direct opposition to parental wishes, the assistance of social services and legal counsel may be required.

Recognition of children as "persons" with inherent rights underscores the necessity for their participation in the decision-making process.[8] Therefore, the traditional emphasis on the child's "best interests" may be insufficient to address the child's "rights," and although the *informed permission* given by parents may be sufficient for ethical purposes and is required for legal purposes, it does not satisfy the strict moral standards of the doctrine of informed consent. Therefore, a specific role has been advocated for children in their own decision making, particularly for older children and adolescents. This concept of pediatric *assent* was articulated by William Bartholome when he wrote, in 1982, that "assent of the child is indeed an idea before its time. It is a fragile idea that can easily be crushed amidst the boulders of consent, autonomy, rights, and competence. It's an idea that is so foreign to adult reality that its central thrust is missed even by astute minds."[9]

Several decision-making models have been proposed as a template for pediatric assent, but they differ primarily on the relative roles assigned to the child and the parents and whether they should be guided by the principle of autonomy or follow a best-interests design.[10] Nevertheless there is broad agreement that, depending on the circumstances, the *assent* of the pediatric patient should be sought as appropriate to their development, age, and understanding in conjunction with informed permission from the parent or legal guardian. Every state has enacted minor consent statutes that seek to determine instances in which children can give their informed consent, as highlighted in a policy statement by the American Academy of Pediatrics (Table 15-1).[11] However, in most instances parent/guardian consent is required by law. Pediatric surgeons have an ethical duty to familiarize themselves with their own institutional guidelines and appropriate local statutes.

For surgical procedures, the essential components of the informed consent process include (1) a surgeon who provides adequate information to facilitate decision making and (2) a competent patient or legal proxy who indicates full understanding of the intervention, including the indications, risks, and possible alternatives, and who voluntarily consents to the proposed intervention.[12,13]

In the unique triadic relationship between the pediatric surgeon, parent, and child, surgeons bring the values and ethical principles of their profession, which give priority to the interests and well-being of their patients and families. In their landmark book, *Surgical Ethics*, McCullough and colleagues[14] present patients' rights related to the surgical encounter, each of which implies a key professional value. They remind us that "(patients have the right) . . . not to be killed intentionally or negligently by the surgeon, not to be harmed by intent or negligence of the surgeon . . . not to be deceived by the surgeon . . . to be adequately informed about the risks and benefits of surgery, to be treated by a knowledgeable, competent practitioner, to have his or her health and well-being more highly valued than the surgeon's own economic interest, and to decide whether to accept treatment under the conditions described."[14]

Prenatal Surgical Consultation

Routine prenatal screening with ultrasonography and biochemical markers now permit detection of major fetal anomalies that may require operative intervention shortly after birth, or rarely, in utero. When a significant fetal malformation is detected by screening, consultation with the pediatric surgeon or other specialists is usually offered to prospective parents. Ethical issues that may arise during the course of a prenatal consultation include (1) the possibility of prenatal intervention or termination of pregnancy; (2) the timing, location, and mode of delivery; and (3) potential postnatal surgical intervention.[15]

The prenatal surgical consultation should be guided by the same ethical principles of autonomy (self-determination), beneficence, and justice, and in addition respect for the woman's choice and her reproductive freedom. The proper role of the pediatric surgeon is not only to give information but also to provide a supportive, caring environment for informed decision making. In theory, a value-neutral norm that promotes objectivity and client autonomy may be considered ideal, but such an approach usually proves insufficient as the moral basis for prenatal surgical consultation. Value neutrality and moral detachment on the part of the surgeon creates an obstacle to forming a professional relationship with prospective parents who are seeking compassion, honesty, and integrity, virtues cited by Pellegrino and Thomasma as being essential components of the physician-patient relationship.[3]

Very few prospective parents consider termination of pregnancy when they present for a prenatal surgical consultation.

TABLE 15-1

Types of Minor Consent Statutes or Rules of Common Law That Allow for the Medical Treatment of a Minor Patient Without Parental Consent*

Legal Exceptions to Informed Consent Requirement	Medical Care Setting
The "emergency" exception	Minor seeks emergency medical care
The "emancipated minor" exception	Minor is self-reliant or independent: • Married • In military service • Emancipated by court ruling • Financially independent and living apart from parents In some states, college students, runaways, pregnant minors, or minor mothers also may be included
The "mature minor" exception	Minor is capable of providing informed consent to the proposed medical or surgical treatment—generally a minor 14 yr or older who is sufficiently mature and possesses the intelligence to understand and appreciate the benefits, risks, and alternatives of the proposed treatment and who is able to make a voluntary and rational choice (*in determining whether the mature minor exception applies, the physician must consider the nature and degree of risk of the proposed treatment and whether the proposed treatment is for the minor's benefit, is necessary or elective, and is complex*)
Exceptions based on specific medical condition	Minor seeks: • Mental health services • Pregnancy and contraceptive services • Testing or treatment for human immunodeficiency virus infection or acquired immunodeficiency syndrome • Sexually transmitted or communicable disease testing and treatment • Drug or alcohol dependency counseling and treatment • Care for crime-related injury

From Committee on Pediatric Emergency Medicine: Consent for emergency medical services for children and adolescents. Pediatrics, 2003. 111: p. 703-706.
*These laws vary by state and the surgeon should refer to the applicable jurisdiction.

In fact, most are seeking the pediatric surgeon's knowledge and reassurance that their unborn fetus can be treated with a good outcome. These prospective parents typically provide the surgeon with their most current fetal ultrasonogram and other diagnostic tests, its gender, and its first and middle names. The stage is therefore set for the pediatric surgeon to forge an ongoing professional relationship that is centered on the care of the future infant and that both parties share in making ethically responsible and medically sound decisions for the fetus.

We suggest the following as guidelines for pediatric surgeons during a prenatal surgical consultation:

1. Empathize with the inevitable grief and sorrow that the prospective parents feel on the recent unexpected and frightening diagnosis of a fetal malformation.
2. Candidly disclose the benefits, harms, and alternatives for the given fetal condition and offer recommendations that balance maternal and fetal interests.
3. Foster an atmosphere that facilitates the exchange of medical information and help the prospective parents make decisions that are consistent with their own beliefs, goals, and values.
4. Promote responsible efforts to improve access to the full range of prenatal services available at high-risk perinatal centers for women from all socioeconomic, ethnic, and cultural groups.

On occasion, ethical conflict may arise if the pregnant woman, in the exercise of her reproductive freedom, chooses a course of action that is inconsistent with conventional pediatric surgical recommendations. For example, a decision on the part of the woman to terminate the pregnancy because of a nonlethal anomaly, such as gastroschisis, could provoke emotional, moral, and professional conflict with the pediatric surgeon. Sadly, termination rates for gastroschisis remain high, particularly in Europe, where 29% of prospective parents in the EUROSCAN study[16] and as much as 44% in another study[17] elected termination for a condition with such a favorable prognosis. Prenatal counseling, when successful, should allay parental anxiety and reduce the rate of unnecessary terminations. Fortunately, other European studies have reported termination rates for gastroschisis of 5% or less.[18,19]

When, despite the objective medical fact of the low lethality of the fetal malformation, the woman insists on termination or other action detrimental to the fetus, it is not clear whether the pediatric surgeon can interfere with her choice. Under usual circumstances, a pediatric surgeon might invoke the power of the state when they believe that a pediatric patient's best interests are not being protected by the parents. However, there is no similar authority to intervene on behalf of the fetus. There has also been some concern that in situations in which maternal and fetal interests diverge, the obstetrician and the pediatric surgeon might be drawn into an ethical conflict as they seek the best interests of the mother and fetus, respectively.[20]

End of Life

Advances in technology and development of new diagnostic and therapeutic interventions have created new life-sustaining treatments that can prolong a patient's life. These "high tech"

measures (e.g., renal dialysis, ventilators, and organ transplantation) as well as new applications of existing therapies (e.g., antibiotics, fluids and nutrition delivered by enteral tubes or intravenous means) and chemotherapy increase the potential to extend life after critical illness. Depending on the therapeutic goal, surgical treatment could correct a surgical anomaly, provide palliation of symptoms, or merely improve selected physiologic parameters. In many cases, attainment of the defined therapeutic goal can allow an infant to develop normally or a child to pursue a meaningful life. However, in some cases the price of success is a relatively poor quality of life and a burden of care that could overwhelm some families. The question therefore is no longer whether pediatric surgeons *can* save the life of an infant with severe malformation or other neonatal disease but whether they *should* save it.[20]

Determination of what constitutes an optimal quality of life and the threshold below which life-saving measures should not be undertaken is a difficult moral, ethical, spiritual, and legal problem. Decisions to withhold life-sustaining treatment are generally made in advance and agreed on by the parents and physicians. However, there are limits to parental authority to make end of life decisions for their children as illustrated in the United States by the Baby Doe case.[21] Baby Doe was born in Bloomington, Indiana in 1982 with Down syndrome and esophageal atresia. The infant died after 6 days when the obstetrician recommended, and the parents agreed, to no surgical intervention. The Surgeon General at the time, C. Everett Koop, himself a pediatric surgeon, publicly expressed disagreement with this decision, which he believed was made on the basis of the infant's mental retardation rather than on the prospect for success after surgery. Several months later, Dr. Koop was again drawn into opposition when the parents of a second infant, "Baby Jane Doe" born with spina bifida cystica, decided not to have operative treatment. This time, a "right-to-life" lawyer and subsequently the federal government brought a court action, but the court ruled that the parents refusal was "a reasonable one, based on due consideration of the medical options available, and on genuine concern for the best interests of the child."[22]

Although several courts upheld the parental decisions in these and subsequent cases, public outcry led to federal intervention. Congress passed the Baby Doe law that specified criteria under which withholding of life-saving treatment can be permissible as follows:

- Child is irreversibly comatose
- Treatment is "virtually futile" in terms of survival
- Treatment would only prolong dying

Although the Baby Doe rules were designed to protect the child's right to life-saving treatment, regardless of the parents' wishes, the intent was not to mandate unnecessary or inappropriate treatments. To the contrary, the Baby Doe law positively directs physicians to make treatment recommendations to parents based on "reasonable medical judgment." Unfortunately, the law has been widely misinterpreted and misunderstood among physicians. In a 1988 survey, one third of pediatricians stated that maximal life-prolonging treatment was not in the best interests of the infants, but because of the Baby Doe law they would provide such treatment.[23] Some critics of the law also complained about federal imposition of medical decisions that would lead to proliferation of severely handicapped children without assurance of the resources needed to care for them.[22]

In both infants and older children, medical advances have created ethical dilemmas in the initiation or withdrawal of medical care for conditions with poor prognosis, particularly in situations in which treatment may prolong survival with an unacceptable quality of life. Although many individuals believe it is "worse" to discontinue life-sustaining treatment than to never institute such treatment, ethicists, moral philosophers, and legal scholars find no ethical or legal distinction between not starting treatment and stopping treatment.

A common situation in the neonatal intensive care unit is when a premature infant with several comorbid factors, such as chronic lung disease and intraventricular hemorrhage, requires surgical exploration for necrotizing enterocolitis or midgut volvulus. Issues that may arise include the appropriateness of extensive small bowel resection and whether care should be withdrawn in the face of poor prognosis. If bowel resection leads to short-bowel syndrome, will the infant be a candidate for intestinal or liver transplantation, or both? This situation typifies an all too frequent ethical dilemma faced by pediatric surgeons. When making decisions to prolong life or to discontinue life-sustaining treatment for an infant with critical illness, the *best interests standard* is generally used to focus on issues that are patient centered and to assess the benefits and burdens of continued treatment for a *particular infant*. In this case the infant's best interests standard would include consideration of the following:

- Severity of the medical condition
- Availability of curative or corrective treatment
- Achievability of medical goals
- Presence of serious neurologic impairments
- All associated medical conditions
- Life expectancy
- Extent of suffering
- Proportionality of treatment benefits to burdens in both the short term and long term

In making these difficult decisions, the medical team must work cooperatively with the parents. and their wishes should be given due consideration. There is an emerging consensus that great discretion should be given to parents in making decisions on nonintervention or withdrawal of life-saving treatment.[24] The guidelines issued in 2007 by The American Academy of Pediatrics encourage a family-centered, patient-oriented approach.[25] When there is disagreement, continued engagement between physicians and parents will often lead to an agreement. Conflict resolution may require transfer of care to another physician or consultation with the institution's ethics committee.

With life-threatening illnesses, such as terminal cancer, in older children and adolescents, parental protective instincts may come into conflict with the child's autonomy to participate in end-of-life decisions. However, older children who are capable of giving assent in ordinary situations are equally competent to do so when forced to confront their mortality. In fact terminal illness may impact the developmental understanding of pediatric patients by accelerating their grasp of serious illness and by promoting their wishes to control decisions about their health care. The stresses of their illness may "make them grow up faster" and make them wiser than their same-age peer group. For example, a 12-year-old child with terminal cancer may ask to discontinue chemotherapy or other unpleasant treatments and request to have "one final special vacation."

Because children cannot give morally or legally valid consent to or refusal of treatment, practice among physicians in the past was to shelter dying children from the truth of their dire circumstances. Current practice, favored by The American Academy of Pediatrics, acknowledges that these patients usually have a much more mature understanding of their situation than previously realized by their physicians and parents and that they should be told the truth about their prognosis and included in discussions about their care.[26,27] These discussions should include the extent of desired life-sustaining treatments, whether a do-not-resuscitate (DNR) or an allow natural death (AND) status is to be invoked, the role of palliative procedures in granting a better quality of life, and their desire for hospice services.

Ethical Issues in Pediatric Bariatric Surgery

Bariatric operations in the pediatric population are increasingly used as an effective means of achieving weight loss and thereby relieving comorbidities such as type 2 diabetes, cardiovascular dysfunction, hypertension, obstructive sleep apnea, and dyslipidemias. These and other unsuspected comorbidities are present in nearly one third of all patients treated at the Center for Healthy Weight and Nutrition at Nationwide Children's Hospital. Morbidly obese children are likely to remain so in adulthood and carry with them the increased risks of premature morbidity and mortality. From a public health perspective, there is a rising childhood obesity epidemic that could dramatically increase the cost of medical care and cause a decline in life expectancy, thereby eroding the gains in longevity achieved during the 20th century in developed countries.

A multidisciplinary approach is currently used in the treatment for morbid obesity. The range of success with these approaches varies, and research is needed to better assess them, particularly in the pediatric population. Medical therapy that includes a comprehensive program of exercise and diet has not been successful in adults over the long term. Few children's hospitals have developed comprehensive medical obesity programs. Thus there is scant evidence in the pediatric literature about the outcomes of such programs. For adults with morbid obesity, surgical therapy is quite popular because it has been successful in achieving weight reduction with acceptable morbidity and mortality rates. Based on the good results in the adult population, it is not surprising that pediatric surgeons are being asked by the public—in particular, eager patients and their parents—to provide bariatric surgery for children and adolescents with morbid obesity.

Roux-en-Y gastric bypass and gastric banding, both performed laparoscopically, are the two bariatric operations performed most frequently in North America and Europe. Although both achieve weight loss, gastric banding does not alter the anatomy and is reversible; gastric bypass alters the anatomy in an essentially irreversible manner. Gastric bypass is very effective in achieving weight loss not only because it reduces the size of the stomach but also because it causes malabsorption. Long-term studies in adults indicate that gastric banding is somewhat less effective in achieving major weight loss but is successful in reducing the comorbid conditions of hypertension and diabetes.

As noted by Caniano,[28] both principle-based ethics (autonomy, beneficence, nonmaleficence, and justice) and virtue-based ethical considerations (trustworthiness, compassion, phronesis, fortitude, integrity, and self-effacement) must be included in order to fully capture the moral complexity of pediatric bariatric surgery. Also, because bariatric surgery remains an innovative treatment, insofar as its long-term consequences for pediatric patients remain unknown, there are additional ethical obligations for evaluation of outcomes and for clinical research. All of these factors must be considered when (1) a pediatric surgeon recommends a bariatric operation to an individual patient, (2) the pediatric patient and her or his family decide to have bariatric surgery, (3) hospitals establish pediatric bariatric programs, and (4) the major professional surgical organizations endorse the performance of pediatric bariatric interventions. The following discussion examines how various ethical principles apply specifically to bariatric surgery.

True *autonomy* for the morbidly obese adolescent considering bariatric surgery is reflected by adequate informed consent. More than most other cases, the balance between parental permission and the child's assent weighs heavily toward the latter. Unfortunately, true autonomy under these settings is under severe pressure from the flurry of information available in the media, lay publications, and the Internet, which often highlight former morbidly obese individuals who became svelte after their intervention. The desire to have a body that is socially acceptable and free of comorbidities may interfere with a deep understanding of the operative risks and the irreversible nature of some of the proposed procedures. The burden of providing informed consent to the adolescent patient and his or her family rests on the surgical team, which should include at the least medical specialists, psychologists, and pediatric surgeons. Interested readers are referred to the guidelines proposed by Raper and Sarwer on the elements of informed consent that constitute the minimum amount of information to be discussed with prospective adolescent patients interested in bariatric treatment and their families.[29]

Beneficence obliges physicians to seek to reverse the physical and psychological derangements that interfere with well-being in morbidly obese children. If nonsurgical interventions—such as calorie-restriction diets, exercise programs, and behavioral therapy—were effective in achieving substantial weight loss with reversal of comorbidities, beneficence would favor these approaches. However, adolescent patients whose body mass index (BMI) exceeds 40 kg/m^2 have only a 3% reduction in BMI after 1 year of intensive medical weight management, a result that is insufficient to reverse comorbidities.[30] However, given the risks associated with bariatric surgery, beneficence warrants that prospective patients undergo thorough assessment of their metabolic and psychological parameters, receive a "reasonable" trial of medical/behavioral weight loss treatment, and continue such treatment if it proves effective. For most patients who are unsuccessful with this approach, bariatric surgery upholds the principle of beneficence in enhancing health and well-being.

The well-known risks of harm during and after bariatric procedures impose an obligation of *nonmaleficence* in recommending treatment choices. Although reported rates of serious short-term risks of bariatric surgery are low, adolescent patients who are eager to lose weight may not appreciate the potential impact of such complications in terms of lengthy hospitalization, reoperative surgery, and other unanticipated problems. Furthermore, assessment of possible harm must include consideration of complications that may develop several years later. Wilde, in a 2004 law review article, observes that physicians trust that morbidly obese adult patients can put all the known risks and complications into perspective before agreeing to a bariatric operation, but it is not clear that pediatric patients and their families have that same perspective given the uncertainty of outcomes decades after the operation.[29a]

The principle of *justice* (also a virtue) requires that each person share equitably in the benefits and risks of health care. Studies have found significant disparities in access to adult bariatric surgery for African Americans, Hispanics, low-income individuals, and males.[30] Similarly, justice is threatened when disparities occur in the manner in which pediatric hospitals and their bariatric programs provide access to and participation in surgical treatments. The mission and values of pediatric hospitals generally include the provision of health care for all patients, regardless of their socioeconomic status. Pediatric obesity in the United States affects one in three socially disadvantaged children, with particularly high rates among African American girls and Hispanic and Native American children of both genders.[31] Children from socially and economically challenged families fare poorly on most childhood health indicators and may not have ready access to medical weight management and bariatric services. The "conscience" of the pediatric hospital system, within the context of its local and regional community, will be the driving force behind distributive justice relative to many children and adolescents with morbid obesity. Organized efforts to support costly multidisciplinary weight management and behavioral therapy programs, as well as bariatric programs, require professional leadership that advocates for equitable access for all children. Any pediatric bariatric program that excludes patients based on lack of insurance or financial resources would violate the principle as well as the virtue of justice.

Surgeons and Industry

There are many benefits to patients and the general public when physicians work together with pharmaceutical, medical device, and biotechnology companies. Much of the development in new tests, drugs, and devices that have vastly improved the quality of medical care have been the direct outcome of industry support for medical education, research, and innovation. In fact, industry funds about 50% of the costs of continuing medical education (CME) programs and 60% of clinical research in the United States.[32,33] However, renewed focus on professionalism in medical education and practice has raised the concern that these relationships may create conflicts of interest (COI), potentially resulting in undue influence on professional judgments. Industry practices that cross the line between patient welfare and profit seeking can induce physicians to perform unnecessary tests and treatments that may be harmful to patients and contribute to rising health care costs.[34] Increasing scrutiny by the public, patient advocacy groups, and Congress has therefore led most medical institutions and professional organizations to adopt stricter COI policies.

From an ethical standpoint, COIs are not inherently immoral or even unethical. However, COIs increase the potential for unethical physician behavior. There are three characteristics of a COI:[35]

1. A fiduciary relationship exists in which a physician acts in a fiduciary role in which they act primarily in the patient's best interest.
2. The fiduciary agent (physician) has self-interests that can be influenced and potentially override the agent's primary concern and obligation to the patient's interest.
3. A relationship with another entity (industry) exists that has the capacity to influence the physician to shift primacy of concern from the recipient of the fiduciary relationship (patient) to one that is motivated by direct or indirect self-interest.

It becomes readily apparent that COIs can exert a corrosive effect on several moral and ethical principles, particularly those of fidelity, beneficence, and nonmaleficence. Of these, fidelity is the most directly applicable to COI. The principle of fidelity establishes the physician's responsibility to carry out duties carefully and completely and in doing so demonstrate loyalty to, and in turn receive the trust of, the patient.[3] COIs erode the trust of the patient and compromise the physician's fiduciary role.

The ethical response to COI may take one or a combination of two forms: disclosure and avoidance. Disclosure of COI tends to dominate policies adopted by many institutions and professional bodies, in keeping with Brandeis' famous maxim that "sunshine is the best disinfectant."[36] However, there are distinct limitations to the power of disclosure alone as an effective antidote to COI. One possible reason is that full disclosure may not be attainable because the primary source of funding can be obfuscated through a labyrinthine maze that could involve front organizations or even accredited medical education companies.[37] Even a full disclosure, while raising the suspicion of bias, is too ambiguous to help the recipient of information from financially conflicted individuals to determine whether bias is present.[38] In fact, disclosure may allow some physicians to maintain or even strengthen their conflicts and has no inbuilt mechanism to actually eliminate bias. Therefore some have proposed that the only true way to eliminate industry bias in physician behavior is to avoid it whenever possible. Physicians, they argue, should avoid situations that unnecessarily introduce COI. However, avoidance is not always practical and may be impossible if physicians and investigators are going to pursue industry-funded research that has the potential to benefit patients.[38] This has produced somewhat of a backlash among those who complain that the new COI rules are too stringent and that the pendulum has swung far in the direction of stifling innovation and jeopardizing patient care.[39]

The 2009 report "Conflict of Interest in Medical Research, Education, and Practice" issued by the Institute of Medicine (IOM) has brought renewed urgency to this issue.[40] The IOM stresses the importance of preventing bias and mistrust rather than trying to remedy damage after it is discovered, and it encourages the enactment of policies and laws that identify, limit, and manage COI without negatively affecting constructive collaborations between the medical profession and industry.

Multiculturalism

With the increasing diversity of modern society, pediatric surgeons are faced with the difficult task of providing care to children from culturally heterogeneous backgrounds. Many pediatric surgeons, like other physicians, may consider themselves culturally competent and perhaps take pride in their personal commitment to providing equitable care to all patients. However, an ever-increasing body of evidence continues to highlight disparities in several areas of health care delivered to ethnic minority populations.[41] A contributing factor to this problem might be a failure among physicians to appreciate and actively counter cultural bias in their own relationships with their patients.

Culture is a term that may have different meanings, but in this context we define culture as the common and accepted way of thinking, feeling, and acting for a group of people. This includes a set of shared beliefs, values, attitudes, patterns of meanings, and behaviors that characterize a group of people. However, we must not restrict the definition of a "group of people" to political borders, religious practices, or physical characteristics. Focusing on such distinctions risks objectifying those whose appearance, language, or national origin is different from the majority into overly simplistic categorical stereotypes.[42]

It may be tempting for physicians, who are socialized by traditional values inherent in Western medical training, to view with suspicion attitudes from other cultures that challenge deeply held normative values. Western attitudes to health are based on a set of assumptions and values about disease and well-being that are not necessarily shared by other cultures. For example, Western medicine views health in biologic terms, with disease being the consequence of disruption of anatomic form or malfunctioning in biologic processes. In contrast, some cultures may ascribe spiritual, superstitious, or metaphysical causes to various illnesses and may have less trust in Western medicine as they pursue an assorted variety of alternative medicine or natural cures. In meeting parents and children whose culture is different, the pediatric surgeon should inquire about their beliefs, goals of treatment, and concerns.[43]

Individuals from minority cultures differ in the extent to which they assimilate the values of the larger society. Some parents will be informed by Western values on some issues, whereas maintaining their own cultural beliefs in others, and individuals from a similar cultural background or even within the same families may disagree on specific issues. Therefore the pediatric surgeon must resist the tendency to assign stereotypes of beliefs or behavior to individuals based on their identification with a cultural group. For example, some immigrant Chinese-American patients and families base their disease management decisions on their concerns for family well-being, family face, and the reciprocal responsibilities required by varied family roles,[44] but not all Chinese-American patients will be motivated by such values.

Along with cultural diversity, language barriers are increasingly encountered in our health system and may contribute to disparities for patients with limited English proficiency (LEP).[45] U.S. Census data shows that, other than English, more than 100 other languages are spoken by 47 million people in the United States, and the proportion of those with limited English proficiency nearly doubled from 4.8% in 1980 to 8.1% in 2000.[46] Fortunately, health disparities due to language barriers can be reduced or eliminated entirely when physicians use the services of trained interpreters.[47,48] Whenever possible, however, pediatric surgeons should avoid using family members or older siblings of the patient for translation to ensure accuracy of transmitted information both to and from the parents and child patient, to avoid translation bias, and to help in reading nonverbal and verbal cues about underlying concerns. A recent study identified specific risks of working with family interpreters, such as imposing their own agenda (rather than the patient's agenda) and controlling the consultation process.[49]

How then does a pediatric surgeon deal with cultural practices that are different from the norm, particularly when they affect parental acceptance of and compliance with recommended treatments? First we must consider that our patients (including children and their parents) experience illness as represented by their personal, interpersonal, and cultural reactions to the disease. Therefore the key is to understand *how* and *why* parents of a particular culture react in a certain way and hold certain attitudes when faced with illness in their children. We previously outlined the following strategies to reduce cross-cultural conflicts: asking questions about the parents' values and listening to their responses, indicating to the parents that their views are important, allowing enough time to deal with the parents whose culture is different, and seeking assistance from "experts" who understand the parents' cultural beliefs when significant differences arise in the course of treatment.[43]

Surgical Error

The 1999 Institute of Medicine (IOM) report "To Err Is Human"[50] focused the spotlight on the high incidence of medical errors and alerted the health care community and general public in the United States on the significant impact medical errors have on patient outcomes. The IOM report estimated that as many as 98,000 patients die each year as a result of medical error. The report also noted that many more patients undergo serious harm from a medical error that prolongs their hospitalization, causes unnecessary suffering, and increases the cost of care. Common examples of errors encountered during surgical treatment include wrong diagnosis, wrong patient (or site) procedures, and retained foreign bodies.

The process of medical decision making may be considered in four phases (1) data gathering, (2) integration or processing of data, (3) confirmation of diagnosis, and (4) treatment.[51] Medical errors are often due to deficiencies in medical judgment rather than knowledge, but other contributing factors include inadequate experience, carelessness, and fatigue. The core problem is often a defect in medical decision making, whether in formulating a diagnosis, choosing an appropriate surgical technique, or in the initial response to an adverse outcome. An analysis of the process of data integration among physicians identified four common sources of error: (1) wrong synthesis (lack of knowledge leading to an incorrect conclusion), (2) premature closure (incomplete consideration of all disease processes), (3) inadequate synthesis (data do not support conclusions), and (4) omission (important diagnostic information was not obtained).[52]

Considerable effort has been directed at establishing patient safety practices that minimize the incidence of errors. In contrast, there has been relatively less attention to how to respond after an error has occurred. Historically in the United States, fear of malpractice litigation has fostered a "code of silence" among physicians that is detrimental to efforts to improve patient safety, breeds mistrust, and fractures the therapeutic relationship between physicians and their patients. However, concern regarding legal liability should not affect the pediatric surgeon's honesty with parents. There is also a "human dimension" to the problem, as the silence, shame, anger, and guilt exacts an emotional toll on everyone involved, including physicians.[53] Research indicates that patients want full disclosure, a sincerely framed apology, and clear admission of responsibility.[54] Most parents desire an explicit acknowledgment that an error had occurred, what the error was, how the error occurred, how the error will affect their child, and what efforts are being made to prevent occurrence of similar errors in the future. Studies indicate that patients were more likely to trust physicians who participated actively in disclosing a serious error. In addition, fears that disclosure of an error will increase the likelihood of a malpractice claim have not been substantiated.[55]

In the United States, most medical institutions, professional organizations, and regulatory agencies consider full disclosure of a surgical error to be an ethical imperative. When a surgical error has occurred, the pediatric surgeon should proceed to inform the patient and parents in clear language about the nature of the error, the anticipated consequences, and how the error will be managed in the patient. This conversation requires that the pediatric surgeon explain how the error occurred, offering an empathetic apology about the commission of the error. The offering of an apology with disclosure of the error is a key step in the process. The apology must acknowledge the error and its consequences; the pediatric surgeon must assume responsibility and communicate regret, shame, or humility for having caused harm and in some cases offer reparation.[56] Most parents want to know that specific action will be taken to prevent the same error from harming another child. In some situations, an offer of compensation or early settlement offers by hospitals can dramatically reduce malpractice claims. In countries with no-fault compensation systems, malpractice claims are much less common. There is a movement in the United States to encourage physicians to offer an apology to patients and families when medical error occurs. More than 30 states in the United States and several Canadian provinces have passed "apology laws" to enhance medical error reporting and medical safety. Such laws make it possible for physicians to be able to use the dreaded phrase "I am sorry," without the statement being construed as an admission of liability.

Now, more than a decade after "To Err is Human," the subject of medical errors has gained wide currency in our society. Language such as adverse events, root cause analysis, disclosure, and risk management are commonly used in the lay press. Medical schools and residency training programs are rapidly adopting simulation modules, virtual patients, and other novel educational strategies to minimize the risk of harm to patients, while meeting needs of educating the next generation of physicians.[53] The opportunity seems ripe for competency-based medical education, initiated by the Accreditation Council for Graduate Medical Education (ACGME), to firmly embrace patient safety. In fact a proposal has been made that the identification of medical error recognition and disclosure be recognized as a *seventh* core competency to be adopted in our medical education.[57]

Innovation and Research

Innovation involves the introduction of a new method, idea, treatment, medication, or device to benefit the individual patient.[58] A surgical innovator is motivated by the belief that the new technique or therapy, or modification of an existing procedure, will improve the care of an individual patient. Such innovations often proceed without prior study and occur in real time. Sometimes the surgeon employs the innovative procedure in a small series of patients, using an iterative process to perfect the technique one patient at a time. In contrast, clinical research involves formal testing of different approaches to treatment with the aim to discover new knowledge that will benefit humankind, although there may be no benefit to individual study subjects. Therefore the results of formal research are generalizable, but the results of innovation initially apply to only a single patient.[59] Despite these distinctions, innovation and research are intertwined, and one cannot proceed effectively without the other.[60]

In pediatric surgery, much advancement has been brought about by research and development of innovative surgical techniques. Pediatric surgeons have been among the most notable surgical innovators, and many of the procedures beneficial to children today, including appendectomy and pyloromyotomy, may never have passed the rigor of randomized trials. Even with the advent of randomized trials, many innovative procedures have been widely adopted without evidence to support their advantage over standard techniques. For example, minimally invasive surgery has become the preferred approach for treating many childhood conditions, although rigorous evaluation of its role has rarely been undertaken.[61] Yet too little regulation creates the potential for abuse and can be harmful and dangerous. For example, some innovative procedures that were intuitively appealing when first proposed such as sympathectomy for Hirschsprung disease and jejunoileal bypass for morbid obesity were subsequently abandoned and may never have been widely used in the first place if a stricter regulatory regimen were in place. Also, some operations have failed to withstand the process of rigorous research evaluation. Recent experience with fetal surgical treatment of congenital diaphragmatic hernia provides a case in point. Thus far all randomized trials comparing prenatal intervention to standard postnatal therapy for congenital diaphragmatic hernia have shown no benefit to prenatal intervention.[62]

The fundamental ethical question is how to balance the need for research and innovation to advance human progress against the potential risks to patients who are the first recipients of the new procedures or the subjects in a clinical trial. Current ethical standards for the conduct of clinical research in the United States are derived from several standards, including the Nuremberg Code, the Declaration of Helsinki, and the Belmont report. Similar standards are in place in most progressive societies. Recent implementation of the Privacy Rule now requires the investigator to protect not only the safety but also the privacy of the research subject. In most institutions, compliance with these requirements is promoted by the institutional review board (IRB). The editors of most pediatric surgery journals have joined a growing coalition of medical journals requiring IRB approval before publication of results of research studies. In contrast, patient protections in innovative surgery are informal and rely primarily on the surgeon's competence and integrity.[59] In considering a new procedure, the surgeon must balance competing ethical principles, and relevant questions include whether it should be performed outside of a formal research protocol, what level of disclosure is needed to achieve an adequate informed consent, what research design meets the desired standard of evaluation, and how the burdens and benefits of such research can be distributed fairly.[63]

Randomized clinical trials (RCTs) are the most effective method to evaluate new procedures, but the specialty of pediatric surgery has lagged behind some other surgical specialties in the numbers of RCTs that guide our practice. Although RCTs compose 3% to 6% of studies reported in adult surgical literature, Moss and colleagues found that a trivial 0.17% of pediatric surgical studies were RCTs.[64] A recurrent obstacle cited for the reluctance among pediatric surgeons to participate in RCTs is the lack of clinical equipoise.[64,65] The meaning of equipoise is often misunderstood. The concept of equipoise was introduced by Charles Fried to express the uncertainty that a physician may have in choosing the best treatment out of competing alternatives.[66] Although this definition is useful in guarding the physician's fiduciary relationship with his or her patient, it could intensify a physician's state of uncertainty about whether a patient should be enrolled in a clinical trial. Freedman subsequently proposed the notion of clinical equipoise (or community equipoise), a state of uncertainty or professional disagreement within a professional group or clinical specialty regarding the relative merits of competing treatments.[67] In declaring clinical equipoise as the basis for participating in a clinical trial, the physician acknowledges that there is a reasonable uncertainty within his profession about the best treatment, even though he or she may have a strong preference for one option. Acceptance of clinical equipoise as sufficient ethical and moral justification for RCTs will increase enrollment in such trials.

Ultimately pediatric surgeons must be conservative guardians in surgical innovation. We agree with McNeally that the terminology of innovation has a seductive connotation of added value that attracts patients seeking the "latest and greatest" treatment.[68] Instead it should be replaced by the term *nonvalidated* as proposed by Levine because it more accurately reflects the ethical and medical hazard entailed in new procedures.[69] The concept of a nonvalidated operation is more transparent and honest because it embodies the fact that the proposed operation has not been subjected to rigorous investigation. This awareness may nudge both parents and pediatric surgeons toward supporting the ideal of RCTs, when a state of clinical equipoise exists about the role of a new procedure, before it is widely imposed on vulnerable and trusting patients and their families.

Conclusion

The ethical principles of beneficence, nonmaleficence, autonomy, and justice, and virtues such as trust, compassion, prudence, justice, courage, phronesis, fortitude, integrity, honesty, and self-effacement provide a sound basis to navigate the moral dilemmas we encounter in pediatric surgery practice and research. Although there is no universal solution to a given ethical problem, we think that an acceptable solution can be reached if these principles are followed. Formal teaching of clinical bioethics has been lacking in most pediatric surgery training programs.[70] Recently, a case-based, practice-oriented ethics curriculum was developed by the American Pediatric Surgical Association (APSA) for pediatric surgery training programs in North America. In addition to all the topics discussed in this chapter, these case studies cover important ethical concerns related to child abuse, conflict resolution, and the disruptive surgeon. The APSA curriculum is an invaluable clinical bioethics learning resource for both trainees and practicing pediatric surgeons and is available on the APSA web site.[71]

The complete reference list is available online at www.expertconsult.com.

SUGGESTED READINGS

Caniano DA. Ethical issues in pediatric bariatric surgery. Semin Pediatr Surg 2009;18:186–192.

Emanuel EJ, Wendler D, Grady C. What makes clinical research ethical? JAMA 2000;283:2701–11711.

Flake A. Prenatal Intervention: Ethical considerations for life-threatening and non-life-threatening anomalies. Semin Pediatr Surg 2001;10:212–221.

Frader JE, Flanagan-Klygis E. Innovation and research in pediatric surgery. Semin Pediatr Surg 2001;10:198–204.

Freedman B. Equipoise and the ethics of clinical research. N Engl J Med 1987;317:141–144.

Hedrick HL, Nelson RM. Handling Ethical conflicts in the clinical setting. Semin Pediatr Surg 2001;10:192–197.

Jasper J, Clark W, Cabrera-Meza G, et al. Whose child is it anyway? Resolving parent-physician conflict in the NICU setting. Am J Perinatol 2003;20:373–380.

Kriezek TJ. Surgical error: ethical issues of adverse events. Arch Surg 2000;135:1359–1366.

Reason J. Human error: models and management. BMJ 2000;320:768–770.

Wu AW, Cavanaugh TA, McPhee SJ, et al. To tell the truth: ethical and practical issues in disclosing medical mistakes to parents. J Gen Intern Med 1997;12: 770–775.

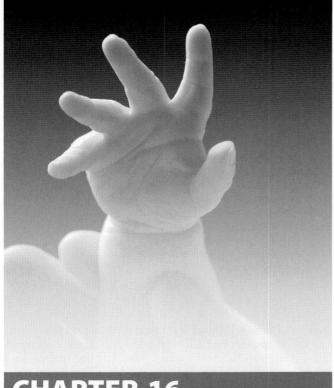

CHAPTER 16

Patient- and Family-Centered Pediatric Surgical Care

Sherif Emil

"I am a mother of a child who was born with trisomy 13. My daughter died at home on April 13, 2010, at age 5, surrounded by her loved ones. She was not supposed to live that long, but she had great determination to beat the odds. During her last few months, I was introduced to the supportive/palliative care service. This program focused on helping her to live life to the fullest—her life, my life, our family's life. I wish there had been this program when she was born. By focusing on the quality of her life, rather than trying to fix things, my daughter would have had less hospitalizations and more special time with us at home. She would have had better pain management and would have been able to live life to the fullest, which I believe she did during those last few months."

Fundraising email sent by Rachel Llanos, mother of Kellie Llanos, a child with trisomy 13 who died at age 5 after a plethora of medical and surgical interventions.

This is the first edition, in the long history of this illustrious textbook, that dedicates a chapter to patient- and family-centered care (PFCC). It is befitting, because the 21st century

has seen the principles of PFCC quickly permeate through all areas of medicine, including pediatric surgery. Some may feel that these principles are self-evident, politically correct terms of what surgeons have always practiced. Although it is true that a competent, empathetic, ethical surgeon with good listening and communication skills is very likely to practice PFCC, the concept is far more than one of competency, empathy, or communication. Over the last 20 years, PFCC has evolved into a health care discipline, with a significant volume of research, publication, and programs. Systematic reviews show that PFCC increases adherence to management protocols, reduces morbidity, and improves quality of life for patients.[1] This chapter aims to introduce surgeons to this relatively new discipline and to emphasize the potential positive impact PFCC can have on pediatric surgical practice.

Definition

The Institute for Patient- and Family-Centered Care (IPFCC) in Bethesda, Maryland is a non-profit organization that was founded in 1992 with a mission to advance the understanding and practice of PFCC and to partner with patients, families, and health care professionals to integrate PFCC concepts in all aspects of health care.[2] The institute defines PFCC as *an innovative approach to the planning, delivery, and evaluation of health care that is grounded in mutually beneficial partnerships among health care providers, patients, and families.* The core concepts of PFCC are (1) respect and dignity, (2) information sharing, (3) participation, and (4) collaboration.[2] In a recent technical report and policy statement, whose lead author is a pediatric surgeon, the American Academy of Pediatrics (AAP) deemed these same concepts essential to professionalism.[3,4] The Institute offers a plethora of resources on its Web site, and partners with practice groups and health care organizations to help integrate these concepts into the health care environment. Some of the contrasts between traditional medical care and PFCC are shown in Table 16-1.

Background

In what is perhaps the oldest pediatric surgical textbook in the English language, published in 1895, D'Arcy Power wrote the following:

> "When an operation has been decided upon, it will generally be found that better results are obtained if the child be removed from its accustomed surroundings and is placed in the charge of those who have special experiences in nursing sick children. Only in very exceptional cases can a mother be trusted to nurse her own child after a serious operation, and in many instances the recovery of a spoilt and fractious child is seriously retarded by the presence of those who love it best. It is therefore acting in the best interests of the child, to recommend that it should be placed in a surgical home, or in the charge of an experienced children's nurse."[5]

This was essentially the paradigm for the surgical care of children in the first half of the 20th century. In 1953, Robert Gross included a section on "psychic preparation" for surgery in his seminal pediatric surgical textbook.[6] He challenged the paradigm of the child's separation from his family by emphasizing that abandonment "can seriously undermine the

TABLE 16-1

Contrasts Between Traditional Care and Patient and Family-Centered Care

Traditional Care	Patient- and Family-Centered Care
Doctor knows what is best for the patient	Doctor and patient/parents together decide what is best for the patient
Exclusion of religious and cultural issues from medical decisions	Inclusion of religious and cultural issues in medical decisions
Psychosocial issues are ignored or approached separately	Psychosocial issues are included in the overall care plan of the patient
Parental role is minimized in overall care	Parental role is optimized in overall care
Parental absence during invasive procedures, resuscitation, or anesthetic induction	Parental presence during invasive procedures, resuscitation, or anesthetic induction
Withholding of information, particularly regarding poor outcomes or complications	Open and transparent information sharing, including admission of error or adverse events
Minimal preoperative preparation	Thorough preoperative preparation
Reactive approach to pain management	Proactive approach to pain management
Separate specialty clinics for complicated diseases	Multidisciplinary clinics for complicated diseases
Outcome studies analyze only physical or biological factors	Outcome studies also analyze quality of life factors pertaining to patient and family

faith of the child in his mother or father."[6] He emphasized the importance of preoperative mental preparation at home and the role parents can play in the child's surgical experience. Dr. Gross's desire for an enhanced familial role probably was far ahead of the resources available at the time, because the same chapter shows a postoperative child shackled to the bed by her wrists and ankles in order to receive intravenous infusion.[6] As pediatric surgeons continued to tackle and win more surgical battles, their attention began to turn to psychosocial issues surrounding pediatric surgical care. In the mid-1990s, Caniano ushered in the field of pediatric surgical ethics, inevitably bringing attention to family dynamics and "the big picture" during fetal consultation, management of congenital anomalies, and pediatric surgical care in general.[7,8] In the last decade, outcome studies for a variety of pediatric surgical conditions started to look at emotional and developmental results on the child, in addition to the physical ones. Recently, these outcome studies have begun to investigate the effects of interventions on parents and caregivers. In one recent study, Zaidi and colleagues investigated the caregiver's perspective after esophagogastric dissociation in neurologically impaired children with severe gastroesophageal reflux disease, arguing for a greater role for this procedure because of the unexpectedly high caregiver satisfaction.[9] Another recent study looked past the typical outcomes of treatment, to analyze the child's emotional quality of life as well as the degree of parenting distress, in two arms of a randomized controlled trial for perforated appendicitis with abscess.[10] These types of studies are bringing to light the concept that successful physical outcomes may not necessarily translate into the best patient and family-centered outcomes. Finally, Paice and colleagues recently raised the possibility of parental presence in the operating theatre.[11] Pediatric surgery has come a long way in 100 years!

Core Concepts

RESPECT AND DIGNITY

All persons should be treated with respect and regard for individual worth and dignity, including sensitivity to gender, race, and cultural differences, as well as maintenance of patient confidentiality when appropriate.[4] Pediatric surgeons, particularly in developed countries, find themselves practicing in increasingly multicultural settings. The forces of immigration and globalization have created many international cities and communities, where people of diverse cultures, faiths, beliefs, and economic circumstances seek surgical care for their children. The parents' background and belief system, in turn, influences their interaction with the medical system; their expectations of medical personnel; and their decisions regarding their children's health care. At times, the surgeon may find himself or herself at odds with the approach or the decision of the child and/or the parents. The surgeon does not have to agree with the family. However, the principle of respect implies recognition that rational people may hold opposing and irreconcilable views.[8] The surgeon can demonstrate respect for the family and acknowledge their dignity by listening carefully, understanding their perspectives, and attempting to see beyond his or her own personal experience. Respect does not imply compromising the surgeon's primary responsibility to his or her patient's welfare. For example, the AAP has repeatedly called for the equal application of legal interventions whenever children are endangered or harmed, without exemption for actions based on religious beliefs.[12,13] It has also opposed religious or cultural practices, such as ritual genital cutting of female minors, that consistently harm children, and it has called on its members to actively dissuade families from carrying out these practices.[14]

COMMUNICATION

We live in the age of information. Accurate and timely information sharing with patients and parents is one of the hallmarks of medical practice in the 21st century. Parents of children undergoing surgery desire comprehensive perioperative information. In fact, Fortier and colleagues recently reported that the vast majority of children older than 7 years also desire comprehensive information about their surgery.[15] The responsibility for providing this information lies mainly with the surgeon, because it has been shown that information acquired from elsewhere (general practitioner, books, popular magazines, Internet) does not necessarily improve the parents' understanding of the child's operative risk.[16] Clinicians may feel an impetus to withhold information, to decrease parental anxiety. This notion has been disproven by strong evidence.[17,18]

Information sharing is often used interchangeably with communication. However, effective communication goes well beyond information sharing, to include understanding, empathy, compassion, transparency, and advocacy. One of the few acts that require more trust than surrendering oneself to a surgeon is surrendering one's child to a surgeon. This intense trust is built on many factors, including the surgeon's reputation and competence, but none more important than effective communication. Good communication skills are essential core competencies that are associated with improved health outcomes, better patient adherence, fewer malpractice claims, and enhanced satisfaction with care.[19] Communication obviously serves the pediatric surgeon well on a daily basis, but certain situations require particular attention to communication if PFCC is to be provided. These include prenatal consultations, planning for correction of congenital anomalies, relaying a diagnosis of cancer, provision of end-of-life care, communicating the death of a child, and transmission of information regarding surgical errors and adverse events.

Prenatal consultation with pediatric surgeons by parents carrying a fetus with a congenital anomaly has become routine in the developed world. Although these consultations have not been proven to improve outcomes, they serve the vital purpose of relaying information to the parents before the stressful events of childbirth. They also help the surgeon establish early rapport with the parents and start building a trusting relationship. Parents are typically interested in more than a description of the anomaly, its treatment, and its potential outcome. They usually seek to learn what the future may hold for their baby, including his or her potential social function and interaction with family and society.[8] Caniano and Baylis stress the importance of compassion in such interactions, particularly in situations where couples may choose to end much-wanted (and sometimes difficultly acquired) pregnancies associated with life-threatening fetal malformations, for which there are no effective surgical interventions.[8] After examining prenatal surgical consultations for congenital diaphragmatic hernia (CDH), Aite and colleagues found that 70% of patients found it difficult to follow the surgeon's explanations or ask questions because of fear and other intense emotions.[20] Interestingly, consultations for lesions associated with better prognoses, such as congenital cystic adenomatoid malformation, were less effective in decreasing parental anxiety than consultations for CDH.[21] The reasons for this were uncertainty about prenatal outcome and lack of a defined management plan.[21] These data point to a possible deficiency in a single prenatal consultation, where the surgeon relays all the pertinent information. Follow-up by the surgeon or ancillary medical personnel after the initial consultation may enhance communication in this regard.

The setting of surgically correctable congenital anomalies, especially in the absence of prenatal diagnosis, presents another communication challenge for the pediatric surgeon. Families, even relatively sophisticated ones, often have never heard of the anomaly and are overwhelmed by the notion that their newborn baby can undergo and survive a major operation.[22] Provision of written and illustrated material can significantly enhance communication.[20-22] Before the operation, families are most interested in the description of the anomaly and its prognosis, whereas after the operation, they are most interested in the recovery process and assessment of the long-term quality of life.[22] Many congenital anomalies produce permanent and profound effects on the family dynamic, with potential marital, social, and financial implications. In an analogy to the five stages of grief described by Elizabeth Kubler-Ross, Drotar and colleagues described five stages of parental reaction after the birth of an infant with a congenital malformation (Table 16-2).[23] Understanding these stages can allow the pediatric surgeon to effectively relate to the family in the immediate perioperative period and beyond.

A new diagnosis of cancer presents a major crisis in the life of the patient and family. Fortunately, most pediatric solid and hematologic malignancies have better prognoses than their adult counterparts. This could be mentioned early in the discussion, because most parents will automatically remember a family member or loved one who died of cancer. The hospital and community resources available to the family should be clearly described, convincing the family that they will not be alone during this difficult experience. The emotional state of the parents is often associated with very poor receptiveness and comprehension on their part when the diagnosis is first relayed.[24] Repetition and constant clarifications of treatment plans and other details are typically necessary. Although information should be shared liberally with the parents, and often the child, the surgeon should remember that hope is not statistical. Hope is often recognized as an important component for healing; therefore, while remaining realistic in the expectation of cure, the surgeon should not try to remove all hope from the patient and family.

Communication with the family when the end of the child's life is in sight, or after the death of a child, presents particular challenges to the surgeon, who often has to deal with his or her own emotions. A sense of failing the child or family can interfere with the surgeon's ability to care for and comfort the family, when cure is no longer possible. The physician needs to find the strength to discuss life-threatening illnesses in an open, sympathetic, and direct manner, because families resent evasive or brief interactions.[25] Researchers at Children's Hospital Boston have identified six parental priorities for end-of-life care in the pediatric intensive care unit—namely, honest and complete information, ready access to staff, communication and care coordination, emotional expression and support by staff, preservation of the integrity of the parent–child relationship, and faith.[26] One can see that most of these priorities relate to communication. The pediatric surgeon's role does not end with the death of a child. The families a surgeon often bonds with the most are the ones whose children's funerals the surgeon has attended. A pillar of American pediatric surgery, Dr. Morton Woolley, chose the subject of a child's death as his last publication, in an attempt to help pediatric surgeons provide appropriate responses when confronted with the death of a child.[27]

Finally, communication, in general, and transparent communication, in particular, is exceptionally important in

TABLE 16-2	
Five Stages of Parental Reaction After the Birth of an Infant with a Congenital Malformation[23]	
Stage I	Shock
Stage II	Denial
Stage III	Sadness and Anger
Stage IV	Adaptation
Stage V	Reorganization

decreasing litigations.[28] The American College of Surgeons Closed Claims Study identified failure to communicate as the major cause of litigation in 22% of claims.[29] The adverse consequences of these failures included medical errors, escalation of the consequences of otherwise nonpreventable adverse events, and anger or mistrust even when the standard of care was met. A policy of transparent disclosure of error with an apology or expression of regret when preventable adverse events were identified, coupled with an offer of reasonable compensation, has been shown to dramatically decrease medicolegal costs.[30]

Effective communication between health care team members is also essential in providing PFCC to complex pediatric patients. In one study, Meltzer and colleagues found that physicians, faced with difficult patients or families, were more likely to distance themselves or refer the family to the psychosocial profession, while nurses were more likely to consult with colleagues.[31] Communication skills and relational abilities in pediatric health care can be significantly improved by formal training.[19]

PARTICIPATION

Surgery is often described in terms of doing things *to* patients, and not *with* patients. It is not surprising, therefore, that the patient's and family's active participation in the surgical experience has constituted the most controversial aspect of PFCC over the past 2 decades, a period that has seen a flurry of research into issues such as preoperative family preparation, parental presence during induction of anesthesia (PPIA), and parental involvement in the choice of potentially anxiolytic preoperative and postoperative maneuvers. Preoperative anxiety in young children undergoing surgery is associated with more pain during the recovery period, as well as higher incidences of emergence delirium, postoperative anxiety and sleep disturbance, and postoperative maladaptive behavior.[32,33] The parents' preoperative anxiety may also influence outcomes. For example, many mothers who exhibit a high desire to be in the operating room are also very anxious, and their children are likely to exhibit high anxiety levels during induction of anesthesia.[34] Interventions to decrease the mother's anxiety during PPIA were found to also decrease the child's anxiety on entrance to the operating room and during introduction of the anesthesia mask.[35] Most of the research, therefore, is aimed at identifying maneuvers that may decrease child and parental anxiety during the perioperative period, outcomes that are understandably difficult to assess. Nevertheless, multiple scales, such as the Motivation for Parental Presence during Induction of Anesthesia (MPPIA),[34] the Yale Preoperative Anxiety Scale (mYPAS),[36] and the Child-Adult Medical Procedure Interaction Scale,[37] have been developed in an attempt to provide some objective data. Chorney and Kain have recently presented a comprehensive model of family-centered pediatric perioperative care.[38] This model covers the preoperative, intraoperative, and postoperative environments, and includes family factors, such as anxiety and previous medical experience, as well as provider and system factors, such as training and organizational policy.[38]

Preoperative Preparation

Most children's hospitals currently have some type of preoperative preparation program for surgical patients. These programs generally include an orientation to the operating room (OR), a description of the anticipated events on the day of surgery, and, in some instances, psychological preparation of the parent and pediatric surgical patient.[39,40] Certain patient factors identified during the preoperative preparation, such as age, previous anesthesia, and anxiety level, have been found to predict poor behavioral compliance during inhaled induction.[41] These factors may help identify children who could benefit from behavioral or pharmacologic interventions. Targeting the parents in such programs is also important, because there is evidence that the parents' anxiety on the day of surgery is highly associated with the child's anxiety.[42] During the preoperative visit, options such as PPIA may be discussed, if available in the institution. These visits also afford the anesthesiologist an opportunity to assess the family as a whole and formulate a plan for induction. For example, a preoperative assessment of the anxiety level of parent and child, in addition to other specific factors, such as age, temperament, and coping style, were found to predict which child-parent pair is likely to benefit from PPIA.[43,44] Kain and colleagues have performed two randomized controlled trials to assess the value of preoperative preparation.[45,46] In the first study, an extensive preoperative program (OR tour + videotape + child-life preparation), produced limited anxiolytic effects, which were seen only in the preoperative period and did not extend to induction or postoperative recovery.[45] In a more recent study, an ADVANCE program (Anxiety reduction, Distraction, Video modeling and education, Adding parents, No excessive reassurance, Coaching, and Exposure/shaping) was compared with three other arms: standard of care, PPIA, and oral midazolam. The ADVANCE program resulted in multiple improved outcomes for children and parents.[46] Children in the ADVANCE group exhibited a lower incidence of emergence delirium, required significantly less analgesia in the recovery room, and were discharged from the recovery room earlier than children in the three other groups.[46] A more recent Brazilian study also showed improvement in anxiety levels and behavior during the postoperative period in children who received preoperative psychological preparation prior to undergoing elective surgery.[40]

Intraoperative Period

The main controversy surrounding PFCC during the intraoperative period is PPIA. PPIA was an almost natural extension of increased parental participation and presence during critical procedures on their children, including trauma resuscitations, emergency room resuscitations, bedside invasive procedures, and cardiopulmonary resuscitations. Many of these situations also involve the pediatric surgeon. This movement has significantly grown in strength in the last quarter century. Parental presence during these procedures, in many institutions, now occurs routinely. Although there are no research studies that point to a patient benefit if the family is present, there appears to be at least a major psychological benefit to the family. Research suggests that families want to be given the option to be present during invasive and resuscitative procedures, and they often choose that option.[47–49] Those who are present generally report favorable experiences.[47] Parents who witnessed a terminal medical event involving their child in the pediatric intensive care unit (PICU) were less distressed than those who did not and felt that their presence helped them cope with their child's death.[48,49] Family presence has not been found to prolong time to computed tomography (CT) imaging or to resuscitation completion for pediatric trauma patients.[50] Uninterrupted care can be delivered with the family present.[51] Physicians and nurses have become increasingly comfortable with family presence in critical situations.[47,52–55] Major professional organizations, including the AAP and the American College of Emergency Physicians, have endorsed the practice.[56–58]

However, many do not see PPIA as a natural extension of parental presence during other clinical scenarios. Critics of PPIA cite decreased OR efficiency, additional staffing requirements, increased cost, and possible medico-legal implications as potential arguments against its practice. There are no data to support these arguments. On the other hand, data regarding positive outcomes of PPIA are also mixed. Kain and colleagues reported several randomized trials of PPIA over the past 15 years.[59–63] In the first study, published in 1996, PPIA did not reduce any behavioral or physiologic measures of anxiety during induction.[59] A benefit was seen in specific subgroups of children when cortisol levels were measured, an outcome of questionable clinical significance.[59] In another study, oral midazolam was superior to PPIA in reducing anxiety and increasing compliance of the child during the perioperative period.[60] Interestingly, that study also showed that parents of children in the midazolam group had lower anxiety scores after separation from their children.[60] In a study comparing oral midazolam alone to oral midazolam plus PPIA, children in both arms exhibited similar levels of anxiety.[61] However, parents in the PPIA arm had lower self-reported anxiety scores and higher satisfaction stores.[61] The physiologic effects of PPIA on parents were specifically investigated in another trial, which found that parents in the PPIA arms, regardless of whether a sedative was also given to their child, manifested a significantly higher physiologic stress response during induction (increased heart rate and skin conductance level), than parents in the control arm.[62] The most recent study investigated the presence of one versus two parents during induction.[63] The presence of two parents did not affect observed child anxiety, but reduced parents' self-reported anxiety.[63] Chundamala and colleagues recently published a comprehensive evidence-based review of the effects of PPIA on parent and child anxiety and concluded that, contrary to popular belief, PPIA does not appear to alleviate parents' or children's anxiety.[64] These authors, from Toronto's Hospital for Sick Children, raise the possibility that PPIA may be driven by market forces and hospital competition in the United States. The use of PPIA has certainly grown in the United States.[65] However, the practice is far more frequent in Britain, where support for PPIA is dramatically higher than in the United States among both anesthesiologists and pediatric surgeons.[66,67] In fact, the practice has become so routine in Britain, that some are raising the possibility of parental presence during the surgical procedure.[11] One would be hard pressed to cite the market as the driving force for PPIA in Britain. Chorney and Kain, with practices in very different health care settings (Halifax, Nova Scotia and Orange County, California), argue that the focus on efficacy data has misguided the debate over PPIA.[38] They stress that PPIA is overwhelmingly preferred by parents, increases parental satisfaction, and improves hospital public relations.[38] Some parents may see it as a basic right.

PPIA is an instrument that may work well for many, but not all, families. Medical personnel are therefore encouraged to respect the family's decisions and preferences.[38] There is undoubtedly a strong demand for this option. The number of parents in our practice who are asking for PPIA is exponentially increasing. The demand is particularly strong among parents whose children have undergone prior surgery with or without PPIA.[68] PPIA is therefore not a passing fad, but rather a practice well on its way to becoming a standard of care.

Postoperative Care

Postoperative care and recovery are facilitated if adequate preoperative preparation is given and a positive intraoperative surgical experience ensues.[38,40,69] A quick reunion with the parents in the recovery room now occurs routinely. Daily, clear updates to the parents of hospitalized children are a must. When pediatric surgery fellows or other house staff are part of a surgical service, a special effort should be made to give the patient and parents clear and nonconflicting information. Inadequate pain management is of utmost concern to the child and parents. This should be addressed appropriately, and preemptively, when possible. If the child is on a treatment protocol or algorithm, the relevant details and end points should be clearly explained to the parents. Support for the parents and the child during recovery at home is also essential. Home health care resources should be mobilized as early as possible to allow the child to continue care at home, when it is deemed appropriate and safe. Clear and detailed discharge instructions should be given both directly and in writing. Some data suggest that many children do not receive optimal pain management at home after day surgery.[70] A follow-up phone call from the surgeon or nurse during the first 72 hours after day surgery is highly appreciated by the parents. In the late 1990s, reports of successful phone follow-up for select pediatric surgical operations, with the intent to provide convenient and cost-effective care, appeared in the literature.[71,72] Following these reports, our service began an active phone follow-up program for the majority of day surgery cases and many simple inpatient cases (e.g., nonperforated appendicitis, pyloric stenosis).[73] This has been extremely popular with parents, because it avoids an unnecessary postoperative visit, while identifying those patients who require or request follow-up. More recently, a 90% satisfaction rate has been reported with a similar strategy.[74]

COLLABORATION

Collaboration can be best defined as a health care environment that regards the parents and family as health care team members, and not spectators. In fact, the family should be seen as the most consistent and permanent member of the health care team, because nurses, ancillary medical staff, social workers, and even the attending staff surgeon may change from time to time. This concept is often referred to in the literature as *partnership*—the physician and health care team partnering with the family to provide the best care possible to the patient. This is not such a new or modern concept. Surgeons who have practiced in missionary settings or underdeveloped countries will attest to the huge role the family plays in the active medical care of the patient.

Partnerships are formed when the health care team values the information given by parents, actively seeks their input in decisions affecting their child, acknowledges their positions

TABLE 16-3

Montreal Children's Hospital Division of Pediatric General Surgery Pledge to Patients and Families

We will treat every child and family with dignity, compassion, and respect.

We will draw on the expertise of the entire team and other hospital services to offer the best care to each child.

We will discuss with patients and families all relevant alternatives for treatment.

We will serve as advocates for each child within the health care system.

We will keep patients and families fully informed of the treatment plan, and address concerns in an open and honest manner.

TABLE 16-4

PFCC Best Practices in Pediatric Surgery

A commitment to respect the culture, faith, and belief system of each family, while always advocating for the child's best interests

A commitment to keeping the patient and family united as long as possible during the perioperative period

Inclusion of family advisors as partners in facility design of surgical waiting rooms and perioperative areas

Inclusion of family advisors in the review and formulation of surgical documents, including preoperative instructions, consent, and discharge forms

Encouragement of families to ask questions, share concerns, and offer feedback to surgeons, anesthesiologists, and surgical staff

Open, honest, and continuous sharing with families of procedural risks and safety precautions

Provision of information to families on how they can actively partner with staff to reduce risks and optimize outcomes

Provision of information to families on pain management and recruitment of their feedback on its efficacy

Provision of information to families on the roles and responsibilities of the members of the surgery team, as well as clear instructions on who to contact for questions and concerns

Open and honest disclosure of surgical complications and adverse events

and concerns, and acts on their feedback. The United States Maternal and Child Health Bureau defines a positive family–provider partnership as a core program outcome.[75] Denboba and colleagues found that a sense of partnership between the families of children with special health care needs and their physicians was associated with improved outcomes across a number of important health care measures.[75] However, poverty, minority racial and ethnic status, and absence of health insurance placed families at elevated risk of being without a sense of partnership.[75] An extra effort, therefore, is needed to build partnerships with certain at-risk populations. Partnerships are also created when parents feel that they have full access to the health care team. Parents who desire to meet with the entire tumor board, fetal diagnosis and treatment group, or any other multidisciplinary treatment team, to obtain comprehensive information, should be encouraged and invited. Partnerships can also be integrated into daily patient care. An example comes from Cincinnati Children's Hospital, where families can choose to be part of attending physician rounds.[76] Integration of the family into multidisciplinary rounds was found to require an additional 2.7 minutes per patient and affect the medical decision-making discussion

in 90% of cases—an excellent investment![77] Collaboration is particularly important in the long-term care of pediatric surgical patients with congenital anomalies, such as imperforate anus or esophageal atresia, which become lifelong chronic medical conditions after repair. Rahi and colleagues recently offered a detailed and practical account of how a support program for children with a newly diagnosed lifelong disability can be built in collaboration with family, counselors, and health care personnel.[78]

Putting It All Together: PFCC in Action

Many individual surgeons, surgical practices, and institutions apply the principles of PFCC intuitively. However, an intentional commitment to PFCC can have a transforming effect on pediatric health care. Our hospital, like most children's hospitals, saw itself as a child- and family-friendly hospital. However, after a visit from a national leader and advocate of PFCC in October 2009, the hospital made a firm commitment to examine its practices and traditions. Such examination showed ample potential for growth in PFCC. Specific actions included the formation of a PFCC working group, with representation from all areas of the hospital, stronger collaboration with the hospital's family advisory forum and their inclusion in planning and policy making, the hiring of a PFCC coordinator to act as a liaison between the hospital and families, and taking PFCC issues into account in the design and building of a new hospital. Within our Division of Pediatric General Surgery, we adopted a new mission statement that reflects a strong commitment to PFCC, as well as a pledge to patients and families (Table 16-3). The mission statement and pledge are included in a color brochure that provides core information about our services and our staff, which is given to all families who come in contact with our division. A color chart containing the names and pictures of all members of the pediatric surgical service, including students, residents, and fellows, is also given to all admitted patients so that families are always clear about the roles of each member of the team. Our surgery and anesthesia departments started to investigate the incorporation of PPIA into the OR culture and to explore other ways of enhancing the role of parents in the operative experience.

A list of 10 PFCC best practices, relating to pediatric surgery, is shown in Table 16-4. These are practical steps that can be taken to apply the principles discussed in this chapter. In addition, the Web site of the IPFCC has many additional concrete examples of PFCC in action from children's hospitals throughout the United States that have been leaders in the adoption of PFCC principles and practices.[2] These principles and practices are as important to the psychosocial aspects of pediatric surgical care in the 21st century as evidence-based medicine is to the biological aspects.

Acknowledgments

The author is grateful to Juliette Schlucter, who is a parent of two chronically ill children and a patient- and family-centered care consultant, for sharing her experience, inspiring this chapter, and reviewing the manuscript.

The complete reference list is available online at www.expertconsult.com.

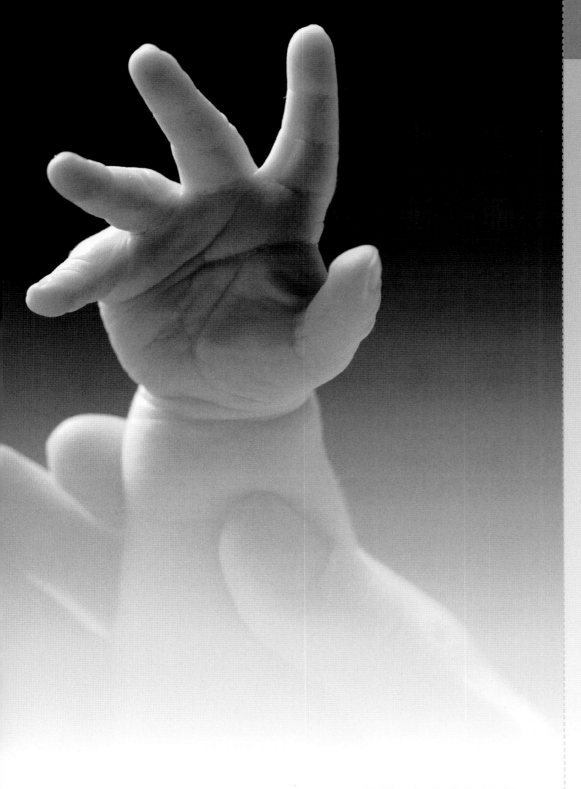

Part II

TRAUMA

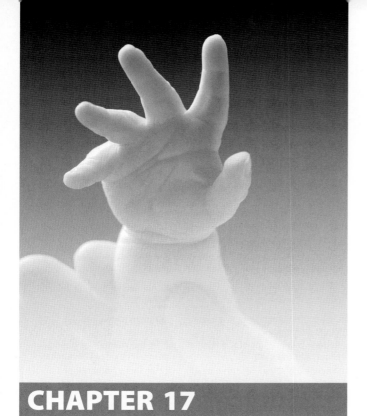

CHAPTER 17

Injury Prevention

Gina P. Duchossois and Michael L. Nance

"If a disease were killing our children in the proportions that injuries are, people would be outraged and demand that this killer be stopped."

—C. Everett Koop

Injury presents the greatest threat to life of all diseases in the pediatric population. More children die each year from injury than all other causes combined.[1] More than one in nine children will require medical attention for an injury each year. Many more children will be injured but not require or seek medical care (Fig. 17-1). The economic costs of injury are staggering. In addition to direct costs for care, there is the additional loss of future productivity as well as loss of productivity by parental caregivers who must provide for the injured child. For the year 2000, these costs were estimated to top $130 billion in total costs, with nearly $25 billion due to direct medical costs.[2] The significance of the costs of injury become even more provocative when one considers the potential financial savings that can be realized from injury prevention strategies (Table 17-1).

William Haddon, in the 1970s, reported his classic characterization scheme (the Haddon "matrix") and approach to injury prevention.[3] This system argued against the traditional idea that injury was an accident, leaving the burden of prevention on the individual. Rather, he suggested that injuries result from predictable events and thus offer an opportunity for systematic intervention and injury reduction. This strategy, which considers injury in pre-event, event, and post-event phases, each offering opportunity for intervention, is still relevant today (Table 17-2). Pre-event (primary) prevention measures seek to prevent the event leading to the injury through education, intervention, and/or safety design measures. For example, crosswalks and count-down timers are effective safety engineering actions to make our roadways safer for pedestrians. Measures aimed at altering the event (secondary) seek to lessen the severity of an injury if it occurs. For example, child safety seats are not designed to prevent a motor vehicle collision but rather minimize (or eliminate) the severity of any injuries if a collision occurs. Finally, post-event (tertiary) injury prevention is the strategy used by most health care providers. It seeks to mitigate the consequences of the injury once it has occurred. For example, management of intractable intracranial hypertension through hemicraniectomy is tertiary prevention. Advances in health care have led to marked improvements in outcome for children with traumatic injuries. However, quite clearly, primary prevention, averting the event altogether, is the optimal approach. Haddon provided 10 countermeasures to use when addressing the prevention of a particular injury (Table 17-3).[4] These concepts can be applied to most any injury and help break down the problem into potentially actionable steps.

Prevention Priorities

Injury prevention resources are finite. As such, priorities for these prevention efforts must be established. These priorities may vary depending on the individual, the community, or perhaps the nation interested in prevention. A variety of factors are integral to the decisions regarding how best to deploy these limited resources. At the individual level, one might favor efforts to minimize in-home injury and "child-proof" the surroundings. A community might work toward pedestrian safety efforts in neighborhoods in which such injuries have been predominant. Finally, a nation (e.g., the United States) might focus efforts to reduce motor vehicle–related injuries, the leading cause of injury death. Simply counting the number of deaths from a particular injury mechanism may not provide an accurate or adequate representation of the burden of injury (by mechanism) in the geographic area of study. For instance, an injury mechanism that is highly lethal (e.g., hanging) but infrequent may not be an optimal prevention target. Nor might efforts to reduce an injury that is common but usually of limited severity (e.g., assault) be the ideal strategy. An injury that is both common and severe would, in most settings, represent the ideal target for mitigation efforts. To help define such injuries, Haider and colleagues used an injury prevention priority score.[5] This calculation takes into account both the frequency of an injury and the mean severity of an injury by mechanism. In a comparison of pediatric populations from two geographically distinct trauma centers, they noted differences in injury patterns. In the inner city, auto/pedestrian injuries achieved the highest priority score, while in the community center, motor vehicle–related injuries ranked highest. Wiebe and colleagues applied this methodology to a national trauma center population and demonstrated that motor vehicle–related injuries, falls, and firearm-related

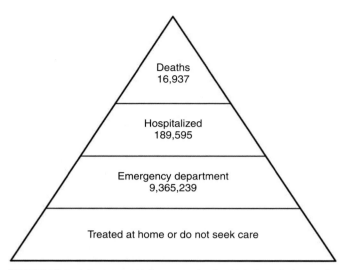

Deaths
16,937

Hospitalized
189,595

Emergency department
9,365,239

Treated at home or do not seek care

FIGURE 17-1 Injury pyramid demonstrating fatal injuries, injuries requiring hospitalization, and injuries resulting in an emergency department visit for children age 0 to 19 years, 2007. (Data from National Center for Injury Prevention and Control.[1])

injuries, respectively, were the highest ranking injury mechanisms (Table 17-4).[7] In addition, Wiebe and colleagues also created additional scores that take into account the relative mortality of an injury mechanism (mortality priority score), the cost of an injury (hospital cost priority score), and the years of productive life lost (years of productive life lost priority score) to further characterize the burden of a particular injury. As suggested by Haider in his original publication, the methodology is easily applied to individual populations, such as that of a trauma center or a county or a state, to help determine how best to deploy prevention

TABLE 17-3
Haddon Measures to Combat Injury and Their Application to Firearm Injury

Haddon Countermeasure	As Applied to Firearm Injury Prevention
Prevent the creation of the hazard in the first place	Eliminate handguns
Reduce the amount of the hazard brought into being	Limit the number of handguns allowed to be sold or purchased
Prevent the release of the hazard that already exists	Install locks on handguns
Modify the release of the hazard that already exists	Eliminate automatic handguns
Separate, in time and space, the hazard and that which is to be protected	Store handguns only at gun clubs rather than at home
Separate, by material barrier, the hazard and that which is to be protected	Keep guns in locked containers
Modify the relevant basic qualities of the hazard	Personalize guns so they can be fired only by the owner
Make that to be protected more resistant to damage from the hazard	Create and market bullet-proof garments
Counter damage already done by the hazard	Provide good access to emergency care in the prehospital period
Stabilize, repair, and rehabilitate the object of the hazard	Provide high-quality trauma care in hospitals

TABLE 17-1
Potential Financial Savings from Selected Injury Prevention Initiatives

Expenditure of $1 Each on:	Savings ($)
Smoke alarms	65
Child restraints	29
Bicycle helmets	29
Prevention counseling by pediatricians	10
Poison control services	7
Road safety improvements	3

From Peden M, OyegbiteK, Ozanne-Smith J, et al: World report on child injury prevention. Geneva, Switzerland, World Health Organization, 2004. Available at http://www.who.int/violence_injury_prevention/child/injury/world_report/en/index.html. Accessed November 12, 2010.

TABLE 17-2
Haddon Matrix Applied to Motor Vehicle Crashes in Children

	Child Factors	Vehicle and Safety Equipment	Physical Environment	Socioeconomic Environment
Pre-event	Age; gender; lack of supervision; risk-taking; impulsive behavior; disobedience; lack of police enforcement	Lack of roadworthiness of vehicle; poor lighting; poor state of brakes; speeding; overloading	Poor road design; lack of public transport; no enforcement of speed limits; no safety barriers; lack of alcohol laws; poor infrastructure for pedestrian safety	Poverty; single-parent family; large family size; poor maternal education; lack of awareness of risks among caregivers, childcare providers, and educators
Event	Size and physical development of child; lack of equipment to protect occupants, or equipment improperly used; underlying conditions in child	Child restraints and seat belts not fitted or incorrectly used; bicycle and motorcycle helmets not used; poor design of vehicle for protection in crashes; no rollover protection	Roadside objects such as trees and poles	Lack of safety culture in the car and on the road
Post-event	Child's lack of resilience; child's general condition; lack of access to appropriate health care; postinjury complications	Difficult access to victim; lack of trained health care and rescue workers	Lack of availability of adequate pre-hospital care, acute care and rehabilitation	Lack of culture of supporting injured people; no first aid given at scene

From Peden M, Oyegbite K, Ozanne-Smith J, et al: World report on child injury prevention. Geneva, Switzerland, World Health Organization, 2004. Available at http://www.who.int/violence_injury_prevention/child/injury/world_report/en/index.html. Accessed November 12, 2010.

TABLE 17-4

Incidence and Characteristics of 13 Injury Mechanisms Presenting to United States Trauma Centers, 2000-2004, and Priority Scores and Priority Rankings by Injury Mechanism

Mechanism	Incidence and Characteristics						Priority Scores and Rankings							
							Mortality		Injury Severity		Hospital Charges		Years of Life Lost	
	N	Median Age (Years)	Median ISS	Median Charges	Median YPLL	Mortality (%)	Mort PS$	Rank	IPPS*	Rank	Charge PS†	Rank	YPLL PS‡	Rank
Motor vehicle traffic	378,029	32	9	$15,941	37	5.0	69.7	1	72.0	1	74.0	1	74.6	1
Suffocation	1,314	28	1	$12,754	48	23.0	63.4	2	38.5	12	48.5	6	53.3	4
Firearm	53,146	26	9	$14,484	48	16.2	59.5	3	55.5	3	54.4	4	57.4	3
Fall	237,500	53	9	$12,922	10	3.5	58.4	4	64.9	2	61.1	2	42.9	11
Drowning/ submersion	945	20	4	$10,777	56	16.5	56.2	5	43.9	10	44.9	10	59.4	2
Pedestrian, other	3,100	32	9	$15,936	36	5.9	44.8	6	53.0	5	54.4	3	44.3	9
Transport, other	45,151	29	9	$14,240	42	2.9	44.5	7	55.1	4	53.5	5	51.2	5
Fire/burn	17,511	28	2	$7,412	23	4.6	44.4	8	41.2	11	39.6	12	35.5	13
Struck by, against	61,962	30	5	$10,367	35	1.5	44.1	9	48.8	6	47.3	8	48.2	7
Cut/pierce	40,574	31	4	$10,477	42	1.9	43.0	10	45.9	8	46.4	9	51.8	6
Machinery	12,221	40	4	$12,442	31	1.8	41.0	11	44.5	9	48.5	7	41.2	12
Poisoning	1,041	32	1	$5,201	38	2.5	41.0	12	38.5	13	34.7	13	45.7	8
Pedal cyclist, other	13,934	17	6	$9,277	34	0.9	40.1	13	48.2	7	42.8	11	43.6	10

From Wiebe DJ, Nance ML, Branas CC: Determining objective injury prevention strategies. Inj Prev 2005;12:347-350.
*Injury prevention priority score.
†Charge priority score.
‡Years potential life lost priority score.
§Mortality priority score.
Note: data based on trauma centers participating in the National Trauma Data Bank surveillance system.
ISS, injury severity score.

resources. Using data to better understand the scope of the problem is essential to designing effective prevention strategies.

INJURY PREVENTION DESIGN STRATEGIES

Effecting behavior change is always a difficult task to accomplish in injury prevention. As the Haddon matrix suggests, a multifaceted approach is necessary when designing effective injury prevention programs. It is important to understand the injury problem, associated risk factors, and the target population. The most successful prevention strategies are those that combine comprehensive methods and models. Most prevention models employ a variety of methods, often referred to as the three "Es": education, engineering (modification of the environment), and enforcement (policy change).[8] The fourth "E" that is often incorporated into prevention strategies is encouragement (e.g., economic incentives).

Education is the most common prevention strategy employed, with the goal of affecting behavioral modification. It is hoped that with understanding of risk will come behavior change. However, increased knowledge through education does not always translate readily into a behavior change. For example, although an adult may realize that using a crosswalk is the safest way to cross a busy street, crossing mid-block is much quicker. This strategy incorrectly assumes the public will voluntarily and preferentially adopt a safe behavior.

Enforcement (policy change) uses the force of the law to increase compliance and change behavior. This strategy is most effective when combined with education. There are many studies highlighting the positive impact that laws can have on injury prevention. As an example, the use of safety belts in motor vehicles increased by 15% after law enforcement agencies began issuing traffic citations.[9] Government regulations and industries have done much to offset poor behavior choices in order to save lives. Safety features have been introduced throughout our everyday lives, from air bags and crumple zones in cars to child-resistant caps on medicines to fire-resistant clothing for children. Other legislation requires an active response from the end user, such as the installation of smoke alarms in the home or wearing a bicycle helmet. Legislation is generally regarded as one of the most powerful tools in injury prevention, and has affected a positive behavior change.

Engineering (modification of the environment or product) is often used because this approach eliminates the need to change behavior in the individual. Effective engineering modifications for pedestrians include the introduction of side-walks, barriers, and pedestrian signs. Engineering is often the most expensive strategy and at times even cost prohibitive. To decrease the likelihood of crossing midblock, a roadway barrier can be put in place to eliminate crossing midblock. The cost to a governmental agency or to a product manufacturer must be weighed against the potential societal benefit in determining efficacy of such prevention strategies.

SELECTED INJURY PREVENTION INITIATIVES

Child Passenger Safety

One of the most dramatic examples of the efficacy of injury prevention strategies is that of child passenger safety efforts (Figure 17-2). Motor vehicle crashes are the leading cause of death for ages 3 to 14 in the United States. However, research has shown that lap/shoulder seat belts and child safety seats, when used, save lives. Vehicle seat belts reduce the risk of fatal injury to front seat occupants of passenger cars by 45%, while child safety seats reduce fatal injury by 71% for infants and 54% for toddlers in passenger cars.[10] The challenge is to make sure every passenger (regardless of age) is properly secured, every single ride.

Studies suggest that efforts to reduce injury risk to children in a motor vehicle should promote use of child restraint systems through a combination of education, distribution programs, and appropriate laws governing use.[11] Pierce and colleagues illustrate the importance of providing ongoing education combined with legislation and enforcement during a booster seat giveaway program in a Head Start program.[12] The program measured the knowledge level of Head Start providers, parents, and students regarding booster seats. It combined education along with the provision of age-appropriate restraints and direct observation following the program. The project was successful in increasing the use of booster seats, although the majority (66%), while restrained, were done so suboptimally. Despite the demonstrated efficacy, child passenger restraint misuse and inappropriate use is common (>72%) and offers additional room for prevention efforts.[13]

In a systematic review of five different interventions designed to increase child safety seat use, Zaza and colleagues demonstrated that the most successful interventions were those that did not stand alone but rather were multifactorial.[14] There was insufficient evidence for education-only programs. However, they identified strong evidence for effectiveness of child safety seat laws and distribution plus education programs. Also, community-wide information plus enhanced enforcement campaigns and incentive plus education programs had sufficient evidence of effectiveness.[14] Based on these findings, as well as other evidence-based programs designed to reduce injury risk to children in motor vehicles, efforts should promote use of child restraint systems through improved laws combined with education and disbursement programs.

Fire Safety

Because the causes for residential fires are multifactorial, efforts to prevent fire-related morbidity and mortality should also consider multiple approaches. A smoke alarm is arguably the single most important piece of safety equipment to prevent fire-related morbidity and mortality. The risk of dying in a residential fire is cut in half when a functioning smoke alarm is present.[15] Two efforts thought to be essential in reducing fire-related injury are the use of smoke alarms and identifying an escape plan for use in the event of a fire; both require action on the part of the resident. Previous research has demonstrated that the most effective and cost-efficient method to distribute smoke alarms is through direct home visits.[16] Harvey and colleagues have proven that direct installation is much more effective than voucher distribution for a free fire alarm.[17]

There are other passive preventive techniques that are also as effective, such as flame-resistant clothing for children. Half of the persons who start reported fires by playing are 5 years of age and younger. Most child-playing home fires are started with matches or lighters.[18] Legislatively, there are a variety of laws and standards that are designed to save lives, such as the requirement of smoke alarms on every level of the home and in every bedroom, sprinkler systems in some dwellings, and cigarette lighter standards. The U.S. Consumer Product

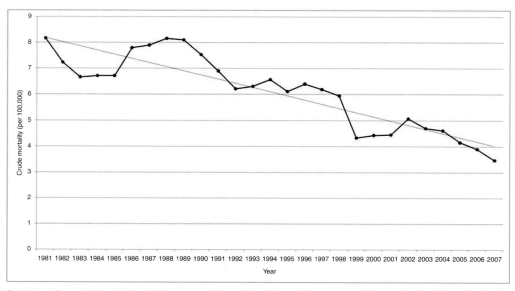

FIGURE 17-2 Decline in crude mortality rate for child occupants (age 0 to 19 years) in motor vehicle crashes for the period 1981 to 2007. (Data from National Center for Injury Prevention and Control.[1])

Safety Commission has issued a safety standard for cigarette lighters, which requires that disposable cigarette lighters be resistant to operation by children younger than the age of 5. In an analysis of this standard, it has been proven to reduce fire injuries, deaths, and property loss by children playing with cigarette lighters and can be expected to prevent additional fire losses in subsequent years.[19] Some states are now enacting novelty cigarette lighter legislation to protect against lighters that are being mistaken for toys. Continued efforts are necessary to maximize prevention efforts.

Firearm Storage

Firearm-related injuries have posed significant prevention challenges. With one of the highest case fatality rates of all injury mechanisms, prevention of the initial exposure is vital. However, with more than 250,000,000 firearms in circulation in the United States, that task is daunting.[20] The presence of a firearm in the home has been shown to increase the risk of unintentional firearm death (3.7-fold), suicide (3.4-fold), and homicide death (1.4-fold) versus households without firearms.[21,22] The effectiveness of educational programs geared to children and firearm use have been questioned. In a classical behavioral study, Hardy and colleagues demonstrated persistence of curious behaviors among children who encountered a firearm despite having undergone prior gun safety education.[23] Efforts to limit access to firearms by children have also had mixed results. A survey of parents visiting pediatrics practices revealed unsafe gun storage practices in 70% (gun unlocked 61%, gun loaded 15%, gun unlocked/loaded 7%, gun locked/unloaded 30%) of the homes.[24] The outcome of strategies geared toward parental firearm storage behaviors was summarized by McGee and colleagues, who did note an improvement in reported storage practices following counseling and education.[25] However, evidence to demonstrate a reduction in injury related to improved safety measures is limited. Grossman and colleagues were able to demonstrate that several factors were associated with a protective effect when examining the risk of youth unintentional and suicide firearm injuries: keeping a gun locked and unloaded, and storing ammunition locked and in a separate location.[26] Although firearm injury mitigation strategies have been of uncertain success, continued efforts are warranted given the ongoing risks that exist.

Helmet Use

Bicycle riding is enjoyed by millions of children and adults every day. Learning to master the technical challenges of a two-wheeled bicycle is a rite of passage for most children. However, because of its popularity and widespread use, bicycle riding is also a common source of injury in the pediatric population. Helmet use has long been advocated to mitigate the risk of serious head injury. Helmet use has been demonstrated to reduce head injury of all types, serious head injury, and facial injury related to bicycle collisions.[27–29]

Both educational initiatives as well as legislative mandates have been used to encourage routine helmet use among pediatric riders. Educational programs promoting use of bicycle helmets have been shown to increase their routine use. Rivara and colleagues demonstrated an increase in helmet use from 5.5% baseline to 40.2% after introduction of a community-wide bicycle helmet campaign.[30] At the same time, the rate of bicycle-related head injuries decreased by 67%. The effects

of bicycle helmet use campaigns seem to be most effective in the younger-aged children and in the higher socioeconomic status populations.[31,32] Parkin and colleagues demonstrated the efficacy of legislative approaches to improving helmet use in children, with a significantly increased observed rate of use from 46% to 68%.[33] Interestingly, the least impact of the legislation was noted in the highest socioeconomic groups. However, these groups also had the highest rates of baseline use, suggesting perhaps the efficacy of prior educational campaigns. A side benefit of mandatory laws may be heightened awareness of riders in areas not covered by helmet use laws. For example, in a Canadian study, the risk of bicycle-related head injury declined 45% in areas with mandatory use but also by 27% in areas without mandated use.[34]

Although a less common issue in the pediatric population, motorcycle helmet use has similarly been shown to reduce the incidence of serious head injury and death related to motorcycle accidents. A Cochrane collaborative reported a reduction in mortality of 42% and serious head injury of 69%.[35] Evidence was lacking regarding helmet use and risk of facial injuries. Mandatory motorcycle helmet use laws frequently are met with stiff opposition from riders, but such laws save lives and reduce serious head injuries.[36]

Pedestrian Injury

Pedestrian injuries in children resulted in 573 deaths (2007) and more than 47,000 injuries (2009) in the United States.[1] The burden of injury globally is far greater where pedestrians represent the largest category of child road traffic casualties.[37] A Cochrane Collaboration review demonstrated the effectiveness of pedestrian education programs geared toward children.[38] Programs included direct education of the child by professionals as well as use of the parents as educators. An improvement in knowledge was exhibited along with changes in baseline pedestrian behaviors, but a correlation with risk reduction was not possible. Most studies have been carried out in developed nations. As pedestrian injuries are increasing in developing nations along with an increase in motor vehicle use, effective prevention strategies are warranted. Somewhat paradoxically, most pedestrian injuries in children occur in optimal driving conditions (daylight hours, dry road conditions, no adverse weather conditions).[39] The majority of child pedestrians struck were crossing the street at the time of injury, frequently obscured by an obstacle.[39,40]

Engineering modifications to vehicles offer tremendous hope. Improving sight lines, optimizing visualization of the area surrounding the vehicle (through mirror placement and use of rear-facing cameras), and design changes to mitigate energy transfer at common impact points (e.g., front bumper) may reduce the burden of injury.[41] Efforts to change the environment, such as "traffic calming" techniques, have demonstrated efficacy.[42,43] The calming measures might include the use of speed humps, lower posted speed limits, traffic circles, installation or enhancement of crosswalks, and use of crossing aids.

Poisoning

Drug overdose death rates in the United States have never been higher. Rates of unintended ingestions have increased roughly fivefold since 1990, a leading cause of death in the pediatric population.[44] In addition, the Drug Abuse Warning Network (DAWN) reports the number of emergency department (ED) visits for legal drugs is now comparable to visits from illegal drugs.[45] Most fatal poisonings in the United States are from drug misuse (i.e., overdose). Overdose may include attempts at self-harm (suicide), assault (intentional), and accidental ingestion (unintentional).[44]

Among children, ED visits for medication poisonings are most common in children less than 6 years of age.[46] Emergency department visits for medication poisonings are twice as common as poisonings from other household products.[47] One of the most effective injury prevention initiatives in poison prevention was the introduction of child-resistant packaging for aspirin and oral prescription medicine that went into effect in the early 1970s.[48]

For children, caustic agents such as household cleaners that are marked with clear warning labels are not the only items in the home that can be dangerous to children. Everyday items such as cleaning supplies and medicines can be poisonous as well and should be kept out of the reach of children. The national poison control hotline (800-222-1222) provides parents and practitioners with readily accessible information about the toxicity and treatments for specific ingestions.

Measuring Success (Programmatic Evaluation)

Measuring the success of an injury prevention program or prevention initiative is imperative. There are many injury prevention programs in the community that appear to be effective. However, without adequate evaluation of the efforts, there is no way to verify if a program is actually achieving the goal of injury mitigation.

The most important aspect of evaluation is an adequate measurement of the problem conducted before, during, and after the intervention. The evaluation process should be dynamic. Assessment is started early, immediately after a program idea is conceived, and should continue through the intervention phase until the program is complete, when one determines whether the program has met its overall goal. In some cases, evaluation may continue for years after the intervention is complete to assess the durability of the desired outcome.

Evaluation is also critical to prove to funding agencies that their support is making a difference. A successful evaluation can also be used to strengthen funding proposals and to continue or replicate the program in other areas. A program that has rigorous, scientifically proven success is much more likely to receive continued funding. The same standards are necessary to publish the work in professional journals and disseminate prevention ideas to professionals in other communities.

Evaluation has four essential stages that are intertwined throughout the planning and intervention phase of a program. These stages are formative, process, impact, and outcome evaluation.[49] A well-designed formative evaluation will give the

TABLE 17-5	
Selected Internet Resources for Injury Prevention	
The American Association of Poison Control Centers	www.aapcc.org
National Fire Protection Association	www.nfpa.org
Safe Kids Worldwide	www.safekids.org
Centers for Disease Control and Prevention	www.cdc.gov
National Center for Injury Prevention and Control	www.cdc.gov/ HomeandRecreationalSafety/ Poisoning/index.html
Consumer Product Safety Commission	www.cpsc.gov

program a better chance at success, along with elucidating areas of improvement. In the formative stage, a targeted issue is identified (e.g., bicycle helmet use to lessen head injury) and may include an assessment of existing resources and deficiencies. During this stage, it is important to identify barriers to success (e.g., age, access to target population, education). Inclusion of community stakeholders at this stage increases the likelihood of long-term success.

Through process evaluation, the second stage, a plan is formulated to measure whether or not the program is reaching the desired audience. This stage typically requires documentation of the number of people reached during the educational or interventional program, for instance, the number of bicycle helmets distributed or the number of students taught bicycle safety. Such data will provide the foundation for sound assessment of the program.

Impact evaluation is a measure of how well the program is progressing toward its goals. It is a measurement of knowledge, attitudes, and beliefs. This assessment may be through direct observation of a particular behavior, or perhaps though survey or questionnaire. Preintervention and postintervention data collection (e.g., observed bicycle helmet use) will provide insight regarding the success of a program.

The final phase, outcome evaluation, measures whether or not the program met its goal of decreasing incidence of injury, morbidity, and/or mortality. Demonstrating long-term success (beyond the intervention stages) is ideal, but such study can be time consuming and resource intensive. However, demonstration of sustained injury reduction is likely to lead to dissemination of practices and ongoing funding.

Injury is the leading cause of death and disability in the pediatric population. Although trauma systems have evolved to provide optimal care, prevention is the preferred approach. Prevention strategies should be tailored to the target population and studied to ensure efficacy. For additional Internet-based injury prevention resources, see Table 17-5.

The complete reference list is available online at www. expertconsult.com.

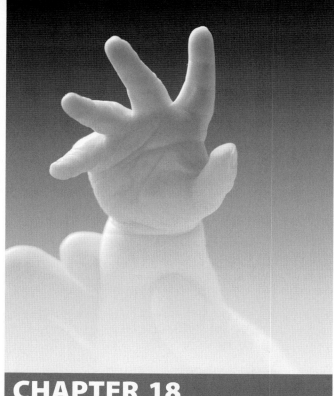

CHAPTER 18

Infants and Children as Accident Victims and Their Emergency Management

Jeffrey R. Lukish and Martin R. Eichelberger

Epidemiology of Childhood Injury

Preventable injuries take an enormous financial, emotional, and social toll on the injured children and their families, but also on society as a whole. Worldwide, childhood injuries are a growing problem. Every year, approximately 875,000 children are killed, and nonfatal injuries affect the lives of between 10 million and 30 million more globally (Fig. 18-1).[1] In the United States, unintentional injury is the leading cause of death among children ages 18 and younger, claiming more than 12,000 child lives annually, or an average of 30 children each day. In addition to the deaths, there were 9.2 million

medical visits for unintentional injury among U.S. children, accounting for 151,319 hospitalizations.[2] More than 16% of all hospitalizations for unintentional injuries among children result in permanent disability.[3]

The unintentional injury fatality rate among children ages 14 years and younger declined 45% in the United States since 1987. Despite this decline, unintentional injury remains the leading cause of death among children ages 1 to 14 years in the United States. In fact, 5,162 children ages 14 years and younger died in 2005 from an unintentional injury, and 6,253,661 emergency room visits for unintentional injuries in this age group occurred in 2006.[4] From 2000 to 2005, the leading cause of fatal unintentional injury among children was transportation-related followed by drowning and airway obstruction injury. Falls were the leading cause of nonfatal, hospital emergency room–treated childhood injury and accounted for 2.8 million visits in 2005.[1]

Leading causes of unintentional injury-related death vary according to a child's age and are dependent on developmental abilities and exposure to potential hazards, in addition to parental perceptions of a child's abilities and injury risk. Falls were the leading cause of nonfatal injury for all age groups less than 15 years. The least progress in the injury death rate decline was among infants less than 1 year of age, who had a decline of only 10%, compared with children in the age groups 1 to 4 years (42%), 5 to 9 years (42%), and 10 to 14 years (40%). Children less than 1 year of age have the highest rate of unintentional injury-related death, with a rate more than twice that of all children. Airway obstruction is the leading killer in this age group. In children, ages 1 to 4 years of age, drowning was the leading cause of injury death followed by transportation-related injury. The lowest rate of unintentional death among children less than 14 years of age is in the group of children 5 to 9 years of age. The most common cause of death in this age group and those children aged 10 to 14 years was motor vehicle occupant injury (Fig. 18-2).[2]

In all age groups, male children are at higher risk for unintentional injury than females. This can be attributed to a variety of factors, including biology (differences in temperament), exposure to risky behavior, gender socialization, and cognitive differences.[3] Race and ethnicity are also important factors in the risk for unintentional injury in children. American Indian and Native Alaskan children have the highest unintentional injury death rate at 15.3 per 100,000, and Asian or Pacific Islanders have the lowest fatality rate at 4.24 per 100,000. African-American and white children have approximately the same fatality rate, which has declined 44% and 48%, respectively, in these groups since 1987. In 1990, Hispanic and non-Hispanic children had similar fatality rates from unintentional injury at approximately 12.11 and 12.48 per 100,000, respectively. Since then, the fatality rate has declined by nearly 40 percent for Hispanic children and only 30 percent for non-Hispanic children. In 2005, 4,229 non-Hispanic children and 922 Hispanic children in the United States died from unintentional injuries. Although the number of fatal injuries among Hispanic children increased, the rate of injuries declined because of the increased population size. These racial and ethnic disparities have more to do with economic conditions than with biologic differences, because living in impoverished communities is a primary predictor of injury. Fatality rates from unintentional injury declined in each of the four regions of

GLOBAL CHILD INJURY DEATH BY CAUSE,
CHILDREN 17 AND UNDER, WORLD, 2004

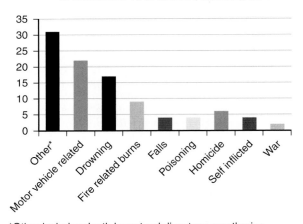

*Other includes death by natural disasters, smothering,
choking, asphyxiation, hypothermia and hyperthermia

FIGURE 18-1 Percentage of fatal injuries in children 17 years of age
and younger worldwide in 2004. (From Peden MM, UNICEF, World Health
Organization: Geneva, Switzerland, World Health Organization, 2008.)

UNINTENTIONAL INJURY DEATH BY CAUSE,
CHILDREN 19 AND UNDER, UNITED STATES, 2005

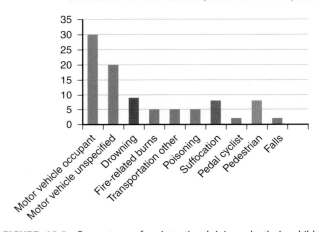

FIGURE 18-2 Percentage of unintentional injury death in children
19 years of age and younger in the United States from 2000 to 2005.
(From Borse NN, Gilchrist J, Dellinger AM, et al: CDC Childhood Injury
Report: Patterns of unintentional injuries among 0-19 year olds in the
United States, 2000-2006. Atlanta, Ga, Centers for Disease Control and
Prevention, National Center for Injury Prevention and Control, 2008.)

UNINTENTIONAL CHILDHOOD INJURY
MORTALITY, 1987–2006

Motor vehicle occupant	↓ 53%
Drowning	↓ 54%
Pedestrian	↓ 64%
Bicycle	↓ 78%
Fire and burn	↓ 73%
Firearm	↓ 94%

FIGURE 18-3 Percentage decrease of unintentional injury mortality in
children 19 years of age and younger in the United States from 1987 to
2006. (From Wallace AL, Cody BE, Mickalide AD: Report to the Nation:
Trends in unintentional childhood injury mortality and parental views.
Washington, DC, National Safe Kids Campaign, April 2008.)

related injuries were highest in some southern states and some
states of the upper plains, while the lowest rates occurred in
states in the northeast region.[1,4]

Over the last 20 years there has been a dramatic reduction
in childhood injury death (Fig. 18-3). These extraordinary
decreases in the injury death rate are due to multifaceted
prevention strategies.

Intentional injury results in a fatal outcome from homicide,
child abuse, or suicide. National and state efforts in this regard
have led to continued reductions, and now these deaths represent a much smaller percentage of fatalities in children in the
United States. Recognition of this intent requires referral to the
child protection service for assessment. The resuscitation of
these children is frequently a challenge, because abuse may
be chronic, which results in a child with a limited physiologic
reserve (refer to Chapter 27 on child abuse).[4]

Resuscitation and Impact
on Outcome

Resuscitation of the injured child includes the actions
necessary to reverse and control the sudden alterations in
physiologic homeostasis that occur as the result of injury.
Children are remarkably resilient; however, the initial period
of stability has been shown to be significantly shorter as age
decreases.[5] Therefore, resuscitation is not complete until
injuries have been definitively treated and the child displays
physiologic stability without continued intervention.

Differences between children and adults with respect to
patterns of injury, physiologic presentation, and management
are important. Physicians who treat injured children must recognize and understand the important distinctions so that the
resuscitation process addresses the special needs of the child.

The principle of a trimodal pattern of trauma-related mortality and morbidity in adults must be modified for children.
In the trimodal model, the first group of injured children dies
very rapidly after injury, within seconds or minutes, because of
injuries to the central or peripheral nervous system and the
central vasculature. Survival can only be improved in this
group through prevention efforts, such as education, social
awareness, and behavior modification. A second peak occurs
from minutes to hours after the injury and is due to mass
lesions in the central nervous system (CNS) (usually subdural

the United States between 1987 and 2005. The largest decrease,
almost 60%, was in the Northeast, while the Midwest had the
smallest decrease, 40%. Since 1987, the South has consistently
had the highest rate of fatality, 10 per 100,000 in 2005, and the
Northeast has had the lowest, 4.56 per 100,000. Geographic
differences in injury fatality rates reflect demographic differences and different levels of exposure to hazardous activities.
At the state level, rates of unintentional injury fatality tend
to be highest in the South, potentially because of large rural
populations with high rates of poverty and limited access
to trauma care. Overall, states with the lowest injury death rates
were in the Northeast. Fire and burn death rates were highest in
some of the southern states. Death rates from transportation-

and epidural hematomas), solid organ injury, or collection of fluid in the pleural and pericardial space. These are the specific injuries that require rapid identification and treatment and are the focus of the advanced trauma life support (ATLS) protocol. Although initial physiologic compensation may have been sufficient to achieve some temporary accommodation, progressive dysfunction and exhausted reserves bring about a critical impairment of oxygen delivery and the child's eventual demise. Advances in the aggressive and systematic delivery of emergency medical services (EMSC) for children have a salutary effect upon preventable death in children. A third mortality peak occurs days to weeks after the initial injury and is the result of complications of injury, such as sepsis and systemic inflammatory response syndrome, leading to multiple organ failure syndrome.[6] This late peak in trauma-related mortality is less frequent in younger children.

Resuscitation Principles

PREHOSPITAL CARE

Systematic management following an injury to a child is essential to survival. The resuscitation process begins when emergency transport personnel first encounter the child in the field. The fate of any given child can turn on the decisions and interventions that transpire during these first crucial moments. In general, children fare worse than adults in the out-of-hospital phase of resuscitation. The injury-adjusted death rate for children is twice that of adults. Similarly, the survival rate for out-of-hospital cardiac arrest in children is only half that of adults.[7] Although part of this discrepancy results from the different causes of cardiac arrest in children and adults, unfamiliarity and inadequate training with children contributes to poor outcome. The failure rate for resuscitation interventions in the field is twice as high in children as adults; the failure rate for prehospital endotracheal intubation of children is close to 50%.[8] Unfamiliarity with pediatric resuscitation skills is understandable; trauma is the most common indication for pediatric ambulance transport, but accounts for less than 10% of total paramedic patient volume in most metropolitan areas.

The most important objectives for emergency personnel in the field are
- Recognition and treatment of immediate life-threatening dysfunction
- Assessment of the mechanism of trauma and extent of injuries
- Documentation of pertinent medical data
- Triage to the appropriate-level pediatric trauma facility

Add to these the additional challenges of comforting a terrified and hurt child, as well as a distraught parent, and the paramedic's task becomes formidable. Consequently, prehospital personnel function best by adopting strict protocols to treat the injured child. The priorities and techniques associated with pediatric field resuscitation are similar to those for emergency department care.

PRIMARY SURVEY AND TREATMENT OF LIFE-THREATENING INJURIES

When the injured child encounters medical personnel, whether in the field or in the emergency room, events transpire in a rapid sequence that is dictated by a systematic protocol to recognize and treat acute injuries. This approach is designed to standardize diagnostic and treatment decisions so that individual variations in patterns of injury do not distract caregivers from recognizing and treating subtle injuries that can have a profound impact upon outcome. This systematic framework comprises a primary survey, a resuscitation phase, and a definitive secondary survey. The primary survey is the initial process of identifying and temporizing injuries that are potentially life-threatening and follows the "ABCDE" sequence (Airway, Breathing, Circulation, Disability, and Exposure). The system relies upon simple observations to assess physiologic derangement and immediate intervention to prevent death.

Airway and Cervical Spine Control

Provision of airway control is perhaps the least controversial of all priorities in pediatric trauma management. The inability to establish and maintain a child's airway, leading to hypoxia and inadequate ventilation, continues to be a common cause of cardiorespiratory arrest and death. Significant clinical hypoxia is suspected when oxygen saturation is less than 95%.

Assessment of the airway includes inspection of the oral cavity; manual removal of debris, loose teeth, and soft tissue fragments; and aspiration of blood and secretions with mechanical suction. If a child is neurologically intact, phonates normally, and is ventilating without stridor or distress, invasive airway management is unnecessary. Airway patency can be improved in the spontaneously breathing child by use of the jaw-thrust or chin-lift maneuvers.

An airway that is unsecured because of coma, combativeness, shock, or direct airway trauma requires endotracheal intubation. A nasopharyngeal or oropharyngeal airway can improve management during bag mask ventilation but are temporizing measures until definitive control is established. In most cases, orotracheal intubation with in-line cervical spine stabilization is the preferred approach to airway control. Although nasotracheal intubation is recommended in nonapneic adult with potential cervical spine injury, this approach is not indicated and poorly tolerated in children.

The pediatric airway anatomy is unique and affects management technique. The child's larynx is anatomically higher and more anterior than that of the adult patient, necessitating an upward angulation of the laryngoscope to place the endotracheal tube properly. Removing the anterior half of the rigid cervical collar allows access to the neck for gentle cricoid pressure. The pediatric epiglottis is shorter, less flexible, and tilted posteriorly over the glottic inlet. Because of this, direct control of the epiglottis with a straight blade is usually necessary for proper visualization of the vocal cords. The vocal cords themselves are more fragile and easily damaged. The narrowest point in the pediatric airway is the subglottic trachea at the cricoid ring, as opposed to the glottis in adult patients. Therefore passage of the endotracheal tube through the vocal cords does not guarantee safe advancement into the trachea or avoidance of subglottic injury. The selection of an appropriate endotracheal tube is an important part of pediatric resuscitation. Internal diameter sizes can range from 3.0 to 3.5 mm in newborns to 4.5 mm at 1 to 2 years of age. After 2 years of age, internal diameter can be estimated by the following formula: internal diameter = age/4 + 4. Approximating the diameter of the patient's little finger is also useful. Because of the narrow subglottic trachea, an uncuffed endotracheal tube is indicated in children 8 years of age or younger (Fig. 18-4).[8,9]

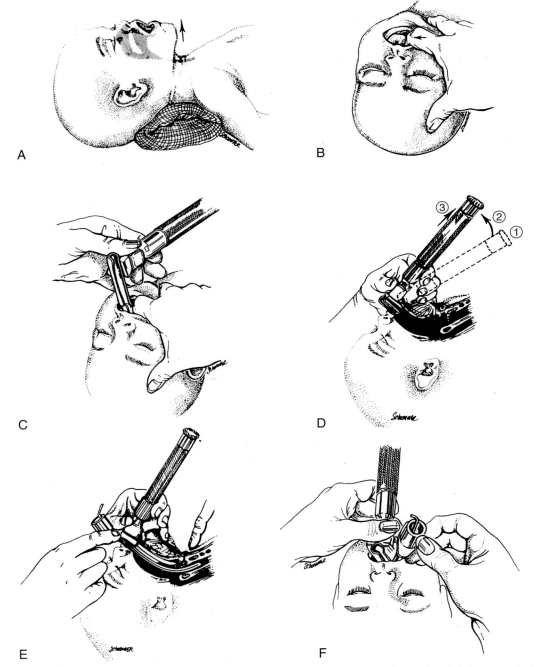

FIGURE 18-4   Endotracheal intubation. **A,** The pediatric larynx and supraglottic space are anterior and angled cephaled compared with the position in adults. A posterior neck roll optimizes visualization of the vocal cords in children. **B,** The tongue is large relative to the space in a child's oral cavity. The tongue should be moved to one side of the oral cavity to facilitate exposure of the posterior pharynx and supraglottic area. **C,** The laryngoscope blade is inserted from the right side of the mouth and slides back along the vallecula. **D,** With the blade in the proper position and the child's neck slightly extended in the sniffing position, lifting the handle (positions 1, 2, and 3) raises the epiglottis and brings the vocal cords into direct vision. **E,** In all except newborns, the straight blade should be placed over the epiglottis to lift it, along with base of the tongue, to expose the larynx. A stylet with the tip curved within the endotracheal tube facilitates successful intubation. **F,** The endotracheal tube is held in place while the laryngoscope is removed and secured after verification of bilateral breath sounds. (From Eichelberger MR: Pediatric Trauma, Prevention, Acute Care, Rehabilitation. St Louis, Mosby, 1993.)

The technique of intubation depends on the urgency of establishing an airway. In the hypotensive, hypoxemic, comatose child, orotracheal intubation is accomplished without delay as an integral part of the resuscitation. In a more elective situation, more attention is given to adequate preoxygenation and premedication. An adequate oxygen saturation (i.e., more than 95%), as measured by pulse oximetry, is attempted by bag-mask ventilation with 100% oxygen. Thoracic trauma can preclude and make attainment of adequate oxygen saturation impossible before intubation. Inducing hypocarbia ($Pco_2 = 28$ to 32 torr) by hyperventilation is advantageous and can reduce intracranial hypertension.

Following preoxygenation using mask ventilation, children should receive atropine sulfate (0.1 to 0.5 mg) to ensure that the heart rate remains high during intubation. It is important to maintain heart rate, because this is directly proportional to cardiac output; stroke volume does not change in a child. Also, the child should be premedicated with intravenous sedatives and muscle relaxants. Appropriate sedatives include short-acting barbiturates, such as thiopental sodium (5 mg/kg), if volume status is normal, or a benzodiazepine, such as midazolam (0.1 mg/kg), if hypovolemia is suspected. Muscle relaxation is achieved with short-acting nondepolarizing agents (vecuronium bromide, 0.1 mg/kg) or shorter-acting depolarizing agents (succinylcholine chloride, 1 mg/kg). The presence of burns and devitalized tissue precludes the use of succinylcholine because of the risk of hyperkalemia. Continuous monitoring of the intubated child with end-tidal carbon dioxide (CO_2) and pulse oximetry is essential to safe resuscitation.

In the rare circumstance, when tracheal intubation is not possible as a consequence of oral maxillofacial trauma or congenital anomaly, a surgical airway is indicated. A surgical crycothyrotomy is the preferred approach in older children (>10 years). Because this crycothyroid membrane is easily exposed through a transverse skin incision, placement of a small, uncuffed endotracheal tube via this incision is possible. The morbidity is less because of the superficial location of the crycothyroid membrane in contrast to an emergency tracheostomy. The crycothyrotomy should be converted to a formal tracheostomy, when the child is stabilized, to avoid subglottic stenosis.

In small children, the cricoid cartilage is a delicate structure and provides the majority of support to the trachea. Injury of this membrane during emergency cricothyrotomy can lead to significant morbidity and lifelong laryngotracheomalacia. To avoid this complication, children younger than 10 years of age should undergo needle cricothyrotomy and jet insufflation of the trachea. A 16- to 18-gauge intravenous catheter is used to access the tracheal lumen through the crycothyroid membrane, and is connected to a 100% oxygen source at a high flow rate of 10 to 12 L/min. Needle-jet ventilation is limited in children by hypercarbia that occurs in approximately 30 minutes; therefore this method is a temporary means of ventilation. Following stabilization of the child, endotracheal intubation or formal tracheostomy is necessary.[9]

Breathing

Compromised breathing and ventilation in the injured child usually results from either head injury (impaired spontaneous ventilatory drive), or thoracic injury (impaired lung expansion). Recognition of the head-injured child is usually clear, while recognition of a thoracic injury that impairs lung expansion requires a detailed survey. The potential seriousness of these injuries is underscored by the fact that mortality rates for thoracic trauma in children approach 25%.[10]

Following thoracic trauma, air, fluid, or viscera can occupy the pleural space. Compression of the pulmonary parenchyma can result in impairment of gas exchange sufficient to produce respiratory distress. In the case of traumatic rupture of the diaphragm, loss of muscular integrity also has a direct effect on lung expansion. The pediatric mediastinum is extremely mobile; as pressure increases in the pleural space, the mediastinum is displaced to the opposite side, causing compression of the contralateral lung. The distortion of mediastinal

vascular structures, along with the elevated intrathoracic pressure, can result in a critical reduction of venous return to the right atrium.

Loss of chest wall integrity from flail chest impairs ventilation and oxygenation. Consequently, paradoxical chest wall movement occurs during inspiration preventing complete lung expansion; treatment is best by assisted positive-pressure breathing. The force required to fracture multiple ribs in a child is enormous and is transmitted to the underlying lung parenchyma, resulting in a pulmonary contusion. Regions of parenchymal hemorrhage and edema impair ventilation-perfusion matching; the decrease in pulmonary compliance can dramatically increase the work of breathing, which can precipitate ventilatory failure.

Recognition of ventilatory compromise is usually not difficult, especially with a high index of suspicion. The sound of air movement at the mouth and nares is assessed, as are the rate, depth, and effort of respirations. On inspection, asymmetric excursion of the chest wall suggests a ventilatory abnormality. Percussion elicits dullness or hyper-resonance, depending on the presence of fluid or air in the pleural space, while breath sounds are decreased. With tension hemopneumothorax, mediastinal shift may be detected by tracheal deviation, displacement of the point of maximal impulse, and distention of neck veins caused by impaired venous return to the heart.

Mechanical ventilatory failure is life threatening and requires immediate treatment during the primary survey. All children require supplemental oxygen by nasal cannula, mask, or endotracheal tube. Endotracheal intubation and assisted ventilation are sufficient to treat hypoventilation caused by head injury, pain from rib fractures, flail chest, and pulmonary contusion. Simple hemopneumothorax may be well tolerated with supplemental oxygen until tube thoracostomy can be performed after the primary survey (Fig. 18-5). In cases of hemopneumothorax, which results in compromised ventilation or hypotension, a thoracostomy tube is required, often combined with endotracheal intubation and intravenous access for rapid fluid infusion. If tension is present, the hemodynamic derangements can be minimized by needle thoracostomy in the second intercostal space at the midclavicular line, followed by definitive thoracostomy tube. When endotracheal intubation has been performed, the child should receive 100% Fio_2 with a tidal volume of 10 to 12 mL/kg at a respiratory rate of 15 to 20 cycles/min. Oxygenation and ventilation should be manipulated to maintain an arterial Po_2 > 80 mm Hg and a Pco_2 of 28 to 32 torr, with a positive end-expiratory pressure (PEEP) not to exceed 5 cm H_2O. The goal is to prevent secondary brain injury by optimizing oxygenation and cerebral perfusion by minimizing intracranial pressure. Children with head trauma are best managed by moderate hyperventilation and hypocarbia (Pco_2 = 30 to 35 mm Hg) to reduce intracranial pressure.[6,9,11]

Tube thoracostomy is accomplished during this phase of resuscitation for symptomatic hemopneumothorax. A chest tube of adequate caliber to evacuate blood and air is inserted into the pleural cavity. The narrow intercostal space of a small child usually limits the size of the tube, but the largest caliber tube that can be placed is preferable (18° F to 20° F). The tube should be placed in the midaxillary line at the nipple level (fourth or fifth intercostal space) to avoid intra-abdominal

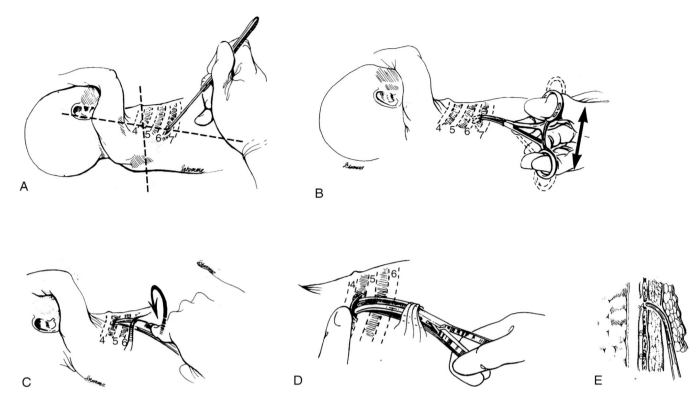

FIGURE 18-5 Thoracostomy tube insertion. **A,** An incision is made in the midaxillary line just below the nipple in a male or inframammary fold in a female (fourth intercostals space). **B,** The dissection is carried out in a cephalad direction, subcutaneously over two ribs. A long subcutaneous track is preferable in a child to minimize air leak around the tube. **C,** The fourth intercostal space is the ideal place for thoracostomy tube placement. **D,** The entrance into the pleural space should be made just over and superior to the rib to avoid injury to intercostal vessels. **E,** Lateral view of the technique. (From Eichelberger MR: Pediatric Trauma, Prevention, Acute Care, Rehabilitation. St Louis, Mosby, 1993.)

placement through an elevated diaphragm. The tube should be directed posterior and cephalad to evacuate both blood and air. The tube is connected to a pleurovac closed-suction drainage system set at −15 cm H$_2$O. Persistent hemorrhage from a thoracostomy tube is uncommon in children; however, drainage of 1 to 2 mL/kg/hour is a sign of ongoing significant bleeding from a vascular or mediastinal injury that requires thoracotomy to identify the source of blood loss and to secure hemorrhage.

Circulation and Vascular Access

The third priority in the sequence of the primary survey is the rapid assessment of circulation and the establishment of venous access. Seriously injured children often have normal vital signs, even with significantly decreased circulating volume as a result of a remarkable cardiovascular reserve. This compensation that occurs in the injured child delays the early hemodynamic signs of hypovolemia until relatively late in their physiologic decline. A high index of suspicion based on the mechanism of injury and continuous careful scrutiny of physiologic parameters and clinical signs is necessary to minimize morbidity.

A reliable sign of adequate perfusion is a normal mental status. As the child is resuscitated, clinical signs of the efficacy of resuscitation should be monitored. Improvement in the following parameters is consistent with hemodynamic stability and success of resuscitation:
- Slowing of the heart rate (<100 beats/min)
- Increased pulse pressure (>20 mm Hg)
- Return of normal skin color
- Increased warmth of extremities
- Clearing of the sensorium (improving Glasgow Coma Scale [GCS] score)
- Increase in systolic blood pressure (>80 mm Hg)
- Urinary output of 1 to 2 mL/kg/hour in infants and 1 mL/kg/hour in adolescents

After establishing an adequate airway, provision of venous access in a hypovolemic child is often a challenge. Two functioning catheters are best in all cases of significant injury. Optimal circumstances would be to achieve venous access above and below the diaphragm, given the potential for extravasation of resuscitation fluids from occult intra-abdominal venous injuries. Nevertheless, in children any peripheral venous access is useful.

Two attempts should be made to place large-bore peripheral IVs in the upper extremities. If percutaneous placement is unsuccessful, insertion of an intraosseous (IO) line is useful in a child less than 6 years of age. If more than 6 years of age, a venous cutdown performed at the ankle is best. The greater saphenous vein is easily exposed through short transverse incisions, 0.5 to 1 cm proximal and anterior to the medial malleoli. The exposed vein can be suspended over a silk ligature, and the largest appropriate intravenous catheter is introduced into the vessel lumen under direct vision. Trans-section or ligation of the vein is not necessary (Fig. 18-6).

Because central venous catheterization can result in significant complications, such as laceration of the subclavian or

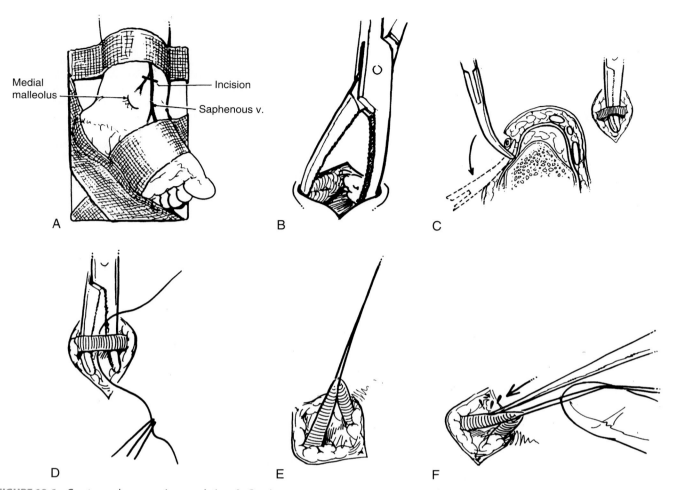

FIGURE 18-6 Greater saphenous vein cannulation. **A,** Consistent emergency venous access is achieved at the ankle, anterior to the medial malleolus via the saphenous vein. **B,** A transverse incision is made anterior to the medial malleolus (1 cm anterior and 1 cm cephalad). Perpendicular dissection in the incision exposes the saphenous vein. **C,** The vein is dissected circumferentially. **D,** A suture ligature is passed around the vessel. **E** and **F,** Gentle traction on the suture facilitates catheterization of the vein. (From Eichelberger MR: Pediatric Trauma, Prevention, Acute Care, Rehabilitation. St Louis, Mosby, 1993.)

femoral artery, this technique is less useful. The femoral route is preferred because of ease of access. If subclavian venous access is necessary, the child should be positioned in the Trendelenberg position, with the head maintained in a neutral position without the placement of a posterior shoulder roll. This position provides optimal cross-sectional area of the subclavian vein in both children and adults.[12]

An intraosseous (IO) line is a simple, reliable, and a safe route for administration of fluids, blood products, and medication. The technique is applicable in children 6 years of age and younger, because of the well-perfused marrow of early childhood. The preferred site for IO insertion is through the flat anteromedial surface of the tibia, about 2 to 3 cm below the tibial plateau. The needle is angled 60 degrees from horizontal and pointed toward the foot. The cortex is penetrated and the marrow cavity detected by aspirating blood and particulate material. Alternative sites include the midline distal femur, 3 cm above the condyles directed cephalad in small children, and the distal tibia above the medial malleolus or the proximal humerus in the adolescent. Specially designed IO needles should be available in the pediatric resuscitation room to facilitate this maneuver; however, a 14- to 16-gauge needle can be used. The complication rate of IO is low but

includes osteomyelitis, cellulitis, fracture, growth plate injury, fat embolism, and compartment syndrome.

As soon as vascular access is established, fluid resuscitation with a bolus of fluid is begun. Generally, isotonic crystalloid solution, such as lactated Ringer solution, is administered in 20 mL/kg increments. If evidence of hypovolemia persists after 40 mL/kg has been given, transfusion of ABO-matched packed red blood cells (RBCs) is initiated in a bolus of 10 mL/kg. Packed RBCs have the desirable qualities of raising colloid oncotic pressure and effecting a more rapid and sustained intravascular expansion than crystalloid. In addition, the red blood cell provides hemoglobin to increase oxygen-carrying capacity. All fluids (crystalloid, colloid, and blood) should be warmed during infusion. This is accomplished by use of a microwave to heat crystalloid solutions and use of a warming device.

It is important to reassess the child's response to resuscitation continually to characterize the nature and extent of the injuries and to avoid the complications of excessive fluid resuscitation. As perfusion is restored, the rate of fluid infusion is gradually reduced to avoid unnecessary fluid administration. Pulmonary edema rarely occurs in normal lungs, but considerable morbidity results from fluid sequestration in a region of pulmonary and cerebral contusion. If hemodynamic stabilization does not occur with crystalloid and blood resuscitation, hemorrhage is likely from an intra-abdominal or pelvic source, cardiac dysfunction because of tamponade, contusion, or tension hemopneumothorax; cerebrospinal injury, such as atlantooccipital disassociation; and profound hypothermia.[9,13]

Disability

A rapid neurologic evaluation is included in the primary survey to identify serious injuries that may have immediate consequences for airway management. A rapid method for describing gross cerebral function is the AVPU pneumonic: alert, voice responsive, pain responsive, or unresponsive. An assessment of pupillary responsiveness and symmetry is also useful. Transtentorial herniation secondary to an expanding intracranial hematoma causes ipsilateral pupillary dilation and loss of light reflex. Direct trauma to the eye is an equally common cause of unilateral anisocoria. Characterization of extremity posturing as decorticate or decerebrate indicates the loss of cortical or global brain function, respectively. In the comatose child with a unilateral fixed and dilated pupil, measures to reduce intracranial pressure (ICP) are imperative. These include early controlled endotracheal intubation to keep the Pco_2 regulated (30 to 35 mm Hg) with moderate hyperventilation, which causes cerebral vasoconstriction and decreases cerebral blood flow. This lowers brain volume and ICP with resulting increase in cerebral perfusion pressure (CPP). The reverse Trendelenburg position, in which the head is slightly elevated by 30 degrees, can also reduce intracranial hypertension but should be employed in children with normal cardiac function.

Exposure

Complete exposure of the child is essential to facilitate a thorough examination and identification of injury. A conscious child does not understand the need for such action, so exposure must be done carefully. A thorough primary survey on a stable child with a normal GCS score can be performed without removing all items of clothing simultaneously. Children are particularly apprehensive about exposing an injury that had previously been covered. Attention to the special sensitivities of the child in this regard frequently results in a more efficient resuscitation.

In a child, hypothermia affects physiologic parameters, such as cognitive function, cardiac activity, and coagulation. It is important to maintain core temperature above 35 to 36 degrees Celsius. A warm resuscitation room preserves core body temperature and minimizes heat loss. Similarly, resuscitation fluid and inhaled gases should be warmed and humidified. Overhead and bed warmers are essential but a radiant warmer is best for the injured infant.

RESUSCITATION PHASE

The cornerstone of resuscitation is continuous reappraisal of the child's response to therapeutic intervention. Deterioration at any point requires repetition of the primary survey. After the ABCs are completed and life-threatening injuries are stable, place a gastric tube and urinary catheter, followed by removal of blood for analysis and establishment of a cardiac monitor.

In children, acute gastric dilation can cause both respiratory compromise and vagus-mediated bradycardia. Gastric decompression to evacuate the stomach and reduce the risk of vomiting and aspiration is important in all injured children, especially those with a decreased level of consciousness. Assessment for a stable midface and for presence of cerebrospinal fluid (CSF) rhinorrhea are important before placement of nasogastric tube for decompression. If abnormal, gastric tube placement is contradicted.

A urinary catheter is also placed following a thorough perineal assessment, including a rectal exam prior to placement. In instances of a high-riding prostate, meatal bleeding, perineal or scrotal ecchymosis, or unstable anterior pelvic fracture, a retrograde urethrogram is indicated before insertion of the catheter.

An electrocardiogram (ECG) is essential to monitor cardiac rhythm, which is rarely abnormal. Secondary abnormalities are occasionally seen and include sinus bradycardia because of advanced shock; or electromechanical dissociation from hypovolemia, tension pneumothorax, or pericardial tamponade; and ventricular fibrillation because of hypothermia or acidosis. Ventricular ectopy, low voltages, and signs of ischemia can accompany myocardial contusion. Beyond evaluating the actual rhythm, diffuse low voltage may be the first indication of hemopericardium.

After vascular access, blood and urine is obtained for laboratory analysis, hemoglobin, urinalysis, and arterial blood gas analysis. Blood alcohol level and a toxicology screen are not routine in children but reasonable in adolescents. Blood should be drawn for typing and crossmatching for possible transfusion.[13,14]

NEURORESUSCITATION

Brain injury is the most common cause of acquired disability and mortality during childhood. It is estimated that 1 in 500 children in the United States sustains a brain injury, 7000 children die from head injury, and 28,000 children become permanently disabled.[15,16] Largely a result of prevention strategy and of regional trauma systems, the overall mortality from severe traumatic brain injury has decreased from approximately 50% in the 1970s to 36% in 2006. In children, the current overall mortality from injury is 3%; the primary cause of death in 70% of the cases is CNS injury. Overall, the outcome for children older than 3 years of age is better than for adults with comparable injuries; however, outcome in young children (<3 years) is often poor.[6,9,17]

Traumatic brain injury can be defined as either primary or secondary. Primary brain injury is the structural derangement of cerebral architecture that occurs from direct, mechanical impact, resulting in cellular and vascular disruption, infarction, or tissues loss. The child's brain is susceptible to injury of deep white matter shear, punctate hemorrhage, brain swelling, and linear, nondepressed skull fractures rather than a mass lesion, such as subdural, epidural, intracerebral hematoma, and depressed skull fractures, which are more frequently encountered in adults. Children, however, have a higher incidence of epidural hematoma, perhaps because the thinner, less rigid skull is more apt to fracture and lacerate the meningeal artery. The proportionally larger size of the cranium in children, along with a less muscular and more flexible ligamentous cervical spine, may account for the increased incidence of diffuse axonal injury in the injured child.

Primary brain injury responds only to prevention efforts, while the secondary brain injury is the target of clinical neuro-resuscitation. Secondary brain injury occurs as a result of decreased cerebral perfusion after the traumatic event. Both diffuse and regional brain swelling impair oxygen and substrate delivery largely as a result of increasing intracranial pressure (ICP) and its effect upon cerebral perfusion pressure (CPP). CPP, ICP, and mean arterial pressure (MAP) are related by the following formula: CPP = MAP − ICP. Resuscitation should optimize CPP by controlling ICP and maintaining MAP. When ICP exceeds venous outflow pressure (as a result of brain swelling), it acts as a Starling resistor and determines the pressure gradient for cerebral blood flow. Normal CPP values and the ideal range of ICP in children with severe brain injury are not clear.[17] Favorable outcomes in children are possible by maintaining the ICP less than 20 mm Hg in all ages and a CPP greater than 45 mm Hg in children younger than 8 years of age and 70 to 80 mm Hg in older childen.[18]

Efforts to reduce secondary brain injury focus upon maintaining a therapeutic ICP and CPP and the normalization of MAP. The most expeditious method is intubation and controlled hyperventilation—initially, by reducing Pco_2 to a range of 30 to 35 mm Hg, while maintaining Po_2 greater than 100 mm Hg, and pH to 7.40 ± 0.05. Hypocarbia and alkalosis promote cerebral vasoconstriction, limiting cerebral blood volume and lowering ICP. The effect is rapid but can be limited in duration by re-equilibration of cerebrospinal fluid (CSF) pH balance. The maximal duration of the effect is unknown but may range from several hours to several days. Current therapy maintains the Pco_2 in the range of 35 ± 5 mm Hg. This regimen avoids excessive hyperventilation, which has been found to be deleterious in severe brain injury by converting borderline regions of cerebral ischemia into infarction.[17] A ventriculostomy is usually placed to allow CSF to drain to further optimize CPP. Repeat computed tomography (CT) of the head is indicated 24 to 48 hours after injury to assess the extent of brain edema, to identify new infarcts, or to demonstrate the development of a new hematoma or large contusion, which may require evacuation. The ventilation and fluid hydration status are reassessed and optimized.

If measures fail to control ICP, then osmotherapy with 20% mannitol rapid bolus intravenous infusion is administered: 0.25 gm/kg to 0.5 gm/kg/dose every 4 to 6 hours. Mannitol is withheld if the serum sodium concentration is greater than 145 meq/L, serum osmolarity is greater than 310 mOsm, urine output is less than 0.5 mL/kg/hour, or blood pressure is low. Mannitol exerts a therapeutic effect by creating a hyperosmolar environment in the cerebral microcirculation; this improves brain oxygen delivery by exerting a diuresis of free water from the cerebral interstitium, which improves red blood cell rheology.[17]

The induction of mild to moderate hypertension may reverse abnormal ICP and raise CPP by improving brainstem microvascular perfusion.[19] Therapy is begun with dopamine 5 to 20 μg/kg/min intravenous infusion with avoidance of cerebral edema.

Hyperthermia and seizures are common after traumatic brain injury and adversely affect efforts to normalize ICP and CPP. Both fever and seizures promote further secondary brain injury by increasing metabolic demand of the compromised brain. Therefore core temperature in children is maintained in the normal range (35° to 36° C) with acetaminophen, 10 mg/kg/dose every 4 to 6 hours. Cooling blankets may be necessary for recalcitrant fever. A single seizure in a child after the injury and resultant normal neurologic assessment does not require treatment. Seizures that occur within 1 week after injury is treated with phenobarbital in children less than 1 year of age, and with dilantin in children greater than 1 year of age. Either drug is administered by one-time intravenous therapy of 10 to 20 mg/kg, followed by daily dosage of 5 mg/kg/day. Treatment is discontinued after 7 days. Children who develop a late seizure require long-term anticonvulsant medication. Whether the comatose child who has not demonstrated seizure activity requires anticonvulsant prophylaxis during the resuscitation process is controversial.[20]

COAGULOPATHY

Dysfunctional coagulation related to injury occurs in several circumstances: extreme hypothermia, massive transfusion, and severe brain injury. Hypothermia causes excessive bleeding by reducing the efficiency of enzymatic processes that cause coagulation. Massive transfusion, defined as the acute administration of blood products equal to or greater than one blood volume (65 to 80 mL/kg) causes coagulopathy by hypothermia. Another mechanism results from storage of blood in anticoagulants containing ethylenediaminetetraacetic acid or citrate (citrate-phosphate-dextrose), both of which chelate calcium and inhibit the calcium-dependent steps of the coagulation cascade. Acute hypocalcemia is another consequence of massive transfusion.

The most common mechanism by which massive transfusion causes coagulopathy, is dilutional thrombocytopenia. Coagulopathy resulting from dilution of clotting factors is much less common because of a much greater functional reserve of these components. As continued hemorrhage depletes circulating platelets and blood is replaced with RBCs, a progressive reduction in the platelet count ensues. With acute injury, a decrease of platelet count to 50,000 can produce surgical bleeding. Such drastic reductions in platelet levels requires a massive transfusion of at least two blood volumes. Platelet levels less than 100,000 signify impending coagulopathy, and levels of 50,000 or less require platelet transfusion. Administration of ABO-matched platelets at an initial dose of 0.1 U/kg raises the platelet level by about 40,000.

Severe head injury is also associated with a coagulopathy unrelated to platelet dilution. Presumably, large concentrations of procoagulant tissue thromboplastin are released from cerebral laceration. These thromboplastins initiate disseminated intravascular coagulation, resulting in a consumptive coagulopathy in which clotting factors and fibrinogen are depleted as well as platelets. Coagulopathy after head injury is a grim prognostic sign. Treatment requires administration of matched fresh frozen plasma at a dose of 15 to 30 mL/kg. Cryoprecipitate contains large amounts of fibrinogen, factor VIII, factor X111, and von Willebrand factor and can be given at a dose of 0.1 U/kg in addition to fresh frozen plasma. Administration of fresh frozen plasma, cryoprecipitate, or both may also be required in the setting of preexisting coagulopathies, such as hemophilia, von Willebrand disease, and advanced liver disease.[9]

It is clear that the coagulopathy associated with traumatic injury is a result of multiple independent but interacting mechanisms. Early coagulopathy is driven by shock and requires thrombin generation from tissue injury as an initiator. Following initiation and further activation of anticoagulant and fibrinolytic pathways, the acute coagulopathy of trauma-shock is propagated by events associated with the care of the traumatically injured child, specifically acidemia, hypothermia, and dilution.[21]

Damage Control

The goal of "damage control" is to reverse the sequelae of shock. Severely traumatized children who require operative intervention are at risk for hypothermia, acidosis, and coagulopathy. In these circumstances, the child may require emergent completion of the surgical procedure using a process of damage control surgery. The fundamentals of damage control in children are the following:

1. Exposure and control of vascular or solid organ hemorrhage
2. Control of contamination from hollow-viscus injury
3. Packing of the abdomen
4. Temporary abdominal closure
5. Transport to the pediatric intensive care unit (PICU)

All measures available for core rewarming should be used in these children. Efficient and rapid abdominal closure is critical. Since the early descriptions of the wound vacuum-assisted closure (VAC) technique, commercially produced products have been developed for managing these open abdominal wounds by temporary abdominal closure.[22] The VAC allows for a rapid abdominal closure as well as minimizing the risk of abdominal compartment syndrome post-operatively in the PICU during the physiologic and biochemical restoration phase. The VAC has also been shown to be of benefit in children with head injury by optimizing cerebral blood flow.

During damage control, blood products should be used in a 1:1:1 ratio of RBC to plasma to platelets. The decision to return to the operating room for formal closure occurs when all aspects of physiology have been restored.[23]

Pain Management

The primary goal of acute pain management is to reduce the stress of the injured child and to improve outcome. Acute pain serves as a noxious stimulus that leads to the activation of the physiologic stress response. The result is a disruption in the neuroendocrine response, which has a profound and deleterious effect upon metabolism, thermoregulation, wound healing, and immunity.

The following are critical elements in the pain management of injured children:
- An experienced interdisciplinary team, lead by a clinician devoted to pain management
- Ensuring the least possible pain
- Recognizing that effective pain management requires constant adjustment
- Recognizing that anxiety needs to be considered and treated, because it may alter the effectiveness of pain treatment
- The ability and knowledge to effectively use all pain therapy in real-time coordination with the rest of the child's supportive care and treatment plans

A team-oriented, protocol-based algorithm that attempts to control pain in this environment will further enhance the overall success of the emergency management of these children.[24]

Conclusion

A systematic approach to the injured child saves lives. Nevertheless, prevention of injury is essential to children.

The unintentional childhood injury death rate has declined nearly 48% during the past 25 years.[4] Among the most notable advances in childhood injury prevention are the declines in death rates for unintentional firearm (94%) and bicycle-related injury (78%). The death rate from fire and burn injury declined 53%, while that of pedestrian injury dropped 64%. Unfortunately, the motor vehicle occupant death rate, particularly among children ages 5 to 9 years, has been slow to decline, and the death rate from airway obstruction injury among infants remains unchanged.

Many factors have contributed to the overall dramatic decline in the unintentional childhood injury death rate. It is clear that the highest priority should be on injury prevention with particular emphasis placed on minimizing injury risk to minorities, younger children, and motor vehicle occupants. Once injury occurs, proper resuscitation can save lives.

The complete reference list is available online at www. expertconsult.com.

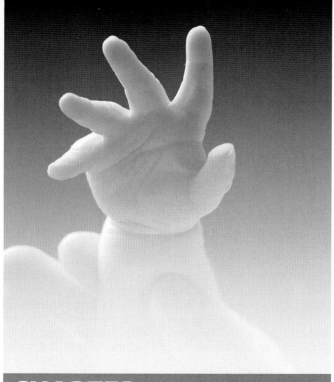

CHAPTER 19

Thoracic Injuries

David E. Wesson and Charles S. Cox, Jr.

Epidemiology and Prevention

Injuries to the chest wall, diaphragm, lungs, and mediastinal structures occur in about 25% of children treated in level I pediatric trauma centers, usually after high-energy blunt or penetrating trauma. Change in velocity, ΔV, is a strong predictor of significant injury for children in motor vehicle crashes.[1] Low-energy mechanisms, such as simple falls from playground equipment, seldom cause chest injury. Thoracic injuries range in severity from minor to rapidly fatal, but virtually all chest injuries can be treated successfully if they are promptly diagnosed and appropriately treated. Although chest injuries are less common than injuries to the abdomen, soft tissues, and extraaxial skeleton, they are more lethal. Because of the impact required, patients who have sustained such injuries have a significant risk of mortality. In fact, thoracic injuries account for a high proportion of all trauma deaths not caused by central nervous system (CNS) injury.

As with most types of pediatric trauma, the male-to-female ratio is between 2:1 and 3:1. Thoracic injuries can be classified by anatomic site (e.g., rib fracture, pulmonary contusion, bronchial laceration), mechanism (blunt or penetrating), or threat to life (immediate or potential). Although most serious blunt injuries to the chest are motor vehicle–related in all age groups, the proportion of children injured as pedestrians is much higher than in adults. The causes of penetrating thoracic injuries in teenagers mimic those in adults—mostly knife and gunshot wounds. BBs or pellets fired from air guns, although often considered to be relatively innocuous, may also be life threatening.[2] The causes of penetrating injuries in preadolescent children include a number of other unusual mechanisms, such as impalement by shards of broken glass or metal rods.[3]

The most common thoracic injuries seen clinically are listed in Table 19-1. Autopsy series, which include prehospital and emergency department deaths, reveal a higher proportion of rapidly fatal, major vascular and cardiac injuries.[4] In adults, rib fractures are by far the most common type of blunt trauma to the chest. In children, pulmonary contusions are the most frequent.[5,6] Tracheobronchial lacerations are more common in children than in adults, whereas the opposite is true for traumatic rupture of the aorta.[7]

The most common thoracic injuries are lung contusion, pneumothorax, hemothorax, and fractures to the ribs, sternum, or scapula. Injuries to the heart, aorta, trachea, bronchi, and diaphragm are much less common but potentially more dangerous. The most common *immediately* life-threatening injuries to the chest are airway obstruction, tension pneumothorax, massive hemothorax, and cardiac tamponade. Open pneumothorax and massive flail chest are rare. The most common *potentially* life-threatening injuries of the chest are myocardial contusion, aortic disruption, ruptured diaphragm, and tracheobronchial disruption. Esophageal rupture is rare.

The relative incidence of blunt and penetrating thoracic trauma varies widely, depending on the amount of violence in the community. Peterson and colleagues[3] reported a large series of adults and children with thoracic trauma. Blunt injuries comprised 81% of thoracic injuries in children 12 years of age or younger; penetrating injuries accounted for 58% of chest injuries in adolescents. In Nakayama's series, 97% of thoracic injuries in children up to 17 years of age were blunt.[6] Meller[8] reported a series in which nearly all wounded teenagers had penetrating injuries. The National Pediatric Trauma Registry reflects the combined experience of many pediatric trauma centers across North America. From 1985 to 1991, more than 25,000 cases were reported to the National Pediatric Trauma Registry, including 1553 cases with thoracic injury.[5] Eighty-six percent of injuries were blunt (mostly motor vehicle related). The remaining 14% were penetrating (mostly stab or gunshot wounds).

The overall mortality rates for blunt and penetrating cases were almost identical at 15% and 14%, respectively.[5] Mortality increases with the number of associated injuries. Most of the deaths in the group that had blunt trauma were caused by associated head injuries, whereas most of the deaths in the group with penetrating injuries resulted from the chest injuries themselves. Overall, thoracic injuries were second only to CNS injuries as the cause of death in the National Pediatric Trauma Registry. Most deaths from chest injuries occur at the scene of the accident or in transit to the hospital and result from fatal injuries to vital organs. Patients with thoracic injuries who reach the hospital alive are potentially salvageable.

Although the ratio of blunt-to-penetrating injuries varies in adults and children, the spectrum of chest injuries and the basic principles of diagnosis and treatment are the same for all ages. The most common injuries—pulmonary contusion, rib fracture, pneumothorax, and hemothorax—can be treated with simple measures, such as tube thoracostomy, oxygen, and analgesia. Approximately 20% of patients with these injuries also require endotracheal intubation and

TABLE 19-1

Epidemiology of Pediatric Chest Injuries

	Hospital for Sick Children	Memorial Hermann Children's Hospital
Ribs/sternum	26%	24%
Pneumothorax/ hemothorax	26%	30%
Heart	1%	1%
Great vessel	1%	1%
Lung	44%	43%
Bronchus/esophagus/ diaphragm	2%	2%

Percentage of the total patients with chest injuries with each type of injury from the trauma registries of two leading pediatric trauma centers: the Hospital for Sick Children, Toronto, Ontario and Memorial Hermann Children's Hospital, Houston, Tex.[101,102]

mechanical ventilation, often for the management of associated head injuries.

Several thoracic injuries virtually always require operation: major airway lacerations, aortic injuries, structural cardiac and pericardial injuries, and esophageal perforations. One of the greatest challenges in thoracic trauma is to recognize the rare cases that need an operation as early as possible during the course of treatment. In Nakayama's series, 2 of 3 patients with penetrating injuries and only 3 of 83 patients with blunt injuries had chest operations.[6] In Peterson's report, 15% of the children with blunt injuries required thoracotomy (about the same as in adult series). Forty percent of those with penetrating injuries required surgery (far higher than in adult series).[3]

Although clinicians are naturally concerned with the needs of individual patients, no consideration of chest injuries in children would be complete without mentioning prevention. Motor vehicle accidents and gunshot wounds cause the vast majority of severe pediatric thoracic injuries. These injuries are all preventable. Increasing the use of seat belts and child restraints would substantially reduce the risk for injury to motor vehicle occupants. Reducing the illegal use of firearms would also have major benefits, especially for teenagers. Chest protectors may be effective in reducing the incidence of chest injuries, including *commotio cordis* in young athletes.[9,10] In combination, these measures would substantially reduce the incidence and severity of pediatric thoracic trauma and the deaths and disabilities which result from it.

Clinical Presentation

The pathophysiology of thoracic trauma and the anatomy and physiology on which management strategies are based differ significantly between children and adults. The most important anatomic factors that distinguish children are the relatively narrow airway, which is prone to obstruction, the anterior and superior position of the glottis, which makes nasotracheal intubation difficult and therefore inappropriate in an emergency, and the short trachea, which increases the risk of endobronchial intubation. The increased oxygen consumption and low functional residual capacity of children predispose them to hypoxia. Because young children rely largely on

their diaphragm to breathe, any increase in intra-abdominal pressure compounds the problem by restricting diaphragmatic excursion.

Children with significant thoracic injuries may present with minimal signs and symptoms. A large adult series from the Maryland Institute of Emergency Medical Services Systems (MIEMSS) found that two thirds of patients with thoracic injuries arrived with stable vital signs.[11] This same finding was reported in children.[8] About 25% of the patients with significant intrathoracic injuries in the MIEMSS series did not have a rib fracture. These "occult" injuries included pneumothorax, hemothorax, myocardial contusion, cardiac rupture, tracheobronchial injury, pulmonary laceration, ruptured diaphragm, and ruptured aorta.

The ribs of a child are more pliable than those of an adult. Consequently, rib fractures are much less common in children. However, it is important to note that because of the elasticity of the chest wall in childhood, severe thoracic injuries may occur without injury to the chest wall or external signs of injury. In Nakayama's series, less than half of the children with significant thoracic injuries had rib fractures.[6] The compressibility of the chest wall may also explain why traumatic asphyxia is almost unique to children and why major airway trauma is so much more common in children than in adults.

The mediastinal structures are more mobile in children than in adults. Therefore tension pneumothorax is more likely to shift the mediastinum, compromising ventilation of the contralateral lung and impairing return of venous blood to the heart.

Diagnosis and Initial Resuscitation

Diagnosis and initial treatment of patients with traumatic chest injury must proceed simultaneously. Although the manifestations of thoracic injury may be immediate or delayed by hours or days, the initial goal should be to rule out injuries that are immediately life threatening, such as airway obstruction, tension pneumothorax, massive hemothorax, and cardiac tamponade.

All injury victims should be managed according to the principles of the Advanced Trauma Life Support (ATLS) Program of the American College of Surgeons.[12] The overall plan is as follows:
1. Primary survey
2. Resuscitation of vital functions
3. Detailed secondary survey
4. Definitive care

All children with thoracic trauma must have supplemental oxygen, two large-bore intravenous lines, and a nasogastric (NG) tube to prevent gastric distention. A NG tube may also reveal an abnormal position of the esophagus or stomach, thereby indicating aortic injury or a ruptured diaphragm. Children with thoracic trauma should be observed closely. Vital signs and oxygen saturation in arterial blood (Sao_2) should be continuously monitored. If the child is intubated, end-tidal carbon dioxide should be monitored continuously or checked frequently. Blood should be available for transfusion. The equipment and skilled personnel needed to address breathing problems and to manage the airway with suction, oral airways, endotracheal tubes, laryngoscopes, and a bag-valve-mask apparatus must always be on hand, especially during transport and diagnostic procedures.

Life-threatening injuries should be identified *and* treated during the initial resuscitation phase of the ATLS protocol. The first priority is to clear and secure the airway. Endotracheal intubation may be required. After intubation, the position of the endotracheal tube must be checked by observing chest excursion, listening for bilateral air entry, monitoring end-tidal carbon dioxide, and obtaining a chest radiograph. A colorimetric carbon dioxide detector may be used to verify endotracheal tube position, especially in the prehospital setting.[13]

The second priority is to ensure adequate ventilation. Tension pneumothorax, if present, should be treated before a radiograph is obtained. Occasionally, open pneumothorax or massive flail chest requires intubation and assisted ventilation during the initial resuscitation. Persistent shock despite adequate fluid administration usually indicates ongoing (most likely abdominal) blood loss. However, if no obvious cause of hypovolemia can be found, the possibility of acute pericardial tamponade should be considered; this disorder can be relieved, at least temporarily, by pericardiocentesis.

The indications for urgent thoracotomy may become obvious at any stage (Table 19-2). The most common indications are massive bleeding, massive air leak, and cardiac tamponade. Emergency room (ER) or resuscitative thoracotomy is a controversial technique that does not seem to have clear indications or contraindications. In the report from MIEMSS,[11] none of 39 adult patients who presented without vital signs in the ER survived after emergency thoracotomy. However, emergency thoracotomy may be lifesaving in children, especially those with penetrating cardiac injuries. Powell and colleagues reported a 26% survival rate in a series of children and adolescents who had ER thoracotomy.[14] These authors recommended thoracotomy in the ER for post-traumatic arrest, or near arrest, in the following three situations:

1. All cases of penetrating thoracic trauma
2. Blunt trauma with acute deterioration but signs of life in the ER
3. Blunt trauma with signs of life at the scene when the scene is in proximity to the hospital

The incision for emergency thoracotomy should be on the left anterolateral chest wall in the fifth interspace. A rib spreader should be used. If evidence of pericardial tamponade exists, the pericardium should be opened longitudinally,

anterior to the phrenic nerve. Cardiac wounds should be controlled by direct pressure and simple suture. If cardiac tamponade is not present, the descending aorta should be cross-clamped. If the patient has massive lung injury, the hilum should be clamped or twisted off (see Treatment later). Patients who respond to these measures should then have definitive repair performed in the operating room.

In most cases of thoracic trauma, the child is physiologically stable. After initial resuscitation, the next step is the detailed secondary survey. To avoid missing a significant injury, a complete and careful assessment is essential. In nearly all cases, a history that suggests significant impact to the chest can be elicited. Therefore it is crucial to obtain as much information as possible regarding the details of the accident. Children involved in motor vehicle accidents, occupants and pedestrians alike, demand especially careful assessment. A history of difficulty breathing also indicates significant thoracic injury.

A systematic physical examination of the chest by inspection, percussion, palpation, and auscultation is the next step of the secondary survey. Tachypnea and tenderness and abrasions of the chest wall are predictive of intrathoracic injury.[15,16] One should look for cyanosis, dyspnea, noisy breathing, tracheal deviation, hoarseness or stridor, subcutaneous emphysema, open or sucking chest wounds, reduced or absent breath sounds, venous engorgement, pulsus paradoxus, and hypotension. Dyspnea and cyanosis suggest inadequate oxygenation. Noisy breathing may result from an injury to the airway or the presence of foreign material, such as blood, mucus, or vomitus. Tracheal deviation implies tension pneumothorax or massive hemothorax. Hoarseness, stridor, or other difficulty with phonation suggests direct laryngeal or tracheal injury. Surgical emphysema suggests a tracheal or bronchial laceration or, on rare occasions, an esophageal perforation. Jugular venous engorgement, hypotension, and pulsus paradoxus greater than 10 mm Hg imply cardiac tamponade. The patient should also be checked for signs of acute aortic coarctation, which can be caused by injury to the thoracic aorta. The most sensitive sign of a significant cardiac injury is hypotension or a large fluid requirement that is not explained by bleeding. A cardiac injury may also cause a loud systolic murmur. Acute congestive heart failure may result from valvular injury or a traumatic ventricular septal defect.

Holmes and colleagues developed a set of clinical predictors for the presence of chest injuries in a group of children less than 16 years old with blunt torso trauma.[17] The strongest predictors were hypotension, increased respiratory rate, abnormal physical examination of the thorax, associated femur fracture, and Glasgow Coma Scale (GCS) less than 15. Ninety-eight percent of proven cases had at least one of these predictors. Inspection and palpation were the most sensitive, but abnormalities detected on auscultation had the highest positive predictive value. This confirms the importance of clinical assessment in children with blunt trauma. The most common injuries were lung contusion, pneumothorax, and rib fracture, in that order.

In recent years, bedside surgeon–performed ultrasonography (US) has proven helpful in assessing abdominal trauma, and US is now a routine part of the clinical assessment of all major trauma cases.[18] US also has a role in chest trauma. It is sufficiently accurate to be clinically useful in diagnosing

TABLE 19-2
Indications for Emergency Thoracotomy
1. Penetrating wound of the heart or great vessels
2. Massive or continuous intrathoracic bleeding
3. Open pneumothorax with major chest wall defect
4. Aortogram indicating injury to aorta or major branch
5. Massive or continuing air leak, indicating injury to a major airway
6. Cardiac tamponade
7. Esophageal perforation
8. Diaphragmatic rupture
9. Impalpable pulse with cardiac massage

pneumothoraces, hemothoraces, and pericardial effusions.[18–20] Recent reports document that surgeon-performed ultrasonography in the emergency department (ED) is an accurate screening test for the presence of a pneumothorax.[19,21]

Because it lacks sensitivity and specificity, clinical assessment is routinely supplemented by diagnostic imaging, usually the key step in identifying those children who need an operation.[22] Plain chest radiographs are routine, although Bokhari suggests that they are not necessary in blunt trauma cases with a completely normal chest physical examination.[15,23] A standard posteroanterior and lateral examination is best, but a supine anteroposterior film will suffice. The chest radiograph should be repeated on arrival at the trauma center even if the patient has been transferred from another hospital. The important signs of chest injury on plain chest radiographs include subcutaneous emphysema, fractures to the rib or other bony structures, hemothorax, pneumothorax, contusion or other parenchymal lesion (e.g., aspiration pneumonia), mediastinal shift or widening, and diaphragmatic rupture.

Computed tomography (CT) gives greater detail than plain radiographs and is more sensitive in the diagnosis of pneumothorax, rib fracture, and pulmonary contusion. It may also help in the diagnosis of ruptured diaphragm. Because chest films are not 100% sensitive, some groups have recommended that CT be used to screen all patients suspected of having a chest injury. However, this is not proven, and plain chest radiographs are still the standard screening tool for chest trauma.[24] The most common injuries identified by CT are pulmonary contusions and lacerations.[25] Many pneumothoraces revealed by CT are either not evident or underestimated on plain films. CT gives greater detail than plain radiographs in pulmonary contusions.[25] Manson concluded that plain radiographs, especially those obtained in the trauma resuscitation room, are only "a gross screening examination" for thoracic injury and recommended dynamically enhanced CT in all cases of significant thoracic trauma diagnosed clinically or by plain radiograph. In such cases, CT will give better definition of the injuries already recognized and may well reveal occult injuries not visible on plain radiographs. Exadaktylos and colleagues support this view.[26] In their experience, CT revealed potentially life-threatening aortic injuries, even when the plain chest radiographs were normal. They recommended routine chest CT in all patients with major chest trauma. Renton and colleagues studied the question of whether CT should replace routine chest radiograph as the initial diagnostic imaging test of choice.[27] They concluded that it should not, mainly because the increased cost was not justified by the relatively few changes in management that resulted from the use of CT scans. They estimated that 200 CTs would have to be done for each clinically significant change in management. In summary, CT should not be used liberally in cases of suspected chest injury.

Occasionally, other diagnostic tests, including ultrasonography, transthoracic or transesophageal echocardiography, bronchoscopy, radionuclide bone scan, angiography, and even video-assisted thoracic surgery are also helpful. Ultrasonography is more sensitive than supine anteroposterior (AP) chest radiographs and equally sensitive to CT in the diagnosis of traumatic pneumothorax.[28] Recent case reports document the use of video-assisted thoracic surgery to diagnose pericardial rupture and herniation of the heart.[29] In cases of suspected child abuse, a radionuclide bone scan helps to detect recent and long-standing rib fractures. Although impractical in most emergencies, MR is very helpful in defining injuries to the thoracic spine, especially when spinal cord involvement is suspected. It may also help identify diaphragmatic injuries in equivocal cases.[30]

For many years angiography has been the gold standard for the diagnosis of injuries to the aorta and its main branches. However, there is a clear trend to use helical CT as the initial test for suspected aortic injury, reserving aortography for proven cases to guide the repair, or, in some reports, eliminating aortography entirely.

Transthoracic echocardiography is a very useful way to diagnose all types of structural heart injury and ventricular dysfunction caused by contusion. Transthoracic echocardiography may reveal intracardiac injuries or pericardial tamponade. Transesophageal echocardiography is a useful screening test for traumatic rupture of the aorta. It can identify the cause of mediastinal hematomas seen on plain radiographs or CT scan.[31]

Pericardiocentesis may be used for diagnosis when cardiac tamponade is suspected and echocardiography is unavailable. All patients with thoracic trauma should have continuous echocardiographic monitoring during assessment in the ER. A full 12-lead echocardiogram should be obtained in cases of suspected cardiac contusion to rule out an arrhythmia. Bronchoscopy should be done in the operating room under general anesthesia in cases of suspected major airway trauma.

Treatment

The treatment of thoracic injuries varies from supportive only (oxygen, analgesia), to simple interventions (endotracheal intubation, ventilation, tube thoracostomy) to operation (minimally invasive, open thoracotomy), depending on the specific structures injured and the severity of the injuries. However, most patients do not require an operation and can be managed with supportive measures, with or without tube thoracostomy.[32]

The ideal location for the incision when an operation is indicated varies depending on the preoperative diagnosis. An anterolateral incision in the fifth interspace, which can be extended across the midline, is best in an emergency. A trapdoor incision, which may be best, has been described for vascular injuries in the upper mediastinum. For esophageal injuries, a right posterolateral thoracotomy gives adequate exposure, except for the most distal thoracic esophagus, which is best viewed from the left. Median sternotomy is best for cardiac injuries. Heart–lung bypass is only rarely needed emergently for such injuries as coronary artery laceration and laceration of the thoracic aorta. Intracardiac injuries to the atrioventricular valves or the atrial or ventricular septae do require bypass, but they can be repaired semielectively. Injuries to the root of the neck or shoulder can be approached through a supraclavicular extension of a median sternotomy.

The concept of damage control, which is now well established for intra-abdominal trauma, can also be applied in selected cases of intrathoracic injury. Nonanatomic resection of the lung to control bleeding and massive air leak, pulmonary tractotomy with a gastrointestinal anastomosis (GIA) stapler for through and through wounds of the lung, en masse pneumonectomy, and hilar twist[33] all may be lifesaving. The latter has been reported in cases of uncontrollable bleeding or air leak from the lung. The inferior pulmonary ligament is divided, and the lower lobe is twisted anteriorly over the upper lobe. This controls the situation so that the patient can be taken back to the intensive care unit (ICU) for stabilization and returned to the operating room (OR) later for definitive control, usually by pneumonectomy. The EndoGIA stapler (Covidien, Mansfield, MA) with vascular staples is very useful for rapid control of major pulmonary vessels in damage control.

BLUNT INJURIES

Chest Wall

Soft Tissue Although seldom clinically important, injuries to the soft tissue of the chest wall suggest the possibility of more serious associated intrathoracic injuries. Soft tissue injuries to the chest wall should be managed according to accepted principles of wound care.

Rib Fractures In childhood, the ribs are strong and pliable. Therefore rib fractures are less common than in adults and flail chest is quite rare. Because rib fractures require a great deal of force, they are an indication of severe injury. Fractures of the first rib suggest the possibility of a major vascular injury, especially to the subclavian artery.[34] First rib fractures may also be complicated by Horner syndrome and thoracic outlet syndrome.

The goal of treatment is to prevent atelectasis and pneumonia while optimizing patient comfort. The treatment of rib fractures includes rest and analgesia. Oral or intravenous narcotics are usually sufficient for pain control. Intercostal nerve blocks may also be helpful. Children rarely experience pulmonary atelectasis from splinting of the chest wall. Rib fractures usually heal spontaneously within 6 weeks. The overall mortality rate for children with rib fractures in the National Pediatric Trauma Registry was 10%.[5]

Rib fractures in infants and toddlers less than 3 years old are often caused by child abuse.[35,36] The likelihood of non-accidental injury in children with one or more rib fractures decreases with increasing age.[36] In cases of child abuse, the typical site of fracture is the neck of the rib near the costotransverse process articulation. Kleinman and colleagues[37] described fractures of the head of the rib in abused infants, which are usually undetectable on radiographs because the head is cartilaginous. Cystic lesions of the ribs that are located posteriorly are another indication of child abuse,[38] as are multiple rib fractures at varying stages of healing.

Flail Chest Flail chest is relatively uncommon in children. It occurs when a segment of the chest wall is destabilized when several adjacent ribs are fractured. The injured chest wall moves paradoxically—*in* during inspiration and *out* during expiration. Ventilation is inefficient because of the paradoxical movement. Flail chest is usually associated with a lung contusion. Chest wall splinting and ineffective coughing often compound the primary injury. This leads to consolidation and collapse of the affected lung, which, in turn, result in a ventilation/perfusion (V/Q) mismatch and hypoxia.

Initial treatment of flail chest includes supplemental oxygen, pain relief (intercostal nerve blocks, oral or intravenous narcotics, or an epidural blockade given as a continuous infusion), and physiotherapy. Fluid therapy must be carefully monitored to avoid pulmonary edema, and intensive care monitoring is advisable. Children with isolated flail chest and no other significant injuries seldom require ventilation. If respiratory failure develops, endotracheal intubation and positive-pressure ventilation with positive end-expiratory pressure may be required for several days. Tracheotomy is rarely necessary. In the National Pediatric Trauma Registry, the overall mortality rate for patients with flail chest was 40%.[5]

Sternal Fractures Sternal fractures are less common in young children than in adults, because the sternum is cartilaginous.

Lung and Airway

Pneumothorax Pneumothorax can result from an injury to the chest wall, the lung parenchyma, the tracheobronchial tree, or the esophagus. High energy is required to produce a pneumothorax; so, it must be considered a marker for other occult injuries.

Simple Pneumothorax Simple pneumothorax may cause chest pain, respiratory distress, tachypnea, decreased air entry on the affected side, and oxygen desaturation. Careful examination may reveal an abrasion of the chest wall, crepitus, or tracheal shift. However, many patients show no clinical signs or symptoms. This underscores the importance of routine chest radiographs for all trauma cases. The radiographic signs include unilateral or asymmetric lucency, a sharp outline of the mediastinum, mediastinal shift, and a visible visceral pleural border away from the chest wall. The diagnosis of simple pneumothorax should be confirmed by chest radiography before treatment.

Simple pneumothoraces should be treated by intercostal chest tube drainage (Fig. 19-1). The best location for chest tube insertion is the fourth or fifth intercostal space (nipple level) in the anterior axillary line. The recommended chest tube sizes are as follows: newborns, 12 to 16 Fr; infants, 16 to 18 Fr; school-age children, 18 to 24 Fr; and adolescents, 28 to 32 Fr. Safe chest tube insertion requires training and experience to minimize complications.[39,40] The chest tube should be connected to an underwater seal on gentle suction and removed when the air leak stops. For most cases, this is the only treatment necessary. A continued or massive air leak suggests injury to the tracheobronchial tree.

A small, asymptomatic pneumothorax may be observed in carefully selected cases. If the patient is to be transferred to another hospital or intubated and ventilated for any reason, or if the pneumothorax exceeds 15%, it should be drained. When in doubt, a chest tube should be inserted.

Open Pneumothorax Open pneumothorax is rare in children. In cases of open pneumothorax, the intrapleural pressure is equal to that of the atmosphere. As a result, the lung collapses and alveolar ventilation decreases. Sucking wounds should be recognized clinically. They may be treated by insertion of a Heimlich valve or applying an occlusive dressing to the wound, taping the dressing on three sides only so that it can act as a flutter valve, and inserting a chest tube in the usual location.

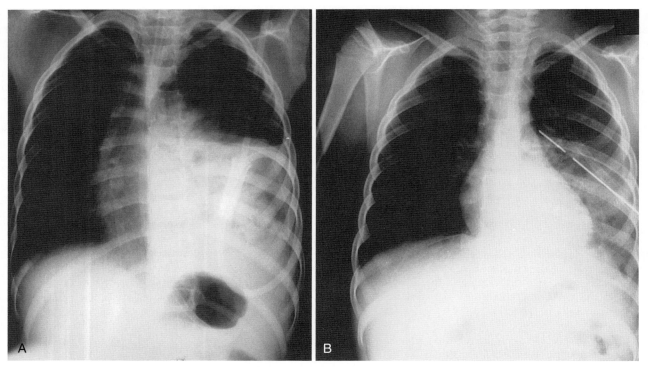

FIGURE 19-1   **A,** Left hemopneumothorax; note the nasogastric tube in situ. **B,** Same patient after insertion of intercostal drain; no other treatment was required. (From Wesson DE: Trauma of the chest in children. Chest Clin North Am 1993;3:423-441. Used with permission.)

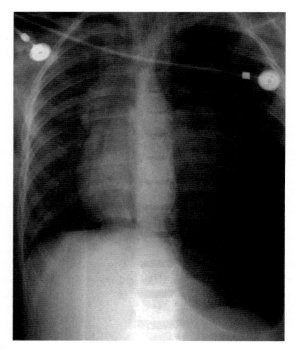

FIGURE 19-2   Tension pneumothorax. Pneumothorax resulting from blunt thoracic trauma in a 4-year-old boy run over by a school bus. He was unconscious when seen in the emergency department, and no breath sounds could be heard in the right chest. The trachea was shifted toward the left. The suspected pneumothorax on the right was treated initially with needle aspiration and then a chest tube inserted. (From Haller JA Jr, Shermeta DW: Acute thoracic injuries in children, Pediatr Ann 1976;5:71-79. Used with permission.)

Tension Pneumothorax   Tension pneumothorax may develop when a one-way valve effect occurs, allowing air to enter the pleural space but not to escape (Fig. 19-2). The underlying cause is usually a pulmonary laceration or an injury to the trachea or a large bronchus. The intrapleural air pressure exceeds that of the atmosphere, collapses the ipsilateral lung, pushes the mediastinum to the opposite side, flattens the diaphragm, impairs ventilation of the opposite lung, and reduces return of venous blood to the heart. The pulse and respiratory rate increase, and the patient becomes severely distressed. The trachea is usually deviated away from the involved side, and the neck veins may become engorged. The ipsilateral side of the chest is hyperresonant to percussion with diminished breath sounds. Frank cyanosis is a late sign. The most important differential diagnosis is pericardial tamponade. However, this disorder can be distinguished from tension pneumothorax, because the trachea is not displaced and the chest is normal to percussion. Tension pneumothorax should be considered when an injured patient, especially one on a mechanical ventilator, suddenly deteriorates for no apparent reason. Both acute gastric dilation and right mainstem intubation may result in diminished breath sounds on the left, and should not be confused with a tension pneumothorax.

The treatment for tension pneumothorax is immediate needle-catheter drainage (without waiting for chest radiographs) through either the second intercostal space in the midclavicular line or the fourth or fifth interspace in the axilla, followed by insertion of a chest tube.

Hemothorax   When enough blood is lost into the thorax to cause shock, the term massive hemothorax is used. Massive hemothorax is more common after penetrating than blunt trauma.

Hemothorax may result from a laceration of an intercostal or internal mammary artery, the lung, or a mediastinal blood vessel. Free bleeding into the pleural space from a major vessel, such as the aorta or one of the pulmonary hilar vessels, is usually rapidly fatal. Most bleeding from the lung stops spontaneously because of the low pressure in the pulmonary circulation. Bleeding from a systemic vessel, such as an intercostal artery, is more likely to cause massive hemothorax producing signs of hypovolemia, mediastinal shift, diminished breath sounds, and dullness to percussion on the affected side. Hemothorax is often associated with pneumothorax (see Fig. 19-1). The treatment is intercostal drainage to prevent a clotted hemothorax and to monitor the rate and total volume of blood loss. It is wise to establish two large-bore intravenous catheters, begin treatment for shock, if present, and obtain blood for transfusion before draining a massive hemothorax, because it may precipitate further bleeding. However, drainage and reexpansion of the lung usually stop the bleeding.

In most cases, intercostal drainage is the only treatment needed. However, thoracotomy may be indicated for the following reasons:

1. Initial drainage exceeds 20% to 25% of estimated blood volume
2. Continued bleeding exceeds 2 to 4 mL/kg/hour
3. Bleeding is increasing
4. The pleural space cannot be drained of blood and clots

Hoth and colleagues reported an increased likelihood of nontherapeutic exploration when thoracotomy is performed for increased chest tube output of blood in blunt trauma.[41] Auto-transfusion may be helpful during surgery for massive intrathoracic bleeding.

Lung

Hematoma and Contusion   Pulmonary contusion is the most common type of blunt injury to the chest in children. Direct force to the lung causes disruption of the parenchyma, bleeding, and edema in a nonanatomic distribution, often without obvious injury to the chest wall. Specific clinical signs or symptoms are seldom evident at presentation, although rib fractures and abrasions over the chest may be present.

Because of the lack of specific physical features, routine chest radiographs are the key to the diagnosis of hematoma and contusion. Pulmonary contusions are usually obvious on plain radiographs taken at admission (Fig. 19-3) and are even more striking on CT, which has shown that they usually lie posteriorly or posteromedially.[25] However, there is no need for a CT when a contusion is obvious on plain films. Pulmonary contusions may be progressive, especially when compounded by edema and atelectasis. Children with pulmonary contusions seldom require mechanical ventilation and almost never develop adult respiratory distress syndrome. The differential diagnosis includes aspiration pneumonia, which can result from aspiration at the scene, en route, during intubation, or with vomiting after admission. It affects the right lower lobe most frequently.

Patients with extensive lung hematomas or contusions should be monitored carefully with continuous SaO_2 measurements, preferably in an intensive care unit. The treatment for these disorders is supportive, with analgesia, physiotherapy, supplemental oxygen, and fluid restriction. Endotracheal intubation and mechanical ventilation are less likely to be needed for children than for adults. Deterioration after admission is unusual.[42] It is important to guard against over-hydration and aspiration of gastric content. The most common complication is infection of the lung. Most pulmonary hematomas and contusions clear within 10 days, unless the lung becomes infected.

Pulmonary contusions may be complicated by pneumothorax, hemothorax, or pleural effusion, all of which may require intercostal drainage. These secondary phenomena are much more common in the presence of concomitant fractures of the bones of the chest wall and may be delayed as long as 48 hours. Therefore serial chest radiographs should be obtained in cases of pulmonary contusion (see Fig. 19-3).

Occasionally, a post-traumatic pneumatocele forms when the injured lung cavitates during healing. Because pneumatoceles usually resolve spontaneously in a few months, treatment is seldom necessary.

Laceration

Pulmonary lacerations are most often seen after penetrating injuries and usually result in a pneumothorax or hemothorax. They may also be caused by rib fractures.

Air embolus is the most serious complication of pulmonary laceration. This diagnosis should be suspected in all children with thoracic trauma who suddenly deteriorate, especially while receiving positive-pressure ventilation in the absence of a pneumothorax. Air embolus may cause focal neurologic deficits. Frothy blood aspirated from an arterial cannula is a telltale sign. Emergency thoracotomy, clamping of the pulmonary hilum, and aspiration of the air from the heart or right ventricular outflow tract may be lifesaving.[43]

Trachea and Bronchi   Injuries to the major airways are uncommon in children. Nearly all are caused by blunt trauma.[5] The most common specific lesions are partial or complete transections of one of the main bronchi and tears of the membranous trachea. Airway injuries usually occur within 2 to 3 cm of the carina and may be rapidly fatal if not recognized and treated promptly.

Some patients with major airway injuries die from respiratory failure before reaching the hospital or shortly thereafter. Most present with dyspnea, which is often caused by tension pneumothorax. Other characteristics of patients with major airway injuries are voice disturbance, cyanosis, hemoptysis, massive subcutaneous and mediastinal emphysema, and failure of expansion of the lung or continuing large-volume air leak despite properly functioning chest tubes. Failure of the lung to expand or a continuous massive air leak after intercostal drainage strongly suggests a major airway injury (Fig. 19-4). Although not common, "dropped lung," in which the lung actually falls to the lower half of the pleural cavity below the level of the injured bronchus, is virtually diagnostic of a major airway injury. Finally, some patients present late with chronic collapse and infection of the involved lung from bronchial obstruction.

Initial management in the trauma room depends on the clinical situation. The initial treatment of airway injuries is to control the airway and breathing according to the ATLS protocol. This may require endotracheal intubation and intercostal drainage. If the patient has a good airway and is well oxygenated, it is prudent not to manipulate the airway by attempting intubation before taking the patient to the OR. Flexible bronchoscopy may facilitate endotracheal intubation

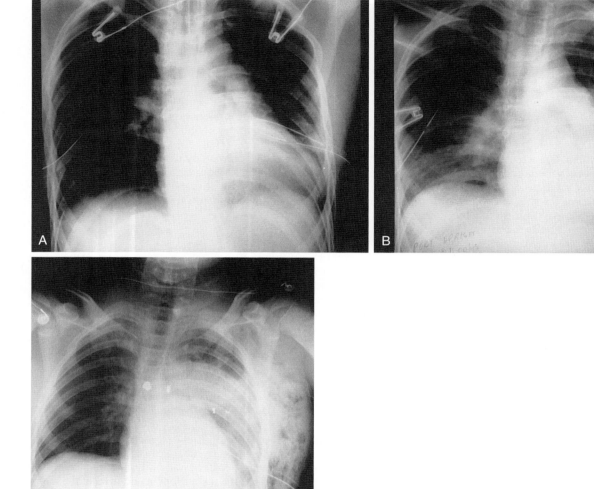

FIGURE 19-3   Pulmonary contusion. **A,** Crush injury with pulmonary contusion; note multiple rib fractures. **B,** Same patient 2 days later; note progression of lesion. **C,** Gunshot wound with pulmonary contusion and surgical emphysema. (From Wesson DE: Trauma of the chest in children. Chest Clin North Am 1993;3:423-441. Used with permission.)

beyond the site of the injury or selective intubation of the uninjured bronchus. High-frequency ventilation may be more effective than conventional methods in the presence of a massive air leak and may facilitate stabilizing the patient for surgical repair.[44]

Helical CT may be a good initial test in stable patients with suspected major airway injuries, but bronchoscopy is more reliable. Bronchoscopy is indicated whenever the lung fails to expand or a massive air leak continues after intercostal drainage. It should be done in the operating room under general anesthesia; a rigid, ventilating bronchoscope should be used. If possible, the patient should be allowed to breathe spontaneously during induction of anesthesia and passage of the bronchoscope. Staff and equipment for thoracotomy must be at hand. In unstable patients or those with possible or confirmed cervical spine injuries, flexible bronchoscopy with the patient awake or through an endotracheal tube may also reveal the lesion. At bronchoscopy, a defect in the wall of the airway may be visible. Other bronchoscopic signs of injury include mucosal disruption or exposed cartilage.

Spontaneous healing is the rule for small lacerations in the membranous trachea and some partial bronchial tears involving up to one third of the circumference.[45] These may be treated nonoperatively. For larger lacerations of the trachea or bronchi, primary surgical repair through a posterolateral thoracotomy is the best way to ensure good long-term results. Distal injuries to a lobar or segmental bronchus may be treated by lung resection rather than direct repair. The right side of the chest allows the best exposure of the trachea, carina, and right main bronchus; the left side gives better exposure for injuries to the distal left main bronchus. In the presence of a massive air leak, it may be necessary to clamp the hilum before attempting to repair the airway. Advancing the endotracheal tube or passing a sterile tube across the surgical field into the distal airway may also be helpful during the repair. Simple, interrupted sutures after debridement of the margins work best. Although lobectomy or pulmonary segmentectomy may be necessary, pulmonary resection is done only as a last resort in unstable patients or when the lung is extensively damaged. The late functional results of pulmonary resection or bronchial repair are usually excellent.[46]

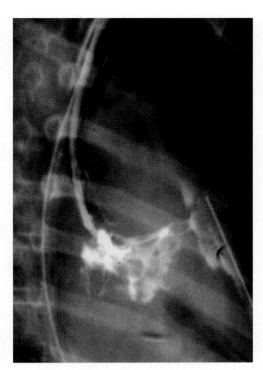

FIGURE 19-4   This patient had a sustained air leak associated with blunt thoracic injury despite adequate chest tube drainage. Blood was noted in the right upper lobe bronchus, and contrast injection demonstrated the location and extent of the leak, which was controlled by the injection of fibrin glue and chest tube drainage. Operative closure or resection is sometimes required.

Asymptomatic pneumomediastinum is often detected on chest CT during the evaluation of the multiple injury patient. Recent studies have demonstrated that there is an exceedingly low incidence of aerodigestive tract injuries presenting with pneumomediastinum alone.[47–49]

Bronchial injuries that are missed initially may seal spontaneously, but there is a risk of stenosis. After months or years, children with spontaneously sealed bronchial injuries may have persistent atelectasis often with pneumonia or frank bronchiectasis in the involved lung caused by a bronchial stricture. The diagnosis can be confirmed by bronchography or bronchoscopy. This type of stricture can be dilated in some cases. Open repair or even resection of the involved lung is usually necessary. One report illustrates that late repair of a completely transected main stem bronchus with preservation of the lung is possible.[50]

Esophagus   The most common causes of esophageal injury are ingestion of caustic liquids and penetrating trauma, which includes iatrogenic instrumentation. Forceful vomiting and retching rarely cause esophageal tears in childhood. External blunt trauma rarely causes esophageal injury. The mechanism of esophageal injury from blunt trauma is believed to be a sudden increase in intraesophageal pressure caused by expulsion of gas from the stomach through the gastroesophageal (GE) junction.

Esophageal perforations cause fever, chest pain, and tachycardia. Occasionally, subcutaneous emphysema develops in the neck. Mediastinal or intrapleural air may be visible on routine chest radiographs or CT. If esophageal injury is suspected, a water-soluble contrast swallow, endoscopy, or both should be done.

When diagnosed within the first 12 hours, esophageal injuries are best treated by primary closure, and drainage. When diagnosed later and for more destructive lesions, they may require salivary diversion by means of a cervical esophagostomy and gastrostomy in addition to thoracic drainage. Alternatively, the repair can be buttressed by a neurovascular intercostal muscle pedicle flap. The flap can be secured akin to a modified Graham closure after primary repair, or it can be used to augment the extramucosal repair.[51] There has been a growing, favorable experience with endoscopic stenting of esophageal perforations/leaks in adults, and this may be an alternative to standard approaches in some circumstances.[52]

Diaphragm   Although rare in children, diaphragmatic injuries can be caused by a forceful impact to the abdomen or by a penetrating missile. It is important to recognize these injuries, because the stomach and bowel may herniate through the defect and strangulate. Ninety percent of diaphragmatic injuries occur on the left side. In blunt trauma, tears are usually in or near the central tendon and oriented radially.

Diaphragmatic injuries are easily missed at initial presentation, especially because they are often associated with other severe injuries. They may be asymptomatic or cause abdominal, thoracic, or ipsilateral shoulder tip pain. Physical examination is rarely helpful in the diagnosis of diaphragmatic injuries. The diagnosis is usually based on the plain chest radiograph, which is the most important diagnostic test (Fig. 19-5). Table 19-3 summarizes the radiographic signs of diaphragmatic injury. Basically, any abnormality of the diaphragm or near the diaphragm on plain chest radiography should arouse suspicion. Chest radiographs are initially normal in 30% to 50% of cases.[53] Therefore repeat radiographs should be obtained if a diaphragmatic injury is suspected.

Because other injuries often dominate the clinical picture, delayed diagnosis of a diaphragmatic injury is common. At first, herniation of abdominal viscera into the chest may not have occurred, especially in patients receiving mechanical ventilation. However, the negative intrathoracic pressure of normal breathing may gradually draw the stomach and bowel up into the chest. This can be recognized on plain radiographs, especially if the stomach herniates with a nasogastric (NG) tube in place. In the absence of an NG tube, acute dilation of the herniated stomach may develop leading to severe respiratory distress.

The diagnosis may be confirmed, if necessary, by contrast upper- or lower-intestinal studies. However, these studies may not be possible in patients with multiple acute injuries. Here, CT with multiplanar reconstruction may be helpful. The signs of diaphragmatic injury on CT include discontinuity of the diaphragm, herniation of intra-abdominal viscera into the chest, and constriction of the stomach as it passes through the defect.[54] In stable patients, MR may also help to establish the diagnosis.

Some patients present late with obstruction or strangulation of the herniated gut. This causes severe abdominal or chest pain (or both), nausea, and vomiting. Primary repair through an abdominal incision is indicated. The usual repair is by open laparotomy, but several recent reports of laparoscopic repair demonstrate the feasibility of this approach.[55,56]

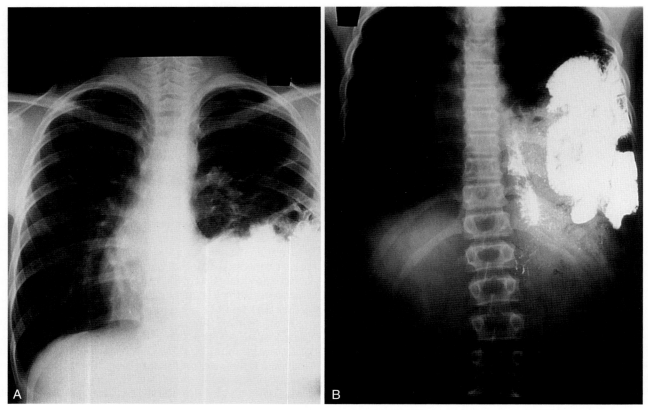

FIGURE 19-5   Ruptured diaphragm. **A,** Plain chest radiograph. **B,** Herniated bowel on gastrointestinal contrast study.

TABLE 19-3
Radiographic Signs of Diaphragmatic Injury

1. Obscured hemidiaphragm
2. Elevated hemidiaphragm
3. Herniated viscera causing abnormal gas pattern above the diaphragm
4. Tip of nasogastric tube curled up into the chest
5. Atypical pneumothorax
6. Platelike atelectasis adjacent to the diaphragm

Heart and Pericardium

Blunt trauma to the heart can produce several types of injury: concussion, contusion, or frank rupture of the myocardium, a valve, or septum.[57,57a] Although rare, disruption or thrombosis of a coronary artery may also occur. A tear of the pericardium may allow herniation of the heart into the pleural space, thereby impairing cardiac function and causing a low output state. Occasionally, blunt trauma to the chest produces occult structural cardiac injuries without gross impairment of cardiac function, bleeding, or cardiac tamponade.[58] These injuries include atrial or ventricular septal defects, mitral or tricuspid insufficiency, and ventricular aneurysm formation. Often, the only sign is a new murmur or a change on the electrocardiogram. The diagnosis can be confirmed by echocardiography or cardiac catheterization. These injuries may be repaired electively once the patient is stable.[58] Follow-up echocardiography should be arranged in all cases of known or suspected injury to the heart.

Several case reports have appeared documenting sudden cardiac arrest in children after a direct blow to the chest.

The term *commotio cordis* has been applied to this entity.[9,10] *Commotio cordis* occurs most often during organized sporting events such as baseball. No contusion or other sign of injury can be found at autopsy, and death has usually been attributed to ventricular fibrillation.

When performing emergency surgery for cardiac trauma, the surgeon should bear in mind a few simple rules:

1. Prepare and drape the entire chest.
2. Place the incision in the left fourth or fifth interspace in an anterolateral direction (except for stable patients undergoing elective repair of known cardiac injuries, which should be repaired through a median sternotomy).
3. Avoid the phrenic nerve when opening the pericardium.
4. Apply direct pressure to control the bleeding.
5. Suture the heart using pledgets as required, avoiding the main coronary arteries.
6. Leave the pericardium open.

Some authors have reported the use of skin staples to control cardiac wounds. Direct suture is preferable. A Foley catheter may be introduced through the defect to control the bleeding during repair.

Although most cardiac injuries can be repaired without cardiopulmonary bypass, this option should be available. During the operation, the surgeon should always check for a thrill, which might indicate a ruptured valve or traumatic ventricular septal defect. Intraoperative trans-esophageal echocardiography may be a useful adjunct to diagnose traumatic septal and valve injuries as well as monitor the integrity of any repair. It is also important to check for intracardiac lesions by listening for new murmurs and performing echocardiography in the postoperative period. Follow-up echocardiography should also be done after discharge.

Myocardial Contusion   Myocardial contusion is the most common type of blunt cardiac injury. It produces focal damage to the heart that can be identified histologically. It can cause life-threatening arrhythmias and cardiac failure. Treatment is aimed primarily at these complications.

Contusion can be distinguished from concussion and *commotio cordis* because the latter do not produce any structural change, even at the microscopic level. Contusions are usually, but not always, associated with an injury to the chest wall. Myocardial contusions may be completely silent or cause an arrhythmia (supraventricular tachycardia or ventricular fibrillation) or hypotension secondary to reduced cardiac output.

Unfortunately, although many tests have been proposed, including electrocardiography, echocardiography, myocardial enzyme determinations (creatine kinase–myocardial band [CKMB], cardiac troponin I, and troponin T), and radionuclide scans, there is no definitive diagnostic test for cardiac contusion. This makes it difficult to define the indications for any of the currently available diagnostic tests and even more difficult to decide on treatment. Tellez and colleagues concluded that a "comprehensive diagnostic evaluation of the heart in all children sustaining multiple injuries from blunt trauma cannot be justified."[59] The simplest test is a 12-lead electrocardiogram, which may reveal reversible changes to ST segments and T waves. Echocardiography may show reduced ejection fraction, localized systolic wall motion abnormality, or an area of increased end-diastolic wall thickness and echogenicity. Swaanenburg and colleagues found that cardiac troponin I and T levels were more accurate and reliable than any of the other diagnostic tests in selecting patients for ICU monitoring.[60–62] They recommended a repeat analysis after admission for patients suspected of having myocardial contusion who have normal values at admission.

A prospective study of 41 children with blunt thoracic trauma, which used a battery of tests that included serum enzyme levels, electrocardiography, echocardiography, and pyrophosphate myocardial scanning, revealed a high incidence of abnormal tests. However, there was little correlation among the tests or between any of the tests and the clinical course.[63] The authors concluded that myocardial contusion is rarely clinically significant in pediatric thoracic trauma. For practical purposes, significant myocardial contusion can be ruled out when findings on 12-lead electrocardiography and echocardiography are normal.

Treatment of myocardial contusion includes electrocardiographic monitoring for 12 to 24 hours, frequent blood pressure determinations and inotropic support as indicated. Complications tend to occur early in the disorder or not at all.[64] Tellez and colleagues recommended cardiac monitoring in the emergency room and intensive care unit to identify arrhythmias and, in patients with arrhythmias and obvious thoracic injuries, serial electrocardiograms and cardiac enzyme tests.[59] Rarely, patients may suffer profound myocardial dysfunction after myocardial contusion. Extracorporeal circulatory support has been useful in isolated cases with marked cardiac dysfunction after blunt trauma.[65] Consideration must be given to left ventricular decompression at the time of circulatory support to prevent distention and subendocardial ischemia.

Myocardial Rupture   Rupture of the heart is usually rapidly fatal. In fact, myocardial rupture is the most common cause of death from thoracic injury. In a population-based autopsy series, Bergman and colleagues found that two thirds of these patients died at the scene of the accident, and one third died in the emergency room.[4] Most cases of cardiac rupture result from high-energy impacts, such as those sustained in motor vehicle accidents or falls from great heights. The atria tend to rupture from impact occurring during late systole; ventricles rupture from impact during late diastole. The right ventricle is the most commonly ruptured site.

Children with myocardial rupture usually present with pericardial tamponade (discussed later). Myocardial necrosis, aneurysm formation, and delayed rupture may also occur.[66] Those with a traumatic atrial septal defect or ventricular septal defect may present with a new murmur without obvious cardiac failure. All patients with chest trauma should be checked carefully for a new murmur before discharge. Any new murmur is an indication for echocardiography. Occasionally, with early diagnosis and repair, patients can survive myocardial rupture.

Valve Injury   Valve injuries are rare but well recognized after blunt trauma.[67,68] Atrioventricular valves are most commonly injured, causing incompetence by damage of the annulus or rupture of the chordae tendinae or papillary muscle (Fig. 19-6). A diastolic murmur, and worsening pulmonary failure out of proportion to the initial pulmonary injury should prompt echocardiography and/or pulmonary artery catheterization to investigate the possibility of a valve injury. This is one type of blunt cardiac injury that can be repaired semielectively.

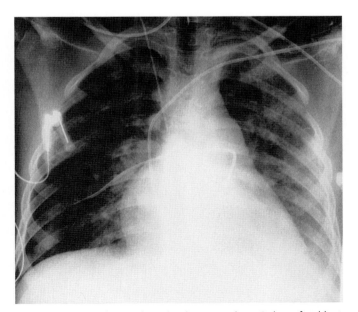

FIGURE 19-6   Cardiomegaly and pulmonary edema 2 days after blunt chest trauma; note Swan-Ganz catheter. Torn mitral valve annulus and chordae tendinae were successfully repaired. (From Wesson DE: Trauma of the chest in children. Chest Clin North Am 1993;3:423-441. Used with permission.)

Pericardial Tamponade Pericardial tamponade can result from an accumulation of blood in the pericardial sac after blunt trauma. The full spectrum of pericardial tamponade—pulsus paradoxus and the Beck triad (elevated jugular venous pressure, systemic hypotension, and muffled heart sounds)—rarely develops in patients with acute trauma. Pericardial tamponade is usually associated with tachycardia, peripheral vasoconstriction, jugular venous distention, and persistent hypotension, regardless of aggressive fluid resuscitation. In fact, pericardial tamponade should be suspected in all cases of unexplained hypotension, especially when it is associated with elevated jugular venous pressure. The best way to confirm the diagnosis is by transthoracic echocardiography, which can be performed by the surgeon at the bedside in conjunction with the FAST (focused abdominal sonography trauma) examination.[20,69]

Treatment of suspected pericardial tamponade begins with control of the airway and breathing plus restoration and expansion of the circulating blood volume. The diagnosis should be confirmed by echocardiography, which is the single best diagnostic tool. However, if the patient is in severe shock, needle-catheter drainage of the pericardial space may be lifesaving (Fig. 19-7). Therefore, in emergency situations or when echocardiography is not available, immediate pericardiocentesis is indicated. The needle should be inserted by the subxiphoid approach at a 45-degree angle upward and toward the left shoulder. A successful tap is confirmed by aspiration of nonclotting blood. A catheter should be inserted and left for repeated aspirations, if necessary, pending definitive treatment. Pericardiocentesis may be complicated by bleeding or damage to the left anterior descending coronary artery. If pericardiocentesis is positive, and does not stabilize the patient, immediate thoracotomy should be performed to relieve the tamponade and control the bleeding.

Pericardial Laceration The pericardium may be torn by blunt trauma. The most common site is on the left, anterior to the phrenic nerve. The heart may herniate through the defect, impairing its function and reducing cardiac output. This type of injury may be recognized on CT or by video-assisted thoracic surgery.[54,70,71]

Aorta and Great Vessels

Traumatic rupture of the aorta and its major branches is uncommon in children.[72] Eddy and colleagues reported that aortic injuries caused 2.1% of all traumatic deaths in children in King County, Washington.[73] Traumatic rupture of the aorta causes a higher proportion of traumatic deaths in adults (approximately 10%) than in children, probably because adult aortas are more brittle and easily torn. Predictors of aortic injury include hypotension, head injury, unrestrained motor vehicle occupant, pelvic fracture, extremity fracture, and other chest injuries. However, it is not clear which mechanism is a reliable predictor. Dyer found mechanism of injury to be "imperfect" and "subjective."[74] Horton found that ΔV greater than or equal to 20 mph and near-side passenger compartment intrusion of greater than or equal to 15 inches correlated strongly with aortic injury.[75]

Traumatic rupture of the aorta occurs with rapid deceleration, which applies shear stress to the wall of the aorta. The most common sites of injury are near the ligamentum arteriosum, the root of the aorta or one of the other main branch points, such as the take-off of the innominate, vertebral or carotid artery. Tears of the distal arch are usually located on the anteromedial aspect of the aorta and oriented horizontally. Children with Marfan syndrome are at risk for aortic dissection following blunt torso trauma.

Although it is usually rapidly fatal, in some cases, the adventitia and pleura contain the blood and prevent

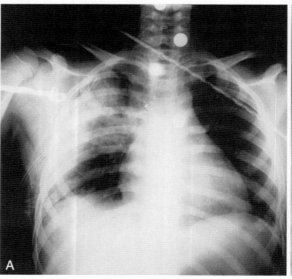
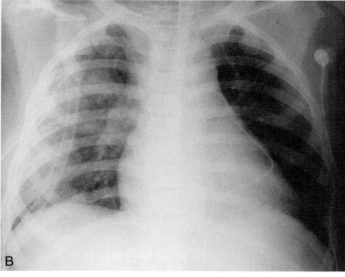

FIGURE 19-7 Pericardial tamponade from blunt chest trauma. The patient was a rear seat passenger in a high-speed frontal collision. Seat belt mark over lower sternum. Shock unresponsive to fluid. Pericardial effusion on transthoracic echocardiography. **A,** Normal heart on plain chest radiograph with evidence of pulmonary contusion. **B,** Chest radiograph after catheter drainage of bloody pericardial effusion. No further treatment was required. (From Wesson DE: Trauma of the chest in children. Chest Clin North Am 1993;3:423-441. Used with permission.)

exsanguination. The natural history of patients who do not exsanguinate immediately is unknown, but imminent rupture in these patients is unlikely. Therefore it is unnecessary to rush them to the OR before stabilization, a full diagnostic workup, and treatment of other injuries. This may require laparotomy, craniotomy, or both before repair of the aorta.

The management of aortic injuries in children is essentially the same as in the adult.[76,77] Diagnosis is difficult, because there may be no clinical evidence of thoracic injury. The acute coarctation syndrome—upper limb hypertension, a difference in blood pressure between the upper and lower limbs, and a loud murmur over the precordium or back—is rare. DelRossi and colleagues reported a series of 27 cases of aortic injury without a single case of coarctation syndrome.[78]

The diagnosis is most often suggested by plain chest radiography, which is sensitive (false negatives, 2% to 7%) but not specific (false positives, 80%). The radiographic signs of traumatic rupture of the aorta are the same as described for adults (Table 19-4 and Fig. 19-8). Nearly all reported cases demonstrate widening of the mediastinum (mediastinum: chest ratio > 0.25) and an abnormal aortic contour.

Until recently, most authors referred to aortography as the gold standard diagnostic test. Many now believe that contrast-enhanced multislice helical CT, which is equally sensitive to aortography, has become the definitive test for diagnosing aortic injury (Fig. 19-9).[74,79–81] If the helical CT is normal, an aortogram is unnecessary. This has substantially reduced the number of negative aortograms done for patients with blunt chest trauma and suspicious plain radiographs. The techniques of helical CT and CT angiography have been reviewed by Melton and Rubin.[79,82] Timing of the contrast injection, as well as the volume and rate of infusion must be carefully controlled to yield optimal results. Helical CT costs about half as much as aortography.[80]

There is still a role for aortography in equivocal cases or to provide more anatomic detail before repair in proven cases.[83] However, many authorities now argue that helical CT alone is sufficient for management of aortic injuries.[79]

Transesophageal echocardiography (TEE) also has a role in the diagnosis of injuries to the descending thoracic aorta, especially for unstable patients in the ICU not able to go to radiology. It is not useful for injuries to the ascending aorta or its branches. Unfortunately, TEE is operator dependent and not universally available. Le Bret and colleagues noted three signs on TEE that are sensitive enough to screen patients for aortic injury.[31] These are increased distance (>3 mm) between the probe and the aorta, double contour of the aortic wall, and an ultrasonographic signal between the aorta and the visceral pleura. The sensitivity for diagnosing traumatic rupture of the

aorta by transesophageal echocardiography in this report was 100%; the specificity was 75%. Le Bret proposed that TEE should be done in all cases of severe chest trauma. TEE is also useful in cases with equivocal findings on CT or aortography to avoid an unnecessary thoracotomy.[84]

Once the diagnosis is proven the treatment options include open repair, endovascular stent graft, or even nonoperative observation in some cases. Aortic surgery carries a significant risk of complications, including intracranial hypertension, which may exacerbate bleeding, left ventricular strain, renal failure, and spinal cord ischemia. When used, heparin may increase the likelihood of bleeding at remote sites of injury.

A small intimal flap may heal spontaneously, but surgical repair after the patient has been stabilized (the bleeding at other locations should be repaired first) through a left posterolateral thoracotomy is the treatment of choice. Surgery may be safely delayed pending repair or control of associated severe injuries to the CNS, extensive burns, septic or contaminated wounds, solid organ injuries likely to bleed with heparinization, and respiratory failure.[85] In such cases, beta blockade to control mean arterial blood pressure and ICU monitoring are essential until repair can be safely accomplished. Esmolol is the preferred beta blocker.

Cardiopulmonary bypass (CPB) should always be available during repair in the event that the injury extends to the aortic root. The left lung should be collapsed and retracted. Care is required when dissecting the aorta for cross-clamping to avoid injury to the branches of the aorta that supply the spinal cord and to the vagus nerve and its recurrent branch. Some partial tears can be repaired primarily; however, repair usually requires placement of a woven Dacron graft, especially when the tear is circumferential. There are three basic ways to perform the operation:

Clamp and sew
Intraoperative shunt
Mechanical circulatory support

The simplest is to "clamp and sew" without a shunt or CPB. This is the fastest method and requires the shortest cross-clamp time; it is adequate if the injury is not too extensive. Razzouk and colleagues reported that the "clamp and sew" technique "is feasible in the majority of patients without increased mortality or spinal cord injury."[86,87] Kwon and colleagues also believe that the clamp technique does not increase mortality or morbidity.[88] However, others strongly disagree. Hochheiser and colleagues reported a lower incidence of postoperative paraplegia after repair with mechanical circulatory support.[89]

Another option is intraoperative shunting with a heparin-bonded shunt. This may reduce the risk of ischemic damage to the spinal cord without the risks of systemic heparinization. However, no controlled studies to prove this exist. The third method is to use mechanical circulatory support during the repair. The most common choice is CPB from the left superior pulmonary vein or left atrium to the femoral artery.[90] Femoral–femoral bypass with direct perfusion of the distal descending thoracic aorta has also been used. CPB is thought by some authorities to reduce the risk of paraplegia, but conventional circuits require systemic heparinization, which can increase the incidence of intracranial hemorrhage; heparin-bonded circuits (including cannulas) are available, and short-term use at higher flows does not require anticoagulation.[91]

TABLE 19-4

Radiographic Signs of Aortic Injury

1. Widened mediastinum (mediastinum:chest ratio > 0.25)
2. Loss or abnormal contour of aortic knob
3. Depression of left main bronchus (>40 degrees below horizontal)
4. Deviation of trachea (left margin to right of T4 spinous process)
5. Deviation of esophagus (nasogastric tube to right of T4 spinous process)
6. Left pleural cap
7. Left hemothorax

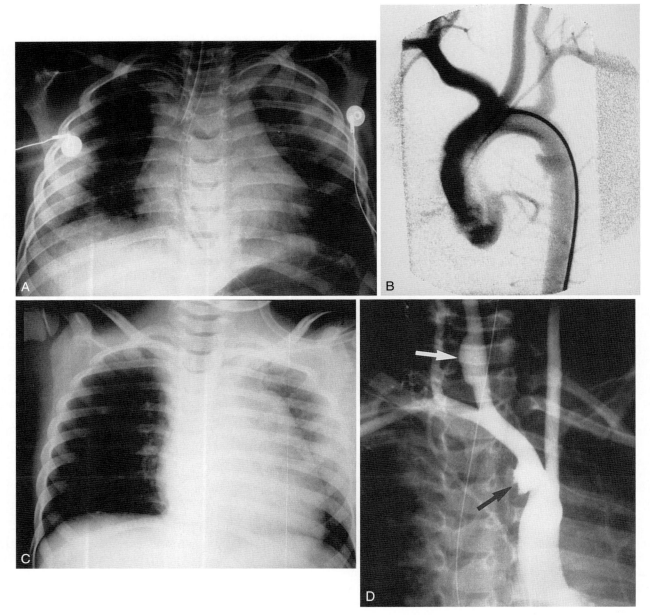

FIGURE 19-8 Traumatic rupture of the aorta and branches. **A,** Widened mediastinum with deviation of the endotracheal and nasogastric tubes to the right. **B,** Same patient as in **A.** Aortic injury was confirmed by aortogram. **C,** Widened mediastinum in a patient who sustained blunt trauma to the chest. **D,** Same patient as in **C.** Innominate artery laceration at its origin (*arrow*). (From Wesson DE: Trauma of the chest in children. Chest Clin North Am 1993;3:423-441. Used with permission.)

The rate of paraplegia after repair of traumatic rupture of the aorta is about 5% to 10%. Individual variations in spinal cord blood supply, cross-clamp time, and intraoperative hypotension are important determinants of spinal cord injury.

There have been several recent reports of transfemoral stent insertion (endovascular stent grafting–thoracic endovascular aortic repair [EVSG–TEVAR]) for injuries to the thoracic aorta in adults. Early results indicate that the results may be better than with standard open repair. Three case series have appeared with remarkably low incidences of paraplegia.[92–94] EVSG–TEVAR has been reported in a small series of children, but there are no reports of long-term results.[77]

Only 1 of 13 patients in Eddy's report, a population-based study that included prehospital deaths, survived traumatic rupture of the aorta.[73] In contrast, DelRossi reported a 75% survival rate in a clinical series.[78] Three of the 21 survivors in Del Rossi's series were paraplegic after repair, but two recovered later. DelRossi found no evidence to support one technique of repair versus the others. However, Fabian and colleagues reported that the clamp and sew technique is more likely to result in paraplegia than repair with bypass, especially if the cross-clamp time is greater than 30 minutes.[95] As is true for many types of injury, outcome also depends on associated injuries.[91] Hormuth reported excellent overall

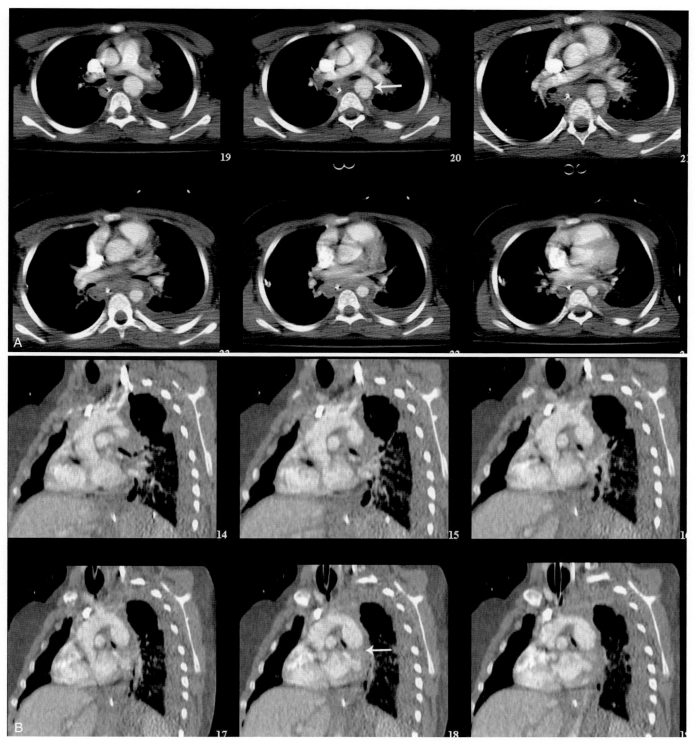

FIGURE 19-9   Helical computed tomography (CT) scan reconstruction showing traumatic rupture of the aorta in a 14-year-old boy. **A,** Transaxial view. Note periaortic hematoma at the isthmus. **B,** Three-dimensional reconstruction. Note interruption of flow at the isthmus.

results in a series of 11 children with thoracic aortic injuries.[76] They repaired isthmus injuries with left heart bypass with direct perfusion of the distal thoracic aorta and arch injuries with hypothermic arrest.

Other thoracic vascular injuries in children are rare, and the majority of injuries are in older children, resulting from penetrating mechanisms.[87] The standard vascular exposure for right subclavian vessel/innominate vessel injuries is a median sternotomy with a supraclavicular or anterior sternocleidomastoid-type neck extension. The choice depends on the injury complex and the potential need for extension distally toward the axilla on more distal injuries. Traditionally, the left subclavian artery was approached through an anterior third intercostal space thoracotomy for proximal control with a supraclavicular approach for exposure of the middle-distal vessel. The proximal left subclavian artery can be controlled by a sternotomy as well, with a type of extension similar to that of right-sided injuries. Alternatively, hemodynamically stable patients have had thoracoscopic proximal control and direct repair performed. More recently, adolescents have undergone endovascular repair/stenting of these injuries. Caution must be exercised in considering the site of injury, because most grafts are not suitable for crossing joints because of an increased risk of thrombosis.

Chylothorax

Injury to the thoracic duct, although rare, causes chylothorax. Most cases resolve spontaneously with nutritional support (total parenteral nutrition or elemental diet with medium-chain triglycerides). Occasionally, ligation of the thoracic duct is necessary.

Traumatic Asphyxia

Traumatic asphyxia, a clinical syndrome that is unique to children, occurs with sudden compression of the abdomen or chest (or both) against a closed glottis.[96] This event causes a rapid rise in intrathoracic pressure, which is transmitted to all the veins that drain into the valveless superior vena cava. Extravasation of blood occurs into the skin of the upper half of the body, sclerae, and possibly the brain. The brain may also be damaged by hypoxia during and after the injury. The clinical features of this disorder include seizures, disorientation, petechiae in the upper half of the body and conjunctivae, and respiratory failure (Fig. 19-10). The treatment is supportive. Most patients recover uneventfully.

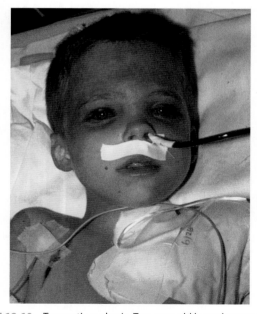

FIGURE 19-10 Traumatic asphyxia. Two-year-old boy who was run over by truck wheel, causing typical plethoric appearance of "traumatic asphyxia." (From Haller JA: Thoracic injuries. In Welch KJ, Randolph JG, Ravitch M, et al (eds): Pediatric Surgery, ed 4. St Louis, Mosby-Year Book, 1986. Used with permission.)

PENETRATING INJURIES

The initial management of penetrating injuries is the same as for blunt trauma: Clear the airway, give oxygen and intravenous fluids, carefully assess the patient, and obtain a plain chest radiograph in every case. An attempt should be made to determine the path of the injury by marking the entry and exit wounds on the plain films. Endotracheal intubation and chest tube insertion should be done as needed during the initial resuscitation. It is important to remember the possibility of a concomitant abdominal injury with any wound below the nipple line. Bronchoscopy is indicated for suspected injury to the major airways; esophagoscopy and water-soluble contrast studies are indicated for suspected esophageal wounds. Echocardiography can be used in stable patients to diagnose suspected heart injuries.

Treatment is also the same as described for blunt trauma. Most of these patients do not require thoracotomy. The most common indications for surgery are massive bleeding, massive air leak, and pericardial tamponade.

Penetrating injuries are more likely to involve the heart, especially with anterior wounds medial to the midclavicular line. These injuries may cause pericardial tamponade or, if the pericardium has a defect, exsanguinating hemorrhage into the chest. Shock is a clear indication for urgent thoracotomy in cases of penetrating wounds to the chest. However, the management of patients who present with normal physiologic parameters and with wounds near the heart is problematic. The most conservative and safest approach is to take all such patients to the operating room for a subxiphoid pericardial window followed by thoracotomy through a median sternotomy, if necessary. Recent reports suggest that early echocardiography may be a very sensitive test for occult cardiac injuries and that this technique may be used to select patients who require a pericardial window, thereby minimizing unnecessary invasive procedures.[20,57,69] In this report, only patients with pericardial effusions on echocardiography underwent subxiphoid pericardial window; if blood was found, a median sternotomy followed. Patients with normal echocardiographs were observed clinically. Harris and colleagues reported a large experience with penetrating cardiac injuries and recommended cardiac ultrasonography in the diagnosis of these injuries in stable patients.[34]

When an operation is required for a penetrating cardiac injury, a Foley catheter placed through the defect may control the bleeding temporarily to facilitate suture of the defect. Median sternotomy is best for known cardiac injuries.

THORACOABDOMINAL INJURIES

Thoracoabdominal injuries can be vexing because of the high mortality from multiple injuries and the need for combined procedures with appropriate sequencing for optimal results. Inappropriate sequencing of thoracic versus abdominal exploration occurs 20% to 40% of the time. The pitfalls are related to the unreliability of abdominal examination, inaccuracy of chest tube output as an indicator of ongoing thoracic bleeding, miscalculation of bullet/knife trajectory, and unreliability of central venous pressure as an index of preload. All of these pitfalls are managed by maintaining a high index of suspicion of occult or underappreciated blood loss in the nonexplored cavity. Prompt changes in initial approaches minimizes delayed intervention, despite initial exploration of the less critical cavity.[97,98]

TRANSMEDIASTINAL INJURIES

Transmediastinal injuries are initially managed according to hemodynamic status. Unstable patients are explored without extensive imaging or diagnostic studies. Stable patients should undergo initial chest radiography; then subsequent imaging or diagnostics depend on those findings/trajectory of the missile. CT imaging of the chest using helical scanners can diagnose most vascular injuries and give high-resolution images of potential aerodigestive tract injuries. Further localization depends on the findings and degree of certainty of the imaging studies.

Complications

Very little information can be found in the literature on the morbidity of chest injuries or the complications after surgery for thoracic injuries in children. The two most common complications of thoracic surgery are pulmonary atelectasis and pneumonia. The most serious is paraplegia, which occurs in 5% to 10% of cases of injury to the thoracic aorta.

Outcome

The risk for death from thoracic injury varies with the type of injury and the number and severity of associated injuries, particularly to the central nervous system. Roux and Fisher reported a series of 100 consecutive children with motor vehicle–related chest trauma in South Africa.[99] Ninety-one pedestrians comprised the largest subgroup. Eight died with a mean Injury Severity Score of 34 compared with 25 among the survivors. Seven of the 8 children who died had fatal head injuries. Thus in blunt injuries to the chest in children, the level of injury reflected in the Injury Severity Score and the presence of concomitant head injuries are the main determinants of survival. Deaths from thoracic injury in children tend to occur in the first few days after the injury, usually from other injuries and not from respiratory failure or sepsis, as is the case in adults.

The overall mortality for chest injuries was 15% in the National Pediatric Trauma Registry—virtually identical to most adult series.[5] Mortality increases with each individual chest injury: 30% for a ruptured diaphragm, 40% for cardiac injury, and 50% for injury to a major vessel.

The morbidity among survivors is remarkably low. DiScala[100] reported that 90% of survivors in the National Pediatric Trauma Registry had no impairment at the time of discharge.

Summary

The following points summarize the management of thoracic injuries in children:
1. Most thoracic injuries can be diagnosed by a combination of clinical assessment and plain chest radiographs.
2. Most heal with medical (not surgical) treatment.
3. Life-threatening thoracic injuries are relatively uncommon.
4. A few thoracic injuries require surgery, but even the most severe can be managed successfully if recognized and treated expeditiously.

The complete reference list is available online at www. expertconsult.com.

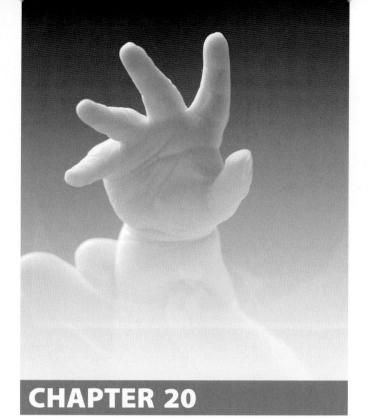

CHAPTER 20

Abdominal Trauma

Steven Stylianos and Richard H. Pearl

Who could have imagined the influence of Simpson's 1968 publication on the successful nonoperative treatment of select children presumed to have splenic injury?[1] Initially suggested in the early 1950s by Warnsborough, then chief of general surgery at the Hospital for Sick Children in Toronto, the era of nonoperative management of splenic injury began with the report of 12 children treated between 1956 and 1965. The diagnosis of splenic injury in this select group was made by clinical findings, along with routine laboratory and plain radiographic findings. Keep in mind that this report predated ultrasonography (US), computed tomography (CT), or isotope imaging. Subsequent confirmation of splenic injury was made in one child who required laparotomy years later for an unrelated condition, when it was found that the spleen had healed in two separate pieces. Nearly half a century later, the standard treatment of hemodynamically stable children with splenic injury is nonoperative, and this concept has been successfully applied to most blunt injuries of the liver, kidney, and pancreas as well. Surgical restraint is now the norm, based on an increased awareness of the anatomic patterns and physiologic responses of injured children. Our colleagues in adult trauma care have slowly acknowledged this success and are applying many of the principles learned in pediatric trauma to their patients.[2]

Review of multiple large trauma databases indicates that 8% to 12% of children suffering blunt trauma have an abdominal injury.[3] Fortunately, more than 90% of them survive.

Although abdominal injuries are 30% more common than thoracic injuries, they are 40% less likely to be fatal. The infrequent need for laparotomy in children with blunt abdominal injury has created a debate regarding the role of pediatric trauma surgeons in their treatment. Recent analyses of the National Pediatric Trauma Registry (NPTR) and the National Trauma Data Bank emphasize the overall "surgical" nature of pediatric trauma patients, with more than 25% of injured children requiring operative intervention.[4,5] Clearly, a qualified pediatric trauma surgeon would be the ideal coordinator of such care.

Few surgeons have extensive experience with massive abdominal solid organ injuries requiring immediate surgery. It is imperative that surgeons familiarize themselves with current treatment algorithms for life-threatening abdominal trauma. Important contributions have been made in the diagnosis and treatment of children with abdominal injury by radiologists and endoscopists. The resolution and speed of computed tomography (CT), the screening capabilities of focused abdominal sonography for trauma (FAST), and the percutaneous, angiographic, and endoscopic interventions of nonsurgeon members of the pediatric trauma team have all enhanced patient care and improved outcomes. This chapter focuses on the more common blunt injuries and unique aspects of care in children. Renal and genitourinary injuries are covered separately in Chapter 21.

Diagnostic Modalities

The initial evaluation of an acutely injured child is similar to that of an adult. Plain radiographs of the cervical spine, chest, and pelvis are obtained after the initial survey and evaluation of the ABCs (airway, breathing, and circulation). Other plain abdominal films add little to the acute evaluation of pediatric trauma patients. As imaging modalities have improved, treatment algorithms have changed significantly in children with suspected intra-abdominal injuries. Prompt identification of potentially life-threatening injuries is now possible in the vast majority of children.

COMPUTED TOMOGRAPHY

CT has become the imaging study of choice for the evaluation of injured children owing to several advantages. CT is now readily accessible in most health care facilities; it is a noninvasive, accurate method of identifying and qualifying the extent of abdominal injury, and it has reduced the incidence of nontherapeutic exploratory laparotomy. CT can be particularly helpful in diagnosing abdominal injuries in intubated, multi-injured children.[6]

Use of intravenous contrast is essential, and "dynamic" methods of scanning have optimized vascular and parenchymal enhancement. The importance of a contrast "blush" in children with blunt spleen and liver injury continues to be debated and is discussed later in the chapter (Fig. 20-1).[7] Head CT, if indicated, should be performed first without contrast, to avoid concealing a hemorrhagic brain injury. Controversy remains regarding the benefits of enteral contrast for diagnosis of gastrointestinal (GI) tract injuries. Many authors conclude that CT with enteral contrast does not

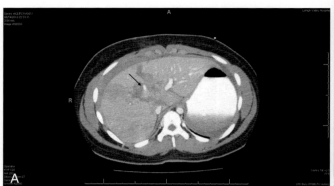
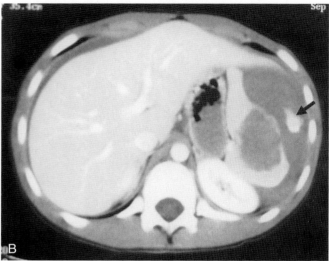

FIGURE 20-1   **A,** Abdominal computed tomography scan demonstrating a significant injury to the right hepatic lobe with intravenous contrast "blush" (*arrow*). This patient had successful angiographic embolization and avoided operation. **B,** Abdominal computed tomography scan demonstrating a significant injury to the spleen with intravenous contrast blush (*arrow*). The patient remained hemodynamically stable and avoided operation.

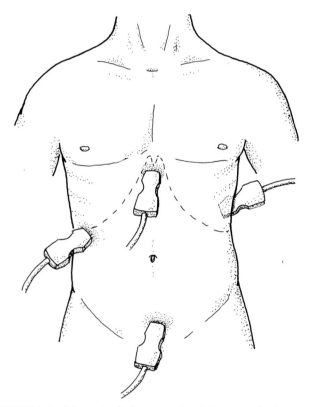

FIGURE 20-2   Schematic of a focused abdominal sonography for trauma (FAST) examination, with emphasis on views of the subxiphoid, right upper quadrant and pouch of Morrison, left upper quadrant and left paracolic region, and pelvic region and pouch of Douglas. (Original illustration by Mark Mazziotti, MD.)

improve diagnosis of GI injuries in the acute trauma setting and can lead to delays in diagnosis and aspiration.[8–12]

Not all children with potential abdominal injuries are candidates for CT evaluation. Obvious penetrating injury often necessitates immediate operative intervention. A hemodynamically unstable child should not be taken out of an appropriate resuscitation room for the performance of CT. These children may benefit from an alternative diagnostic study, such as peritoneal lavage or FAST, or urgent operative intervention. The greatest limitation of abdominal CT in trauma is the inability to reliably identify intestinal rupture.[13] Findings suggestive but not diagnostic of intestinal perforation are pneumoperitoneum, bowel wall thickening, free intraperitoneal fluid, bowel wall enhancement, and dilated bowel.[14] A high index of suspicion should exist for the presence of bowel injury in a child with intraperitoneal fluid and no identifiable solid organ injury on CT.[10] The diagnosis and treatment of bowel injury are reviewed in detail later.

FOCUSED ABDOMINAL SONOGRAPHY FOR TRAUMA

Clinician-performed sonography for the early evaluation of an injured child is currently being evaluated to determine its optimal use. Examination of the pouch of Morrison; the pouch of Douglas; the left flank, including the perisplenic anatomy; and a subxiphoid view to visualize the pericardium is the standard four-view FAST examination (Fig. 20-2). This bedside examination may be a good rapid screening study, particularly in patients too unstable to undergo an abdominal CT scan. Early reports have found FAST to be a helpful screening tool in children, with a high specificity (95%) but low sensitivity (33%) in identifying intestinal injury. However, a lack of identifiable free fluid does not exclude a significant injury.[15] FAST may be useful in decreasing the number of CT scans performed for "low-likelihood" injuries. Repetition of the study may be necessary, depending on clinical correlation, and the finding of free fluid by itself is not an indication for surgical intervention. A recent meta-analysis of FAST in pediatric blunt trauma patients revealed modest sensitivity for hemoperitoneum.[16] The authors concluded that a negative FAST may have questionable utility as the sole diagnostic test to rule out the presence of an intra-abdominal injury. A hemodynamically stable child with a positive FAST should undergo CT.

DIAGNOSTIC PERITONEAL LAVAGE AND LAPAROSCOPY

Diagnostic peritoneal lavage (DPL) has been a mainstay in trauma evaluation for more than 3 decades. However, its utility in pediatric trauma is limited. Because up to 90% of solid organ injuries do not require surgical intervention, the finding of free blood in the abdomen by DPL has limited clinical significance. Hemodynamic instability and the need for ongoing blood replacement are the determinants for operation in patients with solid organ injury in the absence of blood in the abdominal cavity. Additionally, the speed and accuracy of CT have further decreased the indications for DPL in pediatric trauma. The sensitivity of CT in diagnosing solid organ injuries and more subtle injuries to the duodenum, pancreas, and intestines continues to improve. This has relegated DPL to the evaluation of patients with clinical findings suggestive of bowel injury and no definitive diagnosis on CT. In this setting, the presence of bile, food particles, or other evidence of GI tract perforation is diagnostic. Recent literature has suggested that laparoscopy can both diagnose and, in some cases, allow definitive surgical management without laparotomy, further limiting the usefulness of DPL.[17]

Large series using laparoscopy in adults have demonstrated increased diagnostic accuracy, definitive management of related injuries, decreased nontherapeutic laparotomy rates, and a significant decrease in hospital length of stay, with an attendant reduction in costs.[18,19] The extent of feasible operations is directly related to the surgeon's skill with advanced laparoscopic techniques and the patient's overall stability. At the Children's Hospital of Illinois, our two most recent handlebar injuries causing bowel perforation were successfully treated laparoscopically. As with elective abdominal surgery, the role of laparoscopy in trauma will increase substantially as trauma centers redirect their training of residents to this modality and as more pediatric centers report outcome studies for laparoscopic trauma management in children.[20–22]

Solid Organ Injuries

SPLEEN AND LIVER

The spleen and liver are the organs most commonly injured in blunt abdominal trauma, with each accounting for one third of the injuries. Nonoperative treatment of isolated splenic and hepatic injuries in stable children has been universally successful and is now standard practice; however, there is great variation in the management algorithms used by individual pediatric surgeons.[23]

Controversy exists regarding the utility of CT grading and the finding of contrast blush as a predictor of outcome in liver and spleen injury.[24–26] Several recent studies reported contrast blush in 7% to 12% of children with blunt spleen injury (see Fig. 20-1).[27–29] The rate of operation in the blush group approached or exceeded 20%. The authors emphasized that CT blush was worrisome but that most patients could still be managed successfully without operation. The role and impact of angiographic embolization in adults is still debated and has yet to be determined in pediatric spleen injury.[30,31] Initial retrospective studies have found angiographic embolization to be safe and effective in children; however, selection criteria remain undefined.[32]

The American Pediatric Surgical Association (APSA) Trauma Committee analyzed a contemporary multi-institution database of 832 children treated nonoperatively at 32 centers in North America from 1995 to 1997 (Table 20-1).[33] Consensus guidelines on intensive care unit (ICU) stay, length of hospital stay, use of follow-up imaging, and physical activity restriction for clinically stable children with isolated spleen or liver injuries (CT grades I to IV) were defined based on this analysis (Table 20-2). The guidelines were then applied prospectively in 312 children with liver or spleen injuries treated nonoperatively at 16 centers from 1998 to 2000.[34] Patients with other minor injuries, such as nondisplaced, noncomminuted fractures or soft tissue injuries, were included as long as the associated injuries did not influence the variables in the study. The patients were grouped by severity of injury defined by CT grade. Compliance with the proposed guidelines was analyzed for age, organ injured, and injury grade. All patients were followed for 4 months after injury. It is imperative to emphasize that these proposed guidelines assume hemodynamic stability. The extremely low rates of transfusion and operation document the stability of the study patients.

Specific guideline compliance was 81% for ICU stay, 82% for length of hospital stay, 87% for follow-up imaging, and 78% for activity restriction. There was a significant improvement in compliance from year 1 to year 2 for ICU stay (77% versus 88%, $P < 0.02$) and activity restriction (73% vs. 87%, $P < 0.01$). There were no differences in compliance by age,

TABLE 20-1

Resource Use and Activity Restriction in 832 Children with Isolated Spleen or Liver Injury by Computed Tomography Grade

	Grade I (n = 116)	Grade II (n = 341)	Grade III (n = 275)	Grade IV (n = 100)
Admitted to ICU (%)	55.0	54.3	72.3	85.4
No. hospital days (mean)	4.3	5.3	7.1	7.6
No. hospital days (range)	1-7	2-9	3-9	4-10
Transfused (%)	1.8	5.2	10.1*	26.6*
Laparotomy (%)	0	1.0	2.7†	12.6†
Follow-up imaging (%)	34.4	46.3	54.1	51.8
Activity restriction (mean wk)	5.1	6.2	7.5	9.2
Activity restriction (range wk)	2-6	2-8	4-12	6-12

From Stylianos S, APSA Trauma Committee: Evidence-based guidelines for resource utilization in children with isolated spleen or liver injury. J Pediatr Surg 2000;35:164-169.
*Grade III vs. grade IV, $P < 0.014$
†Grade III vs. grade IV, $P < 0.0001$
CT, Computed tomography; ICU, intensive care unit.

TABLE 20-2

Proposed Guidelines for Resource Use in Children with Isolated Spleen or Liver Injury by CT Grade

	Grade I	*Grade II*	*Grade III*	*Grade IV*
ICU days	0	0	0	1
Hospital stay (days)	2	3	4	5
Predischarge imaging	None	None	None	None
Postdischarge imaging	None	None	None	None
Activity restriction (wk)*	3	4	5	6

From Stylianos S, APSA Trauma Committee: Evidence-based guidelines for resource utilization in children with isolated spleen or liver injury. J Pediatr Surg 2000;35:164-169.

*Return to full-contact, competitive sports (e.g., football, wrestling, hockey, lacrosse, mountain climbing) should be at the discretion of the individual pediatric trauma surgeon. The proposed guidelines for return to unrestricted activity include "normal" age-appropriate activities.

CT, Computed tomography; ICU, intensive care unit.

gender, or organ injured. Deviation from the guidelines was the surgeon's choice in 90% of cases and patient-related in 10%. Six patients (1.9%) were readmitted, although none required operation. Compared with the previously studied 832 patients, the 312 patients managed prospectively by the proposed guidelines had a significant reduction in ICU stay ($P < 0.0001$), hospital stay ($P < 0.0006$), follow-up imaging ($P < 0.0001$), and interval of physical activity restriction ($P < 0.04$) within each grade of injury.

From these data, it was concluded that prospective application of specific treatment guidelines based on injury severity resulted in conformity in patient management, improved use of resources, and validation of guideline safety. Significant reductions in ICU stay, hospital stay, follow-up imaging, and activity restriction were achieved without adverse sequelae when compared with the retrospective database. The pendulum continues to swing toward less hospitalization of stable children with solid liver or spleen injury. Retrospective and prospective studies suggest that the APSA guidelines for hospital length of stay can be reduced further.[35,36]

Authors from the Arkansas Children's Hospital reported on an abbreviated protocol based on hemodynamics while "throwing out" the CT grade of injury in 101 patients with isolated spleen or liver injury. Their protocol resulted in a significant reduction in length of stay (3.5 vs. 1.9 days, $P < 0.001$) from that predicted by APSA guidelines.

The attending surgeon's decision to operate for spleen or liver injury is best based on evidence of continued blood loss, such as low blood pressure, tachycardia, decreased urine output, and falling hematocrit unresponsive to crystalloid and blood transfusion. The rates of successful nonoperative treatment of isolated blunt splenic and hepatic injury now exceed 90% in most pediatric trauma centers and in adult trauma centers with a strong pediatric commitment.[35-37] A study of more than 100 patients from the NPTR indicated that nonoperative treatment of spleen or liver injury is indicated even in the presence of associated head injury if the patient is hemodynamically stable.[38] Rates of operative intervention for blunt spleen or liver injury were similar with and without an associated closed head injury.

Not surprisingly, adult trauma services have reported excellent survival rates for pediatric trauma patients; however, an analysis of treatment for spleen and liver injuries reveals alarmingly high rates of operative treatment.[39-41]

This discrepancy in operative rates emphasizes the importance of disseminating effective guidelines, because the majority of seriously injured children are treated outside of dedicated pediatric trauma centers. Mooney and Forbes[37] reviewed the New England Pediatric Trauma Database in the 1990s and identified 2500 children with spleen injuries. Two thirds were treated by nonpediatric trauma surgeons, and two thirds were treated in nontrauma centers. After allowing for multiple patient- and hospital-related variables, the authors found that the risk of operation was reduced by half when a surgeon with pediatric training provided care to children with splenic injuries. In a similar review using the Kids' Inpatient Database (KID) 2000 administrative data set, Mooney and Rothstein[42] found that despite adjustment for hospital- and patient-specific variables, children treated at an adult general hospital had a 2.8 greater chance ($P < 0.003$), and those treated at a general hospital with a pediatric unit had a 2.6 greater chance ($P < 0.013$), of undergoing splenectomy than those cared for at a freestanding pediatric hospital.

Several recent studies provide a basis for ongoing concern regarding disparity of treatment in children with blunt spleen injury.[37,40,42-45] Using large nonselected databases and adjusting for risk, these studies indicate that the disparity is substantial and continuing on a regional and national basis (see Table 20-5).

Todd and colleagues analyzed the Healthcare Cost and Utilization Project's National Inpatient Sample (HCUP-NIS), which contains a sample of discharges from 1300 hospitals in 28 states (representing 20% of all hospital discharges in the United States).[43] Children with splenic injury treated at rural hospitals had a risk-adjusted odds ratio for laparotomy of 1.64 (95% CI, 1.39 to 1.94) when compared with those treated at an urban teaching hospital. The APSA Center on Outcomes compared the treatment of pediatric splenic injury using discharge datasets from four states.[41] The authors found a risk-adjusted odds ratio for laparotomy of 2.1 (95% CI, 1.4 to 3.1) when comparing treatment at nontrauma centers versus centers with trauma expertise. Mooney and colleagues reviewed more than 2600 children with splenic injury from the New England Pediatric Trauma Database and found that similarly injured patients treated by nonpediatric surgeons had a risk-adjusted odds ratio for laparotomy of 3.1 (95% CI, 2.3 to 4.4) when compared with those treated by pediatric surgeons.[37] The last two studies found even greater disparity when comparing the treatment of children with isolated splenic injury as contrasted with those with multiple injuries. Bowman and colleagues used data from the Kids Inpatient Database (KID 2000) of the Healthcare Cost and Utilization Project, sponsored by the Agency for Healthcare Research and Quality.[44] This administrative database represents an

80% sample of non-newborn discharges from 2784 hospitals in 27 states (2.5 million pediatric discharges). The authors found a risk-adjusted odds ratio for laparotomy of 5.0 (95% CI, 2.2 to 11.4) when comparing treatment at general hospitals versus children's hospitals in pediatric patients with splenic injury. Davis and colleagues reviewed discharge data from 175 hospitals in Pennsylvania and found the risk-adjusted odds ratio for laparotomy to be 6.2 (95% CI, 4.4 to 8.6) when comparing treatment at adult trauma centers versus pediatric trauma centers.[45] Although these studies suggest marked differences in the processes of care, administrative datasets do not readily allow risk adjustment for differences in physiologic status at presentation, a potential major limitation (Table 20-3).

Sims and colleagues surveyed 281 surgeons (114 pediatric, 167 adult) regarding their treatment of children with solid organ injury (SOI).[40] For all clinical scenarios, adult surgeons were more likely to operate or pursue interventional radiologic procedures than their pediatric colleagues (relative risk [RR]: 8.6 with isolated SOI, $P < 0.05$; 14.8 SOI with multiple SOI, $P < 0.001$; 17.9 SOI with intracranial hemorrhage,

$P < 0.0001$). Adult surgeons were also more likely to consider any transfusion a failure (13.3% vs. 1.2%, $P < 0.01$) and had a much lower transfusion threshold.

The importance of these data is further amplified by the fact that the overwhelming majority (68% to 87%) of pediatric patients were treated at the facilities or by physicians with the higher likelihood of operation.[37,44,45] In contrast, Stylianos and colleagues found that nearly two thirds of children with splenic injury were treated at institutions with trauma expertise.[41] Trauma centers had a significantly lower rate of operation for both multiple-injury patients (15.3% vs. 19.3%, $P < 0.001$) and those with isolated injury (9.2% vs. 18.5%, $P < 0.0001$) when compared to nontrauma centers (see Table 20-6). The operative rates at both trauma centers and nontrauma centers exceeded published APSA benchmarks (Tables 20-4 and 20-5) for all children with splenic injury (3% to 11%) and those with isolated splenic injury (0% to 3%).

Thus trauma centers and their corresponding state or regional trauma systems may represent rational targets for dissemination of current pediatric trauma guidelines and benchmarks. Broad application of existing APSA guidelines for splenic injury should

TABLE 20-3

Studies Comparing Operative Rates for Pediatric Blunt Splenic Injury

First Author	Study Period	No. Patients	Database	Adjusted Odds Ratio (95% CI) for Operation	Ratio	P value
Todd[43]	1998-2000	2569	HCUP-NIS	1.64 (1.39-1.94) RH vs. UTH	n/a	n/a
Stylianos[41]	2000-2002	3232	State UHDDS	2.1 (1.4-3.1) NTC vs. TC	34:66	<0.0001
Mooney[37]	1990-1998	2631	NEPTD	3.1 (2.3-4.4) NPS vs. PS	68:32	<0.0001
Bowman[44]	2000	2851	KID 2000	5.0 (2.2-11.4) GH vs. CH	87:13	<0.001
Davis[45]	1991-2000	3245	State UHDDS	6.2 (4.4-8.6) ATC vs. PTC	84:16	<0.0001

ATC, Adult trauma center; CH, children's hospital; GH, general hospital; HCUP-NIS, Healthcare Cost and Utilization Project's National Inpatient Sample (1300 hospitals in 28 states; 20% of all hospital discharges in United States); KID 2000, Kids' Inpatient Database of the Healthcare Cost and Utilization Project, Agency for Healthcare Research and Quality (2784 hospitals in 27 states; 2.5 million pediatric discharges); n/a, not available; NEPTD, New England Pediatric Trauma Database; NPS; nonpediatric surgeon; NTC; nontrauma center; PS, pediatric surgeon; PTC, pediatric trauma center; RH, rural hospital; TC, trauma center; UHDDS, Uniform Hospital Discharge Data Set; UTH, urban teaching hospital.

TABLE 20-4

Operative Rate in Children with Splenic Injury[41]

	Trauma Center	Nontrauma Center	P value	APSA Benchmarks
Multiple injuries ($n = 1299$)	15.3%	19.3%	<0.001	11%-17%
Isolated spleen injuries ($n = 1933$)	9.2%	18.5%	<0.0001	0%-3%
TOTAL ($n = 3232$)	12.1%	18.8%	<0.0001	5%-11%

APSA, American Pediatric Surgical Association.

TABLE 20-5

Pediatric Surgery Benchmarks for Operative Rate in Children with Splenic Injury

First Author	Database	Study Period	No. Patients	Operative Rate: Pediatric Surgeon and/or Children's Hospital-PTC	Splenic Injuries
Bowman[44]	KID 2000—AHRQ	2000	363	3%	All
Davis[45]	Pennsylvania Trauma Outcome Study-UHDDS	1991-2000	507	5%	All
Mooney[37]	New England Pediatric Trauma Database-UHDDS	1990-98	866	11%	All
Stylianos[33,34]	APSA Trauma Committee Multicenter Registry	1995-2000	652	3%	Isolated
Mooney[46]	Children's Hospital-Boston Trauma registry	1993-99	82	0%	Isolated

KID2000, Kids' Inpatient Database of the Healthcare Cost and Utilization Project, Agency for Healthcare Research and Quality (AHRQ) (2784 hospitals in 27 states; 2.5 million pediatric discharges); PTC, Pediatric Trauma Center; UHDDS, Uniform Hospital Discharge Data Sets.

encourage conformity of care and result in reduced rates of operative intervention and diminished resource use.

Failure of nonoperative management (NOM) can have serious consequences; therefore patient selection is important.[47] Two recent multi-institutional reviews sought to evaluate the time line and the characteristics of patients who fail NOM.[48,49] There was operation in 120 of 1813 (6.6%) children with solid organ injury in a median time of 2.4 hours with 90% of patients having surgery within 24 hours. Pediatric patients who sustained pancreatic injuries were more likely to fail nonoperative management (odds ratio [OR] 7.49; 95% CI, 3.74 to 15.01) compared with those who suffered other injuries. The patients who failed had higher injury severity scores (ISS; 28 ± 17) than those who underwent successful NOM (14 ± 10, $P < 0.001$). Severely head-injured patients (Glasgow Coma Scale [GCS] = 8) had a higher failure rate for NOM (OR 5.09; 95% CI, 3.04 to 8.52). Factors associated with increased failure rate include bicycle-related injury mechanism, isolated pancreatic injury, more than one solid organ injury, and an isolated grade 5 solid organ injury. The time to failure of NOM peaked at 4 hours and then declined over 36 hours from admission. Thus continued surgical evaluation and assessment during the entire hospital stay is required to limit morbidity and mortality of the pediatric trauma patient.

Summary

If care is to be optimally provided at centers outside of the tertiary pediatric setting, health care providers in these environments need to reassess their approach to the management of pediatric splenic injury, recognizing that the operative rate is presently 4 to 6 times lower for children with splenic injury treated by pediatric surgeons at pediatric facilities than in other environments. It is incumbent upon pediatric trauma centers to do a better job of educating trauma colleagues in nonpediatric trauma centers regarding the optimal care of pediatric patients with splenic injury, so that these results are not limited to highly selected centers. Focusing educational programs and evidence-based management guidelines on centers with higher rates of splenectomy may be the next step to improve the rate of splenic conservation. Although the impact on in-hospital mortality might not be a relevant end point, because it is infrequent, these patients are at higher risk for overwhelming postsplenectomy sepsis and complications related to laparotomy, such as adhesive small bowel obstruction and incisional hernia.

Adult trauma surgeons caring for injured children must consider the anatomic, immunologic, and physiologic differences between pediatric and adult trauma patients and incorporate these differences into their treatment protocols.[50] The major concerns are related to the potential risks of increased transfusion requirements, missed associated injuries, and increased length of hospital stay. Each of these concerns has been shown to be without merit.[51–53]

ASSOCIATED ABDOMINAL INJURIES

Advocates of surgical intervention for splenic trauma cite their concern about missing associated abdominal injuries if no operation is performed. Morse and Garcia reported successful nonoperative treatment in 110 of 120 children (91%) with blunt splenic trauma, of whom 22 (18%) had associated

abdominal injuries.[51] Only 3 of these 120 patients (2.5%) had GI injuries, and each was discovered at early celiotomy done for a specific indication. There was no morbidity from missed injuries or delayed surgery. Similarly, a review of the NPTR from 1988 to 1998 revealed 2977 patients with solid abdominal visceral injuries; only 96 (3.2%) had an associated hollow visceral injury.[52] Higher rates of hollow visceral injury were observed in assaulted patients and in those with multiple solid visceral injuries or pancreatic injuries. Differences in mechanism of injury may account for the much lower incidence of associated abdominal injuries in children with splenic trauma. There is no justification for an exploratory celiotomy solely to avoid missing potential associated injuries in children.

COMPLICATIONS OF NONOPERATIVE TREATMENT

Nonoperative treatment protocols have been the standard for most children with blunt liver and spleen injuries for the past 3 decades. This cumulative experience has allowed us to evaluate both the benefits and the risks of the nonoperative approach. Fundamental to the success of a nonoperative strategy is the early, spontaneous cessation of hemorrhage. Transfusion rates for children with isolated spleen or liver injuries have fallen below 10%, confirming the lack of continued blood loss in the majority of patients.[33,34,53] Rare anecdotal reports of significant delayed hemorrhage with adverse outcomes after solid organ injury continue to appear and cause concern.[47,54–56] Shilyansky and colleagues[56] reported two children with delayed hemorrhage 10 days after blunt liver injury. Both children had persistent right upper quadrant and right shoulder pain despite normal vital signs and stable hematocrits. The authors recommended continued in-house observation until symptoms resolve. The incidence of delayed bleeding after blunt splenic injury was 1 (0.33%) in 303 children reported from the Hospital for Sick Children in Toronto and resulted in a fatality.[47] These rare occurrences lead to caution when determining a minimum safe interval before the resumption of unrestricted activities.

Routine follow-up imaging studies have identified pseudocysts and pseudoaneurysms following splenic injury.[57] Splenic pseudoaneurysms often cause no symptoms and appear to resolve with time. The true incidence of self-limited, posttraumatic splenic pseudoaneurysms is unknown, because routine follow-up imaging after successful nonoperative treatment has been largely abandoned. Once identified, the actual risk of splenic pseudoaneurysm rupture is also unclear. Angiographic embolization techniques can successfully treat these lesions, obviating the need for open surgery and loss of splenic parenchyma (Fig. 20-3).[58] Splenic pseudocysts can achieve enormous size, leading to pain and GI disturbance (Fig. 20-4). Simple percutaneous aspiration leads to a high recurrence rate. Laparoscopic excision and marsupialization are highly effective (Fig. 20-5).

SEQUELAE OF DAMAGE-CONTROL STRATEGIES

Even the most severe solid organ injuries can be treated without surgery, if there is a prompt response to resuscitation.[59,60] In contrast, emergency laparotomy, embolization, or both are

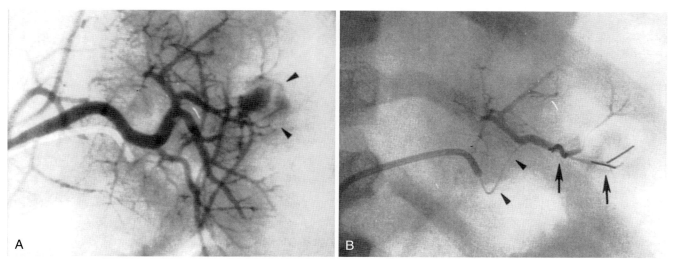

FIGURE 20-3   **A,** Splenic pseudoaneurysm (arrowheads indicate contrast within the pseudoaneurysm) after nonoperative treatment of blunt splenic injury. **B,** Successful angiographic embolization (*arrows* show occlusion of ruptured vessels).

indicated in patients who are hemodynamically unstable despite fluid and red blood cell transfusion (Fig. 20-6). Most spleen and liver injuries requiring operation are amenable to simple methods of hemostasis using a combination of manual compression, direct suture, topical hemostatic agents, and mesh wrapping. In young children with significant hepatic injury, the sternum can be divided rapidly to expose the suprahepatic or intrapericardial inferior vena cava, allowing for total hepatic vascular isolation (Fig. 20-7). Children can tolerate periods of vascular isolation for 30 minutes or longer, as long as their blood volume is replenished. Venovenous bypass may be useful but is rarely available for such rare injuries.[61] With this exposure, the liver and major perihepatic veins can be isolated and the bleeding controlled, permitting direct suture repair or ligation of the offending vessel. Although the cumbersome and dangerous technique of atriocaval shunting has been largely abandoned, newer endovascular balloon catheters can be useful

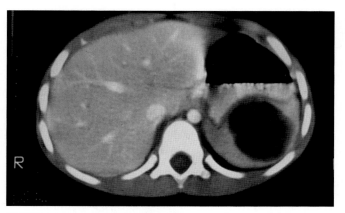

FIGURE 20-4   Computed tomography scan of post-traumatic splenic pseudocyst.

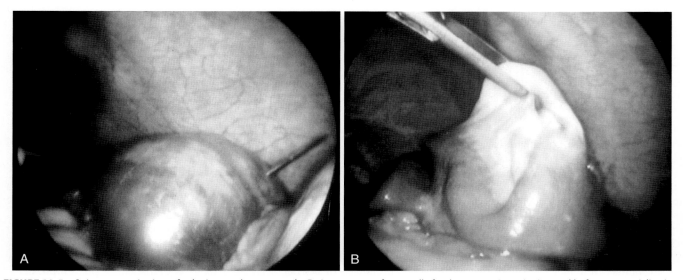

FIGURE 20-5   **A,** Laparoscopic view of splenic pseudocyst capsule. **B,** Appearance of cyst wall after laparoscopic aspiration and before marsupialization.

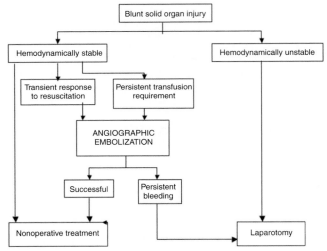

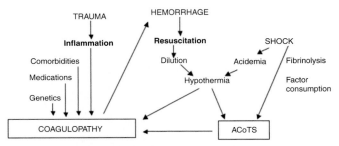

FIGURE 20-8 Acute coagulopathy of trauma and shock (ACoTS). (From Hess JR, Brohi K, Duton RP, et al: The coagulopathy of trauma: A review of mechanisms. J Trauma 2008;65:748-754.)

FIGURE 20-6 Algorithm for selected use of angiographic embolization in patients with blunt solid organ injury. (Modified from M. Nance, Children's Hospital of Philadelphia.)

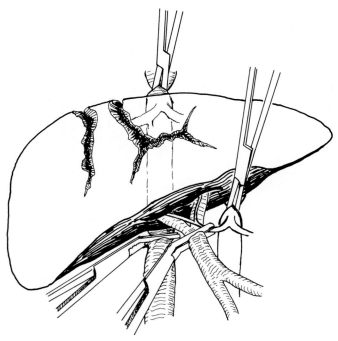

FIGURE 20-7 Total hepatic vascular isolation with occlusion of the portahepatic, suprahepatic, and infrahepatic inferior vena cava and supraceliac aorta (optional). (Original illustration by Mark Mazziotti, MD.)

for temporary vascular occlusion to allow access to the juxtahepatic vena cava.[62]

The early morbidity and mortality of severe hepatic injuries are related to the effects of massive blood loss and replacement with large volumes of cold blood products. The consequences of prolonged operations with massive blood-product replacement include hypothermia, coagulopathy, and acidosis. Although the surgical team may keep pace with blood loss, life-threatening physiologic and metabolic consequences are inevitable, and many of these critically ill patients are unlikely to survive once their physiologic reserves have been

exhausted. A multi-institutional review identified exsanguination as the cause of intraoperative death in 82% of 537 patients at eight academic trauma centers.[63] The mean pH was 7.18, and the mean core temperature was 32° C before death. Moulton and colleagues reported survival in only 5 of 12 (42%) consecutive operative cases of retrohepatic vascular or severe parenchymal liver injury in children.[64]

Maintenance of physiologic stability during the struggle for surgical control of severe bleeding is a formidable challenge even for the most experienced surgical team, particularly when hypothermia, coagulopathy, and acidosis occur. This triad creates a vicious circle in which each derangement exacerbates the others, and the physiologic and metabolic consequences often preclude completion of the procedure. Lethal coagulopathy from a combination of tissue injury, dilution, hypothermia, and acidosis can rapidly occur (Fig. 20-8).[65] Experimental studies have defined the alterations in procoagulant and anticoagulant enzyme processes, platelet activation, and platelet adhesion defects with varying degrees of hypothermia.[66] The infusion of activated recombinant factor VII in children with massive hemorrhage has been promising in several case reports, and experimental studies suggest that recombinant factor VII maintains its effectiveness at hypothermic temperatures[67–70]

Increased emphasis on physiologic and metabolic stability in emergency abdominal operations has led to the development of staged, multidisciplinary treatment plans, including abbreviated laparotomy, perihepatic packing, temporary abdominal closure, angiographic embolization, and endoscopic biliary stenting.[71–74] Asensio and colleagues[75] reported on 103 patients with mostly penetrating grade IV or V hepatic injuries treated between 1991 and 1999. Mean blood loss was estimated at 9.4 L, and mean volume infusion in the operating room was 15 L. Packing of the hepatic injuries was used in 50% of patients at the first operation. Forty percent of patients who survived the initial operative control of hemorrhage had postoperative angiographic embolization (Fig. 20-9). Survival was 63% in grade IV patients and 24% in grade V patients, emphasizing the lethality of such injuries despite a well-choreographed, staged, multidisciplinary approach. Trauma surgeons treating critically injured children must familiarize themselves with these lifesaving techniques.

Hepatic angioembolization can clearly be an important adjunct in the treatment of patients with major liver injury. However, evidence of significant hepatic necrosis and biliary leaks occur in 30% to 40% of patients, thus emphasizing the need for cautious patient selection.[76,77]

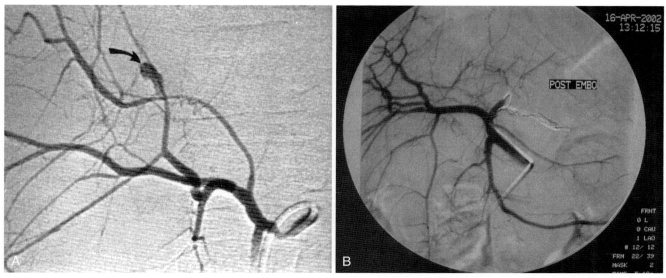

FIGURE 20-9   A, Hepatic artery angiogram in a patient with persistent hemorrhage after initial damage-control laparotomy. The bleeding vessel is identified (*curved arrow*). **B,** Successful embolization was performed.

Abbreviated laparotomy with packing for hemostasis, allowing resuscitation before planned reoperation, is an alternative in unstable patients in whom further blood loss would be untenable. This damage-control philosophy is a systematic, phased approach to the management of exsanguinating trauma patients.[78–80] The three phases of damage control are detailed in Table 20-6. Although controversial, several resuscitative end points have been proposed beyond the conventional vital signs and urine output, including serum lactate, base deficit, mixed venous oxygen saturation, and gastric mucosal pH. Once a patient is rewarmed, coagulation factors are replaced, and oxygen delivery is optimized, he or she can be returned to the operating room for pack removal and definitive repair of injuries. A review of nearly 700 adult patients treated by abdominal packing from several institutions demonstrated hemostasis in 80%, survival of 32% to 73%, and abdominal abscess rates of 10% to 40%.[81,82] Although abdominal packing with planned reoperation has been used with increasing frequency in adults during the past 2 decades, there is little published experience in children.[61,83–88] Nevertheless, we believe that this technique has a place in the management of children with massive intra-abdominal bleeding, especially after blunt trauma. As an example, we reported a 3-year-old child who required abdominal packing for a severe liver injury, making closure of the abdomen impossible.[88] A Silastic silo was constructed to accommodate the bowel until the packing could be removed. The patient made a complete recovery. The combined technique of packing and a silo allowed time for correction of the hypothermia, acidosis, and coagulopathy without compromise of respiratory mechanics. One review reported 22 infants and children (age 6 days to 20 years) with refractory hemorrhage who were treated with abdominal packing.[87] The anatomic site of hemorrhage was the liver or hepatic veins in 14, retroperitoneum or pelvis in 7, and pancreatic bed in 1. Primary fascial closure was accomplished in 12 patients (55%), and temporary skin closure or prosthetic material was used in the other 10. Packing controlled hemorrhage in 21 of 22 patients (95%). Removal of the packing was possible within 72 hours in 18 patients (82%). No patient rebled after the packing was removed; however, 2 patients died with the packing in place. Seven patients (32%) developed an abdominal or pelvic abscess, and all were successfully drained by laparotomy (6 patients) or percutaneously (1 patient); 6 of the 7 patients with abdominal sepsis survived. Overall, 18 patients (82%) survived. Two deaths were due to multisystem organ failure, one to cardiac failure from complex cardiac anomalies, and one to exsanguination after blunt traumatic liver injury. There were no differences in the volume of intraoperative blood product transfusion, time to initiate packing, physiologic status, or type of abdominal closure between survivors and nonsurvivors.

Preperitoneal pelvic packing for hemodynamically unstable patients with pelvic fracture is another unique use of pack tamponade in life-threatening hemorrhage.[89]

Although the success of abdominal packing is encouraging, it may contribute to significant morbidity, such as intra-abdominal sepsis, organ failure, and increased intra-abdominal pressure. Intra-abdominal packs are contaminated by skin and gut flora, but these organisms are not those implicated in

TABLE 20-6	
Damage-Control Strategy in Exsanguinating Trauma Patients	
Phase 1	Abbreviated laparotomy for exploration
	Control of hemorrhage and contamination
	Packing and temporary abdominal wall closure
Phase 2	Aggressive ICU resuscitation
	Core rewarming
	Optimization of volume and oxygen delivery
	Correction of coagulopathy
Phase 3	Planned reoperation(s) for packing change
	Definitive repair of injuries
	Abdominal wall closure

ICU, Intensive care unit.

subsequent patient sepsis.[90] Adams and colleagues[91] evaluated fluid samples from 28 patients with abdominal packing and found peritoneal endotoxin and mediator accumulation even when cultures were sterile. The authors concluded that laparotomy pad fluid accumulating after damage-control laparotomy can contribute to neutrophil dysfunction by enhancing neutrophil respiratory burst and inhibiting neutrophil responses to specific chemotactic mediators needed to fight infection. Thus the known propensity of such patients to both intra-abdominal and systemic infection may be related to changes in neutrophil receptor status and effector function related to the accumulation of inflammatory mediators in the abdomen. Early washout, repetitive packing, and other efforts to minimize mediator accumulation deserve consideration.

It is essential to emphasize that the success of the abbreviated laparotomy and planned reoperation depends on an early decision to use this strategy before irreversible shock occurs. When used as a desperate, last-ditch resort after prolonged attempts at hemostasis have failed, abdominal packing has been uniformly unsuccessful. Physiologic and anatomic criteria have been identified as indications for abdominal packing. Most of these focus on intraoperative parameters, including pH ($\approx$7.2), core temperature ($<35°$ C), and coagulation values (prothrombin time >16 seconds), in a patient with profuse hemorrhage requiring large volumes of blood product transfusion.

The optimal time for reexploration is controversial, because neither the physiologic end points of resuscitation nor the increased risk of infection with prolonged packing are well defined. The obvious benefits of hemostasis provided by packing are also balanced against the potential deleterious effects of increased intra-abdominal pressure on ventilation, cardiac output, renal function, mesenteric circulation, and intracranial pressure. Timely alleviation of the secondary abdominal compartment syndrome may be a critical salvage maneuver for patients. Temporary abdominal wall closure at the time of packing can prevent the abdominal compartment syndrome. We recommend temporary abdominal wall expansion in all patients requiring packing, until hemostasis is obtained and visceral edema subsides.

A staged operative strategy for unstable trauma patients represents advanced surgical care and requires sound judgment and technical expertise. Intra-abdominal packing for control of exsanguinating hemorrhage is a lifesaving maneuver in highly selected patients in whom coagulopathy, hypothermia, and acidosis render further surgical procedures unduly hazardous. Early identification of patients likely to benefit from abbreviated laparotomy techniques is crucial for success.

ABDOMINAL COMPARTMENT SYNDROME

The abdominal compartment syndrome is a term used to describe the deleterious effects of increased intra-abdominal pressure.[92] The syndrome includes respiratory insufficiency from worsening ventilation-perfusion mismatch, hemodynamic compromise from preload reduction resulting from inferior vena cava compression, impaired renal function resulting from renal vein compression, decreased cardiac output, intracranial hypertension resulting from increased ventilator pressures, splanchnic hypoperfusion, and abdominal wall overdistention. The causes of intra-abdominal hypertension in trauma patients include hemoperitoneum, retroperitoneal or bowel edema, and use of abdominal or pelvic

packing. The combination of tissue injury and hemodynamic shock creates a cascade of events, including capillary leak, ischemia-reperfusion, and release of vasoactive mediators and free radicals, which combine to increase extracellular volume and tissue edema. Experimental evidence indicates that there are significant alterations in cytokine levels in the presence of sustained intra-abdominal pressure elevation.[93,94] Once the combined effects of tissue edema and intra-abdominal fluid exceed a certain level, abdominal decompression must be considered.

The adverse effects of abdominal compartment syndrome have been acknowledged for decades; however, abdominal compartment syndrome has only recently been recognized as a life-threatening but potentially treatable entity.[95,96] The incidence of this complication has increased markedly in recent years due to high-volume resuscitation protocols. Measurement of intra-abdominal pressure can be useful in determining the contribution of abdominal compartment syndrome to altered physiologic and metabolic parameters.[97,98] Intra-abdominal pressure can be determined by measuring bladder pressure. This involves instilling 1 mL/kg of saline into the Foley catheter and connecting it to a pressure transducer or manometer through a three-way stopcock. The symphysis pubis is used as the zero reference point, and the pressure is measured in centimeters of water or millimeters of mercury. Intra-abdominal pressures in the range of 20 to 35 cm H_2O or 15 to 25 mm Hg have been identified as an indication to decompress the abdomen. Many prefer to intervene according to alterations in other physiologic and metabolic parameters rather than a specific pressure measurement. Chang and colleagues[97] reported 11 adult trauma patients with abdominal compartment syndrome in whom abdominal decompression using pulmonary artery catheters and gastric tonometry improved preload, pulmonary function, and visceral perfusion. Anecdotally, decompressive laparotomy has been used successfully to reduce refractory intracranial hypertension in patients with isolated brain injury without overt signs of abdominal compartment syndrome.[99]

Experience with abdominal decompression for abdominal compartment syndrome in children is limited.[*] Nonspecific abdominal CT findings in children with abdominal compartment syndrome include narrowing of the inferior vena cava, direct renal compression or displacement, bowel wall thickening with enhancement, and a rounded appearance of the abdomen.[100] Neville and colleagues[101] reported the use of patch abdominoplasty in 23 infants and children, only 3 of whom were trauma patients. These authors found that patch abdominoplasty for abdominal compartment syndrome effectively decreased airway pressures and oxygen requirements. Failure to respond with a decrease in airway pressures or fraction of inspired oxygen was an ominous sign in their series. Several authors have found that abdominal decompression resulted in decreased airway pressures, increased oxygen tension, and increased urine output in children with abdominal compartment syndrome.[95,98,101]

Many materials have been suggested for use in temporary patch abdominoplasty, including Silastic sheeting, Gore-Tex sheeting, intravenous bags, cystoscopy bags, ostomy appliances, and various mesh materials. The vacuum-pack

---

* References 87, 88, 95, 98, 100, 101.

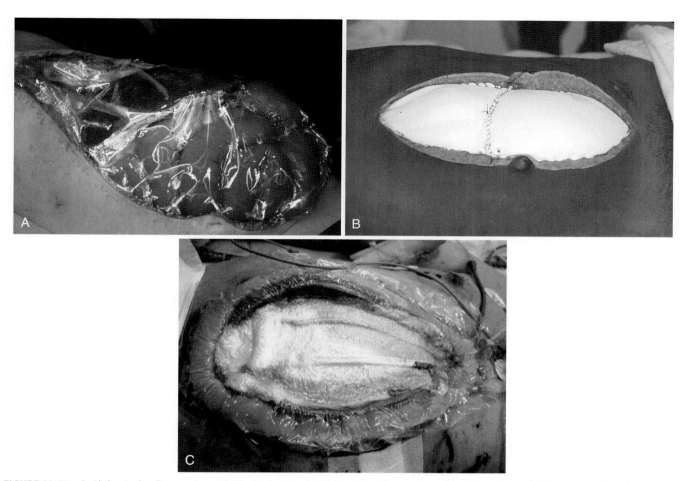

FIGURE 20-10   A, Abdominal wall expansion with Silastic sheeting. **B,** Abdominal wall expansion with a Gore-Tex patch. **C,** Vacuum-pack technique. *(See Expert Consult site for color version of part **C**)*

technique, used successfully in adults, has been an outstanding addition in children (Fig. 20-10).[78,85,102] Use of the vacuum-pack technique at the first trauma laparotomy may limit the early benefits of the open abdomen by resulting in a lower volume reserve capacity.[103]

BILE DUCT INJURY

Nonoperative management of pediatric blunt liver injury is highly successful but is complicated by a 4% risk of persistent bile leakage.[104,105] Radionuclide scanning is recommended when biliary tree injury is suspected.[106] Delayed views may show a bile leak even if early views are normal. Several reports have highlighted the benefits of endoscopic retrograde cholangiopancreatography (ERCP) with placement of transampullary biliary stents for biliary duct injury following blunt hepatic trauma. Although ERCP is invasive and requires conscious sedation, it can pinpoint the site of injury and allow treatment of the injured ducts without open surgery (Fig. 20-11). Endoscopic transampullary biliary decompression is a recent addition to the treatment options for patients with persistent bile leakage. The addition of sphincterotomy during ERCP for persistent bile leakage following blunt liver injury has been advocated to decrease intrabiliary pressure and encourage internal decompression.[105–108] It is important to note that endoscopic biliary stents may migrate or become obstructed and require specific treatment.

Injuries to the Duodenum and Pancreas

In contrast to the liver and spleen, injuries to the duodenum and pancreas are much less frequent, accounting for less than 10% of intra-abdominal injuries in children sustaining blunt trauma. Isolated duodenal and pancreatic injuries occur in approximately two thirds of cases, with combined injuries to both organs occurring in the remainder. The severity of the duodenal or pancreatic injury and associated injuries determines the necessity for operative versus nonoperative management. The "protected" retroperitoneum both limits the chance of injury and increases the difficulty of early diagnosis. Added to this diagnostic dilemma is the frequency of associated intra-abdominal or multisystem injuries, which can mask subtle physical and radiographic diagnostic signs of injury to the duodenum and pancreas.

DUODENUM

In a report on blunt duodenal rupture, Ballard and colleagues[109] reviewed a 6-year statewide (Pennsylvania) experience. Of 103,864 patients registered from 28 trauma centers, blunt injury to the duodenum occurred in 206 (0.2%), of whom only 30 (14%) had full-thickness rupture. The mechanism of injury was car crash in 70%, which included both adults

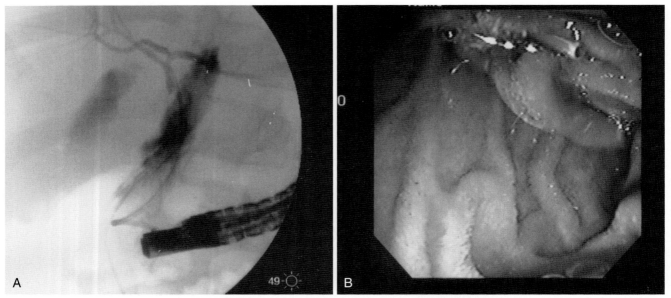

FIGURE 20-11 **A,** Endoscopic retrograde cholangiopancreatography demonstrating several bile leaks after blunt liver injury. **B,** Endoscopic view of transampullary biliary stent.

and children. Of those without significant head injury (26 of 30), 92% either reported abdominal pain or had tenderness or rebound on physical examination. CT was performed in 18 patients; retroperitoneal air or extravasation of contrast was seen in only 26% of scans; an equal number were interpreted as normal. Mortality was 13% and was not affected by a delay in diagnosis or treatment. This study emphasizes the difficulty of analyzing this injury because of the low numbers reported by individual centers (and surgeons). Additionally, the investigators reviewed the range of repairs performed—from duodenal closure to the Whipple procedure—but commented that no definitive recommendations could be made because of the small number of patients and the many centers reporting.

In contrast, a group from Toronto reported a single-center experience in a series of 27 children (mean age, 7 years) sustaining blunt duodenal injuries and treated over a 10-year period.[110] Thirteen children had duodenal perforations (mean age, 9 years), and 14 sustained duodenal hematomas (mean age, 5 years). Associated injuries were seen in 19 patients (10 pancreas, 5 spleen, 4 liver, 2 long bone fracture, 1 central nervous system, 1 renal contusion, 1 jejunal perforation, and 1 gastric rupture). Seventeen patients were transferred from other facilities, with a 4-hour median time to transfer. The median interval from injury to surgery in those sustaining perforation was 6 hours. A comparison of the clinical presentation, laboratory evaluation, and radiographic findings in those with duodenal hematoma versus perforation is presented in Table 20-7. Most patients had abdominal CT scans performed with oral and intravenous contrast (Figs. 20-12 and 20-13). A comparison of CT findings in these patient groups is presented in Table 20-8. These data demonstrate that the clinical presentation is strikingly similar in both groups, with only age and injury severity score achieving statistical significance (but of little clinical relevance in individual patients). However, extravasation of air or enteral contrast into the retroperitoneal, periduodenal, or prerenal space was found in every child with a duodenal perforation (9 of 9) but in none of the 10 who had duodenal hematoma. The authors noted that few previous reports in the literature described these specific CT findings with duodenal injuries in general, and in particular, no previous series of pediatric patients had been reported. The CT scans (or upper GI contrast studies in equivocal cases) showing duodenal narrowing, corkscrewing, or obstruction without extravasation were diagnostic in all cases. In the current series of 14 patients treated nonoperatively, the duration of nasogastric decompression was 12 days (mean), and the length of total parenteral nutrition administration was 18 days (mean). Symptoms resolved in 13 of 14 patients an average of 16 days after injury. The remaining child developed a chronic fibrous stricture requiring operative duodenoplasty 49 days after injury. This child also had a pancreatic contusion.

Desai and colleagues,[111] from St. Louis Children's Hospital, reviewed their experience with 24 duodenal injuries from blunt abdominal trauma. There were 19 duodenal hematomas (15 diagnosed by CT, and 4 by upper GI studies), 17 of which were treated nonoperatively. In those with perforation, 4 of 5 were amenable to simple suture repair. The experiences from Salt Lake City and Pittsburgh emphasize an alarming finding that a common cause of duodenal trauma is child abuse, especially in younger patients.[112,113] Therefore isolated duodenal injures should raise suspicion if the history or mechanism of injury described is inconsistent with the actual injury.

In all these series, patients sustaining duodenal perforation were treated operatively in a variety of ways, depending on the injury severity and the surgeon's preference. We recommend primary closure of a duodenal perforation (whenever possible). Primary closure can be combined with duodenal drainage and either pyloric exclusion with gastrojejunostomy (Fig. 20-14) or gastric drainage with feeding jejunostomy. These surgical options decrease the incidence of duodenal fistula, reduce the time to GI tract alimentation, and shorten hospital stay. When faced with complicated

TABLE 20-7

Presenting Symptoms and Signs in Children with Duodenal Hematoma and Duodenal Perforation

Patient	Duodenal Hematoma	Duodenal Perforation
Number	14	13
Age (yr)	5	9*
ISS score	10	25*
Seat belt worn: number (%)	6 (100)	5 (71)
Presentation		
Pain or tenderness:	10 (71)	12 (92)
number (%)		11 (85)
Bruising: no. (%)	6 (43)	
GCS score	15	15
Associated injuries		
Pancreatic: number (%)	7 (50)	3 (23)
Lumbar spine: no. (%)	1 (7)	4 (31)
Total: number (%)	11 (79)	8 (62)
Laboratory evaluation		
Hgb: mg %/Hct	12.3/0.36	12.1/0.37
Amylase: units (%)	678 (64)	332 (46)

From Shilyansky J, Pearl RH, Kroutouro M, et al: Diagnosis and management of duodenal injuries in children. J Pediatr Surg 1997:32:880-886.
*Statistically significant difference.
GCS, Glasgow Coma Scale; Hct, hematocrit; Hgb, hemoglobin; ISS, Injury Severity Scale.

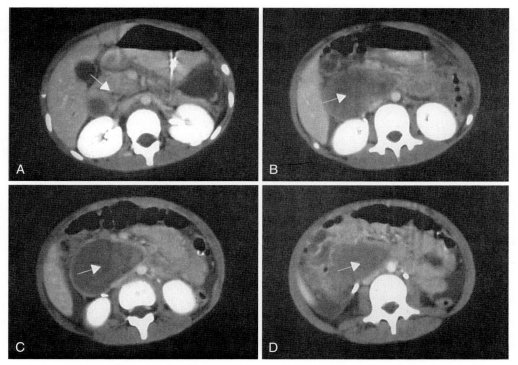

FIGURE 20-12 Abdominal computed tomography findings in an 8-year-old girl who sustained a duodenal hematoma after a fall at a playground. **A,** The *arrow* points to the markedly narrowed duodenal lumen. **B** to **D,** The *arrows* point to the large intramural hematoma. The child was treated with nasogastric suction and total parenteral nutrition. She was eating a regular diet 24 days after her injury.

duodenal trauma, an effective combination is the three-tube technique: duodenal closure (primary repair, serosal patch, or anastomosis) with duodenal drainage tube for decompression (tube 1), pyloric exclusion with an absorbable suture through gastrotomy and gastric tube placement (tube 2), and feeding jejunostomy (tube 3). Several closed suction drains are placed adjacent to the repair. When the duodenum is excluded (by an absorbable suture for temporary closure of the pylorus), complete healing of the injury routinely occurs before the spontaneous reopening of the pyloric channel (Fig. 20-15). Bioprosthetic repair of complex duodenal injury in a porcine model has been reported and could add to operative strategies.[114]

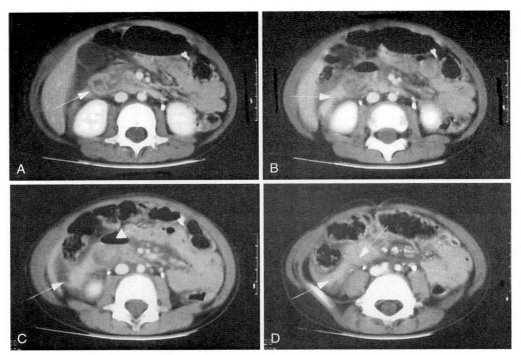

FIGURE 20-13 Abdominal computed tomography findings in a 4-year-old boy with duodenal perforation caused by a motor vehicle accident. **A,** The *arrow* points to the disrupted duodenal wall. **B** to **D,** Arrows point to extravasated retroperitoneal enteral contrast and extraluminal retroperitoneal air. A large defect involving the second and third portions of the duodenum was found. Primary repair, pyloric exclusion, tube duodenostomy, and gastrojejunostomy were performed. The child resumed eating 5 days after injury and went home 4 days later.

TABLE 20-8

Comparison of Computed Tomography Findings in Children with Duodenal Hematoma and Duodenal Perforation

Finding	Duodenal Hematoma (n = 10) Number (%)	Duodenal Perforation (n = 9) Number (%)
Free air	1 (10)*	2 (22)
Free fluid	8 (80)	9 (100)
Retroperitoneal fluid	9 (90)	9 (100)
Bowel wall and peritoneal enhancement	2 (20)	4 (44)
Duodenal caliber change	4 (40)	3 (33)
Thickened duodenum	10 (100)	8 (89)
Mural hematoma	10 (100)	0
Retroperitoneal air	0	8 (89)
Retroperitoneal contrast†	0	4 (57)
Retroperitoneal air or contrast	0	9 (100)

From Shilyansky J, Pearl RH, Kroutouro M, et al: Diagnosis and management of duodenal injuries in children. J Pediatr Surg 1997:32:880-886.
*The child had an associated jejunal perforation.
†Enteral contrast was not administered in two children.

However, no matter what repair the surgeon selects, a summary of the literature demonstrates that protecting the duodenal closure (drain and exclusion) and a route for enteral feeding (gastrojejunostomy or feeding jejunostomy) reduces morbidity and hospital length of stay.[115,116]

The surgical options are listed in Table 20-9 and illustrated in Figures 20-14 and 20-16. Of note, pancreaticoduodenectomy (the Whipple procedure) is rarely required. Although occasionally reported in the literature, pancreaticoduodenectomy should be reserved for the most severe injuries to the duodenum and pancreas in which the common blood supply is destroyed and reconstruction is impossible.

PANCREAS

Injuries to the pancreas are slightly more frequent than duodenal injuries, with estimated ranges from 3% to 12% in children sustaining blunt abdominal trauma. As with duodenal injuries, individual centers frequently have small patient numbers and thus are unable to evaluate their results critically. Recently, two centers (Toronto and San Diego) reported their experience with divergent methods of managing blunt traumatic pancreatic injuries in a series of reports.[117–121] Here we compare these papers and excerpt other authors' experience to make management recommendations.

Canty and Weinman (San Diego)[118] reported 18 patients with major pancreatic injuries over a 14-year period. The mechanism of injury was car or bike crashes. Sixteen of the

18 patients had CT scans on admission. Of these, 11 suggested injury; in 5, the injury was missed. Distal pancreatectomy was performed in 8 patients (44%). In 5 of 6 patients with either proximal duct injuries or injuries missed on the initial CT scan, pseudocysts developed; pseudocysts also occurred in 2 other children who had minimal initial symptoms and no admission CT scans. Of these 7 pseudocysts, 2 resolved and 5 were treated by cystogastrostomy. Two patients, treated more recently, received endoscopic retrograde cholangiopancreatography (ERCP) with duct stenting and experienced resolution of symptoms and complete healing. The authors concluded that distal injuries should be treated with distal pancreatectomy, proximal injuries with observation, and pseudocysts with observation or cystogastrostomy. They also concluded that acute ERCP management with stent placement is safe and effective, and that CT is suggestive but not always diagnostic for the type and location of pancreatic injuries.[117,118]

The experience summarized in three reports from Toronto is markedly different.[119–121] The extensive CT findings suggestive of pancreatic injury are detailed in Table 20-10. In the first brief report, 2 patients with documented duct disruption (by ERCP or cathetergram) had complete duct healing without operative intervention.[119] This was followed by a summary report of 35 consecutive children treated over 10 years (1987 to 1996).[120] Twenty-three had early diagnosis (<24 hours), whereas diagnosis was delayed (2 to 14 days) in 12 patients. Twenty-eight children were treated nonoperatively, and the other 7 had operations for other injuries. In the 28 cases treated nonoperatively, CT was diagnostic, revealing five patterns of injury: contusion, stellate fragmentation, partial fracture, complete transection, and pseudocyst (Fig. 20-17). The patients were placed in three clinical groups based on CT grade (Table 20-11). In these 28 patients, pseudocysts occurred in 10 (2 of 14 in group 1, 5 of 11 in group 2, and 3 of 3 in group 3). No patients in group 1 required drainage, whereas 4 in group 2, and all 3 in group 3 required intervention. These drainage procedures occurred 10 to 14 days after injury. Average time for the initiation of oral feeding was 15 days (11 days for group 1, 15 days for group 2, and 23 days for group 3). Mean hospital stay for all patients treated nonoperatively was 21 days.

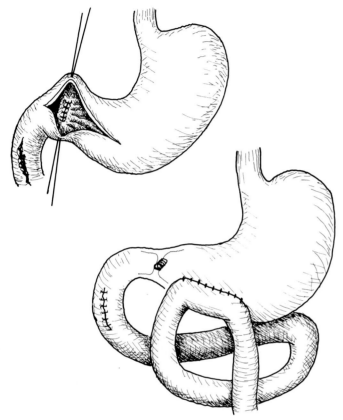

FIGURE 20-14 Lateral duodenal injury treated by primary duodenal repair and pyloric exclusion consisting of closing the pylorus with an absorbable suture and gastrojejunostomy. Closed suction drainage of the repair is not depicted. (Original illustration by Mark Mazziotti, MD.)

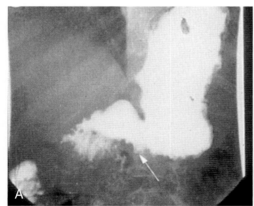
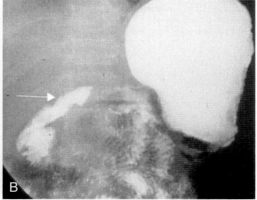

FIGURE 20-15 Upper gastrointestinal study of a 7-year-old girl with duodenal perforation resulting from a motor vehicle accident. Primary repair, pyloric exclusion, retrograde tube duodenostomy, gastrojejunostomy, and feeding gastrostomy were performed. The child tolerated jejunal feeds 6 days after the injury and oral feeds 12 days after the injury. **A,** Six weeks postinjury, an upper gastrointestinal study demonstrated spontaneous closure of the gastrojejunostomy (*arrow*). **B,** A patent pylorus is evident (*arrow*).

TABLE 20-9

Surgical Options in Duodenal Trauma

Repair of the duodenum

Diversion of the gastrointestinal tract (pyloric exclusion or duodenal diverticularization)

Gastric decompression (gastric tube insertion or gastrojejunostomy)

Gastrointestinal tract access for feeding (jejunostomy tube or gastrojejunal anastomosis)

Decompression of the duodenum (duodenostomy tube)

Biliary tube drainage

Wide drainage of the repaired area (lateral duodenal drains)

TABLE 20-10

Summary of Associated CT Findings in Children with Pancreatic Injuries

Associated Finding	Number of Children
Intraperitoneal fluid	21
Lesser sac fluid	20
Focal peripancreatic fluid	20
Retroperitoneal fluid	20
Right anterior pararenal fluid	16
Left anterior pararenal fluid	15
Thickened Gerota fascia (right and left)	16
Mesenteric fluid or hematoma	13
Left posterior pararenal fluid	9
Fluid separating SV and pancreas	7
Fluid surrounding SMV and PV	7
Fluid separating pancreas and duodenum	6

Data from references 119-121.
CT, Computed tomography; PV, portal vein; SMV, superior mesenteric vein; SV, splenic vein.

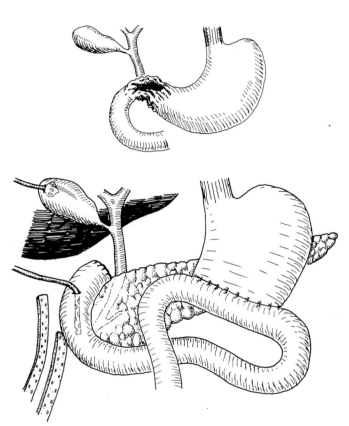

FIGURE 20-16 Duodenal diverticularization for combined proximal duodenal and pancreatic injury. Resection and closure of the duodenal stump, tube duodenostomy, tube cholecystostomy, gastrojejunostomy, and multiple closed suction drains are depicted. A feeding jejunostomy should be strongly considered (not depicted). (Original illustration by Mark Mazziotti, MD.)

A comparison of the San Diego and Toronto protocols is depicted in Figure 20-18. The striking differences in these series are the 100% diagnostic sensitivity of CT in Toronto versus 69% in San Diego and the 44% operative rate in San Diego versus 0% in Toronto. A subsequent study from Toronto reviewed the follow-up on 10 patients with duct transections.[121] Four of these children (40%) developed pseudocysts, three of which were drained percutaneously (Fig. 20-19). The mean hospital stay was 24 days, and all recovered. Follow-up CT in eight of nine patients revealed atrophy of the distal pancreas in six and completely normal glands in two. There was no exocrine or endocrine dysfunction in a mean of 47 months of follow-up. The authors concluded that

following nonoperative management of pancreatic blunt trauma, atrophy (distal) or recanalization occurs in all cases with no long-term morbidity.

Reports from Dallas and Seattle favor early distal pancreatectomy for transection to the left of the spine to shorten hospital stay.[122,123] However, long-term sequelae of adhesive intestinal obstruction and endocrine and exocrine dysfunction were not assessed. Other reports document the efficacy of magnetic resonance pancreatography as a diagnostic tool, early ERCP intervention for diagnosis and treatment with ductal stenting, and the use of somatostatin to decrease pancreatic secretions and promote healing.[124–128] Of note, a large single-center series from Japan reported nonoperative management in 19 of 20 children with documented pancreatic injury (9 contusions, 6 lacerations, and 5 main duct disruptions).[129] In all cases, recovery was complete without surgery. That center's experience with pseudocyst formation and treatment and overall outcome virtually mirrors that of the Toronto report. A recent report from Denver documents their experience with pediatric pancreas injury over an 11-year period.[127] All (n = 18) with grade I injuries were treated nonoperatively. Children with grades II to IV received operative treatment in 14 and nonoperative in 11 cases. They concluded that children undergoing operative treatment had fewer pseudocysts but similar length of stay because of nonpancreatic complications.

These reports from major pediatric trauma centers are clearly in conflict. Some favor and document the efficacy and safety of observational care for virtually all pancreatic injuries, including duct disruption; others advocate aggressive surgical management with debridement or resection. Because proponents supply compelling data for each of these treatments, algorithms reflecting individual hospital or surgeon preference will probably determine which treatment plan is selected. However, it is clear that with simple transection of the pancreas at or to the left of the spine, spleen-sparing distal pancreatectomy can provide definitive care for this isolated injury, with short hospitalization and acceptable morbidity (Fig. 20-20). Laparoscopic techniques may limit perioperative morbidity.[128]

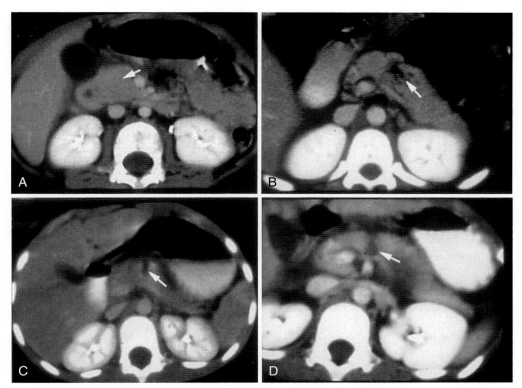

FIGURE 20-17 Computed tomography findings in children with pancreatic trauma. **A,** Contusion. **B,** Stellate fragmentation. **C,** Partial fracture. **D,** Transection. Arrows indicate the specific pancreatic injury.

TABLE 20-11

Proposed Classification of CT Findings in Children with Pancreatic Injuries

Group (Clinical)	Grade (CT)	Pancreatic Injury	Description	Number of Children
1	I	Contusion	Diffuse or focal swelling of the pancreas	14
2	II	Stellate fragmentation	Fluid or blood dissecting within pancreatic parenchyma	2
	III	Partial fracture	Incomplete separation of two portions of the pancreas	1
3	IV	Complete transection	Complete separation of two portions of the pancreas	8
	V	Pseudocyst	Persistent peripancreatic fluid collection	3

Data from references 119-121.
CT, Computed tomography.

With this controversy in mind, we favor conservative therapy whenever possible, including the following:

1. Early spiral CT with oral and intravenous contrast in all patients who, by history, physical examination, or mechanism of injury, may have blunt trauma to the pancreas
2. Documentation of injuries and early ERCP to provide duct stenting in selected cases
3. Nonoperative management with total parenteral nutrition
4. Expectant management of pseudocyst formation
5. Percutaneous drainage for symptomatic, infected, or enlarging pseudocyst (Fig. 20-21)

Injuries of the Stomach, Small Intestine, and Colon

Several different mechanisms cause distinct patterns of injury to these hollow organs. First is a crush injury that occurs as the stomach, jejunum, ileum, or transverse colon is compressed violently against the spine. Hematomas, lacerations, or partial or complete transections can occur with instantaneous or delayed perforation or obstruction. Second, burst injury occurs when rapid compressive forces are applied to a filled and distended hollow viscus, without direct mechanical compression. Shoulder-belt and seat-belt injuries to the GI tract can occur in this fashion. Third is shear injury caused by rapid acceleration–deceleration of an organ that is tethered at one end, such as the ligament of Treitz, ileocecal region, or rectosigmoid junction. With deceleration, the injury is caused by the tearing of tissue at the point of fixation.

Regardless of the mechanism of injury, a perforated viscus causes rapid contamination of the abdominal cavity. On the initial trauma assessment, virtually all neurologically intact patients have some symptoms (pain) and physical findings (tenderness, guarding, rebound). In fact, many reports have documented that the initial and serial physical examinations have a higher degree of diagnostic specificity than US or CT for these injuries.[130–132] In a series from New Mexico

San Diego (OR = 40%)[17]

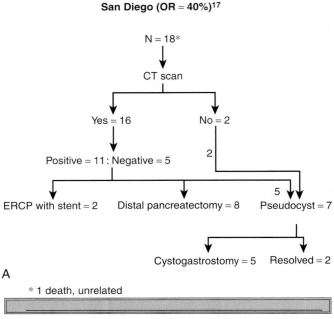

N = 18*

CT scan

Yes = 16   No = 2

Positive = 11 : Negative = 5   2

ERCP with stent = 2   Distal pancreatectomy = 8   5   Pseudocyst = 7

Cystogastrostomy = 5   Resolved = 2

A

* 1 death, unrelated

Toronto (OR = 0%)[126]

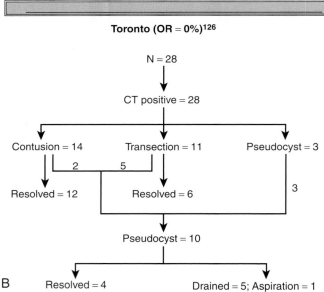

N = 28

CT positive = 28

Contusion = 14   Transection = 11   Pseudocyst = 3

2   5

Resolved = 12   Resolved = 6   3

Pseudocyst = 10

B   Resolved = 4   Drained = 5; Aspiration = 1

FIGURE 20-18 Comparison of protocols in the management of blunt pancreas injury in children. **A,** San Diego. **B,** Toronto. CT, Computed tomography; ERCP, endoscopic retrograde cholangiopancreatography; OR, operating room. (**A,** From Canty TG Sr, Weinman D: Management of major pancreatic duct injuries in children. J Trauma 2001;50:1001-1007; **B,** from Shilyansky J, Sen LM, Kreller M, et al: Nonoperative management of pancreatic injuries in children. J Pediatr Surg 1998;33:343-345.)

reporting 48 patients with small bowel injury, all conscious patients had abnormal physical findings either on presentation or after serial physical examinations.[131] Other diagnostic tests (US, CT, DPL, laboratory tests) were of comparatively less value. These findings were confirmed by a similar series from North Carolina involving 32 children with intestinal injury confirmed at laparotomy; 94% had physical findings suggestive of intestinal injury on admission, with 84% having diffuse abdominal tenderness (peritoneal signs).[132] Prompt diagnosis of these injuries is possible when free air and GI contrast extravasates into the abdominal cavity at the time of the initial injury. However, when partial-thickness lacerations, hematomas, or avulsed

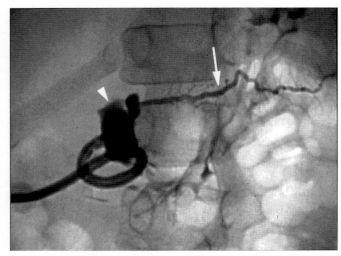

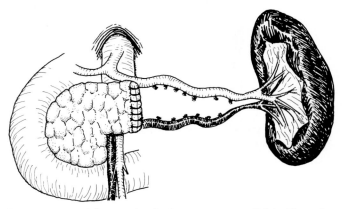

FIGURE 20-19 Contrast study through a percutaneous drain placed into a pancreatic pseudocyst (*arrowhead*) after blunt trauma in a child. Communication with the main pancreatic duct (*arrow*) is demonstrated. The pseudocyst resolved without fistula formation or operative intervention.

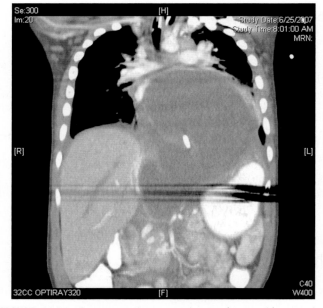

FIGURE 20-20 Spleen-sparing distal pancreatectomy. (Original illustration by Mark Mazziotti, MD.)

FIGURE 20-21 Post-traumatic pancreatic pseudocyst with extension into the mediastinum causing respiratory distress.

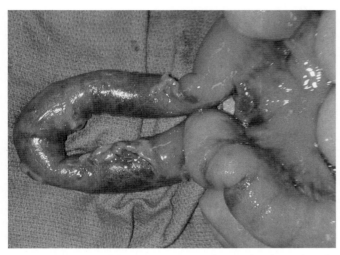

FIGURE 20-22 Small bowel mesentery avulsion with ischemic bowel.

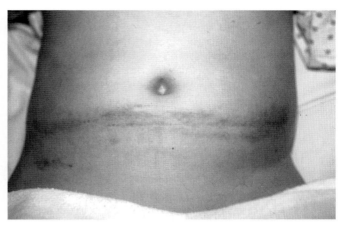

FIGURE 20-23 Seat-belt sign across the lower abdomen.

mesenteric blood vessels occur, progression to full-thickness defects with leakage can be delayed over hours to days (Fig. 20-22). A high index of suspicion is indicated, along with the liberal use of serial physical examinations.

The APSA Trauma Committee recently performed a multi-institutional, retrospective review to determine whether delay in treatment of blunt intestinal perforation adversely affected outcome.[133] Their data in 214 patients suggested that delay in operative treatment up to 24 hours did not have a significant effect on prognosis after pediatric blunt intestinal injury, even when there is peritoneal contamination secondary to perforation.

Injuries to the stomach and small intestine are straight-forward to repair. A full stomach usually ruptures at the greater curvature with a blowout or stellate configuration. Debridement with direct repair is virtually always sufficient. Small intestinal injuries run the gamut from simple laceration to transection to complete avulsion with larger segments of compromised bowel. However, unless the contamination is massive (or other injuries require extensive repair), debridement or resection with anastomosis is usually sufficient. In colon injuries, particularly if there is a delay in diagnosis and significant fecal contamination, colostomy with a defunctionalized distal mucous fistula or a Hartmann pouch is in order. If isolated colon injuries occur and are repaired early, on-table bowel irrigation, bowel anastomosis, and perioperative antibiotic coverage are safe and effective and avoid the complications caused by stomas and reoperation. The critical factors with injuries to the intraperitoneal GI tract are early recognition of the injury; prompt resuscitation; expeditious surgery, with complete removal of contaminated and devitalized tissue; reconstruction or diversion of the GI tract, as clinically indicated; and broad-spectrum antibiotics, with the duration of therapy dependent on the degree of contamination and postoperative clinical course (e.g., normalization of white blood cell count, absence of fever, return of GI tract function). Laparoscopic techniques may limit perioperative morbidity.[17]

SEAT-BELT SIGN

Seat belts, when compared with no restraint, reduce serious injury and death by 50%.[134] Frequent physical examinations and vigilance are required for the subset of injuries caused by lap-belt restraints when children are passengers in high-speed automobile crashes.[130] These children present with visible seat-belt signs on physical examination of the abdomen (Fig. 20-23). Multiple studies have documented increased abdominal injuries to both solid and hollow organs with this finding.[135–137] However, a large retrospective review of 331 child occupants in motor vehicle crashes found that the seat-belt sign had relative risk of only 1.7 for an abdominal injury.[138] An interesting triad of injuries has been noted: abdominal wall contusions or herniation, chance fractures of the lumbar spine, and isolated jejunal or ileal perforations. One report reviewed 95 patients admitted with abdominal trauma, all of whom were wearing seat belts at the time of injury; in 60 of 95, there was a seat-belt sign.[137] Nine (15%) of the 60 patients with the seat-belt sign had intestinal injuries, compared with none of the 35 without the seat-belt sign. The more common injuries described earlier can distract both the patient and the trauma team, causing delay in the diagnosis of serious vascular injuries involving the aorta and iliac vessels.[139–141]

In recent reports from Philadelphia, a database created by the State Farm Insurance Company was used to review 147,985 children who were passengers in motor vehicle crashes.[142,143] In that series, 1967 children (1.33%) had abdominal bruising from seat-belt restraints. Although abdominal wall bruising was infrequent, those with this finding were 232 times more likely to have a significant intra-abdominal injury than were those without a bruise. These data further revealed that 1 of 9 children with an abdominal seat-belt sign had a significant intra-abdominal injury. Therefore, although the seat-belt sign is rare, CT scanning (admission and serial) is mandated when it is present. Optimal ($n = 881$) and suboptimal ($n = 1086$) use of seat-belt restraints was noted. After adjusting for age and seating position, optimally restrained children were more than 3 times less likely (odds ratio 3.51) than suboptimally restrained children to suffer an abdominal injury.

Our recommendation is to admit all children involved in a motor vehicle crash who present with a seat-belt sign, even in the setting of a "normal" FAST and/or abdominal CT. Progression of an intestinal wall crush should be detected with serial examinations with or without repeat imaging.

IMAGING FOR GASTROINTESTINAL INJURY

Imaging of the GI tract has evolved over the past decade, with spiral CT or FAST examinations done by surgeons in the emergency department directly impacting diagnostic accuracy and decision making. Some of the strengths and weaknesses of CT diagnosis have already been discussed. However, the ability to diagnose and treat blunt abdominal trauma in children has clearly been enhanced by this modality. Two studies from Toronto examined these issues. The first, reviewed 12 patients with blunt abdominal trauma evaluated by CT and found that bowel wall enhancement was a sign of either global GI tract ischemia associated with fatal central nervous system injury or bowel perforation when seen with bowel wall thickening and free peritoneal fluid.[144] A follow-up study reviewed 43 patients evaluated over 10 years with surgically confirmed GI tract perforation.[14] Extraluminal air was seen in 47%, with one false-positive. Five CT findings were found to be suggestive but not diagnostic of GI tract perforation: extraluminal air, free intraperitoneal fluid, bowel wall thickening, bowel wall enhancement, and bowel dilation. In every patient who had all five of these findings, bowel perforation was confirmed. However, this occurred in only 18% of the study population. All patients had at least one of these five specific CT findings. There were no false-negative studies. As mentioned previously, although CT scanning is a reliable modality for assessing GI tract perforations, it should not replace and does not improve on diligent serial clinical evaluations. A similar study from Calgary reviewed 145 children with blunt abdominal trauma.[145] CT scans were interpreted as positive for GI tract injury in 20 and negative in 152 (several children had more than one study). The sensitivity of abdominal CT scan was determined to be 0.93 for mesenteric or intestinal injuries requiring surgery, with a negative predictive value of 0.99 in this study population. Therefore CT rarely misses significant mesenteric or intestinal injuries.

The significance of isolated free intraperitoneal fluid in the absence of solid organ injury has frequently been heralded as a sign of intestinal trauma. Hulka and colleagues[146] reported a series of 259 CT scans (all with oral and intravenous contrast) and found only 24 patients (9%) with isolated free intraperitoneal fluid. Among the 16 patients with only a "small amount" of isolated fluid, only 2 required laparotomy. However, 4 of 8 patients (50%) with fluid in more than one location had a bowel injury requiring exploration. These authors also noted that enteral contrast is rarely present to aid in the diagnosis of bowel injury. Similar findings were reported by Holmes and colleagues,[147] with small quantities of intraperitoneal fluid having little clinical significance. In their report, only 8% of abdominal CT scans were positive for isolated intraperitoneal fluid, and in only 17% of these cases was there an identifiable injury. This represented only 7 of the 542 children (1.3%) studied.

Finally, FAST was found to be useful as a screening tool, with high specificity (95%) but low sensitivity (33%), in evaluating intestinal injury.[15] In that study of 89 FAST-negative children, only 20 went on to have CT scans performed, all at the surgeon's request. Without this finding, they all might have had abdominal CT scans. Clearly, FAST can decrease the number of unnecessary CT scans performed, but it cannot detect the specific abdominal organs injured. FAST is therefore of limited value in assessing these injuries. Finally, to come full circle, in a large study from Pittsburgh, 350 children with abdominal trauma were reviewed, with 30 requiring laparotomy (8.5%).[148] There were five false-negative CT scans (26%) in 19 patients who underwent delayed laparotomy (3.5 hours or longer after injury). Those authors concluded that serial physical examination, not CT scanning, is the gold standard for diagnosing GI tract perforations in children. We concur.

Injuries to the Perineum, Anus, and Genitalia

Children present with injuries to the perineum, anus, and external genitalia primarily from two mechanisms: accidental falls and sexual abuse. Accidental injuries are sustained by falling onto blunt or sharp objects in a straddled fashion. These injuries are characterized by bruising, contusion, laceration, or penetration, depending on the object struck and the height of the fall. Accidental injuries frequently involve the external genitalia, urethra, perineal body, and anus but rarely involve the rectum. Conversely, injuries sustained by sexual abuse are commonly rectal or vaginal penetrations from violent, nonconsensual acts or the purposeful insertion of objects into these orifices. Therefore, when examining a child with injuries to the perineum, isolated rectal or vaginal trauma should always be considered child abuse until proved otherwise; conversely, polytrauma to the perineum with genital, perineal, and anal involvement is typically accidental.[149]

Diagnosis of the extent of perineal injury frequently requires examination under anesthesia by means of proctoscopy, sigmoidoscopy, and retrograde urethrogram. After assessing the degree of injury, surgical strategies include repair of urethral injuries (directly or by stenting), urinary diversion with a suprapubic cystostomy, repair of rectal tears, rectal irrigation, placement of drains when required, and, in more complex injuries, fecal diversion by colostomy. After recovery, detailed radiologic confirmation of complete healing (e.g., by intravenous pyelogram, cystogram, urethrogram, contrast enemas) must be performed before reconstruction of fecal continuity or removal of urinary stents or urinary undiversion.

Colorectal and vaginal injuries in personal watercraft passengers highlight another mechanism which should create suspicion and concern.[150] Although rare, pediatric fatalities can occur with rectal impalement from abuse. However, more commonly, rectal insertion of thermometers, Hegar dilators, or enema tubes can cause significant rectal injuries in newborns, requiring surgical repair. We recently treated a 3-day-old infant with perforation of the rectosigmoid junction from frequent enemas required for the treatment of obstipation from cystic fibrosis; laparotomy and colostomy were required. Therefore, in newborns, apparently innocuous rectal manipulation can cause severe injuries requiring surgical evaluation and intervention.

Diaphragmatic Injuries

Traumatic injury to the diaphragm is infrequently observed, even at the largest pediatric trauma centers. At Children's Hospital of Illinois, only two traumatic diaphragmatic injuries were treated from 1998 to 2002 out of more than 800 admissions requiring level I pediatric trauma evaluation. At the Hospital for Sick Children in Toronto, only 15 children with this injury were seen from 1977 to 1998.[151,152] In a similar report, covering 1992 to 2002 at Denver Children's Hospital,

1397 children were admitted and observed for blunt abdominal trauma, 387 had intra-abdominal injuries, but there were only 6 diaphragmatic ruptures (0.5%).[153] The injury is caused by massive compressive forces to the abdominal cavity, creating acceleration of abdominal contents cephalad, rupturing the diaphragmatic muscle. Occasionally, penetrating trauma causes this injury; however, in these cases, the injury is often found incidentally at exploration for other injuries. In the series reported from Toronto, 13 of 15 patients had diaphragmatic rupture from blunt trauma; the mean age was 7.5 years, with the right and left diaphragm equally involved.[152] The diagnosis was made with only a chest radiograph in more than half the patients. Three injuries were missed at the initial evaluation. Because of the force required to cause this injury, multiple associated injuries should be expected. In this report, 81% of patients had multiple injuries, including liver laceration (47%), pelvic fracture (47%), major vascular injury (40%), bowel perfusion (33%), long bone fracture (20%), renal laceration (20%), splenic laceration (13%), and closed head injury (13%). As expected, there were many complications, five deaths, and a mean hospital stay of 20 days. Emergent surgery in children with this constellation of associated injuries should include palpation of both diaphragms as a routine part of the abdominal exploration. Direct suture repair is usually possible after debridement of any devitalized tissue. Pledgeted sutures can be used to buttress the repair and prevent tearing of the muscle, making the closure more secure. If sufficient diaphragm tissue is destroyed, a tension-free closure is optimal using intercostal muscle or a prosthetic patch can be used, similar to the repair of congenital diaphragmatic hernias in newborns.[153] Reports of laparoscopic or thoracoscopic repair of this injury include delayed repairs on stable patients without associated injuries.[154,155] Delayed diagnosis of this injury in infants has been reported, as has renal avulsion into the chest through a traumatically ruptured diaphragm.[156] Because of the infrequent presentation of this injury, one must have a high index of suspicion when the mechanism of injury and the degree and location of other injuries support the possibility of diaphragmatic injury.

Recent advances in the treatment of trauma and the provision of critical care in children have resulted in improved outcomes following major injuries. Much has changed in our understanding of transfusion strategies and coagulation since the previous edition of this textbook.[65,157,158] It is imperative that pediatric surgeons familiarize themselves with current treatment algorithms for life-threatening abdominal trauma. Important contributions have been made in the diagnosis and treatment of children with abdominal injury by radiologists and endoscopists. Clinical experience and published reports addressing specific concerns about the nonoperative treatment of children with solid organ injuries and recent radiologic and endoscopic contributions have made pediatric trauma care increasingly nonoperative. Although the trend is in this direction, the pediatric surgeon should remain the physician of record in the multidisciplinary care of critically injured children. Lucas and Ledgerwood recently posed the provocative question of how we can meet the inherent challenge of teaching the psychomotor skills required for operative hemostasis in an era of nonoperative therapy for most solid organ injuries.[159] As we struggle to meet this challenge, the fact remains that the decision not to operate is always a surgical decision.

The complete reference list is available online at www.expertconsult.com.

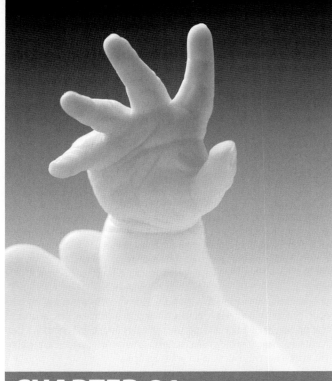

CHAPTER 21

Genitourinary Tract Trauma

Rebeccah L. Brown, Richard A. Falcone, Jr., and Victor F. Garcia

Epidemiology

Injury is the leading cause of death in children and young adults in the United States, with injury to the kidney from either blunt or penetrating trauma being the most common genitourinary tract injury.[1] Almost 50% of genitourinary tract injuries involve the kidney.[2] Blunt abdominal trauma is responsible for 90% of pediatric genitourinary tract injuries,[3] with the kidney being injured in 10% to 20% of all blunt trauma cases.[2,4] Renal injury occurs in about 3% to 6% of patients with penetrating trauma.[5,6] Serious renal injuries are most often associated with injuries to other organs, with multiple organ involvement occurring in 80% to 95% of patients with blunt or penetrating renal trauma.[6,7] The majority of associated injuries are closed-head injuries and extremity fractures.[8] Associated abdominal injuries occur in 42% to 74% of patients and primarily involve the spleen and liver in blunt trauma and the bowel in penetrating trauma.[4,9–12] The majority of isolated renal injuries can be classified as relatively minor injuries. Mortality is rare from isolated renal trauma and is more often attributed to the combined effects of major multisystem trauma.

Mechanisms of Injury

Most blunt renal injuries are due to sudden deceleration forces. Confined within the Gerota fascia, the kidney may be crushed against the ribs or the vertebral column, resulting in laceration or contusion. Direct injury to the renal parenchyma and collecting system may also occur from penetration of sharp, bony fragments of adjacent fractured ribs. Rapid deceleration may cause arterial or venous stretching of the fixed renovascular pedicle.[13] Because the intima of the renal artery is less elastic than that of the media, it is predisposed to laceration, which may lead to subintimal dissection and arterial thrombosis.[14] Mechanisms of blunt renal injury include pedestrian/motor vehicle crashes (60%), falls (22.5%), sports injuries (10%), assault (3.5%), and other causes (4%).[15] Most children who sustain renal injury in motor vehicle accidents are unrestrained;[4] however, violent deceleration with severe flexion-extension as seen with lap belts is a well-recognized mechanism of renal injury associated with a higher risk of renal pedicle avulsion and ureteropelvic junction (UPJ) injury. It is of interest that bicycle crashes are the most common sports-related cause of renal injury in children and are associated with a significant risk of high-grade renal injury.[16] Although there is a perception among pediatric surgeons and urologists that contact sports such as football, hockey, and martial arts incur the greatest risk for renal injury in children,[15] a review by McAleer and colleagues[17] demonstrated that bicycle crashes accounted for 24% of injuries compared with only 5% for contact sports. This may have some impact on the type of counseling that should be provided regarding activity for children after severe renal injury and for those with solitary kidneys. Penetrating genitourinary tract injuries are becoming more common in children and should be suspected with any penetrating injuries to the chest, abdomen, flank, and lumbar regions. Penetrating renal injuries, most commonly due to gunshot wounds (86%) and stab wounds (14%),[6] are more frequently associated with multiorgan injury, higher grades of injury, and higher rates of surgical exploration.[1] For example, in patients with penetrating renal injury, nearly 70% will have grade III or higher injury, whereas with blunt trauma, only about 4% will sustain grade III or higher injury.[1]

Anatomic Considerations

Children are considered to be at increased risk for genitourinary tract trauma owing to unique anatomic differences between children and adults.[3,13,18] In children, the kidneys are larger relative to the size of the child's body and are positioned lower in the abdomen, making them more exposed and vulnerable to injury. They are also less protected because of decreased perirenal fat, weaker abdominal wall musculature, and a poorly ossified thoracic rib cage. Because many pediatric kidneys retain their fetal lobulations, the risk for renal parenchymal disruption and lower pole amputation is increased. Furthermore, the renal capsule and Gerota fascia are less developed than in adults, creating a greater potential for laceration, nonconfined bleeding, and urinary extravasation. Because of the relative mobility of a child's kidney, rapid deceleration is more likely to result in renal pedicle injury and UPJ disruption. In a comparative series of children and adults who sustained blunt renal trauma, Brown and colleagues[3] concluded that although the likelihood of major renal injury was significantly higher in the pediatric population, the severity of trauma was significantly lower.

For similar reasons, preexisting renal disease or congenital renal anomalies may predispose children to an increased risk of genitourinary tract injury from blunt trauma. The reported incidence of preexisting renal disease or congenital genitourinary anomalies in children sustaining renal trauma varies from 1% to 23%.[19–24] Underlying congenital anomalies associated with hydronephrosis (UPJ obstruction), abnormal kidney position (horseshoe kidneys, crossed fused renal ectopia), abnormal kidney consistency (polycystic kidney disease, urinary reflux), and renal tumors such as Wilms' tumor may predispose the kidney to significant injury despite relatively minor forces.[20] Gross hematuria associated with an ostensibly minor trauma should alert the physician to the possibility of an underlying pathologic lesion of the urinary tract and should prompt further radiologic imaging. Although underlying congenital genitourinary anomalies may produce an increased risk of injury in children, they do not appear to be associated with any increased morbidity or long-term disability.[17]

Clinical Features

The evaluation of possible injury to the genitourinary tract is part of the systematic and expeditious assessment required in all seriously injured patients. The mechanism of injury is important to know in order to assess the risk of injury. Direct blows to the abdomen or flank and significant deceleration forces as may occur in motor vehicle crashes and falls should alert the physician to the possibility of renal injury. Penetrating injuries to the abdomen, flank, back, chest, and pelvis should also raise suspicion for injury to the genitourinary tract. Although the presence of abdominal or flank tenderness and flank ecchymosis or mass suggests renal injury, up to 25% of patients with severe renal injury have unremarkable abdominal examinations. Indeed, only 55% of children with significant renal injuries present with tenderness over the injured kidney. Conversely, only about half of children with renal tenderness on examination have a condition more serious than minor renal trauma.[25]

Perineal/scrotal ecchymosis, swelling, laceration, and bleeding are highly suggestive of genitourinary trauma. The presence of blood at the urinary meatus or a boggy mass or upward displacement of the prostate on digital rectal examination in boys requires formal urethrography to evaluate possible injury to the urethra before any attempts at urethral catheterization. However, it should be recognized that the sensitivity of the digital rectal examination for identifying urethral disruption may be quite low (2%),[26] especially in children in whom the prostate may not be fully developed.

Gross hematuria is indicative of genitourinary trauma and mandates further radiologic imaging. Conversely, the absence of hematuria, either gross or microscopic, does not exclude the possibility of significant genitourinary trauma. In fact complete avulsion of the renovascular pedicle and disruption of the UPJ have both been described in the absence of hematuria.[1,8,11,21,27–29]

Fractures of the lower ribs and lumbar spine may be associated with renal trauma, whereas fractures of the pelvis may be associated with bladder and urethral injuries. In a large study using data from the National Trauma Data Bank, Bjurlin and associates[30] reported that about 5% of more than 31,000 patients with pelvic fractures had an associated lower urinary tract injury involving the bladder or urethra, or a combination of both. Aihara and associates[31] found that certain types of pelvic fractures were associated with increased risk for rectal, bladder, or urethral injuries. Rectal injury was associated with widening of the symphysis pubis. Bladder injuries were most commonly associated with widening of the sacroiliac joint, symphysis pubis, and fractures of the sacrum, with widening of the symphysis pubis being the strongest predictor of bladder injury. Urethral injuries were most commonly associated with widening of the symphysis pubis and fractures of the inferior pubic ramus. Fractures involving these locations should heighten suspicion of associated rectal and lower urinary tract injuries and prompt directed diagnostic studies. Gross hematuria in the presence of a pelvic fracture strongly suggests a bladder perforation. Any degree of hematuria in the presence of a pelvic fracture is an indication for cystography.

Diagnostic Evaluation

Although findings on urinalysis (either gross hematuria or microhematuria) may be suggestive of genitourinary tract trauma, the decision to proceed with imaging to assess for injury is usually made before performing urinalysis and is based instead on the clinical scenario and hemodynamic status of the patient. Thus findings on urinalysis are more often than not corroborative rather than diagnostic because imaging usually precedes urinalysis. If, however, urinalysis is obtained early in the course of trauma evaluation, there is great debate regarding the need for further imaging based on this parameter alone. Although most would agree that gross hematuria is an indication for formal diagnostic evaluation, much controversy exists as to whether microscopic hematuria as an isolated finding on urinalysis warrants further radiologic imaging.[9,12,32–41]

It remains unclear what degree of microscopic hematuria, if any, warrants radiographic evaluation in children. Several studies have attempted to answer the question as to whether the adult criteria for imaging of renal trauma, including findings of gross hematuria, microscopic hematuria (>5 red blood cells [RBCs] per high-power field [HPF]) with shock, major associated injuries, significant deceleration injury, and penetrating injury can be applied to children. Although degrees of microhematuria ranging from any degree[36,37] to 20 RBCs per HPF[42] to 50 RBCs per HPF[39] have been reported as significant in the literature, a careful analysis of published reports on 382 children with renal injuries reveals that the application of adult criteria for imaging would have identified 98% to 100% of all renal injuries.[41] One of the pitfalls in applying adult criteria for the imaging of renal trauma in children with regard to the presence or absence of shock is that children are unique in their ability to maintain normal blood pressure in the face of significant hypovolemia and blood loss. In fact only 5% of children with major renal injury have clinical signs of shock.[25] Therefore hypotension itself is not a reliable indicator of the severity of renal injury in the pediatric population. Tachycardia typically precedes hypotension as an early indicator of shock in children and may be a worrisome sign. Accordingly the decision on imaging in children, as in adults, should be based not on isolated findings but rather on the whole clinical picture, including mechanism of injury (direct blow, major deceleration, flexion-extension injury, penetrating trauma), vital signs (tachycardia or hypotension), physical examination findings (abdominal/ flank tenderness, contusion, penetrating injury in vicinity of genitourinary tract), urinalysis (microhematuria or gross hematuria), and associated injuries. In most cases, microhematuria is not an isolated finding. Most children with microhematuria have some other factor, such as mechanism of injury, physical findings, or other associated injuries, that would warrant further imaging, therefore decreasing the likelihood of missed injury.

Abdominal computed tomography (CT) is the standard for radiographic evaluation of abdominal trauma in children and is the most accurate imaging and staging modality for evaluation of renal injury.[43,44] CT with intravenous contrast is highly sensitive and specific for detection of parenchymal contusions/lacerations, perinephric/retroperitoneal hematoma, urinary extravasation, and segmental or major arterial injuries; delineation of nonviable, nonperfused tissue or segmental infarction; and demonstration of other associated intra-abdominal injuries. Since images with multidetector helical CT are obtained before the contrast medium is excreted in the urine, injury of the collecting system may be missed. In patients with significant renal injury detected on the initial images, delayed images 5 to 20 minutes after the contrast injection may identify urine extravasation associated with injury to the collecting system. A plain radiograph may also be suggestive. Delayed images may be omitted to minimize radiation dose if the kidneys are normal or with injury unlikely to be associated with injury to the collecting system and in the absence of retroperitoneal or pelvic fluid.[43,45,46]

CT has replaced the intravenous pyelogram (IVP) in the hemodynamically stable patient. However, a one-shot IVP still remains useful in the hemodynamically unstable patient before emergent surgical exploration to determine the presence of two functional kidneys, the presence and extent of urinary extravasation, and the presence of renal pedicle injury. In children, 2 to 3 mL/kg of nonionic contrast is injected intravenously, followed by an abdominal radiograph immediately and 10 minutes later.[38] It should be recognized that the IVP provides only very basic information and is not useful in staging of renal injuries. In fact, some studies have shown that as many as 20% of patients with significant renal injuries have a normal IVP. Likewise, nonvisualization of the kidney on the IVP does not necessarily correlate with arterial occlusion or injury. Other factors, including renal contusion with vascular spasm, overhydration, and hypotension or hypoperfusion, may produce similar findings in up to half of patients.[47]

Arteriography has been largely supplanted by CT and CT angiography for the diagnosis and staging of renal injury. More invasive than CT, arteriography requires the expertise of an experienced interventional radiologist and may be associated with a formidable risk for arterial injury in small children whose vessels may be prohibitively small, fragile, and difficult to access or cannulate. The current role of arteriography is in the diagnosis of delayed or ongoing renal hemorrhage, renovascular injury, or delayed arteriovenous fistula or pseudoaneurysm formation in which interventional techniques such as selective embolization[48–53] or endovascular stenting[54,55] may be therapeutic.

Ultrasonography, although used extensively in Europe for the assessment of acute renal trauma, has not found widespread acceptance in the United States. Ultrasonography in the trauma patient in the United States is mostly limited to the focused assessment with sonography for trauma (FAST) examination, which is performed primarily to detect the presence of free intraperitoneal fluid. The focused assessment with sonography for trauma examination has not been particularly useful in children except perhaps in the hemodynamically unstable patient with an associated closed-head injury to rapidly exclude the presence of intra-abdominal hemorrhage. In the hemodynamically stable child, CT provides more useful information. Ultrasonography is not particularly sensitive for detecting parenchymal injuries, except in the most experienced hands, and only with close color and pulsed Doppler interrogation can a vascular injury be diagnosed. Therefore, its utility in the acute setting at present remains limited. Ultrasonography may, however, have utility in follow-up of acute renal injuries staged initially by CT to exclude complications of injury, including urinomas, expanding hematomas, abscesses, or pseudoaneurysms, thus reducing radiation exposure.[56]

CT cystography has been found to be equivalent to conventional cystography in terms of sensitivity (95%-100%), specificity (99%-100%), negative predictive value (100%), and positive predictive value (100%) for the detection of the presence or absence of bladder injury and has largely replaced conventional cystography in most major trauma centers.[57–59] An absolute indication for CT cystography is gross hematuria with a pelvic fracture. Other relative indications include gross hematuria alone, microscopic hematuria with pelvic fracture, or microscopic hematuria alone in the context of other clinical indicators of bladder rupture such as suprapubic pain, inability to void, or significant perineal trauma.[60] It is critical that the bladder be fully distended in order to accurately detect bladder injury. Simply clamping a Foley catheter after intravenous contrast agent administration for CT is not adequate and will result in an unacceptably high rate of missed injuries.[59,61] For CT cystography, the bladder is filled in a retrograde fashion by gravity drainage before or after routine abdominal/pelvic CT. The bladder of adolescents should be filled with 300 to 400 mL of contrast medium. The bladder of smaller children should be filled by gravity infusion until the patient becomes uncomfortable or the bladder capacity is reached. In children younger than 2 years of age, the bladder capacity is 7 mL/kg. In children 2 to 11 years of age, the bladder capacity is age in years plus 2 times 30 mL.[62,63] Multiplanar reformatted images are essential to assess the bladder fully for potential injury. If CT cystography is equivocal in any way for either the presence of extravasation of contrast or in differentiating intraperitoneal versus extraperitoneal extravasation, it should be followed by conventional cystography to confirm or exclude injury.[56]

Retrograde pyelography may play a role in the assessment of ureteral and renal pelvic integrity when UPJ injury is suspected. Failure of opacification of the distal ureter on CT should raise suspicion for a ureteral injury[64]; and if insufficient detail is provided by CT, retrograde pyelography is indicated.

Retrograde urethrography is indicated when urethral injury is suspected.[43] A Foley catheter with a minimally inflated balloon is inserted into the fossa navicularis of the distal ure-thra, and approximately 30 mL of contrast medium is instilled under fluoroscopic vision. A normal retrograde urethrogram should demonstrate complete filling of the intact urethra with passage of contrast medium into the bladder. The presence of filling defects or extravasation of the contrast agent indicates urethral disruption. In the presence of hematuria, a cystogram should follow the retrograde urethrogram, even if the retro-grade urethrogram is normal, because 10% to 15% of patients with urethral disruption from a pelvic fracture will have a concomitant bladder injury.[47]

Injury Grading and Scoring Systems for Genitourinary Injuries

In 1989, the American Association for the Surgery of Trauma (AAST) Organ Injury Scaling Committee devised and pub-lished a classification or grading system for genitourinary tract injuries (Table 21-1) to standardize injury descriptions for research and data collection purposes.[65] Figure 21-1 illustrates this grading system. Injuries are graded on a scale from I to V ranging from the most minor injury (grade I) to the most complex (grade V). For the kidney, this grading system has proved highly applicable, and its usefulness as a measure of the seriousness of renal injury and as a predictor of clinical outcomes and nephrectomy has been validated in several subsequent studies.[66–70] For example, patients with a grade I injury require observation only, whereas those with a grade V injury are more likely to require nephrectomy. Those with intermediate injuries (grades II to IV) require individualized therapy, with a trend toward more invasive therapy as injury grade increases. It should be noted, however, these validation studies were composed primarily of adult patients. Thus extrapolation of results may not be entirely applicable to children. Furthermore, the AAST system has been criticized for grouping complex parenchymal injury with major renovas-cular injury in the grade IV and V categories, because manage-ment may be quite different for the same grades of injury. Modifications addressing this issue have been proposed for future iterations of the scaling system. The AAST scaling systems for ureteral, bladder, and urethral injuries (see Table 21-1) have not gained as widespread acceptance and have been used less consistently.

TABLE 21-1

Urologic Injury Scale of the American Association for the Surgery of Trauma

Grade*	Injury Description†
Renal Injury Scale	
I: Contusion	Microscopic or gross hematuria; urologic studies normal
Hematoma	Subcapsular, nonexpanding without parenchymal laceration
II: Hematoma	Nonexpanding perirenal hematoma confined to the renal retroperitoneum
Laceration	<1 cm parenchymal depth of renal cortex without urinary extravasation
III: Laceration	>1 cm parenchymal depth of renal cortex without collection system rupture or urinary extravasation
IV: Laceration	Parenchymal laceration extending through the renal cortex, medulla, and collecting system
Vascular	Main renal artery or vein injury with contained hemorrhage
V: Laceration	Completely shattered kidney
Vascular	Avulsion of renal hilum that devascularizes kidney
Ureter Injury Scale	
I: Hematoma	Contusion of hematoma without devascularization
II: Laceration	≤50% transection
III: Laceration	>50% transection
IV: Laceration	Complete transection with 2 cm devascularization
V: Laceration	Avulsion of renal hilum that devascularizes kidney
Bladder Injury Scale	
I: Hematoma	Contusion, intramural hematoma
Laceration	Partial thickness
II: Laceration	Extraperitoneal bladder wall laceration ≤2 cm
III: Laceration	Extraperitoneal (>2 cm) or intraperitoneal (≤2 cm) bladder wall lacerations
IV: Laceration	Intraperitoneal bladder wall laceration >2 cm
V: Laceration	Intra- or extraperitoneal bladder wall laceration extending into the bladder neck or ureteral orifice (trigone)
Urethra Injury Scale	
I: Contusion	Blood at urethral meatus; urethrography normal
II: Stretch injury	Elongation of urethra without extravasation on urethrography
III: Partial disruption	Extravasation of urethrographic contrast medium at injury site, with contrast visualized in the bladder
IV: Complete disruption	Extravasation of urethrographic contrast medium at injury site without visualization in the bladder; <2 cm of urethral separation
V: Complete disruption	Complete transection with >2 cm urethral separation, or extension into the prostate or vagina

From Moore EE, Shackford SR, Pachter HL, et al: Organ injury scaling: Spleen, liver, and kidney. J Trauma 1989;29:1664.
*Advance one grade for multiple injuries to the same organ.
†Based on most accurate assessment at autopsy, laparotomy, or radiologic study.

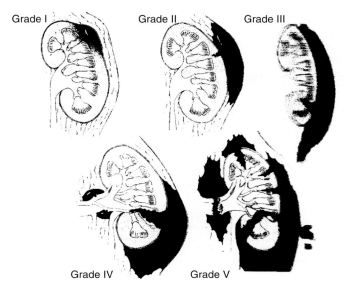

Grade I Grade II Grade III

Grade IV Grade V

FIGURE 21-1 Artist's rendition of the American Association for the Surgery of Trauma grading system for genitourinary tract trauma. (Reproduced with permission from Coburn M: Genitourinary trauma. In Moore E, Feliciano DV, Mattox KL [eds]: Trauma, 5th ed. New York, McGraw-Hill, 2004.)

Management of Specific Injuries

KIDNEY

Blunt Injuries

As with traumatic injuries to the spleen and liver, the vast majority of blunt renal trauma in children can be safely managed nonoperatively.[8,11,35,71–82] Nonoperative management of hemodynamically stable children with blunt renal injury has become the standard of care in most centers, with success rates up to 98%.[77] About 85% of pediatric blunt renal injuries are considered low grade (grades I-III). Since the collecting system remains intact in these lower grade renal injuries, they will invariably heal without further sequelae. Because of disruption of the collecting system and/or vascular pedicle, high-grade injuries (grades IV and V) are associated with increased morbidity and mortality. Grade IV injuries account for about 15% of pediatric renal injuries, whereas grade V injuries with major disruption of the renal pedicle occur in the remaining 5% of children.[*]

Children with minor renal injury (grades I and II) may require brief hospitalization for observation or may be discharged home with clear follow-up instructions. Children with higher grade renal injury (grades III-V) or gross hematuria, or both, are hospitalized and placed on bed rest with close monitoring of vital signs and serial physical examinations and blood cell counts. Traditionally, ambulation is begun once the patient is fully resuscitated and hemodynamically stable, blood cell counts have stabilized, and gross hematuria has resolved. It is not unusual for the bladder outlet or Foley catheter to become occluded with clot in patients with gross hematuria. Decreased urine output, bladder distention, or bladder spasms should alert the clinician to this possibility. Placement of a Foley catheter or irrigation or replacement

of an existing Foley catheter should remediate the problem. Although it is generally suggested that patients maintain a decreased level of activity until the microscopic or gross hematuria resolves, there are no evidence-based guidelines in the literature addressing appropriate length or type of activity restrictions for renal trauma. The time at which healing is adequate to allow return to full activity without risk has not yet been defined. A multi-institutional prospective study is currently under way to address this issue, allowing for immediate ambulation and discharge based on standard criteria rather than on the resolution of hematuria.[83]

Most pediatric and adult series report successful nonoperative management of even the most complex grade IV and grade V injuries, including shattered but perfused kidneys and complex lacerations with extensive perinephric hematoma and urinary extravasation. Although the AAST grading scale appears to have some predictive value on the need for surgery, indications for surgery are based more on hemodynamic stability of the patient and associated injuries, rather than on grade of renal injury based on imaging criteria. The only absolute indication for surgery is hemodynamic instability with ongoing bleeding and transfusion requirements. Radiographic signs of ongoing renal bleeding include an expanding or uncontained retroperitoneal hematoma or complete avulsion of the main renal artery or vein with extravasation as demonstrated by CT or arteriography. Although not an absolute indication for surgical intervention, active extravasation and pooling of contrast-enhanced blood in the arterial phase of the computed tomographic scan should be considered a relative indication for surgical intervention depending on the clinical status of the patient, and the clinician should maintain a low threshold for prompt exploration in patients with this computed tomographic finding. Recent studies would suggest that about 90% of grade IV injuries with urinary extravasation can be successfully managed nonoperatively in the hemodynamically stable patient.[73,78,80,81,84–87]

Although complications are more common with high-grade renal injuries, most complications associated with urinary extravasation are easily treated by percutaneous drainage or endoscopic stent placement, thereby achieving higher rates of renal salvage.[73,84,86,88] Selective nonoperative management of blunt grade V renal injury in both adults[89] and children[80,82] has also been shown to be feasible for hemodynamically stable patients. Henderson and colleagues[80] reported a 73% kidney salvage rate with nonoperative management of 15 patients with grade V injury, whereas Eassa and colleagues[82] reported a 78% kidney salvage rate with nonoperative management of 18 patients with grade V injury. Superselective embolization was used as adjunctive therapy for nonoperative management in a minority of patients with ongoing bleeding and transfusion requirements, thus permitting salvage of traumatized kidneys with a minimally invasive procedure and avoiding a major surgical procedure. An algorithm for the management of blunt renal injuries in children is presented in Figure 21-2.

Penetrating Injuries

Penetrating renal injuries are rare in children. Although there is a role for selective nonoperative management, most gunshot wounds to the abdomen require abdominal exploration because of associated injuries from the blast effect. Retroperitoneal dissection and exploration is indicated only if preoperative or intraoperative assessment suggests a major renal injury

---

[*]References 47,73,76,77,79,83.

ALGORITHM FOR MANAGEMENT OF RENAL INJURIES

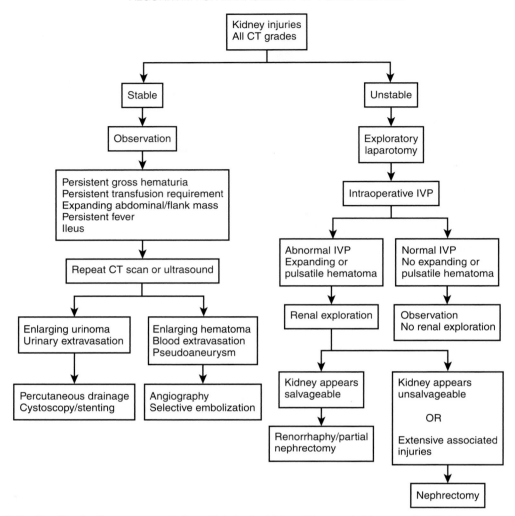

FIGURE 21-2 Algorithm for the management of renal injuries in children. CT, computed tomography; IVP, intravenous pyelogram.

(grade IV or grade V), there is suspicion of significant nonuro-logic retroperitoneal injury (great vessels, duodenum, pancreas, colon), inspection reveals an expanding or pulsatile retroperi-toneal hematoma, or a combination of these conditions exists.[90] McAninch and co-workers[91] classified gunshot wounds involv-ing the kidney into five categories: (1) contusions (18.4%), (2) minor lacerations (13.8%), (3) major lacerations (50.5%), (4) vascular injuries (6.9%), and (5) lacerations combined with vascular injury (10.3%). In a large study of gunshot wounds seen in 206 renal units in 201 patients over a 30-year period, Voelzke and McAninch[92] reported an overall renal salvage rate of 85.4% using a combination of selective observation/bedrest (25%) and various operative techniques including exploration only, mesh repair, omental flap repair, peritoneal patch, renor-rhaphy, vascular repair, and partial nephrectomy. The nephrec-tomy rate was 14.6%. Nonoperative management of renal injury due to gunshot wounds is evolving. In a 4-year pros-pective study by Navsaria and Nicol,[93] 34% of 95 patients with gunshot injuries to the kidney were managed nonopera-tively without laparotomy with a 91% success rate. Selection criteria for nonoperative management included hemody-namic stability, CT for grading of kidney injury and excluding

other associated injuries requiring exploration, and a clinically evaluable patient.

For renal-proximity stab wounds, nonoperative treatment is appropriate in hemodynamically stable patients without associated injuries who have been staged appropriately by triple-contrast CT.[5,94] However, a high index of suspicion for missed ureteral and other associated injuries must be maintained if a nonoperative pathway is chosen.

In a retrospective review by McAninch and co-workers,[95] 55% of renal stab wounds and 24% of renal gunshot wounds were successfully managed nonoperatively with an acceptable complication rate. In the hemodynamically unstable patient with penetrating trauma or in the patient with a retroperito-neal hematoma at laparotomy, a one-shot IVP may be useful to identify renal injury and confirm the presence and function of two renal units to further guide management.

Renovascular Injuries

Major renovascular injuries are rare in children. Carroll and colleagues[96] and Turner and associates[97] reported penetrating trauma as a cause of renovascular injuries in 64% and 68% of their patients, respectively. Conversely, Cass and co-workers[98] identified blunt external trauma as the cause of renovascular injury in 76% of patients. Regardless of the mechanism, these patients tend to have high injury severity scores, large transfusion requirements, and associated life-threatening multisystem injury,[96,98] the management of which supersedes that of renal injury. Knudson and colleagues[99] reported that factors associated with a poor outcome after renovascular injuries include blunt trauma, grade V injury, and attempted arterial repair. Elliott and colleagues[100] similarly demonstrated dismal outcomes for vascular repair of main or segmental renal artery injuries, with functional outcomes similar to nephrectomy. Grade V injuries are associated with severe major parenchymal injuries which contribute to poor function of the revascularized kidney. Patients with grade V main renal artery injuries with severe parenchymal disruption may be better served by immediate nephrectomy provided that a functional contralateral kidney is present. Bruce and associates[101] compared 12 patients with blunt renal artery injuries who underwent operative intervention (9 nephrectomies; 3 revascularizations) with 16 patients who were managed nonoperatively, 1 of whom underwent endovascular stent placement. They concluded that nonoperative management of unilateral blunt renal artery injuries is safe and often successful, with a 6% risk of the development of post-traumatic renovascular hypertension.

The pathogenesis of renovascular injuries due to blunt trauma is thought to be caused by rapid deceleration, which results in stretching of the renal vasculature, disruption of the arterial intima, and arterial thrombosis.[96] Blunt arterial injury occurs more commonly on the left side than on the right side because the right renal artery is longer than the left and may be better able to withstand the stretching caused by deceleration.[96]

Although hematuria may be absent or microscopic in 13% to 56% of patients with renovascular injuries,[1,8,11,96,98] most patients have other symptoms or signs that raise suspicion of a major renal injury and prompt further diagnostic imaging.[11,96] Renovascular injury is suggested on CT by (1) lack of renal enhancement or excretion, often in the presence of normal renal contour; (2) vein enhancement; (3) central hematoma; (4) abrupt cutoff of an enhanced renal artery; and (5) nonopacification of the pelvicaliceal system.[11,96]

The approach to this type of injury depends on the time to diagnosis, the type and extent of the vascular injury, and the extent of the associated injuries.[11,96] Repair of the right renal vein may be difficult owing to its short length and proximity to the inferior vena cava. Nonetheless, injuries to the main renal vein can be repaired in most cases.[96] Laceration of the left renal vein at its origin can be managed by ligation because collateral circulation supplied by gonadal and adrenal veins usually allows for adequate venous drainage.[96,102]

Segmental arteries are difficult to repair and may be managed by ligation with accompanying partial nephrectomy if the area of infarction encompasses more than 15% of the kidney. However, nonoperative management should be considered in any patient with segmental artery occlusion that is not associated with uncontrolled retroperitoneal hemorrhage, extensive urinary extravasation, or other intra-abdominal indications for surgery. This management strategy has been associated with an acceptably low incidence of complications.[96,100,103]

Arterial repair is most appropriate and most successful for renovascular injuries caused by penetrating trauma. Notwithstanding occasional reports of successful revascularization in patients 19 hours after injury,[102] the success of the procedure greatly diminishes after 8 hours of renal ischemia.[96,104,105] Ivatury and co-workers[106] reviewed 40 penetrating renovascular injuries and concluded that salvage of a kidney with a renovascular injury is determined primarily by the nature and extent of associated injuries. Furthermore, they reported that although attempts at renal artery repair are often futile, renal vein injuries are more amenable to repair and have a better prognosis. Nephrectomy, however, remains the procedure of choice in the hemodynamically unstable patient with multiple trauma.

Blunt injuries to the main renal artery are associated with the lowest success rate for complete renal preservation.[11,96,97] Renal artery thrombosis due to blunt trauma is often diagnosed by nonvisualization of the affected kidney on CT. Options for treatment include observation with delayed nephrectomy for complications or attempted vascular repair depending on the timing of the injury.[87] Haas and associates[107] reviewed the management of 12 patients with complete renal artery occlusion secondary to blunt trauma. Renal artery revascularization was attempted in 5 patients with a median warm ischemia time of 5 hours (range: 4.5 to 36 hours). Although 4 of 5 revascularizations were deemed technically successful at the time of operation, 3 patients demonstrated no function and 1 showed minimal function on postoperative renal function scans. Two patients required delayed nephrectomy because of complications, and of the 7 patients who received nonoperative management, significant hypertension developed in 3 patients requiring nephrectomy for blood pressure control. Based on these results, the authors were unable to advocate emergency revascularization for unilateral renal artery occlusion in the presence of a normal functional contralateral kidney unless the patient is hemodynamically stable and warm ischemia time is less than 5 hours. Patients with unilateral injury, complete arterial thrombosis, extensive associated injuries, and a prohibitively long period of renal ischemia may be managed either by primary nephrectomy or expectant nonoperative management depending on the hemodynamic stability of the patient. There are reports of successful endovascular stenting for traumatic renal artery dissection and thrombosis in both children[54] and adults.[55] An attempt should be made to revascularize all patients with bilateral renal artery injury or solitary kidneys.[96,108,109] An algorithm for the management of renovascular injuries is presented in Figure 21-3.

Complications

Although most renal injuries in children can be managed nonoperatively, this type of management is not without complications. If a nonoperative course is chosen, the patient must be carefully monitored. Falling blood counts, ongoing transfusion requirements, and persistent gross hematuria may be indicative of ongoing bleeding. A repeated computed tomographic scan or arteriogram is warranted. An arteriogram may be especially useful because some injuries with ongoing bleeding may be amenable to selective embolization to control the bleeding. Indeed, the success of nonoperative management may be enhanced by angiographic embolization in select

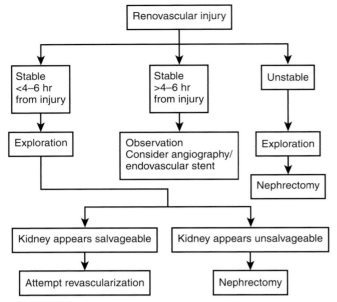

FIGURE 21-3 Algorithm for the management of renovascular trauma in children.

patients.[53,110–112] However, profuse bleeding not amenable to embolization requires emergent operative exploration.

Prolonged ileus, fevers, and an expanding abdominal/flank mass or discomfort may be indicative of persistent urinary extravasation or urinoma, which is the most common complication after renal trauma. Ultrasonography may be used for diagnosis in patients with suggestive symptoms to reduce radiation exposure associated with CT.[56] Most urinomas are asymptomatic and will resolve spontaneously over time in 67% to 90% of patients.[73,81,84,86,87] Accordingly, small, noninfected, stable collections require no treatment other than observation, whereas larger, expanding collections may be managed by percutaneous drainage[73] or endoscopic placement of ureteral stents.[73,81,84,86,87] Traditionally broad-spectrum antibiotics are administered intravenously on an empirical basis, although this practice is not necessarily evidence based.

Delayed renal bleeding is unusual and most commonly occurs within 2 weeks of injury. However, Teigen and coworkers[113] reported two children in whom massive life-threatening hemorrhage developed several weeks after the initial injury diagnosed by arteriography and successfully treated by percutaneous transcatheter embolization.

Perinephric abscesses may be associated with ileus, high fevers, and sepsis. Ultrasonography or CT are diagnostic. Most of these abscesses are successfully treated with intravenous broad-spectrum antibiotics and percutaneous drainage. Multiloculated abscesses not amenable to percutaneous drainage may require operative drainage.

Late complications may include hydronephrosis, arteriovenous fistula, pseudoaneurysm, pyelonephritis, calculus formation, and delayed renal hypertension. Post-traumatic arteriovenous fistula and pseudoaneurysm may be successfully managed by percutaneous endovascular embolization.[48–50,110,111]

The incidence of renal hypertension after trauma is low, occurring in fewer than 5% of patients.[99,114,115] The incidence is thought to be even lower in children. Although hypertension usually occurs anytime from 2 weeks to several months after injury,[107,115] long-term follow-up is essential because onset may be delayed up to 10 to 15 years after injury.[109]

Follow-Up and Outcomes

Evidence-based guidelines for follow-up of children after renal injury are conspicuously lacking in the literature. El-Sherbiny and colleagues[116] studied 13 children with grades III (6 children), IV (4 children), and V (3 children) renal injuries managed nonoperatively with a mean follow-up of 3 years with clinical measures (serial blood pressure measurements, urinalysis, and creatinine determinations), renal scintigraphy and/or CT angiography. Although there were residual morphologic changes noted on imaging in 92% of patients, no patient was hypertensive; all had normal urinalysis results and creatinine levels; and there was no significant functional loss, with all kidneys having a split function of 41% to 50% at final follow-up.

A study by Keller and co-workers[117] similarly evaluated the functional outcome of nonoperatively managed renal injuries in 16 children (grades I-III—4 children; grade IV—9 children; grade V—3 children) as measured by blood urea nitrogen (BUN) and creatinine levels, blood pressure, and technetium-99m-dimercaptosuccinic acid (DMSA) renal scans at 3-month and 1-year follow-up. All injuries were noted to be healed radiographically by ultrasonography or CT at 3 months. Normal to mild impairment (>40% split function) was noted in 56% of injured kidneys, with moderate impairment (30% to 40% split function) noted in 31% of injured kidneys. Severe impairment (< 30% split function) was noted in only 3 children—2 of 9 with grade IV injuries, and 1 of 3 with grade V injury. Furthermore, functional outcome did not change significantly from the 3-month to 1-year follow-up period, and all children, regardless of functional outcome on DMSA scan, remained asymptomatic and normotensive and had normal BUN and creatinine levels.

More recently, Eassa and colleagues[82] performed follow-up CT at a mean time of 8 months in 13 of 14 adult patients with grade V injuries managed nonoperatively and noted reapproximation of shattered parenchymal fragments with separation of individual fragments by thin hypoperfused scars. DMSA scans were obtained in 9 of the 14 patients at a mean time of 3 years—4 patients (44%) showed preserved renal function (>40% split function), with the remaining 5 patients showing variable degrees of renal dysfunction, including 2 with severe dysfunction (split function <30%). No patient was noted to be hypertensive or have elevated creatinine levels or abnormal urinalysis results.

Larger prospective clinical and radiologic outcome studies are warranted to further assess time to healing, incidence of complications, residual function, and long-term outcomes after renal trauma to provide the physician with a more evidence-based approach to appropriate follow-up and counseling for the injured child. At present it is generally recommended that children with severe renal injuries (grades III, IV, and V) be followed with ultrasonography and DMSA renal scans at 3 to 6 months after injury as well as biannual to annual blood pressure monitoring and laboratory tests (urinalysis, BUN, and creatinine determinations) for the first several years after injury. Further imaging is also indicated to look for the onset of any urologic symptoms or development of hypertension.

Operative Management of Renal Trauma

Although most cases of renal trauma in children may be successfully managed nonoperatively, the surgeon should be familiar with techniques of operative management as well. As discussed previously, operative management of renal trauma is generally reserved for hemodynamically unstable patients or patients with severe associated injuries. The patient is usually explored through a generous midline abdominal incision. Although traditionally it has been taught that the surgeon should first gain proximal control of the renal artery and vein before entering the Gerota fascia or the hematoma in order to reduce blood loss and decrease the nephrectomy rate,[118] this approach has recently been challenged. In both retrospective studies[119,120] and a prospective, randomized clinical trial[121] it was concluded that vascular control of the renal hilum before opening the Gerota fascia has no effect on the nephrectomy rate, transfusion requirements, or blood loss but does significantly prolong operative times by up to an hour or more. The nephrectomy rate appears to depend more on the degree of injury rather than on the type of renovascular control.[119]

No matter what the approach, the kidney is exposed and vascular control is obtained at the hilum. With exsanguinating hemorrhage, rapid mobilization of the kidney with digital control of the hilum may be necessary. The left renal vein can be ligated because collateral drainage is provided by the left adrenal and gonadal veins. However, trauma to the right renal vein requires repair. Segmental arteries may be ligated and partial nephrectomy performed if the area of infarction encompasses more than 15% of the kidney. If the patient is hemodynamically stable, the kidney itself is salvageable, and the period of warm ischemia after injury is acceptable (<4–6 hours), renal artery repair and revascularization may be attempted. Otherwise, a nephrectomy should be performed.

If it appears salvageable, the damaged kidney is debrided to viable tissue and intrarenal hematomas are evacuated. Hemostasis should be obtained with absorbable sutures placed in a figure-of-eight pattern. The open collecting system should be closed with fine, absorbable, monofilament sutures because woven sutures may cut through renal tissue. Internal stents may be required if the ureter or renal pelvis has been injured.

The renal capsule should be closed to approximate the renal margins. If the capsule is destroyed, the lacerated margins should be covered with omental pedicle grafts, retroperitoneal fat, or polyglycolic acid mesh. Approximation and covering of renal tissue aids in hemostasis and wound healing and prevents delayed bleeding and extravasation of urine.[92]

Ureter

Ureteral injury is uncommon, accounting for less than 1% of all genitourinary trauma.[122] The rarity of ureteral injury may be attributed to its narrow diameter, mobility, and position in the retroperitoneum where it is well protected by the overlying peritoneal contents, psoas muscles, bony pelvis, and vertebrae. Not surprisingly, associated injuries, most commonly involving kidney, small bowel, colon, liver, and iliac vessels, occur in greater than 95% of patients with ureteral trauma.[123–125]

Anatomically, the ureter is divided into three portions—the proximal ureter extends from the ureteropelvic junction (UPJ) to the point where it crosses the sacroiliac joint; the middle ureter courses across the bony pelvis and iliac vessels; and the distal ureter extends from the iliac vessels to the bladder. The distribution of injuries is fairly equally divided—proximal ureter (37%); middle ureter (31%); distal ureter (32%).[123,124] Ureteral trauma is classified according to the AAST organ injury scaling system by the anatomic location of the injury and by the extent of mural damage (see Table 21-1).[65] The complexity of repair and number of associated injuries have been found to correlate with increasing AAST grade of ureteral injury.[123]

The overwhelming majority of ureteral injuries are due to penetrating trauma from gunshot wounds (94%) or stab wounds (2.5%), with blunt trauma accounting for only 3.5% of all ureteral injuries.[124] Blunt injury may occur by either direct or indirect mechanisms. Direct injuries may result from crush injuries or severe hyperextension or flexion injuries. Direct compression against a transverse process or vertebral body has been described,[126] and an association with traumatic paraplegia has been noted.[127] Patients with congenital ureteral obstruction are also predisposed to injury of the collecting system.[128] Surgical repair is unlikely to be successful if the underlying obstruction is not recognized and treated.

Indirect mechanisms of ureteral injury in children include falls or rapid deceleration. As noted by Boone and colleagues,[129] the UPJ is particularly prone to disruption secondary to these mechanisms. Howerton[130] reviewed 54 cases of ureteral avulsion within 4 cm of the UPJ and found that this type of injury was three times more common in children than in adults.

The clinical diagnosis of ureteral injury can be difficult because of the paucity of early signs and symptoms. For penetrating trauma, any missile tract in the vicinity of the ureter should raise suspicion for ureteral injury, and appropriate diagnostic testing or exploration should be undertaken depending on the clinical status of the patient. For blunt trauma, flank ecchymosis with significant deceleration or a hyperextension-flexion mechanism should alert the clinician to the possibility of ureteral injury. Overall, hematuria is noted in fewer than half of patients with ureteral injury and is thus not a very sensitive indicator of injury.[123–125] Furthermore, absence of hematuria does not exclude injury.

Imaging modalities for diagnosis of ureteral trauma include CT, retrograde pyelography, and IVP. In the setting of blunt trauma or in the hemodynamically stable patient with penetrating trauma, CT is the gold standard for evaluation. With the faster helical CT scanners currently in use, if an injury to the ureter is suspected, it is critical to obtain delayed images during the excretory phase (5 to 20 minutes) so that ureteral extravasation is not missed. Failure of opacification of the distal ureter on CT should raise suspicion for a ureteral injury,[64] and if insufficient detail is provided by CT, retrograde pyelography is indicated.

IVP is used more commonly for penetrating trauma, since emergent exploration may be required because of associated injuries; however, up to 75% of ureteral injuries are missed by IVP.[122,131] Single-shot IVP is often unreliable and non-diagnostic, whereas complete IVP is more accurate but more difficult to obtain in the emergent setting.[125] Abnormal findings on IVP suggestive of ureteral injury include ureteric dilatation or deviation, incomplete visualization of the complete ureter, delayed or incomplete visualization of the kidney, and extravasation of contrast medium.[125]

Delayed diagnosis of ureteral injury occurs in approximately half of patients owing to the subtle nature of the clinical findings, frequent absence of hematuria, lack of sensitivity of radiologic imaging techniques, and high incidence of multisystem injury with concomitant patient instability.[122] Although intraoperative inspection of the retroperitoneum when a missile path is in the vicinity of the ureter may be the most sensitive indicator of injury, a comprehensive review of the literature reveals that 11.1% of ureteral injuries are missed at laparotomy despite preoperative or intraoperative imaging, or both, and intraoperative inspection.[132] Meta-analysis reveals a statistically increased rate of nephrectomy as well as prolonged hospital course when ureteral injury is missed at exploration.[128] Delayed signs of a missed ureteral injury that should prompt further investigation include prolonged ileus, continued high output from surgically or percutaneously placed drains, fever or sepsis, persistent flank or abdominal pain, urinary obstruction, elevated creatinine or BUN levels, and flank mass.[125] Delayed diagnosis results in significantly increased morbidity, including fistula, urinoma, abscess, sepsis, renal failure, and renal loss.[125]

A high index of suspicion for the presence of ureteral injury must be maintained by the clinician in order to avoid missing these highly morbid injuries.

Factors influencing optimal treatment of ureteral injuries include time to diagnosis, associated injuries, degree of injury, and hemodynamic stability of the patient. Many blunt and low-grade ureteral injuries (grades I and II) may be managed nonoperatively with observation and ureteral stenting. The treatment of more complex ureteral injuries is primarily surgical and dictated primarily by the location and mechanism of injury, amount of tissue loss, condition of the local tissues, and stability of the patient. The primary goal is renal preservation with maintenance of urinary drainage from the kidney.

A complex armamentarium of percutaneous and surgical techniques is available to the surgeon to address these injuries.[123-125,133] The most common surgical reconstructive techniques include primary ureteroureterostomy, transureteroureterostomy, and ureteral reimplantation by ureteroneocystotomy.[123] Basic surgical principles of ureteral repair include thorough assessment and staging of injury, adequate mobilization of the ureter taking care to preserve the adventitia, wide debridement to viable tissue, a spatulated tension-free watertight repair over a stent, and adequate drainage of the retroperitoneum.[124] Complex ureteral injury associated with a severely damaged or shattered kidney may be best managed by nephrectomy. In the absence of or with limited renal injury, attempts at primary ureteral repair should be attempted. Proximal ureteral injuries are often short and therefore amenable to debridement and ureteroureterostomy. With disruption of the UPJ, ureteropyelostomy or dismembered pyeloplasty are options for repair. If damage to the renal pelvis is extensive, it should be surgically debrided and closed with ureteral continuity restored by ureterocalicostomy. Middle ureteral injuries can usually be managed by primary ureteroureterostomy, transureteroureterostomy, or a Boari flap and reimplantation. Injuries to the distal ureter are often amenable to a simple ureteral reimplantation (ureteroneocystostomy) or psoas hitch.[123-125,133]

Unstable patients with multiple injuries are best managed by exteriorization of the transected ureter as an intubated ureterostomy or by simple ureteral ligation with intraoperative or postoperative percutaneous nephrostomy.[125] Definitive reconstruction of a long ureteral defect is performed on an elective basis once the patient is stable, and options for reconstruction may include ileal interposition and autotransplantation.[133]

Ureteral injuries in which the diagnosis is delayed or in which secondary leaks occur after primary repair are best managed by percutaneous nephrostomy and antegrade ureteral stenting with later elective surgical correction of stenosis or fistula if encountered. Infected urinomas or abscesses can usually be managed effectively with percutaneous drainage.[125]

Bladder

ANATOMY

Although the bladder in children is located in the extraperitoneal space of Retzius, it is considered an intra-abdominal organ until about the age of 6 years when, as the bony pelvis grows, the bladder assumes a pelvic position and is increasingly protected from injury. The anatomic attachments of the bladder influence the pattern of injury seen after some forms of trauma. The bladder is bound laterally by the internal obturator muscles and the umbilical ligaments. At its base the bladder is attached to the urogenital diaphragm. Denonvilliers fascia or the rectovesical fascia binds it posteriorly. Unlike the rest of the bladder, the dome is mobile and distensible.

CAUSES

Injuries to the bladder are distinctly uncommon in children, accounting for about only 0.05% to 0.2% of all injuries.[134,135] Blunt trauma accounts for the vast majority of injuries to the bladder and usually results from a direct blow to the lower abdomen when the bladder is distended with urine or from a pelvic fracture in which there is shearing of the bladder from its fascial attachments or laceration from a bony spicule. The susceptibility of the bladder to injury is somewhat dependent on the amount of urine contained at the time of injury. Motor vehicle accidents are the most common cause of blunt trauma to the bladder, accounting for about 90% of cases, followed by falls and direct blows to the lower abdomen.[134] There have also been several case reports of bladder injury in children due to nonaccidental trauma.[135] Because of its relatively protected position within the pelvis, considerable blunt force is required to cause bladder injury. Not surprisingly, serious injuries to other intra-abdominal organs are seen in almost half of patients with bladder injuries.[134] Although 60% to 90% of bladder injuries are associated with pelvic fractures, only 2% to 11% of patients with pelvic fractures have concomitant bladder injuries.[134]

CLASSIFICATION AND DEFINITIONS

Bladder injuries due to blunt trauma may be further classified as contusions and extraperitoneal and intraperitoneal ruptures. Extraperitoneal bladder ruptures occur in about 55% to 60% of cases, intraperitoneal ruptures occur in about

25% to 40% of cases, and a combination of the two occurs in about 10% of cases.[136,137] The AAST organ injury grading scale for bladder injuries is shown in Table 21-1.

Contusions are disruptions in the bladder muscular layer without loss of continuity of the bladder wall, whereas ruptures are complete disruptions of the bladder wall with extravasation of urine. Contusions typically resolve without intervention.

Extraperitoneal bladder ruptures are almost invariably associated with pelvic fractures.[134,137]

Nineteen percent of patients (mostly boys) with extraperitoneal bladder ruptures have a concomitant urethral injury, and 8% have an associated intraperitoneal injury.[138] In contrast to extraperitoneal ruptures, intraperitoneal ruptures are infrequently associated with pelvic fractures (Fig. 21-4). These injuries are often caused by compression (burst-type injury) from a suprapubic blow to a distended bladder or sudden, forceful deceleration. Intraperitoneal ruptures most commonly occur at the dome of the bladder, whereas extraperitoneal ruptures are usually caused by bony perforation or shearing forces.[139]

DIAGNOSIS

The hallmark of bladder injury is gross hematuria, which is noted in 95% of cases.[134] Gross hematuria in association with suprapubic pain, inability to void, and pelvic fracture should prompt further investigation to exclude the presence of a bladder injury. Conventional CT and CT cystogram with multiplanar reformatted images are equally accurate for diagnosing bladder rupture.[57,58] Urinary ascites, intra-abdominal sepsis, ileus, abdominal distention, and unexplained abnormal serum electrolyte, BUN, and creatinine levels should alert the clinician to the possibility of a missed intraperitoneal bladder rupture.[134,140]

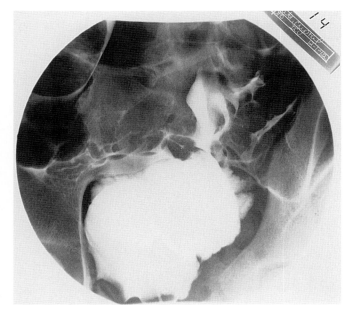

FIGURE 21-4 Voiding cystourethrogram demonstrating intraperitoneal rupture of the bladder. The patient also had bilateral fractures of the superior ischial and inferior pubic rami.

MANAGEMENT

Bladder Contusions

Most bladder contusions heal spontaneously without intervention. If the sacral innervation of the bladder is intact, patients with bladder contusions have excellent outcomes. Patients with a large pelvic hematoma that causes considerable bladder distortion may have difficulty voiding and may benefit from Foley catheter drainage.[134]

Intraperitoneal Rupture

Intraperitoneal ruptures are frequently associated with other significant injuries, necessitating a thorough and deliberate evaluation of the patient. The weakest and most mobile part of the bladder, the dome, is the most common site of intraperitoneal rupture. This type of injury occurs more commonly in younger children. Intraperitoneal rupture is generally associated with a large rent in the dome of the bladder with leakage of urine into the peritoneal cavity.[134]

Intraperitoneal bladder ruptures are best managed by early operative repair through either an open or laparoscopic approach (in select patients).[141,142] For the open procedure the bladder should be approached through a lower midline abdominal incision to avoid lateral contained hematoma. If necessary the rent in the dome of the bladder can be widened to facilitate a thorough examination of the inner aspect of the bladder. Associated extraperitoneal tears can be closed from within by a single running layer of absorbable suture; however, the surgeon must ensure that the patency of the ureteral orifices is preserved. An intravenous injection of indigo carmine or methylene blue may help verify the location and integrity of the ureteral orifices. The dye should be seen exiting the ureteral orifices within 10 minutes. Lacerations extending into the bladder neck should be carefully repaired to reconstruct the sphincteric components and reduce the likelihood of later urinary incontinence. Intraperitoneal bladder injuries are repaired with absorbable suture in two layers.

After the bladder is repaired, a closed-suction drain is placed and brought out through a separate stab incision. Although in the past most surgeons would insert a large-bore suprapubic cystostomy tube instead of or in addition to a transurethral catheter for urinary drainage after repair of an intraperitoneal bladder rupture, more recent literature suggests that transurethral catheter drainage is not only adequate but also preferable. For any degree of bladder injury, transurethral catheters are equally effective, are associated with fewer complications, and may be removed sooner than suprapubic catheters.[143,144]

Urinary drainage is generally maintained for 7 to 10 days. Most surgeons will obtain a cystogram before removal of the urinary drainage catheter to evaluate the integrity of the repair. If no extravasation is documented, the urinary catheter and closed-suction drain can be removed.

Extraperitoneal Rupture

The preferred management of extraperitoneal rupture is transurethral catheter drainage alone. This approach is safe and effective and obviates the need for bladder exploration, manipulation of the extraperitoneal hematoma, and converting a closed pelvic fracture into an open one. At times, the degree of extravasation of contrast medium may be alarming. However, because it is dependent not only on the size of the tear but also on the amount of contrast medium instilled, the degree of extravasation alone may not indicate the severity or extent of the tear in the bladder.[138] In most instances, the tear heals completely and transurethral catheter drainage is successful even with extensive urinary extravasation.[138,139] Almost 90% of extraperitoneal bladder ruptures heal within 10 days and the remainder within 3 weeks.[138] Operative intervention is rarely required. Indications for operative management include failure of the transurethral catheter to provide adequate drainage due to persistent extravasation or clot formation, concomitant vaginal or rectal injury, bladder neck/avulsion injury, or internal fixation of a pelvic fracture to prevent infection of the orthopedic hardware.[134]

Penetrating Injuries

Because of the high likelihood of associated injuries, which often take priority in management, patients with penetrating injuries to the bladder generally require exploratory laparotomy. The peritoneal cavity is opened in the midline, and injuries to the intra-abdominal viscera and major vasculature are addressed first. Attention is then directed to the bladder and the extent of injury is determined. All devitalized bladder tissue and debris from clothing or bony spicules are removed. The integrity of the ureters can be confirmed with intravenous injection of indigo carmine or methylene blue.[134] A diligent search should be made for extravasation, and if necessary the ureters should be intubated.

Bladder mobilization and extensive debridement is unnecessary and invites precipitous bleeding.[134] Large, nonexpanding hematomas should be left undisturbed. The bladder should be entered through the dome. Extraperitoneal defects should be closed intravesically with a single layer of running absorbable suture. A watertight closure is ideal but not essential. With adequate bladder drainage, even a tenuous closure can heal satisfactorily. Intraperitoneal defects should be closed in two layers with absorbable suture to achieve a watertight seal. With rectal or vaginal involvement, once repair is complete, viable tissue should be interposed to avoid overlapping suture lines and subsequent fistula formation.[134] Closed-suction drains are placed as previously described and transurethral catheter drainage is maintained for 7 to 10 days.

Urethra

Although urethral trauma is a secondary consideration in children with potential life-threatening trauma, such injuries account for a disproportionate degree of long-term morbidity. Blunt trauma with disruption of the bony pelvis accounts for most posterior urethral injuries in children. About 5% to 10% of boys with a fractured pelvis will also have an injury to the posterior urethra, usually at the proximal bulbar urethra.[145] Of these cases, 10% to 20% will have an associated bladder rupture[146] and about 27 % will have associated intra-abdominal injuries.[147] Motor vehicle accidents account for 90% of posterior urethral injuries, and the remaining 10% result from falls, crush injuries, or sporting injuries. A lateral pelvic force without pelvic fracture rarely results in urethral disruption. Penetrating injuries involving the posterior urethra are exceedingly rare. Anterior urethral injuries are often encountered after straddle injuries—such as a fall astride a

fence, kicks, or bicycle injuries. Penetrating trauma to the anterior urethra is rare but may be seen with gunshot or stab wounds.[147]

The diagnosis of urethral trauma is relatively straightforward. Symptoms of urethral injury may include the inability to void or the sensation of voiding without passing urine. Blood at the urinary meatus or gross hematuria after trauma strongly suggests urethral injury. Physical examination of the penis, scrotum, and perineum may reveal swelling and ecchymosis. The integrity of and boundaries of the Buck, Colles, and Scarpa fascias indicate the region injured. Digital rectal examination may reveal upward displacement of the prostate or a boggy mass. This, however, may be difficult to assess in young children, so urethral imaging is required to confirm the diagnosis.

If there is suspicion of a urethral injury, blind passage of a transurethral urinary catheter should not be attempted because there is a risk of creating a false passage with the catheter and converting a partial disruption into a complete one. Retrograde urethrography is the imaging modality of choice for diagnosis of urethral trauma. Findings of elongation, filling defect, or extravasation indicate urethral injury. If urethral integrity is demonstrated by retrograde urethrography, the catheter is then advanced and a cystogram is obtained to exclude concomitant bladder injury.

Table 21-1 outlines the classification of urethral injuries, which includes contusions, stretch injuries, partial disruptions, and complete disruptions. A filling defect caused by contusion and hematoma or an elongated urethra without extravasation on retrograde urethrography indicates grade I or grade II injury. Urethral extravasation with bladder continuity indicates partial disruption (grade III). Urethral extravasation with no admission of contrast agent into the proximal urethra or bladder suggests complete disruption (grade IV). Spasm of the periurethral musculature can mimic complete disruption. Figure 21-5 provides an example of injury to the bulbous urethra.

The long-term sequelae of urethral trauma can be devastating and may include impotence, retrograde ejaculation, incontinence, and urethral strictures. Some of these complications may be a direct consequence of the trauma itself or may be related to surgical attempts at repair.

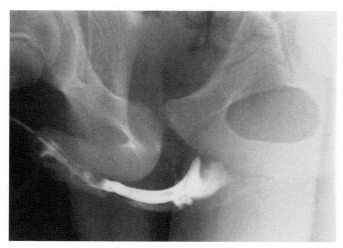

FIGURE 21-5 Extravasation of contrast from the bulbous urethra due to penoscrotal urethral disruption. The posterior membranous and prostatic urethra is intact.

A diagnosis of anterior urethral injury is suggested if the retrograde urethrogram reveals only minimal extravasation with good urethral continuity and if the patient is able to void. Grade I or grade II injury to the anterior urethra usually heals spontaneously without insertion of any indwelling urinary catheters, as long as the patient is able to void. Intermediate-grade anterior urethral injuries may be managed by an indwelling transurethral Foley catheter, whereas more complex injuries are best managed in the initial stages by placement of a suprapubic catheter. Delayed urethral strictures occur commonly and most are amenable to urethroplasty.

Penetrating injuries to the anterior urethra may be managed by exploration and primary repair or suprapubic urinary diversion. Husmann and colleagues[148] reviewed the management of 17 patients with partial transection of the anterior urethra due to low-velocity gunshot wounds and concluded that patients were best managed by aggressive wound debridement, corporeal repair, primary suture repair of the urethra, and placement of a suprapubic catheter. Strictures developed much less frequently with this approach (1 of 8 patients) compared with suprapubic diversion and transurethral catheter stenting (7 of 9 patients). If there is extensive hematoma at the site of injury, it may be more prudent to place a suprapubic catheter, allow the injury to heal, assess for stricture formation by contrast studies or urethroscopy, or both, after more than 3 months, followed by formal urethral reconstruction if indicated.[147]

In children, the majority of posterior urethral injuries may be managed nonoperatively. Grade I or grade II injuries, which may allow spontaneous voiding, are managed without surgery and without an indwelling urinary catheter. Patients who are unable to void are managed by insertion of a small, transurethral Foley catheter. Grade III injuries with minimal extravasation may also be managed by passing a small transurethral Foley catheter under fluoroscopic guidance immediately after the retrograde urethrogram is obtained. If the catheter does not pass easily, however, a suprapubic tube should be placed.

Options for repair of more complex posterior urethral injuries include primary surgical repair with anastomosis of the disrupted urethral ends, delayed primary repair, primary surgical catheter realignment, primary endoscopic realignment with imaging, or suprapubic cystostomy with delayed urethroplasty.

Primary surgical repair involves evacuation of the pelvic hematoma, mobilization of the prostate and urethra, and direct end-to-end anastomosis between the prostatic and membranous urethra. Problems with this approach include increased risk of uncontrolled bleeding from exploration of the injury site with release of the tamponade effect of the hematoma, increased rate of stricture formation, increased risk of impotence due to dissection of the periprostatic and periurethral tissues, and increased risk of incontinence due to damage to the intrinsic urethral sphincter mechanism by dissection, mobilization, and debridement of torn urethral ends.[147]

Primary surgical catheter realignment, despite not requiring direct suturing of the disrupted urethral ends, still requires an open procedure with entry into and evacuation of pelvic hematoma with all of the attendant risks of primary surgical repair. More recently innovative combined transurethral and transvesical endoscopic and interventional radiologic techniques have been introduced to achieve primary alignment

without the risk of exploring the disrupted urethra.[147,149] Furthermore, because there is no manipulation of periprostatic tissues and no additional trauma to the cavernous nerves, there should be no additional risk of erectile dysfunction other than that caused by the injury itself.

Concerns about the impact of primary open surgical repair or catheter realignment on potency and urinary continence led to the introduction of an alternative treatment approach, namely suprapubic cystostomy with delayed urethroplasty. No attempt is made to explore the urethra; rather the urinary stream is simply diverted through a suprapubic cystostomy tube. A stricture is considered inevitable and is repaired several months later. Advantages of this approach include avoiding entry into a fresh pelvic hematoma with risk of blood loss and infection, speed and simplicity of suprapubic tube insertion, and decreased incidence of impotence and incontinence resulting from the avoidance of dissection of the prostate and urethra. Disadvantages include prolonged need for a suprapubic tube with risk of infection and stone formation as well as the nearly 100% risk for urethral strictures, which may be complex and difficult to repair even in the delayed setting. Tunc and colleagues[150] reviewed 77 cases of delayed repair of traumatic posterior urethral injuries and demonstrated adequate urethral continuity in 95%, postoperative incontinence in 9%, and postoperative erectile dysfunction in 16%. They concluded that delayed posterior urethroplasty is a successful treatment option with acceptable morbidity. Although suprapubic drainage with delayed urethroplasty is associated inevitably with stricture formation that may be difficult to repair even in the delayed setting, decreased rates of incontinence and impotence are a definite advantage.

Koraitim[151] reviewed and compared various techniques for repair of complex posterior urethral injuries, including primary repair (37 patients), which was associated with 49% stricture rate, 21% incontinence rate, and 56% impotence rate; immediate and early realignment (326 patients) which was associated with a 53% stricture rate, 5% incontinence rate, and 36% impotence rate; and suprapubic drainage with delayed repair (508 patients), which was associated with a 97% stricture rate, 4% incontinence rate, and 19% impotence rate. After extensive literature review regarding different approaches to management of complex posterior urethral injuries, Holevar and associates[136] in 2004 concluded that these injuries may be treated with either primary endoscopic realignment or suprapubic cystostomy with delayed urethroplasty with similar results. More recent studies in both children and adults, comparing early primary alignment with suprapubic cystostomy and delayed urethroplasty, favor early primary alignment because it may decrease the requirement for subsequent stricture therapy by as much as 50%, resulting not only in fewer strictures but also in strictures that are easier to treat.[152-154] Furthermore, it does not appear to increase the rate of incontinence and impotence.

Urethral trauma in girls is rare, since the urethra is very short and mobile with no significant attachments to the pubic bone.[147,155,156] The usual mechanism of injury involves pelvic fracture incurred during a motor vehicle accident. Straddle injury occasionally results in damage to the urethra. Female urethral injuries may be distal avulsion from the perineal attachment or proximal disruptions and lacerations. The latter type of injury is characteristically associated with other pelvic injuries, including vaginal and bladder neck lacerations.

Perry and Husmann[157] reviewed the evaluation of urethral injuries in girls with pelvic fractures. Blood at the vaginal introitus mandates a meticulous vaginal examination. The urinary meatus must also be carefully examined and its patency confirmed by passage of a catheter. However it is important to note that catheters can often be passed into the bladder even in the presence of a significant urethral injury. Development of vulval edema after removal of the catheter warrants prompt investigation. Because urethrography in young girls is difficult and unreliable, urethroscopy is the preferred diagnostic modality. Delays in diagnosis of urethral injury in girls occur frequently and have devastating consequences.[147,157] Such injury is misdiagnosed in about 50% of cases and can result in life-threatening sepsis and necrotizing fasciitis. Therefore one should have a low threshold for performing urethroscopy when urethral injury is suspected in a young girl.

Treatment is dictated by the extent and location of injury. Urethral injuries that extend into the bladder neck require meticulous repair with reapproximation of the bladder outlet and urethra. Such injuries are encountered about two thirds of the time. Associated vaginal injuries are repaired primarily. Urethral crush injuries that do not involve the bladder neck are managed by extended transurethral Foley catheterization (6 to 8 weeks) or, if necessary, suprapubic catheter drainage. Significant long-term complications associated with pediatric female urethral trauma are common and include urethral stenosis, urethrovaginal fistula, incontinence, and vaginal stenosis.[158] Clearly every effort must be made to promptly detect and aggressively manage this uncommon injury.

External Genitalia

GIRLS

Blunt genital trauma in girls is fairly common. The presenting symptoms are usually the presence of blood in the underpants or on the perineum shortly after injury.[159] Blunt genital trauma most commonly results from straddle injury. The most common types of injury in decreasing order of frequency are lacerations or contusions of the perineal body, vagina, labia, urethra, and rectum. Because of the extreme difficulty of performing a thorough genitourinary examination in an awake, uncomfortable, anxious, and embarrassed child, the majority of patients are best evaluated in the operating room under general anesthesia. Indeed, as many as 76% of patients will have more extensive injuries than can be appreciated in the emergency department.[159]

Management of female genital trauma is dictated by the type and extent of injury.[160] Vulvar hematomas may cause urinary retention and may benefit from placement of a urinary catheter and evacuation of large hematomas. Necrotic contused tissue should be debrided. Lacerations are primarily repaired after hemostasis is achieved. Absorbable sutures are used to preclude the need for removal. Vaginoscopy, urethroscopy, and proctoscopy may be necessary to evaluate the injury more thoroughly.

BOYS

Penile injury resulting from blunt or penetrating trauma is rare in children. All penile injuries, other than very superficial injuries, should be evaluated with retrograde urethrography to exclude concomitant urethral injury. Urethral lacerations should be managed as described in the previous section. The findings of an expanding hematoma, palpable corporal defect, and excessive bleeding suggest cavernosal injuries. When possible these injuries should be repaired primarily. Urinary diversion with a suprapubic tube is occasionally necessary. The preferred method of management of gunshot wounds with a limited extent of injury is debridement of superficial wounds, repair of the cavernosal defects, and primary repair of the urethral injury.[47]

Injury resulting from zipper entrapment of the penis can be addressed in many cases in the emergency department but may require a general anesthetic for release of the penis.[161] Penile strangulation injuries due to constricting bands are managed by division of the constricting band in as atraumatic manner as possible. In children, hair tourniquets are common sources of constriction and may be difficult to remove. Severe strangulation injuries may result in necrosis of the distal penile skin, glans, cavernosum, or urethra. Conservative debridement and urinary diversion may be required.[47] Penile amputation injuries are rare and devastating injuries in children (Fig. 21-6), but reimplantation and reconstructive techniques have been described with variable functional and cosmetic outcomes.[162]

Scrotal injuries may result from penetrating trauma or blunt trauma, or both. High-resolution ultrasonography is useful in the evaluation of these injuries.[163] Ultrasonography of penetrating injuries can identify testicular rupture and extratesticular soft tissue abnormalities as well as the presence and location of foreign bodies.[164] This technique is also useful in distinguishing less serious injuries, such as scrotal hematomas, hydroceles, and hematoceles, from surgical emergencies, such as testicular rupture and infarction. Patients with

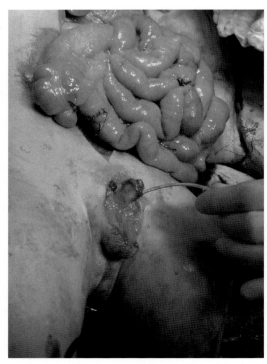

FIGURE 21-6   Penile amputation injury with associated intra-abdominal injury from lawn mower.

hematoceles should be considered for exploration to evacuate the blood from the tunica vaginalis testis because this approach reduces morbidity and hastens recovery. Testicular disruption is managed by debridement and primary closure even if 50% of the parenchyma is destroyed. This approach results in a testicular salvage rate of 30% to 39%.[165] Orchiectomy is reserved for the completely shattered testicle.

The complete reference list is available online at www. expertconsult.com.

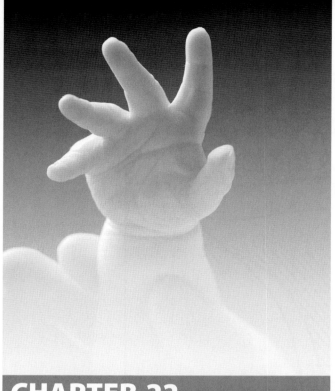

CHAPTER 22

Musculoskeletal Trauma

Richard S. Davidson and B. David Horn

Musculoskeletal trauma is the most common medical emergency in children. The number of cases continues to increase in association with the popularity of motor vehicles, all-terrain vehicles, and power lawn mowers. In a child with multiple injuries, optimal treatment requires a cooperating team of medical professionals with diverse specialties who understand the priorities of each team member. As in all other pediatric specialties, it is important to remember that children are not "little adults." Priority management need not compromise complete patient management.

This chapter reviews the important differences between the musculoskeletal systems of children and adults, and it highlights the principles of evaluation and management in children with musculoskeletal injuries. The treatment of high-priority musculoskeletal injuries is specifically discussed, including open fractures, compartment syndrome, femoral neck fractures, mangled extremities, spine trauma, and suspected child abuse. For details on the management of specific musculoskeletal fractures and injuries of childhood, readers should refer to textbooks on children's fractures.[1-3]

Musculoskeletal Systems of Children and Adults

Differences in the musculoskeletal anatomy and biomechanics of children and adults determine the unique patterns of musculoskeletal injury seen in childhood. Injuries to growing bones are a double-edged sword: They can have a remarkable capacity for healing and remodeling, but they are also subject to the problems of overgrowth and growth disturbance, which can have lifelong consequences.

ANATOMY

The major anatomic distinctions of skeletally immature bones are the physis and the periosteum. Each long bone in a child consists of the epiphysis, physis, metaphysis, and diaphysis (Fig. 22-1). The epiphysis is the end of the bone beyond the physis, or growth plate, and contains the articular cartilage. The secondary center of ossification arises within the epiphysis and progressively enlarges as the cartilage ossifies during skeletal maturation. The physis, or growth plate, provides longitudinal growth of the bone by forming cartilage that is then converted into bone in the metaphysis. The diaphysis, or shaft, is surrounded by periosteum, which generates new bone and provides circumferential bone growth. In younger children, the periosteum also provides structural support to the bone. By adulthood, the growth plate closes, and there is limited potential for remodeling.

BIOMECHANICS

Skeletally immature bones are more porous, less brittle, and better able to tolerate deformation than mature bones. The increased porosity of immature bones stops the progression of a fracture line but weakens the bone under a compressive force. As a result, a greater variety of fractures is seen in children than in adults. A child's bone may undergo plastic deformation, where it bends without fracture; it can buckle under compression, resulting in a buckle or torus fracture; it can fracture like a "green stick," with an incomplete crack on the tension side and a bend on the compression side; or it can fracture completely (Fig. 22-2).

The thick periosteum that surrounds the diaphysis of the bone can minimize or prevent displacement of diaphyseal fractures. The periosteum tears on the tension side of a fracture but often remains intact on the compression side. The intact periosteum can then function as a hinge or a spring, increasing deformity. Depending on the injury, the periosteum may simplify or complicate reduction of a fracture (Fig. 22-3).

In the complex of bone, ligaments, and cartilage in a child, the physis is the weakest part and therefore is the most likely site of failure. An angular force to a joint in a young child is most likely to cause a fracture along the growth plate, whereas in an adolescent or an adult, a ligamentous injury or dislocation would occur; so, it is not uncommon for growth plate fractures to be misdiagnosed as sprains. Frankel and Nordin[4]

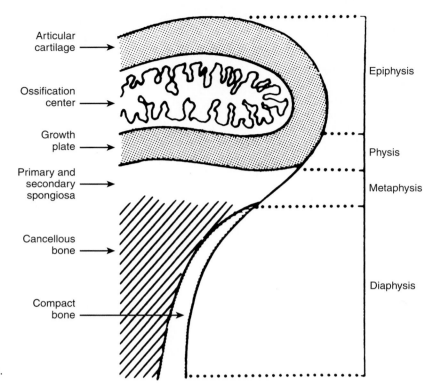

FIGURE 22-1   Anatomy of a child's bone.

Articular cartilage

Ossification center

Growth plate

Primary and secondary spongiosa

Cancellous bone

Compact bone

Epiphysis

Physis

Metaphysis

Diaphysis

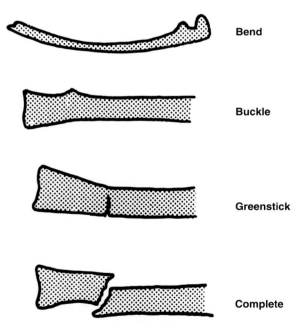

Bend

Buckle

Greenstick

Complete

FIGURE 22-2   Fracture types commonly seen in children. (From Rang M [ed]: Children's Fractures. Philadelphia, JB Lippincott, 1974.)

provide extensive information on the biomechanics of bone. In a fall on an outstretched hand, a young child is unlikely to sprain a wrist; more commonly, a child sustains a fracture through the growth plate of the distal radius. Similarly, instead of spraining an ankle, a child is more likely to sustain a physeal fracture of the distal fibula. Under low-energy forces, these injuries are unlikely to lead to growth disturbance.

The Salter-Harris classification system of fractures involving the physis can guide proper management (Fig. 22-4).[5] Type 1 fractures extend along the entire physis. Type 2 fractures involve part of the growth plate and part of the metaphysis; these fractures are seldom associated with growth arrest except when they occur in the distal femur and proximal tibia. Type 3 fractures involve part of the physis and pass across the epiphysis into the joint. Because of the possibility of incongruity of the joint, type 3 fractures often require open reduction and fixation. Type 4 fractures occur longitudinally, crossing the physis from the metaphysis into the epiphysis. This type of fracture is commonly associated with subsequent formation of a bony bar across the physis, which causes partial growth arrest with subsequent angulation. Open reduction and internal fixation are usually required for type 4 fractures, because joint incongruity and fusion across the physis are common. Type 5 fractures are diagnosed retrospectively, when all or part of the physis fails to grow. It is hypothesized that injury to the physis results from direct compression or local vascular insult. Growth disturbance may result in loss of longitudinal growth or angular deformities. Damage to the physis in high-energy injuries can lead to asymmetric growth in any of the fracture types.

PHYSIOLOGY

Important physiologic differences between the musculoskeletal systems of children and adults are found in healing and remodeling. Growing bones are also at risk for the unique problems of overgrowth and growth disturbance.

Healing in children is rapid and age-dependent. A newborn may achieve clinically stable union of a fracture in 1 week, whereas a similar fracture in an adolescent may take

6 weeks to heal. In children, the rapid healing process partially results from the thick periosteum, which may form its own bone bridge. Except for displaced intra-articular fractures or fractures with gross soft tissue interposition, nonunion of fractures is rare in children.

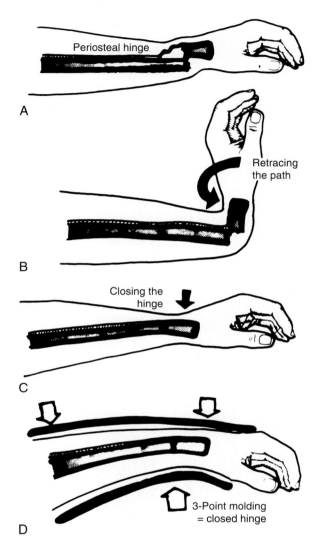

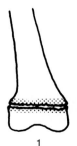
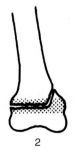

FIGURE 22-3 **A,** In children, the intact periosteum of a fracture prevents reduction by traction. **B,** By retracing the path of injury, the fracture can be reduced. **C,** Closing the hinge. **D,** A cast with three-point molding holds the hinge closed and keeps the fracture reduced. (From Rang M [ed]: Children's Fractures. Philadelphia, JB Lippincott, 1974.)

The bones of children have great potential for remodeling, but limitations must be understood. Remodeling potential is better in younger patients, in deformities closer to the physes, and where angulation is in the plane of motion of the nearest joint. Remodeling does not effectively correct angulation perpendicular to joint motion or rotation. These deformities should be reduced before healing begins (Fig. 22-5).

Growth stimulation may follow fractures of long bones. This can be especially apparent in the lower extremity in children between 2 and 10 years of age. In this group, an average overgrowth of 1 cm can be expected in femur fractures.[6-8] Although discrepancies in leg length are unpredictable, it is often possible to reduce the ultimate inequality by allowing the fracture to heal with a 1-cm overlap in an otherwise anatomic alignment. Most of the growth stimulation occurs within the first year after injury; so, follow-up visits for 1 year are recommended, even after uneventful healing.

Damage to the physis can produce severe shortening, angular deformity, or both. Although this may be caused by the initial trauma, it can also result from failure to obtain anatomic reduction of a physeal fracture or from repeated or overzealous attempts at reduction (Fig. 22-6). Treatment depends on the amount of remaining skeletal growth and the projected difference in limb lengths and may involve timed ablation of the growth plate on the normal limb, shortening osteotomy of the normal limb, or lengthening of the short limb. Angular deformities can also be addressed, taking into consideration the patient's skeletal age and the severity of the deformity.

Evaluation of Musculoskeletal Injuries

CLINICAL ASSESSMENT

The initial assessment of children with multiple injuries may be difficult. Details of the incident may be missing, and the patient's history may be incomplete. The Advanced Trauma Life Support (ATLS) system of assessment involves a primary evaluation to identify and immediately address life-threatening injuries, followed by a secondary evaluation to find and treat other significant injuries. The injuries identified in the secondary evaluation must also be treated in a timely manner to prevent devastating lifelong consequences. Postponing the management of serious musculoskeletal injury for an extended period can be associated with a poor prognosis for return to normal function.

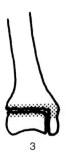
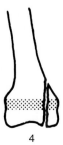
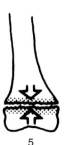

FIGURE 22-4 Salter-Harris classification of epiphyseal fractures. Type 1 involves the entire physis. Type 2 involves part of the growth plate and part of the metaphysis. Type 3 involves part of the physis and passes across the epiphysis into the joint. Type 4 is longitudinal, crossing the physis from the metaphysis into the epiphysis. Type 5 is diagnosed retrospectively when the physis fails to grow. See text for clinical implications of each fracture type.

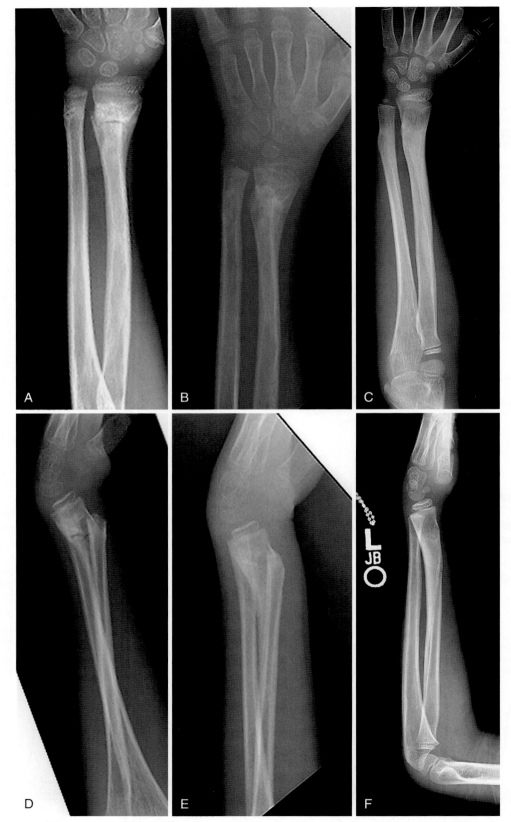

FIGURE 22-5 Forearm radiographs of a 7-year-old boy demonstrating remodeling of a forearm fracture over a 9-month period. **A** to **C,** Anteroposterior plane. **D** to **F,** Lateral plane.

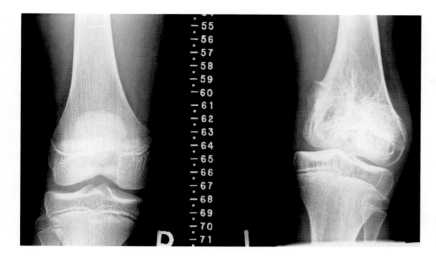

FIGURE 22-6 Anteroposterior radiograph of the knees in a 13-year-old boy shows growth disturbance of the left distal femoral growth plate after a fracture (on right in photo).

The musculoskeletal examination begins with observation of the patient for sites of deformity, swelling, contusions, abnormal color, and open fractures. If a fracture is suspected, confirmatory diagnostic studies may be integrated into the complete physical examination. If such studies cannot be done, it must be assumed that a fracture exists, and the suspected site must be splinted until the fracture is confirmed or ruled out. Splinting may also reduce discomfort and limit further damage to soft tissue. A complete neurovascular examination is essential in any case of suspected limb or spine injury. When an uncooperative patient will not allow an adequate physical examination or, in the case of comatose patients or preverbal children, cannot provide a history, judicial use of special diagnostic studies can be critical.

RADIOGRAPHIC ASSESSMENT

Plain radiography is the first and most widely used test to identify skeletal injury in children, but it can also be a major source of misdiagnosis in this age group. Cartilage, which makes up a large percentage of the child's skeleton, is radiolucent but can fracture. Ossification centers appear at different ages in different locations. The timing of their appearance and their location vary greatly and can suggest fractures.

Confusion most frequently occurs in the elbow, knee, and cervical spine. Comparison of the injured and uninjured limbs can be useful. Plain radiographic soft tissue signs, such as the posterior fat pad sign in elbow injuries, are associated with a high likelihood of underlying fracture (Fig. 22-7).[9] A number of imaging studies are available for the assessment of pediatric musculoskeletal injuries and are injury and age specific. Radiographs may confirm fractures. Ultrasonography is a readily available, noninvasive imaging test that can be used to evaluate the unossified epiphysis, especially in injuries about the elbow.[10] Magnetic resonance imaging (MRI) may also be helpful, especially in evaluating the injured spine, but it may require general anesthesia in a young or uncooperative patient. Computed tomography (CT) scanning is useful in periarticular fractures in children approaching skeletal maturity. For example, ankle physeal fractures with articular extension in children with partially closed physes are best delineated with CT scan.[11] Arteriography may be required to assess vascular injury associated with a fracture. Rarely, proximal tibial physeal fractures and distal humerus fractures through the supracondylar region can be associated with disruption of the blood supply to the distal limb. These injuries require emergent treatment, and an intraoperative arteriogram may be of value in diagnosis and treatment (although in

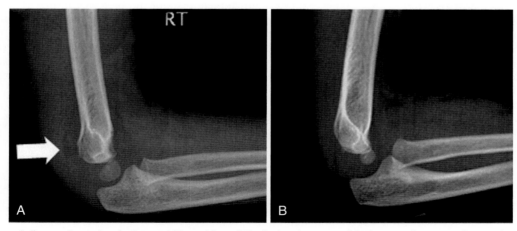

FIGURE 22-7 Lateral elbow radiographs of a 2-year-old boy with a mildly displaced supracondylar humerus fracture and arrow showing a posterior fat pad sign (**A**) and a normal age-matched elbow (**B**).

most situations surgical treatment should not be delayed in order to obtain an arteriogram in the radiology suite).[12] Joint aspiration can identify blood and fat, which indicate an intra-articular fracture that would not be identified on radiographs. Finally, arthrography and arthroscopy may define intra-articular injury to the cartilage and ligaments.

Management of Musculoskeletal Injuries

IMMEDIATE TREATMENT

Priority treatment cannot interfere with complete treatment of an injured child. Proper timing and coordination of management with other disciplines are imperative. Traction or splinting often adequately stabilizes the musculoskeletal injury until other tests and treatments have been completed. Immobilization may also reduce the need for pain medications, which can mask the symptoms of other disorders, such as intra-abdominal injuries, and inhibit diagnosis.

Although there are many types of splints, ranging from plaster to traction bows, the basic principles of fracture management remain the same. The injured part should be splinted as it is found, and the joints above and below the injury should be immobilized without compromising the circulation of the soft tissues. Portable traction splints or custom-molded, well-padded plaster or fiberglass splints can be used in the initial management of fractures. Failure to immobilize the fracture can cause further soft tissue damage from sharp bone ends or the crushing of entrapped neurovascular elements.

DEFINITIVE FRACTURE MANAGEMENT

Adequate stabilization of fracture fragments prevents further soft tissue injury, frequently decreases pain, and facilitates wound care and patient mobilization. Techniques of definitive stabilization in children include splinting, casting, skeletal traction, external fixation, pinning, flexible intramedullary nailing, and plating. The choice of fixation method depends on the child's age, the location of the fracture, the presence and extent of soft tissue injury, and the presence of multitrauma.

Metaphyseal undisplaced or impacted fractures are likely to heal faster than diaphyseal or displaced fractures. Fractures with devitalized bone or soft tissues take longer to heal. Radiographic evaluation in conjunction with clinical judgment and experience is needed when determining the healing time of fractures in children.

Fragments of bone must be held together until they are sufficiently strong to withstand the forces specific to the bone. A satisfactory position must be obtained, without harming adjacent tissue, before the fracture becomes fixed. Fractures in newborns and infants begin to heal within a few days, but fractures in adolescents can be moved freely for 10 to 14 days. Excessive cast padding, resolution of swelling, or a poorly applied cast may permit progressive malposition within the cast. Fractures should be followed with frequent radiographs until union is secure, to avoid displacement. Unstable fractures should be imaged before

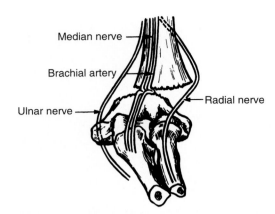

FIGURE 22-8 Supracondylar humerus fracture. Soft tissue and neurovascular structures may become entrapped between bone fragments in these types of fractures.

consolidation to evaluate for loss of alignment. This allows for easier repeat reduction.

In children, the thick periosteum tears on the tension side of a fracture but often remains intact on the compression side. The intact periosteum can then function as a hinge, increasing the success of closed reduction of displaced fractures by three-point molding (see Fig. 22-3). Reduction must be performed gently. Forceful and repeated manipulation of physeal fractures can produce iatrogenic damage and growth disturbances. Entrapment of soft tissue occasionally prevents reduction of an otherwise stable fracture (Fig. 22-8) and requires open reduction and stabilization with internal or external fixation or immobilization in a cast.

In some cases, internal fixation with crossed pins, plates and screws, intramedullary nails, or external fixation with pins in metal outriggers or rods may be useful (Fig. 22-9). The benefits of each of these devices must be weighed against their risks, such as need for future operative removal and the possible disturbance to the growth plate, and should be individualized for each particular clinical scenario. Specific indications for internal and external fixation may include fractures with significant soft tissue injury, fractures in children with closed head injury, those associated with neurovascular injury, and fractures that fail nonoperative treatment. Comminuted and oblique fractures and those with complete tears of the periosteum may also prove to be too unstable for cast immobilization. In cases of intra-articular fractures, such as Salter-Harris types 3 and 4, open reduction and stable internal fixation are frequently necessary to avoid incongruity of the joint or growth disturbance. Fractures associated with neurovascular injury requiring repair should be stabilized first.

High-Priority Musculoskeletal Injuries

Although many musculoskeletal injuries in children can be treated on an urgent rather than an emergent basis, the discussion of some high-priority musculoskeletal injuries in children is warranted. Even in nonurgent cases, it is important to remember that injuries to growing bones can have lifelong consequences.

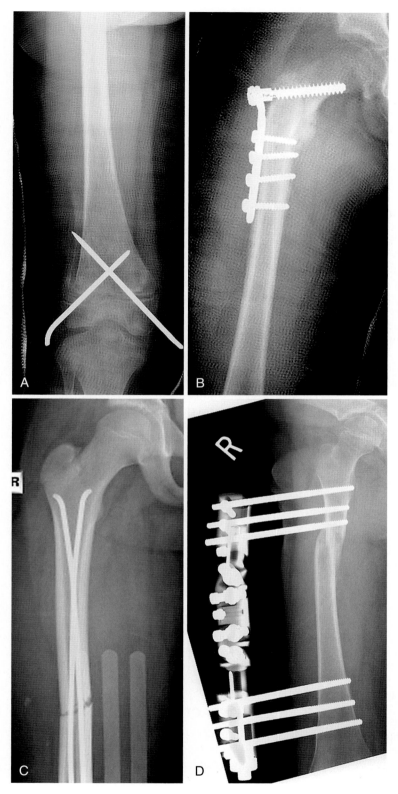

FIGURE 22-9 Anteroposterior radiographs of right femur fractures fixed with a variety of fixation methods. **A,** Salter-Harris type 2 fracture with crossed pins in a 9-year-old girl. **B,** Intertrochanteric fracture with screws and side plate in a 7-year-old boy. **C,** Transverse shaft fracture with elastic intramedullary nails in a 13-year-old boy. **D,** Subtrochanteric fracture with external fixator in an 8-year-old boy.

OPEN FRACTURES AND TRAUMATIC ARTHROTOMIES

Open fractures frequently result from high-energy trauma and communicate with the outside environment, and so are at increased risk for infection.[13–14] The cornerstones of management include recognition, administration of appropriate antibiotics, stabilization of the fracture, and adequate irrigation and debridement of wounds. Open fractures may require multiple surgical procedures to achieve adequate soft tissue coverage and fracture healing.

When a laceration or abrasion is noted in proximity to a fracture, an open fracture must be suspected. Radiographic evidence of air shadows around the fracture may confirm the diagnosis. A sharp fragment of bone can tear through the skin, and the elastic properties of a child's bone can readily straighten the fracture fragments after the force is discontinued. The protruding point of bone can then draw back under the skin, taking debris and bacteria with it into the deep tissues. Minimal signs of injury do not necessarily mean a minimal chance of infection. Wounds should not be probed in the emergency department, where the risk of iatrogenic contamination is high and the likelihood of adequate debridement is low; if necessary, such procedures should be done in the operating room.

The Gustilo system classifies open fractures according to the size and extent of soft tissue damage.[13–15] Type I is an open fracture with a clean wound smaller than 1 cm. Type II is an open fracture with a laceration longer than 1 cm without extensive soft tissue damage, flaps, or avulsions. Type III is an open fracture with extensive soft tissue injury and is further divided into three subtypes: Type IIIA has adequate soft tissue coverage of a fractured bone despite extensive laceration of soft tissue, type IIIB involves extensive soft tissue injury with periosteal stripping that requires grafting or a flap for coverage, and type IIIC is an open fracture associated with arterial injury that requires repair. The risk of infection is related to the severity of the injury: 2% in type I open fractures, 2% to 10% in type II open fractures, and up to 50% in type III open fractures.[15] Wounds should initially be dressed with sterile gauze soaked with antiseptic. Hemorrhage should be controlled by direct pressure. Patients should receive tetanus prophylaxis and antibiotics at recognition of the injury. First-generation cephalosporins cover the gram-positive organisms found in type I and type II injuries. An aminoglycoside is added for type III injuries, and ampicillin or penicillin is added for farm injuries or other massively contaminated wounds to fight potential anaerobic infection.

Each wound must be adequately debrided and copiously irrigated with the patient under general anesthesia. Current evidence suggests that this should be accomplished as soon as the patient is stable, and within 24 hours after injury if possible.[16] Wounds may need to be re-evaluated after 2 or more days for additional debridement. Primary closure or delayed primary closure may be appropriate for some open fractures, whereas grafting or flap coverage is needed for larger soft tissue defects. The goal of debridement is removal of devitalized tissue to avoid the catastrophic consequences of an infection, which may include limb loss or chronic osteomyelitis. Adequate immobilization is necessary for soft tissue healing. For small lacerations, immobilization in a cast that has been windowed for wound inspection may suffice. For larger lacerations, external or internal fixation is often necessary to provide stable fixation with access to the wound.

Joint penetration by a foreign body can cause a diagnostic dilemma. Radiographs can be helpful if they reveal an "air arthrogram." Injection of sterile normal saline into the joint, or saline load test, can also be diagnostic.[17] If the saline load test results in the liquid exiting the wound or laceration, joint penetration has occurred and requires irrigation and debridement in the operating room.

COMPARTMENT SYNDROME

Compartment syndrome occurs when pressure is elevated within a confined fascial space. This causes circulatory compromise and can progress to tissue necrosis. Closed fractures and crush injuries with associated edema may cause compartment syndrome. Forearm and leg compartments are most often involved. Ischemic injury starts when tissue pressure is 30 mm Hg less than mean arterial pressure.[18–19] The pressure within the compartments surrounding a fracture should be measured if compartment syndrome is suspected. Commercially available tissue pressure monitors or other measuring devices, including electronic arterial pressure monitoring devices, can be used.

The diagnosis of compartment syndrome in children can be difficult. Adults with compartment syndrome verbalize extreme pain and demonstrate pain with passive stretch of the muscles within the affected compartments, whereas children often have difficulty communicating their discomfort. The classical signs of compartment syndrome are the five Ps: pain, pallor, paresthesia, paralysis, and pulselessness. These signs are rather unreliable in children and may manifest late in the process. An increasing analgesia requirement is an important sign of compartment syndrome in children.[20]

With early recognition and timely management, full recovery can be achieved. All external compression is removed from the limb, compartment pressures are measured, and, if elevated, the compartments are surgically decompressed. In the forearm, volar and dorsal fasciotomies are required.[19] In the leg, all four compartments (anterior, lateral, deep posterior, and superficial posterior) must be released. This can be accomplished with either a one- or two-incision technique.[18] Without prompt intervention, the result is irreversible damage to soft tissues with loss of function, subsequent contractures, and deformity.[18–19]

FEMORAL NECK FRACTURE

Although rare in children, fractures of the femoral neck and intertrochanteric region require attention (Fig. 22-10). These fractures frequently result from high-energy impact, including traffic accidents and falls from a height, and are associated with a high complication rate from avascular necrosis, coxa vara, nonunion, delayed union, and premature physeal closure.[21] The upper end of the femur lies within the joint capsule. After roughly 4 years of age, blood is supplied primarily by retinacular vessels that course from distal in the neck to proximal in the head. Delay in treatment of a fracture at the

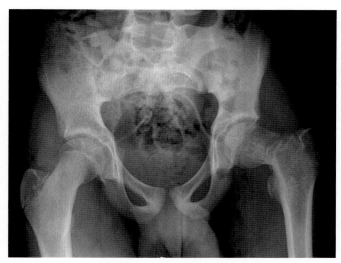

FIGURE 22-10 Anteroposterior pelvis radiograph of a 14-year-old boy shows a displaced left femoral neck fracture that required internal fixation.

  or

FIGURE 22-11 A pediatric backboard should have a torso mattress or an occiput recess to accommodate the child's relatively large head and avoid potentially dangerous cervical spine flexion.

neck is associated with increased risk of avascular necrosis of the head and destruction of the joint and can cause lifelong disability. Early decompression of the hip joint, reduction of the fracture, and internal fixation may minimize the complications.[21]

MANGLED EXTREMITIES

Severely traumatized or mangled extremities in children must be assessed and treated through a multidisciplinary approach on a case-by-case basis. They may involve extensive injury to or segmental loss of skin, muscle, bone, and neurovascular structures. Some limbs may be unsalvageable owing to extensive damage, some can be reconstructed with a resulting dysfunctional limb, and others can be salvaged with a good outcome. The Mangled Extremity Severity Score rates injuries based on objective criteria at initial presentation, including skeletal and soft tissue injury, limb ischemia, shock, and patient age. Although originally developed in a primarily adult population,[22] it can be a useful adjunct to managing lower extremity trauma in children.[23]

Segmental bone loss is rare in children and does not necessitate amputation. If periosteum can be preserved, the potential to reform bone is extensive. Proper techniques of debridement and stabilization, along with adequate time for healing, may produce good results in children. External fixation techniques can allow for bone transport and osteogenesis to replace lost bone and axial deformity.

Power lawn mower injuries are uncommon, preventable injuries that cause significant morbidity in children.[24–26] Direct contact with the blade leads to laceration of tissue, amputation, or devitalizing shredding of the extremity. Such injury can result in damage to the vasculature and growth plate, joint stiffness, infection, or amputation. If salvage is undertaken, treatment follows that of open fractures.

In the case of amputation, preservation of bony length and retention of all viable soft tissue are important for the ultimate functional outcome. Amputation through the diaphysis of a child's bone frequently results in overgrowth of the bony stump through the skin. This is especially true of the fibula, tibia, and humerus and can necessitate cutting back the bone every few years.

SPINE TRAUMA

Injuries of the spine in children can be divided into those affecting the cervical spine and those in the thoracic and lumbar spine. Just as in other parts of the body, patterns of injury to the spine in children differ from those in adults. Radiographic imaging can be challenging. Principles of immobilization are different for children as well.

Cervical spine injuries in children differ from those in adults.[27–28] Children have greater ligamentous laxity and weaker neck musculature. In addition, they have large heads relative to body size; this effect is more pronounced in younger children. Cervical spine injuries in children tend to occur higher in the neck and can be primarily ligamentous or apophyseal without bony fracture.[29] When immobilizing a child on a backboard, the relatively large head should be considered; a child's backboard splint should have a recess for the occiput or a mattress for the torso to maintain the alignment of the cervical spine, avoiding flexion of the neck (Fig. 22-11).[30]

Radiographic evaluation of the pediatric cervical spine can be challenging. Pseudosubluxation, or the apparent forward displacement of C2 on C3 and, less commonly, C3 on C4, is a well-described plain radiographic finding in normal children younger than 8 years.[27,31] Other sources of difficulty in interpreting radiographs include incomplete ossification, epiphyseal variation, and elasticity of the disks and vertebral bodies relative to the neural structures, which allows extensive injury to the soft tissues without evidence of abnormality on plain radiographs or SCIWORA (spinal cord injury without radiographic abnormality). MRI is helpful in evaluating soft tissues in cases of possible cervical spine ligamentous injury in children.[27,32]

Injuries to the thoracic and lumbar spine are rare in children. The growth of vertebral bodies occurs through the apophyses or growth centers on the cranial and caudal ends of the bodies. With compression injury, adolescents are at risk for traumatic displacement of the vertebral apophysis and the attached disk into the spinal canal, especially in the lumbar region.[33] Symptoms are similar to those seen in central disk herniation, including muscle weakness and absent reflexes. This injury requires recognition and emergent surgical decompression.

Lap-belt injuries are flexion-distraction injuries that typically occur in the thoracolumbar region when children violently flex over the seat belt.[28,34] A fracture propagates from the posterior portions of the vertebra to the disks or vertebral body in the front (Fig. 22-12). In addition to the vertebral injury, children can sustain serious abdominal and aortic injuries, and these should be suspected when an abdominal contusion, or the telltale seat-belt sign, is evident in a trauma patient. Lap-belt injuries frequently require immobilization and possible internal fixation.[28]

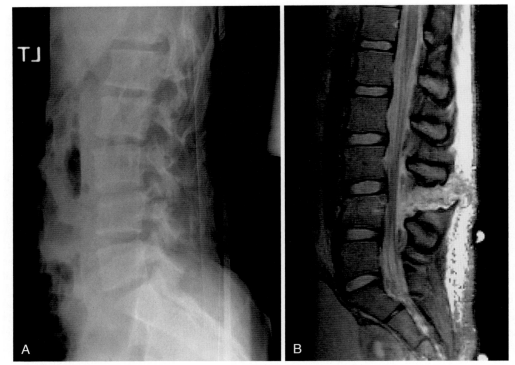

FIGURE 22-12   Lap-belt injury of L4 in a 15-year-old girl without neurologic injury. **A,** Lateral lumbar spine radiograph shows fracture of both the L4 body and the posterior spine. **B,** Sagittal magnetic resonance image of the lumbar spine shows the extensive bony and soft tissue injury.

CHILD ABUSE

The maltreatment of children is a complex medical and social problem, and its recognition is key to management. Fractures before walking age in the absence of metabolic disease or child abuse are rare. Fractures are the second most common manifestation of child abuse after skin lesions.[35] Suspicion of abuse must be raised when there is a discrepancy between history and injury, when multiple fractures are present in different stages of healing, or when bruising, metaphyseal fractures, or long bone fractures appear in children younger than 1 year.[35]

The complete reference list is available online at www. expertconsult.com.

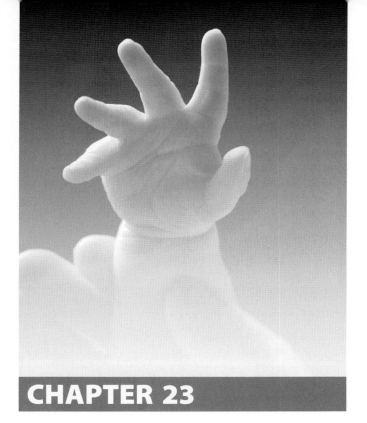

CHAPTER 23

Hand, Soft Tissue, and Envenomation Injuries

Daniel B. Schmid and Michael L. Bentz

Evaluation of pediatric hand and soft tissue injuries requires a systematic approach that includes all relevant organ systems at the site of trauma.[1,2] A high index of suspicion is necessary to make an accurate diagnosis and exclude subtle problems, particularly in toddlers and infants who are unable to cooperate with a detailed examination. Injuries undergo triage according to their threat to life. After triage has taken place, the more peripheral and often more dramatic and distracting injuries can be better defined.[2] The history is important to define baseline function, previous injuries, right- or left-hand dominance, and the mechanism and timing of injury. The initial physical examination must define vascularity and perfusion because an ischemic or poorly perfused extremity necessitates emergent surgical intervention. Other findings can be handled in a less urgent fashion after an orderly assessment is complete. The patient should be examined in a well-lighted area with the parents present to exert a calming influence over a frightened child and thus increase the reliability of findings. This chapter focuses on the acute evaluation and management of hand, soft tissue, and envenomation injuries to provide a foundation for the accurate triage of injured children.[3,4]

Hand and Soft Tissue Injuries

EVALUATION

Vascularity

The goal of the initial examination is to determine the presence or extent of vascular injury, hypoperfusion, or ischemia. Symptoms of ischemia include pallor, paresthesia, paralysis, pain, and lack of pulse. The digits should be pink and warm if the patient has not had hypothermic exposure or proximal tourniquet application. Normal capillary refill time is 3 seconds and is most accurately tested by compressing the lateral aspect of the distal phalanx adjacent to the nail plate. A delayed refill time indicates impaired arterial inflow, whereas a rapid refill time suggests venous hypertension or insufficiency. The pulse should be palpated bilaterally at the radial, ulnar, and brachial arteries. Percutaneous Doppler ultrasonography can be used to qualitatively and quantitatively define inflow if the pulse cannot be detected or if it is asymmetric. An Allen test is important to define the relative contributions of the radial and ulnar arteries to the palmar arches of the hand. The ulnar artery is the dominant source of inflow to the hand and continues into a patent palmar arch in 85% of uninjured hands.[5,6] Significant bleeding noted during the initial evaluation is managed by firm manual compression or, if the time until definitive intervention is expected to be prolonged, by proximal tourniquet application. A hemostat or clamp should not be placed blindly into the wound because lack of blood flow may injure adjacent neural structures. Impaled or retained foreign objects should be left in situ until definitive management is possible because they may staunch the flow of blood from a vascular injury.

Peripheral Nerves

Peripheral nerves should be evaluated after vascular inflow has been assessed. Isolated nerve injuries cause predictable neurologic deficits that manifest as abnormalities in sensation or motor function depending on the location of injury.[7,8] Vascular injuries can also cause neurologic deficits, particularly in subacute wounds; therefore the evaluation of nerve and vascular injuries should generally occur in tandem. A clear concept of cross-sectional anatomy is helpful in visualizing potential at-risk structures.[8] Sensory examination requires a child to cooperate, but even in a young child anhidrosis (loss of sweating function) can be seen and indicates underlying nerve damage.[9,10] In the cooperative patient, evaluating the nerve function at the distal aspect of the hand can be used to screen for a more proximal nerve injury.

The median nerve is responsible for sensation to the three and one-half volar radial digits. The function of this nerve can be tested by a pinprick or, more objectively, by two-point tactile discrimination. Median nerve motor function can be tested by palpating the contraction of the abductor pollicis brevis and opponens pollicis muscles as the patient forms an "O" with the index finger and thumb (Fig. 23-1). The ulnar nerve supplies sensation to the one and one-half ulnar digits. Motor function of this nerve is most accurately tested by palpating the contraction against the force of the first dorsal interosseous muscle while the fingers are spread (Fig. 23-2). There is no radial nerve motor innervation of the intrinsic hand muscles,

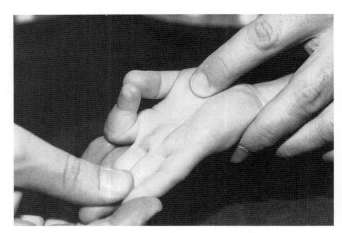

FIGURE 23-1 The ability to form an "O" with the index finger and thumb, with palpable contraction of the thenar muscles, indicates an intact median nerve.

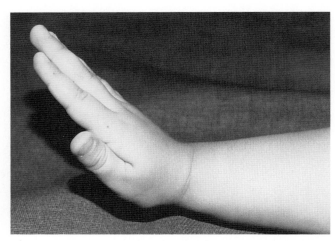

FIGURE 23-3 Digit and wrist extension demonstrates radial nerve integrity because no muscles in the hand are innervated by radial nerves.

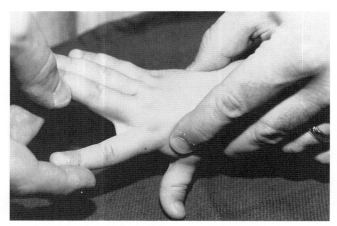

FIGURE 23-2 Digit spread with palpable contraction of the first dorsal interosseous muscle is consistent with an intact ulnar nerve.

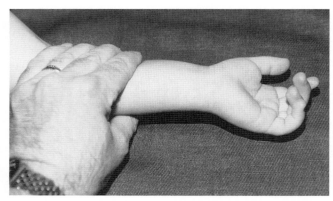

FIGURE 23-4 Forearm compression has failed to cause flexion of the index finger in this patient; this suggests flexor mechanism discontinuity to the index finger.

so the motor function of the radial nerve is best screened by wrist and digit extension (Fig. 23-3). The radial nerves provide sensation to the three and one-half dorsal radial digits of the hand to the level of the distal phalanges, although overlap is common. Serial examination can be helpful, and cooperation and a focused effort are essential for a reliable evaluation. Further, neurologic findings associated with compartment syndrome evolve over time and may not be obvious during the initial examination.[11,12]

Skeleton, Tendons, and Ligaments

Although some skeletal injuries are obvious on routine examination, most require radiographic evaluation. Physical examination findings of fracture include deformity, crepitus, ecchymosis, pain, instability, and swelling. Anteroposterior, lateral, and oblique radiographs should be obtained for all but the most minor injuries to evaluate for fractures, dislocations, and foreign objects. Familiarity with the Salter-Harris classification of pediatric fractures is important because the specific fracture patterns offer prognostic information relevant to subsequent growth (see Chapter 22).[13,14] The presentation of fractures has been well documented.[15–19] Examination and

radiographic appearance are combined to describe the fracture accurately. Open fractures have an associated full-thickness soft tissue injury, whereas closed fractures do not. Simple fractures result in two bone fragments, whereas comminuted fractures involve several fragments. Greenstick fractures involve one cortex and are particularly relevant in children because of their malleable bones. The description of a fracture should also include information regarding length (shortened, elongated, normal), angulation (volar, dorsal, radial, ulnar), rotation (present or absent), and displacement as a percentage of normal alignment.

Tendon injuries can be difficult to diagnose, particularly in young or uncooperative children. In such cases, surgical exploration is necessary to definitely confirm certain injuries. The posture of the hand at rest gives information regarding tendon integrity. In a relaxed position, the hand should form a gentle cascade; this position results from passive tension of the tendons. With compression of the distal forearm, all digits should adopt flexion posturing as a result of the tenodesis effect. A digit that remains extended out of the cascade suggests disruption of the flexor mechanism (Fig. 23-4). The flexor digitorum superficialis tendon to each of the four fingers is tested by holding the adjacent digits in a fixed position and

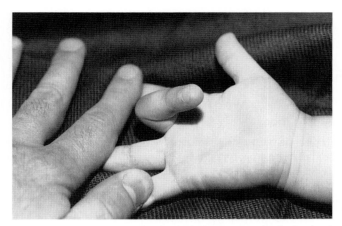

FIGURE 23-5 Function of the flexor digitorum superficialis tendon is tested by demonstrating isolated metacarpophalangeal and proximal interphalangeal joint flexion. Flexor digitorum profundus tendon function is tested by holding the middle phalanx fixed and observing distal interphalangeal joint flexion.

allowing metacarpophalangeal joint flexion (Fig. 23-5). The flexor digitorum profundus and flexor pollicis longus tendons are evaluated by holding the middle phalanx and observing distal interphalangeal joint flexion.

Ligament injuries can be difficult to diagnose, particularly in the presence of associated soft tissue or skeletal injuries.[20] Abnormal joint stability is an indicator of disruption of the ligaments.[15] If the opposite side is uninjured, joint stability should be compared with that side as an indicator of preinjury status. Plain and stress radiographs of an avulsion fracture at the site of ligament insertion can confirm clinical findings.

Soft Tissue

A thorough determination of soft tissue injuries is important for a knowledgeable evaluation of wound healing, but even more so for the evaluation of long-term function and outcome of primary or secondary reconstructive surgery.[21] The amount of soft tissue present in the area of a wound determines the feasibility of primary repair of vascular, neural, and osteoligamentous injuries, and an adequate amount is required for proper healing. The size (measured objectively), shape, location, and general configuration of each wound is recorded, and the mechanism of injury and preinjury status of the patient is established. Obvious foreign objects are removed, although projectiles impaled through an extremity are left in situ until they can be managed definitively. Exposed vital structures as well as associated fractures and tendon injuries are noted.

EARLY TREATMENT

Vascular Structures

Ischemia is one of the few surgical emergencies associated with upper limb trauma. Revascularization is a top priority after the correction of life-threatening injuries. Because irreversible changes start to occur after 4 hours of ischemia, expeditious surgical intervention is mandatory, especially if the ischemic tissue involves muscle. Primary vascular repair is the most effective procedure and is ideally accomplished by debridement, mobilization, and primary anastomosis of

injured segments. Reversed vein grafts, which are frequently performed with foot, forearm, saphenous, or cephalic veins, should be used liberally if tension or lack of tissue prevents easy approximation of adjacent segments. In general, all arteries and veins proximal to the elbow should be repaired. Repair of arterial injuries below the elbow should also be considered to prevent cold intolerance; however, only about half of these repairs remain patent.[22,23] If necessary, the radial artery can be ligated primarily. Once repairs are complete, fasciotomy should be considered if ischemia has been prolonged, soft tissue damage is significant, or adequate postoperative monitoring is not available.[11] Serial examination should then be pursued in an effort to make an early diagnosis of recurrent ischemia or postsurgical thrombosis or bleeding. The role of anticoagulation therapy in this setting is controversial and is based on the surgeon's preference and experience.

Peripheral Nerves

Injury to the peripheral nerves is not an emergency and can frequently be addressed when an adjacent vascular injury is being repaired. When a wound is clean, uninfected, and well vascularized, primary nerves should be repaired in an end-to-end fashion. Such repair can be facilitated through the mobilization of proximal and distal injured segments, which can reduce tension and augment blood flow. If mobilization of the injured segments cannot adequately repair the defect, interpositional nerve grafts, nerve conduits, or vein grafts can be used for definitive reconstruction.[8,24] In such cases, early secondary repair in the first 10 days after injury is optimal. To ensure that the injured area remains intact, the involved limb should be splinted to minimize further proximal migration of the transected nerve before surgery and to relieve anastomotic tension.

Skeleton, Tendons, and Ligaments

When injuries to the skeleton, tendons, or ligaments are diagnosed, restoration of normal or acceptable anatomy followed by appropriate immobilization is indicated. In children, an injury that is suspected but not objectively defined is particularly common. Hand fractures may not be evident on radiographs for several weeks. In this situation, presumptive treatment should be carried out, which usually involves immobilization of the potentially injured area despite equivocal physical examination or radiographic findings. Immobilization is rarely contraindicated in children because it allows protection from further injury, improves pain control, and maintains local anatomy. Use of a splint (instead of a cast) is ideal because it allows swelling into a nonfixed space and limits the possibility of vascular compromise during the acute injury and postreduction periods.

Anatomic reduction of fractures and dislocations can be done at the time of injury or in the following week with good functional results.[25] In the acute setting, excellent anesthesia can be obtained by performing a hematoma block. This is accomplished by injecting 2 to 3 mL of lidocaine 1% without epinephrine into the fracture site. Reduction in the subacute setting most commonly requires a traditional digital block. It must be kept in mind, particularly in smaller children, that the limiting dose of plain lidocaine is 4 mg/kg of body weight. A description of the reduction maneuvers for specific types of fractures is beyond the scope of this chapter, but in general gentle manual traction or finger-trap distraction with simultaneous rotation or derotation allows improvement in many types of fractures and dislocations. Postreduction radiographs should be obtained in most if not all patients before or after immobilization. The specific position of immobilization is less critical for children than for adults because children are less prone to stiffening and tightening of the ligaments. The "position of safety" can always be used at least initially for splinting: the wrist is placed in 30 to 45 degrees of extension, the metacarpophalangeal joints are placed in 70 degrees of flexion, and the interphalangeal joints are left straight. Serial physical and radiographic examinations are tailored to the specific injury and clinical course.

Soft Tissue

After soft tissue and associated vital structure injuries are documented, irrigation of all significant wounds should be performed with normal saline solution, after which foreign objects are removed and tissue that is clearly devitalized is debrided.[26] These procedures may require a local anesthetic, which should be given only after a thorough neurologic examination has been completed. Simple lacerations and small surface area avulsions can be closed primarily using the same layered closure method used for deep or gaping wounds under tension. Suture choice depends on the location, size, and cause of the wound, as well as the patient's age. A smaller child who requires sedation for the primary wound repair will be hypersensitive to suture removal, when sedation is usually not available. In such cases, absorbable sutures reinforced with adhesive strips (Steri-strips) are ideal. Permanent sutures should be used in older or cooperative patients to minimize the inflammatory response and avoid early scarring. The potential for scarring depends on the location of the wound and the mechanism of injury. Scarring can be minimized through judicious wound closure.

Open wounds that cannot be closed primarily require more elaborate intervention. To bridge the gap between injury and wound closure, the wound must be managed and protected. Normal saline wet-to-wet dressings are a simple and effective way to provide limited debridement, allow the initiation of granulation, and prevent desiccation. Povidone-iodine dressings should be reserved for short-term use in infected wounds. Acetic acid solution (0.25%) is appropriate for wounds that have culture documentation of infection with *Pseudomonas* species. Subatmospheric pressure dressings are effective as temporary cover of a contaminated or extensive wound, as a bridge to more extensive soft tissue reconstruction, or for definitive closure of extremity wounds in the pediatric population.[27-29] Quantitative wound biopsies should be reserved for nonthermal burns.

If the skin defect is partial thickness only and no vital structures are exposed, split-thickness skin grafting or skin distraction is appropriate. Split-thickness skin grafts are used for larger wounds, less cosmetically significant wounds, or those in which the wound bed may not be optimal because of infection, inflammation, or ischemia. Full-thickness skin grafts contract less after revascularization and thus are ideal for cosmetically significant areas or where wound contraction is undesirable. Local skin flaps can also be used in such settings, offering a cosmetically favorable replacement of like tissue. These skin flaps can be random if they have no specific blood supply or axial if the blood is supplied by a specific vessel.[30] Regional muscle flaps can be used almost anywhere in the body, especially when highly vascularized tissue of significant bulk is required to cover exposed critical structures and fill dead space. Similar to axial pattern skin flaps, these muscle flaps are used on the basis of a known blood supply, which makes their dissection reliable and safe. Finally, when local tissue is not available or is inadequate to provide wound closure, microvascular free tissue transfer is indicated using specific donor "free flaps" to accomplish specific tasks.[31]

Amputations

Traumatic amputations in children should be considered for replantation by a qualified microsurgical team, given the excellent results obtained when compared with adult series.[32-34] To optimize the chance of success, the amputated part should be wrapped in saline-moistened gauze, sealed in a plastic bag, and placed in a bag of ice and saline solution; the part must not contact the ice directly.

Envenomation Injuries

SNAKEBITES

More than 2700 species of snakes exist; 115 of these species are indigenous to the United States, and only 19 of the 115 species are poisonous.[35] In the United States approximately 8000 bites occur annually from poisonous snakes, half of which occur in children.[36,37] Pit vipers, which are named for the pit located between their eyes and nostrils, account for most bites. Pit vipers include rattlesnakes, copperheads, and cottonmouths (family Viperidae, subfamily Crotalinae).[38] Coral snakes (family Elapidae) represent the other poisonous family. Most bites occur during the summer months in the morning, late afternoon, or evening. Not all bites are associated with envenomation. Signs of envenomation include pain, edema, local tissue necrosis ecchymosis, nausea, vomiting, hypotension, disseminated intravascular coagulopathy, hemolysis, mental status changes, seizures, and death.[39] The severity of signs is proportional to the degree of envenomation. Early intervention includes reassurance and support, immobilization, limb elevation, venous tourniquet application, and rapid transfer to the nearest medical facility. Cryotherapy and wound incision and suction are no longer recommended because of potential damage to vital structures.[40-42] Tetanus immune globulin and toxoid should be given to patients who have had two or fewer immunizations.

The antivenin Fab AV is sheep immunoglobulin immunized with antigen from four snakes—three variety of rattlesnakes and a cottonmouth or water moccasin—that has been shown to be effective after envenomation by all North American rattlesnakes and was found to be safe in children in a small study of 12 subjects.[43-45] Antivenin is administered intravenously only after a skin test has been done to rule out the possibility of an anaphylactic reaction. Four to six vials (4-6 g) of Fab AV is given immediately, with redosing in 1 hour if the patient does not respond.[45] Initial dosing should be followed by aggressive intravenous hydration and close monitoring. A review of 93 patients receiving Fab AV noted immediate allergic reaction in approximately 5% of cases.[46] Because envenomation injuries and the use of antivenom require close monitoring, antivenom administration should not be delayed for skin testing.[47] Fasciotomy should be considered but is seldom required.[48] A review of 227 patients with rattlesnake bites of whom 211 were treated with antivenom showed favorable outcomes in nearly all patients.[47] After initial treatment and baseline testing, patients should be closely observed for at least 12 hours in cases of crotalid envenomation and 24 hours for coral snake bites because of possible delayed-onset neurotoxicity.[49]

OTHER BITE INJURIES

Gila monsters, which are found in the southwestern United States, and their relative the Mexican beaded lizard are active in late spring. These lizards inject venom as long as they cling to the victim. Wounds show edema, but tissue loss is less pronounced than that associated with envenomation by pit vipers; however, systemic signs can ultimately be similar. These injuries are managed by removing the animal from its victim, followed by local and systemic supportive care. Antivenin is not available. Radiographs should be obtained to exclude retained teeth.[50–52]

Black widow spiders are venomous New World spiders; the females are black with an hourglass-shaped red mark on the abdomen.[53–55] Local signs of a bite can be limited and are followed by systemic neuromuscular symptoms of diffuse rigidity and spasm that potentially lead to respiratory arrest approximately 1 hour later. Envenomations by black widow spiders are managed by local care, fluid and cardiovascular support, parenteral calcium gluconate, muscle relaxation, and antivenin.[3,51,55–58]

Scorpion stings in children have serious sequelae. Bark scorpions are the only toxic species in the United States; however, others are common in Mexico and equatorial countries. Local signs of envenomation are minimal, whereas systemic neuromuscular findings are present in the sympathetic and parasympathetic systems. Children are particularly susceptible to the severe cardiorespiratory and neuromuscular dysfunction associated with envenomation. Therapy of scorpion stings includes local wound care, topical ice, specific antivenin, and systemic support, including ventilation, control of tachyarrhythmias, and sedation. Treatment is similar to that for spider bites, although scorpion stings are generally less serious.[55,57,59–61]

Finally, human bite wounds can pose some of the most challenging definitive management problems among all bite-induced injuries.[62,63] Based on the quantitative and qualitative characteristics of oral flora, including the principal pathogen *Eikenella corrodens*, aggressive primary intervention is mandatory to achieve a satisfactory outcome in all these injuries. Thorough irrigation of penetrating bite wounds is mandatory as is broad-spectrum antibiotic coverage followed by frequent wound checks.[64]

The complete reference list is available online at www. expertconsult.com.

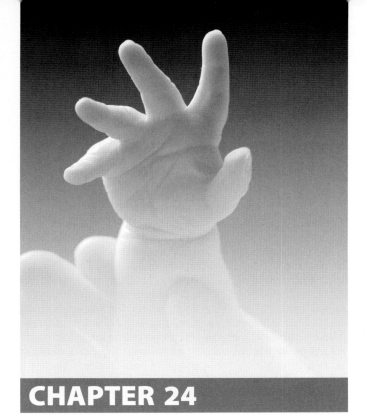

CHAPTER 24

Central Nervous System Injuries

Andrew Jea and Thomas G. Luerssen

Injuries to the brain and spinal cord continue to be major contributors to mortality and morbidity from childhood trauma. Despite over 25 years of intensive clinical research, there is still not a specific medical therapy for traumatic neurologic injury. Nevertheless, there has been a steady and substantial advance in our understanding of the natural history of brain and spinal cord injuries, and accompanying changes in management that continue to be refined and have clearly resulted in improved outcomes.

We are now well into the era of evidence-based medicine, whereby recommendations for disease and injury management are supposed to be derived from critical analysis of scientific research. In the last decade, the management strategies for central nervous system (CNS) injuries have been subjected to this type of analysis, resulting in the publication and continuous updating of practice management guidelines.[1-4] The analysis of the clinical evidence and the development of these recommendations represented a substantial amount of work by many leading experts in the field. Unfortunately, these reviews also uncovered a remarkable lack of strong scientific evidence upon which to develop recommendations, especially in the pediatric age group, so that most of the available recommendations regarding the diagnosis and treatment of neurologic injuries can only be supported by the lowest degree of medical certainty. Nevertheless, these published practice parameters are useful summaries of the current understanding of the various treatments for brain and spinal cord injuries.

Even in the face of limited evidence, we are also learning that "quality improvement" strategies are beneficial in the management of injury. These strategies allow multidisciplinary agreement and reproducible diagnostic and treatment processes that have specific outcomes that can be measured and continuously improved. Thus although there may be variation between centers, approaches within a single center can be uniform and workable for that institution.

Basic Strategy of the Therapy of Central Nervous System Injury

One of the most enduring concepts underlying the management of brain and spinal cord injury is that of primary and secondary injury.[5] The primary neurologic injury involves the immediate disruption of neuronal, axonal, supportive structures, and vascular tissues. The magnitude and location of the primary injury along with the variety of irreversible cellular processes that immediately ensue, which has been referred to as the delayed primary injury, are directly related to the mechanism of the injury. These immediate tissue disruptions are also considered to be self limited and are, by definition, essentially untreatable. Given all of this, one can easily see that the primary brain injury is still the major determinant of injury outcome.

The primary injury triggers a cascade of intracellular and extracellular biochemical changes, both in the region of the injury and systemically, many of which are deleterious and cause acceleration and augmentation of the initial injury. These reactive processes represent the onset of what has been termed the secondary injury. These secondary reactive processes can begin at almost any time after the injury and can persist for some time. The secondary injury results not only in new damage both in the region of the primary injury, but also in areas of previously uninjured brain or spinal cord. It can also cause deleterious effects in other organs and body systems.

Systemic reactions commonly seen after brain or spinal cord injury include alterations in blood pressure and respiration, usually manifested by hypotension and hypoxia. It has been clearly shown that even brief and mild episodes of either hypoxia or hypotension can have profoundly deleterious effects on the outcome of both brain and spinal cord injury.[6-8] Although it is well known that spinal cord–injured patients can be rendered hypotensive by an isolated injury, it is now also clear that isolated brain injury can cause systemic hypotension. Multiple injuries, occult organ injuries, or other causes of exsanguination that result in hypovolemia are not required for this hypotensive response to occur. Of the early systemic complications, it appears that hypotension is much more deleterious to the acutely injured brain than is hypoxia. This is probably also true for the acutely injured spinal cord. Finally, it is clear that these complications can occur very early, frequently, and, in many cases, so briefly that they can go undetected.[9,10]

There are also other common systemic responses, many of which occur shortly after an injury but can also cause further injury even days after the institution of therapy. Hyperthermia, either from fever or as the result of overly aggressive warming, is harmful to the injured brain.[11] Hyperglycemia, which is commonly seen in the stress response and which can be aggravated by fluid administration or attempted nutrition, is also thought to be deleterious to the acutely injured neurons.[12–14]

Tissue disruptions, commonly referred to as cerebral or spinal cord contusions, cause reactive changes in the tissues immediately surrounding the area of injury. A variety of tissue factors, such as those in the kallikrein-kinin system, are released, and these factors can cause disturbances of microcirculation and the blood–brain or blood–spinal cord barrier, which ultimately results in the complex entity that has been generally referred to as post-traumatic edema.[15] There are hypermetabolic responses related to neural-tissue injury that may outstrip the local or regional substrate supply.[16] Excitotoxic amino acids, such as glutamate and aspartate, are released from injured neurons.[17] Post-traumatic seizures, especially prolonged subclinical seizures, may contribute to this response in the injured brain.[18] Along with the reactive biochemical changes, expanding local hemorrhages can cause further compression of adjacent vessels and tissues, resulting in an ischemic penumbra around the acute injury.

Although the systemic and biochemical processes of the secondary injury are complex, it appears that the pathophysiologic end point of all of them is ischemic damage. Ischemic neuronal damage is almost universally seen in the neuropathologic examinations of patients who have suffered traumatic brain and spinal cord injuries.[19,20]

Even though numerous biochemical cascades have been identified and physiologically characterized, and many have been the targets of pharmaceutical intervention, no drug has yet been shown to be specifically effective for CNS injury treatment. Trials of high-dose steroids, calcium channel blockers, free radical scavengers, and glutamate antagonists have been generally negative, although small and specific subgroups of patients were identified in post hoc analyses, which may have benefited from one or another of these therapies. More concerning is that some groups of patients were apparently harmed by the administration of some of these agents.[21] Despite this lack of development of a specific therapy, there has been steady improvement in neurologic outcomes, more so in the arena of brain injury than in spinal cord injury. This trend in improved outcome is almost certainly because of the realization that many of the ischemic processes can be prevented by aggressively applying various systemic manipulations, beginning with the resuscitation phase of the injury and continuing through the acute therapy period.

The essential therapeutic strategies for brain and spinal cord injury are based on preventing ischemic injury by the aggressive support of intravascular volume and blood pressure at all times. The historical idea of restricting fluids to head-injured patients is no longer accepted or acceptable management. The early use of vasopressors for both brain and spinal cord injury is appropriate. Reduction of focal vascular compression by removing mass lesions and aggressively preventing and managing reactive brain or cord swelling to protect perfusion are beneficial. These three relatively simplistic concepts—support of systemic blood pressure, reduction of intracranial pressure to assure cerebral perfusion, and removal of compressive lesions and the prevention of deleterious complications—are still the mainstay of management for brain and spinal cord injuries.

Immediate Issues: Resuscitation and Transport of Injured Children

Effective, supportive, and preventative therapy should begin as quickly after the injury as possible. Goals of the initial resuscitation are twofold: to prevent as much secondary injury as possible and any new primary injury prior to the undertaking of neurodiagnostic studies. One can accomplish the first goal by assuring oxygenated perfusion of the brain and spinal cord, by restoring and maintaining age-appropriate normal blood pressure, and maintaining normal ventilation. These factors are of primary importance and are more important than the administration of any drug. The exact means of accomplishing this goal—the type of resuscitation fluid or the means of assuring ventilation—is probably less important than accomplishing the goal itself. Most current studies indicate that isotonic or slightly hypertonic saline solutions are appropriate fluids for resuscitating and maintaining blood pressure for neurologically injured patients.[2,22,23]

Tissue oxygenation is important; so, adequate airway support and ventilation are required. Early intubation by experienced personnel and using appropriate analgesia and sedation certainly will accomplish this goal. However, the role of intubation of injured children (and adults) in the field is still controversial. This maneuver is associated with a relatively high complication rate and may not be warranted in many situations.[1,24,25]

For patients with possible spinal injuries, prevention of further injury begins with stabilizing the spine. This maneuver involves much more than applying a collar or securing a child to a rigid board. It is important that the normal anatomic alignment be maintained. Very young children have proportionately larger heads and therefore have a tendency for cervical flexion when lying supine.[26] A cervical collar alone does not completely immobilize a child's injured spine.[27] The spine should be immobilized in anatomic position, with the head in a normal relative position to the body. Young children will require some additional elevation of the body so that the head falls back to a truly neutral position. Once these parameters have been achieved, that is, stabilization of the spine in anatomic position and the establishment of support of systemic blood pressure and respiration, the injured child may be transported for definitive diagnosis and therapy of the injury.

Traumatic Brain Injury

EPIDEMIOLOGY

Despite the frequency of head injury in children, epidemiologic data in this area are relatively limited. A study in the United Kingdom indicated that 40% of all patients seen in emergency rooms for the treatment of head injuries were children.[28] It is important, however, to distinguish between head injury and brain injury when discussing outcomes and therapy, although it is probably equally important to group these entities when discussing mechanisms and prevention. Accordingly, population-based studies indicate an average incidence of clinically important head injury in children at about 185 per 100,000, with the incidence generally dropping with increasing age.[29,30] Boys are injured at a rate approximately twice that of girls.

Overall, 85% of the brain injuries sustained in childhood are mild and non–life threatening.[31,32] On the other hand, well over half of all deaths resulting from blunt trauma in children are caused by a brain injury.[33,34]

The severity and mechanism of brain injury are determinants of outcome. The mechanism of injury also depends on age. The most common mechanism resulting in head injury in children is a fall, but the usual falls of childhood rarely cause severe injury. Inflicted injury is by far the leading cause of severe brain injuries in very young children. In older children, severe brain injury is most commonly seen in relation to motor vehicle accidents.

Many accidental brain injuries that occur in children are preventable. Proper use of occupant restraints in motor vehicles can prevent up to 90% of the serious injuries to young children.[35] The implementation of a mandatory child restraint law in Michigan reduced the number of motor vehicle–related injuries in children by 25%.[36] Wearing helmets for bicycle riding as well as for other recreational activities, such as skateboarding, skating, skiing, and horseback riding, should decrease the risk for brain injury,[37–39] although educational programs regarding helmet use have had only limited success so far.[40] Many falls are preventable. Vigilance regarding open windows and stairways, including the use of gates or bars substantially reduces the occurrence of these injuries.

SPECTRUM OF TRAUMATIC BRAIN INJURY

There are many ways to undertake an overview of the major types of traumatic brain injuries. The authors have come to prefer one that includes a relationship of injury types, mechanism, and natural history. The simplest way to do this is by categorizing major injury types as either focal or diffuse. Accepting the caveat that many traumatic injuries are mixtures of focal and diffuse injury, one can still undertake individual management strategies based on the initial appearance of the type of brain injury.

Focal or Diffuse Brain Injury?

Focal injuries include contusions, lacerations, traumatic hematomas, and localized damage resulting from expanding masses, shifts, and distortions of the brain. Diffuse injuries include the spectrum of diffuse axonal injury, which includes what is commonly called cerebral concussion, as well as other diffuse insults, such as global ischemia, systemic hypoxia, diffuse brain swelling, and diffuse vascular injury. Focal injuries are usually immediately apparent on the admitting computed tomography (CT) scans even when they appear to be clinically asymptomatic. In contrast, diffuse injuries may show much less striking changes on early neuroimaging studies, even though the patient may exhibit profound alterations in consciousness and neurologic function. Diffuse injuries may require a series of diagnostic studies to determine the type

and magnitude of the injury. They are also more likely to require prolonged monitoring and management of intracranial pressure.

Focal Brain Injury

Most focal brain injuries are associated with impact-related mechanisms. Because short falls are the most common cause of accidental head injuries in childhood, cranial impacts and resulting focal injuries are also common. Impact mechanisms also result in skull fractures, which are also commonly seen in the pediatric age group. In fact, about 20% of head-injured children who are admitted to the hospital have skull fractures.[41] Despite the frequency of skull fracture in childhood, the majority of children with this injury will not require any treatment. Therefore the clinical importance of most skull fractures is that the fracture serves as an indicator of both the mechanism and the severity of the head injury. Most studies of the importance of skull fractures have determined that finding a skull fracture in a head-injured patient is statistically associated with a higher likelihood of developing an expanding intracranial hematoma or harboring a significant brain injury.[41–45] Furthermore, complex skull fractures, or the occurrence of multiple fractures, are generally associated with higher-energy mechanisms and are therefore associated with more severe injuries to the brain.

As indicated previously, most focal brain injuries are immediately apparent on initial neuroimaging studies and, depending on the size and location, result in focal neurologic dysfunction. The most common focal injury resulting from nonpenetrating mechanisms is a cerebral contusion (Fig. 24-1). These are generally surface lesions related to cranial impacts or brain movement over irregular intracranial surfaces or along the edges of dura. The clinical presentation of cerebral contusions depends mostly upon the extent of the

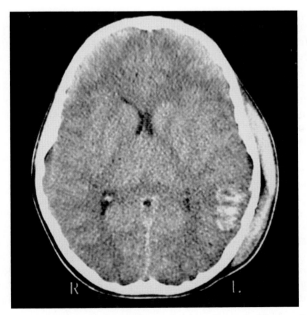

FIGURE 24-1 A cerebral contusion underlying a linear skull fracture (not demonstrated). This was the result of a cranial impact, as demonstrated by the overlying soft tissue swelling and hemorrhage. The patient had no neurologic deficit.

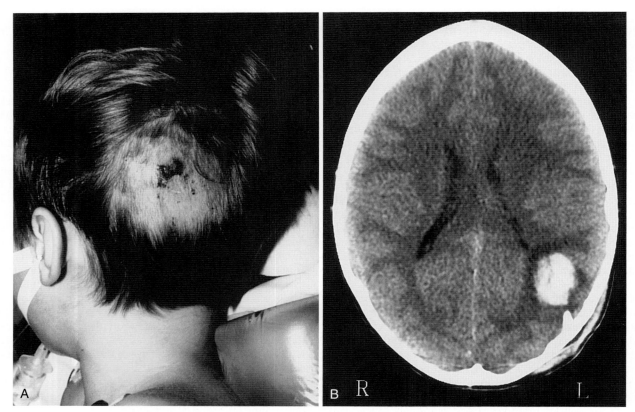

FIGURE 24-2 The occult injury frequently seen with low-velocity cranial penetration in young children is demonstrated. The patient was struck in the left parietal region by a lawn dart, and loss of consciousness did not occur. The lawn dart fell out immediately. The injury was misinterpreted as a minor scalp laceration and was closed with butterfly bandages. Three days later, fever and headache developed. **A,** Appearance of the entry wound before surgical exploration. **B,** Computed tomography shows a compound fracture and intracerebral hematoma. During surgery, hair, dirt, and bone fragments were removed from the cerebral cortex.

initial injury, the amount of associated hemorrhage resulting in mass effect, and the location of the contusion in the brain. Even though cerebral contusions may develop localized swelling, isolated lesions are not generally life threatening. Many cerebral contusions are neurologically silent and only discovered on the initial CT scan, underlying a skull fracture or along the anterior cranial base. When these injuries are symptomatic, they usually cause focal neurologic deficit or seizures. The latter are thought to occur commonly in adults with acute cerebral contusions.[46] However, the incidence of seizures in children with cerebral contusions appears to be no greater than in children with either normal CT scans or epidural hematomas.[47]

Traumatic intracerebral hematomas are unusual lesions in the pediatric age group. The pathogenesis of these hemorrhages is unclear, but it seems to be related to the disruption of central arterial blood vessels. Accordingly, these lesions are associated with more severe mechanisms of injury and with more profound neurologic dysfunction. In many cases, these lesions are part of a larger picture of diffuse axonal injury that is discussed later. Traumatic intracerebral hematomas are distinguished from hemorrhagic contusions by their lack of contact with the surface of the brain.[48] They can be quite large and, because of the location, can leave a child with a profound neurologic deficit. Surgical evacuation can be considered if intracranial pressures are high, but, in the authors' experience, neurologic outcomes are not improved by the evacuation of these hematomas.

Children are prone to nonmissile penetrating injuries of the skull and brain. These injuries usually occur when a child falls onto or is struck by sharp objects, such as nails, pencils, sharp sticks, or lawn toys (Fig. 24-2). One of the major dangers of these injuries is that, unless the offending object remains embedded, the entry wound may be hidden or seem trivial.[49–51] The anterior penetrations of the skull base can be transorbital (through the orbital roof) or through the nose or mouth.

Penetrating injuries can result in focal contusions, intracerebral hemorrhages, and cerebral lacerations, but these lesions are usually silent because of their locations and small size. The deeper penetrations are more likely to be symptomatic, not only because the tissue injury is more extensive but also because of the potential for injuring major vessels. Many penetrating injuries become symptomatic in delayed fashion because of expansion of intracerebral hemorrhage, the recognition of cerebral spinal fluid (CSF) fistula, or by the appearance of symptoms indicating infection. Therefore a very high index of suspicion is required, and careful radiologic studies are called for whenever there is a possibility of subtle cranial penetration. Wood, glass, and residual bits of debris may be difficult to detect on routine imaging studies, including CT scans.[52]

Cranial penetrating injury is also strongly associated with direct cerebrovascular injury.[53] When there is evidence of deep cranial penetration or if there is substantial subarachnoid hemorrhage or focal intracerebral hemorrhage, one should

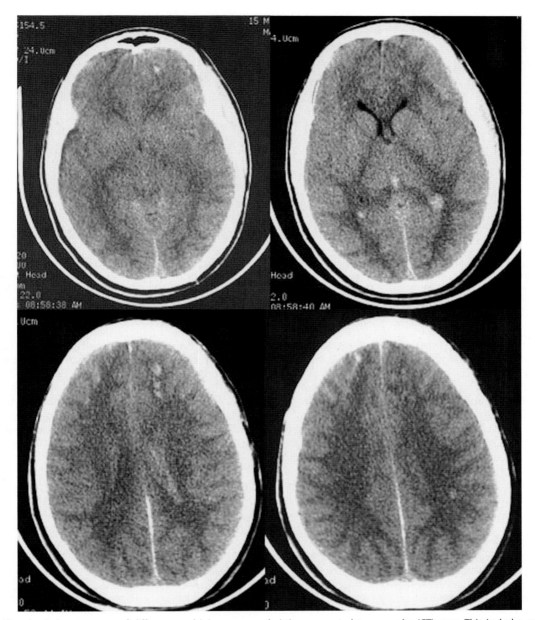

FIGURE 24-3   The classical appearance of diffuse axonal injury on an admitting computed tomography (CT) scan. This includes subarachnoid and intraventricular hemorrhages, brain swelling, and small petechial hemorrhages throughout the brain.

consider magnetic resonance imaging (MRI) with the addition of magnetic resonance angiography or the increasingly useful modality of CT angiography.

Diffuse Brain Injuries

The majority of brain injuries occurring in childhood are diffuse injuries that are characterized by general disturbances of neuronal function that begin immediately at the time of injury, while showing general preservation of brain structure on early CT scans. Diffuse injuries are a direct result of energy dissipation within the substance of the brain or as the result of systemic insults. All of these injuries exist on a continuum from extremely mild—and, apparently, completely reversible—to lethal. Frequently, the different types of diffuse brain injury

occur together, or in sequence, and can act synergistically to affect the neurologic presentation and the outcome.

Diffuse primary brain injuries are generally the result of angular or translational accelerations (or decelerations), with the amount of tissue disruption being roughly proportional to the amount of energy dissipated in the brain substance.[54] As the amount of neuronal disruption increases, the depth and duration of neurologic dysfunction increases and the neurologic outcome worsens. The appearance of certain hemorrhages on the CT scans (specifically, subarachnoid hemorrhage), small but widespread intracerebral hemorrhages and intraventricular hemorrhage, are a typical finding (Fig. 24-3).[55] Finally, although the occurrence of traumatic surgical masses is not characteristic of the diffuse brain injuries, subdural hematomas occur commonly with

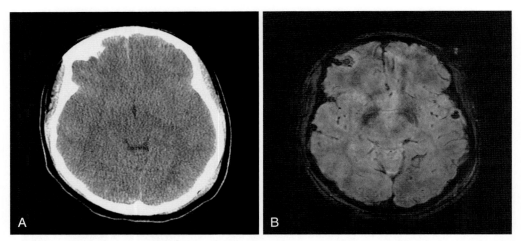

FIGURE 24-4 The importance of imaging in mild traumatic brain injury. Patients with apparently normal consciousness at presentation can suffer widespread cerebral damage when subjected to mechanisms that cause diffuse axonal injury. Cognitive disturbances and neurologic symptoms are common in these patients. **A,** Unenhanced computed tomography scan of conscious patient (GCS 15) showing subarachnoid hemorrhage. **B,** Susceptibility-weighted gradient echo magnetic resonance image (MRI) showing widespread parenchymal hemorrhages characteristic of diffuse axonal injury. (Courtesy Jill Hunter, MD.)

diffuse axonal injury, and some of these hemorrhages need early surgical evacuation. However, subdural hemorrhages are better viewed as another marker of the diffuse brain injury rather than as a mass that should be treated in isolation, such as an epidural hematoma or a hemorrhagic contusion.

Like all brain injuries, diffuse primary brain injuries occur within a spectrum of severity. At one end of the spectrum are the very mild, transient physiologic disturbances of neurologic function (which includes the syndromes commonly referred to as cerebral concussion), while at the other is the progressively more damaging and ultimately lethal entity that is now called diffuse axonal injury (DAI).

The modern view of cerebral concussion is based on the pioneering work of Ommaya and Gennarelli,[56,57] who define concussive brain injuries as a graded set of clinical syndromes with increasing disturbances in the level and content of consciousness. This definition allows specific post-traumatic disturbances commonly seen in children after so-called "mild" head injuries to be included, such as confusion without amnesia, confusion associated with amnesia of varying depths and duration, and the classical loss of consciousness with and without transient sensorimotor paralysis or disturbances of respiration or circulation.

As the amount of energy in the injury mechanism increases, tissue disruption occurs and results in DAI. It is now clear that the most common cause of prolonged coma from mechanical brain injury is DAI. Patients who have suffered DAI are unconscious from the time of injury and remain so for a prolonged period.[58] It is not uncommon to note pupillary changes, skewed gaze, and decerebrate posturing. This constellation of symptoms had historically been called a brainstem contusion in the era prior to MRI. Most comatose patients who appear to show brainstem dysfunction after closed head injury have really suffered DAI.

The appearance of DAI on CT scans depends upon the severity of the injury and the degree of associated hemorrhages. In some cases, the initial CT scan may appear to be normal. Subsequently, the characteristic lesions may be discovered on MRI, varying from some transient signal changes in the deep white structures to widespread hemorrhagic and nonhemorrhagic shears (Fig. 24-4). The characteristic CT scan appearance of DAI is multiple petechial hemorrhages in the deep white matter and central structures. However, the finding of intraventricular hemorrhage or focal subarachnoid hemorrhage specifically located in the prepontine cistern is also strongly suggestive of DAI.

Gunshot Wounds

Children's injuries from firearms are a major public health problem. Recent reports indicate that 10% of all childhood-injury deaths are related to firearms, a number exceeded only by deaths from motor vehicle accidents, drowning, and house fires.[59,60] From the standpoint of management and outcomes, there is little to differentiate gunshot injuries in children from those in adults. Poor outcomes are related to depth of coma, bilateral or transventricular injury, elevated intracranial pressure, and large intracerebral hemorrhages.[61] Aggressive treatment of all patients is recommended, except those with clearly nonsurvivable injuries,[62] although substantial neurologic and cognitive deficits can be expected.[63,64]

In childhood, injuries resulting from nonpowder firearms, such as BB and pellet guns, are more common than true gunshot wounds.[60] Adolescent males have the highest risk of this type of injury.[65] These injuries are generally less severe and therefore carry lower mortality rates. Surgical treatment is not usually required for BB gun injuries. Pellet rifle injuries, being higher velocity and larger caliber missile injuries, are more severe and are probably best treated as true gunshot wounds.

Crush Injuries

Young children are susceptible to the unusual static-loading type crushing injury to the skull, which happens when a heavy object falls on a child or when the child is run over by a vehicle. These injuries are dramatic, both in the clinical presentation and in the radiographic findings (Fig. 24-5), but

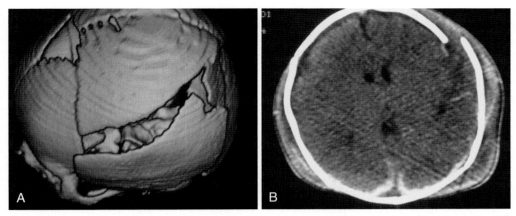

FIGURE 24-5 A crushing type injury in an infant. **A,** This shows a cranial "burst" injury on CT three-dimensional reconstruction of the skull. **B,** Although there is intracranial hemorrhage and dural laceration, the structure of the brain is preserved and decompressed. The child required dural and cranial reconstruction but recovered with minimal deficits.

the neurologic outcomes can be quite good.[66] Multiple skull fractures, including complex basilar skull fractures and facial fractures, are typical. Cerebrospinal fluid leaks and cranial nerve palsies are commonly seen. However, despite the initial appearances of the injury, major cortical structures are often preserved. Therefore, if the child has survived the initial injury, aggressive multidisciplinary management can yield satisfactory long-term functional outcomes.

Inflicted Injuries

The most common cause of severe and life-threatening brain injury in infants is inflicted injury. All physicians involved in the care of injured children should be familiar with the clinical presentations and the characteristic radiographic findings of inflicted injuries. This entity has been reviewed in detail.[67,68] Infants presenting with alteration of consciousness (with or without the new onset of seizures), retinal hemorrhages, and acute intracranial hemorrhages on the CT scan are likely to have suffered nonaccidental injuries, especially if the history of the injury is unknown or reported to be minor. The additional finding of new or healing skeletal fractures or other solid organ injuries are pathognomonic for this injury. All infants who are suspected to have been abused need a comprehensive multidisciplinary evaluation by physicians knowledgeable about the mechanisms and clinical spectrum of inflicted injury.

INITIAL ASSESSMENT OF BRAIN-INJURED CHILDREN

The purpose of the initial assessment of a brain-injured patient is twofold. First, and most important, one establishes a working diagnosis of the type and severity of the injury that directs the selection of initial therapies as well as the planning and coordination of other diagnostic studies and the management of any associated systemic injuries. Second, it establishes a baseline to measure the effects, both positive and deleterious, of the therapies or interventions.

Historically, the main focus of a brain-injured patient's initial assessment was to determine the severity of the injury by scoring the level of consciousness. The most widely used scale for this purpose is the Glasgow Coma Scale Score (GCS),[69]

which, as it was designed, correlates well with outcome. However, with improvements in transportation and field resuscitation of severely injured patients, which usually requires the prehospital administration of analgesics and sedation, a neurologic assessment to determine brain injury type and severity becomes less useful.[70] Furthermore, there is a small but important group of brain-injured patients who present with little or no impairment of consciousness and who subsequently deteriorate from mass lesions or brain swelling.[71–73]

It is now clear that neuroimaging is probably a better predictor of outcome from brain injury than is the clinical examination. Regardless of the apparent level of consciousness, the early radiographic identification of injury types and the institution of appropriate management or monitoring have substantially improved the overall outcome from traumatic brain injury. Furthermore, it is now clear that a head-injured patient who has a completely normal CT scan has an exceedingly low risk of either deterioration or poor outcome. In the authors' experience, the CT scan has become the most important element in diagnosing brain injury early, especially for young children.

The important CT scan findings not only involve the detection of potentially surgical mass lesions but also the search and detection of the constellation of findings typically seen with diffuse brain injury. These are subarachnoid, intraventricular, or intraparenchymal hemorrhage and what may be very subtle early signs of brain swelling, including compression of the perimesencephalic cisterns or shift or compression of the ventricular system. These findings should influence the expectations for outcome and the decisions for monitoring and therapy. Diffuse brain injury severity can be graded by the appearance of the admitting CT scan and can direct therapeutic decision making.[74]

Most current practice parameters regarding the evaluation of head-injured patients include recommendations for an early diagnostic CT scan.[1,2,22,75,76] Essentially, all potentially severely injured patients, that is, patients presenting with an alteration of consciousness, should undergo CT scanning as soon as they are physiologically stable and can be safely transported and maintained in the scanner. Older children with apparently trivial injuries can be observed clinically. However, as mentioned previously, the finding of a normal CT scan after head injury can mitigate further clinical observation and allow return to home sooner. On the other hand, children with the following symptoms should undergo CT scanning as soon as possible: a history of more than a few seconds of unconsciousness; a seizure; clinical signs of cranial impact, skull fracture, cranial penetration, or CSF leak; and headache, persistent vomiting, lethargy, or irritability.[77,78] Finally, children who have been injured in accidents with high-energy mechanisms that result in apparently isolated chest, abdominal, or skeletal injuries should undergo a brain CT scan prior to anesthetic administration or the institution of narcotic analgesia or sedation that would preclude accurate ongoing neurologic examinations.

It should be clear from the previous discussion that plain skull radiography has only a limited and secondary role in the initial evaluation of head injury. CT scanning will detect most clinically important skull fractures. Conversely, skull radiographs provide only limited information about the type and location of any brain injury. MRI is more sensitive than CT scanning for detecting most brain pathology, and it has supplanted CT scanning as the study of choice for many neurologic disorders. Some centers are using "fast" MRI techniques to assess acute brain injury.[79] This may become more common, especially in view of the long-term effects of radiation in children.[80]

Finally, although acknowledging the expanding primary role of neuroimaging in the diagnosis and management of traumatic brain injury, a careful physical and neurologic examination is still extremely important. The entire head should be inspected for indications of impact, scalp injury, cranial deformities, and indications of cranial or orbital penetration. It is necessary to document cranial nerve function, especially pupillary size, shape, and reactivity, which will serve as a comparison for serial examinations. Evidence of anterior basilar skull fractures, manifested by periorbital ecchymoses, nasal hemorrhage, or CSF rhinorrhea, is a contraindication to the placement of nasogastric tubes until the integrity of the anterior cranial skull base can be determined. Retroauricular bruising, hemotympanum, otorrhagia, or CSF otorrhea are indicative of temporal bone fractures. In the circumstance of possible inflicted injury, dilated funduscopic examination by an ophthalmologist is recommended.[81] It is still necessary to document the level of consciousness and any apparent motor or sensory deficits and note the presence of confounders to the examination (such as intubation, medications, swelling, splints, etc.), in the initial evaluation of the head-injured patient.

EARLY MANAGEMENT OF SEVERE BRAIN INJURY

The primary objective of resuscitating brain-injured patients is to preserve cerebral perfusion during transport and evaluation. The ongoing objective of therapy for severe brain injury is to optimize the perfusion of the injured and uninjured brain and create a milieu that minimizes the chance for secondary injury and maximizes the amount of neuronal recovery. One must do this while avoiding or reversing deleterious processes that would result in further neuronal injury or the expansion of hemorrhagic masses, including systemic complications that directly affect an injured brain, such as sepsis, acute lung injury, hyperglycemia, and coagulopathy.

There are a variety of treatment strategies that have been propounded for the treatment of traumatic brain injury. Most of these therapies involve systemic manipulations to achieve what is believed to be either a therapeutic or a protective response. All of the newer therapies have theoretical attractions, and their proponents report outcomes that appear to be better than historical controls. However, at least so far, when these therapies have been tested directly against what could be termed standard therapies, no benefits have been demonstrated. Given this, the treatment recommendations currently in place are essentially descriptions of how to apply the historically standard therapies of controlled ventilation, fluid management, sedation, and control of blood pressure and intracranial pressure (ICP).

To do this, one must understand intracranial dynamics and optimize cerebral perfusion by removing surgical masses and by managing the intracranial pressures, which can be done by safely manipulating, as much as possible, the cerebral blood volumes (arterial and venous), the cerebrospinal fluid volume, and the brain or skull volume.[82] For severely injured patients, and for some less severely injured patients, intracranial pressure monitoring guides the institution and manipulation of therapies. ICP monitoring provides the basis for making many of the important management decisions for brain-injured patients.[83,84]

The application of individual medical therapies is beyond the scope of this chapter. However, it is important to realize that each of the current therapies for elevated intracranial pressure has both general and specific effects, and each has complications associated with its use. The historically common administration of high-dose steroids to brain-injured patients is no longer considered to be beneficial and may, in fact, be harmful. Accordingly, the current guidelines do not recommend that *any* specific therapy—for instance, hyperventilation, osmotic diuretics, or other medications—be administered prophylactically or universally for brain-injured patients. It is also suggested that specific therapies be applied in a logical sequence, guided by ICP monitoring and by frequent reassessments of the responses to the therapy.

The basic level of therapy for severe traumatic brain injury includes controlled ventilation and maintaining normal oxygenation and $Paco_2$ concentrations. Intubated patients should have adequate sedation and analgesia at all times. Intravascular volume should be supported at all times with blood and fluids, maintaining normal hematocrit and electrolyte concentration. Fluid restriction is not recommended. Hypotonic fluids should be avoided in order to avoid any trend toward hyponatremia. The head of the bed may be elevated to reduce intracranial venous pressure as long as normal central venous pressures are maintained by adequate volume replacement. For many severe diffuse brain injuries, this level of therapy may be all that is necessary.

Escalated therapies include the use of CSF drainage, usually by way of a ventricular catheter, osmotic therapy, and mild hyperventilation. Whenever escalation of therapy is considered, one must also escalate the physiologic monitoring for treatment effect and complications. Table 24-1 summarizes the authors' approach to escalating medical therapy for brain injury, based on current treatment guidelines. Others have different strategies, including the use of decompressive craniectomy early in the treatment cascade. As discussed at the outset of this chapter, the available evidence allows many

TABLE 24-1	
Medical Therapies for Traumatic Brain Injury	
Treatment	*Monitoring*
Evaluation and Resuscitation	
Restoration of normal blood pressure	Systemic blood pressure and oxygenation
Intubation and ventilation	Neurologic examination
	End-tidal CO_2
Basic Level Therapy	
Elevating head of bed	Systemic blood pressure and oxygenation
Keeping head in neutral position	Intracranial pressure
Sedation and muscular paralysis	Arterial Po_2, Pco_2, and pH
Mechanical ventilation to maintain $Paco_2$ at 35-40 mm Hg	Weight, urine output, pulse, and pulse pressure
Maintaining normal to slightly increased intravascular volume	Hemogram, serum electrolytes, glucose, and BUN
Normal fluid and electrolyte status (no fluid restriction) avoiding anemia, hyperglycemia	Monitoring and aggressively treating fever and sepsis
Body temperature normal to slightly hypothermic	CT scan
Escalated Therapy	
Ventricular CSF drainage	Ventricular catheter
Osmotic therapy including hypertonic saline	Central venous pressure
Moderate hyperventilation to maintain $Paco_2$ at 30-35 mm Hg	Serum osmolality and electrolytes
Intensive Therapy of Refractory Intracranial Pressure	
High-dose barbiturate therapy	Continuous or compressed spectral EEG
Decompressive craniectomy	Barbiturate levels
Optimized ventilation	Brain oximetry, monitors of cerebral blood flow

BUN, blood urea nitrogen; CSF, cerebrospinal fluid; CT, computed tomography; EEG, electroencephalogram; $Paco_2$, partial pressure of arterial carbon dioxide; Pco_2, partial pressure of carbon dioxide; Po_2, partial pressure of oxygen.

different logical strategies for the management of traumatic brain injury, and each center should develop their own protocols and carefully measure the outcomes and complications.

Surgical decision making for severely injured patients is usually straightforward. Obviously, penetrating injuries, including compound skull fractures, require urgent surgical attention. The removal of large, surgically accessible mass lesions may be the first step in the overall therapeutic management of a severe brain injury. Some centers advocate decompressive craniectomy as an initial therapy. In many cases, such as closed depressed fractures, burst fractures, comminuted cranial, and craniofacial fractures, surgical correction can be performed when the patient is stable or improving from the neurologic injury.

Typically, major surgical therapy for brain injury involves the removal of traumatic intracranial hematomas. The overall incidence of surgical hematomas in childhood is substantially lower than in adults, and the distribution of hematoma types is different. Subdural hematomas are most common in infants but rarely reach a size that requires surgical removal. As discussed at the outset of this chapter, acute subdural hematomas in older children are generally more indicative of a severe diffuse injury (Fig. 24-6). Extradural hematomas are the more common surgical mass in children, especially older children who have suffered cranial impacts (Fig. 24-7). Small epidural hematomas over the cerebral convexity are likely to resolve without surgical removal, that is, those that occur in more limited "spaces" (like the temporal fossa) or the posterior fossa are more concerning, and even small epidurals in these locations may need removal. Large hemorrhagic contusions or traumatic intracerebral hematomas are very rare in the pediatric age group.[32] In summary, the decision to remove a traumatic intracranial hematoma is simply one part of an overall treatment strategy for the brain injury.

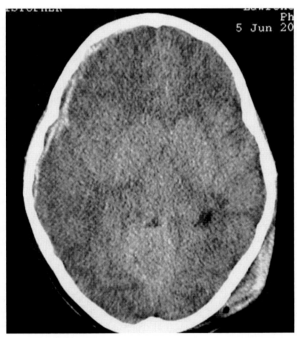

FIGURE 24-6   Acute subdural hematoma. The hemorrhage overlying the hemisphere (left side of image) seems small. Note however, the extensive shift of the brain and the hemispheric swelling that are indicative of severe diffuse injury.

Management of Minor Brain Injuries

The vast majority of children with head injury have trivial, minor, or minimal primary brain injuries. These children will most likely recover without any intervention. However, within this large group, there exists a small fraction of patients who

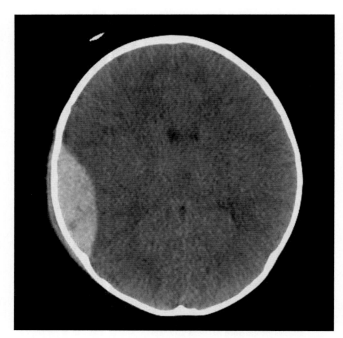

FIGURE 24-7 Acute extradural hematoma. Note the thickness of the hemorrhagic mass but also the lack of shift compared with what is demonstrated with a subdural hematoma shown in Figure 24-6. This lack of swelling and shift is an indication of an uninjured brain responding normally to the expanding mass. As long as this mass is removed prior to onset of coma, mortality and morbidity is essentially nil.

harbor enlarging hematomas or who are in the early stages of brain swelling. These patients face increased risk of delayed but rapid deterioration that will result in death or disability. The focus of evaluating of the apparently minor brain injury is twofold: (1) to identify patients at risk of neurologic deterioration or delayed complications and (2) to prevent either from occurring.[77] In many ways, the diagnosis and management of these patients is more challenging and important than managing severe injuries, because successful intervention results almost universally in good outcomes.[72,73]

There are published recommendations about this issue.[75,85] As with other types of brain injury, early neuroimaging is the lynchpin to accurately diagnose and recognize brain-injured patients at risk for deterioration.[44,86–88] Identification of cisternal compression, hemorrhagic shear, and contusion, or small traumatic hematomas indicates that the patient is at risk for deterioration regardless of their level of consciousness. These patients are candidates for frequent reassessments, including repeat neuroimaging, intracranial pressure monitoring, and even the early application of therapies to control the intracranial dynamics.[89,90] It appears that paying attention to intravenous fluid management is very important, because many children with trivial brain injuries seem to deteriorate in the face of even a mild hyponatremia.[91,92] Therefore maintenance fluids for these patients, as for most patients with brain injury, should be normal saline or its equivalent.[23] One should also pay close attention to maintaining normal intravascular volume and serum electrolyte status.

Identifying patients at risk for deterioration includes the appearance of certain abnormalities on CT scanning, but an even more important finding from the burgeoning literature about CT scanning and head injury is emerging: A completely normal CT scan in a mildly injured patient is associated with essentially no risk of life-threatening deterioration.[93,94] Given this additional information from a normal CT scan, a child with a history of an accidental minor head injury, who has neither a skull fracture nor a history of seizure and who is asymptomatic, may be released to competent caretakers and not be admitted for observation.

For adolescents who suffer cerebral concussion as a result of sporting activities, there are now published guidelines describing how to evaluate and manage these individuals, along with recommendations about when the athlete may return to sporting activities after a concussion.[95–98]

EARLY COMPLICATIONS OF HEAD INJURY

Acute complications of head injury include those related to skull fractures, infectious processes related to cranial penetrations and CSF fistulas, and acute neurologic complications such as post-traumatic epilepsy. As with most aspects of head injury management, the key to optimizing the outcome is recognizing patients with injuries that put them at risk for these complications, followed by appropriate diagnostic studies, monitoring, and, when possible, intervention.

Complications of Skull Fractures

Simple nondepressed or minimally depressed skull fractures will heal spontaneously. Widely diastatic or cranial burst fractures[99] in young children are indications of dural injury and are not likely to heal without surgical reconstruction. With modern neuroimaging, the early identification of these injuries allows elective early repair, thereby avoiding the complication usually referred to in the literature as "growing skull fracture."[100,101] The typical syndrome of an enlarging skull defect and progressive neurologic deterioration, both of which are related to a craniocerebral erosion and enlarging leptomeningeal cyst that appears during the course of months to years after the injury, is completely avoidable with early repair of the dura and skull. However, focal brain injury is commonly seen with severely depressed, diastatic, and cranial burst fractures, and these patients will have an increased incidence of seizures and focal neurologic deficits.

Basilar Skull Fractures

For patients with presumed basilar fractures, the important clinical issue is that these are potentially compound fractures; therefore they place the patient at increased risk for infection. The obvious indication of CSF leaking from the nose or ear is present in only 10% to 20% of cases.[102,103] Therefore one must search for other signs of basilar fracture, which include bilateral orbital ecchymoses or swelling, signs of midface or orbital fracture, hemotympanum, otorrhagia, or the Battle sign, because these are easily missed on routine neuroimaging studies. These patients are at increased risk for developing meningitis, and this risk continues for several weeks after the injury. Given this, and considering that compounding of basilar fractures probably occurs more often than not without any evidence of CSF fistulas, it is necessary for parents and caretakers of children considered to have suffered basilar fractures to be counseled not only about the importance of recognizing CSF rhinorrhea or otorrhea, if it should occur at home, but also about the urgent importance of seeking immediate medical attention for children who develop signs or symptoms even remotely suggestive of bacterial meningitis up to several weeks following the injury. Despite the increased risk of bacterial meningitis, the administration of prophylactic antibiotics has not been shown to be beneficial.[104–106] Some centers are administering pneumococcal vaccine to patients with presumed basilar skull fractures, although it is not yet clear that this reduces the occurrence of pneumococcal meningitis.

Basilar skull fractures are also associated with cranial neuropathies. The olfactory nerve is the most commonly injured of all cranial nerves, and patients with anterior basilar fractures are especially at risk of injuring them. Fractures that occur more posterior along the skull base, or that include the orbit and midface, place the optic nerves at risk. Visual loss may be acute or delayed, and ophthalmologic evaluation and follow-up are warranted. Basilar fractures involving the petrous bone can result in auditory, vestibular, and/or facial nerve injury. These patients may need otologic evaluation and audiometric studies.[107]

Direct Cerebrovascular Injuries

Although traumatic intracranial aneurysms are exceedingly rare after closed head injury, greater than 20% of all post-traumatic aneurysms occur in the pediatric age group.[108] Penetrating injuries, especially stab wounds and deep penetrations, are associated with a high incidence of vascular injury. Suspicion of direct cerebrovascular injuries is raised when there is a large amount of subarachnoid hemorrhage or a focal intracerebral hemorrhage on the CT scan. CT angiography and/or magnetic resonance angiography can screen for injury, but in some cases, diagnostic angiography should be performed. If the studies are not conclusive, early repeat imaging is warranted.

Post-traumatic Seizures

One of the most common complications of brain injury, even mild brain injury, is epilepsy. Most studies indicate that the incidence of post-traumatic seizures is substantially higher in children than in adults.[109,110] Risk factors associated with post-traumatic epilepsy include younger age and increasing injury severity.[47,111] However, it is not clear that the infants with inflicted injuries, who would have a very high incidence of early epilepsy, were excluded from these studies.[112] If one removes this particular group from the analysis, the incidence of post-traumatic epilepsy in children appears to be relatively low.

One must make a distinction between early and late post-traumatic seizures. Early seizures are generally defined as those that occur within the first week after injury. For pediatric patients, this definition would include the so-called impact-related seizure that occurs in up to 10% of mildly head-injured children.[47,113,114] These seizures are usually self limited, and the CT scan is normal. Treatment is not recommended, and the long-term outcome is good.[115,116] This particular syndrome is almost never seen in head-injured adults, in whom early epilepsy is strongly associated with structural brain injury or subdural hematoma.

For severely head-injured children, that is, children in coma or with structural injury on the admitting CT scan, there is limited and conflicting information regarding the clinical significance and the management of early and late post-traumatic epilepsy.[111,117,118] Current recommendations indicate that all severely injured patients who experience recurrent seizures should be treated with anticonvulsant medication. Phenytoin is still the most widely recommended drug for this purpose,[1,119] although newer agents are being introduced and studied.

Postconcussion Syndromes

A syndrome of neurologic dysfunction that seems to be unique to young children has been called the pediatric concussion syndrome. Shortly after what would seem like a mild cranial impact injury, the child exhibits the acute onset of pallor, diaphoresis, and impaired responsiveness. CT scans are normal, and the syndrome appears to resolve as rapidly as it occurs. The underlying mechanism is unknown, although it has been suggested that it may be a variation of post-traumatic epilepsy.[120]

Other much more rarely occurring transient neurologic disturbances have been reported after mild head injury in childhood. This includes transient cortical blindness, speech arrest, ataxia, receptive dysphasia, and prolonged disorientation.[121,122] CT scans are, again, normal, and the symptoms resolve spontaneously. The etiology is not clear.

OUTCOMES FROM TRAUMATIC BRAIN INJURY

There is substantial variability in the reporting of outcomes from childhood head injury. With the exception of infants suffering inflicted head injuries, the overall mortality from head injury in childhood is roughly half of that reported for similarly severe head injury in adults.[2] In larger series of patients, mortalities for head injury in childhood are generally less than 5% for all levels of injury severity and less than 20% for those children who are defined as having severe injuries based either on the GCS or other injury severity scoring systems.[32,117,123] Factors related to poor outcomes include high-energy mechanisms, structural injury, swelling and shift on admitting CT scans, persistent or resistant elevations in intracranial pressure, the presence of chest or abdominal injuries, and systemic complications.

Traumatic brain injury is the leading cause of acquired disability in childhood[124]; children who survive have neurologic and cognitive outcomes related to their age, severity of injury, and amount of permanent structural injury to the brain.[123,125–128] Children who have suffered severe brain injuries are likely to show persistent adverse effects on intellectual function, memory, attention, language, and behavior.[129] It is likely that these deficits have ongoing and perhaps compounding effects on learning and socialization. Given that, it is possible that the overall neurobehavioral outcomes for significant childhood head injury are worse for children than for similarly injured adults.

Outcomes from inflicted brain injuries deserve separate discussion. This particular injury is associated with the highest mortality and morbidity of childhood head injuries. Reported mortalities approach 40%.[130,131] Morbidity is also high, especially if the infant shows evidence of cerebral infarction or hypoxic-ischemic injury.

POSTCONCUSSION SYNDROMES

Mild brain injury—a brain injury with a limited effect on consciousness and with preservation of brain structure—is by far the most common central nervous system injury in the pediatric age group. Greater than three quarters of all childhood head injuries are classified as mild.[32,132] Only recently have pediatric specialists begun paying attention to the long-term outcomes from cerebral concussion in children.[133] Although there is still variability in defining mild head injury and the spectrum of severity within that taxonomy,[134–136] there appears to be two general emerging concepts in the available literature. First, somatic complaints, such as headache, visual disturbances, light and noise intolerance and dizziness, emotional disturbances (such as depression, anxiety, or irritability), and cognitive impairments, including poor school performance, are common in mildly brain-injured children in the days and weeks immediately following the injury.[137] Second, as long as the child did not have any cognitive or behavioral disturbances before the brain injury, all of the early postconcussion symptoms described previously appear to resolve completely during weeks or months.[136]

Spine and Spinal Cord Injury

Spinal cord injuries in children are rare, but the consequences of such injuries can be devastating. As with traumatic brain injury, modern neuroimaging has contributed considerably to the diagnosis and management of traumatic myelopathy. As discussed at the beginning of this chapter, the major therapeutic efforts for spinal cord injury are the same as for brain injury and aim to prevent new primary injury and ameliorate secondary injury. The first objective is accomplished by maintaining anatomic alignment of the vertebral column during the period of resuscitation and evaluation. The second objective is much more difficult[138] but begins with supporting blood pressure and oxygenation.

In general, the diagnostic and therapeutic algorithms for children with spinal and spinal cord injuries are similar to those used for adult patients. Guidelines for the management of spinal cord injury have been published recently and summarize current knowledge.[4] However, there are important differences in clinical presentations, anatomic and radiographic findings, and management for spinal injuries in children, especially very young children. This section will concentrate on those issues.

EPIDEMIOLOGY

Less than 10% of spinal cord injuries[139–142] and approximately 1000 new spine[143] or spinal cord injuries[144] each year occur in children. Vertebral column injuries that do not involve the spinal cord are much more common. In a large recent series, only half of children with vertebral injuries had neurologic deficits.[145]

The mechanisms and pattern of injury are related both to age and gender. In very young children, the male to female ratio is roughly equal. In older children, the more "adult" distribution appears with a male to female ratio of about 4:1. Adolescent boys are most affected.[146] The most common causes of pediatric spine injury include falls, athletic activities, child abuse, diving accidents, and motor vehicle trauma.[146–151] Approximately one half of pediatric spinal injuries are the result of motor vehicle accidents.[152] One quarter of injuries are the result of diving accidents. Prevention efforts directed at those two mechanisms alone would dramatically reduce the rate of spinal injury in children. The remaining major mechanisms of injury—falls, child abuse, and sporting activities—each account for about 10% of reported injuries. Younger children are more likely to be injured as the result of a fall, while older children are more likely to be injured in diving accidents or sports.[153,154]

ANATOMY

Younger children tend to have spinal column injuries in the cervical region, while older children tend to have a distribution of spinal injuries similar to that of adults.[155] Children are more likely to experience spinal cord injury without apparent vertebral fractures or dislocations. These characteristics are generally thought to be related to the anatomic properties of the juvenile spine and are independent of the mechanism of injury. The pediatric spine has several properties that essentially allow significant, self-reducing displacement of the vertebral column. These properties include increased elasticity of the joint capsules and ligaments, shallow- and horizontally-oriented facet joints, anterior wedging of the vertebral bodies, and poorly developed uncinate processes.[156,157] Furthermore, young children have disproportionately larger heads and weaker cervical musculature. All of these elements permit a wider range of flexion and extension and rostrocaudal distraction. The fulcrum of motion is higher in the juvenile spine, which explains the greater incidence of rostral injuries in children. This tendency decreases—and the incidence of more characteristic vertebral fracture and dislocation increases—with increasing age.[158] Finally, it is important to remember that 10% to 15% of spinal injuries in children involve "skip" injuries with vertebral or cord injuries at multiple levels.[145,159] Therefore, and depending on the injury mechanism, when a child is determined to have spinal cord injury or vertebral disruption, the entire spinal axis should be surveyed for other injuries.

Spine fractures in children represent 1% to 2% of all pediatric fractures.[160] Overall, injuries to the thoracic and lumbar spine are uncommon in children. When spine injury does occur, the thoracic region (T2-T10) is most commonly injured, followed by the lumbar region (L2-L5).[161] Trauma to the lower thoracic or lumbar spine in children is rarely associated with spinal cord injury,[160] most often occurring at the cervical spinal cord. Less than 20% of all spinal injuries in children occur below the cervical spine.[162] Pediatric cervical spine injuries are typically soft tissue, ligamentous injuries without associated bony fractures for the aforementioned reasons.

EVALUATION OF SPINE AND SPINAL CORD INJURY

Because spinal cord injury is rare in children, it may be overlooked, especially in the very young and in the presence of multiple injuries. As discussed later, the presence of apparently normal plain radiographic studies will not completely

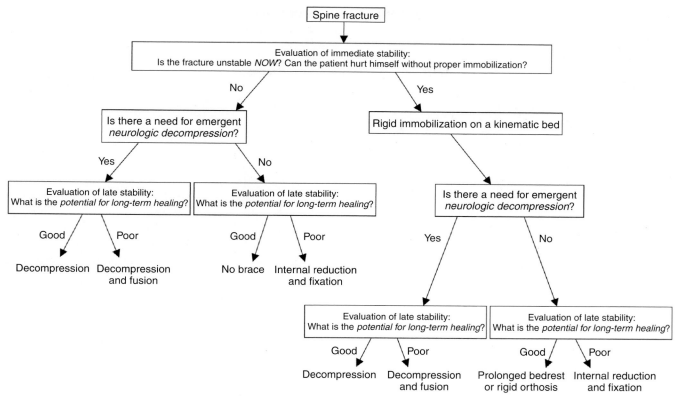

FIGURE 24-8   A systematic approach to spine injuries. Indications for closed or open reduction and decompression and external or internal fixation borne out by answers to three fundamental questions: (1) Is the injury acutely stable or unstable; (2) is there a need for urgent neurologic decompression; and (3) what is the potential for healing with external orthosis?

rule out either vertebral instability or spinal cord injury. Therefore one must have an increased index of suspicion based on injury mechanism and the neurologic presentation. High-energy mechanisms, such as motor vehicle accidents and falls from heights, are more likely to cause spine or spinal cord injury. Until a complete assessment is possible, one should assume that an unconscious patient of any age has a spinal cord injury (Fig. 24-8).

HISTORY

Neck or back pain after a major accident or fall from a significant height may increase suspicion for spine injury. A major accident may include significant vehicular damage, head-on high-speed collision, vehicular rollover, or death at the scene. Accidents that may be associated with spine injuries include those involving the lack of seatbelt use, prolonged extrication, airbag deployment, damage to the steering wheel or windshield, passenger ejection from the vehicle, or passenger space intrusion. Vehicular accidents involving motorcycles, bicycles, or pedestrians have a high association with spine injuries. Transient or persistent symptoms may include pain, weakness, numbness, and tingling. Children can present with torticollis as the result of atlantoaxial rotatory subluxation, which can occur from a minor injury or even a coughing spell. The children are usually neurologically normal. The plain radiographs can be deceiving, but the CT scan of the spine in the axial plane is diagnostic (Fig. 24-9).[163]

PHYSICAL EXAMINATION

Examination should start with a general survey to look for tenderness, swelling, ecchymosis, or a palpable defect posteriorly along the spinous processes. A seatbelt mark across the abdomen or injury of abdominal organs should increase suspicion for any type of thoracic or lumbar fracture.[160] Injuries in the lower thoracic region to upper lumbar region (T11-L1) are notably associated with a significant increase in risk of gastrointestinal injury. Injuries in the lumbar and sacral regions (L2-sacrum) are noted to be associated with risks of orthopedic injuries and gastrointestinal injuries.[146] Any loss of sensation or motor function should be accurately documented. A child with spinal cord injury above the T6 level may present in spinal or neurogenic shock (hypotension and bradycardia), which represents a loss of descending sympathetic tone. This must be recognized early, because pure fluid resuscitation may not be effective and a vasopressor may be needed to restore adequate perfusion.[162]

CLINICAL SPECTRUM OF SPINE AND SPINAL CORD INJURY

Spine injuries must be assessed in terms of immediate and late stability (Table 24-2). Immediate stability refers to the risk of new or further neurologic injury while bearing physiologic loads without immobilization. Late stability implies the potential to heal with proper immobilization based on a specific injury pattern.[164] Management decisions are based on the degree of stability (see Fig. 24-8).

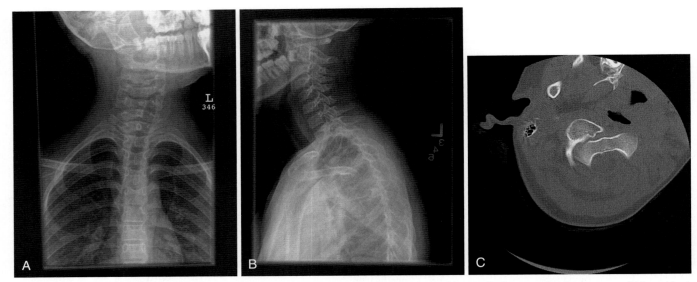

FIGURE 24-9   An example of C1-C2 rotatory subluxation. The patient is a 9-year-old girl with painful torticollis for 3 months after a motor vehicle accident. Anteroposterior (AP) (**A**) and lateral (**B**) cervical spine radiographs confirm torticollis; however, bony details and relationships are obscured at the craniocervical junction. **C,** Axial computed tomography (CT) shows the right C1 lateral mass dislocated and rotated clockwise relative to C2, which is diagnostic of C1-C2 rotatory subluxation.

TABLE 24-2

Common Spine Injuries, Association with Spinal Cord Injury, and Stability

		Stability	
Fracture Type	*Associated Spinal Cord Injury*	*Immediate*	*Late*
Upper Cervical Spine			
Atlanto-occipital dislocation	Common	Poor	Poor
Occipital condyle fracture (Montesano and Anderson type I or II unilateral)	Uncommon	Good	Good
Occipital condyle fracture (Montesano and Anderson type III or type I or II bilateral)	Uncommon (may be associated with cranial nerve deficit; XII most common)	Poor	Fair
C1-2 rotatory subluxation (Fields and Hawkins type I)	Uncommon	Good	Good
C1-2 rotatory subluxation (Fields and Hawkins type II or III)	Possible	Poor	Poor
C1 burst (Jefferson fracture) (sum C1/2 lateral mass overhang < 14 mm)	Uncommon	Good	Good
C1 burst (sum C1/2 lateral mass overhang > 14 mm)	Uncommon	Poor	Poor
Odontoid fracture (d'Alonso and Anderson type I or III)	Uncommon	Good	Good
Odontoid fracture (d'Alonso and Anderson type II)	Possible	Fair	Fair
C2 pars fracture (Effendi type I or II)	Uncommon	Good	Good
C2 pars fracture (Effendi type IIA or III)	Possible	Poor	Poor
Subaxial Cervical Spine			
Unilateral jumped facet	Uncommon	Good	Fair
Bilateral jumped facets	Common	Poor	Poor
Teardrop fracture (flexion-compression)	Common	Poor	Poor
Thoracic and Lumbar Spine			
Compression	Uncommon	Good	Good
Burst	Possible	Fair	Good
Fracture-distraction	Possible	Fair	Good
Fracture-rotation	Common	Poor	Poor

The cardinal sign of a spinal cord injury is neurologic dysfunction below an anatomic spinal motor or sensory level. Complete or severe incomplete cord injuries with motor dysfunction are readily detectable in conscious patients. A spinal cord injury generally presents as symmetrical flaccid paralysis with sensory loss at the same anatomic level. There are strong indirect indicators of spinal cord injury in comatose patients or those with multiple injuries. Cervical spinal cord injuries can cause profound systemic hypotension, a syndrome known as neurogenic shock, which is caused by disruption of sympathetic pathways below the level of injury. Unlike the more common hypovolemic shock, neurogenic shock is suggested

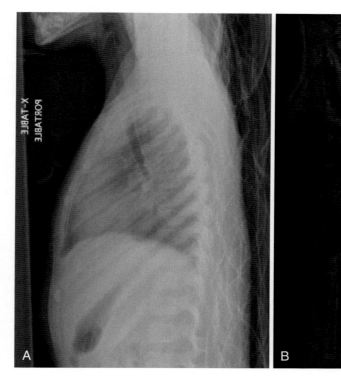

FIGURE 24-10 An example of spinal cord injury without radiographic abnormality (SCIWORA). The patient is a 6-year-old girl who, on neurologic examination, is a T10 complete paraplegic after a motor vehicle accident. **A,** Normal-appearing plain radiograph of the thoracic spine. **B,** Further workup with magnetic resonance imaging (MRI) shows cord signal change *(white arrow)* at the T10 level on the sagittal T2-weighted sequence, indicating a spinal cord injury without evidence of abnormality on the plain radiograph at the T10 level.

by the finding of bradycardia in the face of hypotension. These patients are also vasodilated despite being hypothermic. Hypovolemic shock results in hypotension, tachycardia, and vasoconstriction. Other systemic findings suggesting spinal cord injury include paradoxic respiration, priapism, Horner syndrome, and inability to sweat.

Less severe injuries may present with transient neurologic dysfunction, dysesthesias, focal weakness or sensory loss, or a dissociation of motor and sensory dysfunction, such as Brown-Séquard or central cord syndromes. Any history of transient neurologic dysfunction involving the limbs or bladder, regardless of duration and apparent complete recovery, must be taken as strong evidence for spinal cord injury.

Spinal Cord Injury Without Radiographic Abnormality

Pang and Wilberger defined spinal cord injury without radiographic abnormality (SCIWORA) in 1982 to describe patients who exhibit objective findings of traumatic myelopathy with no evidence of fracture or ligamentous instability on routine screening plain radiography or CT scanning.[165] SCIWORA is essentially an injury of children, especially younger children, and is likely directly related to the biomechanical properties of the juvenile spine outlined previously. As with vertebral injury, there is a tendency toward more rostral injury with younger age. Younger children suffering SCIWORA are more likely to have severe or complete spinal cord injuries than older children. Severe spinal cord injury in older children is more often associated with a vertebral injury than with SCIWORA.[145,166,167]

The diagnosis of this syndrome is complicated by the frequent occurrence of delayed neurologic deficits. Many children with this injury will develop neurologic deficits hours to days after the reported injury and in the absence of any further injury. The mechanism of this delayed deterioration is unknown, but

Pang has speculated that there is repeated injury to an already mildly injured spinal cord either because of the innate normal flexibility of the spine or because of subtle ligamentous injury with increased segmental movement at the injury site.[168] This argument is supported by the observation that recurrent SCIWORA may occur in about 20% of children who are not immobilized and that immobilization of the cervical spine markedly reduces the incidence of this phenomenon.[169]

Finally, this syndrome was initially described before the widespread use of MRI for spinal disease diagnosis. Although it is still true that these children do not have evidence of bony injury or overt instability on plain spine radiographs or CT scans, most (but not all) patients will have evidence of spinal cord and/or ligamentous or other soft tissue injury on MRI (Fig. 24-10).[170–172] Therefore it is essential that all physicians who provide early evaluations of injured children be aware of this disorder and continue to consider the possibility of spine or spinal cord injury, even when the initial radiographic studies may be reported as normal.

INITIAL MANAGEMENT OF SPINE AND SPINAL CORD INJURY

Spine Stabilization

The mainstay of management of spine injury is immobilization of the entire spinal axis in the field. An appropriately sized cervical collar should be used; in the absence of an appropriately sized collar, blocks and tape are effective for immobilizing the head on the backboard.[162] In young children less than the age of 8 years, the disproportionately large head places them in flexion when placed on a neutral board. Proper immobilization requires either a special board with a recess for the occiput, allowing the head to rest in-line with the body, or placement of a thin mattress under the torso relative to the head.[162]

Imaging

Currently, no national guidelines exist for the clearance of the pediatric spine, particularly the cervical spine, after trauma. In addition, no institution-specific spine clearance protocol has been shown to be superior versus another. A meta-analysis conducted and published in 2002 found insufficient evidence to support a standardized, diagnostic protocol.[173]

Radiologically, the integrity of the pediatric spine (especially the cervical spine), may be difficult and time consuming to assess. However, an accurate and timely evaluation is important in pediatric trauma. Younger children present an additional challenge, because they are developmentally unable to communicate crucial symptoms or are unable to cooperate with a detailed neurologic examination.

Most institutional spine clearance protocols require pediatric trauma victims to undergo lateral and anteroposterior (AP) plain radiography of cervical spine, with the addition of an odontoid image for children older than 3 years.[174] An improper radiographic evaluation has been shown to be the leading cause of missed injury and subsequent neurologic deterioration in large series of trauma patients.[175–178]

Performing CT of the cervical spine has recently led to a more efficient evaluation of the cervical spine in adult trauma victims.[179–181] Little is known about the use of CT for evaluating the cervical spine in pediatric victims of acute trauma. However, the number of repeat radiographs required to ascertain that the pediatric cervical spine is free of injury after suspected head trauma has been shown to be significantly decreased when initial CT of the cervical spine is performed at the time of head CT.[182] Including cervical spine CT in trauma protocols for children undergoing workup for traumatic brain injuries may lead to more effective clearance of the pediatric cervical spine; likewise, reconstructing thoracic and lumbosacral spine CTs from chest and abdomen and pelvis CTs in patients undergoing workup for multisystem blunt trauma may effectively clear the pediatric thoracic and lumbosacral spines (Fig. 24-11).

Plain Radiographs In general, plain radiographs are able to detect most osseous injuries of the cervical, thoracic, and lumbosacral spine in children and give an adequate global view of the spine.[162] Flexion/extension radiographs of the cervical spine are important to rule out subluxation in any patient with reported transient neurologic symptoms. Paraspinous muscles will often "splint" the cervical spine, rendering any subluxation undetectable in the acute setting; follow-up radiographs should be performed in 5 to 7 days after muscle spasm subsides.[165]

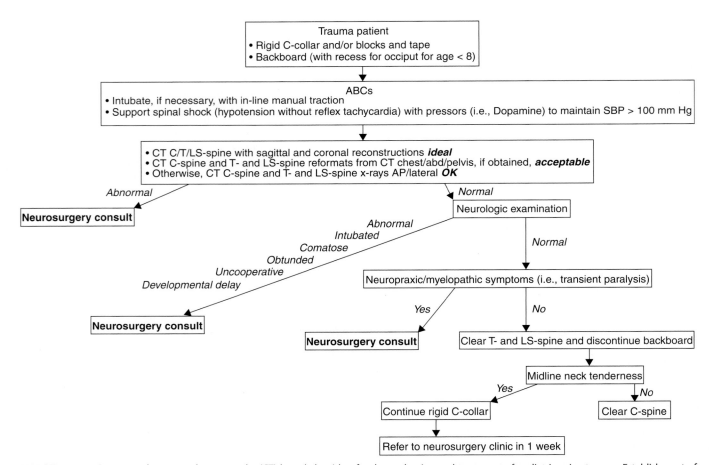

FIGURE 24-11 A proposed computed tomography (CT)-based algorithm for the evaluation and treatment of pediatric spine trauma. Establishment of CT-based protocols to clear the pediatric spine of suspected injury has been shown to decrease the time required to accomplish clearance[178–181,201] and reduce the number of missed injuries.[174,175,178,181,202] ABC, airway, breathing, circulation; abd, abdomen; AP, anteroposterior; C-collar, cervical collar; C-spine, cervical spine; CT, computed tomography; LS-spine, lumbosacral spine; SBP, systolic blood pressure; T-spine, thoracic spine.

Computed Tomography Computed tomography may suggest soft tissue, ligamentous injury, which most often occurs in the pediatric cervical spine. When using atlanto-occipital dislocation as a model for purely ligamentous injury, seen almost exclusively in the pediatric population, lateral cervical spine plain radiographs helped to make the diagnosis in 57% of patients; CT helped make 84% of diagnoses.[173] Another example of purely soft tissue injury in the pediatric population is atlantoaxial rotatory subluxation. Radiographic sensitivity during diagnosis was only 33%, whereas CT sensitivity reached 93% to 95%.[183]

Patients undergoing cervical spine and brain CT simultaneously had statistically significant less repeat or excessive radiographs than patients undergoing brain CT with cervical spine radiographs.[182] Children who underwent initial cervical spine CT did receive approximately 4 to 8 mSv of radiation; however, statistically significant increased risk of fatal cancer from low-dose radiation is in the range of 50 to 100 mSv.[184]

High-quality CT scans, perhaps, are most useful in identifying an occult and, possibly, surgically correctable vertebral fracture or dislocation.[166]

Magnetic Resonance Imaging In the last decade, MRI has become the modality of choice for pediatric patients with apparent spinal cord injury but negative radiographic studies. MRI seems to be very sensitive at detecting ligamentous disruption and instability not seen on plain radiographs or CT.[185] MRI demonstrates the extent of actual damage to the spinal cord, ranging from mild hemorrhage and/or edema to cord transection.[186]

Magnetic resonance imaging findings are prognostic of patient outcome. A normal-appearing MRI suggests excellent recovery of function; major hemorrhage or cord transection on MRI is associated with permanent cord injury.

Magnetic resonance imaging is also useful in ruling out surgical lesions (i.e., those causing persistent cord compression, such as epidural hematoma or traumatic disc herniation).[187–189]

EARLY MANAGEMENT OF SPINAL CORD INJURY

As with traumatic brain injury, it is extremely important to aggressively support systemic perfusion and oxygenation. Because children tend to have more rostral cervical cord injuries, impaired respiratory function is likely to be a concern. Furthermore, gastric dilatation commonly accompanies acute spinal injuries and can add a substantial mechanical barrier to effective respiration; therefore early nasogastric decompression of the stomach should be considered. For midlevel and higher cervical injuries, elective intubation may be needed to support respiration until a comprehensive assessment of the injury is completed. Because endotracheal intubation in a spinal-injured child is technically challenging, it should be performed by an expert who should not manipulate the relative position of the head and neck.

By restoring and supporting systemic blood pressure, one can maintain perfusion of the injured spinal cord. Patients with severe cord injuries, especially in the cervical cord, are most at risk for systemic hypotension. Although a patient can undergo initial resuscitation with intravascular volume loading, neurogenic hypotension should be treated with vasopressors. The resuscitation and maintenance of normal blood pressure in a patient with a spinal cord injury is complicated and may be aided by invasive monitoring of central venous pressure.

The pharmacotherapy of spinal cord injury has been the subject of active research and scientific controversy. The second National Spinal Cord Injury Study (NASCIS-II)[190] recommended that all patients with acute spinal cord injuries be administered high-dose methylprednisolone. Although the recommendations did not officially extend to pediatric patients, most centers applied these treatment recommendations to all age groups. Despite a subsequent study[191] that appeared to confirm the initial findings, the methodology and conclusions of these studies have been seriously questioned.[4,192] Current evidence suggests that administering high-dose steroids to spinal cord–injured patients, including children, is a listed treatment option, albeit one in which the harmful side effects may not justify clinical benefit.[4]

Early surgical therapy is rarely needed. Most pediatric fractures and dislocations can be reduced and maintained in anatomic alignment with a variety of orthotic devices, including a halo brace. Early surgical reduction and fusion is considered only for cases where there is clear neurologic deterioration occurring in the face of irreducible subluxation or compression from bone fragments, extruded disk material, or enlarging hematoma. These issues are unusual in young children. Adolescents suffer injuries similar to adults and can be treated using the surgical recommendations available for adult patients.[4] There is limited scientific information about the advisability and outcomes of operative management of spinal injury in young children, although recent reports indicate that surgical instrumentation is becoming more common.[193,194] Anatomic reduction of deformity, stabilization of clearly unstable injuries, and decompression of neural elements are indications cited for surgical treatment of spinal injury in children. Most of these goals can be accomplished nonoperatively. Current recommendations indicate that most vertebral injuries in young children should be initially treated nonoperatively, reserving surgical management for persistent or progressive deformity or ligamentous instability (see Fig. 24-8).[4]

COMPLICATIONS

Children are subject to all of the complications associated with spine injury, which include skin breakdown, infections, deep venous thrombosis, autonomic dysreflexia, contractures, spasticity, neurogenic bladder and bowel, and progressive spine deformity.[195] However, the single major acute complication of spinal cord injury in children is respiratory; the most common cause of death in the acute phase of injury is respiratory failure.[196] Aggressive pulmonary care is essential, and ventilatory support may be necessary until accessory muscles of respiration can strengthen. Many of the other complications can be avoided or minimized by the early intervention of physiatrists and other rehabilitation specialists.

The incidence of venous thromboembolism in spinal-injured children has been reported, probably incorrectly, to be roughly similar to the incidence reported in adults.[195] However, series involving only pediatric patients indicate that this complication is extremely rare.[197] Therefore specific recommendations for prophylaxis of this possible complication vary widely. For adults, and presumably, for older children and adolescents, thromboprophylaxis for up to 12 weeks after the injury is recommended, using low-molecular-weight or low-dose heparin in combination with rotating beds, pneumatic compression stockings, or electrical stimulation.[4,195]

OUTCOMES

The mortality of spinal cord injury in childhood has been reported at 28%, which is significantly higher than the mortality rate for this injury reported for adults (approximately 15% at 10 years postinjury).[168,198] The majority of these deaths appeared to occur at the scene and would not be affected by current management strategies. For survivors of spine injury, outcomes are related to the level and severity of injury. Complete injuries remain complete, and although limited functional improvement may be seen over time, full recovery is not expected.[145,159,166,167] Children with incomplete spinal cord injuries have a good chance of showing significant functional improvement and even complete recovery.

The cost of long-term care for these injuries is staggering. The lifetime cost of care for a child with a spinal cord injury extends into the millions of dollars.[154,199,200] This cost must be added to the loss of productivity that accompanies these devastating injuries. The adult employment rate for individuals suffering childhood spinal cord injury is about 50%.[195] Factors associated with successful employment are younger age at injury, less severe neurologic impairment, better education, longer duration of living with the sequelae of the injury, and ability to drive independently.

Acknowledgments

Lily Chun provided invaluable assistance in preparing and editing the manuscript.

The complete reference list is available online at www.expertconsult.com.

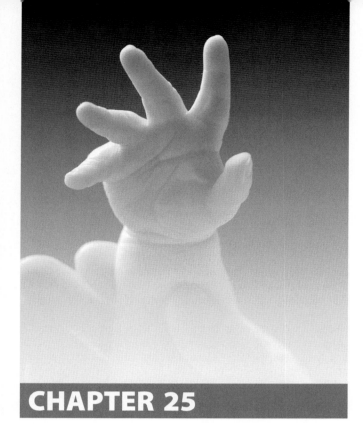

CHAPTER 25

Vascular Injury

Joseph J. Tepas III and Danielle S. Walsh

In the century since Alexis Carrel was awarded the Nobel Prize for his work in devising the surgical technique of vascular transplantation and repair, management of the patient with multisystem injury has emerged as a constantly improving process of recognition, rescue, resuscitation, and repair. Recent combat casualty experience in Iraq and Afghanistan has validated the role of damage control surgery and has stimulated the emergence of increasingly sophisticated systems of care for the severely injured. Although this experience has been forged in the treatment of massive open wounds usually caused by explosive devices, the principles that have been developed are beginning to permeate the process of civilian trauma care. The treatment of vascular injury in particular has been advanced through the use of temporary vascular shunts, permitting the transfer of life- and limb-threatening injuries to centers able to perform reconstruction.[1] Sadly there are also a significant number of pediatric casualties about whom little is known because they were simply the collateral damage of civil war. Reports by pediatric specialists deployed to these theaters validate the incidence and intensity of these injuries and indicate that the same management approaches used in the adults have been equally effective in rescuing children. Also noted has been a significantly better outcome for those children managed by pediatric specialists. In short the war experience has taught us that the basic principles of management of vascular injuries are similar for children and adults.[2]

The pediatric surgeon must approach every injured child with an organized process of assessment based on thorough review of the mechanism of injury, a careful physical examination, and an appropriate strategy for imaging and intervention. The predictive accuracy of clinical examination and better definition of indications and techniques for arteriography have led to more timely operative intervention after effective resuscitation, assessment of associated injuries, and anticipation of reperfusion injury.[3,4] The emergence of endovascular technology has begun moving the acute management of some vascular injuries from the operating room to the angiography suite. At the heart of vascular injury management, however, remains restoration of peripheral perfusion and the technical repair of damaged blood vessels. Although these basic surgical skills are similar for patients of all ages, infants and children have unique characteristics, which can present significant challenges.[5-9]

Epidemiology

As in the adult population, vascular trauma can be classified into torso injuries that involve major truncal vessels and extremity injuries that disrupt peripheral perfusion. Although blunt injury predominates in pediatric trauma overall, our young patients increasingly mirror the adult population as is evidenced by penetrating injury overtaking blunt injury as the cause of most vascular injury.[10,11] Fortunately the incidence of both remains relatively low, although the mortality rates are significant. Archival data in the National Pediatric Trauma Registry (NPTR), demonstrated an incidence of vascular trauma of only 1.3% of registry cases in a 13-year span. However the 13% crude mortality rate for this group was significantly higher than the 2.9% rate for the entire registry, demonstrating the lethality of these injuries. Table 25-1 lists mechanisms of injury and mortality in 1368 children with at least one vascular injury recorded in the registry. Table 25-2 further characterizes these injuries by variability of outcome with body region affected. Penetrating injury accounted for slightly more than half of reported cases and was more likely to require intervention. Blunt traumatic disruption of torso vessels, in contrast, was more likely to be fatal. Two institutional trauma databases from the Medical College of Wisconsin and the University of Miami similarly found a higher incidence of penetrating wounds at 68% and 53%, respectively, in children with vascular injury.[11,12]

A report by Allison and colleagues[13] reviewed management and outcome of 75 truncal vascular injuries encountered in 57 of 10,992 patients 17 years or younger treated at their regional pediatric trauma center between 1997 and 2006. The low incidence (0.7%) and high lethality associated with presenting hemodynamic instability is in accord with the NPTR experience as well as the experience at our University of Florida, Jacksonville regional trauma center with 38 of 3996 (1%) children younger than 14 years treated between 1995 and 2009. Our experience included a 47% incidence of penetrating extremity vascular injury; all these patients survived. Of epidemiologic significance in all these reports is that boys are more likely than girls to sustain vascular injuries of all types, by a margin of 2 or 3:1.[14,15]

TABLE 25-1

Injury Mechanism in 1367 Children in the National Pediatric Trauma Registry II and III

	Proportion	Mortality
Penetrating	52%	10%
Blunt	47%	17%
Crush	1%	8%

Evaluation

General principles of assessment of acute vascular disruption are based on clinical evaluation. Regardless of cause, suspicion of vascular injury should prompt an organized clinical assessment based first on the patient's history. During initial clinical evaluation two immediate questions must be answered. First, is there evidence of disruption of integrity of the circulatory system, and second, is perfusion adequate? Despite the implied causal relationship of these two points, each can be deranged without immediate effect on the other. Prolonged spasm after injury, a common characteristic of childhood vascular trauma, may cause peripheral ischemia in an otherwise anatomically intact vascular tree. Conversely, effective collateral circulation, enhanced by the absence of obliterative vascular disease, may sustain distal circulation despite deranged proximal flow. Thus not every disruption of vascular flow produces immediate peripheral ischemia, and evidence of acute ischemia may not necessarily portend operative vascular injury. Regardless of circumstances, confirmation of restoration of cellular perfusion is the immediate priority in assessing any child with vascular injury.[8]

Children usually do not suffer from atherosclerotic vascular disease. Their vessels are more elastic and usually respond to application of force by stretch and transient deformity rather than rupture. The immediate result of this is an increased potential for intimal tears, which cause flow disruption in an otherwise anatomically intact vessel. The effect of this decreased flow may be acute ischemia or marginal insufficiency that stimulates increased collateralization. Although the former should be easily discernable on clinical examination, the latter can be subtle and clinically silent. The relevance of this is rooted in the mandate that functional and anatomic integrity of the circulation be clinically confirmed and documented in every injured child. Of equal importance is the understanding that unexplainable absence of palpable pulses, especially in the lower extremities, may be the result of preexisting rather than acute injury. If perfusion pressure is suddenly lowered because of other acute injuries, collateral circulation may become inadequate and symptoms of progressive ischemia may emerge.

Frykberg and associates demonstrated the predictive accuracy of "hard signs" of injury and recommended immediate operative intervention for any patient with active bleeding, an expanding hematoma, pulse deficit, or a bruit/thrill.[16] Nonexpanding hematoma, hypotension, peripheral nerve deficit, or a history of bleeding from the wound were considered "soft" signs, which required only clinical observation. Long-term follow-up of this population has confirmed the predictive accuracy of this approach and has validated the authors' initial recommendation that routine arteriography was not necessary for management of proximity injury.[4,17] Reichard and colleagues analyzed the predictive accuracy of clinical signs in their review of 75 children with vascular injury treated at the pediatric trauma service of Cook County Hospital.[18] Part of their report includes comparison to an additional 12 children managed by an "adult" protocol that required traditional arteriography. None of the studies performed for proximity injury alone was abnormal. All 10 children with vascular injury had hard signs. Four of 77 children with no vascular injury also manifested at least one hard sign, yielding a sensitivity of physical examination of 100% and a specificity of 95%. It is of note that these data validate similar recommendations published by Meagher and colleagues in 1979 and emphasize that arteriography for acute injury should be considered only if the risk of performance is outweighed by a threat of ischemia that cannot be defined by history and clinical signs.[16,19–21] Numerous investigators have validated the predictive accuracy of thorough clinical examination and in the process have refined indications for further imaging, particularly arteriography.[3,16] Although the emergence of multidetector computed tomography (CT) and magnetic resonance angiography (MRA)-based angiography has minimized the trauma of arterial vascular access, the additional radiation of CT, the lesser availability of MRA, and the risk of contrast toxicity still mandate a studied decision as to the appropriateness of these imaging studies.[22] Although CT and MRA do not require direct arterial puncture or manipulation of foreign bodies against arterial intima, they do require relatively large boluses of contrast medium and in the case of CT significant radiation exposure. The risk of inappropriate angiography has simply changed in characteristic rather than in magnitude or incidence.

Lineen and colleagues published their review of 78 pediatric patients with suspected vascular injury undergoing CT angiography for 41 penetrating and 37 blunt mechanisms.[12,23] Eleven injuries were identified from the penetrating trauma group, with 100% sensitivity and 93% specificity. Two normal veins were read as abnormal adjacent to missile tracts: one patient had ultrasonography to confirm the integrity of the adjacent vein and the other was observed because the physical

TABLE 25-2

Vascular Injuries (1628) in 1368 Children in the National Pediatric Trauma Registry II and III

Region	ICD-9-CM	Total	Lived	Died (%)	Operated (%)
Neck	900-901	249	196	53 (21)	41
Chest	901-902	161	98	63 (39)	70
Abdomen/pelvis	902-903	374	248	126 (34)	50
Upper Extremity	903-904	497	494	3 (1)	21
Lower Extremity	904-905	326	318	8 (3)	36

examination was normal. Eight injures from blunt trauma were noted with 88% sensitivity and 100% specificity. One injury was listed as "indeterminate" but was confirmed on conventional arteriography as a subclavian artery injury. The authors therefore propose that CT angiography be used as the study of choice when the soft signs of vascular trauma are present on physical examination.

A recent report by Hsu and colleagues defined the clear benefit of CT angiography in assessment of pediatric extremity injuries both acutely and as an essential planning "road map" before definitive reconstruction.[24] In addition to avoiding problems with direct vessel injury, these authors cite the speed and accessibility of CT scanners and the ability of CT to define three-dimensional spatial anatomy as major advantages in assessing the injured child. Three-dimensional reconstructions precisely define level of injury and efficiency of collateral circulation (Fig. 25-1). However they may require a higher volume of contrast medium.

Duplex Doppler and B-mode ultrasonography are emerging, noninvasive, portable technologies that supplement clinical imaging with determination of flow and flow velocity. Their role in the diagnosis of acute injury, however, has not been well established. Because both CT and magnetic resonance imaging (MRI) are limited in accurate identification of spasm, Doppler flow studies can be extremely useful for both diagnosis and follow-up. Transesophageal echocardiography may also provide useful data in the evaluation of thoracic truncal injuries in particular.[25] "One-shot" emergency department arteriography, despite reports of safety and efficacy, has essentially been replaced by CT angiography.[26]

Traumatic Injuries

Traumatic injuries can be divided into those involving the torso (neck and trunk) and those involving the extremities (upper or lower). Each area presents unique challenges to accurate diagnosis and timely management.

TORSO INJURIES

Torso injuries in the cervical region appear to be rare in childhood, although they are more common in metropolitan areas with a higher incidence of pediatric penetrating trauma from missile and stab wounds.[12,23] Cox and associates' review of the operative management of 36 children with vascular injury included 9 children with 11 carotid or jugular injuries.[13,27] Eight of these injuries were penetrating neck wounds. Mortality occurred in 2 of the 3 hemodynamically unstable children. Their updated publication of 2009 identified 14 patients with 20 head and neck vascular injuries, of which 53% were of a penetrating mechanism. Of the 8 children managed in our unit, 5 were victims of penetrating trauma, including all 3 fatalities, each of whom presented with nonsurvivable injuries. Rozycki and colleagues evaluated their proposed algorithm for diagnosis of blunt cervical vascular injury by reviewing injuries associated with a cervicothoracic seat belt sign in 797 motor vehicle accident victims treated over 17 months by the Grady Memorial Hospital Trauma Service.[28] The 3% of patients with carotid injury were all adults. No injuries were missed, and no injuries were noted in children. With the gradual increase

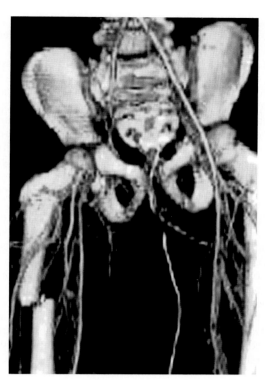

FIGURE 25-1 Computed tomographic angiogram from a 5-year-old hit by a car. He underwent repair of transposition of the great vessels as an infant and was noted to have a pulseless right foot. Evaluation demonstrated a clinically silent femoral artery disruption.

in child restraint law compliance, this potential association between seatbelt marks and significant vascular injury will require continued close follow-up.

Thoracic and abdominal torso vascular injuries are also relatively rare in childhood. This is probably the result of the greater elasticity of young and healthy vessels. Although children are not immune to thoracic vascular disruption, most series that include pediatric patients demonstrate a low incidence compared with adults. The report by Cox and colleagues included abdominal vascular injuries in 39 children and thoracic vascular trauma in 13 patients.[27] Fifty-four percent of the abdominal injuries and 46% of the thoracic injuries stemmed from blunt trauma. A higher percentage of the injuries specific to the aorta were by blunt mechanism, whereas nonaortic injures—such as great vessel, mammary, and pulmonary vein injuries—were from traumatic missiles. In general, clinical reports of aortic injuries seen in children suggest a natural history no different from that of adults. Mortality is extremely high, especially for children with a presenting systolic blood pressure below 90 mm Hg and those with associated severe traumatic brain injuries.[13] Eddy and colleagues reviewed the King County Coroner's records over a 12-year period (1975–1987), and found 13 cases of aortic disruption in children.[29] Only 3 of these children reached a hospital alive, and just 1 child survived. Experience in the NPTR is somewhat more heartening in that 26 of 54 children with aortic ruptures (48%) survived to hospital discharge. This representative sample from multiple contributing hospitals in North America is similar to that reported from a single institution by Cox and colleagues, suggesting that outcome from this catastrophic injury may be better than what has been consistently reported for adults.[27] Major thoracic venous injuries are even less common and are usually associated with major pulmonary disruption.

Because of the preponderance of blunt mechanisms of injury in the pediatric population, especially as the result of vehicular-related mishaps, abdominal vascular injuries can and do occur.[30] Arterial disruption is far less common than venous disruption. Hypotension progressing to frank shock is the most common associated finding, making the decision to explore the abdomen relatively straightforward, although usually there is the expectation of solid viscus derangement as the most likely cause. Fayiga and colleagues reviewed 18 years of experience in operative management of pediatric blunt vascular injury.[31]

Twenty-one major abdominal venous injuries were present in 17 patients and were lethal in 11 of them (65%). None of the abdominal venous injuries was recognized before laparotomy. As in numerous other series, survival was directly related to the presence of hemodynamic stability. Most complications were related to nonvascular injuries. The majority of vascular injuries were repaired directly, which parallels the experience from a similar series of 16 abdominal vascular injuries reported by Cox and colleagues.[27] Interposition grafts were required to repair only one aortic disruption and one superior mesenteric artery transection.

EXTREMITY INJURIES

Vascular extremity injuries are uncommon in children. Most are associated with fractures, although the rising tide of violent crime is also driving an increase in penetrating mechanisms. As in the adult, careful and expeditious clinical examination is the critical starting point. Evidence of diminished peripheral flow may be the result of spasm (discussed in detail further on) with or without associated vascular disruption. In the absence of hard signs of disruption, imaging assessment using ultrasonography or CT angiography may be required to define the cause of distal ischemia. The use of stents for angiographically identified injuries is becoming more common in the adult population. However it is still rare and controversial in children.[32,33] Migration and stent impact on subsequent growth are still undefined, making formal operative repair the recommended option for vascular disruption. Chang's[33] report of use of a stent to treat an axillary arterial and venous stab wound includes follow-up that documents critical stenosis mitigated by adequate collateralization. The authors make a strong case, however, that this approach avoided dissection of a huge hematoma in an anatomic space that is difficult to approach safely. Future elective reconstruction, if required, will be much less difficult and dangerous than operative repair during the acute phase of injury. This experience implies a reasonable role for at least a temporizing if not definitive therapy for some vascular injuries.

Interposition of reversed contralateral saphenous vein remains the treatment of choice for all disrupted segments. Synthetic material should be considered only as a last resort when an autologous vessel cannot be harvested and fabricated into a patch or conduit.[7] Veins should be repaired before arteries. Anastomoses are constructed using monofilament simple sutures.[8] As the repair is being completed, the distal clamp is first released to confirm adequate backflow. The proximal clamp is then released to flush any residual air or

clot before the final sutures are tied. Vasospasm if significant can usually be reduced by gentle mechanical dilation, using coronary artery dilators, topical 2% lidocaine, or papaverine. Investigators emphasize that the high proclivity for prolonged vasospasm can make arterial anastomosis in childhood especially challenging.[31] LaQuaglia and associates described experience in nine children with iatrogenic arterial injuries repaired using microsurgical technique using 9-0 to 11-0 nylon suture.[34] As microsurgical technique continues to evolve and better suture materials become available, this approach will become an increasingly valuable adjunct to the management of major injuries to tiny vessels. If ischemia time has been prolonged longer than 6 hours, the possibility of evolving compartment syndrome should spark consideration for fasciotomy.[35] Children who have undergone repair of injuries should undergo anticoagulation for 48 hours postoperatively. Some authors use heparin, whereas others simply use dextran solutions for 2 to 3 days postoperatively.

Although lower extremity vascular injuries are most commonly associated with fractures and soft tissue avulsions, the rising incidence of violence in our urban youth is increasing the frequency of disruption of groin and femoral vessels.[12] Popliteal injuries are often the result of sport and cycling mishaps associated with a skeletal fracture and warrant particular attention. Initial assessment must confirm the presence of palpable distal pulses and adequate capillary perfusion. Immediate reduction of displaced fracture fragments or subluxed joints will often result in restoration of palpable distal pulses. Reed and colleagues reported their experience with seven children with popliteal arterial injury who underwent immediate operative repair. Four had blunt trauma and three had penetrating injuries.[36] Associated morbidity included three fractures, four severe soft tissue wounds, and one nerve injury. All patients underwent angiography; three cases were intraoperative. Treatment included two primary repairs and four vein graft bypasses. One child required fasciotomy; there were no deaths, amputations, or reoperations. At the time of their report, follow-up ranged between 10 and 42 months. All patients had normal Doppler pressures or distal pulses, or both. These data illustrate the relationship between prompt, aggressive treatment and successful outcome. The potential for development of delayed pseudoaneurysm, which usually requires excision with vein grafting, mandates that every child with an extremity vascular injury be followed for at least 5 years.

Upper extremity vascular injury is most often associated with supracondylar fractures or penetrating trauma. Supracondylar fractures may disrupt brachial arterial flow by direct injury or by compression with or without prolonged spasm.[37] As with the lower extremity, definitive management begins with assessment of adequacy of perfusion and confirmation of integrity of the vessel. Of interest is a recent report that describes the use of the ipsilateral basilic vein as an ideal interposition graft for reconstruction of vessels in which segmental loss has occurred.[38] Axillary stretch injuries, especially when associated with high energy such as vehicular ejection, may disrupt arterial or venous structures, producing a hematoma that is not as precisely definable as those seen with more distal injuries. In addition to signs of obvious blood loss, diffuse edema of the axilla or shoulder region and diminution of peripheral pulses should prompt angiographic confirmation of both the existence and anatomic configuration of the injury. Salvage from damage of upper extremity injuries is generally good, with return of functionality related to the nature of the associated musculoskeletal and neurologic disruption. The incidence of compartment syndrome as a result of prolonged ischemia in the upper extremity is reported to be significantly lower than that for lower extremity injuries. However careful follow-up for adequacy of perfusion and avoidance of potential postischemia muscular contracture must be part of long-term management.

Mangled Extremity

The vast majority of extremity vascular injuries seen in children are associated with axial skeletal disruption. In its most severe form, this combination of bone and soft tissue destruction can result in what has been called the "mangled extremity." It is usually characterized by major soft tissue avulsion that can be associated with significant tissue loss. Initial assessment must consider tissue viability, anticipated limb function, and the need for amputation of a potential source of massive tissue necrosis and sepsis. The Mangled Extremity Severity Score (MESS) has been proposed as an accurate system of evaluation and prediction of limb salvage (Table 25-3). Although originally devised for adults, Fagelman and colleagues demonstrated a predictive accuracy of 93% when it was retrospectively applied to 36 injured children.[39]

Vascular disruption associated with fractures must be immediately addressed so that subsequent axial skeletal repair will produce a viable extremity. Restoration of flow may be achieved by temporary bypass until fracture fixation is achieved. When possible, venous repair should precede arterial repair. Devitalized tissue must be debrided and fasciotomy considered. Nerve function must be evaluated and documented before debating amputation. Although it is true that children do recover amazingly well from what initially appear to be devastating injuries, being permanently disabled by an insensate, immobile extremity is a poor alternative to an active life with a functional and properly fitted prosthesis. The

decision to amputate is therefore based on assessment of limb viability and prediction of limb functionality. The Mangled Extremity Severity Score serves as a reasonable guideline, although the ultimate decision rests with the surgeon, the child's parents, and when possible the child.

Iatrogenic Injury

With continued evolution of increasingly sophisticated methods of imaging for infants and children, the potential for damage to the vascular integrity of a small child or tiny infant remains ever present. There have been numerous reports over the past decade describing this particular problem.[40-43] Many have been case reports of complications from some usually innocuous maneuver of routine care. Demircin and associates, for example, reported an infant with brachial arterial pseudoaneurysm resulting from inadvertent puncture during antecubital venipuncture.[10] The lesion was repaired by direct suture under proximal compression. Gamba and colleagues reviewed their experience with iatrogenic vascular lesions in low-birth-weight neonates. Of 335 infants encountered between 1987 and 1994, 9 (2.6%) were diagnosed with vascular injury.[44] Mean birth weight was 880 g (range 590-1450 g), although mean weight at diagnosis was 1825 g (range 1230-2730 g). Injuries were associated with venipuncture in seven of the nine cases and included six femoral arteriovenous fistulas, two of which were bilateral. One carotid lesion and five femoral arteriovenous fistulas were repaired using microvascular technique. Outcome as determined by follow-up clinical examination and Doppler flow was excellent, leading the authors to emphasize the role of aggressive medical and microsurgical management of these injuries. In 1981 O'Neill and colleagues reviewed their experience with surgical management of 41 infants with major thromboembolic problems associated with umbilical artery catheters.[45] Although the majority of complications were related to emboli distal to the femoral artery, 8 infants required emergency operative intervention for acute aortic obstruction. Four of these operations were transverse aortic thrombectomies; three patients recovered completely. As principles of umbilical artery catheter management have become better established, these problems appear to have become less frequent.

In their analysis of the predictive accuracy of clinical findings in pediatric vascular injury, Reichard and colleagues extolled the accuracy of the ankle-brachial index (ABI) as indicative of inadequate peripheral perfusion.[18] Their data suggest that an ABI less than 0.99 indicates clinically critical vascular injury and reinforce recent reports of intensive care nursery discharge data that suggest the true incidence of vascular injury is far more common than previously thought. In fact, findings reported by Seibert and colleagues suggest that assessment of the peripheral pulses and measurement of the ABI should be part of a routine postdischarge assessment of any infant treated with umbilical artery catheterization.[46]

The increasing use of complex endovascular diagnostic and therapeutic procedures in pediatric patients is also associated with a low but consistent incidence of unplanned iatrogenic damage to vascular structures.[9,42,47] However, with refinement of technique and improving technology, this also appears to be decreasing.[9,48] Morbidity from these iatrogenic

---

TABLE 25-3

Mangled Extremity Severity Score (MESS)

Skeletal/soft tissue injury	
Low energy (stab, simple fracture, pistol or gunshot wound)	1
Medium energy (open or multiple fractures, dislocation)	2
High energy (high-speed crash or rifle gunshot wound)	3
Very high energy (high-speed injury, gross contamination)	4
Limb ischemia	
Reduced/absent pulse, normal perfusion	1*
Pulseless, paraesthesias, poor capillary refill	2*
Cool, insensate, paralyzed, numb	3*
Shock	
Systolic BP always >90 mm Hg	1
Transient hypotension	2
Persistent hypotension	3
Age (yr)	
<30	1
30-50	2
>50	3

*Score doubled for ischemia >6 hours.
MESS >7 = 100% prediction for amputation
BP, blood pressure.

injuries occurs primarily in the neonatal period when small vessel diameter and vasospastic tendencies predispose to ischemia. Long-term consequences of such injuries include soft tissue loss, amputation, limb growth discrepancies, and the ultimate need for surgical reconstruction of these deformities. As CT and MRI-based angiography becomes more common and diagnostic, incidence of injuries directly related to vascular access for traditional angiography may be minimized.

Lin and associates analyzed 1674 diagnostic or therapeutic catheterizations performed in 1431 infants over a 15-year period.[49] Thirty-six procedures were required in 34 children. The authors stratified complications into nonischemic, acute femoral ischemia, and chronic femoral ischemia. Nonischemic lesions included pseudoaneurysms (n = 4), arteriovenous fistulas (n = 5), and groin hematoma (n = 5), and all underwent direct suture repair. Acute femoral ischemic lesions were most common and required a variety of procedures from thrombectomy to patch repair. Seven children presented with chronic femoral ischemia, defined as having evidence of flow disruption more than 30 days after the procedure, at an average of 193 days (range 31-842 days) after the index intervention. All seven children were symptomatic with claudication, leg length discrepancy, or gait disturbance. Operative repair consisted of revascularization using reversed saphenous vein for iliofemoral bypass in five children and femorofemoral bypass in one child. One child required patch only angioplasty. Risk factors for ischemia included age younger than 3 years, need for therapeutic or multiple catheterizations, and catheter size larger than 6 French. The value of this study lies not only in its identification of potentially predictive factors but also in its documentation of the relatively short time interval required for chronic ischemia to become symptomatic.

Children at risk of vascular injury with any abnormal clinical finding must be followed at least 5 years and preferably through at least the start of adolescence. The evolution of limb length discrepancy as a result of disruption of a major vascular structure may not become manifest until years after the precipitating event.[50] Recent reports have suggested that operative revascularization of iatrogenic injury before adolescence will correct some limb length discrepancy; however, these reports have been relatively small series and do not represent consensus.

The femoral artery remains the most common site of iatrogenic injury. As noted previously in the discussion of traumatic injury, efficient collateralization of the pelvis and gluteal region may result in these lesions remaining clinically silent throughout most of childhood. Mourot and colleagues reported their experience with ischemia after femoral arterial line placement in the pediatric burn population.[51] In a group of 234 children who underwent 745 femoral artery catheterizations, 8 patients developed loss of distal pulses, indicating occlusion or spasm of the femoral artery. Five children responded to nonsurgical treatment consisting of catheter removal and systemic heparinization. The other 3 patients required surgical thrombectomy.[51] The authors point out the importance of timely removal of foreign bodies from vessels in ischemic limbs with both vasospasm and occlusion for prevention of tissue loss.

Extracorporeal membrane oxygenation (ECMO) represents another area in which iatrogenic vascular injury may result in long-term consequences. Many authors advocate preferential use of venovenous ECMO over venoarterial ECMO because of uncertainty over the potential long-term consequences of neonatal carotid artery injury.[52] For patients requiring carotid artery cannulation, scientific inquiry continues to ensue over whether carotid artery reconstruction should be performed at decannulation, particularly in the neonatal population. Sarioglu and associates reported their experience in 61 infants with carotid artery cannulation for ECMO. End-to-end carotid artery repair was performed in 32 patients and simple ligation in 29 patients.[53] Early patency rate as evidenced by MRI and ultrasonography was 97%, although 12% appeared stenotic. These authors recommend routine carotid artery repair when technically feasible. Longer term patency after carotid artery reconstruction following ECMO for congenital diaphragmatic hernia was assessed by Buesing and associates in 18 infants.[54] All underwent three-dimensional MRA 2 years after the procedure and the common carotid artery was occluded or highly stenotic in 72% of the patients. All had patent internal carotid arteries and evidence of both intracranial and extracranial collateral vessel development. They also noted that unsuccessful repair of the artery was not predictive of a poor neurologic outcome. They concluded that the benefits of surgical repair are "doubtful" but that longer term assessment is still required. A recent report from Duncan and associates points out two cases of aneurysms at the site of carotid artery repair after ECMO, highlighting a potential complication of repair.[55]

Vasospasm

As is the case with management of traumatic injury, the high proclivity for spasm and the need to differentiate prolonged spasm from arterial disruption remains one of the most challenging components of initial assessment. Prolonged spasm is felt to be the result of intimal injury, which causes derangement of nitric oxide production and disrupts control of arterial wall tension.[56,57] When endothelial-medial contact is lost, as can be caused by shearing friction from an oversized or overzealously placed catheter, underlying vascular smooth muscle is incapable of relaxation.[58] Angiographic confirmation of spasm requires the additional risk of the very mechanism suspected of causing the problem. CT or MRA may be the solution to this clinical conundrum, although dose and concentration of contrast medium must be carefully considered in comparing risk to benefit.

The role of spasm in causing gangrene is controversial despite case reports suggesting cause and effect.[59] From a clinical perspective once spasm has been confirmed to be the sole cause of diminished peripheral perfusion, management must focus on confirmation of evidence of tissue viability and absence of signs of evolving compartment syndrome or peripheral ischemia. Assuming that the basic cause of acute spasm is at least partly related to intimal injury, risk of thrombosis must be a primary consideration. Over the past few years, routine anticoagulation therapy has been supplemented by thrombolytic agents, especially urokinase.[60] Recommended doses of urokinase vary and tend to be empirical. Up to 6000 U/kg/hr have been used in infants with good success and no complications. Most recently, a report by Zenz and colleagues on the use of tissue plasminogen activator suggested that more rapid restoration of flow could be achieved with this drug.[61,62] Some patients may still require operative intervention for thrombectomy after a period of time in a low-flow state.

Digital Ischemia Syndrome

Intravenous catheter-related, ipsilateral digital ischemia may suddenly develop in acutely ill infants or small children with acute infectious disease. It is usually associated with dehydration and hypovolemia. In a review of 104 cases, Villavicencio and González Cerna reported primary involvement of the hand in 68.2% of patients and the foot in the remainder.[63] The age of the patients ranged from 29 days to 36 months; the mean age was 14 months. The infectious process was of respiratory origin in 27.8% of cases, localized to the gastrointestinal tract in 60.5%, and other areas in 11.5%. The most frequently cultured microorganisms were *Escherichia coli, Salmonella, Shigella, Streptococcus, Staphylococcus, Klebsiella,* and *Pseudomonas* species. Digital cyanosis usually occurs shortly after vessel cannulation and is probably the result of vasospasm provoked by the presence of an indwelling catheter. As described earlier, damaged endothelium may stimulate vasoconstriction. Immobilization causes constriction of the limbs and impairs the muscle action that is necessary to assist venous return. Persistence of these conditions increases extravascular pressure and gradually produces microcirculatory failure, leading to necrosis, which begins at the most distal areas of the digits.

Effective treatment requires prompt recognition of persistent cyanosis, correction of the underlying systemic disorder, and immediate removal of the catheter. Anticoagulation therapy should be initiated immediately. Application of nitroglycerin paste has been shown to improve local microcirculation and limit the extent of ischemic necrosis.[64,65] Lesions should be gently washed daily in warm water, and the involved limb should be actively and passively exercised through the full range of motion. Direct heating should be avoided because ischemic tissue burns at lower temperatures. Small pieces of cotton should be placed between fingers or toes; all lesions should be covered with sterile, dry dressings. Areas of dry gangrene do not require surgical removal. If there is concern whether infection is trapped under eschar, the area can be gently elevated at its corners to allow adequate drainage. As is the case with arterial lesions, amputation should not be considered until clear demarcation has occurred.

Conclusion

In summary, although the epidemiology of vascular injury in the pediatric population is considerably different from that encountered in adults, treatment imperatives remain the same. Traumatic injury presents a unique set of characteristics that reflect the epidemiology of pediatric trauma. All vascular injuries, if carefully managed, can exploit the intrinsically healthy status of the child's vascular system and yield optimal results. Iatrogenic injury is the price of miniaturization. It is a recognized tradeoff for the dramatic advances that now make possible many lifesaving procedures. Attention to detail in those most at risk may not eliminate the problem but will at least reduce incidence and raise awareness. Accurate diagnosis, timely revascularization, and aggressive management of reperfusion are essential for complete recovery and normal long-term growth. The key to success is a high index of suspicion, recognition of the unique characteristics listed earlier, and operative intervention using the high level of precision that is the cornerstone of success in the surgical care of children.

The complete reference list is available online at www. expertconsult.com.

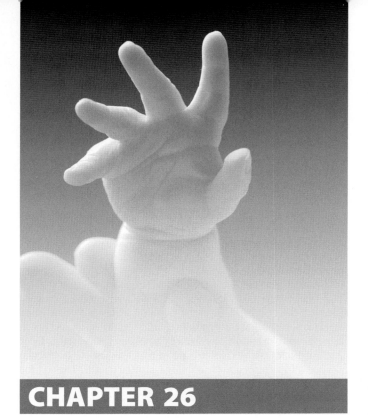

CHAPTER 26

Burns

Dai H. Chung, Nadja C. Colon, and David N. Herndon

The cornerstone of burn management stems from decades-long advances in the understanding of major burn sequelae. In 1944, Lund and Browder introduced a diagram to assess burned areas, allowing a quantifiable assessment of percentage of total body surface area (TBSA) burned.[1] While treating victims of the Coconut Grove fire in Boston in 1946, Oliver Cope and Francis Moore were able to quantitate the appropriate amount of fluid required to maintain the central electrolyte composition after "burn shock."[2] From there, the development of the Parkland formula transformed our approach to fluid resuscitation. In the 1960s, the discovery of efficacious topical antimicrobial agents, such as 0.5% silver nitrate,[3] mafenide acetate (Sulfamylon),[4] and silver sulfadiazine (Silvadene),[5] likewise revolutionized burn wound care, and when used adjunctively with early debridement and grafting, the rates of wound infection and graft failure decreased dramatically. In recent years, continued progress has been made in several areas of burn care. Early surgical excision of eschar and grafting has significantly lowered the incidence of burn wound sepsis and shortened length of hospital stay. The nutritional support with early enteral feeding has been found to blunt the hypermetabolic response that contributes to derangements in gut function and immunomodulation seen with severe burns. Treatment with anabolic agents restores net positive nitrogen balance during prolonged postburn hypermetabolic period. Acute recognition of inhalation injury and effective treatment have also improved overall burn patient outcome. These examples of significant recent advances made in burn care have led to a further decline in burn-related deaths.[6] Today, the overall increase in survival of major burn victims is most evident in the pediatric burn population, where mortality rate is 50% for 98% TBSA burns in children 14 years old and younger and 75% TBSA burns in other age groups.[7]

Hence, burn injuries that were once considered to be uniformly fatal are now survivable, in part because of vigorous efforts to promote evidence-based care of the burned patient. Despite implementation of aggressive prevention measures and legislation, nearly one million people sustain a total of 2 million burn injuries yearly in the United States alone, and one half of these require medical treatment. Approximately 60% of the 40,000 admissions for burn injury are now admitted to hospitals with specialized burn centers.[8] The majority of burns are minor and represent less than 10% TBSA, and although the mortality rate for all burns is 3.7%, mortality increases dramatically with larger TBSA burns (42% to 81% for 60% to greater than 90% TBSA). Although mortality from burn injury increases with advancing age and burn size, the presence of an inhalation injury in patients with a TBSA of less than 20% significantly increases the likelihood of death by 25 times (National Burn Repository 2010). Unfortunately, those at the extremes of age continue to have worse outcomes, likely related to their unique physiology. Burns in children, particularly those less than 5 years of age, represent 17% of total reported burn cases and constitute a large at-risk population in which burn injuries are responsible for nearly 2,500 deaths per year. The percentage of admissions accounting for child abuse–related burn injuries varies, but is estimated to be anywhere from 1% to 25%, with infants and toddlers comprising the majority of these cases.[9]

Accounting for more than 70% of reported instances, the most common etiologies of burn injuries are fire/flame and scalds. Scald burns remain the most common cause of burn injury in children younger than 5 years of age. The majority of scald burns in infants and toddlers are from hot foods and liquids. Hot grease spills are notorious for causing deep burns. Hot tap water burns frequently result in larger TBSA injuries in children and can easily be averted by installing faucet valves that prevent water from leaving the tap if its temperature is greater than 120° F (48.8° C). Children also frequently suffer contact burns to their hands and faces from curling irons, ovens, steam irons, and fireworks. In the adolescent age group, flame burns are more common, often occurring as a result of experimentation with fire and volatile agents. Particular consideration must be given to burn injuries secondary to child abuse, which also represents a significant cause of burns in children. Burns with a bilaterally symmetrical or stocking-glove distribution in conjunction with a delay in seeking medical attention should raise the suspicion of child abuse (Fig. 26-1).

Pathophysiology

As the largest organ in the body, the skin guards against harmful environmental insults, prevents entry of microorganisms, maintains fluid and electrolyte homeostasis, and is critical for thermoregulation. Other important functions include

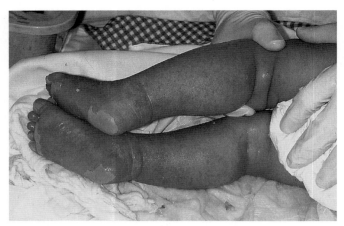

FIGURE 26-1 Scald burn from child abuse of an infant. Bilateral stocking-glove distribution with well-demarcated margins is consistent with a burn injury from abuse.

vitamin D metabolism and processing neurosensory inputs. The total surface area of skin ranges from 0.2 to 0.3 m² in an average newborn to 1.5 to 2.0 m² in an adult, making up nearly 15% of total body weight. The epidermis is composed primarily of epithelial cells, the most abundant of which are keratinocytes. Cells are generated at the stratum basale, from which they divide and migrate upwards through the strata spinosum, granulosum, lucidum, and finally, the stratum corneum. As they move through layers, the keratinocytes begin to flatten out, their nucleus degenerates, and they secrete a matrix made of lipids, cholesterol, and ceramides, which increases cohesion between the cells and is responsible for the barrier characteristic of skin. Once at the stratum corneum, the keratinocytes become corneocytes-anucleate cells that are filled with keratin, and the complete transformation is termed keratinization. Eventually, the corneocytes lose their cohesion and slough off. This entire process of epidermal maturation from the basal layer to desquamation generally takes 2 to 4 weeks.

The basement membrane at the dermoepidermal junction is composed of mucopolysaccharides rich in fibronectin, and the basement membrane functions as a barrier to the passage of macromolecules. The dermis, consisting of fibroblasts that produce collagen and elastin, is subdivided into a superficial papillary dermis and a deep reticular dermis. The papillary dermis is rather functionally active, and because it is this layer that is lost in deeper partial-thickness burns, such injuries tend to heal much more slowly than superficial partial-thickness burns.[10] A plexus of nerves and blood vessels separates the papillary and reticular dermis, and the reticular dermis and hypodermis (subcutaneous tissue) contain skin appendages, such as hair follicles, sweat glands, and sebaceous glands. Therefore burns involving the depth of deep dermis are generally insensate to touch and painful stimuli.

Thermal injury produces coagulation necrosis of the epidermis and a varying depth of injury to the underlying tissue. The extent of burn injury depends on the temperature, duration of exposure, skin thickness, tissue conductance, and specific heat of the causative agent. For example, the specific heat of lipid is higher than that of water, and therefore grease burns often result in much deeper burns than a scald burn

from water with the same temperature and duration of exposure. Thermal energy is easily transferred from high-energy molecules to those of lower energy during contact through the process of heat conduction. The skin generally provides a barrier to the transfer of energy to the deeper tissues, and hence, much of the burn injury is confined to this layer. However, local tissue responses to the zone of the burn injury can lead to progression of the burn injury, with the result being a much deeper burn of the surrounding tissue than initially observed.

Classified according to the depth of injury, burns are described as superficial, superficial partial-thickness, deep partial-thickness, full-thickness, and subdermal (Fig. 26-2). Superficial (*first-degree*) burns, like sunburns, affect only the epidermis and are characterized by erythema, pain, and desquamation that resolve without scarring within 7 to 10 days. Superficial partial-thickness (*second-degree*) burns extend through the epidermis into the papillary dermis and are characterized by blisters, erythema, and edema. These burns blanch with pressure and have a brisk capillary refill. Deep partial-thickness (*second-degree*) burns involve the reticular dermis and exhibit a more sluggish capillary refill. The wound is very moist and edematous with diminished to complete loss of sensation. The tissue injury of full-thickness (*third-degree*) burns extends into the subcutaneous tissue and can have a leathery appearance, whereas that of subdermal (*fourth-degree*) burns extends into the fascia, muscles, and bone.

The early response to a burn can be described as local and systemic. The local phase response is characterized by three zones: coagulation, stasis, and hyperemia (Fig. 26-3). Representing the product of maximal insult, the zone of coagulation is identified by surface tissue necrosis as cells are irreversibly damaged secondary to denaturation and coagulation of constituent proteins and loss of plasma membrane integrity. The area immediately surrounding the necrotic area is called the zone of stasis. In this zone, most cells are initially viable, but tissue perfusion becomes progressively compromised because of the local release of inflammatory mediators, such

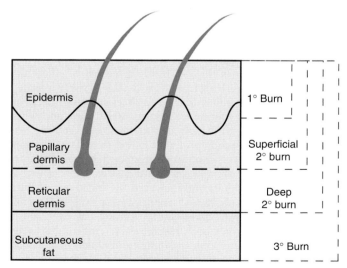

FIGURE 26-2 Depths of burn. First-degree burns are confined to the epidermis. Superficial second-degree burns involve the papillary dermis, and deep second-degree burns involve reticular dermis. Third-degree burns are full-thickness through the epidermis and dermis.

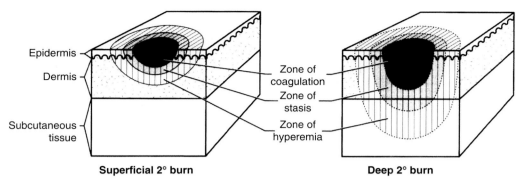

FIGURE 26-3   Three zones of burn injury: coagulation, stasis, and hyperemia.

as thromboxane A_2, arachidonic acid, histamine, oxidants, and cytokines. Their influence on the microcirculation results in the formation of platelet thrombus, neutrophil adherence, fibrin deposition, and vasoconstriction, all of which lead to cell necrosis and progression of the burn injury. However, adequate wound care and resuscitation may reverse this process and prevent extensive cell necrosis.

Thromboxane A_2 inhibitors, antioxidants (vitamins C and E), and bradykinin inhibitors can significantly improve dermal blood flow and thereby limit the expansion of the zone of stasis. Recently, activated protein C, a physiologic anticoagulant with antithrombotic and anti-inflammatory properties, was shown to improve perfusion in the zone of stasis and decrease the area of necrosis in animal models.[11] Similarly, statins are known to have multiple effects, such as decreasing oxidative stress while up-regulating endothelial nitric oxide synthesis, prostacyclins, and tissue-type plasminogen activator. In another animal model study, the administration of simvastatin was shown to increase blood flow and decrease intravascular coagulation, which resulted in salvage of the zone of stasis.[12] Finally, the zone of hyperemia lies peripheral to the zone of stasis and is characterized by vasodilatation with subsequent increased blood flow and edema resulting from the inflammatory response. Tissue within this zone frequently recovers unless affected by severe sepsis or prolonged hypoperfusion.[13]

The mechanisms involved in the response to burns are rather complicated but interconnected. The initial tissue loss sets off a chain of reactive processes, beginning with activation of toxic inflammatory mediators, such as oxidants and proteases, that not only further damages tissue and capillary endothelial cells but also potentiates further tissue necrosis. Both complement and neutrophil activation results in the production of cytotoxic reactive oxygen species and histamine, which mediates progressive vascular permeability.[14] Disruption of collagen cross-linking and loss of cell membrane integrity compromises osmotic and hydrostatic pressure gradients, resulting in local edema and exacerbation of marked fluid shifts.[10] Thus burn wound progression is compounded by the presence of edema, infection, and hypoperfusion.

The burn-induced inflammatory response is not limited to the local burn wound. A massive systemic release of thromboxane A_2, along with other inflammatory mediators (bradykinin, leukotrienes, catecholamines, activated complement, and vasoactive amines) induces a significant physiologic burden on multiple organ systems, particularly the cardiopulmonary, renal, and gastrointestinal systems. Decreased plasma volume resulting from increased capillary permeability with a subsequent plasma leak into the interstitial space can lead to depressed cardiac function. As a result of low cardiac output, renal blood flow can decrease, leading to a diminished glomerular filtration rate. Activation of other stress-induced hormones and mediators, such as angiotensin, aldosterone, and vasopressin, can further compromise renal blood flow, resulting in oliguria. If not promptly recognized and treated, this condition can progress to acute tubular necrosis and renal failure, which contributes to poor outcomes in burn patients.

Burn injury can also affect remote organ systems, such as the gastrointestinal tract. Splanchnic vasoconstriction can cause transient mesenteric ischemia and a rapid onset of atrophy of the small bowel mucosa resulting from increased epithelial apoptosis and decreased epithelial proliferation. Moreover, studies have found that intestinal permeability to macromolecules increases after burns, lending an explanation to how bacterial translocation and subsequent endotoxemia ensue. Burn injury also causes a global depression of immune function. Macrophage production and cytotoxic T-lymphocyte activity are decreased, and neutrophils become impaired in terms of diapedesis, chemotaxis, and phagocytosis. Taken together, these impairments in function contribute to an increased risk for infectious complications after burns.

Acute Management

INITIAL EVALUATION

The burn patient must be immediately removed from the source of burn injury and potential life-threatening injuries quickly assessed and addressed independent of the cutaneous burns, as in the case of a multiple-trauma victim. Burning clothing articles and metal jewelry are quickly removed. Immediate cooling, such as pouring cold water on the burn wound, can minimize the depth of burn injury but must be used with extreme caution in a small TBSA burn because doing so can result in systemic hypothermia. In the case of chemical burns, victims should be promptly removed from the continued exposure to the causative chemical agent(s) and the wounds irrigated with copious amounts of water, taking caution not to spread chemical on burn wounds to adjacent uninvolved skin areas. Attempts to neutralize chemicals are contraindicated, because this process may produce additional heat and further add insult to the initial burn injury.

As with any trauma patient, burn patients are quickly assessed through primary and secondary surveys. Airway, breathing, and circulation status are assessed, and any potential life-threatening conditions should be promptly identified and managed as deemed appropriate. Respiratory symptoms, such as wheezing, tachypnea, or hoarseness, may signify an impending major airway problem. Therefore the airway should be rapidly secured with 100% oxygen support. Oxygen saturation is monitored using pulse oximetry, and chest expansion is observed to ensure adequate and equal air entry. Circumferential full-thickness burns to the chest can significantly impair respiratory function by constricting the chest wall and preventing adequate chest expansion. If necessary, escharotomy should be performed to allow for better chest expansion and subsequent ventilation. Blood pressure may be difficult to obtain in burned patients with charred extremities, and an arterial line may be necessary. One review of femoral artery catheterization in pediatric burn patients found that the complication rate was quite minimal and provided a more accurate measure of hemodynamics.[15] Nonetheless, a change in the pulse rate is a sensitive indicator for intravascular volume status, and therefore the presence of tachycardia should prompt aggressive fluid resuscitation.

The management of the burn patient depends on the depth of the injury. For superficial or first-degree burns, the treatment is focused on symptomatic relief and consists of a topical ointment containing *Aloe vera* along with a nonsteroidal anti-inflammatory agent. Superficial and deep partial thickness burns are also known as second-degree burns. The former heals spontaneously with re-epithelialization occurring within 10 to 14 days. Slight skin pigment discoloration is usually the only significant sequela. Deep partial thickness wounds, on the other hand, heal slowly over several weeks, usually with significant scarring, and generally require surgical debridement and skin grafting for a more rapid recovery and shorter hospitalization. Third-degree burns are synonymous with full-thickness injuries, and because there are no residual epidermal or dermal appendages, these burn wounds heal by re-epithelialization from the burn wound edges. As can be expected, this process is slow, requiring a prolonged hospitalization with an increased risk of burn wound infection. Fourth-degree burns, typically resulting from a profound thermal or electrical injury, involve organs beneath the layers of the skin, such as muscle and bone. The treatment for both third- and fourth-degree burns is similar in that they respond best to early debridement and grafting.

Accurate and rapid determination of burn depth is vital to the proper management of the injury. In particular, the distinction between superficial and deep dermal burns is critical because this can dictate whether the burn can be managed with or without excision and grafting. Early excision and grafting provides better results than nonoperative therapy even for so-called indeterminate burns. Because overall estimates report that clinical depth assessment is accurate in about two thirds of cases, more precise and objective methods to determine burn depth have been investigated.[16,17] One particular study examined the use of laser Doppler imaging in 48 children with burn injury and found that it could accurately predict whether a wound would need grafting or would re-epithelialize in less than 21 days.[18] A similar study reported that wounds healing within 14 days had a significantly higher perfusion on Doppler evaluation than late-healing wounds.[19] Thus laser Doppler flowmetry can be helpful in accurately predicting burn depth and wound healing capacity. Other less frequently used techniques include a punch biopsy with histologic confirmation, fluorescein fluorescence, indocyanine green video angiography, and high-frequency ultrasonography. Reflection-optical multispectral imaging and fiberoptic confocal imaging are two novel, noninvasive techniques that rely on the illumination characteristic of the tissue to determine the depth of the burn, and they may very well become the newest innovation in the field of diagnostics.[16] Ultimately, burn wound biopsy would seem to be the most precise diagnostic tool. However, this is not clinically useful, since it is invasive and can only provide static information of burn wound. It also requires an experienced pathologist to interpret histologic findings. Despite recent diagnostic advances, clinical observation still remains the standard and the most reliable method of determining the burn depth.

The size of the burn is generally assessed by the "rule of nines" in adolescents and adults. The upper extremities and head each represent 9% of the TBSA, and the lower extremities and the anterior and posterior trunks are 18% each. The perineum, genitalia, and neck each measure 1% of the TBSA. A quick rough estimate of the burn size can also be assessed by the use of the patient's palm, which represents 1% TBSA. However, the general use of this rule can be misleading in children, because of different body proportions. Children have a relatively larger portion of their body surface area (BSA) in the head and neck and a smaller surface area in the lower extremities. For instance, an infant's head constitutes 19% of TBSA compared with 9% in an adult. Thus the modified rule of nines takes into account the anthropomorphic differences of infancy and childhood, making it a more accurate assessment of pediatric burn size (Fig. 26-4). Table 26-1 also shows the chart used to estimate the percentage of TBSA burned based on age of patients and area of burns.

Full-thickness circumferential burns to the extremities produce a constricting eschar, which potentially can result in vascular compromise to the distal tissues including nerves. Accumulation of tissue edema beneath the nonelastic eschar impedes venous outflow, first resulting in a compartment syndrome and eventually affecting arterial flow. When distal pulses are absent by palpation or Doppler exam, which is not as a result of global hypoperfusion, escharotomies should be performed to avoid vascular compromise of the limb tissues. With the use of either the scalpel or electrocautery, escharotomies can be performed at bedside along the lateral and medial aspects of the involved extremities (Fig. 26-5). When the hands are involved, incisions are carried down onto the thenar and hypothenar eminences and along the dorsolateral aspects of the digits, taking care to avoid injury to the neurovascular bundle. Because burn wounds requiring escharotomies are typically full-thickness injuries, minimal bleeding is encountered. With prolonged vascular compromise, reperfusion after an escharotomy may cause reactive hyperemia and further edema formation in the muscle compartments. Ischemia-reperfusion injury also releases free oxygen radicals resulting in transient hypotension. If increased compartment pressures are noted, fasciotomy should be performed immediately to avoid permanent ischemic injuries to nerves and soft tissues.

Intravenous (IV) access should be established immediately to infuse lactated Ringer solution according to the

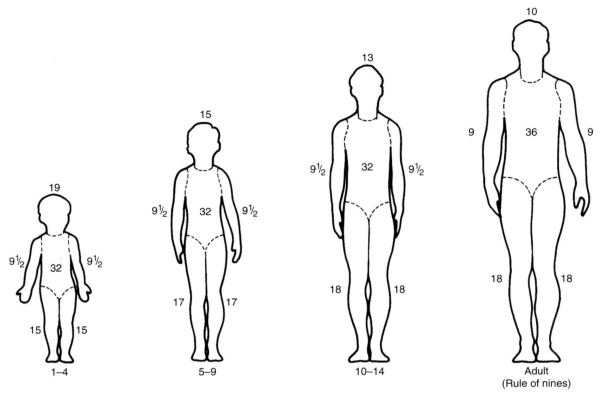

FIGURE 26-4 Modified "rule of nines" for pediatric burn patients. (Adapted from Lee J, Herndon DN: The pediatric burned patient. In Herndon DN [ed]: Total Burn Care, ed 3. Philadelphia, Saunders, 2007, p 487.)

TABLE 26-1

Burn Size Estimates Based on Area of Burn and Age Groups (Value = % Total Body Surface Area)

Area	<1 Year	1-4 Years	5-9 Years	10-14 Years	15 Years	Adult
Head	19	17	13	11	9	7
Neck	2	2	2	2	2	2
Anterior trunk	13	13	13	13	13	13
Posterior trunk	13	13	13	13	13	13
Buttock	2.5	2.5	2.5	2.5	2.5	2.5
Genitalia	1	1	1	1	1	1
Upper arm	4	4	4	4	4	4
Lower arm	3	3	3	3	3	3
Hand	2.5	2.5	2.5	2.5	2.5	2.5
Thigh	5.5	6.5	8	8.5	9	9.5
Leg	5	5	5.5	6	6.5	7
Foot	3.5	3.5	3.5	3.5	3.5	3.5

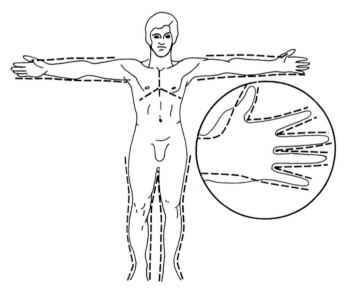

FIGURE 26-5 Escharotomies. The incisions are made on the medial and lateral aspects of the extremity. Hand escharotomies are performed on the medial and lateral digits and on the dorsum of the hand. (With permission from Eichelberger MR [ed]: Pediatric Trauma: Prevention, Acute Care, Rehabilitation, St Louis, Mosby, 1993, p 569.)

resuscitation guideline. Peripheral IV access is preferred, but femoral venous access is an ideal alternative in patients with massive burns, particularly those involving the extremities. When vascular access becomes problematic in small children with burned extremities, the intraosseous route is another alternative option in children less than 6 years of age. However, proper technique must be used to avoid potential injury to the bone growth plate. A nasogastric tube is placed in all patients with major burns in anticipation of a gastric ileus and potential vomiting. In addition, almost immediate implementation

of enteral nutrition by either a gastric or transpyloric feeding tube can mitigate burn-induced small bowel ileus. A urinary catheter should likewise be inserted to accurately monitor urine output as a measure of end-organ perfusion. Initial laboratory tests should include complete blood count, type and

TABLE 26-2

Calculation Formulas for Body Surface Area

Dubois formula	BSA (m^2) = height (cm)$^{0.725}$ × weight (kg)$^{0.425}$ × 0.007184
Jacobson formula	BSA (m^2) = [height (cm) + weight (kg) − 60]/100

BSA, body surface area.

crossmatch for packed red blood cell, chemistry, urinalysis, coagulation profile, and chest radiograph. If inhalation injury is suspected, arterial blood gas with carboxyhemoglobin level should also be determined to guide respiratory therapy.

FLUID RESUSCITATION

Appropriate fluid resuscitation should begin promptly upon securing IV access. Peripheral IV access is sufficient in the majority of small to moderate size burns. Saphenous vein cut-downs are useful in cases of difficult access in larger patients. In children, percutaneous femoral central venous access may be easier and more reliable when confronted with a difficult peripheral IV access situation. Many guidelines exist regarding fluid resuscitation, with the administration of varying concentrations of colloid and crystalloid solutions.[20] The Parkland formula (4 mL of lactated Ringer solution per kg of body weight per percentage of TBSA burned) is most widely used, but children's fluid resuscitation guideline should be based on BSA. Children have a greater BSA in relation to weight, and as a result, weight-based formulas can under-resuscitate children with minor burns and may grossly over-resuscitate with extensive burns. Nonetheless, fluid loss is also proportionally greater in children, and consequently, they may require more fluid per kilogram. TBSA can be assessed using standard nomograms based on height and weight or calculated using formulas (Table 26-2). The Galveston formula (Shriners Hospital for Children) uses 5000 mL/m^2 BSA burn plus 2000 mL/m^2 BSA of lactated Ringer solution given during the first 24 hours after burn, with half the volume administered during the first 8 hours and the remaining half during the following 16 hours (Table 26-3).

Regardless of which guidelines are used, the primary goal of fluid resuscitation is to achieve adequate organ tissue perfusion. Fluid administration should be titrated to maintain a urine output of greater than 1 mL/kg/hr. Approximately 50% of administered fluid is sequestered in nonburned tissues in 50% TBSA burns because of increased capillary permeability that occurs particularly in the first 6 to 8 hours after injury. During this period, large molecules leak into the interstitial space to increase extravascular colloid osmotic pressure. Therefore to maintain intravascular osmotic pressure, albumin is added 12 hours after the injury. Closely mirroring a similar study in adults, one retrospective study of fluid resuscitation in pediatric burn patients noted that patients requiring albumin supplementation took significantly longer to resuscitate (30.5 vs. 22.0 hr) and received significantly more fluid than patients receiving crystalloid only (9.7 vs. 6.2 mL/kg/%TBSA). Although their outcomes were the same, the nature of their injuries was more significant, however, given the greater percentage TBSA full-thickness burn and presence of inhalation injury.[21] After the first 24 hours, 3750 mL/m^2 BSA burned is given to replace evaporative fluid loss plus

TABLE 26-3

Acute Burn Fluid Resuscitation Guidelines

Formula	First 24 Hours	Thereafter
Parkland	Lactated Ringer solution; 4 mL/kg/% TBSA burn: 50% total volume during the first 8 hr after injury and the remaining during the subsequent 16 hr	5% dextrose with Na$^+$, K$^+$ and albumin to maintain normal serum electrolytes and colloid oncotic pressure
Brooke	Lactated Ringer solution (with colloid 0.5 mL/kg/% TBSA burn); 2 mL/kg/% TBSA burn; 50% total volume during the first 8 hr after injury and the remaining during the subsequent 16 hr	Titrate to maintain urine output 0.5-1.0 mL/kg/hr
Shriners-Galveston	Lactated Ringer solution (12.5 g albumin/L added 12 hr after injury); 5000 mL/m^2 BSA burn + 2000 mL/m^2 TBSA; 50% total volume during the first 8 hr after injury and the remaining during the subsequent 16 hr	3750 mL/m^2 BSA burn + 1500 mL/m^2 TBSA; substitute IV fluid volume with enteral formula

IV, intravenous; TBSA, total body surface area.

1500 mL/m^2 BSA per 24 hours for maintenance requirement (Galveston formula). Dextrose containing solution, such as 5% dextrose with {1/4} to {1/2} normal saline is used as the primary solution. Children less than 2 years of age are susceptible to hypoglycemia because of limited glycogen stores, and therefore lactated Ringer solution with 5% dextrose is usually given during the first 24 hours after burns.

Over-resuscitation during the first 24 hours postburn has been shown to be associated with an increased incidence of pneumonia, bloodstream infection, acute respiratory distress syndrome, multiple-organ failure, and death. "Permissive hypovolemia" during burn fluid resuscitation has been shown to improve multiple-organ dysfunction, further suggesting that this is a safe and beneficial approach during the acute burn resuscitation. One recent study reiterated the findings of a prospective clinical study, which reported that the use of high-dose ascorbic acid is associated with a decrease in fluid requirements and an increase in urine output during resuscitation after thermal injury without an increased risk of renal failure.[22] Some interest lies in the use of hypertonic saline as a resuscitative fluid in burn-induced shock and has been shown to be beneficial in treating burn-induced shock.[23] It theoretically should maintain intravascular volume more effectively by removing fluid from the interstitial space by osmosis, resulting in a decrease in generalized tissue edema. However, it is not widely used because of its potential risk for hypernatremia, hyperosmolarity, renal failure, and alkalosis. Importantly, no prospective randomized controlled studies have yet to confirm these end points.[24] Some favor the use of a modified hypertonic solution by adding one ampule of sodium bicarbonate to each liter of lactated Ringer solution during the first 24 hours of resuscitation.

Children often do not exhibit clinical signs of hypovolemia until more than 25% of the circulating volume is depleted and complete cardiovascular collapse is imminent. Thus

American Burn Association Criteria for Major Burn Injury

Second- and third-degree burns > 10% TBSA in patients < 10 or > 50 years of age

Second- and third-degree burns > 20% TBSA in other age group

Third-degree burns > 5% TBSA in any age group

Burns involving the face, hands, feet, genitalia, perineum, and skin overlying major joints

Significant chemical burns

Significant electrical burns including lightning injury

Inhalation injury

Burns with significant concomitant trauma

Burns with significant preexisting medical disorders

Burn injury in patients requiring special social, emotional, and rehabilitative support (including suspected child abuse and neglect)

symptoms of hypovolemia, such as hypotension and oliguria, can be late signs of shock in such children. Tachycardia typically indicates an early sign of hypovolemia, but caution should be used not to overinterpret, because reflex tachycardia caused by postinjury catecholamine response is also common. A lethargic child with decreased capillary refill and cool, clammy extremities requires prompt attention. Measurement of arterial blood pH and base deficit values can also reflect adequacy of fluid resuscitation. Hyponatremia is also a frequent complication in pediatric burn patients after aggressive fluid resuscitation. Although rare, a serious complication, such as central pontine myelinolysis, can occur with rapid correction of hypernatremia.[25] Frequent monitoring of serum chemistry with appropriate correction is required to avoid severe electrolyte imbalance.

After initial first aid and start of appropriate fluid resuscitation, it must be determined whether a burn victim should be transferred to a tertiary burn center. Burn units with experienced multidisciplinary team members are best prepared and experienced to handle major burn patients. In addition to physicians and nurses, respiratory and rehabilitation therapists also play critical roles in the management of acute burn patients. As defined by the American Burn Association, any patients who sustain *major burn injury* should be transferred appropriately to a nearby burn center for further care (Table 26-4).

INHALATION INJURY

Inhalation injury remains the major contributor to mortality in burn patients. The mortality rate of children with isolated cutaneous burns is 1% to 2%, but this can significantly increase to 16% in the presence of inhalation injury.[26] The initial assessment of patients with combined thermal and other traumatic injuries should, as always, center on airway, breathing, and circulation per advanced trauma life support (ATLS) guidelines. The treatment of inhalation injury begins at the scene of the burn accident. The administration of 100% oxygen rapidly decreases the half-life of carbon monoxide. If the respiratory distress is significant, intubation or a surgical airway may be required. Although hypoxemia is usually evident, the initial chest radiograph and arterial blood gas may be normal, but the inhalational injury can evolve for hours.

The diagnosis of an inhalation injury is usually made on the clinical history and physical findings at the initial evaluation. For instance, victims trapped in a house fire with excessive smoke and fumes are likely to have sustained a severe inhalation injury. Common signs include cough, stridor, singed nasal hair, carbonaceous sputum, and a hyperemic oropharynx. Although the immediate injury results in hyperemia, ulceration, and edema, these symptoms may not be obvious until the airway becomes significantly obstructed, in which case the time lapse can exceed 18 hours. Hoarseness and stridor should alert the surgeon to significant airway obstruction, and the airway should immediately be secured with endotracheal intubation. Patients who present with disorientation and obtundation are likely to have an elevated carbon monoxide level (carboxyhemoglobin > 10%). Cyanide toxicity as a result of the combustion of common household items may also contribute to unexplained metabolic collapse. Fiberoptic bronchoscopy remains the gold standard test to confirm a diagnosis of an inhalation injury by demonstrating inflammatory changes in the tracheal mucosa, such as edema, hyperemia, mucosal ulceration, and sloughing. A ventilation/perfusion scan can also identify regions of inhalation injury by assessing respiratory exchange and excretion of xenon gas by the lungs.[27] Together, these complementary diagnostic tools are more than 90% accurate in the diagnosis of inhalation injury.

Smoke inhalation injury can be divided into three different types of injury: thermal (usually restricted to the upper airway), chemical irritation of the respiratory tract, and systemic toxicity resulting from inhalation of fumes, gases, and mists. Although the supraglottic region can be injured by both thermal and chemical insults because of highly efficient heat exchange, tracheobronchial and lung parenchymal injuries rarely occur as a result of direct thermal damage, because the heat disperses so rapidly in the larynx. The heat destroys the epithelial layer, denatures proteins, and activates the complement cascade, leading to the release of histamine and the formation of xanthine oxidase to release reactive oxygen species (ROS) such as superoxide. At the same time, nitric oxide (NO) and reactive nitrogen species (RNS) formation by endothelial cells is propagated by histamine stimulation. Both ROS and RNS cause increased permeability to proteins, resulting in edema formation. In addition, interleukin-8 (IL-8) is also released after injury, leading to the recruitment of polymorphonuclear cells, which further amplify the inflammatory process.[28] Using an ovine model with combined thermal and inhalation injuries, one group found that infusion of 7-nitroindazole, a selective neuronal nitric oxide synthase inhibitor, blocks the inflammatory cascade, as demonstrated by a 40% and 30% respective decrease in IL-8 and myeloperoxidase activity in lung tissue concentrations compared with the injured control group. The treated group also saw a reduction in bronchial injury, peak pulmonary pressures, and shunting.[29] Thus 7-nitroindazole may represent an effective therapy in the management of inhalation injuries.

Hypoxia, increased airway resistance, decreased pulmonary compliance, increased alveolar epithelial permeability, and increased pulmonary vascular resistance may be triggered by the release of vasoactive substances (thromboxanes A_2, C_{3a}, and C_{5a}) from the damaged epithelium.[30] Neutrophil activation plays a critical role in this process, whereby pulmonary function has been shown to improve with the use of a ligand binding to E-selectins (inhibiting neutrophil adhesion) and anti–IL-8 (inhibiting neutrophil chemotaxis). Sloughing of the respiratory cilia impairs the physiologic cleaning process of the airway, resulting in an increased risk of bacterial infections and pneumonia. This may be further complicated by increased bronchial secretions and mucous plugging, which may predispose to distal airway obstruction and atelectasis, thereby impairing pulmonary gas exchange. These exudates, consisting of lymph proteins, coalesce to form fibrin casts that can create a "ball-valve" effect in localized areas of lung, eventually causing barotrauma.

To reduce respiratory complications such as pneumonia, protocols have been instituted in an effort to improve the clearance of tracheobronchial secretions and decrease bronchospasm (Table 26-5). Aggressive pulmonary toilet with physiotherapy and frequent suctioning is an important adjunct. The patient is frequently turned side to side along with chest physiotherapy every 2 hours. In the critically ill patient, high-frequency percussive ventilation has been shown to reduce development of pneumonia through clearance of bronchial secretions. When physiologically stable, the patient is transferred out of bed to a chair, with progressive ambulation to prevent compressive atelectasis. Humidified air is delivered at high flow, while bronchodilators and racemic epinephrine are used to treat bronchospasm. The use of nebulized heparin has been shown to reduce tracheobronchial cast formation, improve minute ventilation, and lower peak inspiratory pressures after smoke inhalation. Inhalation treatments, such as 20% acetylcysteine nebulized solution (3 mL q4h) plus nebulized heparin (5,000 to 10,000 units with 3 mL normal saline q4h), are effective in improving the clearance of tracheobronchial secretion and minimizing bronchospasm, thereby significantly improving reintubation rates and decreasing mortality.[31,32]

The presence of inhalation injury generally requires an increased amount of fluid resuscitation, up to 2 mL/kg/% TBSA burn more than would be required for an equal-size burn without an inhalation injury. In fact, pulmonary edema that is associated with inhalation injury is not prevented by fluid restriction, but rather, inadequate resuscitation may increase the severity of pulmonary injury by sequestration of polymorphonuclear cells.[33] Corticosteroids have not been shown to be of any benefit in inhalation injury. Prophylactic IV antibiotics are not indicated unless there is clinical suspicion of pneumonia. Early pneumonia is usually the result of gram-positive organisms, such as methicillin-resistant *Staphylococcus aureus*, whereas gram-negative organisms, such as *Pseudomonas* and *Acinetobacter,* are responsible for later-onset infection. Antibiotic therapy should be guided by sensitivities and susceptibilities of serial cultures from sputum, tracheal aspirates, or bronchoalveolar lavages.

TABLE 26-5

Inhalation Injury Treatment Protocol

Treatment	Interval and Dosages
Suction and lavage	q2h
Bronchodilators (Albuterol)	q2h
Nebulized heparin	5000-10,000 units with 3 mL NS q4h
Nebulized acetylcysteine	20%, 3 mL q4h
Hypertonic saline	Induce effective coughing
Racemic epinephrine	Reduce mucosal edema

NS, normal saline.

Burn Wound Care

The proper wound care is generally dictated by the accurate assessment of the burn depth and size. First-degree burns require no particular dressing, but the involved areas should be kept out of direct sunlight. They are generally treated with topical ointments for symptomatic pain relief. Superficial second-degree burns are treated with daily dressing changes with topical antimicrobial agents. They can also be treated with application of petroleum gauze or a synthetic dressing to allow for rapid re-epithelialization. Deep second- and third-degree burn wounds eventually require excision of the eschar with skin grafting. Table 26-6 describes various available antimicrobial, synthetic, and biologic dressing products for burn wound care.

TOPICAL ANTIMICROBIALS

Various topical antimicrobial agents have been used for management of burn wounds. None of these agents effectively prevent colonization of organisms that are commonly harbored in the eschar, but instead promote bacteriostasis to limit bacterial burden to less than 10^2 to 10^5 colonies/g of tissue. Routine punch quantitative wound biopsy of burned areas can alert to impending burn wound sepsis and risk of failure of skin graft from infection. The National Burn Repository estimates that 4.4% of deaths after burn injury are attributable to burn wound sepsis. With evidence of multidrug-resistant organisms (MDROs), one study evaluated 47 MDROs and 27 non-MDRO controls versus 11 different topical agents, in which the topical agents were effective against 88% of the non-MDROs but only 80% of MDROs. Mafenide acetate, silver sulfadiazine, and silver nitrate were effective against both gram-negative and gram-positive bacteria, regardless of drug resistance status. Nonetheless, the results reinforce the concern that bacteria are becoming more resistant to antimicrobial regimens.[34]

Silver sulfadiazine (Silvadene; Monarch Pharmaceuticals, Bristol, Tenn.) is the most commonly used topical agent for burn wound dressings. Although it does not penetrate eschar, Silvadene has a broad spectrum of efficacy and mitigates the pain associated with second-degree burns. However, it frequently adheres to the wound surface, thereby traumatizing newly generated epithelial surfaces and delaying healing. Silvadene on fine mesh gauze can be used separately or in combination with other antimicrobial agents, such as nystatin. The combination of Silvadene with nystatin has significantly reduced the incidence of *Candida* infection in burned patients.[35] The most common side effect of Silvadene is leukopenia, which is likely related to margination of white blood cells and is only transient.[36] However, when the leukocyte count falls below 3000 cells/mm^3, changing to another topical antimicrobial agent is warranted.

Mafenide acetate (Sulfamylon; UDC Laboratories, Rockford, Ill.) is more effective in penetrating eschar, and therefore is frequently used in third-degree burns. Fine mesh gauze impregnated with Sulfamylon (10% water-soluble cream) is applied directly onto the burn wound. Sulfamylon has a much broader spectrum of antimicrobial efficacy, including against *Pseudomonas* and *Enterococcus*. It is also available in 5% solution to soak burn wounds, eliminating a need to perform

TABLE 26-6
Burn Wound Dressings

Dressings	Advantages	Disadvantages
Antimicrobial Salves		
Silver sulfadiazine (Silvadene)	Painless; broad spectrum; rare sensitivity	Leukopenia; some gram-negative resistance; does not penetrate eschar; inhibition of epithelialization
Mafenide acetate (Sulfamylon)	Broad-spectrum; penetrates eschar; effective against *Pseudomonas*	Painful; metabolic acidosis (carbonic anhydrase inhibitor); inhibition of epithelialization
Bacitracin/neomycin/polymyxin B	Ease of application, painless, useful on face	Limited antimicrobial property
Nystatin	Effective in inhibiting fungal growth; use in combination with Silvadene, Bacitracin	Cannot use in combination with mafenide acetate
Mupirocin (Bactroban)	Effective against *Staphylococcus,* including MRSA	Cost; poor eschar penetration
Antimicrobial Soaks		
0.5% Silver nitrate	Painless; broad-spectrum; rare sensitivity	No eschar penetration; discolor contacted areas; electrolyte imbalance; methemoglobinemia
Povidone-iodine	Broad-spectrum antimicrobial	Painful; potential systemic absorption; hypersensitivity
5% Mafenide acetate	Broad-spectrum antimicrobial	Painful; no fungal coverage; metabolic acidosis
0.025% Sodium hypochlorite (Dakin solution)	Effective against most organisms	Mildly inhibits epithelialization
0.25% Acetic acid	Effective against most organisms	Mildly inhibits epithelialization
Silver-Impregnated		
Aquacel, Acticoat	Broad-spectrum antimicrobial; no dressing changes	Cost
Synthetic Dressings		
Biobrane	Provides wound barrier; minimizes pain; useful for outpatient burns, hands (gloves)	Exudate accumulation risks invasive wound infection; no antimicrobial property
Opsite, Tegaderm	Provides moisture barrier; minimizes pain; useful for outpatient burns; inexpensive	Exudate accumulation risks invasive wound infection; no antimicrobial property
Transcyte	Provides wound barrier; accelerates wound healing	Exudate accumulation risks invasive wound infection; no antimicrobial property
Integra, Alloderm	Complete wound closure, including dermal substitute	No antimicrobial property; expensive; requires training, experience
Biologic Dressings		
Allograft (cadaver skin), Xenograft (pig skin)	Temporary biologic dressings	Requires access to skin bank; cost
Amniotic membrane	Minimizes dressing changes	Minimal experience; not widely used

frequent dressing changes. Sulfamylon is a potent carbonic anhydrase inhibitor and can therefore cause metabolic acidosis. This side effect can usually be avoided by limiting its use to only 20% TBSA at any given time and rotating application sites every several hours with another topical antimicrobial agent. In addition, the application of Sulfamylon can be painful, which limits its practical use in an outpatient setting, especially with children.

Other agents, such as 0.5% silver nitrate and 0.025% sodium hypochlorite (Dakin solution), are also available as soak solutions. These soak solutions are generally poured onto gauze dressings, which minimizes dressing changes and the potential loss of grafts or healing keratinocytes. Silver nitrate is painless on application and has broad coverage, but its side effects include electrolyte imbalance (hyponatremia, hypochloremia) and dark gray or black stains. Dakin (0.025%) solution is effective against most microbes, including *Pseudomonas*. However, it requires frequent dosing because of inactivation of hypochlorite when coming in contact with protein and can also retard healing cells.[37] Petroleum-based antimicrobial ointments, such polymyxin B, bacitracin, and polysporin, are painless and transparent, allowing easier monitoring of applied burn wounds. These agents are mostly only effective against gram-positive organisms, and their use is limited to facial burns, small areas of partial-thickness burns, and healing donor sites. As with Silvadene, petroleum-based agents can also be used in combination with nystatin to suppress skin *Candida* colonization.

Commercially available dressings containing biologically active silver ions (Aquacel, ConvaTec, Skillman, NJ; Acticoat, Smith & Nephew, Auckland, NZ) hold promise for retaining the effectiveness of silver nitrate but without its side effects. Allowing it to adhere to the wound within 24 hours, the hydrocolloid properties of the Aquacel dressing make it absorbent and non-traumatic to the delicate tissues of the healing wound. Since it can be left without dressing changes for up to 2 weeks, it may be useful in the outpatient management of a burn injury. Similarly, Acticoat has been shown to have improved bacterial clearance, which is related to a sustained release of silver that allows for less frequent dressing changes.[38]

BURN WOUND DRESSINGS

Superficial second-degree burns can be managed using various methods. A topical antimicrobial dressing using Silvadene is most commonly used, but synthetic dressings, such as Biobrane (UDL Laboratories, Rockford, Ill.) and Opsite (Smith & Nephew), offer unique advantages of eliminating frequent painful dressing changes and potential tissue fluid loss. The general principle of these synthetic products is to provide sterile coverage of superficial partial-thickness burn wounds to allow rapid spontaneous re-epithelialization of the involved areas. Biobrane is a bilaminate thin membrane composed of thin semipermeable silicone bonded to a layer of nylon fabric mesh that is coated with a monomolecular layer of type I collagen of porcine origin. This dressing provides a hydrophilic coating for fibrin ingrowth that promotes wound adherence. Its porosity allows for drainage of exudates while remaining permeable to topical antibiotics, and it simultaneously acts as a barrier to the ingress of bacteria and evaporation to prevent dessication.[39] It is supplied in simple sheets or preshaped gloves (Fig. 26-6). After it is placed onto clean fresh superficial second-degree burn wounds using Steri-strips and bandages, the Biobrane dressing dries up and becomes well adhered to burn wounds within 24 to 48 hours. Once adherent, the covered areas are kept open to air and examined closely for the first few days to detect any signs and symptoms of infection. As the epithelialization occurs beneath the Biobrane sheet, it is easily peeled off the wound. When serous fluid accumulates beneath the Biobrane, a sterile needle aspiration can preserve its use. However, once foul-smelling exudate is detected, it should be removed and topical antimicrobial dressings applied. When used as directed, Biobrane has been found to reduce pain levels, fluid loss, healing time, instances of hypothermia, and hospital stay when compared with traditional dressings.[39,40]

Alternatively, Opsite or Tegaderm (3M Pharmaceuticals, St. Paul, Minn.) can also be used to cover superficial partial-thickness burns. Commonly used as postoperative dressings, it is easy to apply and provides an impervious barrier to the environment. It is also relatively inexpensive, and its transparent nature allows for easier monitoring of burn wounds. Despite lacking any special biologic factors (i.e., collagen, growth factors) to enhance wound healing, it promotes spontaneous re-epithelialization process. Biobrane and Opsite are preferred to topical antimicrobial dressings when dealing with small superficial second-degree burn wounds, especially in the outpatient settings to alleviate pain associated with dressing changes. TransCyte (Advanced BioHealing, Westport, Conn.), composed of human fibroblasts that are then cultured on the nylon mesh of Biobrane, is also an alternative option.

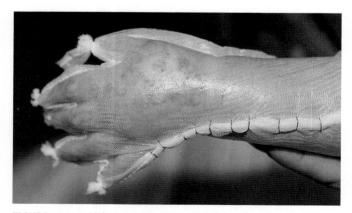

FIGURE 26-6 Biobrane glove for superficial second-degree burn. Biobrane is an ideal synthetic wound coverage for superficial second-degree burns, promoting rapid re-epithelialization without painful dressing changes.

Synthetic and biologic dressings are also available to provide coverage for full-thickness burn wounds. Integra (Integra LifeSciences, Plainsboro, NJ) consists of an inner layer made of a porous matrix of bovine collagen and the glycosaminoglycan chrondroitin-6-sulfate, which facilitates fibrovascular growth. The outer layer is composed of polysiloxane polymer with vapor transmission characteristics similar to normal epithelium. In the treatment of full-thickness burn wounds, Integra serves as a matrix for the infiltration of fibroblasts, macrophages, lymphocytes, and capillaries derived from the wound bed, and it promotes rapid neodermis formation. After the collagen matrix engrafts into the wound in approximately 2 weeks, the outer silicone layer is replaced with epidermal autografts. Epidermal donor sites heal rapidly without significant morbidity.

Although synthetic dermal substitutes have a tremendous potential for minimizing scar contractures with improvement in cosmetic and functional outcome, they are also susceptible to wound infection and must be monitored carefully. The use of Integra for children with large TBSA burns was evaluated for short- and long-term follow-up.[41] Burned children treated with Integra demonstrated significantly decreased resting energy expenditure as well as increased bone mineral content and density, along with improved scarring at 24 months after burn injury, thus validating the use of this dermal substitute in the management of pediatric burned patients.[41] Moreover, some advocate that Integra can be successfully used in extensive postburn scar revisions in younger patients.[42] Recently, the use of Integra with negative-pressure therapy and a vacuum-assisted closure system has been shown to shorten the time between the application of Integra and skin grafting by fixing the dermal substitute to the wound bed and promoting neovascularization.[43] In addition, this method simplifies wound care, evacuates fluid, and provides a sterile covering.

Biologic dressings, such as xenografts from swine and allografts from cadaver donors, can also be used to cover full-thickness burn wounds as a temporary dressing. Alloderm (LifeCell, Branchburg, NJ) is a dermal substitute procured from decellularized cadaveric dermis. This synthetic dermal substitute also has a potential for minimizing scar contractures, particularly at joints, and improving cosmesis and functional outcomes. Particularly useful when dealing with large TBSA burns, biologic dressings can provide the immunologic and barrier functions of normal skin. The areas of xenograft and allograft are eventually rejected by the immune system and sloughed off, leaving healthy recipient beds for subsequent autografts. Although extremely rare, the transmission of viral diseases from the allograft is of potential concern.

Finally, human amnion has been used as a dressing for burns, because it not particularly antigenic. It contains substantial amounts of many growth factors that stimulate epithelial proliferation, but it also minimizes evaporative fluid losses and reduces bacterial counts in the burn wound.[44] Several preservation methods are currently described, including cryopreservation, glycerol preservation, lyophilization, and γ-irradiation. Its use has been limited to dressing partial-thickness burns in specialized areas such as the face. One study compared the use of amnion and traditional topical treatment in pediatric patients with facial burns. Although patients in the amnion group had significantly fewer dressing changes, the overall time to healing, length of stay, and hypertrophic scarring were not different between the two treatment groups. Importantly, the use of amnion was not associated with an increased risk of infection, which suggested that it is a safe alternative dressing for superficial partial-thickness burns.[45]

EXCISION AND GRAFTING

Early excision with skin grafting has been shown to decrease operative blood loss, length of hospital stay and ultimately improve overall survival of burn patients.[46,47] Similar to earlier clinical reports in patients, two separate murine studies found that early excision of full-thickness burns can reduce proinflammatory cytokines, such as IL-6 and tumor necrosis factor-α (TNF-α), in rats with 30% TBSA burn injuries, allowing for abrogation of the systemic inflammatory response.[48,49] Adequate surgical debridement does rely on experience and judgment to determine which tissues are devitalized and should be excised as opposed to those that are still viable. Moreover, aggressive debridement can result in poor functional and cosmetic results, whereas inadequate debridement will often result in infection and poor healing. One group has recommended intraoperative staining of the burn wound with methylene blue to demarcate normal epithelium from granulation tissue and eschar, which can aid in excision. There were no reports of adverse reactions, alterations in skin graft take, or wound healing problems with topical application of methylene blue, though no objective measures of these findings were provided.[50]

Excision and grafting may be staged, with the goal of removing all eschar as early as possible, to not only blunt the inflammatory cascade but also to prevent wound colonization. However, since burn depth from scald burns is more difficult to assess, a more conservative approach is taken with delayed excision. Typically, tangential excision of the full-thickness burn wound is performed 1 to 3 days after burn injury, when relative hemodynamic stability has been achieved. The eschar is sequentially shaved off using a powered dermatome (Zimmer) and/or knife blades (Watson, Weck) until a viable tissue plane is achieved, which is usually characterized by punctate bleeding (Fig. 26-7). Particularly in burns greater than 30% TBSA, early excision of the eschar (usually < 24 hours after

burns) generally decreases operative blood loss resulting from vasoconstrictive substances, such as thromboxane and catecholamines, in the burn wounds. Once the burn wounds become hyperemic 48 hours after burns, bleeding at the time of excision of the eschar can be excessive. Tourniquet and subcutaneous injections of an epinephrine-containing solution can lessen the blood loss, but these techniques can potentially hinder the surgeon's ability to differentiate viable from nonviable tissues. Topical hemostatic agents, such as thrombin, can also be used, but they are expensive and not very effective in preventing excessive bleeding from open wounds. In patients with deep full-thickness burns, electrocautery is useful to rapidly excise eschar with minimal blood loss. The use of Versajet hydrosurgery (Smith & Nephew), which utilizes a high-powered stream of sterile saline for tissue excision, is becoming increasingly popular. Because it is capable of small-scale incremental debridement, the Versajet preserves more dermis than traditional tangential excision techniques and allows for more precise contouring. It has been shown to reduce bleeding and healing times, with improved adherence of biologic dressings.[51] It has the advantage of dermal preservation, which is necessary to minimize hypertrophic scarring and contracture formation, and a significant reduction in bleeding associated with traditional excision. It has been suggested that large TBSA pediatric burn patients receiving blood products have increased morbidity because of being immunocompromised and succumbing to subsequent infections.[52] Thus limiting blood loss and transfusions are critical.

Ideally, the excised burn wound is covered with autograft from donor sites, such as the upper leg, back, or abdomen. For burns less than 20% to 30% TBSA, debrided wounds can be covered at one operation with split-thickness autografts if the wound bed is amenable. It is preferable to use sheets of autografts for better long-term aesthetic outcome, but narrowly meshed autografts (1:1 or 2:1) have the advantage of allowing better drainage of fluid at the grafted sites. However, this also means that they require larger donor areas than more widely meshed grafts. With massive burns, the closure of burn wounds is achieved by a combination of widely meshed autografts (4:1 to 6:1) with an allograft (2:1) overlay (Fig. 26-8). Alternatively, it may be necessary to use only temporary biologic dressings, cadaveric allograft, or a dermal replacement until autologous donor sites are available. Once split-thickness autografts are harvested, the donor sites are dressed with a petroleum-based gauze, such as Xeroform or Scarlet-red (Covidien, Mansfield, Mass.). OpSite can be used to cover donor sites. Repeat grafting is required for large burns, with sequential harvesting of split-thickness autograft from limited

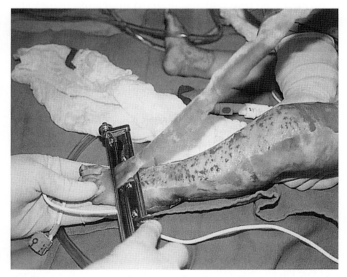

FIGURE 26-7 Tangential excision of eschar. Eschar is excised to the depth of viable, bleeding tissue plane. (With permission from Herndon DN [ed]: Total Burn Care, ed 2. Philadelphia, WB Saunders, 2002, plate 2.) *(See Expert Consult site for color version.)*

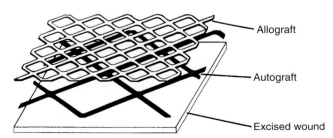

FIGURE 26-8 Schematic diagram of wound covering with 4:1 meshed autograft with 2:1 meshed allograft overlay. (With permission from Eichelberger MR [ed]: Pediatric Trauma: Prevention, Acute Care, Rehabilitation, St Louis, Mosby, 1993, p 581.)

donor sites, until the entire burn wound is covered. As meshed autografts heal, the allografts slough. However, the formation of significant scar remains the major disadvantage of this technique. Therefore the use of widely meshed graft is avoided on the face and hands. Full-thickness grafts that include both dermal and epidermal components provide the best outcome for wound coverage, with less contractures and better pigment match. However, its use is generally limited to small areas because of the lack of abundant full-thickness donor skin.

The limitation of donor sites in patients with burns over massive areas is partially addressed with the use of recombinant human growth hormone (rHGH). Administration of rHGH has resulted in accelerated donor-site healing, allowing more frequent donor-site harvest in a given period of time.[53] The use of rHGH decreased donor-site healing time by an average of 2 days, which ultimately shortened the overall length of hospitalization from 0.8 to 0.54 days per percentage of TBSA burned.[53] These effects from rHGH are thought to result from stimulation of insulin-like growth factor (IGF)-1 release and induction of IGF-1 receptors in the burn wound.[54] Given alone, insulin has been shown to decrease donor-site wound protein synthesis, accelerating healing time from 6.5 to 4.7 days.[55] The decrease in donor-site healing by 1 day between each harvest can significantly impact overall length of hospital stay in patients with massive burns who require multiple grafting procedures. The administration of rHGH in burned children was associated with a 23% reduction in total cost of hospital care for a typical 80% TBSA burn.[53]

The use of cultured keratinocytes from the patient's own skin has continued to generate considerable interest as a potential solution for massively burned patients with limited donor sites. Cultured epithelial autografts (CEA) can theoretically be used to provide complete coverage, but it is wrought with problems in its practical application. Although cultured keratinocytes grow slowly, they are particularly fragile and very susceptible to shear trauma. In noncritically ill patients who are otherwise not sedated, strict bedrest may be necessary to prevent loss of the graft, which consequently delays mobilization and rehabilitation. Thus the successful take rate of CEAs is only 50% to 70%. In one burn center's experience, they recommended CEA in the following subpopulation: large full-thickness burns (>50% TBSA), moderate burns (30% to 50% TBSA) with limited donor-site availability, and burns in which the donor site presents a significant functional or cosmetic issue. They also noted an estimated graft take rate of 72.7% at discharge, but that children had a higher contracture rate than their adult counterparts (90% vs. 57%).[56] It has been reported that there is a significantly longer hospitalization with these grafts in patients with burns of more than 80% TBSA. However, this technology continues to hold promise in treating massive burns.

Hypermetabolic Response

Burn patients demonstrate dramatic increases in metabolic rate. The hypermetabolic response, which is generally greater with increasing burn size, reaches a plateau at 40% in a TBSA burn.[57] The hypermetabolic response to burn injury is characterized by catabolic metabolism, hyperdynamic circulation, insulin resistance, delayed wound healing, and increased risk of infection.[58] These physiologic changes of increased energy expenditure, oxygen consumption, proteolysis, lipolysis, and nitrogen losses are induced by up-regulation of catabolic agents, such as cortisol, catecholamine, and glucagons, which act synergistically to increase the production of glucose, a principal fuel during acute inflammation. Cortisol stimulates gluconeogenesis, proteolysis, and sensitizes adipocytes to lipolytic hormones. Catecholamines stimulate the rate of glucose production through hepatic gluconeogenesis and glycogenolysis, as well as promoting lipolysis and peripheral insulin resistance. Thus serum insulin levels are elevated, but the cells themselves become insulin resistant.[59] The increase in glucagon, which is stimulated by catecholamines, further promotes gluconeogenesis. Recent trials have demonstrated that intensive insulin therapy aimed at maintaining a daily average glucose of 140 mg/dL improves postburn outcomes.[60,61] Patients with intensive insulin treatment have demonstrated improved immune function and decreased sepsis, along with an attenuation of the inflammatory and acute phase response. As such, tight glucose control is thought to be critical in improving the overall recovery of burn patients.

Significant protein catabolism occurs in severe burns. Cortisol is catabolic and is partially responsible for the loss of tissue protein and negative nitrogen balance. In addition, burn injury is associated with decreased levels of anabolic hormones, such as growth hormone and IGF-1, which contribute significantly to net protein loss. The synthesis of protein (essential for the production of collagen for wound healing) and antibodies and leukocytes participating in the immune response, requires a net positive nitrogen balance. Excess catecholamines in postburn patients also contribute to persistent tachycardia and lipolysis. The consequences of these physiologic insults are cardiac failure and fatty infiltration of the liver. The use of a beta blocker, propranolol, has been shown to lower resting heart rate and left ventricular work and decrease peripheral lipolysis without adversely affecting cardiac output or the ability to respond to cold stress.[62,63] Propranolol also increases lean body mass and decreases skeletal muscle wasting. Herndon and colleagues[57] demonstrated that beta blockade using propranolol during hospitalization attenuated hypermetabolic response and reversed muscle-protein catabolism in burned children. Propranolol was given at a standard starting dose (1.98 mg/kg/day) and then titrated to achieve a decrease in the heart rate of approximately 20% from a baseline values. At 2 weeks of treatment, resting energy expenditure and oxygen consumption had increased in the control group. In contrast, patients in the propranolol group had significant decreases in these variables. Concurrent with the decline in energy expenditure, beta blockade also improved the kinetics of skeletal-muscle protein. The muscle protein net balance improved by 82% compared with pretreatment baseline values, whereas it decreased only by 27% in untreated controls.[57] Furthermore, the administration of propranolol to burned children receiving simultaneous human growth hormone has salutary cardiovascular effects, a decrease in the recent release of free fatty acids from adipose tissue, and an increase in efficiency of the liver's handling of secreted free fatty acids and very-low-density lipoproteins. Administration of propranolol has been shown to decrease peripheral lipolysis and fat deposition in the liver of burn patients.[57] A recent report also suggested that administration of propranolol (4 mg/kg/q24h) markedly decreases the amount of insulin necessary to decrease elevated glucose level postburn.[64] The mechanism by which propranolol exerts its effects is still unknown, but it appears to be secondary to increased protein synthesis despite persistent protein breakdown.

Growth hormone and IGF-1 levels are shown to decrease after burn injury. Pharmacologic agents have been used to attenuate catabolism and to stimulate growth despite a burn injury.[65] Growth hormone, insulin, IGF-1/IGF-binding protein-3, testosterone, and oxandrolone improve nitrogen balance and promote wound healing.[66–68] Exogenous administration of rHGH, which increases protein synthesis, has been shown to improve nitrogen balance, preserve lean muscle mass, and increase the rate of wound healing.[69] The anabolic action of growth hormone appears to be mediated by an increase in protein synthesis, whereas IGF-1 decreases protein degradation. Growth hormone also enhances wound healing by stimulating hepatic and local production of IGF-1 to increase circulating and wound-site levels.[70] Plasma growth hormone levels, which are decreased following severe burns, can be restored by administration of rHGH (0.2 mg/kg/day) in massively burned children to accelerate skin graft donor-site wound healing and shorten hospital stay by more than 25%.[71] rHGH in severely burned children has shown to be safe and efficacious. In one randomized prospective trial in pediatric burn patients, rHGH administration led to elevations in serum growth hormone, IGF-I, and IGFBP-3, whereas the percent body fat content significantly decreased when compared with the control group. Long-term administration of 0.1 and 0.2 mg/kg/day rHGH also significantly improved scarring at 12 months postburn.[72] However, it has previously been shown that rHGH is associated with hyperglycemia, along with increased free fatty acids and triglycerides, which limits its clinical applicability. A prospective randomized control trial showed efficacy in rHGH and propranolol treatment in attenuating hypermetabolism and inflammation in severely burned children.[73] In this study, patients receiving rHGH (0.2 mg/kg/day) and propranolol (to decrease heart rate by 15%) for more than 15 days demonstrated significantly decreased percent predicted resting energy expenditure, C-reactive protein, cortisone, aspartate aminotransferase, alanine aminotransferase, free fatty acid, IL-6, IL-8, and macrophage inflammatory protein-1 when compared with controls. Other markers, such as serum IGF-1, IGF-binding protein-3, growth hormone, prealbumin, and IL-7 increased in rHGH/propranolol-treated burned patients.[73] These findings further validate the beneficial role of combination treatment with rHGH and a beta blocker in pediatric burn patients.

In severely burned patients, muscle anabolism can result from administration of submaximum dosages of insulin by stimulating muscle protein synthesis. Insulin administration has also been demonstrated to improve skin graft donor-site healing and wound matrix formation.[74] Testosterone production is greatly decreased after severe burn injury, which may last for months in postpubertal males. Increased protein synthesis with testosterone administration is accompanied by a more efficient use of intracellular amino acids derived from protein breakdown and an increase in inward transport of amino acids. An increase in net protein synthesis is attainable in adults with large burns by restoring testosterone concentrations to the physiologic range.[66] An analog of testosterone with less androgenic effect, oxandrolone (Upsher-Smith Laboratories, Minneapolis, Minn.), has been used in acute and rehabilitating adult burn patients, with promising results regarding weight gained. Oxandrolone, an oral synthetic derivative of testosterone with a lower androgenic/anabolic ratio, has been safely used to improve lean body mass and weight gain in severely burned adults and children. A large prospective double-blind randomized study involving 235 severely burned children (TBSA > 40%) showed that oxandrolone treatment significantly increased lean body mass along with serum total protein, prealbumin levels, and mean muscle strength. Interestingly, the oxandrolone-treated group also had a shorter hospital stay.[75] Similar results were reported in adult burn patient population.[76]

Nutrition

The metabolic rate of patients with burns increases from 1.5 times the normal rate in a patient with 25% TBSA burns to 2 times the normal rate in 40% TBSA burns.[77] Children are particularly vulnerable for protein-calorie malnutrition because of their proportionally lower body fat and smaller muscle mass, in addition to increased metabolic demands. This malnutrition is associated with dysfunction of various organ systems, including the immune system, and delayed wound healing. To ensure that patients remain caught up nutritionally, enteral feeding should be initiated early after a burn injury, especially since early enteral feedings have been shown to decrease the level of catabolic hormones, improve nitrogen balance, maintain gut mucosal integrity, and decrease the incidence of sepsis and overall hospitalization. Feeding tubes are generally placed under fluoroscopy immediately after the initial evaluation of burns, and enteral nutrition is started within hours after burns. Early enteral feedings have been shown to decrease the level of catabolic hormones, improve nitrogen balance, maintain gut mucosal integrity, and decrease overall hospital stay.[78] Although hyperalimentation can deliver sufficient calories, its use in burn patients has been associated with deleterious effects on immune function, small bowel mucosal atrophy with increased incidence of bacterial translocation, and decrease in survival.[79] Enteral nutrition through a feeding tube placed into the stomach or duodenum is always preferred to parental nutrition, and is associated with decreased metabolic rate and decreased sepsis in burn patients.

Several formulas are used to calculate caloric requirement in burn patients. Both Curreri (25 kcal/kg plus 40 kcal/% TBSA burned) and modified Harris-Benedict (calculated or measured resting metabolic rate times injury factor) formulas use the principle of providing maintenance caloric needs plus the additional caloric needs related to the burn size. Similar to fluid resuscitation guidelines, a caloric requirement guideline based on total and burned BSA is more appropriate for pediatric burn patients (Table 26-7).[80] The exact nutrient requirements of burn patients are not clear, but it is generally

TABLE 26-7

Caloric Requirements for Burned Children (Shriners Hospital for Children-Galveston)

Age Group	Daily Caloric Requirements
Infant and toddler	2100 kcal/m² total + 1000 kcal/m² burn
Child	1800 kcal/m² total + 1300 kcal/m² burn
Adolescent	1500 kcal/m² total + 1500 kcal/m² burn

accepted that maintenance of energy requirement and replacement of protein losses are vital. The recommended enteral tube feedings should have 20% to 40% of the calories as protein, 10% to 20% as fat, and 40% to 70% as carbohydrates. Milk is one of the least expensive and best tolerated forms of nutrition, but, to avoid dilutional hyponatremia, sodium supplementation may be needed when milk is used in large quantity. There are also numerous commercially available enteral formulas, such as Vivonex (Nestlé-Nutrition, Vevey, Switzerland) or Pediasure (Abbott Laboratories, Abbott Park, Ill.). One study compared outcomes with the use of Vivonex and milk in 944 pediatric burn patients and found that patients receiving Vivonex had shorter stays in the intensive care unit, a lower incidence of sepsis, and lived significantly longer until death than those receiving milk. Although there was no difference in mortality between the two groups, autopsies demonstrated decreased hepatic steatosis.[81] One report evaluated the efficacy of an anti-inflammatory, pulmonary enteral formula in the treatment of pediatric burn patients with respiratory failure.[82] Based on evidence that the inclusion of dietary lipids (e.g., omega-3 fatty acid, eicosapentaenoic acid) is known to modulate the inflammatory response, and the addition of antioxidants may improve cardiopulmonary function and respiratory gas exchange, this study evaluated the role of a specialized pulmonary enteral formula (SPEF) containing anti-inflammatory and antioxidant-enhanced components in pediatric burn patients. The use of SPEF was shown to be safe in pediatric patients and resulted in an improvement in oxygenation and pulmonary compliance in burned patients with acute respiratory distress syndrome.[82]

Pharmacotherapy

ANALGESIA

Burn wound treatment and rehabilitation therapy produce pain for patients of all age groups. Infants and children do not express their pain in the same way that adults do and may display pain through behaviors of fear, anxiety, agitation, tantrums, depression, and withdrawals. In older children, allowing the child to participate in providing wound care can help the child to have some control and alleviate fear and pain. Various combinations of analgesics with anxiolytic medications are used effectively during procedures and wound dressing changes (Table 26-8). A successful pain management regimen for burned children requires understanding by the entire burn team on how the pain is associated with burn depth and the phase of wound healing. Pain management protocols should be tailored to control background pain as well as that incurred with procedures, such as dressing changes, vascular access placement, and physical therapy. Physical therapy rehabilitation, which is vital to optimize good functional outcome, can more effectively be used if there is appropriate pain control. However, caution must be exercised to prevent any potential injury because of overmedication. Scheduled administration of acetaminophen can often address background pain, and it is not uncommon for dose escalation to occur as patients experience tolerance to a particular pain regimen. Morphine sulfate or fentanyl is frequently used to manage postoperative pain. The use of ketamine (0.5 to 2.0 mg/kg IV) is quite effective and ideal for short procedures, such as dressing changes and vascular access placements. For

TABLE 26-8

Pharmacotherapy Agents

Agent	Dosages	Indications
Morphine Sulfate	0.05-0.1 mg/kg IV or 0.3 mg/kg PO	Acute pain; procedures and dressing changes
Demerol	1-2 mg/kg PO or IV	Acute pain; procedures and dressing changes
Ketamine	1-2 mg/kg IV or 5-7 mg/kg IM	Surgery; procedures and dressing changes
Diazepam	1-2 mg PO or IV	Preoperative; anxiety
Chloral hydrate	250-500 mg PO	Preoperative; insomnia
Midazolam	0.25-0.5 mg/kg PO or IV	Anxiety; used in combination with narcotics
Lorazepam	0.03 mg/kg PO or IV	Background anxiety

burned children requiring deeper sedation and analgesia, a combination of propofol and ketamine has also been shown to be effective. Advanced pain management protocols can be administered safely by those experienced with the use of conscious sedation. Physical therapy, which is vital to optimize good functional outcome, can more effectively be used if there is appropriate pain control. However, caution must be exercised to prevent any potential injury because of overmedication. In children as young as 5 years of age, a patient-controlled analgesia may be used to provide steady-state background infusion of narcotic with additional bolus regimen.[83] Burn injuries are traumatic for the burned child as well as for the family. Burn care professionals must do everything possible to make the experience as tolerable as possible in assisting burn patients to a successful recovery.

As mentioned earlier, the physiologic changes that occur with a burn injury alter metabolism and pharmacodynamics of many medications, including narcotics. In one study, 20 adult patients with a mean burn size of 49% TBSA were compared with a control group after receiving 200 μg of fentanyl. Plasma concentrations were sampled at various times after administration, and it was noted that the burn patients had lower fentanyl concentrations at all time points, with no difference in clearance. This is likely related to the increased volumes of distribution in burn patients, which further suggests that the volume of distribution needs to be carefully considered when administering narcotics and titrating to clinical effect.[84]

SEDATIVES AND ANXIOLYTICS

Ketamine is a commonly used procedural sedative/anesthetic in burn patients. Derived from phencyclidine, it is characterized by dissociative anesthesia and has excellent analgesic properties. Given at a dose of 1 to 2 mg/kg IV or 5 to 7 mg/kg IM, an effect is achieved rapidly with a relatively short duration of action. In addition, ketamine is also frequently used as an anesthetic agent for operative procedures without compromising airway reflexes. The use of ketamine is contraindicated in patients with increased intracranial pressure. Benzodiazepines are commonly used to control burn-related anxiety as well as to enhance the effects of narcotics for pain control. Lorazepam (Ativan) at a dosage of 0.03 mg/kg PO or IV, is an effective anxiolytic agent. It is also useful as a hypnotic agent to improve patient restfulness in the acute care setting. Diazepam (Valium) has a longer duration of action than lorazepam and therefore is useful in more chronic settings. Diazepam also improves muscle relaxation, which can be beneficial to facilitate rehabilitative therapy. Midazolam (Versed) has a rapid onset of action, with peak plasma levels achieved within 30 minutes and a half-life of 2 to 5 hours. It is commonly used to achieve a desired level of sedation for procedures and dressing changes. Because of the anterograde amnesia property, it is used commonly as a premedication agent on operative days.

Dexmedetomidine (DEX) is another adjunct being used in the pediatric population for pain and sedation management. It is a selective α_2-adrenergic agonist that can provide sedation, anxiolysis, and analgesia with less respiratory depression than other sedatives. In one retrospective review of 65 ventilated pediatric burn patients, DEX was continuously infused after loading, and patients were noted to be "adequately sedated," which was in contrast to their sedation failure with opioids and benzodiazepines alone. The patients were successfully extubated while on the DEX infusion, and no patient showed evidence of DEX-induced respiratory depression.[85] In another study, intranasal DEX or oral midazolam was administered to 100 pediatric burn patients preoperatively. Ninety-four percent of the patients who received DEX were appropriately sedated as opposed to 82% in the midazolam group. There were no significant differences in narcotic requirements during the operation, nor increased adverse effects in patients receiving DEX.[86] Thus DEX may prove to be a safe alternative to benzodiazepines in burn patients.

INTRAVENOUS ANTIBIOTICS

The use of perioperative IV antibiotics has significantly contributed to an overall improvement in the survival of major burn patients during the past 2 decades. Bacteria colonized in the burn eschar can potentially shed systemically at the time of eschar excision and contribute to sepsis. Perioperatively, IV antibiotics against *Streptococcus*, *S. aureus*, and *Pseudomonas* are generally administered until quantitative cultures of the excised eschar are finalized. The antibiotic regimen can then be guided by culture results and used under the appropriate clinical conditions. In acute burns, gram-positive cocci are generally the predominate organism involved, but colonization with gram-negative bacteria, and even fungi, are frequently encountered in chronic burn wounds and therefore must be covered with appropriate IV antibiotics during excision and grafting. In addition to burn wound sepsis, graft loss may be attributed to the presence of an infected wound at the time of skin grafting or colonization of the grafted bed shortly after surgery. The most common organisms responsible for graft loss are beta-hemolytic streptococci (*S. pyogenes*, *S. agalactiae, or S. viridans*). They are generally sensitive to third-generation cephalosporin and fluoroquinolones. The emergence of multiresistant bacteria, such as methicillin-resistant *S. aureus*, has become a serious problem for burn centers. Hence, IV antibiotics should be used with diligence, limiting their use for perioperative coverage and treatment of identified sources of infection.

One consideration that should be taken into account is the tissue penetration of IV antibiotics in burned tissue. One study compared the distribution of cephalothin in burned and nonburned tissue, and cephalothin levels were found to be elevated with decreased clearance in both tissues when compared with controls. It was postulated that this resulted from altered blood flow in injured tissue, an increase in capillary leakage, or leakage of albumin-bound cephalothin into the interstitium.[87] This finding suggests that antibiotic pharmacodynamics may need to be re-interpreted in burned patients.

Nonthermal Injuries

CHEMICAL BURNS

Children accidentally come in contact with various household cleaning products. Treatment of chemical burns involves immediate removal of the causative agent and lavage with copious amount of water, with caution for potential hypothermia. Fluid resuscitation is started, and care should be taken to ensure that the effluent does not contact uninjured areas. Decontamination is not performed in a tub, but rather, the wounds are irrigated toward a drain as in a shower. After completion of copious irrigation, wounds should be covered with a topical antimicrobial dressing and appropriate surgical plans made. The rapid recognition of the offending chemical agent is crucial to the proper management. When in doubt, a local poison control center should be contacted for identification of chemical composition of the product involved. The common offending chemical agents can be classified as alkali or acid. Alkali, such as lime, potassium hydroxide, sodium hydroxide, and bleach, are among the most common agents involved in chemical injury.[88] Mechanisms of alkali-induced burns are saponification of fat resulting in increased cell damage from heat, extraction of intracellular water, and formation of alkaline proteinates with hydroxyl ions. These ions induce further chemical reaction into the deeper tissues. Attempts to neutralize alkali are not recommended, because the chemical reaction can generate more heat and add to injury. Acid burns are not as common. Acids induce protein breakdown by hydrolysis, resulting in formation of eschar, and therefore do not penetrate as deeply as the alkaline burns. Formic acid injuries are rare but can result in multiple systemic organ failures, such as metabolic acidosis, renal failure, intravascular hemolysis, and acute respiratory distress syndrome. Hydrofluoric acid burns are managed differently from those of other acid burns in general.[89] After copious local irrigation with water, fluoride ion must be neutralized with topical application of 2.5% calcium gluconate gel. If not appropriately treated, free fluoride ion causes liquefaction necrosis of the affected soft tissues, including bones. Because of potential hypocalcemia, patients should be closely monitored for prolonged QT intervals.

ELECTRICAL BURNS

Three to five percent of all admitted burn patients are injured from electrical contact. Fortunately, electrical burns are rare in children. Electrical burns are categorized into high- and low-voltage injuries. High-voltage injuries are characterized by varying degree of local burns, with destruction of deep tissues.[90] The electrical current enters a part of the body and travels through tissues with lowest resistance, such as nerves, blood vessels, and muscles. Heat generated as electrical current passes through deep tissues with relatively high resistance, such as bone, and damages adjacent tissues that may not be readily visible. Skin is mostly spared because of its high resistance to electrical current. Primary and secondary surveys, including electrocardiography, should be completed. If the initial electrocardiogram is normal, no further monitoring is necessary; however, any abnormal findings require continued monitoring for 48 hours and appropriate treatment of dysrhythmias when detected. The key to management of electrical burns lies in the early detection and proper treatment of injuries to deep structures. Edema formation and subsequent vascular compromise is common to extremities. Fasciotomies are frequently necessary to avoid potential limb loss. Intraabdominal complications can arise from bowel perforation. If myoglobinuria is present, vigorous hydration with administration of sodium bicarbonate, to alkalinize the urine and mannitol to achieve diuresis and as a free radical scavenger, is indicated. Repeated wound exploration and debridement of affected areas are required before ultimate wound closure, because there is a component of delayed cell death and thrombosis. The mechanism of electrical burn injury is to overwhelm the cellular systems that operate at millivolt/milliamp levels, so that cells that survive the initial injury may slowly die during a week's time as ion gradients deteriorate while thrombosis of the microvasculature proceeds. Electrical injuries may also have a thermal, nonconductive component as clothes burn or the electricity flashes. This is treated as if it were a conventional thermal burn. Low-voltage injury is similar to thermal injury, without transmission of electrical current to deep tissues, and usually only requires local wound care.

Outpatient Therapy

The majority of pediatric burns are minor, often resulting from scald less than 10% TBSA or isolated small areas of thermal injuries from contact with hot objects. Such injuries are usually limited to partial thickness of the skin and can be treated on an outpatient basis. After an initial assessment, the burn wound is gently washed with water and a mild bland soap with appropriate pain control. Blisters can be left intact when they are small and not likely to spontaneously rupture, especially when present on the palm of hand. Blisters can provide a natural barrier against the environment and are beneficial in avoiding daily dressing changes. Spontaneous resorption of the fluid occurs in approximately 1 week, concomitant with the re-epithelialization process. Larger areas of blisters should be debrided and topical antimicrobial dressings applied. Silvadene is most commonly used because of its broad-spectrum antimicrobial property as well as its soothing effect on superficial second-degree burns. However, because silver sulfadiazine can impede epithelialization, its use should be discontinued when healing partial-thickness wounds are devoid of necrotic tissue and evidence of re-epithelialization is noted. Alternatively, antimicrobial dressings with triple antibiotic ointment (neomycin, bacitracin, and polymyxin B sulfate) and Polysporin, which do not have any negative effects on epithelialization, are commonly used. For small superficial partial-thickness burns, nonmedical white petrolatum-impregnated fine mesh, porous mesh gauze (Adaptic; Johnson & Johnson, New Brunswick, NJ), or fine mesh absorbent gauze impregnated with 3% bismuth tribromophenate in a nonmedicinal petrolatum blend (Xeroform, Covidien) are usually sufficient without the need for topical antimicrobials.

Superficial burns to the face can be treated with application of triple antibiotic ointment alone, without any dressings. The frequency of dressing change varies from twice daily to once a week, depending on the size, depth of burns, and drainage. Those who advocate twice daily dressing changes base their care on the use of topical antimicrobials whose half-life is about 8 to 12 hours. Others who use petrolatum-based or bismuth-impregnated gauze recommend less frequent, once every 3- to 5-day dressing changes. The use of synthetic wound dressings (e.g., Biobrane) is also ideal for treatment of superficial partial-thickness burns as an outpatient.[91] When applied appropriately to fresh, partial-thickness wounds, Biobrane adheres to the wound rapidly and is very effective in promoting re-epithelialization in 1 to 2 weeks (see Fig. 26-6). Although daily dressing changes are eliminated, Biobrane-covered wounds should still be monitored closely for signs of infection.

Rehabilitation

Rehabilitation therapy is a vital part of burn care. During the acute phase of burn care, splints are used to prevent joint deformities and contractures. By using thermoplastic materials, which are amenable to heat manipulation, splints are fitted individually to each patient. Application of splints at all times, except during an exercise period, can potentially prevent severe contractures that occur in large-burn patients. Patients are mobilized out of bed immediately after the graft takes, and aggressive physical therapy is implemented. After the acute phase, hypertrophic scar formation is of major concern. The burn depth, patient's age, and genetic factors all play an important role in hypertrophic scar formation. In general, deep second-degree burn wounds, requiring 3 weeks or more to heal, will produce hypertrophic scarring. Children are more prone to hypertrophic scar formation than adults, probably because of the high rate of cell mitosis associated with growth. Continuously applied pressure 24 hours a day is the most effective method to minimize the hypertrophic scar formation. Pressure garments should be worn until scars mature, but they may be associated with skin breakdown and patient discomfort. Silicone gel is a commonly used treatment modality, even though its mechanism of action is poorly understood. Silicone treatment is reported to soften, increase elasticity, and improve the appearance of hypertrophic scars, but conflicting results remain in the literature that may be attributed to patient compliance.[92] Nonetheless, scar maturation usually occurs 6 to 18 months after injury. In younger patients, scars mature at a much slower rate. In addition to splints and pressure garments, physical therapy is a crucial component of rehabilitation therapy. Families should be thoroughly instructed on a program of active and passive range-of-motion exercises and muscle strengthening. It is not uncommon for patients to require inpatient or outpatient rehabilitation to return them to a functional quality of life. Burned survivors and families need rehabilitation therapy for extended periods of time both on a physical and psychological level. All must deal with feelings ranging from guilt to post-traumatic stress. A program such as *summer camp for children with burn injuries* has played an important role during the chronic phase of rehabilitation by helping children to improve self-esteem and to promote coping, social skills.[93]

The complete reference list is available online at www.expertconsult.com.

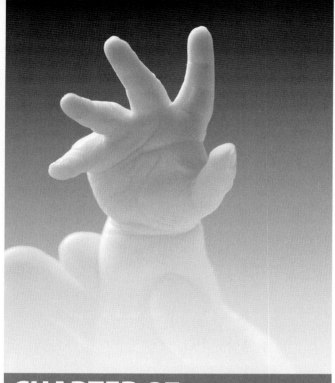

CHAPTER 27

Child Abuse and Birth Injuries

Dennis W. Vane

Child Abuse

Child abuse encompasses physical abuse, sexual abuse, emotional abuse, and neglect. This maltreatment of children has become a significant focus of attention in our society. The media routinely publish accounts of the alleged traumatic and sometimes fatal abuse of children among all socioeconomic classes and levels of celebrity. The myth that child abuse and other violence in the home occur only among the poor and the uneducated has been debunked. Child abuse is a worldwide problem that affects all levels of society. Prevention and effective treatment depend on the timely detection of epidemiologic situations that lend themselves to the maltreatment of children.

Unfortunately, the "minor" status of children leads to the justifiable issue of the relative rights of parents and guardians. In most societies, it is an accepted premise that parents have the authority and responsibility to provide for their children. This is based on the assumption that parents have the best interests of their children in mind when making these decisions. Unfortunately, not all parents are willing or capable of basing their care decisions on their children's best interests; rather, they make these decisions in a more self-centered manner. As a result, these children may become victims of abuse and neglect through actions or the lack of actions by these parents.

Religious and societal "norms" have created barriers to the identification of child abuse victims in many nations. Around the globe, relatively few nations have addressed this problem at all.[1] In the United States and Canada, legislation aimed at identifying child abuse and neglect was enacted beginning in the 1960s.[2] Since that time, the reporting of child abuse to civil authorities has been mandated for almost all professionals dealing with children. The legislation protects the reporting individual from liability (usually by using the phrase "suspicion of" or "injuries consistent with"), supersedes all professional–client privilege, and sometimes even imposes penalties for failure to report abuse.[3]

EPIDEMIOLOGY

In 2007 in the United States, Children's Protective Services investigated 3.5 million reports of child abuse. Of these investigations, 794,000 children were found to be victims of abuse. Thirty percent of all the children were less than the age of 4 years, 20% were between the ages of 4 and 7 years, and 20% were between 8 and 11 years.[4] In about 160,000 children, this maltreatment is considered physically serious or life threatening. Between 1,000 and 2,000 deaths are attributed to child abuse each year in the United States, and 80% of those children are younger than 5 years. Forty percent of the deaths occur in the first year of life and occur in an equal sex distribution.[5] Although deaths occur predominantly in the younger age groups, maltreatment of children is felt to increase with age. In teenagers, the incidence of abuse is thought to be twice that in preschool children; however, that statistic includes sexual abuse.[6] Intentional physical injury is most common in children less than 2 years of age, because they are essentially defenseless victims.[4] Patterns of child abuse occur with differing frequencies over the social strata. Sexual and emotional abuse have no socioeconomic associations, whereas physical abuse and neglect are more frequently associated with poverty.[6] Often, several types of abuse are perpetrated on the same child or within the same family. Additionally, abuse commonly occurs in families with other forms of intrafamilial violence, such as spousal abuse and violence among siblings.[7]

There is no single cause for abuse. However, multiple factors have been described that place a child at high risk to be abused. Commonly, more than one risk factor is present in a family at one time. It is important to remember, however, that the presence of risk factors in a child's environment does not necessarily indicate that abuse has or will occur. It is important to identify those situations where risk factors for child abuse exist. Local family services can often provide assistance to high-risk homes to aid families that may be in crisis. These early interventions potentially reduce or eliminate the risk of abuse.[4]

Risk factors for abuse are generally classified into four broad categories. First, there are the character and personality traits of the caregiver or parent; second, the individual characteristics of the child; third, the family dynamics; and finally, the environment in which the family is living.

Caregiver or Parent

Approximately 80% of all abusers are the parents.[4] Often, the abuser is described as having poor impulse control, antisocial behavior, and low self-esteem. Commonly, they were victims of abuse or witnessed domestic violence in the home themselves. Often, the abuser will have substance abuse problems. In many cases the parent's or caregiver's perception of the child is negative and associated with unrealistic expectations of the child's abilities. The age of the parent is another risk factor—the younger the parent or caregiver, the greater the risk of abuse.

The Child

The profile of the victim related to abuse rates has been studied in great depth.[4] The age of the child clearly impacts the risk, with children less than 3 years of age having the highest rates of abuse. These children require constant care and attention. They are small in stature compared with the adult and clearly are unable to adequately defend themselves. The child may be in a learning phase, such as toilet training, and may not be responding as the caregiver expects. Subsequently, children with cognitive, physical, or emotional disabilities are at significantly greater risk to suffer abuse. This higher risk holds true for premature and low-birth-weight infants as well. Some authors suggest that these factors interfere with appropriate parental bonding early in the child's life.

Family Dynamics

The existing family structure clearly impacts the risk for abuse.[4] A single-parent household significantly increases the risk for abuse, particularly when the father is absent. Households where there are large numbers of individuals living together, including family and nonfamily members, compounds the potential risk for abuse as well. In families where domestic violence has been documented, reports indicate that children suffer a 30% to 60% risk of abuse.

Finally, environmental factors, such as poverty, unemployment, lack of education, and living in high-crime areas, have all been identified as predisposing to potential child abuse. These factors are often coupled with a scarcity of social services to aid these families in these areas, thus adding stress to the dynamics fostering the environment for abuse.[4]

Child abuse is a self-perpetuating social and economic problem. Problems with substance abuse and depression are reportedly 2 to 3 times more likely in abused children than in the general population, and abused children are likely to be far more physically aggressive with their peers.[8,9] It is estimated that approximately 30% of abuse victims eventually abuse their own children.[10] Some authors have suggested that this perpetual cycle of abuse is attributable, in part, to changes in the neuroendocrine system, influencing arousal, learning, growth, and the individual's pain threshold.[10]

What is clear is that the incidence of child abuse is significantly underreported, because professional contact or recognition is often required to identify abuse in the first place. Physicians must recognize not only abuse that has already occurred but also the factors indicating a high potential for abuse, if this dramatic worldwide problem is to be prevented.

Presentation

Physicians must be aware that abused children are often withdrawn and avoid eye contact with their interviewers. Interviewers must be cognizant of the fact that children often respond with answers that they think will please the interviewer; so, care must be taken not to influence the child's responses. Young children are prone to associative fabrication, which may influence or even alter reality. The clinical history in suspected child abuse cases should include a detailed history of

the family situation, unrelated caregivers, substance abuse in the household, and any history of past abuse. Even with these indicators, child abuse is extremely hard to accurately diagnose.

Given the wide spectrum of abuse, presenting symptoms vary accordingly. In the youngest victims, the diagnosis often depends on physical signs, such as bruising, patterned burn injuries, retinal hemorrhages, and long-bone fractures. Among all children, presentations that should raise a high level of suspicion in the clinician include multiple injuries in different stages of healing; injuries not consistent with the history provided by the caregiver; a history that changes when retold, particularly when the incident was "unwitnessed"; and injuries to the perineum. Wisslow[2] provided an excellent summary of the presenting physical injuries in cases of child abuse and neglect (Table 27-1). In children,

---

TABLE 27-1

Signs and Symptoms Suggesting Child Abuse or Neglect

Subnormal growth
  Weight, height, or both less than 5th percentile for age
  Weight less than 5th percentile for height
  Decreased velocity of growth
Head injuries
  Torn frenulum of upper or lower lip
  Unexplained dental injury
  Bilateral black eyes with history of single blow or fall
  Traumatic hair loss
  Retinal hemorrhage
  Diffuse or severe central nervous system injury with history of minor to moderate fall (< 3 m)
Skin injuries
  Bruise or burn shaped like an object
  Bite marks
Burn resembling a glove or stocking, or with some other distribution, suggests an immersion injury
  Bruises of various colors (in different stages of healing)
  Injury to soft tissue areas that are normally protected (thighs, stomach, upper arms)
Gastrointestinal or genitourinary injuries
  Bilious vomiting
  Recurrent vomiting or diarrhea witnessed only by parent
  Chronic abdominal or perineal pain with no identifiable cause
  History of genital or rectal pain
  Injury to genitals or rectum
  Sexually transmitted disease
Bone injuries
  Rib fracture in the absence of major trauma, such as a motor vehicle accident
  Complex skull fracture after a short fall (< 1.2 m)
  Metaphyseal long-bone fracture in an infant
  Femur fracture (any configuration) in a child younger than 1 year
  Multiple fractures in various stages of healing
Laboratory studies
  Implausible or physiologically inconsistent laboratory results (polymicrobial contamination of body fluids, sepsis with unusual organisms, electrolyte disturbances inconsistent with the child's clinical state or underlying illness, wide and erratic variations in test results)
  Positive toxicologic tests in the absence of a known ingestion or medication
  Bloody cerebrospinal fluid (with xanthochromic supernatant) in an infant with altered mental status and no history of trauma

From Wissow LS: Child abuse and neglect. N Engl J Med 1995;332:1425-1431.

essentially any injury can be the result of abuse; however, particular injuries and injury patterns have a high degree of association with abuse.

Traumatic Brain Injury

Head injury is the most common injury associated with child abuse, and is responsible for the majority of deaths.[11-16] Penetrating head injury is rare in abuse victims, and most head injuries occur in younger children.[14] Blunt head injury most commonly manifests as "shaken baby syndrome" or, more accurately, "shaken impact syndrome," in which the insult is caused by an acceleration and deceleration of the brain within the cranial compartment resulting from violent shaking (Fig. 27-1). Recent studies indicate that some sort of contact with an object is necessary for the classical brain injury to occur, but that object may be relatively soft and produce no external indication of trauma (Fig. 27-2).[17] Angular forces created during shaking and eventual percussion against an object result in rotation of the brain within the skull. This causes diffuse axonal injury and tearing of the subdural bridging veins, often resulting in subdural hematoma. Spontaneous

subdural hematoma or its occurrence from unintentional trauma is uncommon in children; so, its presence should raise the suspicion of child abuse (Fig. 27-3). Acute contact with stationary objects results in the characteristic multiple skull fractures associated with repetitive injury. Secondary brain injury is also frequently associated with abuse, resulting in intracranial hemorrhage, anoxia secondary to apnea, hypoperfusion, cardiac arrest, and potentially, herniation of the brainstem.[18] Brain injury secondary to abuse carries a reported mortality rate of 15% to 38%, which is significantly higher than that of similar injuries caused by unintentional trauma.[17] Nonfatal outcomes in abused children with traumatic brain injuries are also significantly worse than in those whose injuries were sustained unintentionally.[19] Nonenhanced computed tomography is considered the most appropriate diagnostic tool for the identification of intentional head injury. Intracranial lesions are easily identified, as are the often associated skull fractures.[20]

Although most commonly seen in younger children, head injury associated with child abuse occurs in older children as well. Whereas external signs of trauma are infrequent in

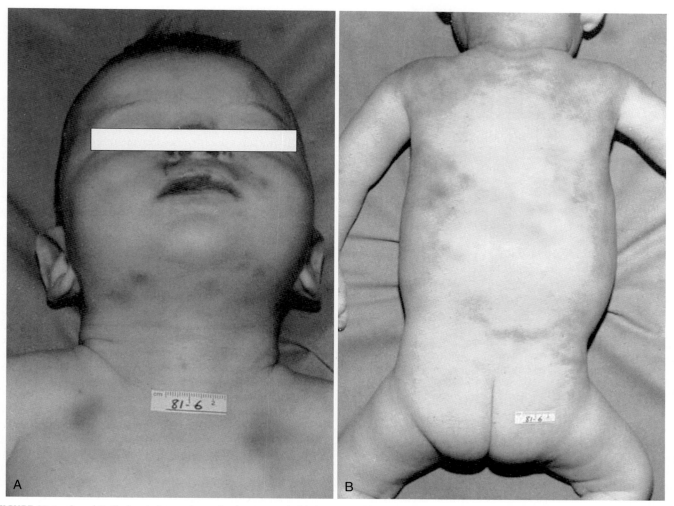

FIGURE 27-1   **A** and **B,** Shaken baby syndrome is often recognizable by external bruising about the chest, shoulders, and neck caused by the fingers and hands. (Used with permission of the American Academy of Pediatrics: Visual Diagnosis of Child Abuse CD-ROM, ed. 3, American Academy of Pediatrics, 2008.)

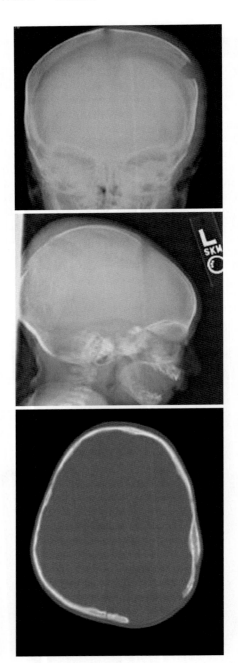

FIGURE 27-2   The radiographs demonstrate a diastatic skull fracture secondary to forcibly striking the child's head against a hard object. These fractures are often associated with later complications from healing and development of leptomeningeal cysts. (Used with permission of the American Academy of Pediatrics: Visual Diagnosis of Child Abuse CD-ROM, ed. 3, American Academy of Pediatrics, 2008.)

younger children, older children usually present with visible injuries secondary to violent external trauma. These injuries are often severe, with poor outcomes.[21]

The identification of retinal hemorrhage has been deemed almost pathognomonic of child abuse[22]; however, recent studies indicate that retinal hemorrhage occurs in cases of nonintentional injury as well, including normal vaginal delivery, which can cause compression of the baby's soft skull.[23,24] The presence of retinal hemorrhage from nonintentional injury is so rare, however, that it should stimulate a high

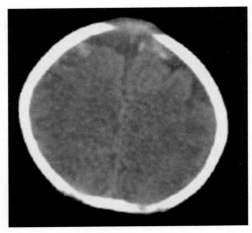

FIGURE 27-3   The computed tomography (CT) scan demonstrates a subdural hematoma in a 6-week-old infant. Subdural hematomas may not present as space-occupying lesions but may cause significant morbidity when evacuated because of significant brain swelling. (Used with permission of the American Academy of Pediatrics: Visual Diagnosis of Child Abuse CD-ROM, ed. 3, American Academy of Pediatrics, 2008.)

level of suspicion for child abuse. When it is identified, the physician should begin an appropriate workup to investigate that possibility.

Fractures

It is postulated that approximately 80% of child abuse cases in the United States are identified radiographically.[25] Fractures secondary to child abuse can be found in any age group, although fractures in older children are more commonly from high-impact unintentional injury.[26] This is the reverse of what is found in younger children where 55% to 70% of fractures associated with abuse occur in children less than 1 year of age; yet, only 2% of unintentional fractures occur in this age group.[12,14,27] The presence of a long-bone fracture in any child younger than 2 years of age has a high association with intentional injury.[28,29] Investigators have historically associated several fracture types with abuse, but it is probably more accurate to state that all fracture types can be associated with multiple causes. Spiral fractures, once reported as the most common type of fracture in abuse victims, have been replaced in more recent studies with single transverse fractures.[30] Spiral fractures are the result of torsional force applied to the extremity secondary to rotation of some sort. Transverse fractures are the result of a direct injury to the bone. This information should be used by the evaluating physician in conjunction with the history of injury to determine whether the history coincides with the presenting injury.

Diaphyseal fractures of the long bones are the most common fractures associated with child abuse, particularly those of the tibia, femur, and humerus. If the child is not ambulatory, the association between these fractures and abuse is extremely high.[30] Epiphyseal-metaphyseal fractures, although much less common than diaphyseal injuries, are reportedly far more specific for intentional injury.[31] The forces required to sustain these injuries greatly exceed the forces normally associated with falls and other minor trauma. Epiphyseal-metaphyseal fractures are also commonly known as corner fractures or bucket-handle fractures.

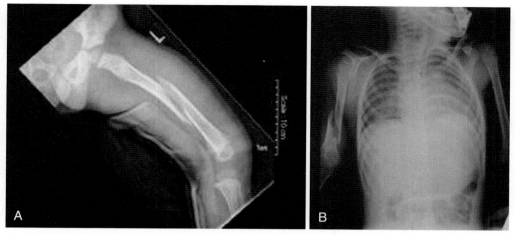

FIGURE 27-4   A, The radiograph demonstrates a fracture of the femur in a 2-year-old child. Femur fractures are highly suspicious in this age group. The parents brought the child in, because it would not bear weight on its leg. **B,** The right humerus fracture in this child was accompanied by significant pulmonary contusions. The history of falling on the arm is inconsistent with this level of injury. (Used with permission of the American Academy of Pediatrics: Visual Diagnosis of Child Abuse CD-ROM, ed. 3, American Academy of Pediatrics, 2008.)

Type 1 fractures of the femur and humerus have a high association with abuse when encountered outside of the neonatal period.[32] This is particularly true if the history of injury does not contain significant high-force violent trauma. These injuries require considerable force to occur and, when nonintentional, are commonly associated with significant soft tissue damage and other injuries. Other types of Salter-Harris injuries do not appear to have a strong association with intentional abuse (Fig. 27-4).

Clavicular fractures can also be associated with abuse, but there is a low specificity. Clavicular fractures of either end, rather than the midshaft, are usually the result of significant traction or the trauma of shaking.[15] Rib fractures, in contrast, have an extremely high association with abuse. It is postulated that the relatively elastic rib cage in children prevents most fractures secondary to accidental trauma. When fractures of the ribs do occur, the association with abuse is high—up to 82%.[33] In general these fractures occur at the posterior segment of the rib near the costovertebral junction (Fig. 27-5).

Spinal fractures are rare in children, as is cord injury. The difficulty in diagnosing vertebral body injuries and the relatively protected spine make any association with abuse difficult to determine. Suffice it to say that any injury of the spine or spinal cord requires an extremely violent force, and the cause must be carefully investigated.

It is critical for any physician treating children to investigate all fractures, particularly in the younger age groups. Minimal trauma does not commonly cause fractures, except when associated with other pathology. Getting an accurate history is critical. The presence of multiple fractures associated with a history of minimal trauma always requires an investigation for potential child abuse. The identification of multiple fractures, particularly when the age of the fractures is different, is almost pathognomonic of abuse. When abuse is suspected, skeletal surveys are indicated. The American College of Radiology has published standards for these surveys.[34]

Burns

Burns are a fairly common indication of child abuse, representing approximately 20% of pediatric burn injuries. Most commonly, the victims are less than 2 years of age.[35] Abuse

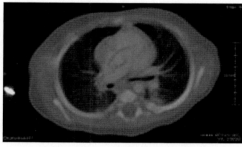

FIGURE 27-5   Posterior rib fractures in children are rare results of accidental injury. Their presence most commonly indicates intentional injury. (Used with permission of the American Academy of Pediatrics: Visual Diagnosis of Child Abuse CD-ROM, ed. 3, American Academy of Pediatrics, 2008.)

victims often have characteristic patterns of burn infliction of which physicians should be aware.[36] Common patterns include circumferential burns, particularly when the burns are on more than one extremity; "pattern" burns or branding; burns to the buttocks, genitalia, or perineum; and punctate or cigarette burns (Figs. 27-6 and 27-7). Burn victims who are abused are usually younger than unintentional burn victims and have a history of being burned in the bathroom.[37] The demographics of intentionally burned children are striking. These children are often being raised by single mothers or are in foster care, they are in homes where other children have previously been removed because of abuse, and there is an almost 40% chance that past abuse has already been investigated.[37]

With burns, the history of injury is critical and is often inconsistent with the burn pattern. The burn itself often exhibits uncharacteristic features, such as lack of splash marks from falling liquids, consistent depth throughout the burn rather than the normal "feathering" of depth, and larger surface areas than expected based on the history. These burns, which are often the result of immersion, present with clear lines of demarcation, indicating that the child was unable to move during the incident and was probably restrained. Inflicted burns to the buttocks and perineum often occur in children being toilet trained when a caregiver becomes frustrated about an

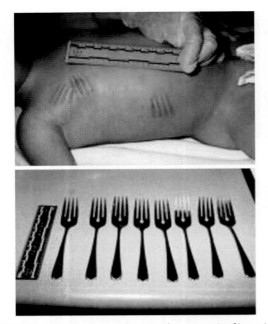

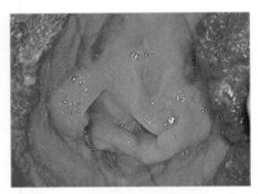

FIGURE 27-8 Total lateral disruption of the hymen pictured here indicates forceful penetration. (Used with permission of the American Academy of Pediatrics: Visual Diagnosis of Child Abuse CD-ROM, ed. 3, American Academy of Pediatrics, 2008.) *(See Expert Consult for color version.)*

FIGURE 27-6 Pattern burns are almost pathognomonic of intentional injury. In this case, the silverware found in the home directly matches the injury seen here. (Used with permission of the American Academy of Pediatrics: Visual Diagnosis of Child Abuse CD-ROM, ed. 3, American Academy of Pediatrics, 2008.) *(See Expert Consult for color version.)*

150° F. That is certainly more time than anyone would keep his or her hands immersed volitionally.

Flame burns, while not usually the result of a direct intentional infliction, often do represent potential abuse by neglect or an unsafe habitation. These types of injuries require a high degree of suspicion and may warrant reporting.

A complete history and physical examination are necessary in any child seen for burns or the suspicion of abuse. Other signs of abuse are often discernible, such as healed or healing fractures or, possibly, perineal injuries. Additionally, recent data indicate that some burn injuries mimic chronic skin conditions.[38] Thus a high level of suspicion must be maintained when clinicians see lesions that do not present in characteristic locations or do not respond to normal therapy. Given the high incidence of recurrence in burn injury, physicians must ensure that the child is discharged to a safe environment.[39]

Thoracoabdominal Injury

Fortunately, significant thoracoabdominal injury secondary to child abuse is uncommon, estimated to occur in about 5% of abused children.[40] Unfortunately, thoracoabdominal injury is the second leading cause of death in these children, following head injury, and has a significantly higher associated mortality than similar unintentional injury.[25,40] Any type of blunt or penetrating abdominal injury can be caused intentionally.[6,34,41–43] Injuries commonly result from severe blows to the abdomen or chest cavity, and as previously stated, rib fractures in children should raise the suspicion of abuse.[33] Most important, the clinician must ascertain the history of injury to determine whether the injury is consistent with the mechanism described. For example, recent reports indicate that a simple fall down a flight of stairs does not generate the force or dynamics necessary for a hollow viscus perforation.[44] Similarly, significant head injury requires a mechanism generating more force than simply rolling out of bed. Studies indicate that a child must fall at least 3 feet onto a hard surface to sustain a skull fracture. This includes wood floors, tile, or cement. Falls on to carpets and mattresses provide adequate cushioning to make a fracture unlikely from this height.[45–47]

Treatment of intentionally inflicted intra-abdominal injuries follows the algorithms of unintentional injuries. Mortality from these intentional injuries exceeds those found with unintentional injuries, mainly because of delay in presentation. Specific organ injuries, such as to the pancreas, carry with

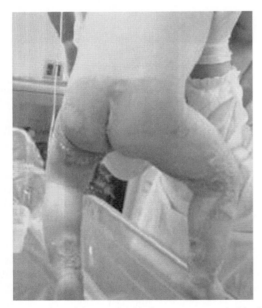

FIGURE 27-7 Bilateral foot and ankle burns accompanied by burns to the perineum indicate abuse. These burns are commonly seen in children being toilet trained, who are in the care of a nonbiologic parent. (Used with permission of the American Academy of Pediatrics: Visual Diagnosis of Child Abuse CD-ROM, ed. 3, American Academy of Pediatrics, 2008.) *(See Expert Consult for color version.)*

"accident." Burns on the dorsum of the hand are suggestive of abuse, whereas burns to the palm are more likely unintentional. Children, similar to adults, explore with the palmar surface, not the back of the hand. The depth of burn is also important. It takes approximately 1.5 seconds to cause a second-degree burn in adult skin immersed in water at

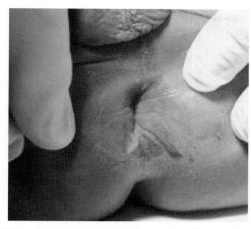

FIGURE 27-9   Lacerations of the anal area, often first noted as blood in the underwear, indicate penetration. (Used with permission of the American Academy of Pediatrics: Visual Diagnosis of Child Abuse CD-ROM, ed. 3, American Academy of Pediatrics, 2008.) *(See Expert Consult for color version.)*

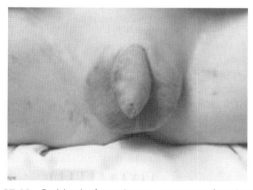

FIGURE 27-10   Bruising in the perineum, scrotum, and penis secondary to intentional injury. (Used with permission of the American Academy of Pediatrics: Visual Diagnosis of Child Abuse CD-ROM, ed. 3, American Academy of Pediatrics, 2008.) *(See Expert Consult for color version.)*

them an increased association of hollow viscus injury versus those of unintentional injury patterns. These associations should prompt a high degree of suspicion for abuse.[49,50]

Injuries to the perineum should always lead to a consideration of child abuse. Aside from burns to the perineum, discussed previously, injuries in this area resulting from abuse tend to be penetrating. Rectal or vaginal trauma resulting in laceration should routinely be investigated, as should lacerations in the penile and scrotal region (Figs. 27-8 to 27-10). Abuse may involve retained foreign bodies as well. The physician should always investigate anal and vaginal orifices that appear to be dilated, particularly those that may result in incontinence. Signs of abuse to the perineum are often chronic, and areas of scar and old lacerations should be noted.

The radiographic and diagnostic workup for children suffering thoracoabdominal abuse is identical to that for unintentional injury. Recommendations for appropriate scans and diagnostics have been updated by the American Academy of Pediatrics.[51] Management of these injuries is also the same as for unintentional thoracoabdominal injuries.[42,52]

Birth Injuries

Birth injury is estimated to occur in 6 to 8 of every 1000 live births in the United States, but it is responsible for about 2% of the perinatal mortality.[53] Injury most commonly occurs in babies with macrosomia but can also be associated with fetal organomegaly, mass lesions, prematurity, protracted labor, precipitous delivery, breech presentation, and cephalopelvic dissociation. The development and widespread use of prenatal ultrasonography, along with other advances in perinatal care, have allowed the early identification of many of these factors, together with recommendations for the delivery of such high-risk infants.[54]

SOFT TISSUE INJURY

The most common birth injury encountered is injury to the soft tissue. This can present as a hematoma (often cephalohematoma), simple cutaneous bruising, or fat necrosis manifesting as subcutaneous masses. These lesions resolve spontaneously within months and require no treatment other than reassurance of the parents. Less commonly, lacerations secondary to instrumentation may occur. These lacerations can usually be closed with adhesive strips or cutaneous glue rather than sutures. Suturing may be necessary, however, when adhesive closure cannot achieve the appropriate cosmetic result. Fine material should always be used, and healing is usually excellent. Lacerations are rarely deep, but if they are, standard precautions for wound exploration should be followed.

Torticollis has been ascribed to birth trauma or intrauterine malpositioning.[55] The cause is debatable, because torticollis has been found in infants who were delivered by cesarean section, as well as in those delivered vaginally. The classical presentation is a small, firm mass in the body of the sternocleidomastoid muscle. The head is tilted toward the mass, with the face classically turned to the contralateral side. Physical therapy performed by the parents is successful in the vast majority of cases, and surgical intervention is rarely indicated. Facial asymmetry may result in untreated lesions. Torticollis has been misdiagnosed as a malignancy in the neck. Careful examination and taking a complete history can often prevent this error.[56]

FRACTURES

The most common fracture associated with birth trauma is clavicular, occurring in about 2.7 of every 1000 births.[57] The fracture is noticed when the infant does not move the arm or swelling occurs over the clavicle. The fracture is commonly in the midshaft and generally requires no treatment, although some authors recommend figure-of-eight splints or pinning the baby's shirtsleeve to the chest on the affected side.[58] Occasionally, because of shoulder dystocia, the clavicle may be intentionally fractured.[59]

Fractures of the humerus usually occur in either the shaft or the proximal epiphysis. Epiphyseal fractures are difficult to diagnose because of a lack of ossification points in the neonatal epiphysis. Associated neurologic findings may be noted with fractures of the humerus, including Erb palsy and radial nerve palsy.[59,60] Shoulder dislocation is most likely not related to birth trauma but rather to intrauterine causes or therapy for Erb palsy.[61] Distal fractures and dislocations of the radial head may also occur and are often associated with breech delivery.[62,63] Proximal fractures of the humerus can be successfully treated by bandaging the arm to the chest in a neutral position for epiphyseal injuries and by strapping the arm to the chest with an abduction device or possibly a posterior splint for shaft fractures.[64]

Birth trauma can cause fractures of the femur at almost any location. Breech delivery and high birth weight are predisposing factors.[65] Presentation consists of abnormal rotation of the lower extremity, pain, or swelling. Treatment involves application of a traction device, spica cast, or both.[66] Reduction should be close to anatomic, because overgrowth and remodeling of the femur are not usually dramatic.[67]

NEUROLOGIC INJURY

Brachial plexus injury is the most common neurologic birth injury.[68] Approximately 21% of these injuries are associated with a shoulder dystocia at birth. Erb palsy (C3 to C5) is the most common of the brachial plexus injuries and usually resolves spontaneously, with little residual effect. Presentation involves a lack of motion of the affected shoulder, with the limb adducted and internally rotated to the prone position. Distal sensation and hand function are usually normal. Even after aggressive physical therapy, about 2% of cases are permanent.[69] Lower injuries of the C6 to T1 cervical roots (Klumpke palsy) present with a lack of hand and wrist function. These lesions may be accompanied by Horner syndrome, with the associated physical findings. Microsurgical repair has been described for recalcitrant brachial plexus injuries, with relatively good success, but this should be reserved only for infants failing aggressive physical therapy.[70] Phrenic nerve paralysis is a commonly associated finding and should be investigated whenever brachial plexus injury is identified. Isolated brachial plexus injury can cause significant shoulder abnormalities, and therapy should not be delayed.[71]

Phrenic nerve injury can also occur in isolation.[53] Treatment of phrenic nerve injury depends on the severity of the respiratory embarrassment experienced by the child. Asymptomatic injuries should not be treated; injuries resulting in respiratory impairment should be treated with diaphragmatic plication or other procedures designed to reduce the paradoxical movement of the diaphragm with respiration.[21]

Certainly the most devastating neurologic birth injuries involve the central nervous system. Lesions of the cervical spine are rare but are devastating when they occur. The cause of injury is usually a vaginal delivery with a breech or transverse lie.[72] As with all cervical spine injuries, high lesions require mechanical ventilation, and lower lesions have devastating physical sequelae. Survival is poor in neonates with complete transection. Partial injury may mimic cerebral palsy.[73]

Subdural, subarachnoid, intraventricular, and intraparenchymal bleeds have also been associated with birth trauma. Outcome is dependent on the extent of the lesion and the presentation. Usually these lesions are secondary to vacuum extraction,[74,75] which is also implicated as the cause of subgaleal cephalohematoma. Although most hematomas resolve without incident or sequelae, approximately 25% have been reported to cause death in affected neonates.[76] Traction injury to the internal carotid artery has also been reported in difficult births. Outcome from these injuries is varied and depends on the extent of vascular damage and collateral perfusion.[77] Similarly, direct injury to the optic nerve has been described.[78]

The most common central nervous system injury during childbirth is anoxic brain damage, and the resultant "cerebral palsy." The cause is controversial, but difficult delivery is a common association.

Treatment of neurologic birth trauma is usually expectant, with aggressive physical therapy. Recalcitrant peripheral injuries have responded to surgical repair.

THORACOABDOMINAL INJURY

Injuries to the chest are believed to be the result of pressure on the thoracic cavity. Pneumothorax, pneumomediastinum, and chylothorax have been described.[53,79] Perforation of the esophagus or cricopharyngeus can also occur. In most cases of birth trauma to the chest, expectant observation is indicated. The clinical course dictates the need for operative intervention. High perforations of the esophagus and cricopharyngeus can usually be treated by observation or occasionally drainage.[53] Lower lesions require drainage or operative repair. With early identification, results are excellent. Perforation of the esophagus can also result from placement of a gastric tube in the neonatal period. The management of these lesions remains controversial and varies from immediate intervention to expectant observation, based on the child's clinical situation.

Liver hematoma is the most common intra-abdominal injury secondary to birth trauma (Fig. 27-11). The usual presentation is anemia, but it can also be shock.[80] Diagnosis is usually made by ultrasonography, but a thorough investigation may be necessary to rule out other hepatic masses in a newborn. Treatment is usually expectant and includes volume resuscitation and correction of any hypothermia or coagulopathy. Occasionally, operative intervention is necessary when the baby is unstable or continued hemorrhage occurs. Hemostatic agents appear to be more helpful than attempts at suture repair in stopping hepatic bleeding in newborns.[81] In any case, control of hepatic hemorrhage is very difficult in this age group.

Splenic injury is rare and presents much like hepatic injury. Intra-abdominal blood may be the only presenting sign, and,

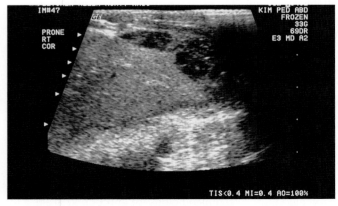

FIGURE 27-11 Ultrasonography of the abdomen clearly demonstrates this hepatic hematoma caused by birth trauma, which resolved spontaneously. Lesions such as this can be followed by ultrasonography; if they persist, other causes, such as neoplasm, must be investigated.

as in hepatic injury, other pathology must be ruled out.[82] Treatment includes expectant observation and correction of coagulopathy or hypothermia. Operative intervention is difficult and usually results in splenectomy. Hemostatic agents may also be useful.

As with splenic injury, injury to the adrenal glands is uncommon because of the relative protection provided by the thoracic ribs. The presentation may be hemorrhage or adrenal insufficiency in severe cases. Injury can also be identified from calcifications found on a radiograph taken later in life. As with all intra-abdominal solid organs, investigation of hematomas requires a workup to rule out other pathology, such as underlying tumor.

The complete reference list is available online at www. expertconsult.com.

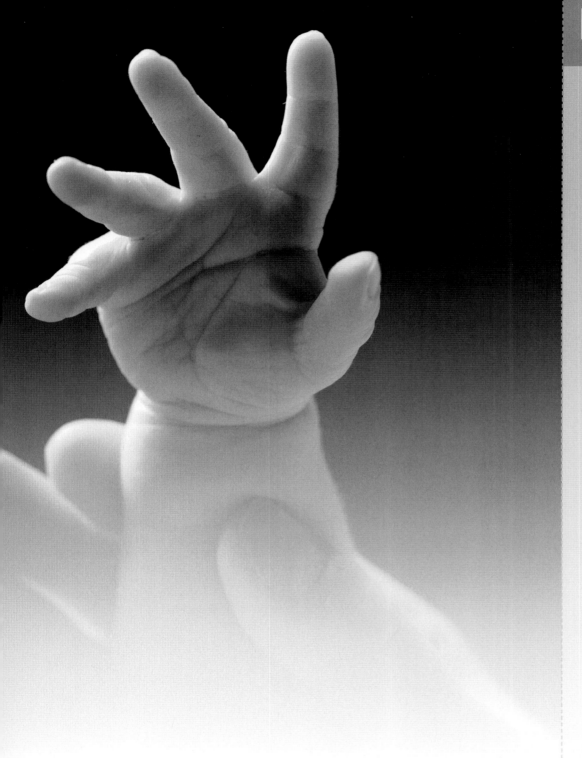

Part III

MAJOR TUMORS OF CHILDHOOD

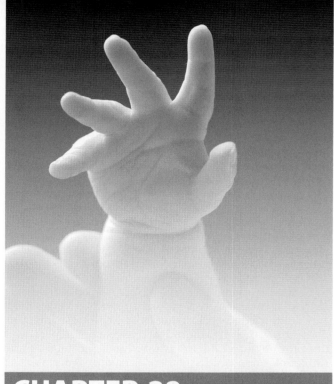

CHAPTER 28

Principles of Pediatric Oncology, Genetics of Cancer, and Radiation Therapy

Matthew J. Krasin and Andrew M. Davidoff

A number of milestones in the evolution of cancer therapy have come from the field of pediatric oncology. The first clear evidence that chemotherapy could provide effective treatment for childhood malignancy occurred in 1950 when Farber reported temporary cancer remission in children with acute lymphoblastic leukemia (ALL) treated with the folic acid antagonist aminopterin.[1] The first successful use of a multidisciplinary approach to cancer treatment occurred in the 1960s and 1970s through the collaborative efforts of pediatric surgeons, radiation therapists, and pediatric oncologists aiming to improve the treatment of Wilms' tumor in children.[2] Such a multidisciplinary approach is now used throughout the field of oncology. The successful use of a combination of chemotherapeutic agents to cure Hodgkin disease and ALL during the 1960s led to the widespread use of combination chemotherapy to treat virtually all types

of cancers. Since the late 1980s, neuroblastoma has been the paradigm for the use of therapies of variable intensity, depending on risk stratification determined by clinical and biological variables, including molecular markers. Other advances in pediatric oncology have included the development of interdisciplinary, national cooperative clinical research groups to critically evaluate new therapies, the efficacy of dose-intensive chemotherapy programs in improving the outcome of advanced-stage solid tumors, and the supportive care necessary to make the latter approach possible. The development and application of these principles and advances have led to substantially increased survival rates for children with cancer and profound improvements in their quality of life.

Additionally, advances in molecular genetic research in the past 3 decades have led to an increased understanding of the genetic events in the pathogenesis and progression of human malignancies, including those of childhood. A number of pediatric malignancies have served as models for molecular genetic research. Chromosomal structural changes, activating or inactivating mutations of relevant genes or their regulatory elements, gene amplification, and gene imprinting may each play a role in different tumor types. In some instances, these genetic events occur early in tumorigenesis and are specific for a particular tumor type, such as the chromosomal translocation t(11;22)(q24;q12) in Ewing sarcoma; other aberrations occur in a variety of different tumor types and are almost always associated with additional genetic changes, such as chromosome 1p deletion in neuroblastoma and Wilms' tumor. Some alterations involve oncogenes—genes that, when activated, lead directly to cancer—whereas others involve tumor suppressor genes, whose inactivation allows tumor progression. The result of alterations in these genetic elements, regardless of the mechanism, is disruption of the normal balance between proliferation and death of individual cells. These discoveries have highlighted the utility of molecular analysis for a variety of purposes, including diagnosis, risk stratification, and treatment planning; the understanding of syndromes associated with cancer; genetic screening and genetic counseling; and prophylactic treatment, including surgical intervention. Soon, treatment regimens are likely to be individualized on the basis of the molecular biological profile of a patient's tumor. In addition, molecular profiling will lead to the development of new drugs designed to induce differentiation of tumor cells, block dysregulated growth pathways, or reactivate silenced apoptotic pathways.

Epidemiology and Survival Statistics

Cancer in children is uncommon; it represents only about 2% of all cancer cases. Nevertheless, after trauma, it is the second most common cause of death in children older than 1 year. Each year, approximately 130 new cases of cancer are identified per million children younger than 15 years (or about 1 in 7000). This means that in the United States, about 9,000 children younger than 15 years are diagnosed with cancer each year, in addition to 4,000 patients aged 15 to 19 years.[3] Leukemia is the most common form of cancer

TABLE 28-1
Frequency of Cancer Diagnoses in Childhood

Type of Cancer	Percentage of Total
Leukemia	30
Brain tumors	25
Lymphoma	15
Neuroblastoma	8
Sarcoma	7
Wilms' tumor	6
Osteosarcoma	5
Retinoblastoma	3
Liver tumors	1

in children, and brain tumors are the most common solid tumor of childhood (Table 28-1). Lymphomas are the next most common malignancy in children, followed by neuroblastoma, soft tissue sarcomas, Wilms' tumor, germ cell tumors, osteosarcoma, and retinoblastoma. A slightly different distribution is seen among 15- to 19-year-olds, in whom Hodgkin disease and germ cell tumors are the most frequently diagnosed malignancies; non-Hodgkin lymphoma, nonrhabdomyosarcoma soft tissue sarcoma, osteosarcoma, Ewing sarcoma, thyroid cancer, and melanoma also occur with an increased incidence.

In general, the incidence of childhood cancer is greatest during the first year of life, peaks again in children aged 2 to 3 years, and then slowly declines until age 9. The incidence then steadily increases again through adolescence. Each tumor type shows a different age distribution pattern, however. Variations by gender are also seen. For example, Hodgkin disease, ALL, brain tumors, neuroblastoma, hepatoblastoma, Ewing sarcoma, and rhabdomyosarcoma are more common in boys than in girls younger than 15 years, whereas only osteosarcoma and Ewing sarcoma are more common in boys than in girls older than 15 years. However, girls in the older age group have Hodgkin disease and thyroid cancer more frequently than boys do. Distribution also varies by race: White children generally have a 30% greater incidence of cancer than do black children. This difference is particularly notable for ALL, Ewing sarcoma, and testicular germ cell tumors. The probability of surviving childhood cancer has improved greatly since Farber induced the first remissions in patients with ALL. In the early 1960s, approximately 30% of children with cancer survived their disease. By the mid-1980s, about 65% of children with cancer were cured, and by the mid-1990s, the cure rate had increased to nearly 75%.[4] Currently, greater than 80% are cured. These great strides have resulted from three important factors: (1) the sensitivity of childhood cancer, at least initially, to available chemotherapeutic agents; (2) the treatment of childhood cancer in a multidisciplinary fashion; and (3) the treatment of most children in major pediatric treatment centers in the context of a clinical research protocol using the most current and promising therapy. Although progress in the treatment of some tumor types, such as ALL and Wilms' tumor, has been outstanding, progress in the treatment of others, such as metastatic neuroblastoma and rhabdomyosarcoma, has been modest. Therefore there is still a need for significant improvement in the treatment of childhood cancer.

Molecular Biology of Cancer

During normal cellular development and renewal, cells evolve to perform highly specialized functions to meet the physiologic needs of the organism. Development and renewal involve tightly regulated processes that include continued cell proliferation, differentiation to specialized cell types, and programmed cell death (apoptosis). An intricate system of checks and balances ensures proper control over these physiologic processes. The genetic composition (genotype) of a cell determines which pathway(s) will be followed in exerting that control. In addition, the environment plays a crucial role in influencing cell fate: Cells use complex signal transduction pathways to sense and respond to neighboring cells and their extracellular milieu.

Cancer is a genetic disease whose progression is driven by a series of accumulating genetic and epigenetic changes influenced by hereditary factors and the somatic environment. These changes result in individual cells acquiring a phenotype that provides them with a survival advantage compared with surrounding normal cells. Our understanding of the processes that occur in malignant cell transformation is increasing; many discoveries in cancer cell biology have been made by using childhood tumors as models. This greater understanding of the molecular biology of cancer has also contributed significantly to our understanding of normal cell physiology.

NORMAL CELL PHYSIOLOGY

Cell Cycle

Genetic information is stored in cells and transmitted to subsequent generations of cells through nucleic acids organized as genes on chromosomes. A gene is a functional unit of heredity that exists on a specific site or locus on a chromosome, is capable of reproducing itself exactly at each cell division, and is capable of directing the synthesis of an enzyme or other protein. The genetic material is maintained as DNA formed into a double helix of complementary strands. The cell must ensure that replicated DNA is accurately copied with each cell division or cycle. DNA replication errors that go uncorrected potentially alter the function of normal cell regulatory proteins. The molecular machinery used to control the cell cycle is highly organized and tightly regulated.[5] Signals that stimulate or inhibit cellular growth converge on a set of evolutionarily conserved enzymes that drive cell-cycle progression. Various "checkpoints" exist to halt progression through the cell cycle during certain environmental situations or times of genetic error resulting from inaccurate synthesis or damage. Two of the most well-studied participants in the cell-cycle checkpoint system are TP53 and retinoblastoma (RB) proteins.[6] In normal circumstances, cells divide and terminally differentiate, thereby leaving the cell cycle, or they enter a resting state. Inactivation of the effectors of cell-cycle regulation or the bypassing of cell-cycle checkpoints can result in dysregulation of the cell cycle, a hallmark of malignancy.

Signal Transduction

Signal transduction pathways regulate all aspects of cell function, including metabolism, cell division, death, differentiation, and movement. Multiple extracellular and intracellular signals for proliferation or quiescence must be integrated by the cell, and it is this integration of signals from multiple pathways that determines the response of a cell to competing and complementary signals. Extracellular signals include growth factors, cytokines, and hormones; the presence or absence of adequate nutrients and oxygen; and contact with other cells or an extracellular matrix. Signaling mediators often bind to membrane-bound receptors on the outside of the cell, but they may also diffuse into the cell and bind receptors in the cytoplasm or on the nuclear membrane. Binding of a ligand to a receptor stimulates the activities of small-molecule second messengers—proteins necessary to continue the transmission of the signal. Signaling pathways ultimately effect the activation of nuclear transcription factors that are responsible for the expression or silencing of genes encoding proteins involved in all aspects of cellular physiology.

Receptors with tyrosine kinase activity are among the most important transmembrane receptors. Several important transmembrane receptors with protein kinase activity have been identified and grouped in families on the basis of structural similarities.[7] These families include the epidermal growth factor receptors (EGFRs), fibroblast growth factor receptors, insulin-like growth factor receptors (IGFRs), platelet-derived growth factor receptors (PDGFRs), transforming growth factor receptors, and neurotrophin receptors (TRKs). Abnormalities of members of each of these families are often found in pediatric malignancies and therefore are thought to play a role in their pathogenesis. Characteristic abnormalities of these receptors often form the basis of both diagnostic identification of certain tumor types and, more recently, targeted therapy for tumors with these specific abnormalities.

Programmed Cell Death

Multicellular organisms have developed a highly organized and carefully regulated mechanism of cell suicide to maintain cellular homeostasis. Normal development and morphogenesis are often associated with the production of excess cells, which are removed by the genetically programmed process of cell death called apoptosis. Apoptosis limits cellular expansion and counters cell proliferation. Apoptosis is initiated by the interaction of "death ligands," such as tumor necrosis factor-α (TNF-α), FAS, and TNF-related apoptosis-inducing ligand (TRAIL), with their respective receptors. This interaction is followed by aggregation of the receptors and recruitment of adapter proteins to the plasma membrane, which activate caspases.[8] Thus the fate of a cell is determined by the balance between death signals and survival signals.[9]

An alternative to cell death mediated by receptor–ligand binding is cellular senescence, which is initiated when chromosomes reach a critical length. Eukaryotic chromosomes have DNA strands of unequal length, and their ends, called telomeres, are characterized by species-specific nucleotide repeat sequences. Telomeres stabilize the ends of chromosomes, which are otherwise sites of significant instability.[10] With time and with each successive cycle of replication, chromosomes are shortened by failure to complete replication of their telomeres. Thus telomere shortening acts as a biological clock, limiting the life span of a cell. Germ cells, however, avoid telomere shortening by using telomerase, an enzyme capable of adding telomeric sequences to the ends of chromosomes. This enzyme is normally inactivated early in the growth and development of an organism. Persistent activation or the reactivation of telomerase in somatic cells appears to contribute to the immortality of transformed cells.

Malignant Transformation

Alteration or inactivation of any of the components of normal cell regulatory pathways may lead to the dysregulated growth that characterizes neoplastic cells. Malignant transformation may be characterized by cellular de-differentiation or failure to differentiate, cellular invasiveness and metastatic capacity, or decreased drug sensitivity. Tumorigenesis reflects the accumulation of excess cells that results from increased cell proliferation and decreased apoptosis or senescence. Cancer cells do not replicate more rapidly than normal cells, but they show diminished responsiveness to regulatory signals. Positive growth signals are generated by proto-oncogenes, so named because their dysregulated expression or activity can promote malignant transformation. These proto-oncogenes may encode growth factors or their receptors, intracellular signaling molecules, and nuclear transcription factors (Table 28-2). Conversely, tumor suppressor genes, as their name implies, control or restrict cell growth and proliferation. Their inactivation, through various mechanisms, permits the dysregulated growth of cancer cells. Also important are the genes that regulate cell death. Their inactivation leads to resistance to apoptosis and allows the accumulation of additional genetic aberrations.

Cancer cells carry DNA that has point mutations, viral insertions, or chromosomal or gene amplifications, deletions, or rearrangements. Each of these aberrations can alter the context and process of normal cellular growth and differentiation. Although genomic instability is an inherent property of the evolutionary process and normal development, it is through genomic instability that the malignant transformation of a cell may arise. This inherent instability may be altered by inheritance or exposure to destabilizing factors in the environment. Point mutations may terminate protein translation, alter protein function, or change the regulatory target sequences that control gene expression. Chromosomal alterations create new genetic contexts within the genome and lead to the formation of novel proteins or to the dysregulation of genes displaced by aberrant events.

Genetic abnormalities associated with cancer may be detected in every cell in the body or only in the tumor cells. Constitutional or germline abnormalities either are inherited or occur de novo in the germ cells (sperm or oocyte). Interestingly, despite the presence of a genetic abnormality that might affect growth regulatory pathways in all cells, people are generally predisposed to the development of only certain tumor types. This selectivity highlights the observation that gene function contributes to growth or development only within a particular milieu or physiologic context. Specific tumors occur earlier and are more often bilateral when they result from germline mutations than when they result from sporadic or somatic alterations. Such is often the case in two pediatric malignancies, Wilms' tumor and retinoblastoma. These observations led Knudson[11] to propose a "two-hit" mechanism of carcinogenesis in which the first genetic defect, already present in the germline, must be complemented by an additional spontaneous mutation before a tumor can arise. In sporadic cancer, cellular transformation occurs only when two (or more) spontaneous mutations take place in the same cell.

Much more common, however, are somatically acquired chromosomal aberrations, which are confined to the malignant cells.

TABLE 28-2

Proto-oncogenes and Tumor Suppressor Genes in Pediatric Malignancies

Oncogene Family	Proto-oncogene	Chromosome Location	Tumors
Growth factors and receptors	ERBB2	17q21	Glioblastoma
	TRK	9q22	Neuroblastoma
Protein kinase	SRC	7p11	Rhabdomyosarcoma, Osteosarcoma, Ewing sarcoma
Signal transducers	H-RAS	11p15.1	Neuroblastoma
Transcription factors	c-MYC	18q24	Burkitt lymphoma
	MYCN	2p24	Neuroblastoma

Syndrome	Tumor Suppressor Gene	Chromosome Location	Tumors
Familial polyposis coli	APC	5q21	Intestinal polyposis, colorectal cancer
Familial retinoblastoma	RB	13q24	Retinoblastoma, osteosarcoma
WAGR*	WT1	11p13	Wilms' tumor
Denys-Drash†	WT1	11p13	Wilms' tumor
Beckwith-Weidemann‡	WT2 (?)	11p15	Wilms' tumor, hepatoblastoma, adrenal
Li-Fraumeni	TP53	17q13	Multiple (see text)
Neurofibromatosis type 1	NF1	17q11.2	Sarcomas, breast cancer
Neurofibromatosis type 2	NF2	22q12	Neurofibroma, neurofibrosarcoma, brain tumor
von Hippel-Lindau	VHL	3p25-26	Renal cell cancer, pheochromocytoma, retinal angioma, hemangioblastoma

*WAGR: Wilms' tumor, aniridia, genitourinary abnormalities, and mental retardation.
†Denys-Drash: Wilms' tumor, pseudohermaphroditism, mesangial sclerosis, renal failure.
‡Beckwith-Weidemann: multiple tumors, hemihypertrophy, macroglossia, hyperinsulinism.

These aberrations affect growth factors and their receptors, signal transducers, and transcription factors. The general types of chromosomal alterations associated with malignant transformation are shown in Figure 28-1. Although a low level of chromosomal instability exists in a normal population of cells, neoplastic transformation occurs only if these alterations affect a growth-regulating pathway and confer a growth advantage.

Abnormal DNA Content

Normal human cells contain two copies of each of 23 chromosomes; a normal diploid cell therefore has 46 chromosomes. Although cellular DNA content, or ploidy, is accurately determined by karyotypic analysis, it can be estimated by the much simpler method of flow cytometric analysis. Diploid cells have a DNA index of 1.0, whereas near-triploid (also termed *hyperdiploid*) cells have a DNA index ranging from 1.26 to 1.76. The majority (55%) of primary neuroblastoma cells are triploid or near triploid (e.g., having between 58 and 80 chromosomes), whereas the remainder are near diploid (35 to 57 chromosomes) or near tetraploid (81 to 103 chromosomes).[12] Neuroblastomas consisting of near-diploid or near-tetraploid cells usually have structural genetic abnormalities (e.g., chromosome 1p deletion and amplification of the *MYCN* oncogene), whereas those consisting of near-triploid cells are characterized by three almost complete haploid sets of chromosomes with few structural abnormalities.[13] Of importance, patients with near-triploid tumors typically have favorable clinical and biological prognostic factors and excellent survival rates compared with those who have near-diploid or near-tetraploid tumors.[14]

Chromosomal Translocations

Many pediatric cancers, specifically hematologic malignancies and soft tissue neoplasms, have recurrent, nonrandom abnormalities in chromosomal structure, typically chromosomal translocations (Table 28-3). The most common result of a nonrandom translocation is the fusion of two distinct genes from different chromosomes. The genes are typically fused within the reading frame and express a functional, chimeric protein product that has transcription factor or protein kinase activity. These fusion proteins contribute to tumorigenesis by activating genes or proteins involved in cell proliferation. For example, in Ewing sarcoma the consequence of the t(11;22)(q24;q12) translocation is a fusion of *EWS*, a transcription factor gene on chromosome 22, and *FLI-1*, a gene encoding a member of the ETS family of transcription factors on chromosome 11.[15] The resultant chimeric protein, which contains the DNA binding region of *FLI-1* and the transcription activation region of *EWS*, has greater transcriptional activity than does *EWS* alone.[16] The EWS–FLI-1 fusion transcript is detectable in approximately 90% of Ewing sarcomas. At least four other *EWS* fusions have been identified in Ewing sarcoma; fusion of *EWS* with *ERG* (another ETS family member) accounts for an additional 5% of cases.[17] Alveolar rhabdomyosarcomas have characteristic translocations between the long arm of chromosome 2 (75% of cases) or the short arm of chromosome 1 (10% of cases) and the long arm of chromosome 13. These translocations result in the fusion of *PAX3*

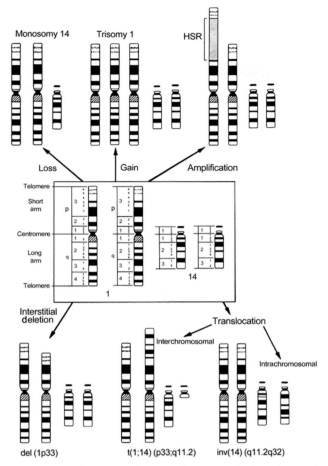

FIGURE 28-1 Spectrum of gross chromosomal aberrations using chromosomes 1 and 14 as examples. HSR, homogeneously staining regions. (From Look AT, Kirsch IR: Molecular basis of childhood cancer. In Pizzo PA, Poplack DG [eds]: Principles and Practices of Pediatric Oncology. Philadelphia, Lippincott-Raven, 1997, p 38.)

TABLE 28-3

Common, Recurrent Translocations in Soft Tissue Tumors

Tumor	Genetic Abnormality	Fusion Transcript
Ewing sarcoma/primitive neuroectodermal tumor	t(11;22)(q24;q12)	FLI1-EWS
	t(21;22)(q22;q12)	ERG-EWS
	t(7;22)(p22;q12)	ETV1-EWS
	t(17;22)(q12;q12)	E1AF-EWS
	t(2;22)(q33;q12)	FEV-EWS
Desmoplastic small round cell tumor	t(11;22)(p13;q12)	WT1-EWS
	t(11;22)(q24;q12)	FLI1-EWS
Synovial sarcoma	t(X;18)(p11.23; q11)	SSX1-SYT
	t(X;18)(p11.21; q11)	SSX2-SYT
Alveolar rhabdomyosarcoma	t(2;13)(q35;q14)	PAX3-FKHR
	t(1;13)(p36;q14)	PAX7-FKHR
Malignant melanoma of soft part (clear cell sarcoma)	t(12;22)(q13;q12)	ATF1-EWS
Myxoid liposarcoma	t(12;16)(q13;p11)	CHOP-TLS(FUS)
	t(12;22)(q13;q12)	CHOP-EWS
Extraskeletal myxoid chondrosarcoma	t(9;22)(q22;q12)	CHN-EWS
Dermatofibrosarcoma protuberans and giant cell fibroblastoma	t(17;22)(q22;q13)	COL1A1-PDGFB
Congenital fibrosarcoma and mesoblastic nephroma	t(12;15)(p13;q25)	ETV6-NTRK3
Lipoblastoma	t(3;8)(q12;q11.2)	?
	t(7;8)(q31;q13)	?

From Davidoff AM, Hill DA: Molecular genetic aspects of solid tumors in childhood. Semin Pediatr Surg 2001;10:106-118.

(at 2q35) or *PAX7* (at 1p36) with *FKHR*, a gene encoding a member of the forkhead family of transcription factors.[18] The *EWS-FLI-1* and *PAX7-FKHR* fusions appear to confer a better prognosis for patients with Ewing sarcoma and alveolar rhabdomyosarcoma, respectively.[19,20] Translocations that generate chimeric proteins with increased transcriptional activity also characterize desmoplastic small round cell tumor,[21] myxoid liposarcoma,[22] extraskeletal myxoid chrondrosarcoma,[23] malignant melanoma of soft parts,[24] synovial sarcoma,[25] congenital fibrosarcoma,[26] cellular mesoblastic nephroma,[27] and dermatofibrosarcoma protuberans.[28]

Proto-oncogene Activation

Proto-oncogenes are commonly activated in transformed cells by point mutations or gene amplification. The classical example of proto-oncogene activation by a point mutation involves the cellular proto-oncogene *RAS*. RAS-family proteins are associated with the inner, cytoplasmic surface of the plasma membrane and function as intermediates in signal transduction pathways that regulate cell proliferation. Point mutations in *RAS* result in constitutive activation of the RAS protein and therefore the continuous activation of the RAS signal transduction pathway. Activation of RAS appears to be

involved in the pathogenesis of a small percentage of pediatric malignancies, including leukemia and a variety of solid tumors.

Gene amplification (i.e., selective replication of DNA sequences) enables a tumor cell to increase the expression of crucial genes whose products are ordinarily tightly controlled. The amplified DNA sequences, or amplicons, may be maintained episomally (i.e., extrachromosomally) as double minutes-paired chromatin bodies lacking a centromere or as intrachromosomal, homogeneously staining regions. In about one third of neuroblastomas, for example, the transcription factor and proto-oncogene *MYCN* is amplified. The *MYCN* copy number in neuroblastoma cells can be amplified 5-fold to 500-fold and is usually consistent among primary and metastatic sites and at different times during tumor evolution and treatment.[29] This consistency suggests that *MYCN* amplification is an early event in the pathogenesis of neuroblastoma. Because gene amplification is usually associated with advanced stages of disease, rapid tumor progression, and poor outcome, it is a powerful prognostic indicator.[30,31] The cell surface receptor gene *ERBB2* is another proto-oncogene that is commonly overexpressed because of gene amplification, an event that occurs in breast cancer, osteosarcoma, and Wilms' tumor.[32]

Inactivation of Tumor Suppressor Genes

Tumor suppressor genes, or antioncogenes, provide negative control of cell proliferation. Loss of function of the proteins encoded by these genes, through deletion or mutational inactivation of the gene, liberates the cell from growth constraints and contributes to malignant transformation. The cumulative effect of genetic lesions that activate proto-oncogenes or inactivate tumor suppressor genes is a breakdown in the balance between cell proliferation and cell loss because of differentiation or apoptosis. Such imbalance results in clonal overgrowth of a specific cell lineage. The first tumor suppressor gene to be recognized was the retinoblastoma susceptibility gene *RB*. This gene encodes a nuclear phosphoprotein that acts as a "gatekeeper" of the cell cycle. *RB* normally permits cell-cycle-progression through the G_1 phase when it is phosphorylated, but it prevents cell division when it is unphosphorylated. Inactivating deletions or point mutations of *RB* cause the protein to lose its regulatory capacity. The nuclear phosphoprotein gene *TP53* has also been recognized as an important tumor suppressor gene, perhaps the most commonly altered gene in all human cancers. Inactivating mutations of the *TP53* gene also cause the TP53 protein to lose its ability to regulate the cell cycle. The *TP53* gene is frequently inactivated in solid tumors of childhood, including osteosarcoma, rhabdomyosarcoma, brain tumors, anaplastic Wilms' tumor, and a subset of chemotherapy-resistant neuroblastoma.[33–35] In addition, heritable cancer-associated changes in the *TP53* tumor suppressor gene occur in families with Li-Fraumeni syndrome, an autosomal dominant predisposition for rhabdomyosarcoma, other soft tissue and bone sarcomas, premenopausal breast cancer, brain tumors, and adrenocortical carcinomas.[36] Other tumor suppressor genes include Wilms' tumor 1 *(WT1)*, neurofibromatosis 1 *(NF1)*, and von Hippel-Lindau *(VHL)*. Additional tumor suppressor genes are presumed to exist but have not been definitively identified.

Epigenetic Alterations

As stated previously, the hallmark of cancer is dysregulated gene expression. However, not only do genetic factors influence gene expression but epigenetic factors do as well, with these factors being at least as important as genetic changes in their contribution to the pathogenesis of cancer. Epigenetic alterations are defined as those heritable changes in gene expression that do not result from direct changes in DNA sequence. Mechanisms of epigenetic regulation most commonly include DNA methylation and modification of histones, although the contribution of microRNAs (miRNA), a class of noncoding RNAs, is becoming increasingly recognized.

DNA Methylation   DNA methylation is a reversible process that involves methylation of the fifth position of cytosine within CpG dinucleotides present in DNA. These dinucleotides are usually in the promoter regions of genes; methylation of these sites typically causes gene silencing, thereby preventing expression of the encoded proteins. This process is part of the normal mechanism for imprinting, X-chromosome inactivation, and generally keeping large areas of genomic DNA silent, but it may also contribute to the pathogenesis of cancer by silencing tumor suppressor genes. However, both abnormal hypomethylation and hypermethylation states exist in human tumors, resulting in both dysregulated expression and silencing, respectively, of affected genes. These modifications of the nucleotide backbone of human DNA are becoming increasingly recognized in human cancer, both for their frequency and importance. For example, promoter

methylation resulting in silencing of caspase 8, a protein involved in apoptosis, likely contributes to the pathogenesis of *MYCN*-amplified neuroblastoma[37] as well as Ewing sarcoma.[23]

Histone Modification   Histones are the proteins that give structure to DNA and, together with the DNA, form the major components of chromatin. The functions of histones are to package DNA into a smaller volume to fit in the cell, to strengthen the DNA to allow replication, and to serve as a mechanism to control gene expression. Alterations in histones can mediate changes in chromatin structure. The compacted form of DNA, termed heterochromatin, is largely inaccessible to transcription factors and therefore genes in the affected regions are silent. Other modifications of histones can cause DNA to take a more open or extended configuration (euchromatin), allowing for gene transcription. The N-terminal tails of histones can be modified by a number of different processes including methylation and acetylation, mediated by histone acetyl transferases (HAT) and deacetylases (HDAC), and histone methyltransferases (HMT). Each of these processes alters histone function, which, in turn, alters the structure of chromatin and therefore the accessibility of DNA to transcription factors. Methylation of the DNA itself can also effect changes in chromatin structure.

MicroRNA   As stated above, miRNAs are a group of small, regulatory noncoding RNAs that appear to function in gene regulation. These miRNAs are single-stranded RNA fragments of 21 to 23 nucleotides that are complementary to encoding mRNAs.[25] Their function is to down-regulate expression of target mRNAs; it is estimated that miRNAs regulate the expression of about 30% of all human genes.[38] These miRNAs regulate gene expression primarily by incorporating into silencing machinery called RNA-induced silencing complexes (RISC). MiRNAs are involved in a number of fundamental biological processes, including development, differentiation, cell-cycle regulation, and senescence. However, broad analyses of miRNA expression levels have demonstrated that many miRNAs are dysregulated in a variety of different cancer types, including neuroblastoma and other pediatric tumors,[39] frequently losing their function as gene silencers/tumor suppressors. The activity of miRNAs, like gene expression, is also under epigenetic regulation.

METASTASIS

Metastasis is the spread of cancer cells from a primary tumor to distant sites and is the hallmark of malignancy. The development of tumor metastases is the main cause of treatment failure and a significant contributing factor to morbidity and mortality resulting from cancer. Although the dissemination of tumor cells through the circulation is probably a frequent occurrence, the establishment of metastatic disease is a very inefficient process. It requires several events, including the entry of the neoplastic cells into the blood or lymphatic system, the survival of those cells in the circulation, their avoidance of immune surveillance, their invasion of foreign (heterotopic) tissues, and the establishment of a blood supply to permit expansion of the tumor at the distant site. Simple, dysregulated cell growth is not sufficient for tumor invasion and metastasis. Many tumors progress through distinct stages that can be identified by histopathologic examination, including hyperplasia, dysplasia, carcinoma in situ, invasive cancer, and disseminated cancer. Genetic analysis of these different stages of tumor progression suggests that uncontrolled growth results from progressive alteration in cellular oncogenes and inactivation of tumor suppressor genes, but these genetic changes driving tumorigenicity are clearly distinct from those that determine the metastatic phenotype.

Histologically, invasive carcinoma is characterized by a lack of basement membrane around an expanding mass of tumor cells. Matrix proteolysis appears to be a key part of the mechanism of invasion by tumor cells, which must be able to move through connective tissue barriers, such as the basement membrane, to spread from their site of origin. The proteases involved in this process include the matrix metalloproteinases and their tissue inhibitors. The local environment of the target organ may profoundly influence the growth potential of extravasated tumor cells.[40] The various cell surface receptors that mediate interactions between tumor cells and between tumor cells and the extracellular matrix include cadherins, integrins (transmembrane proteins formed by the noncovalent association of alpha and beta subunits), and CD44, a transmembrane glycoprotein involved in cell adhesion to hyaluronan.[41] Tumor cells must decrease their adhesiveness to escape from the primary tumor, but at later stages of metastasis, the same tumor cells need to increase their adhesiveness during arrest and intravasation to distant sites.

ANGIOGENESIS

Angiogenesis is the biological process of new blood vessel formation. This complex, invasive process involves multiple steps, including proteolytic degradation of the extracellular matrix surrounding existing blood vessels, chemotactic migration and proliferation of endothelial cells, the organization of these endothelial cells into tubules, the establishment of a lumen that serves as a conduit between the circulation and an expanding mass of tumor cells, and functional maturation of the newly formed blood vessel.[42,43] Angiogenesis involves the coordinated activity of a wide variety of molecules, including growth factors, extracellular matrix proteins, adhesion receptors, and proteolytic enzymes. Under physiologic conditions, the vascular endothelium is quiescent and has a very low rate of cell division, such that only 0.01% of endothelial cells are dividing.[42–44] However, in response to hormonal cues or hypoxic or ischemic conditions, the endothelial cells can be activated to migrate, proliferate rapidly, and create tubules with lumens.

Angiogenesis occurs as part of such normal physiologic activities as wound healing, inflammation, the female reproductive cycle, and embryonic development. In these processes, angiogenesis is tightly and predictably regulated. However, angiogenesis can also be involved in the progression of several pathologic processes in which there is a loss of regulatory control, resulting in persistent growth of new blood vessels. Such unabated neovascularization occurs in rheumatoid arthritis, inflammatory bowel disease, hemangiomas of childhood, ocular neovascularization, and the growth and spread of tumors.[45]

Compelling data indicate that tumor-associated neovascularization is required for tumor growth, invasion, and metastasis.[46–49] A tumor in the prevascular phase (i.e., before new blood vessels have developed) can grow to only a limited size, approximately 2 to 3 mm^3. At this point, rapid cell proliferation is balanced by equally rapid cell death by apoptosis, and a nonexpanding tumor mass results. The switch to an angiogenic phenotype with tumor neovascularization results in a decrease in the rate of apoptosis, thereby shifting the balance to cell proliferation and tumor growth.[50,51] This decrease in apoptosis occurs, in part, because the increased perfusion resulting from neovascularization permits improved nutrient and metabolite exchange. In addition, the proliferating endothelium may supply, in a paracrine manner, a variety of factors that promote tumor growth, such as IGF-I and IGF-II.[52]

In experimental models, increased tumor vascularization correlates with increased tumor growth, whereas restriction of neovascularization limits tumor growth. Clinically, the onset of neovascularization in many human tumors is temporally associated with increased tumor growth,[53] and high levels of angiogenic factors are commonly detected in blood and urine from patients with advanced malignancies.[107] In addition, the number and density of new microvessels within primary tumors have been shown to correlate with the likelihood of metastasis, as well as the overall prognosis for patients with a wide variety of neoplasms, including pediatric tumors such as neuroblastoma and Wilms' tumor.[54,55]

Molecular Diagnostics

The explosion of information about the human genome has led not only to an improved understanding of the molecular genetic basis of tumorigenesis but also to the development of a new discipline: the translation of these molecular events into diagnostic assays. The field of molecular diagnostics has developed from the need to identify abnormalities of gene or chromosome structure in patient tissues and as a means of supporting standard histopathologic and immunohistochemical diagnostic methods. In most instances, the result of genetic testing confirms light microscopic- and immunohistochemistry-based diagnosis. In some instances, however (e.g., primitive, malignant, small round cell tumor; poorly differentiated synovial sarcoma; lipoblastic tumor), molecular analysis is required to make a definitive diagnosis.

The molecular genetic methods most commonly used to analyze patient tumor material include direct metaphase cytogenetics or karyotyping, fluorescence in situ hybridization (FISH), and reverse transcriptase polymerase chain reaction (RT-PCR). Additional methods, such as comparative genomic hybridization, loss of heterozygosity analysis, and complementary DNA (cDNA) microarray analysis, may eventually become part of the routine diagnostic repertoire but are currently used as research tools at referral centers and academic institutions. Each standard method is summarized in Table 28-4. As with any method, molecular genetic assays have advantages and disadvantages, and it is important to understand and recognize their limitations.

The value of molecular genetic analysis of patient tissue is not limited to aiding histopathologic diagnosis. Many of the most important markers provide prognostic information as well. *MYCN* amplification in neuroblastomas,[13] for example, is strongly associated with biologically aggressive behavior. Amplification of this gene can be detected by routine

TABLE 28-4

Comparison of the Cytogenetic and Molecular Methods Routinely Used as Aids in Pathologic Diagnosis of Soft Tissue Tumors

Method	Purpose	Advantages	Disadvantages
Cytogenetics	Low resolution analysis of metaphase chromosomes of cells grown in culture	Does not require a priori knowledge of genetic abnormalities Available in most diagnostic centers	Requires fresh, sterile tumor tissue for growth in culture Low sensitivity; will only detect large structural abnormalities No histologic correlation Slow and technically demanding (takes up to several weeks to perform)
In situ hybridization	Detection of translocations, amplifications, and gene deletions by hybridization of nucleic acid probes to specific DNA or mRNA sequences	Can be applied to chromosomal preparations as well as cytologic specimens, touch preparations, and paraffin sections Morphologic correlation is possible Multiple probes can be assayed at the same time Rapid (usually only requires 2 days)	Cannot detect small deletions or point mutations Interpretation can be difficult, especially with formalin-fixed, paraffin-embedded material Only a limited number of specific nucleic acid probes are available commercially
PCR and RT-PCR	Extremely sensitive detection of DNA sequences and mRNA transcripts for the demonstration of fusion genes, point mutations, and polymorphisms	Highest sensitivity and specificity of all the molecular diagnostic techniques DNA sequencing of PCR products can confirm result and provide additional information Requires minimal tissue Versatile; can be applied to fresh tissue as well as formalin-fixed, paraffin-embedded tissue Morphologic correlation is possible The presence of normal tissue will usually not affect test results Rapid (usually requires 3-5 days)	Formalin-fixation diminishes sensitivity Combinatorial variability within fusion gene partners requires appropriate redundant primer design to avoid false-negative test results Extreme sensitivity requires exacting laboratory technique to avoid false-positive test results

From Davidoff AM, Hill DA: Molecular genetic aspects of solid tumors in childhood. Semin Pediatr Surg 10: 2001;106-118.
PCR, polymerase chain reaction; RT-PCR, reverse transcriptase polymerase chain reaction.

metaphase cytogenetics or by FISH, and current neuroblastoma protocols include the presence or absence of *MYCN* amplification in their stratification schema. Some fusion gene variants are also thought to influence prognosis. In initial studies, two examples noted to confer relatively favorable prognoses are the type 1 variant fusion of *EWS-FLI1* in Ewing sarcoma or primitive neuroectodermal tumor[20] and the *PAX7-FKHR* fusion in alveolar rhabdomyosarcoma.[19]

New technologies are emerging that permit accurate, high-throughput analysis or profiling of tumor tissue: Gene expression can be analyzed by using RNA microarrays, and proteins by using proteomics. These approaches identify a unique fingerprint of a given tumor that can provide diagnostic or prognostic information. Proteomic analysis can also identify unique proteins in patients' serum or urine; such a profile can be used for early tumor detection, to distinguish risk categories, and to monitor for recurrence. Additional types of "omics" that are currently being used to evaluate tumor or patient specimens include transcriptomics (RNA and gene expression), metabolomics (metabolites and metabolic networks), and pharmacogenomics (how genetics affects host drug responses). Information from each of these areas of investigation provides an increasingly precise and unique perspective on the biology, clinical behavior, and responsiveness to specific therapeutic interventions of individual patient tumors. It is through these analyses that personalized therapy is likely to be realized. In addition, it is anticipated that with the identification of new, critical components of oncogenesis and tumor progression will come new "druggable" targets for cancer therapy. Drugs that act on these targets will not only be effective anticancer agents but, because of their specificity, will also have a broader therapeutic window, thereby improving safety and minimizing toxicity.

Childhood Cancer and Heredity

Advances in molecular genetic techniques have also improved our understanding of cancer predisposition syndromes. Constitutional gene mutations that are hereditary (i.e., passed from parent to child) or nonhereditary (i.e., de novo mutations in the sperm or oocyte before fertilization) contribute to an estimated 10% to 15% of pediatric cancers.[56] Constitutional chromosomal abnormalities are the result of an abnormal number or structural rearrangement of the normal 46 chromosomes and may be associated with a predisposition to cancer. Examples are the predisposition to leukemia seen with trisomy 21 (Down syndrome) and to germ cell tumors with Klinefelter syndrome (47XXY). Structural chromosomal abnormalities include interstitial deletions resulting in the constitutional loss of one or more genes.

Wilms' tumors may be sporadic, familial, or associated with specific genetic disorders or recognizable syndromes. A better understanding of the molecular basis of Wilms' tumor has been achieved largely through the study of the latter two types of tumors. The WAGR syndrome (Wilms' tumor, aniridia, genitourinary abnormalities, and mental retardation) provides an easily recognizable phenotype for grouping children likely to have a common genetic abnormality. Constitutional deletions from chromosome 11p13 are consistent in children with

WAGR syndrome[57] and also occur in approximately 35% of those with sporadic Wilms' tumor.[58] A study of a large series of patients identified the gene deleted from chromosome 11p13 as *WT1*.[59] This gene encodes a nuclear transcription factor that is essential for normal kidney and gonadal development[60] and appears to act as a tumor suppressor, but its precise role is unclear at this time. Aniridia in patients with WAGR syndrome is thought to occur after the loss of one copy of the *PAX6* gene located close to *WT1* on chromosome 11.[61] Denys-Drash syndrome, which is characterized by a very high risk of Wilms' tumor, pseudohermaphroditism, and mesangial sclerosis leading to early renal failure, is associated with germline mutations in the DNA binding domain of *WT1*.[62] The mutated WT1 protein appears to function by a dominant negative effect. Only 6% to 18% of sporadic Wilms' tumors have *WT1* mutations.[62,63]

In another subset of patients with Wilms' tumor, there is loss of genetic material in a region distal to the *WT1* locus toward the telomeric end of chromosome 11 (11p15).[39] It has therefore been suggested that there is a second Wilms' tumor susceptibility gene, tentatively named *WT2*, in 11p15. Loss of heterozygosity at this locus has also been described in patients with Beckwith-Wiedemann syndrome, a congenital overgrowth syndrome characterized by numerous growth abnormalities as well as a predisposition to a variety of malignancies, including Wilms' tumor.[64]

Neurofibromatosis type 1 (NF1) is one of the most common genetic disorders. The NF1 protein normally inhibits the proto-oncogene *RAS*, but in patients with NF1, mutation of one copy of the gene combined with deletion of the other permits uncontrolled RAS pathway activation. These patients are then susceptible to myelogenous disorders, benign tumors, gliomas, and malignant peripheral nerve sheath tumors. An inherited predisposition to pediatric cancers is also associated with Li-Fraumeni syndrome (which results from mutations which inactivate the *TP53* gene and put patients at risk for osteosarcoma, rhabdomyosarcoma, adrenocortical carcinoma, and brain tumors, among other tumors), familial retinoblastoma (which results from mutations that inactivate the *RB* gene and put patients at risk for osteosarcoma as well as retinoblastoma), familial adenomatous polyposis, and multiple endocrine neoplasia syndromes. Another set of inherited risk factors is represented by mutations of DNA repair genes (so-called caretaker genes), as seen in xeroderma pigmentosa and ataxia-telangiectasia.[65] Understanding these complex syndromes and their pathogenesis is important in efforts to screen for early detection and, possibly, for prophylactic therapy.

Recently, the germline mutation associated with hereditary neuroblastoma has been identified as activating mutations in the tyrosine kinase domain of the anaplastic lymphoma kinase (*ALK*) oncogene on the long arm of chromosome 2 (2p23).[66] Further molecular studies have revealed that common genetic variation at chromosome bands 6p22[1] and 2q35[67] are associated with susceptibility to, and likely contribute to the etiology of, high-risk neuroblastoma, providing the first evidence that childhood cancers also arise because of complex interactions of polymorphic variants. Finally, the same group has also shown that inherited copy number variation at chromosome 1q21.1 is associated with neuroblastoma, implicating a neuroblastoma breakpoint family gene in early neuroblastoma genesis.[68]

Genetic Screening

Along with an increased understanding of the molecular basis of hereditary childhood cancer has come the opportunity to identify children who are at high risk of malignancy and, in some cases, to intervene before the cancer develops or when it is still curable. Two examples include familial adenomatous polyposis and familial thyroid cancer.

Familial adenomatous polyposis is an autosomal dominant inherited disease in which hundreds to thousands of adenomatous intestinal polyps develop during the second and third decades of life. Mutations of the adenomatous polyposis coli (*APC*) gene on chromosome 5q21 occur in approximately 80% of kindreds of persons who have the disease.[69,70] These mutations initiate the adenomatous process by allowing clonal expansion of individual cells that, over time, acquire additional genetic abnormalities that lead to the development of invasive colorectal carcinoma.[71] Prophylactic colectomy is recommended for patients with this germline mutation, although the most appropriate timing for this intervention in children with familial adenomatous polyposis is controversial. These patients are also at increased risk of hepatoblastoma.[72]

Medullary thyroid carcinoma (MTC) is a rare malignancy that may occur sporadically or as part of two syndromes: multiple endocrine neoplasia (type 2A or 2B) syndrome or familial MTC syndrome. In children, MTC is much more likely to occur in association with a familial syndrome. An apparently 100% association between germline *RET* mutations[73] and MTC guides the recommendation for prophylactic thyroidectomy in affected patients. There is no effective adjuvant treatment other than surgery for MTC, highlighting the need for early intervention. Patients with germline *RET* mutations should also be screened for pheochromocytoma, which occurs in 50% of patients with multiple endocrine neoplasia type 2A, and hyperparathyroidism, which occurs in 35% of such patients, although these entities generally arise in older patients beyond the pediatric age range.[74] In addition, patients who are at risk for MTC or have newly diagnosed MTC, as well as their relatives, should be screened for the germline *RET* mutation so that appropriate surgical and genetic counseling can be given.

General Principles of Chemotherapy

Cytotoxic agents were first noted to be effective in the treatment of cancer in the 1960s, after alkylating agents, such as nitrogen mustard gas, used during World War II, were observed to cause bone marrow hypoplasia. Chemotherapy is now an integral part of nearly all cancer treatment regimens. The overriding goal of cancer chemotherapy is to maximize the tumoricidal effect (efficacy) while minimizing adverse side effects (toxicity). This goal can be difficult to achieve, however, because the dose at which tumor cells are affected is often similar to the dose that affects normal proliferating cells, such as those in the bone marrow and gastrointestinal tract. Despite the early promise of chemotherapy and the observation that most tumor types are initially sensitive to chemotherapy, often exquisitely so, the successful use of chemotherapy is often thwarted by two factors: the development of resistance to the agent and the agent's toxicity to normal tissues. Nevertheless, chemotherapy remains an integral part of therapy when used as an adjunct to treat localized disease or as the main component to treat disseminated or advanced disease.

A number of principles and terms are essential to the understanding of chemotherapy as a therapeutic anticancer modality. Adjuvant chemotherapy refers to the use of chemotherapy for systemic treatment following local control generally by surgical resection or radiation therapy of a clinically localized primary tumor. The goal in this setting is to eliminate disease that is not detectable by standard investigative means at or beyond the primary tumor's site. Neoadjuvant chemotherapy refers to chemotherapy delivered before local therapeutic modalities, generally in an effort to improve their efficacy; to treat micrometastatic disease as early as possible, when distant tumors are smallest; or to achieve both of these aims. Induction chemotherapy refers to the use of chemotherapeutic agents as the primary treatment for advanced disease. In general, chemotherapy given to children with solid tumors and metastatic disease at the time of first examination has a less than 40% chance of effecting long-term, disease-free survival. Exceptions include Wilms' tumor with favorable histologic features, germ cell tumors, and paratesticular rhabdomyosarcoma, but most children with metastatic disease are at high risk of disease recurrence or progression. Combination chemotherapy refers to the use of multiple agents, which generally have different mechanisms of action and nonoverlapping toxicities, that provide effective, synergistic antitumor activity and minimal side effects.

The mechanisms of action and side effects of commonly used agents are listed in Table 28-5. Alkylating agents interfere with cell growth by covalently cross-linking DNA and are not cell-cycle specific. Antitumor antibiotics intercalate into the double helix of DNA and break the DNA strands. Antimetabolites are truly cell-cycle specific, because they interfere with the use of normal substrates for DNA and RNA synthesis, such as purines and thymidine. The plant alkaloids can inhibit microtubule function (vinca alkaloids, taxanes) or DNA topoisomerases (camptothecins inhibit topoisomerase I; epipodophyllotoxins inhibit topoisomerase II), and these actions also lead to breaks in DNA strands. Topoisomerases are a class of enzymes that alter the supercoiling of double-stranded DNA. They act by transiently cutting one (topoisomerase I) or both (topoisomerase II) strands of the DNA to relax the DNA coil and extend the molecule. The regulation of DNA supercoiling is essential to DNA transcription and replication, when the DNA helix must unwind to permit the proper function of the enzymatic machinery involved in these processes. Thus topoisomerases maintain the transcription and replication of DNA.

The common toxic effects of these agents are also listed in Table 28-5. Most toxicity associated with chemotherapy is reversible and resolves with cessation of treatment. However, some chemotherapeutic agents may have lifelong effects. Of particular concern is that certain drugs can lead to a second malignancy. Most notable is the development of leukemia after the administration of the epipodophyllotoxins and cyclophosphamide.[75]

Finally, understanding the metabolism of chemotherapeutic agents is important. Certain agents require metabolism at a specific site or organ for their activation or are eliminated from the body by a specific organ (see Table 28-5). The processes of activation and elimination require normal organ function (e.g., the liver for cyclophosphamide); therefore children with liver or kidney failure may not be able to receive certain agents.

RISK STRATIFICATION

Major advances in the variety of chemotherapeutic agents and dosing strategies used to treat pediatric cancers in the past 30 years are reflected in improved patient survival rates. Regimen toxicity (including late effects, which are particularly important in the pediatric population) and therapeutic resistance are the two main hurdles preventing further advancement. As more information about diagnostically and prognostically useful genetic markers becomes available, therapeutic strategies will change accordingly. With molecular profiling, patients can be categorized to receive a particular treatment on the basis of not only the tumor's histopathologic and staging characteristics but also its genetic composition. Some patients whose tumors show a more aggressive biological profile may require dose intensification to increase their chances of survival. Patients whose tumors do not have an aggressive biological profile may benefit from the lower toxicity of less intensive therapy. Such an approach may allow the maintenance of high survival rates while minimizing long-term complications of therapy in these patient populations.

The paradigm for the use of different therapeutic intensities on the basis of risk stratification drives the management of pediatric neuroblastoma. There is increasing evidence that the molecular features of neuroblastoma are highly predictive of its clinical behavior. Most current studies of the treatment of neuroblastoma are based on risk groups that take into account both clinical and biological variables. The most important clinical variables appear to be age and stage at diagnosis, and the most powerful biological factors appear to be *MYCN* status, ploidy (for patients younger than 1 year), and histopathologic classification. These variables currently define the Children's Oncology Group risk strata and therapeutic approach, which are further refined by determining whether there is 1p/11q LOH. At one extreme, patients with low-risk disease are treated with surgery alone; at the other extreme, patients at high risk for relapse are treated with intensive multimodality therapy that includes multiagent dose-intensive chemotherapy, radiation therapy, and stem cell transplantation. Other factors, such as 17q gain, caspase 8 inactivation, and TRKA/B expression, are currently being evaluated and may help further refine risk assessment in the future. The management of other solid pediatric tumors is also shifting to risk-defined treatment. For example, the current protocol for the management of patients with Wilms' tumor includes risk stratification and therapy adjustment based on molecular analysis of the primary tumor for 16q and 1p deletions.

TARGETED THERAPY

Another major change in the approach to the treatment of cancer has been the concept of targeted therapy. Until recently, the development of anticancer agents was based on the empirical screening of a large variety of cytotoxic compounds without particular regard to disease specificity or mechanism of action. Now, one of the most exciting prospects for improving the

TABLE 28-5

Common Chemotherapeutic Agents

Class of Drug	Agent	Synonyms	Brand Name	Mechanism of Action	Common Toxic Effects	Site of Activation	Method of Elimination	Susceptible Solid Tumors
Alkylating agents	Carboplatin	CBCDCA	Paraplatin	Platination, intrastrand and interstrand DNA cross-linking	A, H, M (esp. thrombocytopenia), N/V		R	BT, GCT, NBL, STS
	Cisplatin	CDDC	Platinol	Platination, intrastrand and interstrand DNA cross-linking	A, N/V, R (significant), ototoxicity, neuropathy		R	BT, GCT, NBL, OS
	Cyclophosphamide	CTX	Cytoxan	Alkylation, intrastrand and interstrand DNA cross-linking	A, N/V, SIADH, M, R, cardiac, cystitis	Liver	H, R (minor)	Broad, BMT
	Ifosfamide	IFOS	Ifex	Alkylation, intrastrand and interstrand DNA cross-linking	A, CNS, N/V, M, R, cardiac, cystitis	Liver	H, R (minor)	Broad
	Dacarbazine		DTIC	Methylation	H, N/V, M, hepatic vein thrombosis	Liver	R	NBL, STS
	Temozolomide	TMZ	Temodar	Methylation	CNS, N/V, M	Spontaneous	R	BT
	Nitrogen Mustard	Mechlorethamine	Mustargen	Alkylation, intrastrand and interstrand DNA cross-linking	A, M (significant), N/V, mucositis, vesicant, phlebitis, diarrhea		Spontaneous hydrolysis	BT
	Melphalan	L-PAM	Alkeran	Alkylation, intrastrand and interstrand DNA, cross-linking	M, N/V, mucositis, diarrhea		Spontaneous hydrolysis	NBL, RMS, BMT
	Busulfan		Busulfex	Alkylation, intrastrand and interstrand DNA cross-linking	A, H, M, N/V, P, mucositis		R	BMT
Antimetabolites	Cytarabine	Ara-C	Cytosar	Inhibits DNA polymerase, incorporated into DNA	M, N/V, diarrhea, CNS	Target cell	Biotransformation	Limited
	Fluorouracil	5-FU	(Several)	Inhibits thymidine synthesis, incorporated into DNA/RNA	CNS, N/V, M, cardiac, diarrhea, mucositis, skin, ocular	Target cell	Biotransformation, renal (minor)	GI carcinomas, liver tumors

Continued

TABLE 28-5

Common Chemotherapeutic Agents—cont'd

Class of Drug	Agent	Synonyms	Brand Name	Mechanism of Action	Common Toxic Effects	Site of Activation	Method of Elimination	Susceptible Solid Tumors
	Mercaptopurine	6-MP	Purinethol	Inhibits thymidine synthesis, incorporated into DNA/RNA	H, M, mucositis	Target cell	Biotransformation, renal (minor)	Limited
	Methotrexate	MTX	Trexall	Blocks folate metabolism, inhibits purine synthesis	CNS, H, M, R, mucositis, skin		R, H (minor)	OS
Antibiotics	Dactinomycin	Actinomycin-D	Cosmegen	DNA intercalation, strand breaks	A, H, M, N/V, mucositis, vesicant		H	RMS, Wilms'
	Bleomycin	BLEO	Blenoxane	DNA intercalation, strand breaks	P, skin, mucositis		H, R	GCT
Anthracyclines	Daunomycin	Daunorubicin	Cerubidine	DNA intercalation, strand breaks, free radical formation	A, M, N/V, cardiac, diarrhea, vesicant, potentiate XRT reaction		H	Limited
	Adriamycin	Doxorubicin	Adriamycin	DNA intercalation, strand breaks, free radical formation	A, M, N/V, cardiac, diarrhea, mucositis, vesicant, potentiate XRT reaction		H	Broad
Plant Alkaloids Epipodophyllotoxins	Etoposide	VP-16	VePesid	Topoisomerase II inhibitor, DNA strand breaks	A, M, N/V, mucositis, neuropathy, diarrhea		R	Broad
	Teniposide	VM-26	Vumon	Topoisomerase II inhibitor, DNA strand breaks	A, M, N/V, mucositis, neuropathy, diarrhea		Degraded	Broad
Vinca alkaloids	Vincristine	VCR	Oncovin	Inhibits tubulin polymerization, blocks mitosis	A, SIADH, neuropathy, vesicant		H	Broad

Drug	Abbrev	Trade name	Mechanism	Toxicity			Tumors
Vinblastine	VLB	Velban	Inhibits tubulin polymerization, blocks mitosis	A, M, mucositis, vesicant		H	GCT
Taxanes							
Paclitaxel		Taxol	Interferes with microtubule formation	A, M, cardiac, mucositis, CNS, neuropathy			
Docetaxel		Taxotere	Interferes with microtubule formation	A, neutropenia, cardiac, mucositis, CNS, neuropathy			
Camptothecins							
Topotecan	TPT	Hycamtin	Topoisomerase I inhibitor, DNA strand breaks	A, H, M, N/V, mucositis, diarrhea, skin		R	NBL, RMS
Irinotecan	CPT-11	Camptosar	Topoisomerase I inhibitor, DNA strand breaks	A, H, M, N/V, diarrhea	H, GI	H, R (minor)	NBL, RMS
L-Asparaginase	Erwinia	Elspar	L-Asparagine depletion, inhibits protein synthesis	CNS, H, coagulopathy, pancreatitis, anaphylaxis		degraded	Limited
Corticosteroids			Nuclear receptor–mediated apoptosis	avascular necrosis, hyperglycemia, hypertension, myopathy, pancreatitis, peptic ulcers, psychosis, salt imbalance, weight gain	H	H, R (minor)	BT
Miscellaneous							

Toxic effects: A, alopecia; CNS, central nervous system toxicity; H, hepatotoxicity; M, myelosuppression; N/V, nausea and vomiting; P, pulmonary toxicity; R, renal toxicity; SIADH, syndrome of inappropriate antidiuretic hormone; XRT, x-ray therapy.
Solid tumors: BMT, conditioning for bone marrow transplantation; BT, brain tumor; EWS, Ewing sarcoma; GCT, germ cell tumors; NBL, neuroblastoma; OS, osteosarcoma; RMS, rhabdomyosarcoma; STS, soft tissue sarcoma; W, Wilms' tumor.

therapeutic index of anticancer agents, as well as overcoming the problem of therapy resistance, involves targeted therapy. As the molecular bases for the phenotypes of specific malignancies are being elucidated, potential new targets for therapy are becoming more clearly defined. The characterization of pathways that define malignant transformation and progression has focused new agent development on key pathways involved in the crucial processes of cell-cycle regulation, receptor signaling, differentiation, apoptosis, invasion, migration, and angiogenesis, which may be perturbed in malignant tissues. Information about the molecular profile of a given tumor type can be assembled from a variety of emerging methods, including immunohistochemistry, FISH, RT-PCR, cDNA microarray analysis, and proteomics. This information can then be used to develop new drugs designed to counter the molecular abnormalities of the neoplastic cells. For example, blocking oncogene function or restoring suppressor gene activity may provide tumor-specific therapy. In addition, molecular profiling may lead to the development of drugs designed to induce differentiation of tumor cells, block dysregulated growth pathways, or reactivate silenced apoptotic pathways.

Some agents target alterations in the regulation of cell proliferation. Trastuzumab (Herceptin) is a monoclonal antibody that binds to the cell surface growth factor receptor ERBB2 with high affinity and acts as an antiproliferative agent when used to treat ERBB2-overexpressing cancer cells.[76] Pediatric high-grade gliomas that overexpress EGFR may be amenable to a similar therapeutic agent, gefitinib (Iressa), a small-molecule inhibitor of EGFR (ERBB1).[77] In addition, small-molecule tyrosine kinase inhibitors, such as imatinib (Gleevec), designed to block aberrantly expressed growth-promoting tyrosine kinases—ABL in chronic myelogenous leukemia[78] and c-KIT in gastrointestinal stromal tumors[79]—are being evaluated in clinical trials. Imatinib may also be useful in treating pediatric tumors in which PDGF signaling plays a role in tumor cell survival and growth. Also of potential therapeutic utility are small-molecule inhibitors that recognize antigenic determinants on unique fusion peptides or one of the fusion peptide partners in tumors that have chromosomal translocations (e.g., sarcomas). Tumors that depend on autocrine pathways for growth (e.g., overproduction of IGF-II in rhabdomyosarcoma or PDGF in dermatofibrosarcoma protuberans) may be sensitive to receptor blocking mediators (e.g., antibodies to the IGF-II or PDGFR).

Other agents target alteration of the cell death and differentiation pathways. Caspase 8 is a cysteine protease that regulates programmed cell death, but in tumors such as neuroblastoma, DNA methylation and gene deletion combine to mediate the complete inactivation of caspase 8, almost always in association with *MYCN* amplification.[80] Caspase 8-deficient tumor cells are resistant to apoptosis mediated by death receptors and doxorubicin; this resistance suggests that caspase 8 may be acting as a tumor suppressor. However, brief exposure of caspase 8–deficient cells to demethylating agents, such as decitabine, or to low levels of interferon gamma can lead to the reexpression of caspase 8 and the resensitization of the cells to chemotherapeutic drug-induced apoptosis. Histone deacetylase also seems to have a role in gene silencing associated with resistance to apoptosis[81]; therefore histone deacetylase inhibitors, such as suberoylanilide hydroxamic acid (SAHA), are also being tested for the treatment of certain

pediatric malignancies. Finally, cells with alterations in programmed cell death as a result of the persistence or reactivation of telomerase activity, which somatic cells normally lose after birth, can be targeted by various telomerase inhibitors.

Several methods of targeting tumor cell differentiation are being used for the treatment of neuroblastoma. Treatment with 13-cis-retinoic acid, a vitamin A derivative that signals through receptors that mediate transcription of different sets of genes of cell differentiation, including *HOX* genes, is now standard of care for maintenance therapy in patients with high-risk neuroblastoma.[82,83] Also, different neurotrophin receptor pathways appear to mediate the signal for both cellular differentiation and malignant transformation of sympathetic neuroblasts to neuroblastoma cells. Neurotrophins are expressed in a wide variety of neuronal tissues and other tissues that require innervation. They stimulate the survival, maturation, and differentiation of neurons and exhibit a developmentally regulated pattern of expression.[84,85] Neurotrophins and their TRK tyrosine kinase receptors are particularly important in the development of the sympathetic nervous system and have been implicated in the pathogenesis of neuroblastoma. Three receptor–ligand pairs have been identified: TRKA, TRKB, and TRKC, which are the primary receptors for nerve growth factor, brain-derived neurotrophic factor (BDNF), and neurotrophin 3 (NT-3), respectively.[84] TRKA appears to mediate the differentiation of developing neurons or neuroblastoma in the presence of nerve growth factor ligand and to mediate apoptosis in the absence of nerve growth factor.[85] Conversely, the TRKB-BDNF pathway appears to promote neuroblastoma cell survival through autocrine or paracrine signaling, especially in *MYCN*-amplified tumors.[86] TRKC is expressed in approximately 25% of neuroblastomas and is strongly associated with TRKA expression.[87] Studies are ongoing to test agonists of TRKA in an attempt to induce cellular differentiation. Conversely, blocking the TRKB-BDNF signaling pathway with TRK-specific tyrosine kinase inhibitors such as CEP-751 may induce apoptosis by blocking crucial survival pathways.[66,86] This targeted approach has the attractive potential for increased specificity and lower toxicity than conventional cytotoxic chemotherapy.

Inhibition of Angiogenesis

Because tumor growth and spread appear to be dependent on angiogenesis, inhibition of angiogenesis is a logical anticancer strategy. This approach is particularly appealing for several reasons. First, despite the extreme molecular and phenotypic heterogeneity of human cancer, it is likely that most, if not all, tumor types, including hematologic malignancies, require neovascularization to achieve their full malignant phenotype. Therefore antiangiogenic therapy may have broad applicability for the treatment of cancer. Second, the endothelial cells in a tumor's new blood vessels, although rapidly proliferating, are inherently normal and mutate slowly. They are therefore unlikely to evolve a phenotype that is insensitive to an angiogenesis inhibitor, unlike the rapidly proliferating tumor cells, which undergo spontaneous mutation at a high rate and can readily generate drug-resistant clones. Finally, because the new blood vessels induced by a tumor are sufficiently distinct from established vessels to permit highly specific targeting,[88,89] angiogenesis inhibitors should have a high therapeutic index and minimal toxicity. The combination of conventional chemotherapeutic agents with angiogenesis inhibitors appears to be particularly effective.

The first clinical demonstration that an angiogenesis inhibitor could cause regression of a tumor came with the use of interferon alpha in a patient treated for life-threatening pulmonary hemangioma.[90] An increasing number of natural and synthetic inhibitors of angiogenesis, which inhibit different effectors of angiogenesis, have since been identified, and many of these agents have been tested in clinical trials. Examples include drugs that directly inhibit endothelial cells, such as thalidomide and combretastatin; drugs that block activators of angiogenesis, such as bevacizumab (Avastin), a recombinant humanized anti-VEGF antibody, or "VEGF trap"; drugs that inhibit endothelium-specific survival signaling, such as Vitaxin, an anti-integrin antibody; and drugs with nonspecific mechanisms of action, such as celecoxib and interleukin-12 (IL-12).

Immunotherapy

The immune system has evolved as a powerful means to detect and eliminate molecules or pathogens that are recognized as "foreign." However, because tumors arise from host cells, they are generally relatively weakly immunogenic. In addition, malignant cells have evolved several mechanisms that allow them to elude the immune system. These mechanisms include the ability to down-regulate the cell surface major histocompatibility complex molecules required for activation of many of the immune effector cells, to produce immunosuppressive factors, and to variably express different proteins that might otherwise serve as targets for the immune system in a process known as antigenic drift. Nevertheless, because of the large number of mutations and chromosomal aberrations occurring in cancer cells, which results in the expression of abnormal, new, or otherwise silenced proteins, it is likely that most, if not all, cancers contain unique tumor-associated antigens that can be recognized by the immune system. Examples include the fusion proteins commonly found in pediatric sarcomas and the embryonic neuroectodermal antigens that continue to be produced by neuroblastomas.

Recruiting the immune system to help eradicate tumor cells is an attractive approach for several reasons. First, circulating cells of the immune system have ready access to even occult sites of tumor cells. Second, the immune system has powerful effector cells capable of effectively and efficiently destroying and eradicating targets, including neoplastic cells. Initial efforts to recruit the immune system to recognize and destroy tumor cells by using cytotoxic effector mechanisms that are T-cell dependent or independent focused on recombinant cytokines. Cytokines act by directly stimulating the immune system[66] or by rendering the target tumor cells more immunogenic.

Neuroblastoma has been a popular target for immunotherapy in the pediatric population. Although a particular neuroblastoma antigen has not been defined, murine monoclonal antibodies have been raised against the ganglioside GD2, a predominant antigen on the surface of neuroblastoma cells. These antibodies elicited therapeutic responses,[37,91] but with substantial toxicity, particularly neuropathic pain.[92] Because the induction of antibody-dependent cell-mediated cytotoxicity with anti-GD2 antibodies is enhanced by cytokines, such

as granulocyte-macrophage colony-stimulating factor[92] and interleukin-2 (IL-2),[93] current antineuroblastoma antibody trials are evaluating the use of a humanized, chimeric anti-GD2 antibody (ch14.18) with these cytokines and a fusion protein (hu14.18:IL2) that consists of the humanized 14.18 antibody linked genetically to human recombinant IL-2. A recently completed randomized phase III trial using ch14.18 alternating with cycles of granulocyte-macrophage colony-stimulating factor (GM-CSF) or interleukin-2 added to maintenance therapy of cis-retinoic acid demonstrated a significant improvement in 2-year event-free survival for those who received immunotherapy in addition to retinoic acid.[94]

General Principles of Radiation Therapy

Radiation therapy is one of the three primary modalities used to manage pediatric cancers in the modern era. Radiation therapy is delivered to an estimated 2000 or more children per year for the primary treatment of tumor types as diverse as leukemia, brain tumors, sarcomas, Hodgkin disease, neuroblastoma, and Wilms' tumor.[95] Delivery of radiation therapy in the pediatric setting differs from that in the adult setting because of the balance between curative therapy and an anticipated long life span during which long-term morbidity may result from the therapy.

CLINICAL CONSIDERATIONS

Radiation therapy for the management of pediatric cancer is most frequently combined with surgery and chemotherapy as part of a multidisciplinary treatment plan. The sensitive nature of pediatric tumors requires the use of a combined therapy approach to maximize tumor control while minimizing the long-term side effects of treatment. Radiation may be delivered preoperatively, postoperatively (relative to a definitive surgical resection), or definitively without surgical management. Systemic therapy may also be integrated into this management approach.

Definitive Irradiation

Definitive radiation therapy is an alternative local approach to surgical resection of primary solid tumors. It is often the only local therapeutic approach for children and adolescents with leukemia or lymphoma.[96,97] Definitive radiation therapy for rhabdomyosarcoma has been used as an alternative to surgical resection, which has potentially greater morbidity; it has achieved high rates of local tumor control while allowing preservation of function.[38] The Ewing sarcoma family of tumors may also be considered candidates for definitive radiation therapy as an alternative to surgery. With careful patient selection, excellent local tumor control rates can be maintained while reducing or avoiding the morbidity associated with difficult surgical resections.[98,99]

Preoperative Irradiation

Targeting of a localized tumor is straightforward in the preoperative setting; the tumor has clearly defined margins undisturbed by a surgical procedure. The volume of normal, healthy tissues receiving high doses of radiation may be reduced, because the areas at risk for disease involvement can be better defined. Preoperative radiation therapy has been used rarely in the management of Wilms' tumor to decrease the chance of tumor rupture[100] and in the management of nonrhabdomyosarcoma soft tissue sarcoma and Ewing sarcoma to facilitate surgical resection.[101,102] One of the limitations may be the slightly higher incidence of postoperative wound complications noted in the sarcoma population.[102]

Postoperative Irradiation

Postoperative radiation therapy combined with surgical resection is the most common application of adjuvant radiation treatment in the United States. Despite some degree of difficulty in targeting, a postoperative approach allows a review of tumor histology from the complete tumor specimen, including identification of the tumor margins and the response to any previous therapy. Wound healing complications appear to be reduced with this approach, and the radiation dose can be more accurately tailored to the pathologic findings after primary resection.

Interactions of Chemotherapy and Radiation

Most children's cancers are managed with systemic chemotherapy. In children receiving radiation therapy as well as systemic chemotherapy, issues of enhanced local efficacy and enhanced local or regional toxicity need to be considered. Solid tumors that are frequently treated with combined chemotherapy and radiation therapy include Wilms' tumor, neuroblastoma, and sarcomas. These tumors are subdivided into those in which chemotherapy is given concomitantly with radiation therapy[103,104] and those in which it is given sequentially, before or after radiation therapy.[83,100,105] When delivering radiation therapy concurrently with or temporally close to a course of chemotherapy, several issues must be considered.

Chemotherapeutic Enhancement of Local Irradiation

Several systemic chemotherapeutic agents used against pediatric tumors may enhance the efficacy of radiation therapy when delivered concomitantly. Cisplatin, 5-fluorouracil, mitomycin C, and gemcitabine, for example, are well-known radiation sensitizers.[106–108] Concomitant delivery of any of these drugs with radiation therapy may require that they be administered at a dose and schedule different from those typically used when the drugs are delivered alone. Despite the potential of increased toxicity, significant improvements in local tumor control have been shown in randomized studies of concomitant drug and radiation therapy.[106,107]

Irradiation Combined with Agents Having Limited or No Sensitizing Effect

In the management of pediatric malignancies, radiation is often combined with systemic therapy not to increase its local efficacy but to allow continued delivery of systemic therapy to control micrometastatic or metastatic disease. Agents combined with radiation therapy in this setting are common in the management of pediatric sarcomas and include ifosfamide and etoposide, which are delivered concurrently with radiation therapy for Ewing sarcoma, and vincristine and cyclophosphamide, which are delivered concurrently with radiation therapy for rhabdomyosarcoma.[103,104] Although local toxicity may be increased by such an approach, this risk is often outweighed by the benefit of continuously delivered systemic therapy, particularly in tumors associated with a high incidence of micrometastatic disease.

Agents That Increase Radiation Toxicity

Several agents significantly increase the local toxicity of radiation. For this reason, these agents are not given concomitantly with irradiation and are often withheld for a period after the completion of radiation therapy. The two most notable agents are doxorubicin and actinomycin, both of which can induce significant skin and mucosal toxicity when delivered concurrently with radiation therapy.[38,109] The camptothecins (including irinotecan and topotecan) also potentiate mucosal toxicity when delivered concurrently with radiation therapy.[110,111] Although this increase in toxicity suggests a possible increase in local efficacy, this benefit has not been noted with current treatment approaches and chemotherapeutic dosing guidelines. For this reason, these agents are avoided during the delivery of radiation therapy and are withheld for 2 to 6 weeks after the completion of treatment.

The current era of systemic therapy continues to broaden with the availability of many new agents that target molecular pathways. It is important to consider the possibility of new toxicities when combining novel agents with a known therapy such as radiation.

FRACTIONATION OF RADIATION THERAPY

Conventional, external beam irradiation is delivered in a fractionated form. Fractionation implies daily doses of radiation delivered 5 days per week and amounting to the prescribed dose for a particular tumor type. Radiation delivered once daily at a fraction size between 1.5 and 2.0 Gy on 5 days per week is considered "conventionally" fractionated. This daily dose is well tolerated by normal tissues adjacent to the tumor and appears to effect local tumor control in many tumor systems. Though adult malignancies may be treated with increased doses per fraction to overcome the radioresistance of many carcinomas (termed hypofractionation), nearly all the literature describing radiation therapy, its efficacy, and its toxicity in children is based on conventional fractionation.

RADIATION THERAPY TREATMENT TECHNIQUES

Traditional Radiation Therapy

The planning and delivery of traditional, or conventional, radiation therapy are based on nonvolumetric imaging studies (i.e., conventional radiographs). Patients are positioned in a manner that allows the orientation of radiation beams from the conventional directions: anterior, posterior, and lateral. Limitations of this approach are related to the ability of conventional radiographs to accurately convey the location of tumor-bearing tissue. Although treatment beams are oriented around the tumor, adjacent normal tissues also receive high doses of radiation. Depending on the accuracy of the delineation of adjacent normal tissues on radiographs, the dose to those tissues may not be known. Radiation is delivered by a photon beam generated by a linear accelerator.

Focal Radiation Therapy

Focal radiation therapy comprises a group of techniques that deliver radiation to a defined volume, usually delineated by computed tomography (CT) or magnetic resonance imaging (MRI). Relatively low doses may be incidentally delivered to surrounding normal tissues. Radiation therapy may be described as image guided when four criteria are met: (1) three-dimensional imaging data (CT or MRI) are acquired with the patient in the treatment position; (2) imaging data are used to delineate and reconstruct the tumor volume and normal tissues in three dimensions; (3) radiation beams can be freely oriented in three dimensions in the planning and delivery processes, and structures traversed by the beam can be visualized with the eye of the beam; and (4) the distribution of doses received by the tumor volume and any normal tissue is computable on a point-by-point basis in three-dimensional space. Several different methods of delivering image-guided photon radiation are currently in use and are discussed here.

Conformal Radiation Therapy

The delivery of three-dimensional conformal radiation therapy allows specific targeting of tumor volumes on the basis of imaging studies performed with the patient in the treatment position. This method of delivery uses multiple fields or portals, with each beam aperture shaped to the tumor volume, and it is performed daily. Beam modifiers, such as wedges, are used to conform the radiation beam to the tumor and to ensure that the tumor volume receives a homogeneous dose. Conformal radiation therapy has been intensively studied in adults with head and neck cancer, lung cancer, and prostate cancer and has been shown to excel when the target volume is convex and crucial structures do not invaginate the target volume. Available data demonstrate that it has low toxicity despite high doses of radiation to the target volume.[112]

Intensity-Modulated Radiation Therapy

Intensity-modulated radiation therapy is another method of delivering external beam radiation that requires imaging of the patient in the treatment position and delineation of target volumes and normal tissues. Radiation is delivered to the target as multiple small fields that do not encompass the entire target volume but collectively deliver the prescribed daily dose. Intensity-modulated radiation therapy differs from conformal radiation therapy in that it (1) increases the complexity and time required for the planning and delivery of treatment, (2) increases the amount of quality-assurance work required before treatment is delivered, (3) increases dose heterogeneity within the target volume such that some intralesional areas receive a relatively high dose, and (4) can be used to treat concave targets while sparing crucial structures that invaginate the target volume. The last point holds promise for better protecting normal tissue and reducing late toxic effects. Preliminary data from adult patients given intensity-modulated radiation therapy demonstrate its potential for reducing treatment toxicity when applied to pediatric brain tumors and other adult tumors.[113]

Proton Beam Radiation Therapy

Proton radiation therapy and other approaches using heavy charged particles have been investigated at a limited number of centers. The primary benefit of therapy with proton or other heavy charged particle beams is the capacity to end the radiation beam at a specific and controllable depth. This may allow the protection of healthy, normal tissues directly adjacent to tumor-bearing tissues.[114] However, the use of proton therapy has been limited because of the expense of constructing a suitable treatment facility. Several new facilities have opened in the United States, and pediatric malignancies are always noted as one of the tumors systems on which the centers will focus their research efforts. With appropriately designed studies and comparisons with current state-of-the-art focal radiation therapy delivered with photon beams, a determination of the potential benefits of this treatment modality may be made.

Brachytherapy

Brachytherapy is a method of delivering radiation to a tumor or tumor bed by placing radioactive sources within or adjacent to the target volume, usually at the time of surgical resection and under direct vision. Planning of the dose to be delivered to the target volume is accomplished after resection and may use CT or MRI studies; the appropriate strength of the radioactive source is determined prospectively. Sources commonly used in children include iridium 192 and iodine 125. Brachytherapy may consist of either low dose-rate treatments (approximately 40 to 80 cGy per hour) or high dose-rate treatments (approximately 60 to 100 cGy per minute). Low dose-rate treatments are delivered during a period of days, often while the patient remains hospitalized, whereas high dose-rate treatments are divided into fractions and delivered on several days during 1 to 2 weeks. The primary advantage of brachytherapy is that a radiation source can be placed into or adjacent to the tumor, often at the time of resection. Preoperative planning and cooperation between the surgical and radiation oncology teams are necessary to ensure the appropriate and accurate implementation of brachytherapy. Nonrhabdomyosarcoma soft tissue sarcomas and some rhabdomyosarcomas are the pediatric tumors most commonly treated with brachytherapy.[115,116] Most other pediatric solid tumors are not amenable to brachytherapy, however, because of the tumor's behavior (e.g., radioresistance) or its anatomic location (e.g., retroperitoneal).

Intraoperative radiation therapy has been used intermittently after resection in the management of localized tumors.[117] Although of limited availability in the United States, intraoperative radiation therapy has the distinct advantage of allowing the operative tumor bed to be visible in the operating theater while radiation is delivered, thereby enhancing the accuracy of delivery and providing the opportunity to displace or temporarily move mobile crucial structures (e.g., bowel, bladder) from the field of delivery. The primary limitation of intraoperative radiation therapy is that it can deliver only a single fraction of radiation, usually in the 10 to 20 Gy range. Radiation tolerances of normal tissues that cannot be removed from the treatment field must be respected and may limit the ability to deliver an effective treatment dose.

PALLIATIVE RADIATION THERAPY

Despite substantial success in the management of pediatric cancer, some children experience disease recurrence and ultimately die from their malignancy. Palliative radiation therapy is often a valid intervention for these patients.[118] The ultimate goal of a palliative approach is to maintain quality of life for patients who will not survive their disease by palliating their symptoms while minimizing the number of disruptive interventions they must undergo. Painful sites of disease, particularly those with bony involvement, and symptoms resulting from compression of vital structures, including spinal cord, peripheral nerves, and respiratory tract are often palliated with radiation. A palliative course of therapy is highly individualized, and its success or failure depends on the histologic diagnosis, previous therapy, duration of symptoms, and symptom(s) being treated.

ACUTE AND LATE TOXICITIES OF RADIATION THERAPY

The treatment-related effects of radiation therapy, both acute and chronic, are well described for pediatric and adult patients, but unfortunately, their incidence and relation to the dose and volume of treatment are poorly characterized.[119] Historically, treatment-related effects have been classified as acute or late; an arbitrary time point of 90 days after the completion of treatment defines the division between the two classifications. Current guidelines for assessing adverse events related to treatment no longer recognize this arbitrary distinction, but the use of early and late time points is instructive in the discussion of radiation-related effects. Essentially all such effects originate from within the confines of the treatment beams, usually the high-dose regions of treatment. The most common early and late treatment-related effects arising from radiation are listed in Table 28-6. Despite the arbitrary nature of the division into early and late effects, this classification distinguishes effects from which the patient is likely to recover completely from those that are likely to be permanent. Early treatment-related effects, if managed appropriately, will resolve as normal, healthy tissues adjacent to the tumor-bearing tissues, gradually recovering from the effects of radiation. The period of recovery can range from days to months, but the patient is often left with minimal sequelae. Treatment-related effects that are observed later, after the completion of radiation therapy, are more likely to be chronic or permanent. They appear to be related to the normal healing response of healthy irradiated tissue, resulting in the formation of an unwanted effect such as fibrosis. Many late treatment effects can be managed but are not reversible. For children receiving curative therapy, long-term effects are a primary concern and are best managed with a preventive approach. Some of the long-term effects of treatment in children should be ameliorated by limiting the volume of normal tissue irradiated at high doses and by implementing approaches that minimize the radiation dose to adjacent healthy tissues.

TABLE 28-6

Radiation-Related Adverse Events in Children and the Associated Radiation Doses

Organ/Site	Acute	Chronic	Dose Relation	Reference
Skin	Erythema Desquamation	Atrophy Hyperpigmentation	Doses more than 40 Gy increase incidence of moist desquamation	121
Subcutaneous tissue	Edema	Fibrosis	—	
Mucosa	Mucositis	Ulceration	—	
Central nervous system	Headache Edema	Necrosis Myelitis Decline in cognition	2.5% incidence of brainstem necrosis with doses of 59.4 Gy Reduction in intelligence quotient with younger age and doses of radiation to the supratentorial brain more than 30 Gy	122, 123
Eye	Conjunctivitis	Cataract Retinopathy Dry eye	43% incidence of cataract with doses of total body irradiation of $\geq$ 12 Gy	124
Thyroid	—	Hypothyroidism	20% incidence at $\leq$ 21 Gy; 61% incidence when > 21 Gy	125
Heart	—	Pericarditis Myocarditis Valvular disease	2.5% incidence of pericarditis at doses of 30 Gy to the heart	126, 127
Lung	Pneumonitis	Pulmonary fibrosis	Increasing risk of pneumonitis with volume of lung receiving 24 Gy and bleomycin chemotherapy	128
Bowel	Nausea Diarrhea	Necrosis	—	
Kidney	—	Nephritis Renal insufficiency	—	
Bladder	Dysuria Urgency Frequency	Hemorrhagic cystitis	—	
Muscle	Edema	Fibrosis Hypoplasia	Acute edema in adjacent muscle receiving doses above 40 Gy Volume of jaw muscles > 40 Gy increases chronic fibrosis	129
Bone	—	Hypoplasia Fracture Premature physis closure	Increasing reduction in growth above 35 Gy, but effects seen even at 23.4 Gy Weight-bearing bones in patient radiated for sarcomas have a 29% incidence of fracture	130–132

General Principles of Stem Cell Transplantation

Infusion or transplantation of hematopoietic cells capable of reconstituting the hematopoietic system is used in two broad instances. First, hematopoietic stem cell transplantation (HSCT) can be used to replace missing or abnormal components of a defective hematopoietic system. Second, HSCT can be used to reconstitute elements of the hematopoietic system destroyed by intensive chemotherapy or radiation therapy for solid tumors or disorders of the hematopoietic system itself. The transplanted cells can be the patient's own (i.e., autologous), in which case the cells are obtained before the administration of myelosuppressive therapy, or they may come from a donor (i.e., allogeneic) who is generally a histocompatibility leukocyte antigen (HLA)–identical sibling, a mismatched family member, or a partially matched unrelated donor. The latter two circumstances require immunosuppressive and graft engineering strategies to permit successful engraftment and avoid graft-versus-host disease. Hematopoietic progenitor cells are usually obtained from the bone marrow or peripheral blood. They are the crucial component of the transplant, because they are capable of self-renewal and therefore long-term production of cells of the various hematopoietic lineages. Occasionally, when available, banked umbilical cord blood may be used as the source of hematopoietic stem cells (HSCs). In general, although autologous cells are the safest to use for HSCT, they may be contaminated with tumor cells. Graft-versus-host disease, which may occur with allogeneic HSCT, can be life threatening, but a modest graft-versus-host reaction may be beneficial if directed against the host's tumor cells.

Bone marrow is normally harvested from the posterior iliac crest to a total volume of 10 to 20 mL/kg body weight of the recipient. Peripheral blood stem cells are harvested after their mobilization with recombinant granulocyte colony-stimulating factor, given daily for up to a week before harvest. The exact nature of the crucial cellular component responsible for the reconstitution of the hematopoietic system is unknown, but the number of cells having the surface marker CD34 has been shown to be related to the rate of engraftment.[120] Before HSCT, the recipient receives a preparative (or "conditioning") chemotherapeutic regimen. This treatment serves several purposes, including killing residual tumor cells, providing immunosuppression for allogeneic HSCT, and providing "space" in the marrow into which transplanted HSCs can engraft. Before reinfusion, the HSC product may be manipulated ex vivo to enrich it for putative progenitor cells (e.g., CD34$^+$ or CD133$^+$ cells), using positive or negative selection methods to facilitate hematopoietic reconstitution; to remove donor T lymphocytes, thereby decreasing the risk of graft-versus-host disease in allogeneic HSCT; or to purge contaminating tumor cells from the product used in autologous HSCT.

Complications of HSCT can be significant. The most common early complication is infection, which results from the transient but profound immunosuppression of the patient, combined with the breakdown of mucosal barriers. Another common complication is veno-occlusive disease, which is characterized clinically by painful enlargement of the liver, jaundice, and fluid retention. Ultrasound examination shows reversal of flow in the portal vein. Liver biopsy samples show a classic histologic appearance of obliterated hepatic venules and necrosis of centrilobular hepatocytes. There is no specific treatment for this condition; only supportive care can be given, and mild or moderate veno-occlusive disease is self limited. Other acute complications of HSCT include graft-versus-host disease, a process mediated by donor T cells targeting host cells with antigenic disparities, and graft failure. Late complications include chronic graft-versus-host disease, endocrine insufficiency, secondary malignancies, growth failure, and other sequelae related to the use of total-body irradiation as part of some preparatory regimens. Nevertheless, despite the toxicity, HSCT is now an integral part of successful therapy for many high-risk malignancies in children.

Clinical Trials

As previously stated, the past 40 years have seen a significant increase in overall survival rates for children with cancer. This increase has been achieved through the development of new drugs and treatment approaches, improved supportive care, and better diagnostic modalities to permit earlier cancer detection. The benefits of these advances have been confirmed by carefully designed and analyzed clinical trials. Because childhood cancer is relatively rare, excellent organization and planning of these trials are essential. In the United States and other participating countries, clinical trials are largely conducted by the Children's Oncology Group, with smaller pilot studies being run by large individual institutions or small consortia.

Clinical trials are generally divided into three phases. Phase I studies are designed to evaluate the potential toxicity of a new diagnostic or therapeutic agent. Small numbers of patients are usually required for a phase I study, which typically uses a dose-escalating design in which cohorts of patients are observed for signs of toxicity before they advance to higher doses. The end point of this type of study is generally a determination of the safety of the agent or the maximum tolerated dose (or both). However, the increasing number of biologic reagents being introduced and tested may require a shift to the assessment of the optimal biologic dose. Enrollment in a phase I toxicity study is often restricted to patients whose disease has not responded to conventional, or standard-of-care, therapy. Phase II trials are conducted to determine whether a new agent or treatment approach is sufficiently efficacious to warrant further study. Phase II agents are often given to newly diagnosed patients before they begin or just after they complete standard therapy. The testing of new agents in an "upfront window" (i.e., before standard therapy) has been shown not to have an adverse effect on the efficacy of delayed standard therapy. Finally, phase III studies are designed to compare the efficacy of an experimental therapy with that of standard therapy. They are best done as prospective, randomized trials, but often, because of small patient numbers, a phase III study is done by comparing the efficacy of an experimental therapy with that of standard therapy given to historical control subjects. It is through such systematic assessment of the risks and benefits of new therapies that approaches are rejected or accepted as the new standard of care and the field of pediatric oncology is advanced.

Conclusion

Advances in molecular genetic research in the past 3 decades have led to an increased understanding of the genetic events in the pathogenesis and progression of human malignancies, including those of childhood. A number of pediatric malignancies serve as models for the molecular genetic approach to cancer. The pediatric experience highlights the utility of molecular analysis for a variety of purposes. Demonstration of tumor-specific translocations by cytogenetics, FISH, and RT-PCR confirms histopathologic diagnoses. Detection of chromosomal abnormalities, gene overexpression, and gene amplification is used in risk stratification and treatment planning. Elucidation of pathways involving tumor suppressor genes has increased our understanding of syndromes associated with cancer and has led the way for genetic screening and counseling and prophylactic surgical intervention. And in the near future, translation of the molecular profile of a given tumor will form the basis of a new therapeutic approach. Treatment will be tailored such that patients with biologically high-risk tumors receive intensified regimens to achieve a cure, whereas patients with biologically low-risk tumors may experience a cure and benefit from the lower toxicity of nonintensive therapy. Elucidation of the complex molecular pathways involved in tumorigenesis will also encourage the production of targeted anticancer agents with high specificity, efficacy, and therapeutic index.

The complete reference list is available online at www. expertconsult.com.

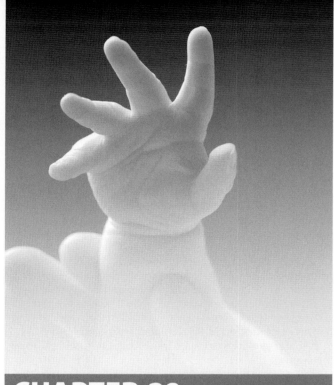

CHAPTER 29

Biopsy Techniques for Children with Cancer

James D. Geiger and Douglas C. Barnhart

The importance of biopsy techniques in the management of children with cancer has increased as the use of preoperative chemotherapy has become commonplace for many childhood cancers. Historically, definitive diagnosis was made at the time of surgical resection of the primary tumor. Currently, many children will undergo percutaneous, minimal access surgical, or open incisional biopsy rather than initial resection. Moreover, with increasing understanding of the molecular changes associated with these malignancies, definitive diagnosis can be accomplished with smaller specimens. This should allow a decrease in the morbidity associated with establishing the diagnosis of solid malignancies in children.

Ironically, this progression to less invasive biopsy has complicated rather than simplified the selection of technique in individual cases, as multiple factors must be considered. Percutaneous needle biopsy,[1,2] minimal access surgical biopsy,[3] and open biopsy have all been demonstrated to be effective in safely establishing initial diagnosis as well as verification of recurrent or metastatic disease. However, the success of these techniques is obviously dependent upon local institutional experience, which

must be considered in the selection. In addition, it is critical to realize that many of the advances in risk stratification and improved therapy of pediatric malignancies has been facilitated by the development of large accessible tumor banks and the associated biology studies. Without large biopsy specimens, these tumor banks and the development of research cell lines would not have been possible. For a number of tumors, including neuroblastoma and Wilms' tumor, collection of such specimens remains important to further our understanding of the disease.

Biopsies may be required in a variety of settings including primary diagnosis, determination of metastatic disease, and assessment for viable tumor in residual masses after therapy. Therefore a biopsy must be considered as a component of the overall plan of care and not simply as a surgical procedure. It is, therefore, essential that the surgeon have a thorough understanding of the therapeutic plan prior to performing a biopsy. This is well-illustrated in the current management of a child with a Wilms' tumor and a solitary pulmonary nodule. Standard therapy for a pulmonary metastasis is lung irradiation. It could, therefore, be important to histologically confirm this metastasis by excisional biopsy prior to proceeding. This approach is complicated, however, by a current Children's Oncology Group research question of whether children in whom the pulmonary lesions respond completely after 6 weeks of chemotherapy can be spared lung irradiation and more intensive chemotherapy. In this research protocol setting, resection of this solitary lesion would be contraindicated, because it would commit the child to lung irradiation and more intensive medical treatment.

Current pediatric oncology protocols use risk-stratified treatment regimens.[4] Information needed from biopsy specimens is disease specific. The surgeon must be knowledgeable about the stratification schema that will be used for multimodality therapy to select the biopsy method that will be least morbid and yet yield all essential information. This concept is demonstrated by considering two patients with abdominal masses suggestive of neuroblastoma with apparent bone marrow involvement as they would be treated under the current Children's Oncology Group schema. The first patient is less than 1 year of age. This patient's treatment group could be low, intermediate, or high risk. Risk group assignment will require MYC-N amplification status, Shimada histology status, and DNA ploidy to determine stratification. This will require sampling of the primary lesion with an adequate sample of the tumor to allow Shimada staging. In contrast, an older child with similar presentation would be classified as high risk, regardless of any of the previous factors. Therefore one could confirm the diagnosis and assign a risk group with bone marrow biopsy alone.[5] Clearly, knowledge of the multimodality therapy decision making is essential in selection of biopsy technique.

Handling of Specimens

Historically most diagnoses were made based on hematoxylin and eosin histology performed on permanent sections. This was supplemented by immunohistochemistry, which could similarly be performed on formalin fixed specimens. There has been extensive progress made in the molecular diagnosis of childhood malignancies, including recognition of genetic aberrations, which has both diagnostic and prognostic significance.[6–9] Techniques used to detect these changes include reverse transcriptase–polymerase chain reaction (rt-PCR),[10] fluorescence in situ hybridization (FISH), microarray analysis, and flow cytometry. Inappropriate specimen handling can preclude these analyses. For example, phenotypic classification of lymphoma cannot be performed using flow cytometry on formalin-fixed lymph nodes. Given the rapidly evolving field of molecular diagnosis, it is essential that the surgeon consult with the pathologist regarding specimen handling prior to performing the biopsy. Additionally, if the patient is eligible for a research protocol, care must be taken to assure the specimen is handled in accordance with the protocol requirements. This requires a coordinated effort by the surgeon, medical oncologist, and pathologist.

Percutaneous Needle Biopsy

Fine-needle aspiration was first introduced as a technique to obtain specimens for cytopathology by Grieg and Gray in 1904. Jereb and colleagues reported success with the use of needle biopsy for the diagnosis of pediatric solid tumors in 1978.[11] Subsequently, extensive experience from multiple institutions has confirmed the accuracy and safety of both needle aspiration and core needle biopsy techniques. The appeal of these techniques is that they both may provide diagnosis without requiring a significant delay in therapy and can be performed as outpatient procedures. Needle biopsies are often performed under either general anesthesia or sedation. In selected older children, some sites may be biopsied under local anesthesia alone.[12]

Percutaneous needle biopsies may be performed by palpation in the extremities and other superficial locations such as lymph nodes. However, deeper biopsies require guidance with either ultrasonography or CT scan. Ultrasonography that can be supplemented with Doppler mode allows clear identification of large vessels and other structures and provides real-time visualization as the needle is advanced.[13] Some core needle devices also deposit a small air bubble that allows verification of the site that was biopsied. CT scan, on the other hand, allows clear visualization of aerated lung and is not obscured by bowel gas.[14] It also allows measurement and planning of depth of biopsy.[1] Decision making regarding image guidance is made in conjunction with the radiologist, and ideally, biopsies should be performed with both modalities available if required.

Fine-Needle Aspiration Biopsy

Fine-needle aspiration biopsy (FNAB) holds the obvious appeal of being the least invasive of all biopsy techniques. It is typically performed using a 22- to 25-gauge needle with multiple passes into the lesion if necessary. Successful diagnosis using FNAB requires coordination with an experienced cytopathologist. To improve the diagnostic yield, the specimens should be examined immediately by the cytopathologist. Additional aspirations may be taken if initial samples are inadequate.[15] Large series with fine-needle aspirates in both children and adults have confirmed the safety of the technique.[16,17]

Historically, diagnosis using fine-needle aspiration was based primary on cytologic appearance with conventional stains and light microscopy. Successful diagnosis using FNAB is dependent upon the availability of an experienced cytopathologist. In adult patients with the higher prevalence of carcinomas, FNA is a popular method for confirming the presence of malignancy in suspicious lesions. Often, in these adult cases, a diagnosis of carcinoma and primary site are sufficient to make initial treatment decisions. However, given the fact that multimodality therapy is histiotype-specific in pediatric patients, FNAB has been used less frequently in children. Recent application of molecular techniques and electron microscopy to supplement light microscopy has increased the histiotype specificity of FNAB and may lead to increased application in pediatric solid malignancies.[18,19] FNAB has been used in several pediatric settings with sufficient data reported for consideration.

The use of FNAB in the evaluation of thyroid nodules in adults is well-established. Although thyroid nodules are less common in children, the techniques and interpretation of FNAB are similar to those used in adults.[20] Given the good degree of specificity, FNAB may be considered a standard component of evaluation of thyroid nodules in children.[21]

Another relatively straight forward application and interpretation of fine-needle aspirate biopsy is in the verification of metastatic or recurrent disease in the setting of a previously characterized primary tumor.[22] In this context, the verification of the presence of malignant cells may be sufficient to guide further clinical decisions. This least invasive biopsy method is particularly appealing in these patients who may already be immunologically or physiologically compromised.

There is a limited body of literature on the use of FNAB in the diagnosis of sarcomas. Osteosarcoma has been diagnosed by the use of fine-needle aspirates, with definitive diagnosis being obtained in 65% to 92% of patients. The technique is as accurate in children as it is in adults.[23] The use of FNAB in soft tissue tumors has been facilitated by the recognition of cytogenetic abnormalities and fusion proteins that are specific to these tumor types.[17,19,24] However, caution should be exercised in the use of FNAB in this setting, because the reported series come from a limited number of institutions with extensive experience in cytologic interpretation. The use of FNAB in diagnosing sarcoma has not gained widespread use.

Fine-needle aspiration has not been widely used for the diagnosis of small, round, blue cell tumors of childhood. However, with the increasing availability of ancillary studies, such as electron microscopy, immunocytochemistry, DNA ploidy, cytogenetics, and fluorescent in situ hybridization, its use may become more common.[25] Use of FNAB for the evaluation of head and neck masses in children has been reported to have good sensitivity and specificity.[26,27] The results of these series, however, should be interpreted with caution, because the majority of aspirates diagnosed as reactive lymphadenopathy and the number of new malignant diagnoses was small. In addition, false-negative FNAB diagnosis occurred frequently in patients ultimately diagnosed with lymphoma in other series (not specifically isolated to the head and neck).[15]

Core Needle Biopsy

The advantage of core needle biopsy versus fine-needle aspiration is that it provides a sample sufficient in size to allow histologic examination rather than only cytologic examination. In addition, it can provide sufficient tissue for molecular evaluation. Despite the widespread use of this technique in adults, its application in children has not been as common.

Various core needle devices may be used. These typically range in size from 14 to 18 gauge. These needles are designed so that a cutting sheath advances over the core of the needle to obtain a biopsy that is protected within the sheath as the needle is withdrawn. This cutting sheath may be advanced either manually (e.g., Tru-Cut, Baxter Travenol, Deerfield, Ill.) or by a spring-loaded firing system (e.g., Biopty, Bard Urological, Murray Hill, NJ) (Fig. 29-1). There are no data directly comparing the quality of specimens obtained with these two systems in pediatric malignancies. The faster deployment of the spring-loaded systems may result in less crush artifact, which

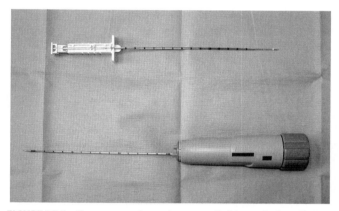

FIGURE 29-1   Two commonly used core needle biopsy devices. The upper device is a 14-gauge Tru-Cut needle (Allegiance, Cardinal Health). It is advanced into the region of interest, and then the inner needle is advanced. The outer sheath is manually advanced over the inner needle to obtain a core. The lower device is a 16-gauge Monopty biopsy device (Bard). It is spring-loaded and is activated after the tip is advanced into the region of interest. The spring-loaded mechanism automatically sequentially advances the obturator and the cannula.

has been demonstrated in pediatric kidney biopsies. Regardless of the system used, visual inspection of the core biopsy is necessary to verify adequate sampling. The number of passes required with a core needle is dependent upon the purpose of the biopsy and the consistency of the tissue being biopsied. For primary tumor diagnosis, multiple cores are typically required to obtain sufficient tissue for biological studies. Alternatively, in pulmonary lesions evaluated for metastatic disease, a single pass was usually sufficient in most series.

Several large series have demonstrated the utility of core needle biopsies in children. The larger, more recent series are summarized on Table 29-1. The three most common scenarios for which percutaneous biopsies in children with malignancies are used are diagnosis of primary tumors, evaluation for possible recurrent disease, and evaluation of pulmonary lesions.

Success with core needle biopsy has been demonstrated in a wide variety of anatomic locations. These include neck, mediastinum, lung, peritoneal cavity, liver, retroperitoneum, kidney, adrenal, pelvis, and extremities.[1,2,12,13,28] Core needle biopsies have been demonstrated to be effective in obtaining adequate tissue for both primary diagnoses and confirmation of recurrence in these series. In the largest series of pediatric oncologic core needle biopsies, multiple passes were typically performed (median = 6 and maximum = 17). With this repetitive sampling, adequate diagnostic tissue was obtained for histologic and biological studies, obviating the need for operative biopsy in a wide variety of pediatric cancers. No patients in these series suffered procedure-related deaths or required operative therapy for procedural complications.[28]

The other common use of percutaneous core biopsies in pediatric oncology patients is in the evaluation of pulmonary nodules. Pulmonary nodules can be biopsied under either CT scan[29] or ultrasound guidance, often determined by the size and location of the lesions.[30] These procedures may be performed under either sedation or general anesthesia with

TABLE 29-1

Series of Percutaneous Biopsies in Children

Author (Year)	Number of Children	Number of Biopsies (Total/Malignancy)	Method	Diagnostic Yield	Comments
Skoldenberg (2002)[13]	110	147/84	US-guided core biopsies of wide range of tumors for initial diagnosis and evaluation for recurrence	89%	
Hayes-Jordan (2003)[52]	32	35/23	US- or CT-guided core needle biopsies of pulmonary lesions under general anesthesia	80%	Patients with nondiagnostic biopsy underwent repeat core needle or thoracoscopic biopsy; 10% small pneumothorax or hemothorax—none required drainage
Cahill (2004)[29]	64	75/24	CT-guided core or FNAB of pulmonary lesions with sedation or general anesthesia	85%	One false negative for Ewing sarcoma; one tension pneumothorax required drainage
Fontalvo (2005)[30]	33	38/32	US-guided core needle of peripheral pulmonary lesions with general anesthesia and controlled ventilation	84%	Included small lesions (24% < 5 mm); 10% pneumothorax—none required drainage (series partially overlaps with Hayes-Jordan, 2003)
Garrett (2005)[28]		202/202	US-/CT- or fluoroscopic-guided core needle biopsies of wide range of tumors for initial diagnosis and evaluation for recurrence	93% overall 98% initial diagnosis 88% suspected recurrence	Multiple passes typically taken (median = 6); accomplished diagnosis, including biological studies without operative biopsies

CT, computed tomography; FNAB, fine-needle aspiration biopsy; US, ultrasonography.

controlled ventilation. Typically, general anesthesia would be used in younger children or in children with smaller or deeper pulmonary lesions. Current series report success in more than 80% of lesions, including lesions less than 1 cm in size. Surprisingly, pneumothoraces are relatively uncommon, occurring in only 10% of children. The majority of these are managed without placement of a thoracostomy tube.

Needle tract recurrence represents an oncologic complication specific to this biopsy technique. Estimates of this complication in adults vary widely, ranging from 3.4% in hepatocellular carcinoma[31] to 1:8500 in thoracic tumors.[32] Obviously, the incidence of this complication is influenced by several factors. Immunologic, chemotherapeutic, and radiotherapeutic effects will decrease the likelihood of needle tract recurrence. The larger needles used for core needle biopsies are associated with a greater risk than the fine needles used for aspiration.[33] The cases series cited previously report no needle track recurrences in children.

Minimal Access Surgery

Laparoscopy and thoracoscopy have become commonplace in general pediatric surgery, and both techniques are now used in cancer diagnosis and therapy. Gans and Berci first reported experience with multiple endoscopic techniques in children in 1971.[34] Interestingly, one of the chief applications for laparoscopy, which they advocated, was for guidance of biopsy of metastatic implants. Subsequently, the application of both laparoscopy and thoracoscopy has grown in the initial diagnostic technique for childhood malignancies and for the assessment of refractory or metastatic disease.

LAPAROSCOPY

Laparoscopy affords several advantages for the evaluation of the abdominal cavity in children with childhood cancer. First, it provides the opportunity to completely examine the peritoneal cavity. A systematic examination of all peritoneal surfaces can be performed. The entire length of the bowel may be examined along with mesenteric lymph nodes. Multiple biopsies can easily be obtained. The second chief advantage of laparoscopy is decreased physiologic stress in children who may already be critically ill. Finally, as in all minimally invasive procedures, postoperative pain is reduced and recovery is hastened.[35] The main disadvantages of laparoscopy are the limited ability to assess retroperitoneal structures and the loss of tactile evaluation of deep lesions.

Diagnostic laparoscopy with biopsy has been used in several settings in the management of children with solid malignancies.[3,35] Biopsies obtained using laparoscopic techniques have a high rate of success in yielding diagnostic tissue.[3,36] Laparoscopy allows the surgeon to obtain larger tissue samples than may be obtained with core needle biopsy. This is particularly relevant if larger samples are required for biological studies. In the initial diagnosis, laparoscopy aids in the identification of site of origin of large abdominal masses. Laparoscopy has been shown to be superior to computerized tomography in assessing intraperitoneal neoplasms and for the evaluation of ascites. For example, laparoscopy allows direct assessment of whether a pelvic mass arises from the ovary or bladder neck, which may be difficult to distinguish by

radiographic studies. Direct visualization with laparoscopy has been used to assess the resectability of hepatoblastoma. During the course of treatment, laparoscopy may be used to assess new metastatic disease or to assess initial tumor response as a second-look procedure.[3]

One area of concern with the use of laparoscopy in oncology has been the issue of port-site recurrence. There are relatively limited data on this issue in children. The Children's Cancer Group retrospective study of 85 children noted no port-site recurrences.[3] A survey of Japanese pediatric laparoscopic surgeons reported 85 laparoscopic and 44 thoracoscopic procedures with no port-site recurrences.[37] It should be noted, however, that 104 of these tumors were neuroblastomas, with many being detected by mass screening. The general applicability of this data may, therefore, be limited. A port-site metastasis has been reported in a child with Burkitt lymphoma.[38] Given the difference in tumor biology between adult adenocarcinomas and pediatric neoplasms, which often have a marked response to neoadjuvant therapy, it is difficult to draw conclusions from the adult literature. Certainly additional surveillance for this issue in pediatric tumors is merited.

Laparoscopy in children is typically performed under general anesthesia to facilitate tolerance of pneumoperitoneum. The only absolute contraindication to laparoscopic evaluation is cardiopulmonary instability, which would preclude safe insufflation of the peritoneal cavity. The supine position is used most commonly and affords a complete view of the peritoneal cavity. To facilitate visualization, a 30-degree laparoscope is used along with at least two additional ports for manipulation and retraction. Ascites should be collected for cytologic analysis and all peritoneal surfaces inspected. Incisional biopsies can be performed using laparoscopic scissors. Hemostasis is achieved with a combination of electrocautery and hemostatic agents (as discussed later in the section on open incisional biopsy) or by tissue approximation via laparoscopic suturing. Biopsy specimens are typically retrieved using a specimen bag. This reduces the chance of specimen destruction during retrieval and may decrease the risk of port-site recurrence. Cup biopsy forceps can be used to obtain specimens as well. Core needle biopsies can be directed by laparoscopy and be used to sample retroperitoneal, intraperitoneal, or hepatic masses. For deep-seated lesions, such as intrahepatic lesions, laparoscopic ultrasonography can be used to guide biopsy procedures and to compensate for the inability to palpate tissues.[39,40]

Complications associated with laparoscopic diagnosis and treatment of solid tumors in children are infrequent. The need for conversion to unplanned open operation has similarly been low.[3,35,41,42]

Thoracoscopy

The initial experience with thoracoscopy in children was reported by Rodgers in 1976 and included two oncology patients (Ewing sarcoma and recurrent Hodgkin lymphoma).[43] Since this initial report, thoracoscopy has become widely used for the evaluation of thoracic lesions in children for several reasons. Postoperative pain associated with thoracoscopic biopsy or resection is markedly decreased compared with that seen with thoracotomy. Moreover, thoracoscopy allows near-complete visualization of all parietal and visceral pleural

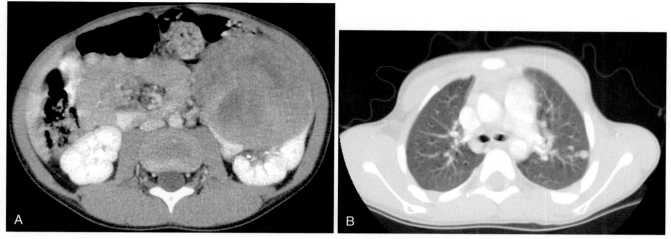

FIGURE 29-2 Computed tomography (CT) scans obtained at the time of diagnosis of a new abdominal mass in a 5-year-old boy. **A,** Abdominal and pelvic CT scan shows a large left-sided renal mass. **B,** Chest CT scan demonstrates a single 8-mm pulmonary nodule in the left upper lobe. No other pulmonary lesions were identified. At the time of nephrectomy, a thoracoscopic excisional biopsy of the lung lesion was performed. Final pathology of the kidney demonstrated a stage II-favorable-histology Wilms' tumor, and the lung pathology showed a hyalinized granuloma.

surfaces, which cannot be accomplished with a thoracotomy. Additionally, in most children the mediastinum does not contain a significant amount of adipose tissue and, therefore, can be inspected thoracoscopically.

Although primary neoplasms of the lung are rare in children, pulmonary lesions are often a confounding issue in the treatment of children with cancer.[44] The most common tumor to have early pulmonary metastases is Wilms' tumor. Pulmonary metastases are also common with bone and soft tissue sarcomas, hepatic tumors, teratocarcinomas, and melanomas. Thoracoscopy is frequently used to evaluate for the presence of metastases either at the time of initial diagnosis or after follow-up imaging. Difficulty in distinguishing an opportunistic infection versus new metastatic disease is a common clinical scenario during the course of therapy. In areas with endemic granulomatous disease, thoracoscopy can also be helpful at the time of diagnosis (Fig. 29-2; case with histoplasmosis granuloma with new diagnosis of a Wilms' tumor). The diagnostic accuracy for thoracoscopic biopsies in this setting is very high.[41,44,45]

Mediastinal lesions may also be biopsied or resected using thoracoscopy.[46,47] Thoracoscopy provides clear visualization of both the anterior and posterior mediastinum, even in small children; therefore we prefer it rather than mediastinoscopy for evaluation of mediastinal lesions in children.

The only absolute contraindications to thoracoscopy are complete obliteration of the pleural space and the inability to tolerate single-lung ventilation when complete collapse of the lung is required.

Thoracoscopy in children is typically performed under general anesthesia with mechanical ventilation. Visualization is facilitated by single-lung ventilation if possible and supplemented with insufflation. In older children, this may be accomplished with a double-lumen endotracheal tube and, in smaller children, by mainstem intubation of the contralateral side. If selective ventilation is difficult to achieve or poorly tolerated by the patient, low-pressure insufflation (5 to 8 cm of water pressure) with carbon dioxide assists with visualization.

The anesthesiologist must monitor for any adverse effects from this controlled tension pneumothorax. It can be evacuated rapidly if need be, but it is typically well tolerated. The child is positioned in the lateral thoracotomy position. Hyperextension of the chest increases the intercostal spaces and will facilitate movement of the thoracoscopy ports. This positioning should be adjusted for mediastinal lesions. For anterior lesions, a more supine position is used, and for posterior lesions the patient is positioned more prone. The initial port is placed in the midaxillary line using blunt dissection. Additional ports are placed under thoracoscopic guidance at sites based upon the location of the lesion of interest. A 30-degree thoracoscope is helpful to achieve complete visualization of all pleural surfaces. Complete inspection is also facilitated by the use of multiple port sites.

Careful correlation with cross-sectional imaging is essential to successful thoracoscopic sampling, particularly of smaller lesions. Pleural-based or subpleural pulmonary lesions are often apparent when the lung is deflated. These can be resected using endoscopic stapling devices and retrieved using specimen bags. Identification of deeper lesions is more challenging. Complete collapse of the lung allows identification of larger lesions. Biopsy of smaller lesions can be based on anatomic location if the location by CT scan is specific, such as apical, lingular, or basilar. CT-guided localization may be performed immediately before surgery to assure correct identification of the area of concern. The lesion may be marked by injection with methylene blue or, preferably, stained autologous blood, which is less prone to diffuse.[48,49] Lesions can be concomitantly marked with placement of a fine wire[50] or microcoils,[51] which can facilitate identification under intraoperative fluoroscopy. These localization techniques have been very effective in obtaining accurate biopsies in children.[48,49,52] Intrathoracic ultrasonography may be helpful in localizing deeper parenchymal lesions.[53] However, this technique is not widely used, and assessment of its efficacy in children is limited.

After sampling of tissues of interest is completed, the pneumothorax may be evacuated with a small catheter to form a water seal. Unless extensive pulmonary biopsies are performed or the lung is otherwise diseased, a thoracostomy tube is often not required. Most children may be discharged the next day, and chemotherapy may be started promptly.[49]

Thoracoscopic techniques are highly effective in achieving diagnosis. Most pediatric series report a rate of success in obtaining accurate diagnostic tissue in almost all cases.[3,41,44,52] Complications during diagnostic thoracoscopy are rare. Pneumothorax or persistent air leakage may occur in children with underlying parenchymal lung disease or those requiring high-pressure ventilatory support.[52]

Open Incisional Biopsy

Incisional biopsy remains the gold standard regarding the quality of tissue sampling if complete excision is not to be performed. Laparotomy or thoracotomy allows large samples to be obtained under direct vision, which can provide improved diagnosis compared with needle biopsies. For example, in the National Wilms' Tumor Study Group-4, open biopsy was more successful than core needle biopsies at identifying anaplasia in children with bilateral Wilms' tumor. Correlation with preoperative imaging allows multiple samples to be obtained if there is inhomogeneity within the tumor, which would raise concerns about sampling error.

The ability to obtain larger specimens is beneficial not only in providing tissue for molecular diagnosis and prognosis, but in providing samples for tissue banking and creation of cell lines. Samples obtained from these biopsies have provided the clinical material that allowed the development of the molecular diagnosis and prognosis techniques referred to earlier in this chapter. Further stratification of risk to allow more precise risk-based therapy remains a major focus for pediatric oncology trials. Finally, specimens that are tissue-banked from these larger specimens may be used for investigational therapies, such as tumor vaccines.

Several important factors should be considered in performing an open biopsy. The initial biopsy should consider the ultimate operative treatment of the tumor. For example, the incision for biopsy of an extremity mass should be oriented parallel to the axis of the limb, and care should be taken to avoid undermining subcutaneous or fascial planes. This allows subsequent wide local excision to be performed with minimal additional resection of tissue because of the biopsy. Likewise, testicular masses should only be biopsied through an inguinal approach, because a scrotal biopsy incision could require the addition of a hemiscrotectomy to the subsequent orchiectomy. Laparotomy for biopsy should be planned to allow subsequent resection through extension of the same incision.

Significant distortion of anatomic relations can occur with large retroperitoneal tumors and attention must be paid to avoid injury to structures, such as ureters or the bile duct, which may be distended over the mass. The most common intra-abdominal tumors in children tend to be vascular, and bleeding from the biopsy site is the most common serious complication. Strategies to reduce perioperative hemorrhage include normalization of coagulation parameters preoperatively and adequate operative exposure. Cauterization of the tumor capsule may help control bleeding, but we have found direct pressure after packing the biopsy site with oxidized cellulose combined with procoagulants, as described later, to be more efficient than generous cautery applied to the base of the biopsy site. If possible, closure of the tumor capsule can help with hemostasis.

Supplements to achieving hemostasis include topical agents and fibrin sealants. Commercially available topical products include gelatin foam pads, microfibrillar collagen, and oxidized cellulose, which is available as fabric and cottonoid. Fibrin sealants are composed of fibrinogen, thrombin, and calcium, which are mixed as they are delivered to the tissue to rapidly form a fibrin clot.

Conclusion

Prior to performing a biopsy of a potential malignancy, the surgeon should consider the likely possible diagnoses. The biopsy should then be planned so that adequate tissue is obtained and preserved to determine not only diagnosis but also risk stratification. Percutaneous, minimal access surgical, and open surgical techniques each have an appropriate place in the evaluation of potential pediatric malignancies. The use of these techniques in a systematic, stepwise fashion is appropriate in some patients. The selection of the appropriate biopsy technique should be driven by both the specific question to be answered by the biopsy and individual institutional experience and resources. Planning an operative biopsy must account for the anticipated operative approach for definitive resection.

The complete reference list is available online at www. expertconsult.com.

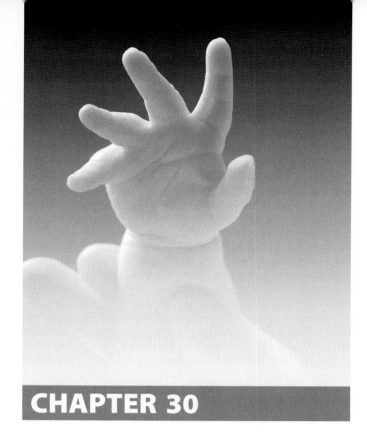

CHAPTER 30

Wilms' Tumor

Peter F. Ehrlich and Robert C. Shamberger

Renal tumors account for 6.3% of cancer diagnoses for children younger than 15 years of age, with a reported incidence of 7.9 per million. Including adolescents younger than 20 years of age, this drops slightly to 4.4% of cancer diagnoses, with an incidence of 6.2 per million.[1] Renal tumors include Wilms' tumor (WT) (also referred to as nephroblastoma or renal embryoma), renal cell carcinoma (RCC), clear cell sarcoma of the kidney (CCSK), rhabdoid tumor of the kidney (RTK), congenital mesoblastic nephroma, cystic renal tumor, and angiomyolipoma.[2,3] WT is by far the most common, accounting for approximately 91% of all renal tumors in childhood. CCSK and RTK were originally considered subtypes of WT, but are now recognized as separate tumors. RCC comprises 5.9% of renal malignancies in children and adolescents.[1,4]

The treatment strategy for children with renal tumors evolved in conjunction with the definition of these pathologic subtypes. Treatment is based on traditional risk factors, stage and histology, and, more recently, on genetic markers. The goal of "risk-based management" is to maintain excellent outcomes but at the same time spare children with low-risk tumors intensive chemotherapy and radiation, with their long-term side-effects, and to intensify therapy for children with high-risk tumors in an effort to increase their survival. Despite these advances, children with rhabdoid, renal cell carcinoma, and anaplastic tumors still do poorly. This chapter reviews the most frequent renal tumors in children, including their biologic properties, multidisciplinary therapies, and future challenges.

Wilms' Tumor

WT is the most common primary malignant renal tumor of childhood and comprises 6% of all pediatric tumors.[5,6] Outcomes for children with WT improved dramatically over the last 50 years, with long-term survival in both North American and European trials approaching 85% (Fig. 30-1). Survival rates for many of the low-stage tumors are 95% to 99%.[7,8] Current treatment protocols for children with WT were developed through a series of multidisciplinary cooperative group trials in both North America and Europe by the Children's Oncology Group (COG), formerly the National Wilms' Tumor Study Group (NWTSG), and the Société Internationale d'Oncologie Pédiatrique (SIOP). Their series of well-designed prospective randomized studies provide a large body of evidence-based knowledge to establish the optimal surgical, radiotherapy, and chemotherapy treatments for tumors based on the early studies on stage and histology and, more recently, also on cytogenetic and response-based factors. There are differences between the approaches of these two groups that affect staging and risk classification that are critical to understand when considering outcomes that will be discussed later in the chapter (Table 30-1).

History

WT is named after Carl Max Wilhelm Wilms, a German pathologist and surgeon. He was one of the first to propose that tumor cells originate during the development of the embryo. He published his findings in 1897 and 1899 in an influential monograph titled "Die Mischgeschwülste der Niere," which described seven children with nephroblastoma as part of a monograph on "mixed tumors."[9,10] Although reports of successful excision of renal tumors in children appeared in the end of the 19th century, his name has been indelibly applied to them. Dr. Thomas Jessop (1837 to 1903), probably performed the first successful nephrectomy at the General Infirmary in Leeds, England, on June 7, 1877, on a 2-year-old child with hematuria and a tumor of the kidney.[11,12]

At the beginning of the 20th century, survival for a child with WT was 5%. Surgery was the first effective treatment for nephroblastoma and continues to be a critical component of successful multimodality therapy. Although surgery at that time was the only option for cure, it carried a significant operative mortality. In 1916, radiation therapy was added by Friedlander.[13] In the late 1930s, Ladd described removing renal tumors in selected children. His technique included a large transverse transabdominal approach with early ligation of the renal vessels and removal of the surrounding Gerota fat and fascia. This modification improved the outcome in children with nonmetastatic nephroblastoma to a 32.2% survival at 3 years, with an operative mortality reduced from 23% to 7%. The basic tenets of this operative procedure described by Ladd are used today, with the exception of early ligation of the renal vessels.[12–15]

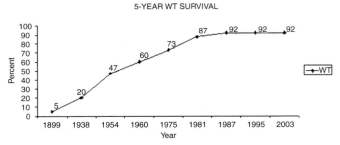

FIGURE 30-1 This graph shows the improved survival of children with Wilms' tumor (WT) over time.

Epidemiology

In the United States, there are 500 to 550 cases of WT per year. It is the second most common malignant abdominal tumor in childhood after neuroblastoma. The risk of developing WT in the general population is 1:10,000.[16] The incidence is slightly elevated for American and African blacks compared with whites and is significantly lower in Asians. The mean age at diagnosis is 36 months, with most children presenting between the ages of 12 and 48 months. Tumors tend to occur about 6 months later in girls than in boys. WT is rare at greater than 10 years and at less than 6 months of age. Tumors can be unilateral or bilateral (Figs. 30-2 and 30-3). Bilateral Wilms' tumors (BWT) occur in 4% to 13% of patients.[5,17–19] Children

with congenital syndromes associated with WT, such as Beckwith-Wiedemann, have a higher risk of developing BWT.

Congenital anomalies, either isolated or as part of a congenital syndrome, occur in about 10% of children with WT.[20] WAGR syndrome (WT, aniridia, genitourinary malformation, mental retardation) is a rare genetic syndrome associated with a chromosomal defect in 11p13. Children with WAGR syndrome are at a 30% higher risk of developing WT than a normal child. Because of the presence of aniridia, most children with WAGR syndrome are diagnosed at birth. Children with WAGR account for about 0.75% of all children with WT.[21]

Beckwith-Wiedemann syndrome (BWS) is a congenital disorder of growth regulation, affecting 1 in 14,000 children. Children with BWS have visceromegaly, macroglossia, omphalocele, and hyperinsulinemic hypoglycemia at birth. They also have an increased risk of tumor development. The risk is greatest in the first decade of life and thereafter approaches that of the general population. Three large studies of children with BWS reported tumor frequencies of 7.1% (13/183), 7.5% (29/388), and 14% (22/159).[22–25] The most frequently observed tumors in BWS are WT and hepatoblastoma, which comprise 43% and 12% of reported cancers, respectively.[22,26] Denys-Drash syndrome (DDS) (nephropathy, renal failure, male pseudohermaphroditism, and WT) is also associated with an increased risk of WT. Some investigators have recommended prophylactic nephrectomy in children with this syndrome once they develop renal failure.[27,28] Other

TABLE 30-1

Children's Oncology Group (COG) and Société Internationale d'Oncologie Pédiatrique (SIOP) Staging Systems

COG Wilms' Tumor Staging

Stage	Criteria
I	The tumor is limited to the kidney and has been completely resected. The tumor was not ruptured or biopsied prior to removal. There is no penetration of the renal capsule or involvement of renal sinus vessels.
II	The tumor extends beyond the capsule of the kidney but was completely resected with no evidence of tumor at or beyond the margins of resection. There is penetration of the renal capsule or invasion of the renal sinus vessels.
III	Gross or microscopic residual tumor remains postoperatively, including inoperable tumor, positive surgical margins, tumor spillage surfaces, regional lymph node metastases, positive peritoneal cytology, or transected tumor thrombus. The tumor was ruptured or biopsied prior to removal.
IV	Hematogenous metastases or lymph node metastases outside the abdomen (e.g., lung, liver, bone, brain).
V	Bilateral renal involvement is present at diagnosis, and each side may be considered to have a stage.

SIOP Staging

Stage	Criteria
I	The tumor is limited to the kidney or surrounded with a fibrous pseudocapsule, if outside the normal contours of the kidney. The renal capsule or pseudocapsule may be infiltrated with the tumor, but it does not reach the outer surface, and it is completely resected. The tumor may be protruding (bulging) into the pelvic system and dipping into the ureter, but it is not infiltrating the walls. The vessels of the renal sinus are not involved. Intrarenal vessels may be involved.
II	The tumor extends beyond the kidney or penetrates through the renal capsule and/or fibrous pseudocapsule into the perirenal fat, but it is completely resected. The tumor infiltrates the renal sinus and/or invades blood and lymphatic vessels outside the renal parenchyma, but it is completely resected. The tumor infiltrates adjacent organs or vena cava, but it is completely resected. The tumor has been surgically biopsied (wedge biopsy) prior to preoperative chemotherapy or surgery.
III	There is incomplete excision of the tumor, which extends beyond resection margins (gross or microscopic tumor remains postoperatively). Any positive lymph nodes are involved. Tumor ruptures before or during surgery (irrespective of other criteria for staging). The tumor has penetrated the peritoneal surface. Tumor implants are found on the peritoneal surface. The tumor thrombi present at resection, margins of vessels or ureter are transected or removed piecemeal by surgeon.
IV	Hematogenous metastases (lung, liver, bone, brain, etc.) or lymph node metastases are outside the abdominopelvic region.
V	Bilateral renal tumors present at diagnosis. Each side has to be substaged according to above classifications.

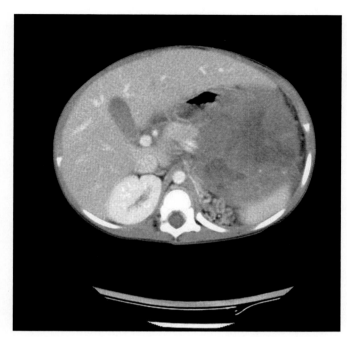

FIGURE 30-2 A computed tomography (CT) scan of a unilateral Wilms' tumor.

syndromes associated with WT include hemihypertrophy and Perlman syndrome. Urologic abnormalities, such as hypospadias, cryptorchidism, and nephromegaly, are also associated with WT.

Molecular Biology and Genetics

A number of important advances in WT development have occurred since the early 1990s. A detailed description is beyond the scope of this chapter. Table 30-2 summarizes some of the key genes and more detailed references are cited.[29–56] There

are several candidate genes that are been investigated and evaluated or are being evaluated in the clinical setting. These are described later.

LOSS OF HETEROZYGOSITY AND DNA PLOIDY

Loss of heterozygosity (LOH) refers to loss of genetic material and allelic uniqueness. LOH was found initially in children with WT on chromosomes 11p (33% of tumors), 16q (20%), and 1p (11%). A major aim of the fifth National Wilms' Tumor Study (NWTS-5) was to determine if tumor-specific LOH for chromosomes 11p, 1p, or 16q was associated with an adverse prognosis for children with favorable-histology (FH) WT, a finding suggested in earlier retrospective studies.[34] Chromosomes 11p, 16q, and 1p were prospectively evaluated. Results demonstrated that outcomes for patients with LOH at 1p and 16q were at least 10% worse than those without LOH (Figs. 30-4 and 30-5). These findings are used as determinants of therapy on the current renal tumor studies of the COG.

A similar but smaller study was reported from the United Kingdom (United Kingdom Children Cancer Study Group Wilms Tumor trials 1 to 3) in which a comparable incidence of LOH for 16q (14%) and 1p (10%) was found, but in this study there was no association between poor outcomes and LOH at 1p.[42] The reasons for the different results are unclear; possible explanations include a smaller sample size of the British study or that the larger doses of doxorubicin used in the U.K. studies served to eliminate part of the adverse impact on prognosis.

Analyses from patients with WT have also identified recurrent deletions and translocations involving the short arm of chromosome 7.[43,48,55] Studies suggest a locus of interest between 7p13 and 7p21, perhaps the *POU6F2* gene at 7p14.[57–59] Clinical correlates of 7p LOH have not been published, and so the exact prognostic role of this possible Wilms' locus, if any, has yet to be determined.

Another aim of NWTS-5 was to determine whether DNA ploidy status is associated with worse outcome in children

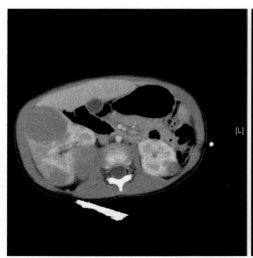 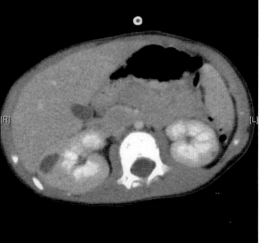

FIGURE 30-3 Two computed tomography (CT) scans of bilateral Wilms' tumor at presentation and after 6 weeks of chemotherapy.

TABLE 30-2

Summary of Current Genes Being Investigated in Wilms' Tumor

Gene(s)	Location	Function	Clinical Relevance
WT1	11.13	Tumor Supressor Functions in normal kidney development	WAGR syndrome Deletions Denys-Drash point mutation
WT2	11p15.5	Several gene loci IGF-2 Cell growth and encodes an embryonal growth factor that is highly expressed in fetal kidney and WT Genomic imprinting	BWS syndrome Genomic imprinting
Cadherin-associated protein β1 gene[4]	3p21	Cellular adhesion protein that also associates with members of the T-cell factor (TCF) family of transcription factors to promote expression of growth-related genes such as c-MYC and CYCLIN D1	Highly correlated with WT1 genes
WTX	Xq11.1	WTX inhibits the Wnt signal transduction to promote post-translational modification and degradation	Unknown
Familial Wilms' genes	17q and 19q13.3-q13.4	Unknown	Unknown

BWS, Beckwith-Wiedemann syndrome; IGF, insulin growth factor; WAGR, Wilms' tumor, aniridia, genitourinary malformation, mental retardation.

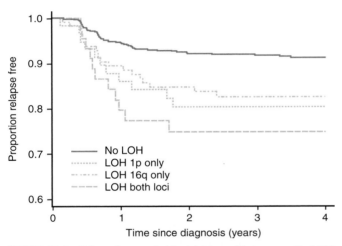

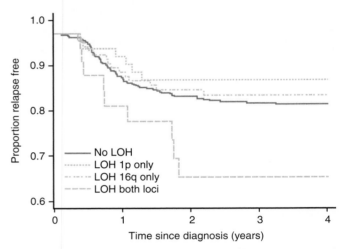

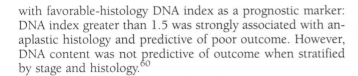

FIGURE 30-4 Relapse-free survival by joint loss of heterozygosity (LOH) at chromosomes 1p and 16q for stage I/II favorable-histology Wilms' tumor patients. (From Grundy PE, Breslow N, Li S, et al: Loss of heterozygosity for chromosomes 1p and 16q is an adverse prognostic factor in favorable-histology Wilms tumor: A report from the National Wilms Tumor Study Group. J Clin Oncol 2005;23:7312-7321.)

FIGURE 30-5 Relapse-free survival by joint loss of heterozygosity (LOH) at chromosomes 1p and 16q for stage III/IV favorable-histology Wilms' tumor patients. (From Grundy PE, Breslow N, Li S, et al: Loss of heterozygosity for chromosomes 1p and 16q is an adverse prognostic factor in favorable-histology Wilms tumor: A report from the National Wilms Tumor Study Group. J Clin Oncol 2005;23:7312-7321.)

with favorable-histology DNA index as a prognostic marker: DNA index greater than 1.5 was strongly associated with anaplastic histology and predictive of poor outcome. However, DNA content was not predictive of outcome when stratified by stage and histology.[60]

TP53 GENE

The TP53 gene is located on chromosome 17. The Tp53 protein is a negative regulator of cell proliferation and a positive regulator of apoptosis in response to DNA damaging agents. TP53 is the most common mutated gene associated with human cancer. Li-Fraumeni syndrome is a multicancer predisposition syndrome that has constitutional TP53 mutations.[61] However, WT rarely develops in Li-Fraumeni syndrome, and the majority of WT develop in the presence of wild-type TP53.[62] TP53 mutations in WT are almost exclusively found in tumors with anaplastic histology. Seventy-five percent of

anaplastic WT have TP53 mutations. In the current COG study, one of the aims of the high-risk protocol is to study the incidence and association of TP53 mutations.

Clinical Presentation

Most children with WT present with an asymptomatic abdominal mass, often discovered by either a parent or pediatrician. Nonpalpable tumors are typically discovered by ultrasonography during evaluation for abdominal pain. Gross hematuria has been reported in 18.2% of patients and microscopic hematuria in 24.4%. Ten percent of children with WT have coagulopathy, and 20% to 25% present with hypertension because of activation of the renin-angiotensin system.[63] Fever, anorexia, and weight loss occur in 10%. Extension of tumor thrombus into the renal vein can obstruct the spermatic vein and result in a left varicocele and, in rare cases, tumor extension into the atrium may produce cardiac malfunction. Tumor rupture and hemorrhage are also infrequent events that can present as an acute abdomen.

The differential diagnosis for an abdominal mass includes neuroblastoma, hepatoblastoma, rhabdomyosarcoma, and lymphoma. Neuroblastoma is the most common solid abdominal tumor in children. One clinical observation to help distinguish between WT and neuroblastoma is that children with neuroblastoma are often ill because of extensive metastatic disease at presentation. In contrast, children with WT are generally healthy toddlers with a palpable abdominal mass.

Diagnosis

After an abdominal mass is identified, radiographic imaging is performed to determine the anatomic location and extent of the mass. Ultrasonography (US) is a good screening examination of a mass to determine its site of origin and to assess for possible intravascular or ureteral extension. About 4% of WT present with inferior vena cava (IVC) or atrial involvement and 11% with renal vein involvement.[5,6] Embolization of a caval thrombus to the pulmonary artery can be lethal, and the presence of a thrombus must be identified preoperatively to prevent this occurrence. US is a sensitive technique to identify vascular extension.[64,65] A computed tomography (CT) scan of the abdomen will confirm the renal origin of the mass and determine whether there are bilateral tumors. Early generations of CT scans missed 7% to 10% of bilateral lesions. Hence, contralateral exploration of the kidney was recommended in NWTSG protocols to assess for bilateral lesions.[66] A recent review of children with bilateral WT, however, demonstrated that only 0.25% of bilateral tumors were missed with modern helical CT scans, all of which were small.[67] Based on these results, bilateral exploration is not recommended in current protocols from the COG. Although magnetic resonance imaging (MRI) avoids radiation exposure, it has not been shown to be superior to CT scanning in standard assessments. MRI is currently being evaluated as a method to help distinguish nephrogenic rests from WT and may be the preferred method to follow children with bilateral WT after resection.

The common sites of metastatic spread are the lungs and the liver. Therefore, in addition to abdominal imaging, pulmonary imaging must be performed. In NWTS-4 and NWTS-5, 13% of patients (575 of 4,006) with unilateral favorable-histology tumors presented with pulmonary disease. Initially this was routinely evaluated based upon a chest radiograph. In current protocols, it is based upon CT scans.

[18]F-fluorodeoxyglucose positron emission tomography (FDG PET) has not been fully delineated in pediatric cancers.[65] It is recognized that FDG PET has an established role in Hodgkin lymphoma and increasingly in sarcomas in children, but its role in WT is unclear.[68,69]

Screening

Screening is reserved for children at risk for developing WT. This includes children with genetic syndromes such as BWS, idiopathic hemihypertrophy (IHH), WAGR, DDS, and Perlman syndrome. Renal ultrasound examination is the preferred modality to screen for WT. It is widely available, noninvasive, does not involve radiation exposure, and generally does not require use of sedation. It is recommended that children be scanned every 3 to 4 months. Debaun and colleagues assessed the cost effectiveness of screening for WT and hepatoblastoma in children with Beckwith-Wiedemann syndrome (BWS).[70] In this analysis, screening a child with BWS from birth until 4 years of age resulted in a cost per life-year saved of $9,642, while continuing until 7 years of age resulted in a cost per life-year saved of $14,740, although it is not truly established that the rate of cure or event-free survival (EFS) is higher based on this early monitoring protocol. Three retrospective studies have evaluated screening in children at risk for WT. One study from the United Kingdom of 41 children with WT and aniridia, BWS, or IHH showed no difference in outcome or stage distribution between screened and unscreened populations.[71] In a second study of BWS/IHH, Choyke and colleagues demonstrated that evaluation by US every 3 months until age 8 years in 12 children with BWS lowered the proportion of patients with late-stage tumors to 0%, which was significantly reduced compared with the 42% incidence of late-stage tumors in 59 unscreened patients with BWS/IHH.[72] A third study analyzed the impact of surveillance in children with aniridia, BWS, and IHH who had developed WT.[73] There was a higher proportion of stage I tumors identified in children who underwent routine screening than in those who did not. Although ultrasonography is easy, false-positive results have been reported and have led to unnecessary investigations and surgery in patients who had benign lesions, such as cysts, nephrogenic rests, or foci of renal dysplasia, supporting the use of either MRI or CT to further define the lesions before surgical intervention.[72–74] The U.K. Wilms' Tumor Surveillance Working Group suggests that surveillance should be offered to children who are at a greater than 5% risk of WT.[75]

Children with Perlman syndrome are at a significantly increased risk of WT; therefore surveillance specifically for WT is warranted. Based on a review by Tan and colleagues, there is currently insufficient evidence to justify tumor surveillance in Sotos, Weaver, Proteus, and Bannayan-Riley Ruvalcaba syndromes or the syndrome of macrocephaly-cutis marmorata telangiectatica congenita. Of interest, children with Klippel-Trenaunay syndrome (KTS) had been considered to be at increased risk for developing WT. In a 2004 study by Fishman and colleagues, the risk of developing WT in children was assessed using the NWTSG database.[76] The risk of WT in children with KTS was no different than in the general population, and thus routine ultrasonography surveillance is not recommended.

Pathology

Tumor histology is a major determinant of therapeutic stratification for children with WT. The diagnostic classification of pediatric renal tumors has benefited from central review of tumors from patients treated in the cooperative group trials.[77] This success has enabled the introduction of disease-specific and risk-based therapy. For example, clear cell sarcoma of the kidney (CCSK) and malignant rhabdoid tumor (MRT) were initially considered to be variants of WT and were managed with chemotherapeutic agents for WT, but they are now considered distinct entities with separate therapies.

WT are embryonal tumors containing components seen in normal developing kidneys. The classic WT consists of three elements: blastemal, stromal, and epithelial tubules. Tumors contain various proportions of each of these elements. Triphasic patterns containing blastemal, stromal, and epithelial cell types are the most characteristic, but biphasic and monophasic lesions occur.[78] Less frequently, abnormal mucinous or squamous epithelium, skeletal muscle, cartilage, osteoid, or fat are found in WT.[79]

When the tumors are monophasic, they can be very invasive and difficult to distinguish from other childhood tumors, such as primitive neuroectodermal tumor, neuroblastoma, and lymphoma. Monophasic undifferentiated stromal WT look like sarcomas, such as clear cell sarcoma of the kidney, congenital mesoblastic nephroma, or synovial sarcoma. Other WT may have differing amounts of skeletal-muscle differentiation, from well-differentiated (rhabdomyomatous) to poorly differentiated (rhabdomyoblastic) skeletal muscle. A WT that is entirely tubular and papillary can be difficult to distinguish from papillary renal cell carcinoma.[79]

WT are divided into two groups: those with "favorable" histology and those with "unfavorable" histology. Favorable-histology tumors comprise 90% of the unilateral and bilateral tumors.

Anaplastic histology is considered unfavorable histology along with the CCSK and rhabdoid tumors. Unfavorable histology is found in about 10% of childhood renal tumors. It is rare in the first 2 years of life (2%), then increases in patients older than 5 years to 13%. It is also more frequent in nonwhite (African-American and Latino populations) than in white patients.[80] In a report by Bonadio and colleagues, 30.1% of anaplastic tumors occurred in the nonwhite population. In a multivariate analysis, older age, being nonwhite, and lymph node positivity were the significant predictors of anaplastic WT histology. Finally, anaplasia has been strongly associated with the presence of *TP53* mutations.[81]

Different treatment protocols for children with anaplastic versus favorable-histology tumors were first used in NWTS-3. Anaplasia is defined by multipolar polyploid mitotic figures, marked nuclear enlargement (giant nuclei with diameters at least 3 times those of adjacent cells), and hyperchromasia.[82] Focal anaplasia is defined as the presence of one or a few sharply localized regions of anaplasia within a primary tumor, the majority of which contain no nuclear atypia. The cells must not be present in any sites outside of the kidney. Tumors with diffuse anaplasia must have at least one of the following four criteria. Anaplastic cells outside of the kidney, presence of anaplasia in a random kidney biopsy, anaplasia in more than one region of the kidney, and anaplasia in one region, with extreme nuclear pleomorphism in another site. The difference between focal and diffuse anaplasia has been demonstrated to have prognostic significance.[83] Anaplasia is a marker of resistance to therapy, not of tumor aggressiveness.[78,82,84] Although associations between histologic features and prognosis or responsiveness to therapy have been suggested, with the exception of anaplasia (unfavorable histology), none of these features have reached statistical significance and therefore have not been used to determine therapy.[78,84]

The classic WT is triphasic, but some tumors can have dominant blastemal, stromal, and epithelial elements. Stromal dominant tumors are associated with intralobar nephrogenic rests, and epithelial dominant tumors have been associated with perilobar nephrogenic rests.

PRETREATED TUMORS AND PATHOLOGY

Tumors that have been treated with chemotherapy before resection differ in their histopathologic findings from tumors resected primarily. In the SIOP-9 study, the most common subtype of tumors resected without neoadjuvant chemotherapy was triphasic mixed histology (45.1%), followed by blastemal (39.4%) and epithelial dominant (15.5%), whereas in tumors that received preoperative chemotherapy, the most common histology was regressive (37.6%), followed by mixed (29.4%), stromal (14%), blastemal (9.3%), and epithelial predominant (3.1%); 6.6% of tumors were completely necrotic.[85,86] The SIOP risk classification uses these histologic findings as prognostic indicators to determine further therapies (Table 30-3). In addition, chemotherapy may produce tumor differentiation.[82,86,87] Anderson evaluated the histologic changes in tumors from 15 BWT patients that did not decrease in size radiographically following chemotherapy.[88] One had complete necrosis, 4 had rhabdomyomatous differentiation, and 10 had mature stromal differentiation. Despite their absence of regression in size, these patients had favorable outcomes, especially if there was rhabdomyomatous differentiation.

In SIOP-9, 10% of patients had postchemotherapy tumors that were completely necrotic. These patients had excellent outcomes. The SIOP-9 study also demonstrated that preoperative chemotherapy extensively ablates the blastemal component of WT.[87,89,90] The frequency of tumors with dominant blastemal components was markedly reduced (to 7.7%) by preoperative treatment compared with the no-treatment group (36%). Furthermore, this response is clearly an important prognostic factor. If predominant blastemal elements persist after initial therapy, the tumors were found to be highly aggressive. In SIOP-9, 5 of 16 (31%) of the postchemotherapy blastemal predominant tumors recurred, compared with none of the tumors that were predominantly epithelial or stromal after chemotherapy. Prior SIOP studies have also shown the prognosis for the purely blastemal group (after preoperative chemotherapy) to be inferior to that for the epithelial and stromal dominant tumors.

TABLE 30-3

Revised International Société Internationale d'Oncologie Pédiatrique Working Classification of Renal Tumors of Childhood (2001)

Stage	Risk	Histology
I	Low	Mesoblastic nephroma Cystic partially differentiated nephroblastoma
II	Intermediate	Nephroblastoma epithelial type Nephroblastoma stromal type Nephroblastoma mixed type Nephroblastoma regressive type Nephroblastoma focal anaplasia type
III	High	Nephroblastoma blastemal type Nephroblastoma diffuse anaplasia type Clear cell sarcoma of the kidney Rhabdoid tumor of the kidney

In the SIOP studies, postchemotherapy risk stratification and stage are used to determine additional therapy after resection. This categorization is different than the risk stratification used for tumors resected primarily in North America. *Low-risk* tumors are those that are completely necrotic following preoperative chemotherapy. *Intermediate-risk* tumors include all histologies other than completely necrotic, rhabdoid, anaplastic, or blastemal (less than 66%) dominant. *High-risk* tumors are those with diffuse anaplasia, rhabdoid, and blastemal dominance (greater than 66%) after chemotherapy (see Table 30-3).

NEPHROGENIC RESTS AND NEPHROBLASTOMATOSIS

Nephrogenesis in the normal kidney is usually complete by 34 to 36 weeks' gestation. Nephrogenic rests (NR) are "areas of metanephric (embryonal tissue) persisting after the 36th week of life." The presence of multiple or diffuse nephrogenic rests is termed nephroblastomatosis.[91] Diffuse hyperplastic perilobar nephrogenic rests (DHPLNR) represent a unique category of nephroblastomatosis in which the rests form a thick rind around the kidney. The rests that cause the greatest diagnostic challenge are those that are actively proliferating or hyperplastic, and can be mistaken for WT. Hyperplastic NR can produce masses as large as conventional WT. Complicating things further is the fact that neoplastic induction of NR can occur. The diagnosis of DHPLNR is often made based on radiographs (Fig. 30-6). Histologically, a rest consists of predominantly small clusters of blastemal cells, but tubules and stromal components can be present. NRs are classified by their growth phase and location: perilobar or intralobar. Perilobar nephrogenic rests are limited to the periphery (subcapsular) of the lobes, while intralobar rests occur within the renal lobes and have an irregular margin. The growth phase of a rest is divided into (1) incipient or dormant nephrogenic rests that show few well-formed tubular structures but no evidence of proliferation and no mitoses, (2) hyperplastic nephrogenic rests that are composed of epithelial elements with nodular expansive growth, and (3) sclerosing rests that consist of stromal and epithelial elements with few blastemal nephrogenic elements (Fig. 30-7).

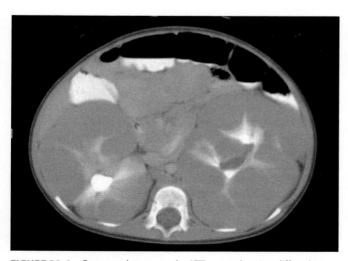

FIGURE 30-6 Computed tomography (CT) scans showing diffuse hyperplastic perilobar nephrogenic rests.

NRs are considered precursor lesions to WT; however, only a small number develop clonal transformation into a WT. A child with a WT and NRs in the resected specimen is at increased risk of developing a metachronous tumor in the other kidney.[92] For a child less than 1 year of age, this risk is very significant, and these children need to be followed very carefully with sequential US examinations. A patient who has a unilateral tumor and a presumed nephrogenic rest is thought to be at increased risk of developing a metachronous tumor, but data to support that assumption does not exist. The prevalence of NRs in unilateral WT has been reported to be 28% to 41% in unilateral WT and close to 100% in bilateral WT.[93] Pathologic distinction between NR and WT can be very difficult. To make the diagnosis, it is critical to examine the juncture between the lesion and the surrounding renal parenchyma to distinguish between the two entities. Most hyperplastic NRs lack a pseudocapsule at the periphery, while most WT will have this feature. An incisional biopsy is of limited value, because it is uncommon for it to contain the interface between the lesion and the adjacent kidney. This is particularly true for patients with DHPLNR. In a study by Perlman and colleagues, pathology alone was insufficient to establish the diagnosis of DHPLNR in 21 of 33 cases that underwent biopsy at the time of initial diagnosis.[94] In addition, because rests are found within and adjacent to WT, a biopsy may result in the inadvertent pathologic diagnosis of WT. Alternatively, a small WT may be present within a large field of nephroblastomatosis, obscuring it for biopsy. Taken together, in these situations where a renal mass could be a tumor or a rest where a biopsy is performed, Perlman and colleagues suggest using the term "nephrogenic process, consistent with a WT or a nephrogenic rest."

Staging

The COG/NWTS and SIOP staging systems are fundamentally different. In COG/NWTS protocols, initial surgical resection is recommended in most cases. Thus for unilateral tumors, the pathology of the tumor is established prior to administration of chemotherapy or radiotherapy. In contrast, SIOP protocols generally recommend chemotherapy followed by nephrectomy, and surgicopathologic staging is assessed at that time.

The COG/NWTS staging system has evolved as features associated with prognosis have been defined. A very important concept for this staging system is that there is a local stage and a disease stage. Local staging refers to the abdominal disease

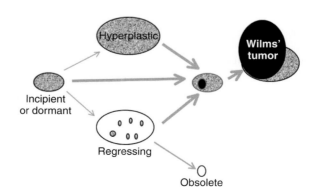

FIGURE 30-7 Cartoon of growth phases and classification of nephrogenic rests.

only, whereas disease stage considers both the local and distant hematogenous metastatic disease. Both factors determine therapy; the use of local radiation therapy to the tumor bed is based on the local stage, and the use of additional chemotherapy is based on both stage III local disease or distant metastasis.[95] The current COG and SIOP staging systems are shown in Table 30-1.

Treatment

The successful treatment for children with WT has been the direct result of prior multidisciplinary studies from cooperative group trials, including the NWTSG, SIOP, and the United Kingdom Children's Cancer Study Group (UKCCSG), that have defined the key components to therapy. These trials have identified several prognostic factors used for risk stratification in current protocols, including biologic markers. This section will review these prognostic factors, operative therapy, chemotherapy, and radiotherapy (with a focus on COG studies).

PROGNOSTIC FACTORS

The current prognostic factors used in COG trials are histology, stage, age, tumor weight, response to therapy, and loss of heterozygosity at 1p and 16q. The two most important continue to be the histology and the stage of the tumor.[7,8,96]

  Histology: The details and prognostic significance of tumor pathology have been previously discussed in the Pathology section.

  Stage: The tumor stage is determined by the results of the imaging studies and both the surgical and pathologic findings at nephrectomy (see Table 30-1).

  Rapid response: This is a prognostic category being evaluated in patients who have stage IV disease that is based on lung metastasis alone. The goal in these patients is to avoid lung radiation. Response to therapy is also being assessed in bilateral disease.

  Loss of heterozygosity: LOH (described previously) at both 1p and 16q are now used as determinants of therapy on the current COG renal tumor studies.[96]

OPERATIVE THERAPY

Surgical therapy is a primary component in the multidisciplinary treatment of WT or other neoplastic renal lesions. Irrespective of whether surgery is performed as a primary therapy or in a delayed fashion after chemotherapy, there are a number of fundamental tasks that are required of the surgeon. These are (1) safe resection of the tumor, (2) accurate staging of the tumor, (3) avoidance of complications that will "upstage the tumor" (rupture or unnecessary biopsy), and (4) accurate documentation of operative findings and details of the procedure in the operative note. Intraoperative events that negatively affect patient survival include tumor spill, failure to biopsy lymph nodes, incomplete tumor removal, failure to assess for extrarenal tumor extension and surgical complications.[97-99]

Technical Concerns: Unilateral Tumors

Ladd and Gross established the basic principles for resection of a presumed malignant tumor of the kidney, including wide abdominal exposure, resection of the surrounding Gerota fat and fascia to remove potential sites of lymphatic spread and early control of the renal vessels.[12,100] Lymph node sampling is now established as crucial for accurate staging.[101] Understaging the extent of the tumor can increase a child's risk of relapse, and overstaging will result in increasing the intensity of chemotherapy or radiation. A transverse transabdominal or thoracoabdominal incision provide the best exposure and are associated with fewer complications than a flank incision.[98,102-104] The thoracoabdominal incision is best for large tumors, to optimize visualization of the plane between the tumor and the diaphragm to avoid rupture from excessive traction on the tumor. Intraoperative events that negatively affect patient survival include tumor spill and inadequate staging.[97-99]

Early examination for involvement of the liver, renal vein, or IVC or peritoneal surfaces is important, as is identification of preoperative rupture of the tumor. Routine exploration of the contralateral kidney for bilateral disease was mandated in NWTS-1 to NWTS-5. In 1995, Ritchey and colleagues reviewed the accuracy of imaging in assessing bilateral disease from NWTS-4 (1986 to 1994). He found that bilateral tumors were missed in 7% of children by using the preoperative imaging studies. Thus, for NWTS-5, routine contralateral exploration was mandated. In 2005, Ritchey and colleagues did a follow-up study to look at what happened in those patients whose lesions were missed by imaging on NWTS-4. The size of the missed lesions was less than 1 cm in six patients and 1 to 2 cm in three patients. Management of missed lesions included enucleation in two cases, biopsy in six, and no surgery in one. No patient underwent irradiation. The postoperative chemotherapy regimen consisted of doxorubicin, dactinomycin, and vincristine in six children, and dactinomycin and vincristine in three. Median follow-up was 9 years. There were no recurrences in any kidney with a missed lesion. All nine patients were alive and disease free at last follow-up. The results of this study in conjunction with the advances in imaging quality means that routine contralateral exploration in the presence of a negative CT is not mandated.[66,67] If a clear contralateral lesion is present, then the child should be treated on the bilateral protocol. If studies suggest a possible contralateral lesion on the kidney, the contralateral kidney should be formally explored prior to nephrectomy.

Ladd and Gross stressed the need for early vascular ligation prior to the development of chemotherapy. This is no longer practiced because of the risk of injury to the vessels, particularly to the superior mesenteric artery in large left-sided tumors. The tumor should be mobilized by opening the lateral peritoneal reflection and reflecting the colon and its mesentery off the anterior surface of the kidney. For right-sided tumors, a Kocher procedure is also helpful. When ligating the renal pedicle, it is best to ligate the renal artery first if it can be safely identified, to avoid increasing the venous pressure within the tumor, which can result in rupture of the capsule. Vascular control in most cases is best completed after the tumor is fully mobilized.[99,105,106] The renal vein should be palpated prior to ligation to be certain there is no venous extension of the tumor. The adrenal gland may be left in place if it is not abutting the tumor; but, if the mass arises in the upper pole of the kidney, the adrenal gland should be removed with the neoplasm. The ureter is ligated and divided as low as possible.[107] The tumor and kidney should be handled gently throughout the operation to avoid rupture, which will increase the intensity of therapy and risk for local recurrence.[99,105,106]

Pathologic assessment of hilar and regional lymph nodes is critical to accurately stage a child with a renal tumor.[97,99] Routine lymph node sampling from the renal hilum, the pericaval, or para-aortic areas must be performed. Simply looking at the lymph nodes to determine whether they are positive is highly inaccurate.[108] Unfortunately, failure to sample lymph nodes (whether dealing with a unilateral or bilateral tumor) is the major technical error noted in WT surgery.[97] Furthermore, studies have demonstrated a higher risk of recurrence in children who did not have their lymph node status documented at the time of nephrectomy.[12,99,109]

WTs tend to displace rather than invade the surrounding vessels. This feature of WT has two implications. First, the surgeon must be certain of the identity of the vessels to ligate.[102] Second, most organs can be dissected away from the tumor, because actual invasion is rare. When actual invasion is identified, radical en bloc resection (e.g., partial hepatectomy or colectomy) is not warranted as primary therapy.[98,99] WTs are very chemosensitive, and, in these situations, prior adjuvant therapy will result in a lower rate of complications than a multiorgan resection.[98] A small section of diaphragm, psoas muscle, or tip of the pancreas, however, is acceptable.

Recent reports have suggested that hepatic metastasis should be resected at presentation.[110,111] To address this question, the COG renal tumor study group reviewed outcomes for patients with different sites of metastasis and found no significant difference in outcome for patients with liver versus lung metastasis. Primary resection of liver metastases prior to adjuvant therapy is not currently recommended.[112]

Spill

"Spill" refers to a break in the tumor capsule during operative removal, whether accidental, unavoidable, or by design. Studies have shown a higher risk of recurrence in patients who had tumor spill or rupture, irrespective of the cause or extent of the soiling.[97–99] Spill is also considered to have occurred if the renal vein or ureter are transected where they contain tumor. In COG protocols, spill is also considered to have occurred if a preoperative or intraoperative needle/open biopsy was performed. This is not the case for those patients treated following Société Internationale d'Oncologie Pédiatrique protocols: Fine-needle or Tru-Cut needle biopsy is allowed in this study; however, incisional biopsies are considered as ruptures, automatically stage III, and are contraindicated. "Rupture" refers to either the spontaneous or post-traumatic rupture of the tumor preoperatively, with the result that tumor cells are disseminated throughout the peritoneal or retroperitoneal space.[101] Bloody peritoneal fluid may be a sign of rupture, and a thorough examination of the tumor surface is mandated. Rupture is also considered to have occurred if the tumor penetrates the kidney capsule, with open neoplastic tissue surface being in free communication with the peritoneal cavity. If found, all of these situations make the child stage III and must be carefully documented in the operative note.

Unresectable Tumors

There are clinical situations where it is agreed that primary nephrectomy is contraindicated. These are when (1) there is extension of tumor thrombus above the level of the hepatic veins; (2) the tumor involves contiguous structures, whereby

the only means of removing the kidney tumor requires removal of the other structures (e.g., spleen, pancreas, and colon but excluding the adrenal gland); (3) there are bilateral tumors; (4) the tumor is in a solitary kidney; or (5) there is pulmonary compromise resulting from extensive pulmonary metastases. Studies conducted by the cooperative groups have shown that pretreatment with chemotherapy almost always reduces the bulk of the tumor.[113–116] This makes tumor removal easier and may reduce the incidence of surgical complications.[117] Preoperative chemotherapy does not result in improved survival rates, and it may result in the loss of staging information and changes the histology of the tumor as noted previously.[118,119]

SPECIAL CONSIDERATIONS

Management of Tumor Extension in the Renal Vein, Inferior Vena Cava, and Atrium

WT patients may present with tumor extension through the renal vein to the IVC and even up to the right atrium. This is found in 4% to 11% of children. Surgical treatment is dependent on the extent of vascular invasion. Extension is usually asymptomatic, and many are detected preoperatively by US, CT, and/or MRI scans. However, those that extend just into the renal vein may only be detected at operation because of compression and distortion of the veins by the tumor, reinforcing the need to palpate the renal vein and IVC at the start of nephrectomy before any mobilization of the kidney that might dislodge the thrombus.[106,120,121] As noted previously, a primary resection when tumor thrombus extends into the inferior vena cava at the level of the liver or higher is discouraged. COG protocols recommend that these patients be managed initially with preoperative chemotherapy. This approach will often achieve significant shrinkage and regression of the intravascular thrombus, facilitating subsequent surgical removal.[106,122] The severity and number of operative complications are reduced with preoperative chemotherapy for those with vascular extension above the hepatic veins. Alternatively, if the tumor extends only into the renal vein or renal vein and IVC below the level of the liver, the tumor and thrombus can, in most cases, be removed en bloc with the kidney.

Control of renal veins and cava above and below the tumor with vessel loops is necessary, using standard vascular surgery techniques. The tumor should not be transected, if possible, because this will result in spill and upstaging of the patient. In some cases, the tumor may be adherent to the vessel wall. A similar technique used for removing plaque for a carotid endarterectomy is helpful to lift the tumor off the vein wall. It must be stated in the operative report if the intravascular tumor extension was removed en bloc or if tumor was transected, as well as if the tumor thrombus is removed completely and if there is evidence of either adherence to or invasion of the vein wall. If, after preoperative chemotherapy, the tumor still extends above the hepatic veins, cardiopulmonary bypass is generally needed to remove the vascular extension of the tumor.

Management of Tumor Extension in the Ureter

Extension of WT into the ureter is a rare event.[107] In NWTS-5, the incidence of ureteral extension was 2%. Preoperative imaging detected ureteral extension in only 30% of these patients; the rest were discovered at operation. Clinical presentations included gross hematuria, passage of tissue per urethra, hydronephrosis, and a urethral mass. The diagnosis should be suspected in these patients, and cystoscopy with retrograde ureterogram may aid in preoperative diagnosis. If extension of tumor into the ureter is detected or suspected, the ureter should be resected with clear margins.

Horseshoe Kidney, Single Kidney, and Nonfunctioning Kidney

A WT in a horseshoe kidney presents unique challenges. Children with a tumor in a horseshoe kidney are treated as unilateral tumors, NOT as bilateral tumors. Children with horseshoe kidneys and WT must be carefully imaged prior to any surgery.[123] The blood supply to horseshoe kidneys is quite variable and must be carefully imaged prior to surgery.[123] At the time of operation, the blood supply to the kidney as well as the location of the ureters must be identified and isolated. Exposure and mobilization of the kidney on the side of the tumor is carried out as in unilateral resection. The side of the kidney containing the tumor, the isthmus, and the ipsilateral ureter are resected. As with other unilateral procedures, the lymph nodes are sampled for staging purposes. Children with a single kidney, or a situation where a tumor occurs in one kidney but the second kidney is nonfunctioning, should be managed using a renal-sparing approach, with preoperative chemotherapy to facilitate surgery and preserve more renal tissue.

Patients with Wilms' Tumor Treated Only with Surgery

NWTS-5 evaluated a subset of very-low-risk patients with favorable-histology tumors who might be treated without chemotherapy. The criteria for this arm of the study was stage I FH in patients who had lymph nodes biopsied, had a specimen weight of less than 550 g, and who were less than 2 years of age. Seventy-five patients were enrolled before closure of the study, and 8 developed recurrent disease (lung involvement in 5 and the operative bed in 3). Three other patients developed metachronous contralateral WT. Stringent stopping rules for the study were designed to ensure closure of this arm of the study if the 2-year EFS was 90% or less based on the expectation that approximately 50% of the surgery-only children would be salvaged after recurrence, thus attaining the 95% predicted survival of these children treated with vincristine and dactinomycin (EE-4A). This limit was exceeded on June 14th, 1998, and this arm of the study was closed when the 2-year disease-free survival estimate reached 86.5%.[124] Subsequent patients were treated with EE-4A. A recent long-term follow-up study of the surgery-only cohort and the EE-4A group, with a median follow-up of 8.2 years, reported the estimated 5-year EFS for surgery only was 84% (95% confidence interval [CI]: 73% to 91%); for the EE-4A patients it was 97% (95% CI: 92% to 99%, $P = 0.002$). One death was observed in each treatment group. The estimated 5-year overall survival (OS) was 98% (95% CI: 87% to 99%) for surgery only and 99% (95% CI: 94% to 99%) for EE-4A ($P = 0.70$).[125] The surgery-only EFS was less than for EE-4A, consistent with the earlier report. The salvage rate for the surgery-only cohort, however, exceeded that seen with children who had received two-drug chemotherapy, which had been predicted to be 50%. Thus 85% of the infants avoided any chemotherapy, while those who did receive it

for relapse were treated with three agents (DD-4A). A current study in the COG is assessing this cohort again and is evaluating biologic markers for this very-low-risk group.[126]

Neonatal Tumors

Neoplastic renal lesions in the neonate are rare and include benign and malignant tumors.[127,128] Acute and long-term toxicity from therapy is a considerable concern in infants. The distribution of tumors is age dependent. In the perinatal period, congenital mesoblastic nephroma (CMN) is the leader, accounting for greater than 50% of the renal tumors, followed in rank by WT, RTK, and CCSK.[127–131] WT, CMN, and rhabdoid tumor of the kidney (RTK) are the principal neoplasms of the kidney occurring after 3 months, when CMN accounts for less than 10%. An international retrospective study of 750 neonatal renal tumors in children less than 7 months of age found that 63.4% were WT.[127] Eighty-two percent of these were stage I/II. In contrast, RTK presented with advanced disease (53% stage III/IV). RTK accounted for nine of eleven tumors presenting with metastases. Outcomes paralleled older children, with excellent results for neonates with WT (5-year OS of 93.4%) and poor for RTK (5-year OS of 16.4%).[127]

Acquired von Willebrand Disease in Children with Wilms' Tumor

von Willebrand disease (vWD) is an inherited coagulation disorder characterized by mucocutaneous bleeding, a prolonged bleeding time (BT), and a reduced level of functional von Willebrand factor (vWF). Secondary laboratory abnormalities include a decreased level of procoagulant factor VIII (FVIII) and activity of ristocetin cofactor (FVIII:RCoF) activity.[132] Acquired vWD has been reported in patients with WT and other malignancies and has important implications for the surgeon.[133,134] A single prospective study of 50 WT patients found the incidence of acquired vWD was 8%.[134] However, the true incidence and prevalence in WT is unknown, because a full bleeding history and factor levels are rarely obtained. Until recently, the literature has suggested that, when identified, the bleeding has been clinically insignificant, characterized by epistaxis, hematuria, gingival bleeding, and easy bruising.[135] Recent reports of profuse intraoperative bleeding that only stopped after ligation of the renal vessels have contradicted this assumption.[136,137] Despite normalization of FVIII and vWF activity and antigen levels prior to surgery, during surgery profuse intraoperative bleeding occurred, requiring multiple transfusions with FVIII, FFP, cryoprecipitate, platelets, and packed red blood cells.[136] Immediately after ligation of the renal vessels, all abnormal bleeding stopped, with normalization of FVIII and vWF antigen activity.

The mechanism of acquired vWD in WT is unknown. Tumor adsorption of vWF has been reported in other malignancies; however, this was not seen in the WT cases where intraoperative bleeding was significant. vWF inhibitors, rapid abnormal clearance of vWF, and coagulopathy related to elevated levels of hyaluronic acid and consequent blood hyperviscosity have also been proposed.[138,139] Why some cases had intraoperative bleeding and others do not is also not known. Baxter[136] suggests that these tumors may be more hypervascular, but this is not proven. The risk of intraoperative bleeding highlights the importance of recognizing acquired vWD in children with WT. In all cases, the initial sign was a prolonged prothrombin time (PT) and partial thromboplastin time (PTT). When found, this should mandate acquiring a further history for bleeding and factor analysis. Although correction of factor levels prior to surgery appears to help in most cases, it does not guarantee that significant intraoperative bleeding will not occur. In the case reports of profound intraoperative bleeding, it was observed that, once the renal vessels were ligated, the bleeding ceased. Thus preoperative embolization should be considered as a management strategy. Alternatively, preoperative chemotherapy may also be a safe option.

BILATERAL WILMS' TUMOR

Bilateral Wilms' tumors BWT occur in 4% to 13% of patients (see Fig. 30-3).[5,17–19] Unfortunately, outcomes for children with bilateral tumors have not been as good as those of children with unilateral tumors. In NWTS-5, the 4-year OS was 80.8% for a child with favorable histology and 43.8% for a child with anaplastic histology.[84] In 1998, the United Kingdom Children's Cancer Study Group published their experience with BWT patients treated between 1980 and 1995.[140] In 57 patients, conservative surgical treatment with initial biopsy was followed by chemotherapy and delayed tumor resection, while 13 underwent initial surgical resection followed by chemotherapy. Overall survival was 69%, with similar survival in the patients with initial surgery versus neoadjuvant chemotherapy. BWT with an unfavorable histology was associated with a poor prognosis, with only one of seven patients surviving. Renal failure was seen in 6% of the survivors who were conservatively treated and in 20% of the survivors who underwent initial resection. In 2004, Weirich reported BWT outcomes from SIOP-9. Twenty-eight patients were evaluated. Although therapy was individualized, all 28 patients with BWT were treated with preoperative therapy. Overall survival at 5 years was 85.1% (95% CI: 71.6% to 98.6%; four deaths), and relapse-free survival was 80.5% (95% CI: 65.2% to 95.8%; five relapses).[141]

Renal failure is another concern of children with BWT (Figs. 30-8 and 30-9). The etiology of renal failure in WT patients is multifactorial.[142–144] Factors that contribute to renal failure include intrinsic progressive renal disease related to a genetic predisposition, inadequate renal parenchyma after one or more tumor resections, the nephrotoxic effects of

chemotherapy and radiation, and the potential for hyperfiltration injury to the remaining renal parenchyma. Ritchey defined the incidence and etiology of renal failure in patients treated on NWTS-1 to NWTS-4. BWT was the greatest risk factor for renal failure (16.4% for NWTS-1 and NWTS-2, 9.9% for NWTS-3, and 3.8% for NWTS-4). Other risk factors identified were Denys-Drash syndrome, metachronous tumor, progressive disease in patients with bilateral tumors requiring bilateral nephrectomies and radiation nephritis.[144] Breslow reported the 20-year end-stage renal disease (ESRD) outcomes in children treated for WT (see Figs. 30-7 and 30-8).[142] The major risk factors he identified for renal failure were BWT and congenital syndromes—Denys-Drash, WAGR, and genital urinary anomalies (hypospadias or cryptorchidism). Thus preservation of renal tissue without sacrificing long-term survival is of particular importance for those with BWT.

Despite 40 years of clinical trials for WT, it was not until 2009 that a formal BWT trial was opened by COG. Several prior reports contributed to the development of this protocol. Shamberger and colleagues examined 38 of 188 patients with BWT with progressive or nonresponsive disease (PNRD).[145] The mean duration of chemotherapy was 7 months; 36 patients were treated with two regimens of chemotherapy, and 21 patients received three. Patients with PNRD fell into two categories: first, patients with anaplasia whose tumors were not sensitive to the therapy administered (4 patients); second, patients who had tumors with very mature rhabdomyomatous or differentiated stromal elements (14 patients) and 1 with complete necrosis. A second study from Anderson looked at the histologic changes in BWT patients who did not respond to chemotherapy and the relationship between these changes and prognosis.[146] Their results mirrored those of the NWTS study. Fifteen patients whose tumors did not respond were evaluated. One had complete necrosis, 4 had rhabdomyomatous differentiation, and 10 had mature stromal differentiation. Despite not radiographically responding to chemotherapy, these patients had favorable outcomes. Patients in these studies fell into two categories. First, there were patients with anaplasia whose tumors were not sensitive to the therapy administered. Anaplastic tumors respond poorly to chemotherapy and, once the diagnosis of anaplasia is made, a complete resection is needed.[84,140,147,148] Second,

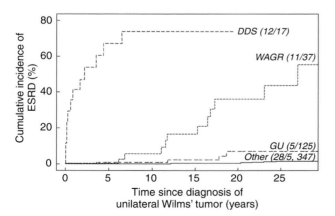

FIGURE 30-8 Kaplan-Meier plot of renal failure rates at 20 years of age in children with a unilateral Wilms' tumor (WT). DDS, Denys-Drash syndrome; ESRD, end-stage renal disease; GU, genitourinary; WAGR (syndrome), Wilms' tumor, aniridia, genitourinary malformation, mental retardation.

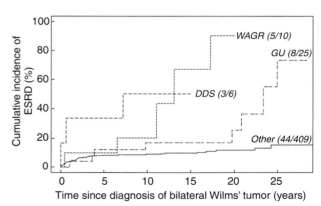

FIGURE 30-9 Kaplan-Meier plot of renal failure rates at 20 years of age in children with bilateral Wilms' tumor (BWT). DDS, Denys-Drash syndrome; ESRD, end-stage renal disease; GU, genitourinary; WAGR (syndrome), Wilms' tumor, aniridia, genitourinary malformation, mental retardation.

there were patients who had tumors with very mature rhabdo-myomatous or differentiated stromal elements and complete necrosis, all of whom had an excellent outcome. Again these patients are best served with resection.[146] Therefore if the bilateral lesions do not respond radiographically to therapy, it is critical to establish whether this is due to anaplasia or mature histology.

Hamilton and colleagues have demonstrated the difficulty in identifying anaplasia in patients with BWT.[148] Twenty-seven patients with anaplasia were reviewed from NWTS-4. Discordant pathology between the kidneys was seen in 20 patients, highlighting the importance of obtaining tissue from both kidneys. Seven children who were eventually found to have diffuse anaplasia had core needle biopsies, which failed to establish the diagnosis in all of these cases. Anaplasia was identified in only three of nine patients who had an open wedge biopsy and in seven of nine patients by partial or complete nephrectomy. Thus percutaneous biopsies rarely establish the diagnosis, and open biopsies were successful in only a third of the cases.

An important question is to determine how long to treat a child who has BWT with chemotherapy before intervening surgically. In SIOP-9, patients with unilateral tumors were randomized to receive either 4 or 8 weeks of dactinomycin and vincristine preoperatively. There was an average 48% reduction in tumor volume after 4 weeks that increased to 62% after 8 weeks of chemotherapy.[116,149] A review by the German Pediatric Hematology Group (GPOH) of their patients with BWT reported that maximum tumor shrinkage occurred in the first 12 weeks of chemotherapy.[150]

The two principal aims of the COG BWT study are to improve 4-year event-free survival and to prevent complete removal of at least one kidney in 50% of patients with BWT by using preoperative chemotherapy. This is a response-based protocol starting with chemotherapy, followed by evaluation at 6 and 12 weeks with definitive surgical therapy in all patients by 12 weeks (see Fig. 30-3). This protocol does not mandate an initial tissue diagnosis because bilateral renal tumors in children are invariably WT; biopsy does not change the therapy in most cases; anaplasia is hard to diagnose, and the biopsy will effectively increase the stage of the tumor and its risk for local recurrence.[148] In the current COG protocol, local spill of the tumor is designated as stage III. This classification was changed because of the finding of an increased incidence of abdominal recurrences in NWTS-4 patients with tumor spill.[99] First, for patients with BWT, the initial regimen will consist of regimen vincristine, actinomycin D, doxorubicin (VAD) (vincristine [VCR], dactinomycin [DACT], doxorubicin [DOX]), a more intensive combination of drugs based on regimens used with good results and minimal toxicities by both SIOP and the UKCCSG WT groups, which enables patients to receive two doses of DOX, in addition to six of VCR and two of DACT, during the first 6 weeks of therapy.[151] It differs from the standard three-drug regimen, DD-4A, in which the DOX and DACT are administered in separate cycles.[152] The three-drug chemotherapy regimen of VAD was chosen to give an enhanced therapy for possible stage III disease, because patients rarely have a lymph node biopsy before initiation of therapy. Second, it was elected to enhance the chemotherapy rather than administer radiotherapy, which might increase the occurrence of radiation nephritis in the remaining kidney. Third, a more intensive therapy was selected for treatment

to avoid the use of a sequential regimen of increasing intensity, which was seen in the review of the prior cohort of NWTS-4 BWT patients.

CHEMOTHERAPY

In 1963, Farber first reported that dactinomycin had activity against WT.[153] Today, dactinomycin continues to be part of the backbone of therapy for children with WT. Other active chemotherapeutic agents have been identified subsequently, including vincristine, doxorubicin, and cyclophosphamide. Clinical trials conducted by NWTSG and SIOP have evaluated, stage by stage, different chemotherapeutic protocols to assess the efficacy of various combinations and duration of therapy.[105,154–159] In NWTS-4, 4-year event-free survival and overall survival averaged 90% for patients with favorable histology.[154,159] Therefore NWTS-5 focused on evaluating biologic markers of prognosis, such as LOH, developing more effective therapy for recurrent disease, and reducing therapy in children with low-risk tumors.

Treatment on the current COG protocols for favorable-histology WT is determined by stage, histology, and LOH. For children with favorable-histology stage I and II tumors without LOH, 18 weeks of vincristine and dactinomycin (regimen EE-4A) is recommended. Results from NWTS-5 showed these children had an overall survival of 98.4% and 98.7%, respectively. For children with FH stage III and IV tumors without LOH, 24 weeks of vincristine, dactinomycin, and doxorubicin is recommended (regimen DD-4A). For those patients who have positive LOH at both loci (1p and 17q), treatment will be intensified. If they are stage I or II and LOH positive, they will receive DD-4A, and if they are stage III and IV LOH positive, they will receive vincristine, dactinomycin, and doxorubicin with alternating cycles of cyclophosphamide versus etoposide (regimen M). Dosing modifications are made for children less than 12 months of age.

Anaplastic tumors have been less successfully treated. NWTS-3 and NWTS-4 were the first studies to prospectively evaluate the benefit of additional/different chemotherapy therapy for these tumors. One randomized arm compared 15 months of vincristine, dactinomycin, and doxorubicin, with or without cyclophosphamide. For patients with stage II to IV diffuse anaplastic histology, the addition of cyclophosphamide resulted in a 4-year relapse-free survival estimate of 54.8% when treated with cyclophosphamide compared with 27.2% when treated without it (P = 0.02).[160] In NWTS-5, patients with focal anaplasia or diffuse stage I were treated with EE-4A. This was based on prior historical data, with a goal of reducing therapy. Unfortunately, the 4-year event-free and overall survival estimates for stage I (focal or diffuse) anaplastic WT were lower than previous studies (EFS 69.5% and OS 82.6%). Thus therapy with EE-4A is inadequate. Patients with focal anaplasia stage II to IV were treated with DD-4A. Children with stage II to IV diffuse anaplastic WT were treated with vincristine, doxorubicin, and cyclophosphamide (VDC) alternating with cyclophosphamide and etoposide (CyE) (regimen I). The 4-year event-free survival estimates for stage II to IV diffuse anaplastic WT on NWTS-5 were 82.6%, 64.7%, and 33.3%, respectively, with similar overall survival.[84] The current protocols and chemotherapy agents for unilateral tumors are shown in Table 30-4.

TABLE 30-4

Current Children's Oncology Group Chemotherapy Regimens for Unilateral Wilms' Tumor

Regimen	Agents
EE-4A	Vincristine and dactinomycin
DD-4A	Vincristine, dactinomycin, doxorubicin, and radiation therapy (XRT)
Regimen I	Vincristine, dactinomycin, doxorubicin, cyclophosphamide (CPM1), and etoposide (ETOP), as well as radiation therapy (XRT)
Regimen M	Vincristine, dactinomycin, doxorubicin, cyclophosphamide, and etoposide; radiation therapy also to be administered as part of this regimen
Revised UH-1	Vincristine, dactinomycin, doxorubicin, cyclophosphamide, carboplatin, etoposide, and radiation
Revised UH-2	Vincristine, dactinomycin, doxorubicin, cyclophosphamide, carboplatin, etoposide, irinotecan, and radiation therapy (XRT)
Vincristine/irinotecan window therapy	Vincristine and irinotecan in conjunction with revised UH-1 or revised UH-2, depending on response

Recurrent Tumor

Treatment of recurrent disease in children with WT is challenging. Recurrence occurs in 15% of patients with favorable histology tumors and in 50% with anaplastic histology. Recurrence is most frequent within 2 years of the initial diagnosis and most common in the lungs, tumor bed, and liver.[161] Less common sites are bone, brain, and distant lymph nodes.

Recurrent disease is treated by chemotherapy, surgery, and radiotherapy. NWTS-5 evaluated two protocols for recurrent disease, avoiding use of agents included in the primary protocols. Stratum B was for patients with stage I and II disease initially treated with EE-4A. The chemotherapy for this relapse protocol was regimen I (alternating courses of vincristine/doxorubicin with cyclophosphamide), in addition to surgical resection and radiation therapy. Event-free survival at 4 years was 71.1%, and 4-year overall survival was 81.8% for all patients and was 67.8% and 81.0%, respectively, for those who relapsed only to their lungs.[162] Stratum C was for patients initially treated with DD-4A.[163] The chemotherapy protocol for this group was alternating cycles of cyclophosphamide versus etoposide and carboplatin versus etoposide. Four-year event-free survival and overall survival were 42.3% and 48.0%, respectively, for all patients and were 48.9% and 52.8% for those who relapsed in the lungs only. Bone marrow transplantations have been performed for patients with recurrent disease, with reported event-free or disease-free survival rates of 36% to 60% in these small series.[164-166] At present, there is no open relapsed study in SIOP or COG, because the groups are awaiting new and more effective agents for treatment of this disease.

RADIOTHERAPY

Analogous to surgery and chemotherapy, the cooperative group trials have refined the indications for radiotherapy. In addition, technologic advances have helped to deliver irradiation with increased efficacy and less toxicity to surrounding tissues. The three principle fields for radiotherapy for renal tumors are whole abdominal, flank, and lung (metastatic lung disease). All five NWTSG studies and the current COG studies use radiotherapy as part of the multimodality treatment for advanced-stage tumors.

In 1950, Gross and colleagues demonstrated the efficacy of radiotherapy as an adjuvant therapy prior to the advent of chemotherapy. In this series, nephrectomy with postoperative radiation improved survival to 47%.[167] Favorable histology tumors are generally very radiosensitive. NWTS-1 to NWTS-3 helped define the indications, timing, and dose of radiotherapy. NWTS-1 established that irradiation provided no advantage in children younger than 24 months with stage I FH tumors who also received 15 months of dactinomycin.[168] That study also demonstrated that in stage III tumors with local tumor spill or previous biopsy, there was no need for irradiation of the whole abdomen, thus sparing patients the associated toxicity.[169] NWTS-2 showed that radiotherapy could be avoided in all children with stage I WT if they received vincristine and dactinomycin.[170] NWTS-3 established that radiotherapy could be avoided in children with stage II tumors given vincristine and dactinomycin and also demonstrated that children with stage III favorable-histology tumors who received 10.8 Gy radiotherapy and vincristine, dactinomycin, and doxorubicin had similar tumor control to those who received 20 Gy with vincristine and dactinomycin. This was an important finding, because it eliminated the need for an age-adjusted dose schedule and significantly reduced the recommended dose of radiation.[157]

Timing of radiation following nephrectomy was assessed on NWTS-2, where a delay of 10 days or more before initiation of radiotherapy was associated with a higher rate of abdominal relapse, particularly among patients with unfavorable-histology tumors and a small radiation field.[157,168,169] A recent review of this issue from NWTS-3 and NWTS-4 data confirmed this observation.[171] Thus, in the COG protocols, it is recommended that abdominal irradiation be delivered as soon as practical after nephrectomy and not later than 14 days after surgery. The current recommendation for radiation therapy for COG protocols is shown in Table 30-5.

In contrast to FH tumors, the ideal dose for patients with anaplastic tumors is unknown. Anaplastic tumors are more resistant to chemotherapy and seem to be more resistant to radiotherapy as well. Anaplastic tumors have not demonstrated a radiation dose response between 10 Gy and 40 Gy.[160]

The radiotherapy strategy for patients with anaplastic histology (AH) on NWTS-5 included no irradiation for stage I AH tumors and 10-Gy radiotherapy for AH stage II and III in conjunction with nephrectomy and regimen I. The outcomes for both of these treatment strategies were suboptimal. Stage 1 patients had a 4-year EFS and overall survival of only 69.5% and 82.6%, respectively. Stage II, III, and IV patients had a 4-year OS after immediate nephrectomy, irradiation, and regimen I chemotherapy of 82.6%, 64.7%, and 33.3%, respectively.[84] EFS was similar to OS in all groups. Fifty percent of stage III recurrences were local, suggesting that the dose of 10 Gy was not adequate. These results form the basis for the current COG study that recommends the addition of irradiation for patients with stage I anaplasia and augmentation of irradiation for patients with stage III anaplasia.

For liver metastases, only those that are unresectable at diagnosis are irradiated. The treatment portal includes that portion of the liver known to be involved as identified by CT or MRI studies. The whole liver is treated in children with diffuse metastases.

TABLE 30-5

Radiotherapy for Favorable-Histology Wilms' Tumor

Treatment Site	Clinical Presentation and Dose (Gy)	
Flank irradiation All instances of soilage will be classified as Stage III and require abdominal radiation. Flank radiation is given to all Stage III patients with three exceptions (the patients meeting any of these exceptions requiring whole abdominal radiation).	Stage III favorable histology Recurrent Wilms' tumor	10.8 10.8
Whole abdomen irradiation (WAI)	Abdominal stage III Preoperative tumor rupture Peritoneal metastases are found at initial surgery A large intraoperative tumor spill affecting areas outside the tumor bed as determined by the surgeon/treating institution.	10.5
	Abdominal Stage III Diffuse unresectable peritoneal implants	21
Liver irradiation Patients with residual tumor will receive supplemental irradiation with 5.4 to 10.8 Gy.	Focal metastases Diffuse metastases	19.8 19.8

Lung Radiotherapy

Historically, pulmonary metastases were diagnosed based on lesions found on routine chest radiographs and were treated with whole lung radiation. For COG studies, it is delivered in eight treatments of 12 Gy. From NWTS-5, the 5-year EFS (95% CI) for stage IV category was lung only 76% (72% to 80%) (513 patients) and liver and lung 70% (57% to 80%) (62 patients).[172] Advances in imaging have changed the assessment of lung disease from plain radiograph to widespread use of chest computed tomography. Lesions are detected on CT scan that are not found on standard radiographs.[173–175] Thus more lesions are being identified. Complicating the use of radiation therapy is the fact that it is a major cause of long-term morbidity, particularly to the lung and heart, producing congestive heart failure, pulmonary fibrosis, and second malignancy.[176–178] Recent studies suggest that the management for pulmonary nodules should be reexamined. In SIOP-9, by 70 days of therapy, resolution of pulmonary nodules on CT scan in children with FH tumors was a favorable prognostic indicator.[179] In SIOP-9, many of these patients were spared whole lung irradiation, if complete resolution of pulmonary metastases occurred after 6 weeks of prenephrectomy chemotherapy with vincristine, dactinomycin, and doxorubicin with or without surgical excision of residual metastases. The 5-year relapse-free survival (RFS) for stage IV patients receiving preoperative chemotherapy was 62.5%.[179] The results of this study have been controversial. The United Kingdom Children's Cancer Study Group (UKCCSG) Wilms Tumor Study 1 followed a similar protocol; yet, their 6-year EFS was only 50%.[180] In their second study, UKCCSG-Wilms Tumor Study (UKWT2), the majority of children with lung metastases received whole lung irradiation (WLI), and the 4-year survival rate improved to 75%.[181] A COG study of patients with pulmonary lesions detected by CT only (as opposed to CT and chest radiograph) and treated with only two chemotherapeutic agents showed an inferior outcome compared with those treated with three drugs *irrespective* of whether or not they received pulmonary radiation.[172] A fourth study examined the value of biopsy prior to treating patients with lesions detected only by CT.[175] Two thirds of the children had tumor on biopsy, suggesting that histologic evaluation may be valuable in directing therapy. The current COG study is evaluating the use of radiographic response to chemotherapy to predict the need for whole lung irradiation. Those patients with stage IV favorable-histology WT with pulmonary metastases who have complete CT resolution of the pulmonary lesions after 6 weeks of vincristine/dactinomycin/doxorubicin chemotherapy will continue the same chemotherapy without whole lung irradiation. Those who do not have resolution of pulmonary metastases by week 6 will have the addition of cyclophosphamide and etoposide to the other three drugs and will receive whole lung irradiation.

LATE EFFECTS

The increasing numbers of survivors of WT have led to a better understanding of adverse medical conditions related to treatment of their disease that can develop over time.[182] Treatment for WT impacts renal function (discussed earlier), pregnancy, cardiac and pulmonary function, and second malignancies may develop.[178,183–187]

Pregnancy

Treatment for WT impacts reproductive capacity and increases the risk of complications during pregnancy. The National Wilms' Tumor Long-Term Follow-Up Study evaluated 700 maternal/offspring pairs.[188] If a woman had received flank radiation for unilateral WT, the dose of radiation correlated with increased risk of hypertension, fetal malposition, and premature labor. The children were also more at risk for low birth weight and prematurity (birth before 37 weeks). Premature labor was seen in 10.2% of women who did not receive flank radiation and 22% of those who received 35Gy (P = 0.001). Radiation therapy to the abdomen has resulted in absent/abnormal function of the ovaries, a small uterus, and premature menopause.[189–193] Male infertility is not at risk unless alkylating agents were used.

Secondary Malignancies

Patients who have been treated for pediatric cancer are known to have an increased risk of second malignancies. This is in part due to treatment with known carcinogens, such as alkylating agents and radiotherapy.[183,194,195] An international cohort of 13,351 children with WT diagnosed before 15 years of age, from 1960 to 2004, was established to determine the risk of second malignant neoplasms (SMN).[178] One hundred and seventy-four solid tumors and 28 leukemias were found in 195 people. Median survival after a secondary malignancy was diagnosed 5 years or more from WT was 11 years; it was 10 months for leukemia. Age-specific incidence of secondary solid tumors increased from approximately 1 case per 1,000 person-years at age 15 years to 5 cases per 1,000 person-years at age 40 years. The cumulative incidence of solid tumors at age 40 years was 6.7%. In those patients whose

WT was diagnosed after 1980, there was a lower age-specific incidence rate for second tumors compared with those treated before 1980. Paradoxically, the incidence of leukemia was higher in those diagnosed after 1990. This may be due to decreasing use of radiation therapy and increasing intensity of chemotherapy in modern protocols for treatment of WT.

Congestive Heart Failure

Congestive heart failure has been identified as a significant morbidity in children treated with doxorubicin, and this is exacerbated in patients who receive thoracic radiation. The cumulative frequency of congestive heart failure in patients treated on NWTS-1 to NWTS-4 was 4.4% at 20 years for patients treated initially with doxorubicin, but that percentage is expected to be lower with current cumulative doses.[184,185,196] The relative risk of congestive heart failure was found to be increased in females (risk ratio [RR] = 4.5; $P = 0.004$), and by cumulative doxorubicin dose (RR = $3.2/100 \text{ mg/m}^2$; $P < 0.001$), lung irradiation (RR = 1.6 for every 10 Gy; $P = 0.037$), and left abdominal irradiation (RR = 1.8/10 Gy; $P = 0.013$).[185] Preliminary results suggest that cardiotoxicity is lower with current radiation doses, but patients still have a substantial lifetime risk of developing cardiac disease.[183,196]

Thoracic

Radiotherapy (RT) has been implicated as a major contributor to late complications. Acute lung injury is relatively uncommon, occurring in a minority of children.[197] The late effects of pulmonary RT include pneumonitis and restrictive lung disease, scoliosis, kyphosis, reduced lung capacity, and secondary tumors. In girls, breast hypoplasia and cancer have been described.[176,177] Paulino and his colleagues reported on the late complications of pulmonary RT in 55 long-term survivors of WT.[176] Two thirds of the patients had at least one complication. Forty-three percent had scoliosis or kyphosis, and 10% developed benign chest tumors (osteochondromas). Secondary tumors were noted in three patients within the lung field (two osteogenic sarcomas of the rib and one breast cancer), and all succumbed to these tumors. Pulmonary function was examined by Attard-Montalto and colleagues.[177] Subjectively, 63% percent of patients had mild to moderate exercise intolerance, and objective measurement of vital capacity and total lung capacity was decreased compared with age and height predicted values in all. All of the females had breast hypoplasia. In another study of long-term survival of females, all developed breast hypoplasia and one had breast cancer.[198]

Other Renal Tumors

CLEAR CELL SARCOMA OF KIDNEY

CCSK accounts for 3% of renal tumors reported to the COG studies. Each year, approximately 20 new cases of CCSK are diagnosed in the United States. CCSK was recognized as a distinct clinicopathologic entity by Kidd in 1970.[199] CCSK has been described as nests of ovoid, epithelioid, or spindled cells separated by fibrovascular tissue with a "chicken wire" pattern of small blood vessels. Most tumors show evidence of this "classical" pattern, but other reported histologic patterns seen include myxoid, sclerosing, cellular, epithelioid, palisading, spindle-cell, storiform, and anaplastic patterns.[200] Immunohistochemistry is used to exclude other renal tumors. CCSK is nonspecifically vimentin and Bcl-2 positive. Gene-expression profiling studies demonstrate the expression of neural markers (e.g., nerve growth factor receptor), expression of member genes of the Sonic Hedgehog pathway and the phosphoinositide-3-kinase/Akt cell proliferation pathway.[201,202] Recently, a translocation t(10;17) and deletion 14q have also been described in CCSK, suggesting that they may play a role in its pathogenesis.[203] CCSK is characterized by bone and brain metastases and the increased tendency for late recurrences. Long-term follow-up of CCSK patients is needed because 30% of relapses occurred more than 3 years after diagnosis, and some occurred as late as 10 years after diagnosis.[204] The tumor is generally unilateral and unicentric, with solid and, occasionally, cystic areas. On NWTS-1 to NWTS-3, treatment for CCSK was the same as for WT, and the outcomes were poor. In NWTS-4, patients were treated with vincristine, dactinomycin, doxorubicin, and RFS, and overall survival was improved versus NWTS-3 (RFS 71.6% versus 60.2% at 8 years, $P = 0.11$; OS 83% versus 66.9% at 8 years, $P < 0.01$).[204] To further improve survival, patients on NWTS-5 with CCSK were treated using regimen I (see Table 30-2), because etoposide and cyclophosphamide were active against CCSK in preclinical models.[205] Four-year OS for stage I patients was 100%. Stage II, III, and IV had 4-year OS of 88.9%, 94.8%, and 41.7%, respectively. LOH was not found in most cases of children with CCSK and is not predictive of outcomes. In the current COG study, patients with CCSK are treated according to the high-risk study. Patients with stage I disease will continue to be treated with regimen I but will not receive radiation therapy. The need to minimize unnecessary therapy in patients with stage I CCSK is highlighted by the fact that treatment-related deaths in the Argani series outnumbered tumor-related deaths, two versus one.[200] In addition, none of the stage I patients from NWTS-5 have relapsed, with a median follow-up of more than 4 years. To improve survival for children with higher-stage disease, they will be treated with revised UH-1 (see Table 30-4).

RHABDOID TUMOR OF THE KIDNEY

RTK was initially described in 1978 as a "rhabdomyosarcomatoid" variant of WT.[206] Haas used the term "rhabdoid tumor" in 1981, because of the absence of muscle differentiation.[207] RTKs have been reported to occur throughout the body, including the brain, liver, soft tissues, lung, skin, and heart. RTK accounts for 2% of all renal tumors, and it is the most aggressive and lethal of all pediatric renal tumors. Clinical features that help distinguish an RTK from WT clinically include the presence of hypercalcemia and diffuse lymphatic and hematogenous spread in a young infant. Tomlinson and her colleagues reviewed 142 patients with RTK from NWTS-1 to NWTS-5.[208] Age at diagnosis was found to be a highly significant prognostic factor for survival of children with RTK. Infants have a dismal prognosis, whereas older children have a slightly more favorable outcome. Higher tumor stage and presence of a central nervous system (CNS) lesion were also predictive of a poor rate of survival. Unfortunately, these tumors tend to present at an advanced stage and are resistant to chemotherapy.[209] RTK is associated with second primary tumors in the brain, including cerebellar medulloblastomas, pineoblastomas, neuroblastomas, and subependymal giant cell astrocytomas.[210]

Grossly, the tumors are solid, unencapsulated, and often have extensive hemorrhage and necrosis. The tumors are very invasive. Microscopically, they consist of sheets of cells showing nuclear pleomorphism and characteristic morphologic features of open vesicular nuclei, prominent nucleoli, and scattered hyaline eosinophilic cytoplasmic inclusions composed of intermediate filaments in a "whorled" pattern. At present, no single immunohistochemical stain or profile is considered to represent a diagnostic criterion. Recently, genetic abnormalities of the *hSNF5/INI1* tumor suppressor gene on chromosome 22 have been shown to be characteristic for both renal and extrarenal rhabdoid tumors; the gene is important for chromatin remodeling. For all other renal tumors, except RTK, immunohistochemical staining for the wild-type integrase interactor 1 (INI-1) protein shows nuclear positivity. In renal and extrarenal rhabdoid tumors, this is absent.[211] This antibody is being evaluated for its diagnostic utility in the current COG renal tumor study.

Both SIOP and COG/NWTSG have reported poor outcomes for children with RTK.[208,212] The outcomes by stage from NWTS-5 are stage I = 50.5%, stage II and III = 33.3%, stage IV = 21.4%, stage V = 0%. Children with RTK, on the current COG study, will be treated using revised UH-1 if they are stage I to IV and have no measurable disease after surgery. If they have measureable disease (stage III, IV), they will receive a vincristine/irinotecan "window," followed by revised UH-2 if they have a partial or complete response (see Table 30-2). The rationale for this treatment strategy was based on reviewing the outcomes from the intergroup rhabdomyosarcoma (IRS) studies and several case reports that documented the successful treatment of advanced or metastatic rhabdoid tumor of the kidney.[213–215]

RENAL CELL CARCINOMA

RCC in childhood accounts for 5% to 8% of all pediatric and adolescent renal malignancies. They are more common than clear cell sarcoma of the kidney and malignant rhabdoid.[1] The median age at presentation in children is 9 years. By age 15, RCC becomes as common as WT (Fig. 30-10). In the pediatric population, there have been limited therapeutic studies with no randomized controlled trials. Similar to WT, children with RCC generally present with an asymptomatic abdominal mass, although hematuria is a frequent finding.[216] Imaging studies cannot differentiate RCC from other solid renal tumors. RCC in children can be divided into two broad pathologic groups.[217] The first is the classical clear cell histology. This includes the adult-type RCC with 3p25 (VHL locus) genetic abnormalities and tumors in patients with tuberous sclerosis. In addition, there is a unique genetic subtype of clear cell that presents in adolescents and young adults, accounting for nearly one third of all cases. These tumors are characterized by the chromosomal translocations involving the *TFE3* gene on Xp11.2[217–219] or the *TFEB* gene on 6p21.[220,221] The abnormal gene fusions produce protein dysregulation and result in overexpression of either *TFE3* or *TFEB* transcription factors, which contribute to tumor pathogenesis. Immunohistochemistry can detect aberrant expression for TFE3 or TFEB and can thus be useful in establishing the diagnosis.[221,222] In addition, these translocation-positive RCCs have been described as second malignancies following previous chemotherapy.[223,224]

The second subgroup of pediatric RCCs are the papillary RCCs.[225–227] Papillary renal cell carcinoma appears more frequently than classical clear cell. Other RCC cell types include chromophobe or collecting duct types.[228] Renal medullary carcinomas are rare, but highly aggressive, malignancies that are associated with sickle cell hemoglobinopathy.[229,230] Approximately 25% of pediatric RCCs are not able to be classified because of atypical histologic features.[217]

Complete tumor resection is the most important determinant of outcome in RCC.[228] Younger age at diagnosis is also a favorable prognostic factor. It has been suggested that regional lymph node involvement does not portend the same grave prognosis as it does in adult renal cell carcinoma; however, because this impression was reached based on only 13 patients, further evaluation is required.[231] Data collected from RCC patients enrolled on NWTS-5 showed 5-year OS survival rates by stage: stage I 92.5%, stage II 73%, stage III 55%, and stage IV 9%. Similar to adult RCC, prognosis worsens with increasing stage, although direct comparisons of adult and pediatric data are confounded by the finding that most reviews of pediatric RCC used the modified Robson staging system rather than the tumor-node-metastasis (TNM) system. Neither chemotherapy nor radiation therapy have demonstrated activity in adult or pediatric patients with metastatic RCC. To address this lack of knowledge and experience, for the first time these tumors will be addressed in a COG protocol. To enable comparison with adult tumors, the staging system proposed by the World Health Organization will be used. The relatively good survival rate for children with localized RCC combined with the relative inefficacy of the known adjuvant therapies support treating children without adjuvant therapy. However, the provision of adjuvant chemotherapy is at the discretion of the local physicians. A major future thrust will be to identify novel agents with activity against RCC.

CONGENITAL MESOBLASTIC NEPHROMA

Congenital mesoblastic nephroma (CMN) is the most frequent renal neoplasm of newborns and young infants, accounting for 5% of all renal tumors.[129,232–234] The median age at diagnosis is 2 months. In 1967, Bolande and colleagues were the first to describe the tumor as a separate entity from WT.[234] CMN are firm on gross examination, and the cut surface has the yellowish gray trabeculated appearance of a leiomyoma. To date,

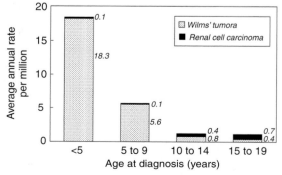

RENAL CANCER AGE-SPECIFIC INCIDENCE RATES BY TUMOR SEER 1975-1995

FIGURE 30-10 Incidence of renal cell carcinoma and Wilms' tumor by age. SEER, Surveillance, Epidemiology, and End Results (Program).

three histologic subtypes have been described. The classical type, first identified by Bolande (24% of cases), cellular type (66% of cases), and mixed type (10% of cases) showing both classical and cellular patterns.[235] The classical variant is characterized by leiomyomatous histology, with spindle cells in bundles, rare mitoses, and the absence of necrosis. It is histologically similar to infantile myofibromatosis. The cellular variant consists of solid, cellular, sheetlike growth pattern of oval or round cells with little cytoplasm and frequent mitoses and necrosis, which resembles infantile fibrosarcoma. The mixed type of congenital mesoblastic nephroma features areas resembling both classical and cellular morphologies.[235–237] The relationship between mixed CMN and the two main histologic subtypes is not clear.[238]

The observation that classical CMN is similar to infantile myofibromatosis and cellular CMN resembles infantile fibrosarcoma suggests that these may be two distinct entities, and genetic studies provide evidence in support of this hypothesis. Cellular CMN is characterized by the t(12;15) translocation, resulting in the *ETV6-NTRK3* fusion gene, a genetic change that has not been identified in classical CMN, but is characteristic of infantile fibrosarcoma.[238,239] This led to the hypothesis that cellular CMN is an intrarenal occurrence of infantile fibrosarcoma, whereas classic CMN reflects intrarenal fibromatosis. The cloning of the resulting gene fusion has allowed the development of molecular detection assays for this subtype of congenital mesoblastic nephroma. The absence of the fusion product in classical congenital mesoblastic nephroma correlates with its demonstrated absence in infantile myofibromatosis. The challenge then is to explain the existence of the mixed lesions.

Clinically, most children with CMN have an excellent prognosis and are cured with a radical nephroureterectomy with lymph node sampling.[236,240] However, CMN tends to grow into the hilar and perirenal soft tissue, and recurrence or metastases are seen.[241,242] In 1973, the first reports of local recurrences in children with CMN appeared in the literature.[243–245] Since then, metastasis to the lung, liver, brain, and heart have been reported.[245–249] Recurrence and metastatic disease has lead to a debate concerning the need for adjuvant therapy to prevent these rare events in a subset of patients versus the risks of this therapy in infants.[237,241]

Subsequent investigations demonstrated that recurrences were seen preferentially in either the cellular or the mixed subtypes. Other suggested risk factors for recurrence included age (more than 3 months of age), stage (stage III resulting from incomplete surgical resection), and vascular invasion.[250,251] In 2006, the German Pediatric Oncology Group published their experience with 50 children with CMNs, suggesting that a subgroup of children more than 3 months of age with stage III cellular CMN tends to develop recurrences more often supporting the earlier findings.[252] Alternatively, Perlman and colleagues evaluated 396 cases of CMN from the database of the J.B. Beckwith Developmental Renal Tumor Collection.[253] Thirty CMNs were known to have recurred (7.6% overall recurrence rate and 9.3% recurrence rate for tumors with a cellular histologic component). Recurrences took place within 1 year of diagnosis (range, 2 to 11.5 months); 20 were local, 8 were metastatic, and 2 were both local and metastatic. None of the classical CMNs recurred, including 18 that were known or suspected to have residual disease. Recurrences were confined to tumors with a cellular component

or cellular and mixed, which had the same risk of recurrence. Stage III disease was the second factor associated with recurrence. Intrarenal and renal sinus vascular invasion correlated with increased potential for recurrence; however, the correlation did not achieve independent statistical significance. Other clinical or pathologic features previously suggested as prognostic factors, including age at diagnosis, were not proven to be of additional prognostic significance. This study concluded that the most important risk factors for recurrence in CMNs are the presence of a cellular histologic component and stage III disease. However, in none of these reports has the efficacy of adjuvant therapy been established.

SOLITARY MULTILOCULAR CYST AND CYSTIC PARTIALLY DIFFERENTIATED NEPHROBLASTOMA

Cystic renal tumors are a diagnostic and therapeutic challenge (Fig. 30-11). Cystic nephroma (CN), cystic partially differentiated nephroblastoma (CPDN), and cystic WT (CWT) are a spectrum with CN at the benign end, CWT at the malignant end (these must have both a solid and cystic component), and CPDN in the intermediate position. The three types cannot be differentiated using imaging techniques and can be confused with cystic clear cell sarcoma and cystic mesoblastic nephroma.[254] Multicystic dysplastic kidney can generally be distinguished radiographically from the other entities, because it lacks any normal renal parenchyma that the other lesions should contain.[255]

CYSTIC NEPHROMA

CN is an uncommon benign renal lesion that occurs most commonly in children younger than 24 months of age, with a male to female ratio close to 2:1. A second peak incidence occurs in adults around 30 years of age, with an 8:1 female to male predominance.[255–258] Grossly, these masses are

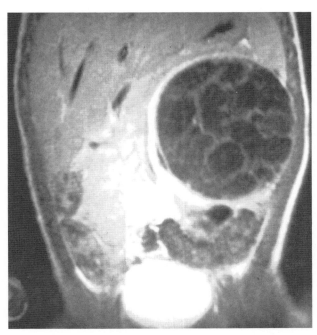

FIGURE 30-11 A magnetic resonance scan of a cystic nephroma.

well-encapsulated multilocular tumors composed of various-sized cysts with thin septations that compress the normal kidney. Microscopically, the identifying feature is that of mature well-differentiated cell types within the septa of the cyst wall. There are no blastemal or embryonal elements.[254,255] Most cases are unilateral, but some are bilateral.[259] Although CN is benign, cases have been reported with pleuropulmonary blastoma as well. The relationship between these two entities is undefined.[260,261]

CYSTIC PARTIALLY DIFFERENTIATED NEPHROBLASTOMA

Cystic partially differentiated nephroblastoma is a multilocular cystic WT composed entirely of cysts separated by delicate septa. The majority of these lesions occur in the first 2 years of life.[256,262,263] Cystic partially differentiated nephroblastoma is usually well circumscribed and sharply demarcated from the adjacent normal kidney. It can be large (up to 18 cm in diameter) and may produce visible abdominal distention. This neoplasm is composed entirely of variably sized cysts; unlike CN, the septal stroma contains small foci of blastema, primitive or immature epithelium, and/or immature-appearing stromal cells.[264,265] In addition, skeletal muscle fibers are commonly present in cystic partially differentiated nephroblastoma.

Both COG/NWTSG and SIOP have reported their experiences with CN and CPDN.[262,266,267] In the NWTSG study, 21 patients were evaluated.[262] Thirteen patients received chemotherapy, and 8 patients did not. In the chemotherapy group, the distribution by stage was 10 children with stage I, 2 children with stage II, and 1 child with stage V. The 8 no-chemotherapy patients were all stage I with a 100% survival. The SIOP evaluated 14 patients with diagnoses of cystic nephroma (7 patients) and cystic partially differentiated nephroblastoma (7 patients). Two patients received preoperative chemotherapy. Primary nephrectomy was performed in 12 patients. Two patients underwent partial nephrectomy. In 1 child, postoperative chemotherapy was administered. None of the patients had progression of disease or recurrence. Overall survival was also 100%.[267] There is some concern about doing partial nephrectomies because of recurrences after incomplete excision as well as distinguishing this tumor from other malignant lesions.[267,268]

The complete reference list is available online at www.expertconsult.com.

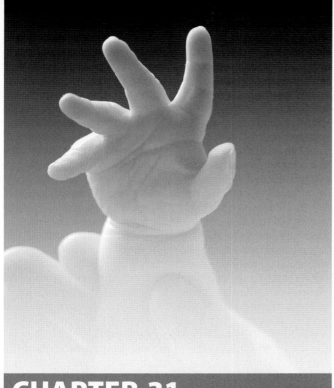

CHAPTER 31

Neuroblastoma

Barrie S. Rich and Michael P. La Quaglia

Neuroblastoma is one of the most common solid tumors in infancy and childhood. This is a neoplasm of neural crest origin, arising in the adrenal medulla and along the sympathetic ganglion chain from the neck to the pelvis. The clinical course is quite variable, because this highly malignant tumor demonstrates unusual behavior. Although instances of spontaneous regression and tumor maturation from a malignant to a benign histologic form have been observed,[1–7] the disease is progressive in many cases. Survival in children with other malignancies, such as Wilms' tumor, rhabdomyosarcoma, acute lymphocytic leukemia, germ cell tumors, Hodgkin disease, and non-Hodgkin lymphoma, has been significantly improved by the intensive use of combined treatment modalities, but the outlook for many children with advanced neuroblastoma remains dismal.[1,5,8–12] This neoplasm exhibits great heterogeneity in its behavior and represents a significant challenge to practitioners.

Primitive neuroblasts can be identified in the fetal adrenal gland in the 10th to 12th intrauterine week. The nodules increase in number by 20 weeks' gestation but gradually diminish in number toward the end of gestation. Neuroblastoma in situ in the adrenal gland is seen in 1 of every 260 neonates who die of congenital heart disease and in as many as 1 in 39 infants who die from other causes in the first 3 months of life. The clinical incidence of the tumor is approximately 1 in 7,500 to 10,000 children.[1,10,13,14] Neuroblastoma is responsible for 10% of all childhood tumors and 15% of all cancer deaths. There are 700 cases diagnosed annually in the United States. Approximately 40% of cases are diagnosed by 1 year of age, 75% by 7 years, and 98% by 10 years.[1] More than half the patients are younger than 2 years at the time of diagnosis.[15] Neuroblastoma is slightly more common in boys than in girls, with a male-to-female ratio of 1.2:1.0.[1,10] It is the most common intra-abdominal malignancy in newborns, and the most frequently diagnosed malignancy in children less than 1 year of age.[16]

The embryonal nature of neuroblastoma has been well documented by its identification on prenatal ultrasonography, and the tumor has been known to invade the placenta during the antenatal period, though this is a rare occurrence.[17–24] More than 55 cases of antenatally discovered neuroblastoma have been reported in the literature since the original description by Fénart and colleagues in 1983.[25] The masses are usually identified during ultrasound examinations performed after 32 weeks' gestation. The earliest reported instance was observed at 18 weeks' gestation.[26]

Mothers of infants with congenital neuroblastoma occasionally experience flushing and hypertension during pregnancy as a result of catecholamine released from the fetal tumor in utero.

Neuroblastoma has been described in twins on many occasions, and familial occurrences in both mother and child and father and son have been reported.[23,27,28] Concordance for neuroblastoma in twins during infancy indicates that hereditary factors may be predominant in this age group, whereas discordance in older twins suggests that a random mutation may be more important for this population. The median age for the occurrence of familial neuroblastoma is 9 months, in contrast to 18 months in the general population. Maris and colleagues[29] observed that 20% of patients with familial neuroblastoma have bilateral or multifocal tumors and reported evidence for a hereditary neuroblastoma predisposition locus on chromosome 16p12-13. Neuroblastoma has been observed in infants with Beckwith-Wiedemann syndrome, neurofibromatosis (von Recklinghausen disease), Hirschsprung disease, central hypoventilation syndrome (Ondine's curse), and fetal alcohol syndrome, and in offspring of mothers taking phenytoin (fetal hydantoin syndrome) for seizure disorders.[30–34] Mutations in the *PHOX2B* gene, which is often seen in congenital central hypoventilation disorder, have been documented in those with familial neuroblastoma, and in 2.3% of those with sporadic neuroblastomas.[35] Recently, it has been determined that genetic mutations in the anaplastic lymphoma kinase (*ALK*) gene explain most hereditary neuroblastoma. However, activating mutations of this gene can also be somatically acquired.[36] This discovery has initiated the development of therapy based on *ALK* inhibition.[37] Although it is unlikely that environmental factors play an important role in causing this tumor, neuroblastoma has been noted among infants of mothers receiving medical therapy for vaginal infection during pregnancy and with paternal occupational exposure to electromagnetic fields.[1]

Neuroblastoma may occur at any site where neural crest tissue is found in the embryo. The neuroblast is derived from primordial neural crest cells that migrate from the mantle layer of the developing spinal cord. Tumors may arise in the neck, posterior mediastinum, retroperitoneal (paraspinal) ganglia, adrenal medulla, and pelvic organ of Zuckerkandl.[5,10,14,38] In 75% of cases, the tumor is located in the retroperitoneum,

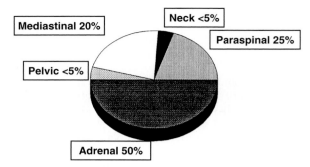

FIGURE 31-1 Distribution of cases of neuroblastoma at each of the primary tumor sites. Primary tumors most commonly occur in the adrenal gland.

in either the adrenal medulla (50%) or the paraspinal ganglia (25%). In 20% of cases, the primary tumor is in the posterior mediastinum. Less than 5% of tumors occur in the neck or pelvis (Fig. 31-1).[1,5,10,14] Primary intracranial cerebral neuroblastoma also occurs.[39,40] In addition, a teratoma in an infant may occasionally contain foci of neuroblastoma. Rare cases of neuroblastoma arising in the bladder have also been reported.[41]

The fate of the neuroblasts can follow 1 of 3 clinical pathways: (1) spontaneous regression, (2) maturation by differentiation from neuroblastoma to a benign ganglioneuroma, or most frequently, (3) rapid progression to a highly malignant tumor that is often resistant to treatment.

Mass Screening

In an effort to identify early cases of neuroblastoma that were amenable to cure, mass screening programs were initiated in Japan in 1985, evaluating urinary vanillylmandelic acid (VMA) and homovanillic acid (HVA) levels in infants at 6 months of age. These studies identified a large number of infants with neuroblastoma. The survival in these cases was exceptionally high compared with the survival in patients who present with clinical disease diagnosed by conventional methods. The Japanese screening effort doubled the actual incidence of neuroblastoma in infants younger than 1 year of age, but neither decreased the number of cases observed in older children nor improved the survival of children older than 1 year of age.[1,42–44] Sawada and colleagues[43,44] reported a 96% survival rate in 170 cases of neuroblastoma identified by screening. These observations suggest that neuroblastomas identified by screening were most likely biologically favorable tumors that spontaneously regressed.[43] However, a small number of screened patients have had tumors with unfavorable biologic markers and a poor prognosis, and a few screened patients who tested negative at 6 months of age later (at 12 to 18 months of age) developed highly aggressive neuroblastomas.[45]

In general, mass screening has provided important information regarding the natural history of this enigmatic tumor and has identified a group of tumors that clearly regress and represent a biologically favorable form of tumor, in contrast to that noted in older children.[7] Prospective, population-based, controlled screening trials in Quebec minimized the rate of false-positive cases, but had an overall sensitivity of only 45%. The results were similar to the findings in Japan.[46] A German study offered screening to 2.6 million infants between 9 and 18 months of age. This effort identified 149 cases of neuroblastoma in 1,800 screened infants, demonstrating a predictive value of 8%.[47] The German investigators estimated that two thirds of the tumors detected by screening would have regressed spontaneously. The potential risks were highlighted by the fact that all 3 children who died in the group detected by screening had localized disease and succumbed from complications of treatment. These studies in North America, Japan, and Europe suggest that screening may result in an overdiagnosis of neuroblastoma and the performance of unnecessary therapies.[48] However, the results observed in screening studies are valuable and should help minimize treatment in the substantial subset of infants diagnosed with early-stage neuroblastoma that has an excellent chance of either maturing or spontaneously regressing.[49] Because of compelling medical and psychological reasons, especially among parents in false-positive cases, neuroblastoma screening was discontinued in many countries.[50,51] Following the cessation of screening elsewhere in the world, the Ministry of Health in Japan discontinued its mass screening program in April 2004.[52]

Clinical Presentation

Neuroblastoma is a tumor with multiple clinical manifestations related to the site of the primary tumor, the presence of metastases, and the production of certain metabolic tumor byproducts. In 50% to 75% of reported cases, patients present with an abdominal mass. The tumor may be hard, nodular, fixed, and painful on palpation. Generalized symptoms include weight loss, failure to thrive, abdominal pain and distention, fever, and anemia.[1,5,10,14] Hypertension is found in 25% of cases and is related to the production of catecholamines by the tumor. Instances of hypercalcemia have been observed in association with neuroblastoma, and hemoperitoneum caused by sudden spontaneous rupture of the neoplasm has also been reported.[53,54]

Neoplasms arising in the upper mediastinum or neck may involve the stellate ganglion and cause Horner syndrome, which is characterized by ptosis, miosis, enophthalmos, anhydrosis, and heterochromia of the iris on the affected side.[5,10,14] Metastases to the bony orbit may produce proptosis or bilateral orbital ecchymosis—often referred to as "panda eyes" or "raccoon eyes" (Fig. 31-2). The latter finding in a child

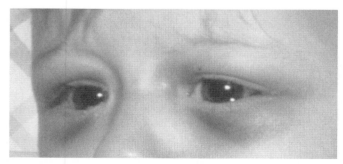

FIGURE 31-2 Child with bilateral orbital ecchymoses ("panda eyes" or "raccoon eyes") resulting from orbital metastases from neuroblastoma.

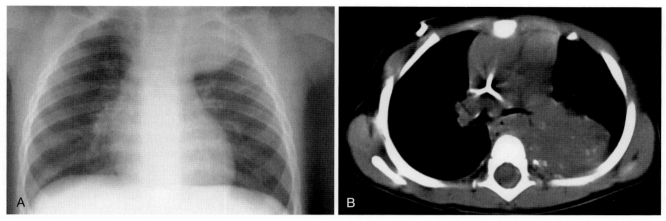

FIGURE 31-3 A, Plain chest radiograph shows the presence of a left upper thoracic tumor. **B,** Computed tomography scan documents a mass in the posterior mediastinum that contains calcium, suggestive of a neuroblastoma.

without a history of trauma should always raise the index of suspicion for the presence of a malignancy. Mediastinal tumors may be associated with respiratory distress because of the tumor's interference with lung expansion and dysphagia caused by extrinsic pressure on the esophagus (Fig. 31-3).[10,55–57] Mediastinal and paraspinal retroperitoneal lesions may manifest with paraplegia related to tumor extension through an intervertebral foramen, resulting in a dumbbell- or hourglass-shaped lesion that may cause extradural compression of the spinal cord.[14,58–61] In a few patients, cauda equina syndrome has also been observed. Pelvic tumors may be associated with bladder and bowel dysfunction. They are usually palpable on rectal examination. They must be differentiated from presacral teratoma, yolk sac tumor, nonosseous Ewing tumor, and pelvic rhabdomyosarcoma.[5,10]

Anemia is often related to bone marrow invasion by the tumor. Excessive catecholamine production by the tumor may result in flushing, sweating, and irritability. Acute cerebellar ataxia, characterized by opsomyoclonus and nystagmus ("dancing eye syndrome"), has been observed.[62–66] This syndrome is seen more frequently (>60%) in patients with primary mediastinal tumors, in patients with stage I or II disease, and in infants younger than 1 year of age.[62,66] In addition, they are often more histologically mature. The involuntary muscular contractions and random eye movements are unrelated to metastases. The cause is suggested to be an autoimmune phenomenon related to an antigen–antibody complex involving antibodies that cross-react with Purkinje cells in the cerebellum.[62,64,66,67] Poor school performance and learning deficits may occur as sequelae.[64,65] The survival rate for patients who present with opsomyoclonus and nystagmus is approximately 90%. Presence of the dancing eye syndrome in patients who present with advanced tumors and N-myc overexpression, however, is associated with a poor outcome.[68] Despite tumor resection and adrenocorticotropic hormone treatment, the neurologic symptoms in survivors (including learning disabilities and attention deficits) may persist for many years.[63–65]

Infants with neuroblastoma, ganglioneuroblastoma, and, occasionally, benign ganglioneuroma may present with intractable diarrhea characterized by watery, explosive stools and hypokalemia.[69–71] The diarrhea is related to the production of vasoactive intestinal polypeptide (VIP) by the tumor.[10,69–71] Tumors associated with this syndrome often have somatostatin receptors and are differentiated, low-risk tumors. Serum VIP levels can serve as a tumor marker; the tumor often does not secrete catecholamines. These observations suggest that somatostatin receptor expression is a favorable prognostic factor.[72,73]

Children with advanced neuroblastoma frequently show evidence of protein-calorie malnutrition associated with immunoincompetence, based on anergy to a variety of skin test antigens.[74,75] Rickard and colleagues[74,75] demonstrated that patients with stage IV neuroblastoma who were malnourished at diagnosis had more treatment delays and a significantly worse outcome than adequately nourished counterparts with similar disease severity. These findings suggest that a nutritional assessment at diagnosis should be a component of the patient's staging.[74] In addition, Van Eys and colleagues[76] and Rickard and colleagues[74,75] showed that significant nutritional depletion occurs with multimodal cancer therapy and that total parenteral nutrition can replete and maintain the patient's nutritional status during intensive tumor therapy. In another study, Sala and colleagues[77] reported that the incidence of malnutrition in children with advanced neuroblastoma was 50%. They stressed the importance of nutritional status and its possible influence on the course of the disease and survival. Of interest is a study from Toronto, Canada, that implies that mandatory folic acid fortification of flour—initially intended to reduce the incidence of neural tube defects—was associated with a 60% decrease in the incidence of neuroblastoma in the province of Ontario.[78]

Neuroblastoma may spread by direct extension into surrounding structures, lymphatic infiltration, or hematogenous metastases. Regional and distant lymph nodes, liver, bone marrow, and bone cortex are frequently involved.[5,10,11,79–81] Patients with bone cortex metastases have an ominous prognosis. Bone metastases occur in sites containing red marrow and involve the metaphyseal areas of long bones in addition to the skull, vertebral column, pelvis, ribs, and sternum.[1,5,10,11] Bone lesions may cause extreme pain and may be first identified when a child refuses to walk because of leg pain. Hematogenous metastases to the brain, spinal cord, and heart are unusual. Brain metastases usually manifest in older children with headaches and seizures.[8,82] Lung metastases are found on chest radiographs in only 4% of patients.[83] This may be the result of direct extension to the lung from mediastinal lymph nodes or diffuse hematogenous spread, presenting with a radiographic pattern that may be confused with pulmonary edema or interstitial pneumonia.[83] Lung involvement by intralymphatic metastases (not seen on chest radiographs) may be noted at autopsy. Occasionally, patients with advanced disease present with a bleeding diathesis related to thrombocytopenia from extensive involvement of bone marrow and interference with hepatic production of clotting factors by liver metastases. Multiple subcutaneous skin nodules and hepatomegaly may occur in infants with stage IV-S neuroblastoma.

Diagnosis

Diagnosis of neuroblastoma is made through a variety of imaging and isotopic studies, serum and urine determinations, and histologic and genetic evaluation of tumor tissue. On the plain abdominal radiograph, approximately 50% of cases may show finely stippled tumor calcification.[10,11,14] Radiographs also may show displacement of bowel gas by a mass. Paraspinal widening is commonly found with celiac axis tumors. Chest radiographs may show a posterior mediastinal tumor, a paraspinal widening above the diaphragm from extension of an abdominal tumor, or a primary thoracic tumor. The diagnostic workup of patients with retroperitoneal tumors includes an initial upright radiograph of the abdomen, an ultrasound examination to distinguish a cystic from a solid lesion, and an evaluation for potential obstruction or compression of the inferior vena cava. As a rule, obstruction of the inferior vena cava in patients with neuroblastoma suggests the presence of an initially unresectable lesion.[10,84] Computed tomography (CT) can demonstrate tumor calcification in approximately 80% of cases (Fig. 31-4).[14,85] With CT studies using contrast enhancement, one can often distinguish kidney and liver from adrenal and paraspinal lesions and evaluate for

intracranial extension of skull metastases.[10,85,86] Magnetic resonance imaging (MRI) is extremely useful in detecting intraspinal tumor extension and, in some instances, the tumor's relationship to major vascular structures. Helical (spiral) CT with three-dimensional reconstruction is also a useful method of evaluating this latter relationship. Abdominal CT is performed with intravenous contrast material, so that an intravenous urogram can be acquired during the same study.[84] In most instances, paraspinal or adrenal neuroblastoma causes lateral or downward displacement of the ipsilateral kidney or ureter (or both). A separate intravenous urogram is not necessary. Metaiodobenzylguanidine (MIBG) also images both soft tissue and bony disease. A recent study for the International Neuroblastoma Risk Group (INRG) task force proclaims MIBG the most sensitive and specific imaging modality for staging purposes for neuroblastoma, in addition to recognizing response to treatment, especially when a semiquantitative scoring method is used.[87] A long bone survey, isotopic bone scintigraphy (using the bone-seeking isotopes technetium and ^{131}I-MIBG), and multiple bone marrow aspirates are also obtained.[10,11,84,85] Isotopic bone scans are also used to identify bone metastases; they show a close correlation with the radiographic skeletal survey and are occasionally more sensitive.[85] False-positive bone scans can occur in cases of recent bone trauma or inflammation. The bone-seeking isotopes are picked up by metastatic foci in the bone and by the punctate calcifications in the primary tumor (Fig. 31-5).[10,14] Demonstration of the bone-seeking isotope in a retroperitoneal or posterior mediastinal mass suggests that the lesion is a neuroblastoma. Although angiography was once performed to evaluate many childhood tumors, this test is rarely used today because vascular structures can be readily identified with less potential morbidity by other imaging studies such as helical CT or magnetic resonance angiography (Fig. 31-6).

Because neuroblastoma is a tumor derived from neural crest cells, it may secrete hormonal products and is likely a member of the amine precursor uptake and decarboxylation (APUD) family of tumors. More than 90% of children with neuroblastoma have tumors that produce high levels of catecholamines or their byproducts. Quantification of

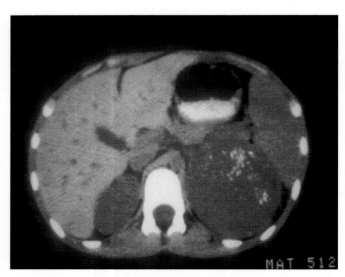

FIGURE 31-4 Abdominal computed tomography shows a retroperitoneal mass with stippled calcification, consistent with neuroblastoma.

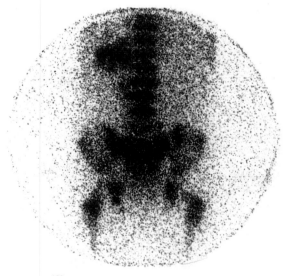

FIGURE 31-5 ^{123}I-MIBG scintiscan shows the presence of bone metastases and uptake of the isotope in a primary tumor in the adrenal gland.

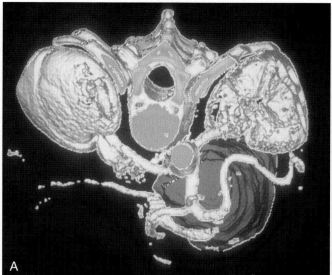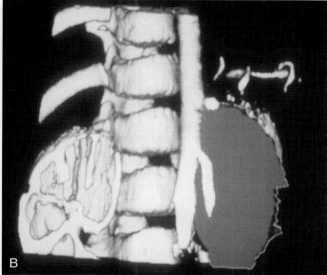

FIGURE 31-6 Helical computed tomography scan with three-dimensional reconstruction of a neuroblastoma arising near the celiac axis. **A,** Anterior view indicates that the tumor does not involve the branches of the celiac axis. **B,** Lateral view demonstrates that the superior mesenteric artery passes through the tumor.

catecholamine byproduct secretion is best done by 24-hour urine collection.[86] Adrenaline, noradrenaline, dopamine, metanephrine, HVA, VMA, and vanillylglycolic acid levels are determined. Children with immature, more undifferentiated tumors tend to excrete higher levels of certain byproducts (e.g., HVA).[14] Patients with more mature tumors excrete more VMA. In rare instances, however, the tumor does not secrete excessive catecholamines. Prasad and colleagues[88] suggested that these are parasympathetic neuroblastomas that secrete increased levels of acetylcholine and fail to metabolize tyrosine to dopamine. Patients with advanced malignancy have elevated urine concentrations of cystathionine and homoserine; increased serum levels of neuron-specific enolase, ferritin, and lactic dehydrogenase; and, in 25% of cases, sera positive for carcinoembryonic antigen.[89–93] Hann and colleagues[89] reported that 63% of patients with stage IV disease had high serum ferritin levels, which was predictive of a poor prognosis, especially in girls older than 2 years. A number of studies showed that neuroblastic tumors produce increased serum levels of neuron-specific enolase.[90,92] Zeltzer and colleagues[93] documented that neuron-specific enolase levels are elevated in 96% of patients with metastatic disease and that high serum levels are associated with a poor prognosis, particularly in infants. Elevated serum lactic dehydrogenase levels are also associated with a poor prognosis in localized neuroblastoma.[91] Although these observations are of historical interest, none of these serum levels are independent prognostic factors, nor are they currently used to determine treatment. Although histologic examination of tissue is the key to the conclusive diagnosis of neuroblastoma, in advanced disease, rosettes of tumor cells in bone marrow aspirate and increased urinary excretion of VMA or other catecholamine byproducts are often considered indicative of the diagnosis. Immunologic analysis of bone marrow aspirate may be more sensitive than conventional analysis in detecting tumor cells.[94] Serial immunocytologic analysis of peripheral blood samples has also identified circulating neuroblasts, documenting tumor dissemination.

Staging

Various staging schemes for neuroblastoma were used in the past. In 1988, an international staging system was devised, establishing a common set of criteria that could be used worldwide and would permit the accrual of large numbers of cases and allow valid comparisons of data (Table 31-1).[95] This system takes into account tumor size and location relative to the midline, in addition to the presence and degree of metastatic disease. It depends on the extent of surgical resection of the primary tumor in patients with nonmetastatic disease. Recently, the INRG developed a new staging system that takes into account pretreatment imaging of the tumor and bone marrow morphology, instead of surgical resection, which is dependent upon the approach of the surgeons and thus varies from institution to institution; this system appears in Table 31-2.[96] The aim of this system is to better evaluate pretreatment risk based on image-defined risk factors, and was developed to be used in tandem with the international system. In contrast to the International Neuroblastoma Staging System (INSS), infiltration across the midline is not included in this classification system.[96] Prospective analyses to validate this new system are ongoing.

Pathology and Histology

The pathologic classification of neuroblastoma has been revised, and histologic features of the tumor that have important prognostic value have been established.[97–99] Previously, the Shimada classification system was used. The Shimada

TABLE 31-1

International Neuroblastoma Staging System

Stage	Description
I	Localized tumor confined to area of origin; complete excision, with or without microscopic residual disease; ipsilateral and contralateral lymph nodes negative (nodes attached to primary tumor and removed en bloc with it may be positive)
IIA	Unilateral tumor with incomplete gross excision; ipsilateral and contralateral lymph nodes negative
IIB	Unilateral tumor with complete or incomplete excision; positive ipsilateral, nonadherent regional lymph nodes; contralateral lymph nodes negative
III	Tumor infiltrating across the midline with or without lymph node involvement; or unilateral tumor with contralateral lymph node involvement; or midline tumor with bilateral lymph node involvement or bilateral infiltration (unresectable)
IV	Dissemination of tumor to distant lymph nodes, bone, bone marrow, liver, or other organs
IV-S	Localized primary tumor as defined for stage I or II with dissemination limited to liver, skin, or bone marrow (limited to infants younger than 1 yr)

From Brodeur GM, Pritchard J, Berthold F, et al: Revision of the international criteria for neuroblastoma diagnosis, staging and response to treatment. J Clin Oncol 1993;11:1466-1477; Brodeur GM, Seeger RC, Barrett A, et al: International criteria for diagnosis, staging, and response to treatment in patients with neuroblastoma. J Clin Oncol 1988;6:1874-1881.

TABLE 31-2

The New International Neuroblastoma Risk Group Staging System

Stage	Description
L1	Localized tumor not involving vital structures as defined by the list of image-defined risk factors and confined to one body compartment
L2	Locoregional tumor with presence of one or more image-defined risk factors
M	Distant metastatic disease (except stage MS)
MS	Metastatic disease in children younger than 18 months with metastases confined to skin, liver, and/or bone marrow

Note: Patients with multifocal primary tumors should be staged according to the greatest extent of disease as defined in the table.
Reprinted from Monclair T, Brodeur GM, Ambros PF, et al: The International Neuroblastoma Risk Group (INRG) Staging System: An INRG Task Force Report. J Clin Oncol, 2009 10;27:298-303, with permission. © American Society of Clinical Oncology.

TABLE 31-3

Modified Shimada Pathologic Classification of Neuroblastic Tumors

	Age	Favorable Histology	Unfavorable Histology
Stroma-rich appearance	All	Well differentiated (ganglioneuroma) Ganglioneuroblastoma, intermixed	Ganglioneuroblastoma, nodular
Stroma-poor appearance (i.e., neuroblastoma)	Age < 18 months	MKI < 4%	MKI > 4% or undifferentiated
	Age 18-60 months	MKI < 2% and differentiating	MKI > 2%, or undifferentiated or poorly differentiated
	Age > 5 years	None	All

From Shimada H, Chatten J, Newton WA Jr, et al: Histopathologic prognostic factors in neuroblastoma: Definition of subtypes of ganglioneuroblastoma and an age-linked classification of neuroblastoma. J Natl Cancer Inst 1984;73:405-416; Shimada H, Stram DO, Chatten J, et al: Identification of subsets of neuroblastomas by combined histopathologic and N-myc analysis. J Natl Cancer Inst 1995;87:1470-1476.
MKI, mitotic karyorrhexis index.

system divided neuroblastic tumors into age-related favorable and unfavorable histologic categories, based on whether the tumor exhibited a stroma-rich or stroma-poor appearance (Table 31-3).[98] Stroma-rich tumors are characterized by extensive Schwannian stroma and signs of neuroblastic differentiation (i.e., developed nuclear and cytoplasmic features of ganglion cells). Stroma-poor tumors contain immature, undifferentiated neural crest cells and have a high mitotic karyorrhexis index (MKI). The MKI refers to nuclear fragmentation and is determined by the sum of the number of necrotic tumor cells; the number of cells with mitosis; and the number of cells with malformed, lobulated, or pyknotic nuclei per 5,000 cells examined. The MKI varies with age; a high MKI value in infants younger than 18 months is greater than 200/5,000 cells, and for those older than 18 months it is greater than 100/5,000 cells. All patients older than 5 years have unfavorable

histology. Stroma-poor tumors often have *MYCN* amplification, a high MKI, and a dismal outcome. A report by Shimada and colleagues[99] documented that both histology and *MYCN* amplification provided prognostic information that was independent of staging. Neuroblastomas with *MYCN* amplification have a characteristic histopathologic phenotype and a rapidly progressive clinical course.

The International Neuroblastoma Pathology Classification (INPC) adopted the Shimada classification with some minor modifications.[90,100–102] This age-linked classification is both prognostically significant and biologically relevant. The current system subdivides the undifferentiated subtype into undifferentiated and poorly differentiated tumors; changes the name of "stroma-rich, well-differentiated" tumors to "ganglioneuroma intermixed"; and adds a descriptive Schwannian, stroma-dominant character to ganglioneuroma.[103] There is also a ganglioneuroblastoma nodular (GNBn) group that is both Schwannian stroma rich/stroma dominant and stroma poor. Age remains a critical prognostic factor, and the grade of differentiation and MKI have different prognostic effects, depending on the patient's age at diagnosis. Favorable tumors are those that are poorly differentiated in children younger than 1.5 years of age, differentiating in children younger than 5 years of age, ganglioneuroblastoma intermixed, and ganglioneuroma. MKI is low (in those less than 5 years of age) or intermediate (in those less than 1.5 years of age) in this group as well. Unfavorable tumors are those that are undifferentiated or poorly differentiated in children older than 1.5 years, or any subtype of neuroblastoma in children older than 5 years. Patients with high MKI, or patients older than 1.5 years with an intermediate MKI, also have an unfavorable prognosis.[101] Although the presence of calcification was thought to favorably influence survival, further studies demonstrated that calcification does not have an independent prognostic impact.[97,103] Favorable Shimada histology was associated with an 85% survival rate, compared with 41% for unfavorable histologic

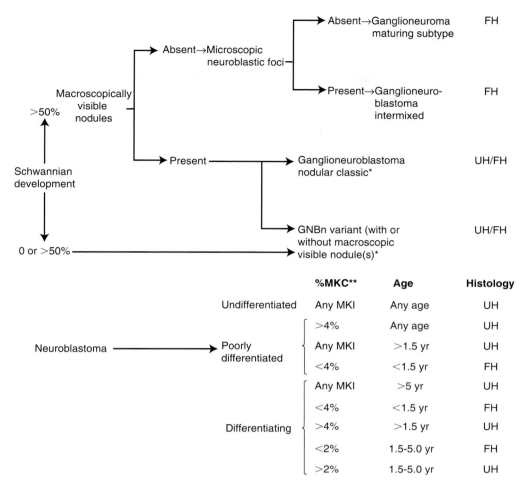

FIGURE 31-7 International Neuroblastoma Pathology Classification. FH, favorable histology; GNBn, ganglioneuroblastoma nodular; MKI, mitotic karyorrhexis index; %MKC, mitotic and karyorrhectic cells; UH, unfavorable histology; *classic GNBn (single, macroscopically visible, usually hemorrhagic nodule in stroma-rich, stroma-dominant tissue background; **MKC 2%, 100 of 5,000 cells; MKC 4%, 200 of 5,000 cells. (From Peuchmaur M, d'Amore ES, Joshi VV, et al: Revision of the International Neuroblastoma Pathology Classification: Confirmation of favorable and unfavorable prognostic subsets in ganglioneuroblastoma, nodular. Cancer 2003;98:2274-2281.)

types. All GNBn cases were initially classified as unfavorable tumors. Umehara and colleagues[104] were the first to define subsets of these specific neoplasms that exhibit different behavior. Peuchmaur and colleagues[105] recently revised the INPC by dividing GNBn cases into two prognostic subsets—favorable and unfavorable. The favorable type was associated with an 86% event-free survival, whereas the unfavorable type (two thirds of cases) had only a 32% event-free survival. Children with the favorable subset of GNBn have an overall survival of greater than 90%, compared with 33.2% for those with the unfavorable GNBn subset (Fig. 31-7).[106] Large cell neuroblastoma has been identified as a distinct phenotype with aggressive clinical behavior.[107] These tumors have unfavorable histologic features, including monomorphous undifferentiated neuroblasts, a low incidence of calcification, and a high MKI. Immunohistochemical studies showed that large cell neuroblastoma cells stained positive for neuron-specific enolase, prodrug gene products, and tyrosine hydroxylase, and were negative for CD99.[107]

On gross examination, neuroblastoma usually appears as a highly vascular purple-gray mass that is often solid but occasionally cystic. The tumor has an easily ruptured, friable pseudocapsule that may lead to significant hemorrhage during operative manipulation. The tumor is often necrotic, especially the undifferentiated form. Mature tumors (ganglioneuromas) have a more solid consistency and frequently have a fleshy white color. The histologic pattern may be quite variable. Primitive stroma-poor neuroblastomas may be indistinguishable from other small, blue round cell tumors, such as Ewing tumor, rhabdomyosarcoma, or primitive neuroectodermal tumors. The neuroblast is a small round cell consisting predominantly of the nucleus without much cytoplasm. Immature, undifferentiated tumors are characterized by closely packed small spheroid cells without any special arrangement or differentiation.[108] Nuclei may appear cone shaped and are hyperchromic. Rosette formation may be observed and is considered a sign of early tumor differentiation (Fig. 31-8). The center of each rosette is formed by a tangle of fine nerve fibers. More mature-appearing, stroma-rich tumors may contain cells that resemble normal ganglion cells, with an admixture of histologic components characterized by abundant nerve filaments, neuroblastic rosettes, and ganglion cells all seen in a single microscopic field.[28,109] On electron microscopy, neurofibrils and electron-dense, membrane-bound neurosecretory granules may be observed. The neurosecretory granules may be the site of conversion of dopamine to norepinephrine.

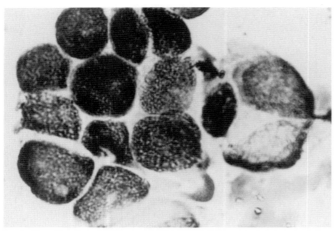

FIGURE 31-8 Histologic appearance of rosettes of neuroblastoma cells from a bone marrow aspirate, an early sign of tumor differentiation.

These ultrastructural findings and genetic identification of the tumor tissue can usually separate neuroblastoma from other small cell tumors. Segregation of neuroblastoma from other tumors can also be achieved by immunohistochemical staining that is positive for neurofilament proteins (S-100), synaptophysin, neuron-specific enolase, ganglioside GD2, chromogranin A, and tyrosine hydroxylase staining for these markers is negative in other small round cell tumors.[110]

Instances of spontaneous maturation from a highly malignant, undifferentiated neuroblastoma to a ganglioneuroblastoma, and subsequently to a benign ganglioneuroma, have been observed. Ambros and colleagues[111] reported that maturing neuroblastomas consist of both Schwann cells and neuronal cells, including ganglion cells. Schwann cells have normal numbers of chromosomes and triploid flow cytometry, in contrast to other neuronal cells, including ganglion cells.[102] These observations suggest that Schwann cells may be a reactive population of normal cells that invade a neuroblastoma, recruited or attracted by trophic factors, and may be responsible for tumor maturation and serve as an antineuroblastoma agent.[112,113] Schwann cells also produce angiogenesis inhibitors that induce endothelial cell apoptosis and may limit tumor growth by restricting angiogenesis.[1,114]

Biologic and Genetic Alterations

Unique oncogenes are observed in tumors, such as *MYCN* and *RAS* oncogenes.[1,8] Amplification of *MYCN* (> 10 copies) is associated with advanced disease, tumor progression, and a poor outcome, especially in children older than 1 year.[1,8,95,98,115,116] The *MYCN* proto-oncogene is located on the short arm of chromosome 2p24. Double minutes and long, nonbanding staining regions have been observed at this site and may represent amplified cellular genes. Studies have determined that the MycN protein binds DNA and leads to an increase in the level of endogenous Mdm2 mRNA and protein expression, with consequent p53 inhibition. This modification of Mdm2 levels by N-myc may partially explain its role in the aggressiveness of neuroblastoma.[117,118] Approximately 30% of patients with neuroblastoma have tumors with *MYCN* amplification. More than 90% of patients with *MYCN* amplification have rapidly progressive disease and are resistant to therapy.

Cellular DNA content is a predictor of response to chemotherapy in infants with unresectable neuroblastoma. DNA flow cytometry studies evaluating tumor ploidy indicate that children with diploid tumors have a worse outcome than those with aneuploid (hyperdiploidy or triploidy) tumors.[1,10] Similar to *MYCN* status, DNA ploidy is of prognostic value independent of stage and age, and the two factors (*MYCN* status, and ploidy) together provide important complementary prognostic information for infants.[1,111] DNA ploidy flow cytometry correlates well with response to chemotherapy and outcome. *MYCN* amplification is commonly associated with chromosome 1p deletion and diploidy.[119,120] Diploid tumors are commonly associated with an unbalanced gain of chromosome 17q, even in the absence of *MYCN*.[1,6,116,120] The most common cytogenetic abnormalities in neuroblastoma are 1p deletion and 17q gain.[119] Both abnormalities are poor prognostic factors and are associated with worse outcomes.[1,6,121–123] Allelic loss of 11q and 14q and gains of 4q, 6q, 11q, and 18q have also been observed (Table 31-4).[1]

TABLE 31-4		
Genetic Alterations in Neuroblastoma		
Genetic Feature	**Associated Factor**	**Risk Group**
MYCN amplification	Diploidy or tetraploidy, allelic loss of 1p, high Trk-B, advanced stage (III, IV)	High
Allelic gain 17q	More aggressive tumor associated with *MYCN* amplification	High
Gain at 4q, 6p, 7q, 11q, 18q	Occurs concurrently with *MYCN* amplification	Risk related to *MYCN* status
Allelic loss 1p36	Often associated with *MYCN* amplification	High
Allelic loss 11q	Few associated with *MCYN* amplification; correlates with LOH 14q	Intermediate decreased survival in patients without *MYCN* amplification
Allelic loss 14q	Correlates with LOH 11q, inverse relationship with allelic loss 1p and *MYCN* amplification	Intermediate
Predisposition of 16p12-13	Familial neuroblastoma, multifocal and bilateral neuroblastoma	Low
Association with chromosome 10 (*RET*-oncogene)	Hirschsprung disease	Variable
Association with 11p15.5	Beckwith-Weidemann syndrome	Low

Note: This table does not include changes in the genetic expression of TRK-A, TRK-B, and TRK-C; the multidrug-resistant protein gene; telomerase; or others that are covered elsewhere in this chapter.
LOH, loss of heterozygosity.

High expression of the neurotropin Trk-A (a high-affinity nerve growth factor receptor) is associated with a good prognosis and is inversely related to N-myc.[116,124] Trk-A is observed in young infants and in those with stage I and stage IV-S tumors, and indicates a very favorable outcome.[116,124] Trk-A is associated with neural cell differentiation and tumor regression and may play a role in angiogenic inhibition. Trk-A downregulates angiogenic factor expression and decreases the number of microvessels in neuroblastoma tumor cell lines. Multivariate analysis, however, suggests that N-myc expression is a more important independent prognostic factor. The low-affinity nerve growth factor receptor gene is another proto-oncogene that has a prognostic effect similar to Trk-A and probably influences cellular maturation.[1,8,125] In contrast, high expression of Trk-B with its ligand BDNF may provide an autocrine survival pathway in unfavorable tumors, particularly those with *MYCN* amplification, possibly by providing a tumor cell survival or growth advantage.[1,126,127] The Trk-B–BDNF pathway also contributes to enhanced angiogenesis, tumorigenicity, cell survival, and drug resistance.[1,126] These patients have more advanced disease, are usually older than 1 year, and have a dismal outcome.[1,126,127] Trk-C expression has also been identified in neuroblastoma and is usually observed in lower-stage tumors that do not express N-myc.[1,128] A recent report identified targets of *TRK* gene expression, and recognized upregulation of proapoptotic factors and angiogenesis inhibitors. Conversely, Trk-B expression was associated with upregulation of genes related to invasion and therapy resistance. Its activation is associated with increased proliferation, migration, angiogenesis, and chemotherapy resistance of neuroblastoma cells.[126,129]

Another gene has been cloned, the multidrug resistance (MDR)-associated protein gene, that is associated with chemotherapy resistance, overexpression of N-myc, and a poor outcome.[130] The prognostic role of the *MDR* gene (*MDR-1*) in neuroblastoma is controversial.[130,131] High levels of the *MDR*-associated protein gene (located on chromosome 16), however, are associated with a poor outcome. This effect is independent of stage, N-myc expression, and Trk-A status.[130] Similarly, elevated P-glycoprotein levels are associated with progressive disease and a poor outcome.[132,133] Telomerase is increased in tumor cells and maintains cell viability by preserving the telomeres that protect the end of chromosomes.[1,134] There is an inverse relationship between telomerase levels and outcome in neuroblastoma and a direct correlation between telomerase levels and *MYCN* amplification.[1] CD44 is a glycoprotein found on the cell surface of a number of tumors, including neuroblastoma. High expression of CD44 is associated with a favorable outcome and is usually found in well-differentiated tumors. In contrast, Nm23 overexpression is observed in instances of advanced and aggressive neuroblastoma.[135] The ganglioside GD2 is found on human neuroblastoma cell membranes, and increased levels are associated with active disease and tumor progression. Gangliosides inhibit the tumor-specific immune response, and GD2 has become a target for immunotherapy.[136]

Evaluation of the relationship between tumor angiogenesis and outcome in infants with neuroblastoma demonstrates that increased tumor vascularity characterized by microvessel density correlates with advanced disseminated disease and the likelihood of metastases.[137–140] Angiogenesis is associated with *MYCN* amplification, unfavorable histology, and poor outcome. Neuroblastoma produces angiogenic factors that induce blood vessel growth, including vascular endothelial growth factor (VEGF), platelet-derived growth factor (PDGF-A), stem cell factor, and their respective receptors— Flk-1, PDGFR, and c-Kit.[141] Komuro and colleagues[142] demonstrated that high VEGF-A expression correlated with stage IV disease and suggested that it could be a target for antiangiogenic therapy. Kaicker and colleagues[143] noted that vascular endothelial growth factor VEGF antagonists inhibit angiogenesis and tumor growth in experimental neuroblastoma in athymic mice with xenograft neuroblastoma cell line NGP. They also found that thalidomide suppressed angiogenesis and reduced microvessel density but not tumor growth. Kim and colleagues[144] and Rowe and colleagues[145] also demonstrated inhibition of tumor growth in experimental neuroblastoma models using antiangiogenic strategies. Imatinib mesylate, a compound used to treat patients with gastrointestinal stromal tumors, has been shown to decrease the growth of neuroblastoma in vivo and in vitro, decrease cell viability, and increase apoptosis (by ligand-stimulated phosphorylation of c-Kit and PDGFR) in a severe combined immunodeficiency (SCID) mouse model.[141] Davidoff and colleagues[138] demonstrated that gene therapy using in situ tumor cell transduction with retroviral vectors can deliver angiogenesis inhibitors for the Flk-1 receptor and restrict tumor-induced angiogenesis and tumor growth.

The Bcl-2 family of proteins is responsible for relaying apoptotic signals that influence tumor cell regression and is expressed in most neuroblastomas. The *BCL-2* gene produces a protein that prevents apoptosis. The level of Bcl-2 expression is high in advanced cases associated with a poor outcome and low in cases demonstrating tumor apoptosis (regression) and differentiation. High Bcl-2 expression may also play a role in acquired resistance to chemotherapy.[146] Subgroups of the Bcl family include Bcl-xL, which inhibits apoptosis, and Bcl-xS, which induces natural cell death. VEGF upregulates Bcl-2 expression and promotes neuroblastoma cell survival by altering apoptosis and its regulation proteins.[147] Elevated caspase levels (enzymes responsible for apoptotic signaling) are associated with an improved outcome in neuroblastomas that demonstrate favorable biologic features.[1] It has been shown that CpG–island hypermethylation inactivates caspase-8, TRAIL apoptosis receptors, the caspase-8 inhibitor, in addition to other proapoptotic factors.[148,149] In view of this finding that gene hypermethylation leads to resistance patterns, demethylating agents, including decitabine, are currently being investigated in preclinical studies.[150]

Neuroblastoma in Infancy

For many years, the age of the patient and the stage of disease at the time of diagnosis were the two key independent variables determining prognosis in children with neuroblastoma. Evans and colleagues[3] and others found that infants younger than 1 year and those with stage I, II, or IV-S disease had a significantly better outcome.[5,11,34,151,152] Historically, patients older than 1 year and those with advanced disease (stages III and IV) did poorly. The worst survival data were observed in patients older than 1 year with stage IV disease and metastases to cortical bone.[1,5,11,14,153]

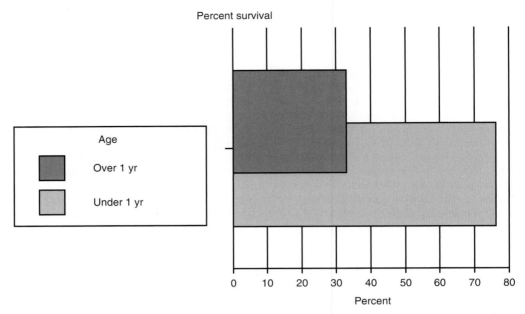

Percent survival

Age

Over 1 yr

Under 1 yr

Percent

FIGURE 31-9 Bar graph demonstrates the improved survival in infants with neuroblastoma who are younger than 1 year.

However, recent reviews have confirmed that 18 months serves as a better cutoff to predict outcome.[154–157]

Infants younger than 18 months at diagnosis have a significantly improved outcome. At the Riley Hospital for Children (Indianapolis, IN), the survival rate was 76% for infants younger than 1 year and only 32% for older patients (Fig. 31-9).[4] This favorable outlook for patients younger than 1 year extends across all stages, including infants with stage IV metastatic disease. The incidence of stage IV lesions in infants younger than 1 year is 30% compared with 60% to 70% in older patients.[4]

Infants with stage IV disease respond better to chemotherapy than do older children; 50% of infants have a complete response to treatment compared with 22% of older children.[158] This observation suggests that resolution of metastases may have a greater impact on length of survival than does the surgical excision. Further, this implies that surgical resection is beneficial in some infants and should be attempted when disseminated disease is controlled by chemotherapy. However, more intensive chemotherapy regimens and bone marrow transplantation (BMT) may be necessary to achieve a cure, especially in highly selected infants presenting with adverse biologic markers.

Stage IV-S

The most unusual group of patients with neuroblastoma is those infants younger than 18 months with stage IV-S disease. This stage is characterized by hepatomegaly produced by extensive metastatic disease, subcutaneous metastases, and positive bone marrow with a primary tumor that would otherwise be classified as stage I or II. Stage IV-S cases account for approximately 30% of patients with neuroblastoma recognized in the first year of life.[4]

Some infants succumb from complications of their stage IV-S disease rather than progression of the tumor. Complications of severe hepatomegaly include respiratory insufficiency,

caused by significant elevation of the diaphragm by the large, tumor-filled liver; coagulopathy; and renal compromise resulting from abdominal compartment syndrome produced by the mass (Fig. 31-10).[4,151,159–161] Vomiting may occur because of a change in the gastroesophageal angle related to the diaphragmatic elevation, resulting in gastroesophageal reflux, protein-calorie malnutrition, and aspiration pneumonia. Total parenteral nutrition may be a useful therapeutic adjunct.[74–76] Most fatalities in stage IV-S cases occur in infants younger than 2 months with severe symptoms related to hepatomegaly, who do not tolerate therapy as well as do older infants.[4,162] Symptomatic hepatomegaly caused by tumor infiltration may benefit from low-dose radiation to the liver in the range of 600 to 1,200 Gy, administered in doses of 100 to 150 Gy/day.[4,5,159] Although some early reduction in the size of the liver is seen, and peripheral edema may resolve in a few weeks, complete resolution may take 6 to 15 months.[4] Resolution of the liver mass is probably related more to the natural course of stage IV-S disease than to radiotherapy. Administration of low-dose cyclophosphamide 5 mg/kg per day is a reasonable treatment alternative. Although some investigators advocate the insertion of a Dacron-reinforced Silastic sheet to create a temporary ventral abdominal wall hernia to accommodate the enlarged liver and reduce intra-abdominal pressure, mortality resulting from septic complications has been observed.[4,159,163] To reduce the risk of infection, Lee and Applebaum[164] recommend the use of an internal polytetrafluorethylene patch to create a temporary ventral hernia. The graft can be removed in stages as the bulk of the hepatic mass regresses over time.

Survival of infants with remote metastases is greater than 80%, often without specific treatment. Most patients with stage IV-S disease (>90%) have favorable genetic and biologic factors, including high Trk-A expression, no *MYCN* amplification, favorable histology, and no evidence of allelic loss of chromosome 1p. This suggests that the majority of stage IV-S tumors undergo spontaneous regression. Although most patients with stage IV-S disease do well, Wilson and

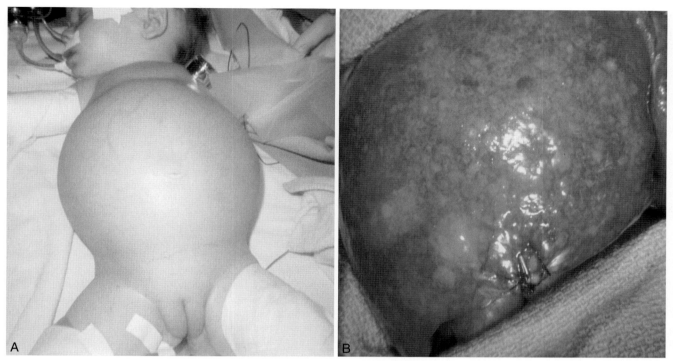

FIGURE 31-10 **A,** Six-week-old infant presented with abdominal distention and hepatomegaly. **B,** Appearance of the liver at laparotomy. There were multiple metastatic nodules, and the biopsy confirmed the diagnosis of stage IV-S neuroblastoma.

colleagues[161] reported 18 cases with a heterogeneous tumor presentation and a survival rate of only 50%, including 3 patients with *MYCN* amplification. The presence of adverse genetic and biologic prognostic factors suggests that this subset of patients (<10%) requires more aggressive therapy. Of interest is that infants with multiple subcutaneous nodules seem to have the most favorable outlook. This may be because of increased immunologic activity as a result of tumor being present in multiple sites.[4] Increased uptake of major histocompatibility complex (MHC) class I antigen by neuroblastoma cells in vitro and in vivo may influence the outcome favorably.[165] Infants with stage IV-S disease have normal levels of MHC class I surface antigen expression, whereas those with stages I to IV have low levels.[165] Sugio and colleagues[166] reported that down-modulation of MHC class I antigen expression is associated with increased amplification of the *dMYCN* oncogene in patients with advanced disease.

In 2000, Nickerson and colleagues[162] described 80 infants with stage IV-S disease from the Children's Cancer Group (CCG). Fifty-eight cases were managed without specific therapy. All 44 asymptomatic patients survived without treatment. Symptomatic patients were treated with cyclophosphamide 5 mg/kg per day for 5 days and hepatic radiation at a dose of 4.5 Gy over 3 days. Five of six deaths occurred in symptomatic infants younger than 2 months. Event-free 5-year survival was 86%, and overall survival was 92%. Early intervention is imperative for stage IV-S patients with life-threatening complications (e.g., hepatosplenomegaly, coagulopathy, renal failure).[4,162] Surgical resection did not alter outcome. More aggressive chemotherapy is also required in those cases in which the tumor demonstrates more than 10 copies of *MYCN*, chromosome 1p deletion, or other adverse biologic

markers.[4,162,167] Amplification of *MYCN* may be observed in 1 of 12 patients with stage IV-S tumors who develop progressive disease and die, despite having a favorable prognostic stage. In 2003, Schleiermacher and colleagues[167] reported on 94 infants with stage IV-S neuroblastoma in France; they observed an 88% overall survival and recommended a more intensive regimen using cisplatin and etoposide for those who require therapy. Some infants with stage IV-S disease have survived without resection of the primary tumor (in some, the primary tumor may not be identified).

Cystic Neuroblastoma

Cystic neuroblastomas are relatively rare and are often identified on prenatal ultrasound examinations.[168] They characteristically occur in the adrenal gland, and almost all are diagnosed in early infancy (Fig. 31-11). Few are calcified, and only 10% are associated with elevation of urinary VMA and HVA levels.[169] They display a benign behavior and a favorable outcome. Some evidence suggests that they often regress and undergo spontaneous involution.[26] Some investigators have recommended observation alone, with close serial sonographic monitoring during the first few months of life. Operative resection should be reserved for tumors that fail to regress or that increase in size. Adjuvant chemotherapy is rarely required after resection. The Children's Oncology Group (COG) has performed a prospective study of observation alone for cases of perinatal neuroblastoma, with strict criteria for enrollment, including tumor volume (<16 mL, if solid, or <65 mL, if cystic). Results from the study are not yet available.

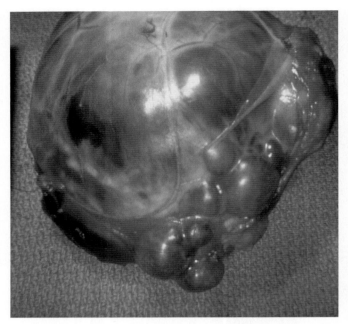

FIGURE 31-11 Photograph of a cystic neuroblastoma of the adrenal gland in a 5-month-old baby who required complete excision. The patient was managed by surgery alone and is a long-term survivor.

Multifocal and Bilateral Neuroblastoma

Bilateral neuroblastoma is relatively uncommon, occurring primarily in familial cases and young infants with alterations at the predisposition locus on chromosome 16p12-13.[29] Therapy has included observation alone; unilateral resection, with observation of the second (smaller) lesion or enucleation; and bilateral adrenalectomy, with postoperative hormonal replacement. Some bilateral tumors resolve spontaneously, while others persist and enlarge, requiring surgical intervention. The prognosis is generally good for these tumors, and most of the children survive. Occasionally these infants have other sites of multifocal disease. Tumor enucleation has been performed in cases with favorable biologic markers to preserve adrenal function. Hiyama and colleagues[170] described multifocal neuroblastoma in 8 of 106 cases (7.5%). Seven of eight cases had favorable histology, and all expressed Trk-A1 mRNA and the Ha-ras p21 protein. None of the tumors had *MYCN* amplification or elevated telomerase levels. Four had near-triploid DNA on flow cytometry, and all 8 had a proliferative index (percentage of cells in the S phase) of less than 25%. Four patients were treated with multistage resections. Five had bilateral neuroblastoma and were treated with tumor enucleation. All survived and are free of recurrence, and none require steroid replacement. The authors reviewed 53 additional cases of multifocal disease and noted that 18 had a family history of neuroblastoma and 25 were detected incidentally. Because of the excellent prognosis in patients with favorable biologic features, Hiyama's group recommended conservative surgical excision (enucleation) using minimally invasive surgical techniques.[170]

Risk Stratification and Risk-Based Management

During the past 2 decades, a number of biologic and genetic factors have been identified that are important prognostic indicators and currently define therapy in North America. Based on the INSS, the use of the INPC, and the identification of numerous biologic and genetic characteristics as risk factors and predictors of outcome, a risk-based management system has been developed to determine treatment.[1,10,100–103] Newer treatment protocols individualize treatment using risk factors as predictors of outcome in an effort to maximize survival, minimize long-term morbidity, and improve the quality of life. Current protocols now categorize patients as low, intermediate, and high risk based on their prognostic factors (Table 31-5). Good outcomes are associated with stage I, II, and IV-S patients who are younger than 18 months and have hyperdiploid DNA flow cytometry, favorable histology, less than 1 copy of *MYCN*, high Trk-A expression, and absence of chromosome 1p abnormalities. In contrast, a poor prognosis is predicted in children older than 18 months with advanced tumors (stages III and IV), more than 10 copies of *MYCN*, low Trk-A expression, diploid DNA ploidy, allelic loss of 1p36, and unfavorable histology.

The site of the primary tumor was also considered predictive of survival by some investigators. Patients with tumors in cervical, pelvic, and mediastinal locations had an improved outlook compared with children with retroperitoneal (paraspinal or adrenal) tumors. Breslow and McCann[153] and Koop and Schnaufer,[152] however, suggested that the improved outlook in these cases can be explained by the patient's age and stage of disease. Despite these conflicting views, Filler and colleagues,[56] Young,[57] and Adams and colleagues[171] reported that site is a beneficial prognostic indicator for mediastinal lesions, and Haase and colleagues[5] noted the same for pelvic tumors, regardless of other factors.

Some early reports concerning neuroblastoma suggested that the more mature and differentiated the tumor, the better the prognosis.[108] Others noted that a more mature histology may be associated with the same dismal outcome as in patients with undifferentiated neuroblasts.[152] In patients with metastatic disease, the presence of more mature elements seemed to improve the outlook and was associated with increased survival.[9,11] Shimada and colleagues[101] subsequently classified the histopathology of neuroblastoma into favorable and unfavorable types, characterized by a stroma-rich appearance for the former and a stroma-poor appearance for the latter. The Shimada classification was also age related. The impact of Shimada histology class on prognosis proved to be important, especially when associated with other prognostic biologic variables, particularly amplification of the *MYCN* oncogene and allelic loss on the short arm of chromosome 1p (1p36).[99] The current INPC (which embraced and modified the Shimada classification) further divided cases into subsets of favorable and unfavorable histologic types and is a highly significant independent predictor of prognosis.[98,102,103,105,172] *MYCN* amplification is seen in approximately 30% of neuroblastoma cases and has an important role in modulating the malignant phenotype in neuroblastoma.[1,124,173] The prognostic value of *MYCN* status is independent of tumor stage and patient age. *MYCN* amplification is associated with a poor response to treatment,

TABLE 31-5
Neuroblastoma Risk Groups*

Risk Group	INSS Stage	Age	MYCN Amplification Status[†]	DNA Ploidy[‡]	INPC (Modified Shimada) Histology
Low	1	Any	Any	Any	Any
Low	2a/2b	Any	Not amplified	Any	Any
High	2a/2b	Any	Amplified	Any	Any
Intermediate	3	< 547 days	Not amplified	Any	Any
Intermediate	3	≥ 547 days	Not amplified	Any	FH
High	3	Any	Amplified	Any	Any
High	3	≥ 547 days	Not amplified	Any	UH
High	4	< 365 days	Amplified	Any	Any
Intermediate	4	< 365 days	Not amplified	Any	Any
High	4	365 to <547 days	Amplified	Any	Any
High	4	365 to <547 days	Any	DI = 1	Any
High	4	365 to <547 days	Any	Any	UH
Intermediate	4	365 to <547 days	Not amplified	DI > 1	FH
High	4	≥ 547 days	Any	Any	Any
Low	4 s	< 365 days	Not amplified	DI > 1	FH
Intermediate	4 s	< 365 days	Not amplified	DI = 1	Any
Intermediate	4 s	< 365 days	Not amplified	Any	UH
High	4 s	< 365 days	Amplified	Any	Any

*Courtesy Children's Oncology Group—Table 109.4 Children's Oncology Group Neuroblastoma Risk Stratification.
[†]MYCN nonamplified = 1 copy, amplified = greater than 1 copy.
[‡]DNA index > 1 (aneuploid) or = 1 (diploid).
DI, DNA index; FH, favorable histology; INPC, International Neuroblastoma Pathology Classification; INSS, International Neuroblastoma Staging System; UH, unfavorable histology.

rapidly progressive disease, and a dismal outcome. Although attempts to stimulate tumor maturation with nerve growth factor, adrenergic agonists, papaverine, prostaglandins, exogenous cyclic adenosine monophosphate, and hyperthermia were successful in the laboratory setting, there was minimal clinical evidence of their usefulness.[14,109,174–177] The use of retinoids as a promoter of differentiation, however, has rekindled interest in this concept and has been successful in prolonging survival in advanced cases during clinical trials.[174] The addition of cis-retinoic acid to the treatment protocol for high-risk cases of neuroblastoma following BMT or peripheral stem cell transplantation is now standard practice.[1]

A new pretreatment classification system based on 13 prognostic factors has recently been developed by the INRG, aiming to create international consensus for risk stratification. These factors include age, INRG stage, histology, DNA index, MYCN amplification status, and presence of 11q abnormality; they classify patients into 1 of 16 groups. Each group is categorized as very low, low, intermediate, and high risk, based on event-free survival rates of more than 85%, more than 75% to less than or equal to 85%, greater than or equal to 50% to less than or equal to 75%, or less than 50%, respectively.[178]

For low-risk patients, surgical excision of the tumor is usually curative and avoids the risks associated with chemotherapy. Intermediate-risk patients are usually treated with surgery and chemotherapy. Studies aimed at minimizing treatment regimens for this group of patients are ongoing. The poor prognosis in high-risk patients justifies a much more intense treatment regimen, including combination chemotherapy followed by complete surgical excision (if possible), radiotherapy to achieve local control, myeloablative treatments with bone marrow rescue, and biologic therapy.

Operative Management

Initial surgery for extensive stage III and IV tumors should be limited to biopsy of tumor tissue, staging, and placement of a vascular access device. There is an increased rate of surgical complications when complete resection is attempted during initial surgery, with no improvement of survival.[179] After 4 or 5 cycles of chemotherapy, second-look surgery is performed. Although opinions vary regarding resection in high-risk patients, most investigators agree that complete gross resection, which is associated with excellent local control and improved outcome,[179,180] should be the goal of second-look procedures. Complete surgical removal of the primary tumor remains an essential component of treatment in the vast majority of cases.

During resection, adequate intravenous access is important because these tumors are quite vascular, and blood loss may be significant. Blood pressure must be carefully monitored intraoperatively to detect sudden hypertension caused by excessive catecholamine release from the tumor.

The surgical approach depends on the characteristics of the primary tumor. For upper abdominal lesions, particularly those involving major midline vessels, thoracoabdominal exposure is advantageous and well tolerated. The goal of resection is a complete dissection of the vasculature and should include the primary tumor site, in addition to all regional lymph nodes. Neuroblastoma often adheres to or surrounds the great vessels, and special care should be taken to identify and spare the blood supply to important visceral structures, such as the branches of the celiac axis and superior mesenteric artery.

In most children with localized disease, all or most of the tumor can be removed successfully. En-bloc contiguous resection of normal surrounding structures, such as the spleen, stomach, pancreas, and colon, almost always can be avoided. In some cases, it is impossible to separate an adrenal or paraspinal neuroblastoma from the ipsilateral kidney, so nephrectomy may be necessary. It is important to excise any suspicious para-aortic and perirenal lymph nodes for staging purposes. A routine retroperitoneal lymph node dissection is usually not performed. The margins of the tumor resection are marked with titanium clips to guide the port if radiation is required and will reduce the scatter effect noted with other types of metal clips on follow-up CT scanning.

Because neuroblastoma may have a friable pseudocapsule, careful handling of the tumor during dissection is important to avoid tumor spill and hemorrhage. Primary adrenal tumors may be fed by a number of small arteries. The major venous drainage is usually constant, directly to the inferior vena cava on the right side, and into the left renal vein and

subdiaphragmatic vessels on the left. Inferiorly located paraspinal and primary pelvic tumors often require careful dissection to separate the lesion from the bifurcation of the aorta and inferior vena cava. The tumor frequently extends into the intervertebral foramina (Fig. 31-12).

Minimally invasive surgical techniques have also been employed for selected cases of neuroblastoma.[180] Adrenal tumors initially detected by mass screening have been excised laparoscopically by a number of investigators.[181,182] Yamamoto and colleagues[49] described three cases of adrenal neuroblastoma in which the lesions were less than 20 mm in diameter. They used a 5-trocar technique and kept the intra-abdominal pressure for the pneumoperitoneum less than 4 mm Hg. The well-encapsulated tumors were completely excised; they were placed in a plastic bag and removed through the 10-mm trocar site. All had favorable

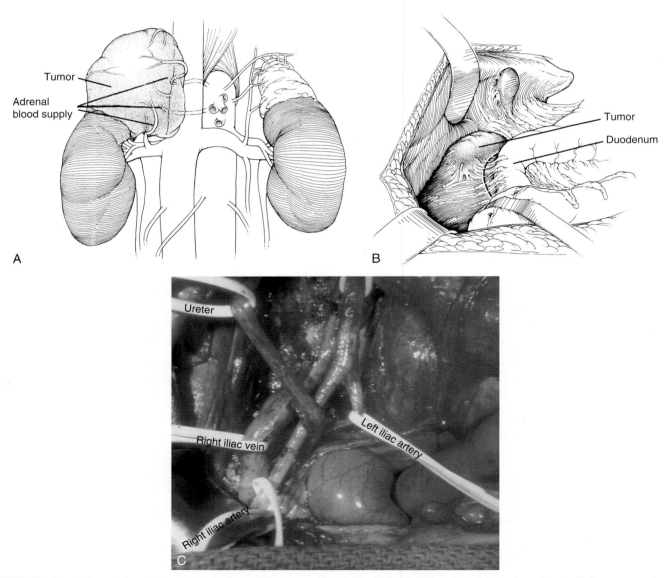

FIGURE 31-12 **A,** Lower retroperitoneal paraspinal neuroblastoma and its relationship to the bifurcation of the aorta and ureter. **B,** Tumor may extend into the vertebral foramina. **C,** Photograph of the operative field after resection of a right-sided pelvic neuroblastoma. Note the vascular loops placed around the iliac arteries, right iliac vein, and ureter to facilitate a safe dissection.

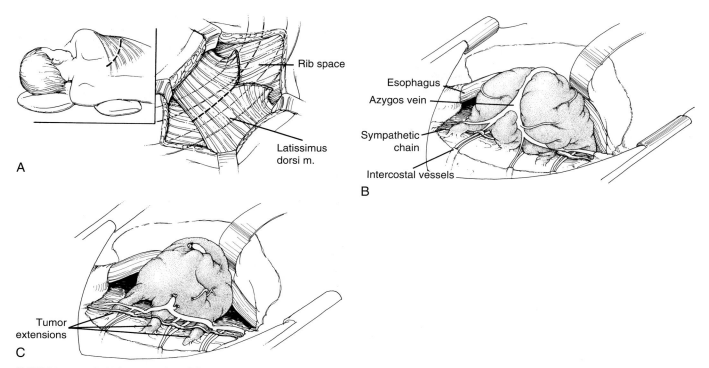

A, Right posterolateral thoracotomy incision used for the excision of a posterior mediastinal neuroblastoma. (Labels: Rib space, Latissimus dorsi m.) **B,** Relationship of the tumor to surrounding tissues. (Labels: Esophagus, Azygos vein, Sympathetic chain, Intercostal vessels) **C,** The tumor is mobilized and retracted anteriorly, exposing numerous intervertebral extensions. (Label: Tumor extensions)

FIGURE 31-13 **A,** Right posterolateral thoracotomy incision used for the excision of a posterior mediastinal neuroblastoma. **B,** Relationship of the tumor to surrounding tissues. **C,** The tumor is mobilized and retracted anteriorly, exposing numerous intervertebral extensions. The tumor extensions are divided at the vertebral foramina, leaving small remnants of residual tumor behind. This does not adversely influence the outcome.

histology, and none had *MYCN* amplification. No recurrences were observed. This and other reports suggest that, in selected cases, laparoscopic biopsy and tumor excision are both safe and effective.[181–183]

Mediastinal tumors are usually approached through a standard posterolateral thoracotomy incision. Excision of the pleura and the endothoracic fascia around the tumor usually allows entry into an appropriate plane of dissection. Mobilization of the tumor from the rib edges is accomplished with both sharp and blunt dissection. It is important to identify and either ligate or clip intercostal blood vessels feeding and draining the tumor. The tumor may be attached to a number of sympathetic ganglia and intercostal nerves and often extends, in one or more areas, into the intervertebral foramina (Fig. 31-13).[56,57,171,184] It may be impossible to remove every bit of tumor at the foraminal sites. Small primary tumors have been successfully removed by thoracoscopic techniques. Thoracoscopy is also useful in obtaining tissue for biopsy.

In patients with neurologic symptoms (including paraplegia) associated with dumbbell tumors, prompt MRI and an urgent laminotomy to excise extradural tumor and relieve cord compression are recommended before attempting intrathoracic resection of the tumor. The mediastinal resection can be delayed a short time to allow the patient's neurologic symptoms to improve. If extradural tumor is present on imaging studies but the patient is asymptomatic, chemotherapy is initiated and may shrink the tumor and avoid the need for laminotomy or laminectomy at the time of resection of the thoracic tumor. The choice of therapy for intraspinal tumor extension is still somewhat controversial. Plantaz and colleagues[59] reviewed 42 patients in France and recommended initial chemotherapy followed by surgical removal of residual disease. Yiin and colleagues[61] described 13 cases of neuroblastoma

with symptomatic spinal cord compression and neurologic deficits. All the patients were treated initially with chemotherapy: 3 recovered, 4 improved, and 6 worsened and became paraplegic. Two of the six recovered after laminectomy. The authors recommended spinal cord decompression for patients who have neurologic deterioration on chemotherapy. Sandberg and colleagues[60] described the treatment of 46 patients with epidural or neural foraminal tumor involvement. Nine were low-risk patients with normal neurologic examinations who remained neurologically intact following operation or chemotherapy. Four low-risk patients with high-grade spinal cord compression improved or remained stable after surgical intervention, but 2 patients who were treated with chemotherapy had worsening deficits. Eleven of twelve high-risk patients with normal neurologic examinations and without radiographic high-grade spinal cord compression were treated with chemotherapy and had no neurologic deterioration. Of 16 high-risk patients with high-grade spinal cord compression, 7 of 10 were treated initially with chemotherapy, and all 6 who underwent initial surgery improved or remained stable. Spinal deformities occurred in 12.5% (2 of 16) treated nonsurgically and in 30% (9 of 30) who underwent surgery. The authors concluded that patients with high-risk tumors and spinal involvement but normal neurologic examinations should be offered chemotherapy, with the understanding that a small percentage may require operations for progressive neurologic deficits. Chemotherapy may be avoided in patients with low-risk tumors who can be offered a potentially curative procedure. Patients and their families should be made aware that operative intervention may be associated with subsequent spinal deformity in as many as 30% of cases.[60]

Cervical neuroblastoma is often localized and has a favorable outcome.[185] In a study of 43 cervical neuroblastomas,

Haddad and colleagues[186] identified four risk factors that were associated with increased operative morbidity: adherence to vascular structures, tumor size, friability, and dumbbell tumors. Imaging studies may show a solid mass with vascular displacement and narrowing.[187] Tumors arising in the neck or upper mediastinum often involve the stellate ganglion. If not present preoperatively, resection may result in postoperative Horner syndrome.[14,188] This is a relatively minor consequence outweighed by complete tumor excision and survival, but the patient's family should be made aware of this possible complication. Special attention should be given to protecting the brachial plexus and the phrenic, vagus, and recurrent laryngeal nerves.

Aggressive surgical management is occasionally associated with late complications in survivors, including ipsilateral atrophy of the kidney following adrenal resection and ejaculatory problems following pelvic tumor excision.[188] Of interest is the very favorable outlook noted in patients with stage III and IV tumors arising in the pelvis following complete tumor resection.[10]

Chemotherapy

Although multiagent chemotherapy has significantly improved the survival rate of patients with many different types of tumors (e.g., Wilms' tumor), chemotherapy has no such effect in infants and children with resectable localized neuroblastoma with favorable biologic and genetic characteristics. For locoregional disease that does not have *MYCN* amplification, surgical resection alone is all that is necessary.[5,10,189] Patients with locoregional disease with poor prognostic biologic and genetic factors, however, are at higher risk and should be treated more aggressively with multiagent dose-intensive chemotherapy, in addition to a variety of therapies thereafter. Patients with stage IV disease who are younger than 18 months at diagnosis receive low-dose chemotherapy, in addition to surgery.[190]

Patients with stage IV disease who are *MYCN* amplified or older than 18 months at diagnosis remain the most difficult population to treat. Historically, these patients received cyclophosphamide, vincristine, and dacarbazine.[9,190,191] Patients in whom this treatment regimen failed received doxorubicin and teniposide (VM-26). Although these chemotherapy regimens did not effectively increase the cure rate of patients with stage IV disease, such treatment reduced the size of the primary tumor, often cleared the bone marrow of tumor cells, and was occasionally associated with histologic maturation from malignant neuroblastoma to benign ganglioneuroma.[9,11] Unfortunately, only 40% of patients with stage IV disease demonstrated a complete response to chemotherapy; 30% had a partial response; and 30% were unresponsive.[9] When the clinical estimation of response was subjected to confirmation by laparotomy, many patients thought to be responders to chemotherapy actually had persistent tumor not identified by preoperative testing.[15,76,172]

Numerous studies confirmed the limited effectiveness of chemotherapy regimens in patients with metastatic disease.[9,73] Using cell kinetic data, Hayes and colleagues[192] demonstrated that the proliferating fraction of the tumor cell population in neuroblastoma is exceedingly small. A large pool of nonproliferating resting cells is resistant to chemotherapy. Timed sequential administration of cell cycle–specific and nonspecific drugs (cyclophosphamide and doxorubicin, or cisplatin with teniposide or doxorubicin) was subsequently tested and resulted in improved response rates.[71,192] This improvement led to more aggressive, more intensive treatment protocols using multiple agents.

Currently, this patient population receives aggressive multimodality therapy, including induction chemotherapy to attain remission, followed by surgery and radiotherapy to further achieve local control. This treatment is followed by consolidation of remission with myeloablative therapy, autologous stem cell transplant, 13-cis-retinoic acid, and, possibly, the addition of immunotherapy.

The purpose of induction chemotherapy is to reduce tumor burden throughout the entire body, both at the primary site and at sites of systemic disease. Multiple agents are often used, including cyclophosphamide, ifosfamide, doxorubicin, cisplatin, carboplatin, etoposide, topotecan, and vincristine. These agents are now given as dose-intensive regimens.

Radiotherapy

Neuroblastoma is a radiosensitive tumor, so radiotherapy remains an important part of the treatment regimen for patients with neuroblastoma. In general, in the management of neuroblastoma, radiotherapy is administered after both induction therapy and surgery, when minimal disease remains. It has also been used for bulky metastatic disease after a response is seen with chemotherapy, and for palliation in patients with refractory end-stage disease or painful metastases.[193–195] At our institution, a regimen that includes dose-intensive chemotherapy, surgery, and a dose of 2100 cGy of hyperfractionated radiotherapy to the primary site in patients with stage IV neuroblastoma resulted in a local control rate of greater than 90%.[46]

Although it is useful, external-beam radiotherapy is associated with considerable toxicity in growing children, resulting in growth disturbance, bony deformity, endocrine deficiency, hypoplastic soft tissue changes, skin atrophy, and, of greater concern, secondary malignancies in the radiation portal. Techniques used to decrease radiation-induced toxicity include hyperfractionation of the radiation dose, which usually does not reduce the desired antitumor effect, and avoiding the simultaneous administration of chemotherapy agents that may enhance the radiation effect. Brachytherapy and intraoperative radiotherapy can better confine the radiation effect to the target tissue and spare surrounding normal tissues.[196,197] Although early local control can be achieved, only 38% of patients with stage IV disease given intraoperative radiotherapy survived after 3 years. Some patients still require supplemental external-beam radiotherapy; postoperative ureteral stricture, renal artery stenosis, and neuropathies have been described.[5] Haas-Kogan and colleagues[196] described an experience using intraoperative radiotherapy in 23 cases of high-risk neuroblastoma and noted that this technique was effective only in patients who had gross total resection of the primary tumor.[196] All patients with partial tumor resection had recurrence, despite radiotherapy, and subsequently died. There are few data to support the efficacy of this therapy. Intraoperative radiotherapy is sometimes cumbersome to perform, especially in institutions that do not have an operative suite in the radiotherapy department or radiotherapy equipment (including linear accelerators) in the operating room. Under these circumstances, after attempted tumor resection, the patient has to be transported under general anesthesia for the radiation treatment.

Children with refractory advanced neuroblastoma with widespread involvement often suffer severe pain due to metastases. Kang and colleagues[194] employed targeted radiotherapy using submyeloablative doses of ^{131}I-MIBG to achieve disease palliation. The treatment stabilized disease, relieved pain, or improved performance status, with 31% of patients showing an objective response to treatment. They concluded that this modality is useful for treating end-stage neuroblastoma. Deutsch and Tersak[193] described the use of radiotherapy (300 to 1000 cGy) for palliative treatment of symptomatic metastases to bone. The most common treatment sites were the skull, spine, hip, and femur. In their study, 29% of patients survived 1 year or longer (range, 1 to 52 months); only 8% survived more than 3 years.

Targeted radiotherapy with MIBG has also been used in combination with myeloablative chemotherapy and proton therapy for recurrent and refractory neuroblastoma. Proton therapy has the advantage of delivering radiation more precisely than conventional radiotherapy. As it becomes more widely available, it may play a greater role in the management of children with neuroblastoma requiring radiation treatment.[1]

Myeloablative Therapy

Myeloablative therapy, using near-lethal doses of phenylalanine mustard (melphalan) with autologous bone marrow rescue, has been shown to improve the tumor response rate. A combination of melphalan, doxorubicin, teniposide, and low-dose total-body irradiation followed by autologous BMT resulted in a relapse-free rate of 40% and, if deaths resulting from toxicity were excluded, there was a 2-year survival rate of 34% in patients with stage IV disease.[198] An alternative treatment was developed that relies on myeloablative chemotherapy using escalating doses of drugs given by constant infusion, followed by autologous (purged) bone marrow infusion but without total-body irradiation.[199]

Currently, stem cells are harvested during the induction phase of treatment, and stored for later use during the consolidation phase of treatment.[200] Chemotherapeutic agents used for this phase of treatment include carboplatin, etoposide, and melphalan. Peripheral blood stem cell infusion is used to reconstitute the marrow after myeloablative treatment. Immunoglobulin G levels are monitored and replaced with gamma globulin. Sulfamethoxazole and fluconazole are given prophylactically to avoid opportunistic *Pneumocystis carinii* and fungal infection.

The use of purged, peripheral blood hematopoietic stem cells has shown to have survival benefits over the use of allogeneic cells, mainly because of a higher toxic death rate and an increased incidence of graft-versus-host disease in the latter group.[94,201] Patients with high-risk stage IV disease have a better outcome with BMT, especially if they have amplification of the *MYCN* oncogene.[37,94,124] Preliminary reports are demonstrating improved event-free survival with rapid sequential tandem transplant consolidation therapy. This has initiated the ongoing COG phase III trial testing single versus tandem transplant as consolidation therapy.[201] However, to date, there

are no prospective studies examining the use of myeloablative therapy in addition to dose-intensive induction therapy.[190] At our institution, the addition of myeloablative chemotherapy to dose-intensive chemotherapy did not decrease the rate of systemic or central nervous system recurrence.[202]

The addition of 13-cis-retinoic acid (isotretinoin), a biologic response modifier that causes tumor differentiation and decreases bone marrow tumor involvement, was shown to be useful.[199] Retinoids serve as multistep modulators of the MHC class I presentation pathway and sensitize neuroblastomas to cytotoxic lymphocytes.[202–204] In a phase III randomized trial in high-risk patients, Reynolds and colleagues[203,204] showed that high-dose pulse therapy with 13-cis-retinoic acid given after completion of intensive chemoradiation (with or without autologous BMT) significantly improved event-free survival. A CCG phase III randomized trial showed the use of 13-cis-retinoic acid after myeloablative chemotherapy had superior event-free survival in patients with remission, and this protocol is now commonly used for these particular patients.[199] A newly developed retinoid, fenretinide, has completed a COG phase I trial, and different oral formulations are being tested in the hopes of improving its bioavailability.[189,205]

Immunotherapy

In the 1970s and 1980s, it was suggested that tumor regression in neuroblastoma involved an immunologic mechanism, resulting from an unusual tumor–host relationship.[206–208] Lymphocytes from children with neuroblastoma were observed to inhibit colonies of neuroblasts in culture but not cells from other tumors.[207] Sera from patients with progressive disease contain a blocking antibody that prevents a lymphocyte-mediated cytotoxic response and inhibits lymphocyte blastogenesis to phytohemagglutinins.[209,210] Lymphocytes from patients with neuroblastoma also have a decreased systemic and in situ natural killer activity.[211] In experimental studies, operative electrocoagulation and hyperthermia resulting from high-intensity focused ultrasonography induced immunity in mice with neuroblastoma.[206,207] A major problem is that advanced neuroblastoma cells are MHC class I deficient and evade immunorecognition.

The mainstay of current immunotherapy for neuroblastoma involves GD2. GD2 is a surface glycolipid antigen that is copiously found on all neuroblastoma cells. Raffaghello and colleagues[212] employed an anti-GD2 antibody in nude mice with neuroblastoma and noted increased long-term survival and decreased metastatic spread in a dose-dependent manner in treated mice compared with controls. Cheung and colleagues[213] suggested that immunotherapy using ganglioside GD2 monoclonal antibody should be directed at minimal disease and must be used in conjunction with dose-intensive chemotherapy to be effective. Kushner and colleagues[214] described the treatment of seven patients who relapsed with widespread disease after initial treatment with surgery alone for locoregional neuroblastoma. They received dose-intensive chemotherapy; anti-GD2 3F8 antibody; and targeted radiotherapy using ^{131}I-labeled 3F8, if they had assessable disease, or 3F8, granulocyte-macrophage colony-stimulating factor, and 13-cis-retinoic acid, if they were in remission. Five of the seven patients remained in remission between 4 and 8 years later.[214] The same group reported that high-dose cyclophosphamide, irinotecan, and topotecan were effective in achieving remission and inducing an immunologic state conducive to antibody-based passive immunotherapy (using 3F8 antibody) in resistant neuroblastoma.[215] Further studies have been completed that continue to show improved outcomes with the use of this antibody.

In contrast to 3F8, which is a mouse-derived monoclonal antibody, ch14.18 is a chimeric human/murine anti-GD2 antibody, and it has shown positive results in both phase I and II clinical trials (German NB90 and NB97 studies). Preliminary results from the COG randomized phase III trial using ch14.18 plus cytokines after autologous stem cell transplant versus control showed improved survival in the treatment group.[216]

Dendritic cells are potential targets for immunotherapy. They can enhance growth and differentiation of CD40-activated B lymphocytes, directly affect natural killer cell function, and act as antigen presenters.[217,218] Redlinger and colleagues[218] noted that advanced neuroblastoma impairs dendritic cell differentiation and function in adoptive immunotherapy. It has been shown that neuroblastoma-derived gangliosides inhibit dendritic cell function. Interleukin-12 (IL-12) is a potent proinflammatory cytokine that enhances the cytotoxic activity of T lymphocytes and resting natural killer cells.[217] In a murine model of neuroblastoma, Shimizu and colleagues[219] demonstrated that IL-12–transduced dendritic cell vaccine (with an adenoviral vector expressing IL-12) led to a complete and sustained antitumor response. Tumor regression was associated with a high infiltration of dendritic cells and viable T cells.

Additional Therapies

^{131}I-MIBG infusion provides a way to specifically deliver radiotherapy to neuroblastoma cells, because it is taken up by more than 90% of neuroblastomas. The use of this treatment alone results in a response in 18% to 37% of patients with refractory or relapsed disease.[220] Rapamycin (mTOR) plays a significant role in cell growth and persistence of neuroblastomas, and phase II trials investigating rapamycin (mTOR) inhibitors are ongoing. Early results reveal a benefit in patients with recurrent neuroblastoma.[221] Additionally, trials are examining targeted therapies for the AKT pathway, as activation of AKT correlates with worse event-free and overall survival.[222–224] Biologic agents, such as histone deacetylase inhibitors, tyrosine kinase inhibitors, IGF-1 receptor inhibitors, N-myc inhibitors, ALK inhibitors, and various antiangiogenic agents, are also being investigated in ongoing clinical trials. The use of bisphosphonates is being explored as a possible treatment for bone metastases. Tumor vaccines and techniques of adoptive immunotherapy are also being evaluated in clinical trials.

Summary and Future Directions

This common pediatric malignancy remains an enigma because of the high variability in tumor behavior. The primitive neuroblastic tumor may follow one of three possible pathways: spontaneous regression (apoptosis); differentiation and maturation to a benign ganglioneuroma; or, more commonly, tumor proliferation and rapid malignant progression. Fetal ultrasonography and infant screening programs have clearly demonstrated that some tumors spontaneously regress. Age-related histopathologic studies have clarified that some tumors (those with favorable histology) differentiate and mature, whereas others (those with unfavorable histology) are undifferentiated neoplasms that respond poorly to treatment and have a rapidly progressive course and fatal outcome.

Recognition of important biologic (and genetic) characteristics can help to categorize these tumors into risk groups (low, intermediate, and high) that determine future treatment protocols. Risk-based management permits individualized care for each patient based on age, INSS stage, INPC histology, and biologic and genetic characteristics that affect the behavior of each tumor.[1,10,102] This avoids unnecessary and potentially harmful treatment in patients categorized as having low-risk tumors and who may do well with surgery alone (and occasionally observation alone in highly selected cases). It allows the physician to reserve the most intensive treatment protocols for children with the highest-risk tumors and the most guarded prognosis. At present, the outlook is best in low-risk patients: infants younger than 18 months; patients with localized tumors that can be completely excised (stages I and II) with favorable INPC histology and low-risk biologic and genetic factors; and infants with stage IV-S disease. Infants with cystic or small solid neuroblastomas detected on prenatal sonograms also have a very favorable outcome. In patients with stage IV-S disease and those with cystic, multifocal, or bilateral tumors and favorable biologic characteristics, observation alone may be feasible. Close sonographic monitoring of these cases in the first year of life is important to ensure that the tumor shrinks and undergoes regression. Increase in tumor size is an indication for operative intervention.

Despite some improvements in outcome using high-intensity treatments, the outlook for patients with advanced neuroblastoma remains dismal, and less than half survive. A better understanding of factors influencing tumor regression and differentiation and tumor–host immune interactions is required. In children with high-risk tumors, identifying additional tumor markers and targeting effective monoclonal antibodies against the tumor, developing improved techniques to clear the bone marrow of tumor cells, using new and more effective chemotherapy regimens, and using growth factors (e.g., other biologic tumor modulators) to promote regression and differentiation may control disease progression and improve the outlook for this highly malignant tumor. Molecular profiling of the genetic changes that occur in neuroblastoma will likely permit a more precise classification system to predict outcome and further define the choice of specific therapy, which may include targeting the genes, proteins, and signaling pathways responsible for malignant progression of the tumor.[1] Also of concern are the long-term effects of neuroblastoma treatment, which include cardiac and renal toxicity, scoliosis, adverse effect on growth and development, delayed sexual maturation, learning disabilities, and occurrence of second neoplasms including renal tumors.[1,225,226]

The complete reference list is available online at www.expertconsult.com.

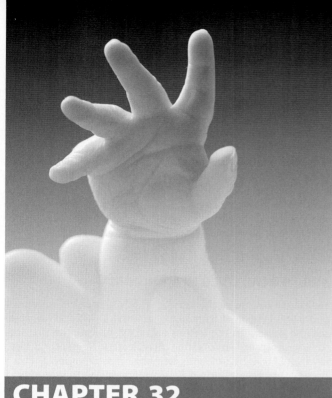

CHAPTER 32

Nonmalignant Tumors of the Liver

Wolfgang Stehr and Philip C. Guzzetta, Jr.

Primary liver tumors constitute less than 3% of tumors seen in the pediatric population, and only one third of those tumors are benign.[1] Benign tumors may be epithelial (focal nodular hyperplasia, hepatocellular adenoma), mesenchymal (hepatic hemangioma, mesenchymal hamartoma), or other (teratoma, inflammatory pseudotumor). Nonparasitic cysts, although not technically neoplasms, are also discussed in this chapter. One of the more interesting aspects of benign liver tumors in children is their predilection to occur in patients with other conditions, and this phenomenon will be discussed with each tumor type.

Clinical Presentation

Most children with benign liver tumors present with a painless right upper quadrant abdominal mass or hepatomegaly. Symptoms of gastrointestinal compression, such as constipation, anorexia, or vomiting, may also be present. If the mass is painful, the pain is usually dull and aching and is caused by expansion of the liver capsule or compression of the normal surrounding structures. Jaundice and weight loss are uncommon except in infants with symptomatic hemangiomas, and those signs should raise the suspicion that the lesion is

malignant. Acute abdominal pain may be caused by bleeding into the mass or into the peritoneum,[2] particularly in hepatocellular adenomas, although this problem is rarely seen in children. Children may present with congestive heart failure (CHF) and thrombocytopenia, which is known as Kasabach-Merritt syndrome when associated with a vascular anomaly such as a liver hemangioma.[3] Cutaneous hemangiomas are seen in about half the children with a liver hemangioma,[4,5] and the rapid enlargement of the liver with a diffuse liver hemangioma can cause abdominal compartment syndrome and respiratory distress.[4] CHF without significant thrombocytopenia can also be seen with liver arteriovenous malformation (AVM)[6] or mesenchymal hamartoma.[7] Fetal hydrops has been identified by prenatal ultrasonography in some fetuses with liver hemangiomas[8] or mesenchymal hamartoma.[9]

Diagnosis

LABORATORY TESTS

Serum alpha fetoprotein (AFP) is present in very high concentrations at birth (48,000 ± 35,000 ng/mL) and rapidly declines to adult levels of less than 10 ng/mL by 8 months of age (Table 32-1).[10] Thus in infants younger than 8 months, AFP levels must be interpreted in the context of this dramatic change. Markedly elevated AFP levels in a child with a liver mass almost certainly means that the mass is malignant, although milder elevation may be encountered with some benign lesions, such as mesenchymal hamartoma[11] or teratoma.[12] As mentioned previously, significant thrombocytopenia associated with a liver mass is usually part of the Kasabach-Merritt syndrome resulting from a liver hemangioma. Hypothyroidism may also occur in multiple or diffuse forms of liver hemangioma[13]; thyroid function tests should be done routinely in these children, because hypothyroidism significantly impacts their management.[14]

IMAGING TECHNIQUES

The initial imaging study in a child presenting with an abdominal mass should be a supine radiograph of the abdomen, looking for calcifications within the mass. The next imaging study should be an abdominal ultrasonogram with Doppler spectral analysis, followed by computed tomography (CT) with intravenous contrast (Fig. 32-1).[15] Magnetic resonance imaging (MRI) may be indicated, depending on the sonogram and CT scan results, especially when surgical resection is planned and more detailed information about the vascular anatomy relative to the tumor is desired or in infants with hemangiomas in whom another diagnosis is being considered because the MRI appearance may be diagnostic. Arteriography is reserved for children with a liver hemangioma, an AVM, or, rarely, a mesenchymal hamartoma with CHF, when embolization of the blood supply to the tumor is needed for treatment. The use of percutaneous biopsy under sonogram or CT guidance in children with benign tumors is generally discouraged, unless excision of the tumor would pose a major risk to the child, because establishing a diagnosis on the basis of a small sample may be problematic for the pathologist and because resection is the proper

TABLE 32-1
Normal Serum Alpha Fetoprotein (AFP) Levels of Infants by Age

Age	No. of Patients	AFP Level ± SD (ng/mL)
Premature	11	138,734 ± 41,444
Newborn	55	48,406 ± 34,718
Newborn to 2 weeks	16	33,113 ± 32,503
2 weeks to 1 month	43	9452 ± 12,610
1 month	12	2645 ± 3080
2 months	40	323 ± 278
3 months	5	88 ± 87
4 months	31	74 ± 56
5 months	6	46.5 ± 19
6 months	9	12.5 ± 9.8
7 months	5	9.7 ±?7.1
8 months	3	8.5 ± 5.5

From Wu JT, Book L, Sudar K: Serum alpha fetoprotein (AFP) levels in normal infants. Pediatr Res 1981;5:50.

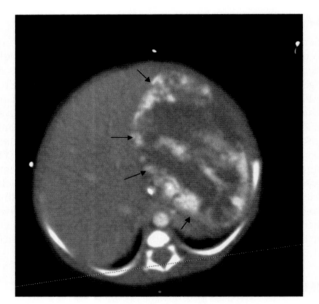

FIGURE 32-1 Contrast-enhanced abdominal computed tomography scan of a 4-day-old infant with a large focal hemangioma of the left hepatic lobe. Note the central area of necrosis.

therapy for most of these tumors, with the exception of liver hemangiomas. The findings on imaging studies are discussed in the sections on each individual tumor.

Hepatic Hemangioma

Hepatic hemangiomas are the most common benign liver tumor in children and are more common than all other benign liver tumors combined. Most of these lesions are identified in the newborn period or during prenatal ultrasound screening.[8] To facilitate discussion about treatment and prognosis, a new subtype classification was delineated in 2007.[4] This classification designates the hemangioma as either focal, multiple, or diffuse and eliminates confusing terms such as infantile hepatic hemangioendothelioma.

FOCAL LIVER HEMANGIOMA

Focal lesions vary in size but can be as large as 8 cm in diameter.[5] They are usually asymptomatic. Some of the children will have cutaneous hemangiomas as well. On MRI, there is a solitary liver lesion that is hypodense on T1-weighted sequences and hyperintense on T2-weighted sequences compared with normal liver. CT scan similarly shows contrast enhancing in the periphery of the mass with little contrast in the center (see Fig. 32-1). These lesions seldom need treatment, may be a hepatic form of hemangioma similar to the cutaneous rapidly involuting congenital hemangioma (RICH), and have generally regressed spontaneously by 1 year of age.[4,5]

MULTIFOCAL LIVER HEMANGIOMA

Multifocal lesions are generally widely dispersed, spherical, and homogeneously enhancing lesions on MRI. Flow voids may be present in the lesions and may indicate the presence of arteriovenous shunts that may lead to congestive heart failure (CHF).[15] Cutaneous hemangiomas are almost always present in these children.[5] Treatment by corticosteroids of patients with CHF is highly successful,[4,5] but if steroids fail to control CHF, embolization of the shunts may be necessary.[6,16] Children with this lesion may have evidence of hypothyroidism, and thyroid function tests (TFT) should be obtained in all children with multifocal lesions. Prognosis is excellent with 100% survival in one series.[5]

DIFFUSE LESIONS

Diffuse lesions frequently replace nearly all of the liver with lesions showing centripetal enhancement on MRI or CT. The clinical course is more complicated and potentially lethal. Massive hepatomegaly may lead to abdominal compartment syndrome, multisystem organ failure, and death. Severe hypothyroidism may develop because of overproduction of type III iodothyronine deiodinase; therefore TFT must be obtained.[13] Despite the large tumor burden, CHF is rare. If corticosteroid therapy does not result in rapid improvement, then liver transplantation should be considered early,[17] because the prognosis is otherwise poor.[4] Medical therapy with vincristine has shown some success,[18] but this option is often limited by the rapid clinical deterioration of children with diffuse lesions. Interferon therapy has been abandoned because of the risk of spastic diplegia in infants.[19] Survival for all children with the diffuse form of liver hemangioma is approximately 75%.[5,13]

ARTERIOVENOUS MALFORMATION

An AVM may occur within the liver parenchyma or outside the liver between the hepatic artery and the portal venous system. Similar to patients with diffuse liver hemangiomas, patients with hepatoportal AVMs usually present before 6 months of age, many in the newborn period, with hepatomegaly, CHF, and a bruit over the liver.[21] In older children and adults, hepatic AVM may occur as part of hereditary hemorrhagic telangiectasia, also known as Osler-Weber-Rendu disease.[15,22] Angiography is diagnostic, and embolization is therapeutic in some patients, but it is necessary to eliminate the extensive collaterals for successful closure of the AVM.[15,21] Fatal complications from the embolization of liver

AVMs have been reported in adults.[23] Steroids have no place in the management of these lesions, and AVMs not managed successfully with embolization may be controlled with ligation of the hepatic artery.[24,25]

MESENCHYMAL HAMARTOMA

Mesenchymal hamartoma (MH) usually presents as a painless right upper quadrant abdominal mass in a child younger than 2 years.[20,26,27] Some patients may have evidence of CHF,[7] and, similar to liver hemangiomas, MH has been diagnosed prenatally.[20,9] Edmondson[28] proposed that MH arises from a mesenchymal rest that becomes isolated from the normal portal triad architecture and differentiates independently. The tumor grows along bile ducts and may incorporate normal liver tissue. Because the blood vessels and bile ducts are components of the mesenchymal rest, the biologic behavior of the tumor varies with the relative predominance of these tissues within the loose connective tissue stroma (mesenchyma) that surrounds them. Thus the tumor may present as a predominantly cystic structure (Fig. 32-2) that enlarges rapidly because of fluid accumulation,[29] or it may be predominantly vascular and present with CHF.[7] Von Schweinitz and colleagues[30] suggested that fat-storing (Ito) cells of the immature liver may be involved in the development of MH. There are reports of chromosomal translocations within mesenchymal hamartomas.[31]

Serum AFP levels are usually normal in children with MH, but they may be mildly elevated.[20,11,32] The radiographic features of these tumors are consistent and distinguishing; abdominal sonography and CT demonstrate a single, usually large, fluid-filled mass with fine internal septations and no calcifications.[33]

Management must be tempered by the understanding that MH usually follows a benign course,[34] although there have been reports of malignant transformation.[35,36] In general, complete operative resection is the procedure of choice, if it can be accomplished safely. Huge lesions or those that involve both lobes may be treated by unroofing and marsupializing the cysts, although the lesion may recur after incomplete resection.

MH is an entity distinct from the liver hamartomas associated with tuberous sclerosis. The latter are smaller, multifocal lesions that may be associated with angiomyolipomas in other locations, such as the kidney; they are rarely symptomatic and usually present in children older than 2 or 3 years. These hamartomas have little clinical significance, but their presence may be helpful in diagnosing tuberous sclerosis.[37]

HEPATOCELLULAR ADENOMA

Although isolated lesions are encountered in childhood, hepatocellular adenoma (HCA) is most commonly observed in adults in association with the use of anabolic corticosteroids or estrogen. HCA has been described in children treated with anabolic steroids and multiple blood transfusions for chronic anemia,[38] and it is expected in children with type I glycogen storage disease.[39] Bianchi[40] proposed several mechanisms for the development of HCA in patients with type I glycogen storage disease, including (1) regional imbalance in insulin and glucagon metabolism, because these hormones are important in the regulation of hepatocyte proliferation and regeneration; (2) response to glycogen overload; and (3) oncogene activation. A giant hepatocellular adenoma has also been reported in a child treated with oxcarbazepine for a seizure disorder.[41]

Microscopic examination of adenomas reveals hepatocytes in sheets and cords oriented along sinusoids without a ductal component. The cells have glycogen-filled cytoplasm and small nuclei without mitoses. Adjacent liver and vessels are compressed but not invaded. Children usually do not have coexisting cirrhosis.[38] The histologic pattern is similar to that of a well-differentiated hepatocellular carcinoma, and development of hepatocellular carcinoma within an unresected HCA has been reported.[42,43]

In children, HCA generally presents as an asymptomatic hepatic mass. The mass is solid on ultrasonography and CT. Liver enzyme and AFP levels are normal. A feature unique to this lesion is its propensity for intraperitoneal hemorrhage from spontaneous rupture. In adults, intraperitoneal bleeding is almost always seen in patients receiving estrogen therapy, and tumor regression may occur with the cessation of hormone administration. In patients with glycogen storage disease and HCA, tumor regression may occur with the correction of metabolic disturbances.[40] Because of the known association between HCA and hepatocellular carcinoma, resection of HCA is recommended when it occurs in a child who is not receiving steroids and does not have glycogen storage disease. If resection cannot be accomplished without substantial risk, observation of the lesion while monitoring the serum AFP level may be appropriate. If the AFP level begins to increase or the lesion is significantly symptomatic, and if the risk of resection is unacceptably high, liver transplantation may be the best alternative.

FOCAL NODULAR HYPERPLASIA

Focal nodular hyperplasia (FNH) in children presents as an irregularly shaped, nontender liver mass. It is frequently found incidentally at laparotomy for another cause or on radiographic studies performed for another indication. The female-to-male

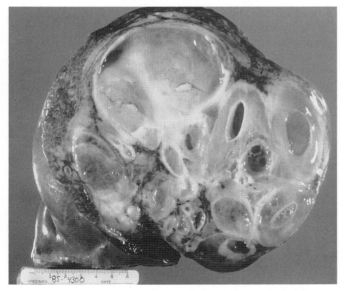

FIGURE 32-2 Cross section of a pathology specimen of a left hepatic lobectomy for mesenchymal hamartoma in a 10-month-old male infant.

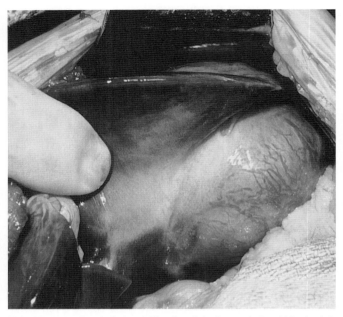

FIGURE 32-3 Surgical view of focal nodular hyperplasia within the left lobe of the liver in a 2-year-old child treated by left lateral lobectomy.

ratio for FNH is approximately 4:1.[44] FNH is occasionally seen with vascular malformations and hemangiomas in the liver,[45] as well as in children with type 1 glycogen storage disease,[46] and it has been postulated that the lesions represent an unusual response to injury or ischemia.[28] On abdominal sonography, the lesions may be isoechoic, hypoechoic, or hyperechoic compared with normal liver parenchyma, and multiple lesions may occur in 10% to 15% of patients. The classic central scar may not be seen on ultrasonography. CT typically shows a hypervascular lesion with a dense stellate central scar. Conventional arteriography or magnetic resonance angiography show a hypervascular mass with feeding arteries entering the periphery and converging on the central portion of the tumor. Some cases of fibrolamellar hepatocellular carcinoma are radiographically indistinguishable from FNH, which is a cause for concern if the diagnosis is being made without a biopsy.[47] There are reports of adult patients who have FNH and hepatocellular carcinoma simultaneously.[48]

On gross examination, the lesions are nonencapsulated, occasionally pedunculated, and quite firm (Fig. 32-3). Microscopic examination shows proliferation of hepatocytes and bile ducts and the pathognomonic central fibrosis. These lesions rarely become malignant or hemorrhage. Therefore expectant therapy is appropriate when removal might be associated with significant morbidity, the child is asymptomatic, and the diagnosis has been made conclusively by radiographic studies, normal AFP levels, and biopsy.[49]

TERATOMA

There have been fewer than 25 case reports of hepatic teratoma in children invariably younger than 1 year.[12,50] Calcification is usually present within the teratoma, helping to differentiate it from other tumors. Some have met the criteria for an intrahepatic fetus in fetu.[51] Serum AFP levels may be elevated with a teratoma, but only mildly elevated in

comparison with the levels seen with hepatoblastoma. Resection is the procedure of choice for a teratoma because of the risk of malignancy in any immature elements of the tumor.

INFLAMMATORY PSEUDOTUMOR

Inflammatory pseudotumor of the liver is rare and generally seen in children older than 3 years but has been reported in younger children as well. Because this lesion is predominantly solid, it is difficult to differentiate it from other benign or malignant tumors by imaging studies. Invariably, the serum AFP level is normal. Fever, leukocytosis, and high C-reactive protein level in a child with a solid liver mass and normal AFP level are suggestive of an inflammatory pseudotumor of the liver thought to be an inflammatory reaction to some insult, although the instigating cause is usually unknown. It is difficult to diagnose this lesion without a large biopsy. Most children undergo resection, which is curative.[52,53]

NONPARASITIC CYSTS

Nonparasitic cysts of the liver are rare and occur more commonly in adults than in children. Although they may be present and symptomatic at birth, most are asymptomatic and are identified incidentally at autopsy or laparotomy. Symptoms are related to abdominal distention or displacement of adjacent structures. Nonparasitic cysts occur with equal frequency in males and females[54] and are generally unilocular lined by cuboidal or columnar epithelium characteristic of bile ducts. The cyst fluid is typically clear or brown, and bile is rarely present. Pathologic studies suggest that nonparasitic cysts arise from congenital or secondary obstruction of peribiliary glands. These glands normally arise from the ductal plate at the hepatic hilum around the 7th week of gestation and continue to proliferate until adolescence.[54] Symptomatic cysts can be effectively treated by simple unroofing, marsupialization,[55] or sclerotherapy.[56] If biliary communication is suspected, cholangiography may identify the source and allow the communicating ductule to be oversewn.

Cystic dilatation of the intrahepatic ducts may also present as a mass, although jaundice and cholangitis are often associated with this problem. Resection of the affected lobe is the preferred therapy.[57] If mesenchymal hamartoma appears to be completely cystic on imaging, it may be misdiagnosed as a nonparasitic cyst. Post-traumatic bile cysts result from ductal disruption and intrahepatic accumulation of bile. These lesions can be treated by percutaneous drainage or, in some cases, by biliary sphincterotomy to reduce the bile duct pressure and lessen the biliary leak.[58] Resection is rarely necessary for post-traumatic cysts. Multiple parenchymal cysts associated with hereditary polycystic kidney disease are generally asymptomatic and so small that they do not require intervention.

Epidermoid cysts differ from other nonparasitic cysts, in that the lining epithelium is squamous rather than cuboidal. This histologic characteristic has led to the theory that these lesions may be foregut bud anomalies trapped in the hepatic substance. Although they are rare, there has been a report of malignant degeneration. Thus resection is the appropriate management.[59]

The complete reference list is available online at www. expertconsult.com.

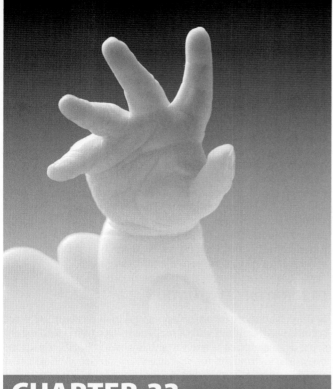

CHAPTER 33

Malignant Liver Tumors

Rebecka L. Meyers, Daniel C. Aronson,
and Arthur Zimmermann

Historical Context

One hundred and thirteen years ago, the first case report of a hepatoblastoma (HB) was published in the English literature in 1898 by Misick in Prague.[1] He reports "A Case of Teratoma Hepatis" in a 6-week-old boy who died of respiratory problems. Autopsy showed a large tumor that occupied the lower half of the right liver lobe. Cysts, cartilaginous, and bony deposits were seen, as well as venous tumor infiltration. It was therefore not surprising that the tumor was described as a teratoma, with tissue representatives of the three embryonic germ cell layers. More than 60 years later in 1962, Willis introduced the term hepatoblastoma for this type of tumor that he defined as "an embryonic tumor that contains hepatic epithelial parenchyma."[2] At that time, hepatoblastoma usually was not distinguished from hepatocellular carcinoma (HCC). Through the work of Ishak and Glunz in 1967, morphologic criteria were defined for HB and HCC that were refined in the decennia that followed.[3,4]

Modern treatment dates to 1975 when Exelby published a landmark paper that has been cited in most reviews dealing with liver tumors in children. He reports the results of a survey of the American Academy of Pediatrics Surgical

Section documenting the 1974 treatment practices and outcomes for liver tumors in children.[5] Through questionnaires sent to the members of the Surgical Section of the American Academy of Pediatrics (AAP), data on liver tumors in children operated upon during the previous 10 years were requested. From 110 replies, 375 liver tumors were reported, of which 252 were malignant (129 HB, 98 HCC), and 123 were benign. All patients with HB underwent primary surgical exploration, with biopsy only in 43 children and a subsequent attempt at definitive resection in 86. Seventy-eight of the 86 children in whom resection was attempted had complete excision of the tumor and 45 (60% of those resected) survived. Excessive blood loss was the most common complication during and immediately after operation, after which cardiac arrest occurred in 9 patients. There were 8 deaths in the operating room and 17 deaths in the immediate postoperative period attributable to the operation. Fifteen HB patients had irradiation of the liver; 53 patients had chemotherapy using a wide variety of agents. It was apparent that no cures were obtained from irradiation and/or chemotherapy in the absence of complete surgical resection. The overall survival for HB was 35%; for HCC it was 13%. With incomplete surgical excision no patient survived. There was no evidence that radiation therapy or chemotherapy controlled disease that could not be completely excised surgically. At this time, before the introduction of cisplatin-based chemotherapy and modern surgical techniques, it seemed that complete operative excision carried a high risk of morbidity, even mortality, but offered the only chance of cure.

The field has progressed considerably since Exelby's 1975 survey. With the introduction of cisplatin-based chemotherapy regimens in the 1980s, overall survival for HB increased from 35% to 70%[6] and has increased further to nearly 80% in the most recent trials.[7] Although our sophistication with chemotherapy and antiangiogenic regimens for both HB and HCC continues to evolve, the primary advantage of chemotherapy has been in a neoadjuvant setting to shrink the tumor and enable surgical resection. Although pediatric HCC is more likely to respond to chemotherapy than its adult counterpart, most HCC remains largely chemoresistant, and treatment efforts often focus on slowing tumor progression with the newest antiangiogenic agents. Complete surgical excision remains the cornerstone for cure in both HB and HCC as evidenced by the recent improvements in survival achieved with complete hepatectomy and liver transplantation.[8–10]

Diagnosis

CLINICAL PRESENTATION

Most liver tumors present with an asymptomatic abdominal mass palpated either by a parent or pediatrician.[11] In the youngest children (infants and toddlers) the most common malignant tumor is hepatoblastoma, which presents as an asymptomatic right upper quadrant or epigastric abdominal mass. Some children may have fatigue, fever, pain, anorexia, and weight loss. Rarely, HB may present with abdominal pain and hemorrhage after post-traumatic or "spontaneous" rupture of a previously occult tumor. Hepatocellular carcinoma and hepatic sarcomas are more common in older children and are more likely to present at an advanced stage. Nonspecific symptoms of inanition or respiratory failure may appear insidiously. As the cancer grows, the pain in the abdomen may progress to shoulder or back pain and becomes more pronounced. The child may develop progressive anorexia and vomiting and appear thin and sickly. Tumor growth may compress or obstruct the normal hepatic architecture causing (1) ascites secondary to occlusion of the portal or hepatic veins, (2) gastrointestinal (GI) bleeding or splenomegaly from the portal hypertension of portal vein occlusion, or (3) jaundice, scleral icterus, and pruritus from obstruction of the biliary tree.[12] Symptoms of biliary obstruction are most common with biliary rhabdomyosarcoma.[13]

DIFFERENTIAL DIAGNOSIS

Differential diagnosis of a pediatric liver mass includes malignant tumors, benign tumors, and a wide assortment of congenital and acquired lesions of the liver, listed as "other masses" in Table 33-1. For many of the "other masses" listed in Table 33-1, the key to the diagnosis might lie in the underlying medical condition. For example, one might expect to see a bacterial hepatic abscess in a child with chronic granulomatous disease, a fatty deposit in the liver of a child with hyperlipidemia, or perhaps an inspissated bile lake in a child with biliary atresia as shown in Figure 33-1. Organizing intrahepatic hematoma should be suspected in any child with a history of hepatic trauma or in newborns with sepsis and coagulopathy, especially if there is a history of perinatal birth trauma or hemodynamic collapse requiring cardiopulmonary resuscitation. Congenital liver cysts are rare and represent a spectrum ranging from large simple cysts, intrahepatic choledochal cyst, and ciliated hepatic foregut cyst. Acquired cysts might be due to a bacterial, hydatid, or amoebic abscess. A simple, asymptomatic congenital liver cyst may be safely observed.[14] If infectious or large and symptomatic, cyst drainage, marsupialization, or excision may be needed to relieve pain and prevent risk of rupture. Recent literature suggests a risk of squamous cell carcinoma arising later in life in those congenital hepatic cysts with a ciliated epithelial lining (ciliated hepatic foregut cyst), and therefore these should probably be excised rather than observed or marsupialized.[15,16]

Neoplastic liver masses, including benign and malignant tumors, account for about 1.0% to 1.5% of all pediatric tumors.[17] Age at presentation is often the key to differential diagnosis (Table 33-2).[18] In newborns, the most common tumor is infantile hepatic hemangioma.[19] Infantile hepatic hemangioma is to be distinguished from the much rarer kaposiform hemangioendothelioma that may present in the extremities, chest, or retroperitoneum. Kaposiform hemangioendothelioma of the retroperitoneum may present with Kasabach-Merritt phenomenon and progress to obstruct the porta hepatis.[20] Hepatoblastoma is most commonly diagnosed between 4 months and 4 years of age. Benign tumors in toddlers are mesenchymal hamartoma and focal nodular hyperplasia. Hepatocellular carcinoma and hepatic adenoma are seen in older children. The other tumors listed in Table 33-2 are rare. Although the most common benign tumors often show classical distinguishing features on computed tomography, imaging is *not* usually a reliable way to differentiate benign from malignant tumors.[21]

LABORATORY EVALUATION

Routine laboratory investigation should include complete blood count; many children with a malignant liver tumor will exhibit some degree of anemia and thrombocytosis.[22] In HB, the thrombocytosis is thought to be caused by tumor production of thrombopoietin, interleukin-6, and interleukin-1B.[23–25] Additional laboratory tests include a liver panel (albumin, transaminases, glutamyl transferase, alkaline phosphatase, total and conjugated bilirubin), lactate dehydrogenase, tumor markers (alpha-fetoprotein [AFP], beta-human chorionic gonadotropin [beta-HCG], ferritin, carcinoembryonic antigen [CEA], catecholamines), and viral titers (hepatitis A, B, and C, Epstein-Barr virus).[18]

The most important tumor marker is the serum AFP. AFP will be elevated in 90% of children with hepatoblastoma and in 50% of children with HCC.[26] Although AFP is elevated in most children with hepatoblastoma, increased AFP is *not* pathognomonic for a malignant liver tumor. European, German, and American multicenter trials have all concluded that hepatoblastomas that fail to express AFP at diagnosis (diagnosis AFP level less than 100) are biologically more aggressive with a worse prognosis.[27–31] Rarely, the opposite has been reported—a case of well-differentiated, fetal-type, favorable prognosis hepatoblastoma that did not express AFP.[32] AFP levels must be interpreted with caution in neonates, because AFP is the major protein produced by the fetal liver

---

TABLE 33-1

Differential Diagnosis of Pediatric Liver Masses

Malignant Tumors	*Benign Tumors*	*Other Masses*
Hepatoblastoma	Mesenchymal hamartoma	Vascular malformations
Hepatocellular carcinoma	Biliary cystadenoma	Arteriovenous malformation
Sarcoma	Focal nodular hyperplasia	Blue rubber nevus syndrome
Biliary rhabdomyosarcoma	Infantile hemangioma	Congenital/acquired cysts
Angiosarcoma	Hepatic adenoma	Simple
Rhabdoid	Nodular regenerative hyperplasia	Ciliated foregut cyst
Undifferentiated	Teratoma	Polycystic liver disease
Metastatic/other	Inflammatory myofibroblastic tumor	Choledochal cyst
Wilms' tumor		Inspissated bile lake/biliary atresia
Neuroblastoma		Parasitic cysts
Colorectal		Amoebic
Carcinoid tumor		Abscess
Kaposiform hemangioendothelioma		Bacterial
Hemophagocytic lymphohistiocytosis		Chronic granulomatous disease
Langerhans' cell histiocytosis		Hematoma
Megakaryoblastic leukemia		Fatty liver

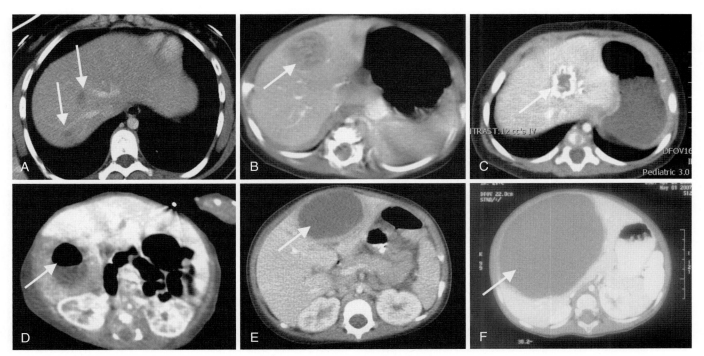

FIGURE 33-1 Differential diagnosis: examples of non-neoplastic liver masses and cysts. **A,** Multiple small bacterial abscesses in a child with chronic granulomatous disease. **B,** Inspissated bile lake in a child with biliary atresia and cholangitis. **C,** Organizing hematoma in a newborn with sepsis and coagulopathy. **D,** Infarction of right lobe liver and hepatic abscess (with air fluid level) in a premature baby with necrotizing enterocolitis. **E,** Acquired cyst is an amoebic abscess in a toddler with fever. **F,** Congenital cyst is a ciliated foregut cyst in an infant with abdominal distension and feeding difficulties.

TABLE 33-2		
Age at Presentation, Most Common Liver Tumors of Childhood		
Age Group	*Malignant*	*Benign*
Infant/toddler	Hepatoblastoma 43% Rhabdoid tumor 1% Malignant germ cell 1%	Hemangioma/vascular 14% Mesenchymal hamartoma 6% Teratoma 1%
School age/adolescent	Hepatocellular (including transitional cell tumors) 23% Sarcomas 7%	Focal nodular hyperplasia 3% Hepatic adenoma 1%

From Von Schweinitz D: Management of liver tumors in childhood. Semin Pediatr Surg 2006;15:17-24.

and is thus produced in high amounts in the normal newborn. AFP may be especially high in neonates after hepatic damage and during regeneration of liver parenchyma. The half-life of AFP is 5 to 7 days, and levels fall throughout the first several months of life so that by 1 year of age the AFP should be less than 10 ng/mL.[33] Moreover, there are many reports of benign tumors, especially infantile hemangioma and mesenchymal hamartoma, in children presenting with high AFP levels.[34–36]

The other tumor markers useful in differential diagnosis are beta-HCG elevated in germ cell tumors, ferritin elevated in HCC and metastatic neuroblastoma; CEA elevated in HCC and metastatic colorectal, lactate dehydrogenase elevated in many malignant tumors, catecholamines elevated in metastatic neuroblastoma, hepatitis C in HCC, and Epstein-Barr viral titers in lymphoproliferative disease or lymphoma.

RADIOLOGY

The radiographic appearance of the most common benign and malignant liver tumors is shown in Figure 33-2. Mesenchymal hamartoma is classically multicystic with the complex cysts separated by thick vascular septae. Focal nodular

hyperplasia is generally well demarcated with a characteristic central stellate scar. Infantile hemangioma classically will demonstrate bright peripheral contrast enhancement. Infantile hepatic hemangioma may be focal, multifocal, or diffuse, as shown in Figure 33-2 in its diffuse form. Hepatoblastoma appears as a large multinodular expansile mass, usually unifocal, but occasionally multifocal. The tumor is generally well demarcated from the normal liver but is not encapsulated. HB may invade hepatic veins, disseminate to the lungs, or penetrate the liver capsule to reach contiguous tissues. An initial ultrasonogram will identify the liver as the organ of origin; additional testing, usually a contrast-enhanced abdominal computed tomography (CT) scan, is aimed at determining the extent of involved parenchyma and the presence or absence of macrovascular compression, displacement, or invasion. Metastatic liver tumors compared with primary malignant liver tumors have been reported to be more hypoechogenic on ultrasonography (US) and have less vessel invasion and contrast enhancement on abdominal CT.[37]

In hepatoblastoma and hepatocellular carcinoma, contrast-enhanced abdominal CT or magnetic resonance imaging

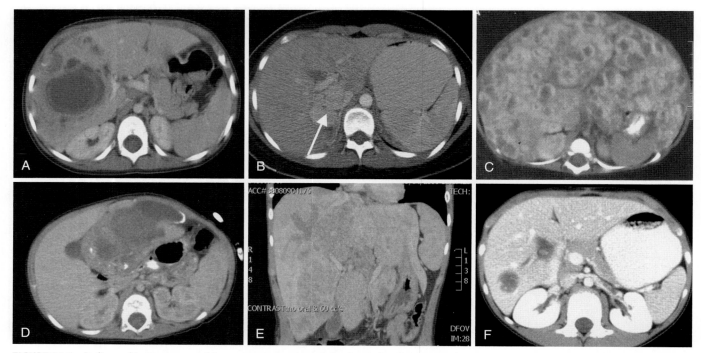

FIGURE 33-2 Radiographic appearance of the most common hepatic benign and malignant neoplastic masses of the liver in children. **A,** Mesenchymal hamartoma, a complex multicystic mass with solid septae. **B,** Focal nodular hyperplasia with *arrow* pointing to classic stellate central scar. **C,** Diffuse infantile hepatic hemangioma with multiple nodules showing peripheral contrast enhancement. **D,** PRETEXT 2 hepatoblastoma. **E,** PRETEXT 4 +P hepatocellular carcinoma with involvement of main portal vein. **F,** Metastatic tumor, two nodules of metastatic colorectal carcinoma in right anterior and posterior sections.

(MRI) outlines the anatomic extent of the tumor, clarifies its relationship to the central venous structures, and evaluates for multicentricity.[38] The radiographic appearance of the tumor at diagnosis is used to assign the tumor *Pretreatment Extent* of tumor (PRETEXT) (Fig. 33-3). The radiographic appearance of the tumor after preoperative (neoadjuvant) chemotherapy has been called *Post-treatment Extent* of tumor (POST-TEXT).[39] A chest CT scan is an essential part of the initial radiographic evaluation, to rule out metastatic pulmonary disease. In children with HB, about 20% present with metastatic disease in the lungs. In HCC, the number of children who present with advanced disease is quite high and pulmonary metastases at diagnosis have been reported as high as 50% in some series.[40]

Malignant Liver Tumors

After neuroblastoma and Wilms' tumor, primary tumors of the liver are the third most common intra-abdominal neoplasms in children.[41] HB is the most frequent liver tumor in children in Western countries, whereas in Asia and Africa, hepatocellular carcinoma (HCC) occurs more frequently than HB, probably as a consequence of the higher prevalence of hepatitis B infection on those continents.[42,43] Other less common malignant pediatric liver tumors are listed in Table 33-1.

HEPATOBLASTOMA

Epidemiology, Biology, and Genetics

Hepatoblastoma accounts for about 80% of the malignant liver tumors in children.[12,44] In the United States, the incidence of HB has increased from 0.6 to 1.2 cases per million population in the last 2 decades.[44] It comprises 1% of all

pediatric malignancies and affects mostly young children between 6 months and 3 years old, but cases in neonates and school-age children are also seen.

Researchers at the University of Minnesota are conducting a large epidemiologic study, termed the "HOPE" study, aimed at elucidating possible environmental and genetic risk factors that might account for the increasing incidence of HB seen over the past 2 decades.[45] The HOPE study (hepatoblastoma origins and pediatric epidemiology) can be reached at www.cancer.umn.edu/hopestudy. A leading theory is that the increased incidence is due to the growing prevalence of premature birth and very-low-birth-weight (VLBW) babies. Both prematurity and very low birth weight have been associated with an increased risk for HB. The association between HB and prematurity or VLBW was first shown in Japan and has since been confirmed in multiple studies.[45–49] No association has yet been found between prematurity as a risk factor and the age at which the tumor diagnosis is eventually made or the histologic subtype of the tumor. Unproven, but postulated, environmental risk factors include occupational exposure of the father to metals, such as welding and soldering fumes, petroleum products, and paint.[50] The list of possible iatrogenic exposures of the premature or VLBW baby in the neonatal care unit includes light, oxygen, irradiation, electromagnetic fields, plasticizers, medications, and total parenteral nutrition.[51]

HB is also associated with fetal alcohol syndrome and hemihyperplasia (formerly termed hemihypertrophy).[52] Hemihyperplasia is associated with an increased risk of embryonal tumors, primarily Wilms' tumor and HB. Curiously, although there is clinical overlap between hemihyperplasia and Beckwith-Weidemann syndrome, the genetic abnormalities seen in HB patients with Beckwith-Weidemann syndrome are not

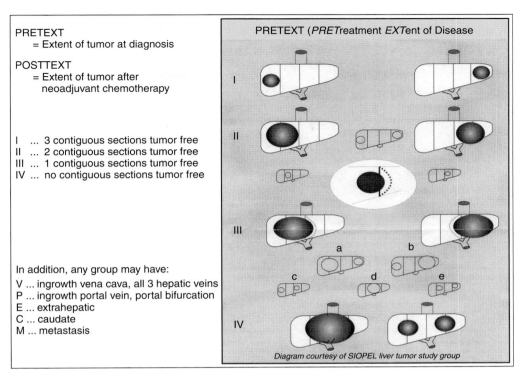

FIGURE 33-3 PRETEXT.

seen in those with hemihyperplasia.[53] In addition to Beckwith-Weidemann syndrome, a number of other genetic syndromes have been associated with an increased risk of HB, including familial adenomatous polyposis (FAP), Li-Fraumeni syndrome, trisomy 18, and others as shown in Table 33-3.[54–68] Familial case reports of HB with familial adenomatous polyposis are striking and suggest a role in the pathogenesis of HB for chromosomes 5 and 11.[56,69] Additional screening for cases in familial adenomatous polyposis kindred families is recommended by testing for germline mutations in the adenomatous polyposis coli (APC) tumor suppressor gene.[55,70] Germline APC mutations are not commonly seen in children with sporadic HB.[71] The association between Beckwith-Weidemann syndrome and HB is so strong that experts recommend that children with Beckwith-Weidemann syndrome be screened with abdominal ultrasonography and AFP at regular intervals until they reach the age of 7 years.[72] The genetic abnormality in HB patients with Beckwith-Weidemann syndrome is mapped to the 11p15.15 locus and suggests the presence of a tumor suppressor gene at this location.[73] Additional biological markers may include trisomy 2, 8, 18, 20, and translocation of the NOTCH2 gene on chromosome 1q12-21.[61] Up-regulation of insulin-like growth factor 2 may be mediated by overexpression of PLGA1 oncogene, a transcriptional activator on the 8q chromosome.[74]

One of the most provocative genetic findings has been the association between HB and mutations of beta-catenin and activation of the WNT/beta-catenin signaling.[75–77] Microarray analysis of WNT/beta-catenin and MYC signaling has defined two tumor subclasses resembling distinct phases of liver development and characterized by a discriminating 16-gene signature. The highly proliferating tumor subclass showed gains of chromosome 8q and 2p and up-regulated MYC signaling.[78,79] Histologic subtypes of hepatoblastoma have also

been characterized by different patterns of WNT and NOTCH pathway activation in DLK+ precursors.[80] The authors speculate that HB may arise from proliferating bipotential precursors with WNT activation most prevalent in embryonal and mixed histologic subtypes and NOTCH activation more prevalent in the differentiated pure fetal subtype.[80] In addition, deregulation of MAPK signaling pathway and antiapoptotic signaling is preferentially up-regulated in aggressive epithelial HB with a small cell undifferentiated component.[81] These gene expression signatures may provide prognostic and diagnostic markers, perhaps even therapeutic targets, in the future.[80,81]

Other genetic markers that have been associated with biological behavior include multidrug-resistance genes and the Hedgehog pathway.[82–85] Increased expression of multidrug-resistance genes is seen in response to chemotherapy in many childhood tumors, and this seems to be particularly true in HB.[82] Chemotherapy has been shown to induce overexpression of the multidrug-resistance gene MDR1, MDR-associated protein MRP1, and lung-related protein (LRP).[84]

Pathology

According to the World Health Organization (WHO) Tumor Classification, hepatoblastoma is defined as a malignant tumor with divergent patterns of differentiation, ranging from cells resembling fetal epithelial hepatocytes, to embryonal cells, and with differentiated tissues, including osteoid-like material, fibrous connective tissue, and striated muscle fibers. In fact, the morphology of HB seems to reflect distinctive phases of hepatogenesis, recapitulating cell lineages derived from endoderm fated to become mature liver cells.[86] The neoplastic offspring of these cell systems is present in HB in a variety

TABLE 33-3

Genetic Syndromes Associated with Pediatric Liver Tumors

Disease	Tumor	Chromosome	Gene	Reference
Familial adenomatous polyposis (FAP)	HB, HCC, adenoma	5q21.22	APC	Thomas 2003[54] Hirschman 2005[55]
Beckwith-Wiedemann syndrome (BWS)	HB, Infantile hemangioma	11p15.5	P57KiP2, WNT, others	Steenman 2000[56] Fukuzawa 2003[57]
Li-Fraumeni syndrome	HB, undifferentiated sarcoma	17p13	TP53, others	Fraumeni 1969[58]
Trisomy 18	HB	18	—	Bove 1996[59] Maruyama 2001[60]
Other trisomies	HB	2, 8, 20	—	Tomlinson 2006[61]
Glycogen storage disease type I-IV	HB, HCC, adenoma	Several	—	Siciliano 2000[62]
Hereditary tyrosinemia	HCC	15q23-25	Fumarylaceto-acetate hydrolase	Demers 2003[63]
Alagille syndrome	HCC	20p12	JAG1	Keefe 1993[64]
Progressive familial intrahepatic cholestasis (PFIC)	HCC	18q21-22, 2q24	F1C1, BSEP	Alonso 1994[65]
Neurofibromatosis	HCC, schwannoma, angiosarcoma	17q11.2	NF-1	Kanai 1995[66]
Ataxia telangiectasia Hepatocellular carcinoma	HCC	11q22-23	ATM	Geoffroy-Perez[67]
Fanconi anemia	HCC, adenoma	1q42, 3p, 20q13	FAA, FAC	Touraine 1993[68]

HB, hepatoblastoma; HCC, hepatocellular carcinoma.

of proportions, used as the basis of HB classifications, of which the current International Society of Pediatric Oncology (epithelial) liver tumor study group (SIOPEL) classification is shown in Table 33-4. Untreated HB presents as a lobulated mass up to more than 20 cm in diameter, being solitary tumors in 80% of the patients and located to the right lobe of the liver in about 60%. The lesions usually show an expanding growth pattern, but conglomerated masses with satellite nodules are also observed. The color of the cut surfaces is variegated in many HB, partly caused by necrosis and hemorrhage, with the exception of fetal HB, which has the tan color of normal liver. The gross presentation of HB postchemotherapy is characterized by firm and well-delineated and sometimes multinodular masses with whitish fibrotic areas and calcifications.

Histologically, the epithelial components range in their differentiation from a small cell undifferentiated (previously termed anaplastic) phenotype, resembling other cellular blue tumors, to cells that are close to mature hepatocytes (the fetal phenotype). The current, histology-based classification is not consistent regarding cellular differentiation, because one subtype (macrotrabecular) reflects a growth pattern rather than a distinct differentiation step. The fetal subtype, occurring in a purely fetal and a so-called crowded fetal variant, displays the highest level of differentiation. Pure fetal histology HB is associated with both a diploid DNA complement and a low proliferative activity. About 20% of epithelial HB shows a mixture of fetal and less differentiated, embryonal-type cells, with a more pronounced mitotic activity. The macrotrabecular subtype (less than 5% of the tumors) reveals a growth pattern with large cell plates consisting either of fetal-embryonal or hepatocyte-like cells. The latter variant, macrotrabecular type 1 (MT-1) is difficult to distinguish from hepatocellular carcinoma and may have an unfavorable biology.[18] Undifferentiated HB mostly occurs as a small cell neoplasm not associated with elevated serum AFP (small cell undifferentiated [SCU] HB), but variants with larger cells also occur. HB-SCU forms a complex group of tumors in that at least part of the lesions seem to have a relation to rhabdoid tumors and are INI1 protein negative.[87,88]

A large proportion of HB (about 45% when examined after chemotherapy) reveal a mixed epithelial and mesenchymal (MEM) phenotype (HB-MEM; see Table 33-4). Osteoid-like bone tissue is a common mesenchymal (heterologous) component. The same epithelial components as found in the wholly epithelial HB subtypes occur in variable expression. The relative proportions of the components in HB-MEM undergo marked changes subsequent to chemotherapy. After exposure to chemotherapy, often the osteoid dominates the histologic pattern. A small proportion of HB-MEM exhibit unusual tissues, such as glianeuronal, enteric, or melanocytic tissues. These tumors are termed HB-MEM with teratoid features. It has to be emphasized that this term is descriptive and does not imply that these neoplasms are germ cell tumors. The prognostic significance of these histologic types and subtypes is currently under study in large trials.

TABLE 33-4

Classification of Hepatoblastoma Histologic Subtype*

Hepatoblastoma, Wholly Epithelial Type

Fetal

Embryonal/mixed fetal and embryonal

Macrotrabecular (MT)

Small cell undifferentiated (SCU; formerly anaplastic)

Hepatoblastoma Mixed Epithelial and Mesenchymal Type (HB-MEM)

Without teratoid features

With teratoid features

Hepatoblastoma, Not Otherwise Specified (HB-NOS)

*This is the classification used by the SIOPEL (International Society of Pediatric Oncology [epithelial] liver tumor study group). Classification systems used by American, German, and Japanese study groups vary.

So far, a prognostic relevance has been worked out for the fetal subtype (favorable)[89] and for HB-SCU (unfavorable).[30,31,90] An unfavorable histology of HB-SCU is also present in cases where the SCU feature is expressed in a focal pattern only.[91] In addition to the lesions listed in Table 33-4, an increased number of variants of HB, or lesions thought to be related to HB, have been described, leading to the concept of *tumor families.*[92]

PRETEXT, STAGING, AND RISK GROUP STRATIFICATION

"Risk Group" stratification determines treatment for hepatoblastoma (HB) in current multicenter group trials. As shown in Table 33-5, The Children's Oncology Group (COG) has low, intermediate, and high-risk treatment groups, whereas SIOPEL defines a standard-risk and a high-risk group. COG continues to use traditional COG (Evans) stage I to IV, and prognostic factors (pure fetal and small cell undifferentiated histology and AFP < 100) to assign risk groups. Although COG does not currently use PRETEXT to assign risk group, it does use PRETEXT to define surgical guidelines, where it determines whether or not a tumor should be resected at diagnosis. The timing of resection will determine the tumor stage for all nonmetastatic tumors. In contrast, SIOPEL uses PRETEXT and prognostic factors to define risk groups.

PRETEXT (see Fig. 33-3) was devised by SIOPEL 1.[93] Subsequent SIOPEL trials (SIOPEL 2, and SIOPEL 3) have used PRETEXT as a tool to stratify treatment, define risk categories, and report outcomes in HB. Although the risk stratification schema differs somewhat between groups, the three other major multicenter pediatric liver tumor study groups, Children's Oncology Group (COG), German Pediatric Oncology Hematology (GPOH), and the Japanese Pediatric Liver Tumor (JPLT) have all chosen to adopt PRETEXT in their current and future protocols. Although PRETEXT has been found to have a slight tendency to overstage patients, it is postulated to show good interobserver agreement (reproducibility.) PRETEXT may also be used to monitor the effect of preoperative therapy when it is applied serially to assess tumor response to neoadjuvant chemotherapy.[28] In North America, COG uses PRETEXT to define surgical resectability (i.e., surgical resection guidelines)

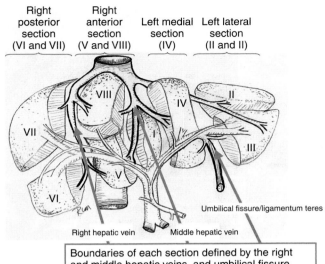

Right posterior section (VI and VII)   Right anterior section (V and VIII)   Left medial section (IV)   Left lateral section (II and II)

Boundaries of each section defined by the right and middle hepatic veins, and umbilical fissure

Right hepatic vein   Middle hepatic vein   Umbilical fissure/ligamentum teres

FIGURE 33-4   PRETEXT is distinct from Couinaud 8–segments (I to VIII) anatomic division of the liver. PRETEXT defines four "sections." Boundaries of each section defined by the right and middle hepatic veins, and umbilical fissure.

in its current HB protocol (AHEP 0731). Building upon the Couinaud 8–segment anatomic structure of the liver, the PRETEXT system divides the liver into four parts, called "sections" (Fig. 33-4). The left lobe of the liver consists of a lateral (Couinaud segments II and III) and medial section (segment IV), whereas the right lobe is divided into an anterior (segments V and VIII) and posterior section (segments VI and VII). Couinaud segment I is the caudate lobe and when involved is shown in PRETEXT with the annotation "C."

As shown by the examples in Figure 33-5, the tumor is classified into one of the following four PRETEXT groups depending on the number of liver sections that are free of tumor: PRETEXT I, three adjacent sections free of tumor; PRETEXT II, two adjacent sections free of tumor (or one section in each hemiliver); PRETEXT III, one section free of tumor (or two sections in one hemiliver and one nonadjacent section in the other hemiliver); and PRETEXT IV, no tumor free sections. Extrahepatic growth and gross vascular involvement is

---

TABLE 33-5

Hepatoblastoma Staging and Risk Stratification

Traditional COG (Evans) Staging System	Current COG Risk Stratification	Current SIOPEL Risk Stratification
Stage I: complete gross resection at diagnosis with clear margins	Very low risk: pure fetal histology, resected at diagnosis (stage I/II); see resection guidelines below*	
Stage II: complete gross resection at diagnosis with microscopic residual disease at the margins of resection	Low risk: any histology resected at diagnosis (stage I/II); see resection guidelines below*	Standard risk: PRETEXT I, II, III
Stage III: biopsy only at diagnosis, or gross total resection with nodal involvement or tumor spill or incomplete resection with gross intrahepatic disease	Intermediate risk: stage III tumors (includes SCU histology)	
Stage IV: metastatic disease at diagnosis	High risk: stage IV tumors, AFP < 100 at diagnosis	High risk: PRETEXT IV, metastasis at diagnosis, SCU histology, AFP < 100 at diagnosis

*COG surgical guidelines recommend resection of tumors at diagnosis (stage I/II) based upon PRETEXT. PRETEXT I and PRETEXT II resected at diagnosis if there is an anticipated greater than 1-cm surgical margin based upon preoperative imaging.
AFP, alpha-fetoprotein; COG, Children's Oncology Group; PRETEXT, pretreatment extent (of tumor) staging system; SCU, small cell undifferentiated; SIOPEL, International Society of Pediatric Oncology (epithelial) liver tumor study group.

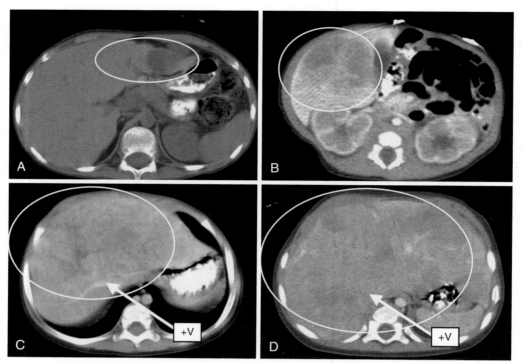

FIGURE 33-5   Examples of PRETEXT for hepatoblastoma risk stratification. **A,** PRETEXT I, left lateral section. **B,** PRETEXT II, right anterior and right posterior sections. **C,** PRETEXT III, +V: left lateral section, left medial section, and right anterior section with invasion of all three hepatic veins (+V). **D,** PRETEXT IV, +V, +P: tumor involves all four sections and invades vena cava and portal bifurcation.

indicated by adding one or more of the following: V, vena cava or all three hepatic veins involved; P, main portal or *both* portal branches involved; C, involvement of the caudate lobe; E, extrahepatic contiguous growth (e.g., diaphragm or stomach), and M, distant metastases (mostly lungs, otherwise specify).[39]

Treatment Strategy, Chemotherapy, and Surgery

In the treatment of hepatoblastoma, complete surgical resection remains the cornerstone of curative therapy. And yet, as has become increasingly clear in recent large multicenter trials, surgery alone cannot cure patients who present with advanced disease. More than half of the patients present with either an initial unresectable tumor or with distant metastases. In the early years when these children were treated with surgery alone, there was a 30% relapse rate in those patients whose tumor could be completely resected. Evidence that HB is a chemosensitive tumor began to accumulate in the early 1970s when responses were seen to combinations of cyclophosphamide, vincristine, 5-fluorouracil, and actinomycin-D,[94] but not until the introduction of cisplatin and doxorubicin–containing regimens in the 1980s was there a major impact of chemotherapy on survival.[6] Twenty years later, cisplatin remains the backbone of current chemotherapy regimen. In fact, in the most recent study of standard-risk HB by SIOPEL, SIOPEL 3, treatment results with cisplatin monotherapy were comparable to those achieved with cisplatin/doxorubicin combination chemotherapy (PLADO).[7] Chemotherapy may reduce tumor volume, making the tumor resectable, and may lead to the complete disappearance of lung metastases. The tumor response rate to the present cisplatin-containing chemotherapy regimens varies from 70% to 90%, according to the different series.[7,31,95–100] Neoadjuvant (preoperative)

chemotherapy not only makes the tumor "smaller" and consequently more likely to be completely resected, but also more solid, less prone to bleeding, and better demarcated from the remaining healthy liver parenchyma.[101,102] Also, when chemotherapy is given as soon as possible after diagnosis, occult (micro)metastases in the lung have no delay in treatment. No matter how small the primary tumor, SIOPEL recommends preoperative chemotherapy in ALL patients as shown in Figure 33-6. This approach is hypothesized to increase the number of patients for whom complete surgical resection will be feasible, to reduce the surgical morbidity of resection, and to provide more time for making definitive surgical plans, including liver transplantation when indicated.[103,104] Because of the large number of countries participating in the SIOPEL studies, standardization of both sophisticated surgical approaches and supportive care measures has been difficult; therefore the use of preoperative chemotherapy in every case has permitted patients from countries with limited resources to participate in these studies.

In contrast to the SIOPEL approach, the North American "legacy groups" Children's Cancer Group (CCG) and Pediatric Oncology Group (POG) (now COG) and the German Study Group (GPOH) have historically recommended primary surgery, *whenever prudently possible*, as the initial treatment. The decision about which tumors are "resectable," and which ones are not, has been subjectively made by the treating surgeon; hence, the approach has been criticized for being highly variable. Because traditional Evans staging relies on the surgical resection decision at diagnosis (see Table 33-5), and because this is a surgeon-initiated subjective decision, the stage has often depended more on the surgeon than on the tumor. Figure 33-6 shows the North American strategy in COG study AHEP0731, which recommends tumor resection

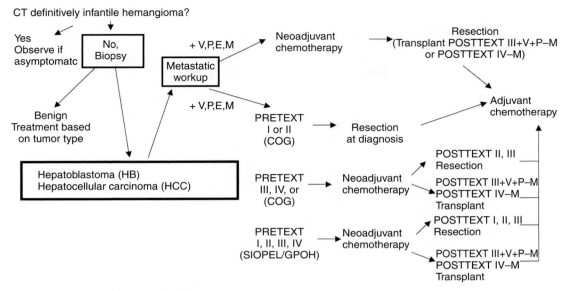

PRETEXT = Extent of disease at diagnosis
POSTTEXT = Extent of disease after neoadjuvant chemotherapy

FIGURE 33-6   Pediatric malignant liver tumor: simplified treatment algorithm. COG, Children's Oncology Group; CT, computed tomography; E, extrahepatic contiguous growth; GPOH, German Pediatric Oncology Hematology (study); M, metastasis; P, main portal or *both* portal branches involved; SIOPEL, International Society of Pediatric Oncology International Society of Pediatric Oncology (epithelial) liver tumor study group; V, vena cava or all three hepatic veins involved.

at diagnosis dictated by PRETEXT-defined surgical guidelines (PRETEXT I and II). Tumors can be resected by straightforward segmentectomy or lobectomy, and are resected at diagnosis. Following these guidelines, approximately one third of HB patients can successfully achieve a gross total resection of tumor at diagnosis, and among them it is possible to identify some that require minimal or no chemotherapy.[89,105] Although it has been debated, postsurgical complications do *not* appear to be more frequent with this approach in the modern era.[30,96,106,107] The potential to reduce cumulative chemotherapy exposure with upfront resection in PRETEXT I and II tumors is important given the ability of HB to develop resistance to standard chemotherapy.[32,82,84] Recent data on magnitude of AFP response actually suggest that the majority of chemotherapy tumor kill probably occurs in the first two cycles.[104]

The strategy in the German trials HB 89 and HB 94 was similar to that used in North America, that is, resection at diagnosis, when feasible, at the discretion of the operating surgeon. In a review of these studies, 30% of children with primary tumor resection had macroscopic or microscopic residual tumor.[31] Despite the larger number of advanced HB in the neoadjuvant chemotherapy group, an incomplete tumor resection was performed in only 18%. Based upon this statistically significant difference, GPOH adopted neoadjuvant chemotherapy for all patients in their latest trial, HB 99, and recommends against any surgical consideration of atypical, nonanatomic, or wedge resection.[18,98]

Surgical guidelines in the current COG trial, AHEP-0731 *do not* leave the decision about surgical resection at diagnosis up to the subjective discretion of the individual surgeon; objective resection guidelines are part of the protocol. PRETEXT is used to define which tumors should be resected at diagnosis (see Fig. 33-6). Resection at diagnosis is recommended for stage I/II only when segmentectomy or a facile, nonextended

lobectomy will predictably yield a complete resection, that is, PRETEXT I or II tumors with at least 1 cm of clear margin anticipated upon review of diagnostic radiographic imaging. A POSTTEXT IIId tumor is a central tumor that may be best resected by mesohepatectomy in the hands of an experienced liver surgeon (Fig. 33-7). Transplantation is preferred in any tumor that invades the major vascular inflow (POSTTEXT +P) or outflow (POSTTEXT +V). If the PRETEXT (and POSTTEXT) suggests the need for major vascular reconstruction, which is sometimes called extreme resection (a resection performed in a patient who would otherwise meet criteria for liver transplantation) or liver transplantation, a referral for transplantation evaluation is advisable. Accuracy of PRETEXT is moderate (because of difficulty in differentiating tumor vessel compression from vessel ingrowth) with a slight tendency to overstage.[28] Nevertheless, good interobserver agreement has been reported, and comparing PRETEXT with POST-TEXT allows for an objective analysis of tumor response to chemotherapy.[39] The predictive value for survival using PRETEXT is excellent, and combining PRETEXT with traditional COG staging yields additional predictive value.[28,30]

Postoperative (adjuvant) chemotherapy is currently recommended by *all* study groups, for *all* patients with one small exception. Stage I pure fetal histology (PFH) in INT-0098 and COG P9645 received reduced or no chemotherapy[89,96,97] and has a 5-year event-free survival (EFS) and overall survival (OS) of 100% and 100%, respectively. Thus no chemotherapy is recommended for pure fetal histology patients resected at diagnosis in COG AHEP-0731. Cisplatin remains the backbone of the chemotherapy regimen, but the drug combinations differ somewhat between study groups. COG currently uses cisplatin/5-FU/vincristine (C5V) for low-risk tumors, C5V + doxorubicin for intermediate risk, and will investigate new agents (irinotecan) with upfront window

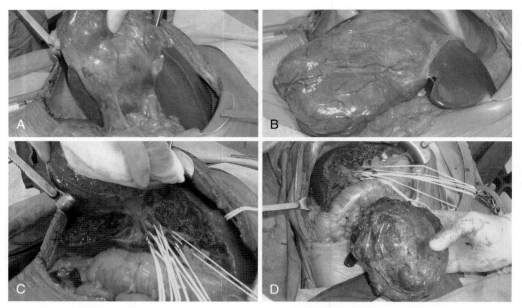

FIGURE 33-7 Central PRETEXT IIId hepatoblastoma: resection with mesohepatectomy versus complete hepatectomy and transplantation, depends upon extent of macroscopic vessel involvement. **A,** Central hepatoblastoma involving left medial and right anterior sections (PRETEXT IIId). **B,** Resection with right or left trisegmentectomy would leave very little residual normal liver. **C,** Much of the normal liver can be saved by mesohepatectomy if the portal vessels are *not* encased and a good margin can be obtained. If tumor encases or invades the portal vessels, complete hepatectomy and transplantation is recommended. **D,** Frozen section shows negative margins. *(See Expert Consult site for color version.)*

therapy in high-risk tumors.[42] SIOPEL 3 compared cisplatin monotherapy with PLADO for standard risk[95] and used SUPERPLADO for high risk.[7] The current SIOPEL 4 high-risk study uses an intensified platinum regimen.[99] The recent GPOH trial HB-94 used IPA (ifosfamide/cisplatin/doxorubicin),[31] and the ongoing GPOH trial HB99 uses IPA for standard risk and carboplatin-VP-16 for high risk.[98] The recent Japanese trial JPLT-2 has used CITA (cisplatin/THP-Adriamycin [doxorubicin]) for standard risk and ITEC (ifosfamide/carboplatin/doxorubicin/etoposide) + HACE (hepatic artery chemoembolization) for high-risk patients.[108] Irinotecan, with or without doxorubicin, has been used in both North America and Europe for patients with relapse.[109,110]

In terms of overall survival rates, the results of the different study groups are generally comparable, projecting 3-year overall survival rates, regardless of the first therapeutic modality used, of 62% to 70% (Table 33-6).[7,31,95–100] The improved results in the high-risk group achieved in SIOPEL 3 highlight some important lessons learned over the past 2 decades. (1) With standard treatment, about 25% of patients who present with metastatic disease are ultimately cured, and alternative chemotherapy and surgical resection of pulmonary metastatic disease should be considered in patients who do not show an excellent early response to chemotherapy. (2) The presence of a positive microscopic margin may not portend a poor prognosis in patients who have had an excellent response to chemotherapy. (3) Liver transplantation or extreme resection (i.e., mesohepatectomy and major venous resection and reconstruction) should be considered in every child with unresectable HB (about 15% of cases).[9,10,102,111–113]

The current COG trial, AHEP-0731, is a risk-stratified study that seeks to diminish toxicity in low-risk patients, increase survival in intermediate-risk patients, and identify new agents(s) in high-risk patients.[107] Very-low-risk patients

with pure fetal histology (PFH) hepatoblastoma resected at diagnosis receive no chemotherapy. Low-risk patients who have non-PFH histology resected at diagnosis receive two adjuvant cycles of cisplatin, 5-flouorouracil, and vincristine (C5V), a reduction from the standard four cycles of chemotherapy used in previous COG trials. For intermediate-risk patients with stage I SCU, stage II SCU, or any stage III hepatoblastoma the chemotherapy regimen will add doxorubicin to the C5V therapy (C5VD). High-risk patients with metastatic tumor or initial AFP less than 100 ng/mL will be treated with an upfront window of a novel agent (irinotecan) preceding the backbone therapy with C5VD.

Liver Transplantation for Hepatoblastoma

In 1968, Starzl reported the first long-term survivor of liver transplantation, a child with hepatoma. From that time until the cluster of papers published by Al-Qabandi, Reyes, Pimpalwar, Molmenti, and Srivastin from 1999 to 2002,[114–118] most descriptions of the use of transplantation in hepatoblastoma were anecdotal case reports. Largely because of early negative experience with liver transplantation in the treatment of adult hepatocellular carcinoma, liver transplantation for the treatment of hepatic malignancy developed a reputation as a dreaded, last resort, heroic, and even potentially ethically inappropriate intervention. The biology of pediatric hepatoblastoma has proven to be very different from that of adult hepatocellular carcinoma, with cisplatin-based chemotherapy proven to be of significant value in a number of randomized trials. This availability of effective chemotherapy led credence to the bold statement by Reyes in his landmark paper in 2000 [115] that "in these children with unresectable tumors, the historical barrier of "unresectability" can be redefined with the concept of 'total liver resection' and salvage orthotopic liver transplantation (OLT)." Thus beginning about 2000, liver transplantation began to be offered to more and

TABLE 33-6

Summary Results Recent Hepatoblastoma Cooperative Trials

Study	Chemotherapy	No. of Patients	Outcomes
INT0098 (CCSG, POG)[96]	C5V vs. CDDP/DOXO	Stage I/II: 50 Stage III: 83 Stage IV: 40	4-Year EFS/OS Stage I/II: 88%/100% vs. 96%/96% Stage III: 60%/68% vs. 68%/71% Stage IV: 14%/33% vs. 37%/42%
P9645 (COG)[97]	C5V vs. CDDP/CARBO	Stage I/II: pending publication Stage III: 38 Stage IV: 50	1-Year EFS* Stage III/IV C5V: 51%; CDDP/CARBO: 37% *Study closed early due to inferior results CDDP/CARBO arm
HB94 (GPOH)[31]	Stage I/II: IFOS/CDDP/DOXO Stage III/IV: IFOS/CDDP/DOXO + VP/CARBO	Stage I: 27; II: 3; III: 25; IV: 14	4-Year EFS/OS Stage I: 89%/96%; II: 100%/100%; III: 68%/76%; IV: 21%/36%
HB99 (GPOH)[98]	SR: IPA HR: CARBO/VP16	SR: 58 HR: 42	3-Year EFS/OS SR: 90%/88% HR: 52%/55%
SIOPEL 2[95]	SR: PLADO HR: CDDP/CARBO/DOXO	PRETEXT: I: 6; II: 36; III: 25; IV: 21; Mets: 25	3-Year EFS/OS SR: 73%/91% HR: IV: 48%/61% HR mets: 36%/44%
SIOPEL 3[7,99]	SR: CDDP vs. PLADO HR: SUPERPLADO	SR: PRETEXT I: 18; II: 133; III: 104 HR: PRETEXT IV: 74; +VPE: 70; mets: 70; AFP < 100: 12	3-Year EFS/OS SR: CDDP 83%/95%; PLADO 85%/93% HR: overall 65%/69%; mets 57%/63%
JPLT-1[100]	Stage I/II: CDDP (30)/THPA-DOXO Stage III/IV: CDDP (60)/THPA-DOXO	Stage I: 9; II: 32; IIIa: 48; IIIb: 25; IV: 20	5-Year EFS/OS Stage I: ?/100%; II: ?/76%; IIa: ?/50%; IIIb: ?/64%; IV: ?/77%

C5V, cisplatin; CARBO, carboplatin; fluorouracil and vincristine; CCSG, Children's Cancer Study Group; CDDP, cisplatin; COG, Children's Oncology Group; DOXO, doxorubicin; EFS, event-free survival; GPOH, German Pediatric Oncology Hematology; JPLT, Japanese Pediatric Liver Tumor (study); IFOS, ifosfamide; HR, high risk; IPA, ifosfamide, cisplatin, Adriamycin; mets, metastatic disease; OS, overall survival; POG, Pediatric Oncology Group; PRETEXT, pretreatment extent (of tumor) staging system; SIOPEL, International Society of Pediatric Oncology (epithelial) liver tumor study group; SR, standard risk; SUPERPLADO, CDDP/CARBO/DOXO; THPA, THP-adriamycin; VP, etoposide; +VPE mets, *Vena Cava*, *Portal vein*, *Extrahepatic metastatic disease*.

more children as part of a planned treatment algorithm. With increased experience defining the optimal timing of transplantation, the outcomes with liver transplantation for hepatoblastoma have blossomed.

Transplantation Outcomes for Hepatoblastoma In the past decade, more than a score of reports have appeared in the literature championing the potential role of liver transplantation in the treatment of unresectable pediatric hepatoblastoma (Table 33-7).[113-130] Transplantation, although potentially lifesaving, carries attendant consequences, including perioperative morbidity and mortality and the subsequent need for lifetime immunosuppression. The experience from Birmingham, United Kingdom illustrates contemporary experience, with 5-year disease-free survival of 100% when primary transplantation was performed in patients with a good response to chemotherapy, 60% after primary transplantation in patients with a poor response to chemotherapy, only 50% in patients with transplantation as a second option or "rescue transplantation," and 0% in patients not undergoing surgery.[116] In SIOPEL 1, overall survival at 10 years was 85% with a primary transplantation but only 40% for the children who underwent a rescue transplantation.[120] In a collaborative report of the world experience of liver transplantation for hepatoblastoma,[120] the overall survival rate at 6 years was 82% for 106 patients who received a primary transplantation, but only 30% for 41 patients who underwent a rescue transplantation.

Indications and Contraindications for Transplantation in Hepatoblastoma The following criteria are currently used by COG and SIOPEL to select potential candidates for transplantation: (1) multifocal PRETEXT IV, multifocal tumor in all four liver sections at diagnosis; (2) unifocal PRETEXT IV, with neoadjuvant chemotherapy often these tumors will "downstage" to a POST-TEXT III and become amenable to conventional resection by trisegmentectomy; (3) POSTTEXT III+V, proximity of the tumor to the vena cava or all three major hepatic veins makes adequate tumor clearance without impaired venous outflow doubtful; (4) POSTTEXT III+P, proximity of the tumor to the portal venous bifurcation or both major branches of the portal vein makes adequate tumor clearance without impaired portal venous inflow doubtful; (5) Intrahepatic relapse or residual tumor after previous attempt at resection, known as rescue transplantation. Although these guidelines are very useful, some uncertainty and controversy remains regarding the management of multifocal tumors, patients with venous involvement who might be candidates for extreme resection, patients who present with pulmonary metastasis, and patients who are referred with relapse or residual tumor and require rescue transplantation.

Transplantation for Multifocal Hepatoblastoma Both COG and SIOPEL currently recommend that all patients with multifocal PRETEXT IV tumors should undergo liver transplantation, even if one of the liver sections is apparently clear of tumor nodules after preoperative chemotherapy (Fig. 33-8). Microscopic foci of viable tumor are seen in explant livers despite the apparent radiographic disappearance of tumor nodules from these areas after preoperative chemotherapy.[131] In addition, multiple series have shown excellent results from primary transplantation and poor

TABLE 33-7

Contemporary Outcomes Transplantation for Hepatoblastoma

	No. of Patients	Survival (%)	Follow-up (years)
Al-Qabandi et al, J Pediatr Surg, Birmingham, UK[114]	8	75	
Reyes et al, 2000, J Pediatr, Pittsburgh, Pa[115]	12	83	0.1-15.4
Pimpalwar et al, 2002, J Pediatr Surg, Birmingham, UK[116]	12	83	0.1-9.2
Molmlenti et al, 2002, Am J Transplant, Dallas, Tex[117]	9	55	0.5-16
Sinivasan et al, 2002, Transplantation, London, UK[118]	13	85	0.1-9
Chardon et al, 2002, Transplantation, Paris/Brussels[113]	4	75	1.1-2
Cillo et al, 2003, Transplant Proc, Padua, Italy[119]	7	57	0.2-9
Otte et al, 2004, Pediatr Blood Cancer,[120] SIOPEL 1 + "World Experience"			
Primary transplantation	106	82	
Rescue transplantation	41	30	
Tiao et al, 2005, J Pediatr, Cincinnati, Ohio[111]	9	80	
Mejia et al, 2005, Clin Transplant, San Antonio, Tex[121]	10	70	3.7-18
Kasahara et al, 2005, Am J Transplant, Kyoto[122]	14	71	3.5 ± ?
Chen et al, 2006, J Pediatr Gastroent Nutr, St Louis[123]	7	85	0.6-18
Avila et al, 2006, Eur J Pediatr Surg, Madrid[124]	11	82	1-14
Austin et al, 2006, J Pediatr Surg, UNOS database[125]	135	69	
Cassas-Medley et al, 2007, J Pediatr Surg, Dupont, Del[126]	8	75	0.6-4.4
Beaunoyer et al, 2007, Pediatr Transplant, Stanford, Calif[127]	15	86	3.3 ± 3.5
Faraj et al, 2008, Liver Transplant, London, UK[128]	25	78	0.9-14.9
Browne et al, 2008, J Pediatr Surg, Chicago, [129]	14	71	3.8 ± ?
Kalicinski et al, 2008, Ann Transplant, Warsaw[130]	6	66	

SIOPEL, International Society of Pediatric Oncology (epithelial) liver tumor study group; UNOS, United Network for Organ Sharing.

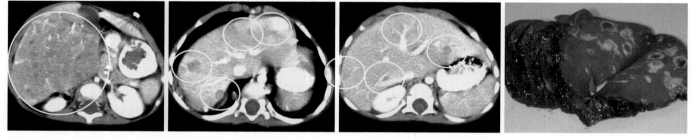

FIGURE 33-8 PRETEXT IV multifocal hepatoblastoma. In the presence of extensive multifocal tumors, microscopic satellites should be assumed, and no distance of surgical margin can ensure complete surgical excision. Extensive multifocal tumors are best treated by complete hepatectomy and liver transplantation. *(See Expert Consult site for color version.)*

results from rescue transplantation.[116,120,124,126,129] In a recent series from Padova, predictors of failed conservative therapy included multifocality.[132]

Major Venous Involvement: Transplantation versus Extreme Resection Aggressive resections, less than total hepatectomy, may be successful in select patients with tumor encroachment on the vena cava or main portal vein. Complex extensive resection, with vascular reconstruction if necessary, depends upon surgical expertise and a careful evaluation of the degree of vascular involvement and realistic ability to achieve complete, *and safe*, resection.[133,134] Poorly planned or executed operations risk excessive bleeding, inflow or outflow vascular obstruction, biliary leakage or stricture, cholangitis, and/or hepatic failure. Although most agree that extreme resection of tumors without liver transplantation will avoid the need for long-term immunosuppression,[102,113,132,133,135–137] outcomes with these techniques have not been rigorously reported. Current recommendations for referral of high-risk

patients with hepatoblastoma to centers that have the ability to do an extreme resection, with liver transplantation as an immediately available safety net, should result in an improved ability to compare the outcomes of these two approaches.[*]

Transplantation for Hepatoblastoma with Pulmonary Metastasis at Diagnosis An absolute contraindication to liver transplantation is persistent pulmonary metastases non-responsive to neoadjuvant chemotherapy and not amenable to surgical resection. Stable or progressive disease in the face of neoadjuvant chemotherapy is a relative contraindication to transplantation.[10,133] Lung metastases that disappear completely with chemotherapy, or with a combination of chemotherapy and surgical resection, do *not* pose a contraindication, yet the risk of post-transplantation pulmonary relapse is substantial, and therefore the use of liver transplantation for children with metastatic disease remains controversial.

* References 9,10,112,131,137,138

TABLE 33-8

Liver Transplantation in Children with Hepatoblastoma and Pulmonary Metastasis at Diagnosis, Review of Literature (Meyers and Otte,[9] 2010)

Pulmonary Metastasis at Diagnosis	No. of Patients	Post-transplantation Pulmonary Relapse	Alive without Evidence of Tumor	Died of Other Causes
Lung lesions disappeared with chemotherapy	24	9 (38%)	14 (58%)	1 (4%)
Pretransplantation pulmonary metastasectomy	8	3 (38%)	5 (62%)	
TOTAL	32	12 (37%)	19 (60%)	1 (3%)

Patients listed in table have been separately reported in the following series during the past 10 years: Perilongo, 2004[95]; Casanova, 2009[99]; Schnater, 2002[101]; Al-Qabandi et al, 1999[114]; Reyes et al, 2000[115]; Avila et al, 2006[124]; Cassas-Medley, 2007[126]; Superina et al, 1996[139]; Nathan 2009[140]; Otte, 2009.[141]

Table 33-8 shows the accumulated cases in the literature and presented at national and international meetings during the past 10 years.* Overall survival appears to be about 60% with no large difference in outcome when there is lung metastasis with complete radiographic resolution on chemotherapy versus pulmonary metastasectomy. Some centers do AFP imaging pretransplantation, PET-CT pretransplantation, median sternotomy with manual palpation of both lungs pretransplantation, and lobectomy rather than metastasectomy if the lung has more than four nodules in the same lobe.[142]

Rescue Transplantation for Local Relapse Hepatoblastoma

Multiple series have shown superior outcome after primary transplantation (about 80% overall survival) when compared with rescue transplantation (about 30% to 40% overall survival).[116,120,124,126,129] The basis for this is undoubtedly multifactorial, but two important reasons are (1) the likelihood of chemotherapy resistance in relapsed tumors and (2) the debilitated state of the patients when transplanted in the face of end-stage disease.

Type of Allograft and Immunosuppression

There is a trend to improved survival of children receiving a live-donor liver transplantation (LDLT).[120,121,128] When a living donor is available, pretransplantation chemotherapy can be scheduled optimally, with a rapid decision towards transplantation.[121] Whether living donor grafts might require less immunosuppression as suggested by Gras,[143] or whether alternative immunosuppression using rapamycin (sirolimus), a drug with both antineoplastic and immunosuppressive properties, will have any impact in children with hepatoblastoma remains to be seen. Many worry that the toxicity of chemotherapy might be potentiated by immunosuppression, but this has *not* been the experience at high-volume centers. With such a small number of patients in each of the individual series reported to date, it is not possible to make a clear recommendation at this time.

Pediatric Liver Unresectable Tumor Observatory (PLUTO)

SIOPEL, together with support from COG, GPOH, and the Study of Pediatric Liver Transplantation (SPLIT), has established a worldwide electronic registry for liver transplantation for childhood liver tumors (hepatoblastoma, hepatocellular carcinoma, and diffuse infantile hemangioma).[9,10,141,144] The link to obtain a password to register patients on this database can be accessed through the PLUTO Registry website: http://pluto.cineca.org/access.

---

* References 95, 99, 101, 114, 115, 124, 126, 139–141.

New Agents and Treatment Modalities

Hepatic Arterial Chemoembolization (HACE), Transarterial Chemoembolization (TACE)

HACE and TACE are different acronyms for the same interventional radiologic procedure, also sometimes referred to as transcatheter arterial chemoembolization. This technique continues to be quite popular in China where recent experience in infants and children showed a mean tumor shrinkage of 59%, mean decrease in AFP of 60%, mean tumor necrosis in the surgical specimens of 87%.[145] Widespread use has been somewhat limited by toxicity, which includes fever, pain, nausea, vomiting, transient coagulopathy, and, most worrisome, pulmonary oil (Lipiodol) embolism.[145–147] Pulmonary oil embolism is infrequent, and although fatalities have been reported, the clinical course is usually self-limited oxygen desaturation for 24 to 48 hours and pulmonary infiltrate for about a week.[148] Chemotherapeutic cocktails have included various combinations of cisplatin, doxorubicin, doxorubicin-eluting beads, vincristine, pirarubicin, mitomycin, and Lipiodol, followed by gelatin foam particles or stainless steel coils, and radioactive microspheres.[131,145–148] There are scattered case reports of cure without the need for surgical resection,[149] although it is most often used not as a definitive treatment, but rather as palliation for large unresectable tumors in the presence of uncontrolled metastatic disease.[145]

Ototoxicity

Both SIOPEL and COG have put considerable effort into investigations trying to decrease the significant ototoxicity induced by the use of cisplatin-based chemotherapy in young patients, especially infants. The risk of cisplatin causing bilateral moderate to severe high-frequency hearing loss is significantly increased in children younger than 5 years of age.[150] The COG 9645 trial failed to reduce ototoxicity with the agent amifostine.[151] The recently opened SIOPEL 6 study will investigate sodium thiosulfate[152] as an agent to decrease the cisplatin-induced ototoxicity. The current COG trial, AHEP0731, attempts to reduce ototoxicity by limiting the extended use of cisplatin in the low-risk patients.

Hepatoblastoma Risk Stratification and International Collaboration

Current data suggest that pure fetal histology and PRETEXT I and II tumors have a favorable prognosis.[28,30,89] Risk factors that seem to portend a worse outcome include metastatic disease at diagnosis (COG Stage IV, PRETEXT +M), PRETEXT IV, AFP < 100 at diagnosis, small cell undifferentiated histology and possibly macrotrabecular and/or extensive multifocal histology.[18,30,90,153] In 2007, SIOPEL, GPOH, and COG decided to embark on a mutual project that was called the *Childhood Hepatic Tumors International Collaboration* (CHIC). The complete databases of these groups are in the process of being united to address prognostic questions requiring increased statistical power. To identify these common data points for prognostication and risk stratification, data regarding prognostic factors (i.e., histology AFP, stage, multifocality, biological markers) can thus be studied in much larger patient groups in which the clinical outcome is known. These developments are the starting point of a new trans-Atlantic converging cooperation on a large intercontinental scale that will be of eventual benefit for children with liver tumors.

New Agents, Tumor Relapse The prognosis for a patient with recurrent or progressive hepatoblastoma depends on many factors, including the site of recurrence, prior treatment, and individual patient considerations. It was recently shown that in patients who initially received only cisplatin/5-FU/vincristine cure may be possible with a multidrug relapse regimen including doxorubicin.[109] Surgical resection of pulmonary relapse is possible and has been reported to produce long-term cure, but does not carry as good a prognosis as resection of pulmonary metastatic lesions present at diagnosis that simply fail to completely resolve on chemotherapy.[154–156] If possible, isolated metastases should be resected completely in patients whose primary tumor is controlled.[138,142,157] Success with autologous peripheral blood stem cell transplantation with a double conditioning regimen has been reported in a child with pulmonary relapse after liver transplantation.[158] Irinotecan has been used in chemotherapy relapse regimens with some success.[159] In recurrent refractory disease, phase I and II clinical trials may be appropriate and should be considered. Multidrug chemotherapy resistance is a key factor for the poor outcome of relapsed HB. Novel gene-directed treatment approaches, such as adenovirus-mediated cytosine deaminase/5-fluorocystine suicide gene therapy, may offer hope for treatment of these chemotherapy-resistant tumors in the future.[82,83] Information on current COG trials can be found at www.childrensoncologygroup.org.

HEPATOCELLULAR CARCINOMA

Epidemiology, Biology, and Genetics

In Western countries, hepatocellular carcinoma occurs approximately half as often as hepatoblastoma (HB) or in 23% of all primary pediatric liver tumor cases, most often in school-age children and adolescents. Although described previously, it was not until 1967 that childhood HCC was identified by Ishak and Glunz[3] as an entity to be distinguished from HB. In 1974, Exelby and colleagues[5] analyzed the clinical course of childhood HCC and found an overall dismal outcome.

HCC occurs predominantly in the setting of underlying liver disease and cirrhosis. Compared with adults, in children cirrhosis is less commonly part of the antecedent process, while congenital or acquired disorders of the liver, such as metabolic disease, are common.[17] Table 33-9 shows the conditions that are associated with HCC in children.[43,66,160–175] Patients with tyrosinemia seem to be a particularly high risk and should be vigilantly screened with serial AFP and imaging.[174] In East Asia and Africa, HCC is more common than HB because of the widespread prevalence of hepatitis B and C.[43] In Taiwan, where HCC is most often seen in carriers of the hepatitis B virus, vaccination

TABLE 33-9

Conditions Associated with Hepatocellular Carcinoma in Children

Alpha-1 antitrypsin deficiency[160]
Anomalous abdominal venous drainage[161]
Alagille syndrome[162]
Biliary atresia[163]
Congenital hepatic fibrosis[164]
Familial polyposis/Gardner syndrome[165]
Focal nodular hyperplasia[166]
Hemochromatosis[167]
Hepatic adenoma[168]
Hepatitis B and C[43]
Glycogen storage disease (type I and III)[169]
Methotrexate therapy[166]
Neurofibromatosis[66]
Oral contraceptives[170]
Parenteral nutrition–associated liver disease (PNALD); total parenteral nutrition (TPN) cholestatic liver failure[171]
Progressive familial intrahepatic cholestasis (PFIC)[172,173]
Tyrosinemia[174]
Wilms' tumor/Bloom syndrome[175]

programs targeted against hepatitis have led to a significant decrease in the incidence of HCC.[42] In contrast to hepatitis B, the cirrhosis and the subsequent development of HCC in the hepatitis C population usually takes several decades to develop.[176] The genetic syndromes associated with HCC are shown in Table 33-3.[54,55,62–68]

Pathology

In the pediatric age group, more than two thirds of HCC occur in children older than 10 years of age, but only 0.5% to 1% of all HCC manifest before 20 years of age, and very few HCCs are diagnosed in children less than 5 years old. About 20% to 35% of children with HCC have underlying chronic liver disease. It is still disputed whether classical (adult-type) HCC in the pediatric age group is the same or a different disease with respect to HCC in adult patients. It is currently suggested that HCC forms a tumor family, consisting of adult-type HCC and its variants, fibrolamellar HCC, and a novel entity occurring in older children and young adolescents, transitional liver cell tumor (TLCT).[92]

HCC presents grossly as solitary or multiple (multifocal) lesions. Solitary tumors display four main growth patterns, that is, expanding (or pushing) mass lesions, pedunculated (or hanging) lesions, invading tumors with poor delineation, and multifocal tumors resembling metastatic disease. These growth patterns exert a considerable influence on the surgical resectability of the tumors. The color of the cut surfaces of HCCs depends, apart from bleeding and necrosis, on differentiation features of the tumor cells, for instance bile synthesis and accumulation.

The microscopic features of pediatric classical HCC are similar to or the same as those in adult patients. Many tumors exhibit a trabecular growth pattern with intervening sinusoid-like vascular channels and a reduced reticulin network. Regarding grading, Edmondson and Steiner developed a system comprising a scale of I to IV.[177]

Fibrolamellar Hepatocellular Carcinoma (FL-HCC) This tumor usually arises in noncirrhotic livers of adolescents or young adult patients and is encountered more frequently in Western countries.[178] Overall, FL-HCC accounts for less than 10% of all HCCs. Recent data show that FL-HCC has biological features similar to that of adult-type HCC. FL-HCC shows vascular invasion in up to 35% of cases, frequently metastasizes into locoregional lymph nodes (about 50% of cases), and tends to show unusual spreading patterns, including intraperitoneal spread. FL-HCC is typically a solitary lesion that has a predilection for the left liver lobe (two thirds; unusual for hepatic primary tumors). It reveals well-defined margins and a central scar in 70%. The cut surface often shows a firm, tan to brown tissue with radiating septa, sometimes closely resembling focal nodular hyperplasia. The leading cell is a large and polygonal, hepatocyte-like cell with a granular cytoplasm of large vesicular nuclei. These cells form strands embedded in the typical fibrosclerotic stroma that may form a central stellate scar. A considerable proportion of the tumor cells contain large, ground glass–like inclusions, the so-called pale bodies, which are helpful in bioptic diagnosis. Periodic acid–Schiff (PAS)-positive globular inclusions in part contain alpha-1-antitrypsin and other glycoproteins. Typically, cells of FL-HCC show marked immunostaining for cytokeratin 7.[92]

Transitional Liver Cell Tumor (TLCT) Transitional liver cell tumor is a recently identified liver neoplasm that occurs in older children and young adolescents. The term transitional had been proposed to denote a putative intermediate position of the tumor cells between hepatoblasts and more mature hepatocyte-like cells. TLCT are highly aggressive lesions that have a treatment response pattern clearly different from hepatoblastoma.[179] The usual presentation is that of a large or very large solitary hepatic tumor (mostly in the right liver lobe), commonly associated with very high serum AFP levels. Grossly, the tumors display an expanding growth pattern and sometimes exhibit a large central necrosis. Histologically, the tumor cells vary between HCC-type cells and cells found in hepatoblastoma, sometimes with formation of multinuclear giant cells. The lesions markedly express beta-catenin, typically in a mixed nuclear and cytoplasmic pattern.[180]

PRETEXT and Staging

Children's Oncology Group staging for hepatocellular carcinoma does not use risk stratification and simply follows the traditional COG stage I, II, III, and IV shown in Table 33-5. Nevertheless, discussions with colleagues describing the extent of tumor involvement of the liver are based upon PRETEXT to aid in making key decisions about surgical resectability.

Treatment Strategies

Hepatocellular carcinoma is relatively chemotherapy resistant and therefore carries a poor prognosis with a dismal rate of cure.[181,182] Complete surgical resection or hepatectomy and transplantation for tumor localized to the liver is often the only hope. Unfortunately, HCC is most often advanced at diagnosis, and cure is rarely possible in the setting of metastatic disease. Even with aggressive attempts at surgical resection, tumor relapse is common and tumor-free survival rates of not more than 25% to 30% can be achieved. These mostly depend on the extent of disease, and the main prognostic factor for childhood HCC is resectability. The first multicenter clinical trials on pediatric liver tumors were conducted in North America by the Children's Cancer Study Group (CCSG) and POG, some of which included HCC in addition to HB.[181] These studies confirmed the poor response of HCC to chemotherapy and radiation and the dismal rate of cure in the majority of patients.

The North American cooperative study (INT-0098) as well as SIOPEL 1[181,182] used pre-operative chemotherapy in an attempt to increase surgical resectability for children and adolescents with HCC, because this is the foundation for curative therapy of liver tumors. Of the 46 patients entered onto INT-0098, only 8 had completely resected tumors (stage I) at study entry, 25 had unresectable tumors (stage III), and 13 presented with metastatic disease (stage IV). Patients were randomized to receive cisplatin with either doxorubicin or 5-fluorouracil and vincristine. No differences were seen in response or survival rates between the two treatment regimens. Seven of the 8 stage I patients (88%) with complete tumor excision at time of diagnosis, followed by adjuvant cisplatin-based chemotherapy, survived. This is a significant improvement when compared with only 12 of 33 patients (36%) treated before the consistent use of adjuvant chemotherapy. This result suggests that adjuvant chemotherapy may be of benefit for patients with completely resected HCC. However, because one third of these initially resected patients have fared well without any additional chemotherapy, the question of the necessity for adjuvant chemotherapy will only be answered in a randomized trial. In contrast, outcome was uniformly poor for patients with advanced-stage disease. The 5-year event-free survival for stage III and IV patients was 23% and 10%, respectively (Table 33-10).

Hepatocellular carcinoma patients have been treated in three consecutive studies of the German Society for Pediatric Oncology and Hematology (see Table 33-10).[26] In the first study, HB89, neoadjuvant and adjuvant chemotherapy consisted of conventionally dosed ifosfamide, cisplatin, and doxorubicin (IPA), which did not show any substantial benefit.[26] Of the registered 12 patients, only 4 with resectable tumor survived. In the second study (HB94), patients with nonresectable HCC received conventionally dosed carboplatin and etoposide in addition to IPA, which seemed to produce at least short-term benefit.[26] Of the registered 25 patients, 9 had locally unresectable and 11 metastatic HCC. Three of the 9 and 1 of the 11 patients survived free of disease in addition to 4 of 5 patients with resectable tumor (total 8 of 25 = 32%).

Results of SIOPEL 1, 2, and 3 are shown in Table 33-10.[182,183] Only 2 of the 39 patients entered onto the SIOPEL-1 study underwent complete resection of the tumor at diagnosis, followed by chemotherapy, while the remaining 37 patients had preoperative chemotherapy with cisplatin and doxorubicin. Metastases were identified in 31% of the patients, and extrahepatic tumor extension, vascular invasion, or both in 39%. Although partial tumor response to chemotherapy was observed in 49% (18 of 37) of the patients, complete tumor resection was achieved in only 36% (14 of 39) of the patients. Outcomes of patients on this study were also unsatisfactory, with a 5-year event-free survival of 17%. All long-term survivors had complete surgical excision of their tumor. Twenty-one patients were enrolled on the subsequent

TABLE 33-10

Summary Results Hepatocellular Carcinoma Cooperative Trials

Study	Chemotherapy	No. of Patients	Outcomes
INT0098 (CCSG, POG)[181]	CDDP/DOXO	Stage I: 8 Stage II: 0 Stage III: 25 Stage IV: 13	5-Year EFS/OS Stage I/II: 88%/88%; III: 8%/23%; IV: 19%/34%
HB89 (GPOH)[26]	CDDP/DOXO	Stage I/II/IIIa: 6 Stage IIIb, IV: 6	5-Year DFS Stage I/II/IIIa: 50%; IIIb, IV: 17%
HB94 (GPOH)[26]	CDDP/DOXO	Stage: I/II/IIIa: 5 Stage IIIb, IV: 20	5-Year DFS Stage I/II/IIIa: 60%; IIIb, IV: 25%
HB99 (GPOH)[26]	CDDP/DOXO	Stage: I/II/IIIa: 14 Stage IIIb, IV: 27	5-Year DFS Stage I/II/IIIa: 71%; IIIb, IV: 15%
SIOPEL 1[182]	CDDP/DOXO	PRETEXT: I, 1; II, 14; III, 11; IV, 13, +VPEM, 8	5-Year EFS/OS 17%/28%
SIOPEL 2[182]	CDDP/DOXO	PRETEXT: I, 1; II, 3; III, 1; IV, 7; +VPEM, 5	5-Year EFS/OS 23%/23%
SIOPEL 3[183]	CDDP/DOXO	PRETEXT: I, 4; II, 22; III, 14; IV, 21; +VPEM, ?	3-Year EFS/OS 10%/16%

CARBO, carboplatin; CCSG, Children's Cancer Study Group; CDDP, cisplatin; DFS, disease-free survival; DOXO, doxorubicin; EFS, event-free survival; GPOH, German Pediatric Oncology Hematology (study); IFOS, ifosfamide; IPA, ifosfamide, cisplatin, Adriamycin; OS, overall survival; POG, Pediatric Oncology Group; PRETEXT, pretreatment extent (of tumor) staging system; SIOPEL, International Society of Pediatric Oncology (epithelial) liver tumor study group; VP, etoposide; +VPEM, Vena cava, Portal vein, Extrahepatic, Metastatic disease.

study SIOPEL 2. Data were available for 17 of these. One patient died 17 days after diagnosis from massive GI bleeding and never received treatment. Thirteen of the 16 treated patients received preoperative chemotherapy with cisplatin, carboplatin, and doxorubicin. Partial response to preoperative chemotherapy was observed in 6 of 13 cases (46%). Gross total tumor resection was achieved in 8 patients (47%), 3 at the time of diagnosis and 1 through liver transplantation. Nine tumors (53%) never became operable. One patient was lost to follow-up just before planned surgery. Four of the patients having resection of their tumors were alive at a median follow-up time of 53 months (range of 35 to 73 months). Twelve patients died because of progressive disease and one from surgical complications. The three-year overall survival for this study was 22%.

In comparing the results of these studies, the outcome for patients with HCC has shown no significant improvement, despite the progress in surgical techniques, chemotherapy delivery, and patient support. It seems obvious that a new treatment approach is needed to increase the rate of cure of childhood HCC.

In adults, fibrolamellar type of hepatocellular carcinoma has been traditionally associated with a higher resection rate and better survival when compared with the typical pathologic variant of HCC both in adolescents and young adults.[184,185] The higher resection rate for children and adolescents with the fibrolamellar variant of HCC was not supported by the studies reported by either Katzenstein[181] or Czauderna.[182] Patients with the fibrolamellar variant did not have a better outcome when compared with those with typical HCC, the 5-year event-free survival was 30% compared with 14%, respectively ($P = 0.18$), although the median survival was longer for patients with the fibrolamellar variant.

Given the poor response of HCC to chemotherapy and radiation, the mainstay of treatment is surgery. This means that, in contrast to hepatoblastoma, a primary radical tumor resection has to be attempted whenever possible using all available techniques in order to achieve this goal.[26] Therefore in school-age children and adolescents with a primary liver

tumor the surgeon has to be prepared to perform highly sophisticated liver surgery after confirmation of the diagnosis by pathologic investigation of intraoperative frozen sections. Patients with the clinical constellation for advanced HCC should always be treated in consultation with a specialized center with experience in childhood liver surgery.

Liver Transplantation for Hepatocellular Carcinoma in Children

Outcomes, Indications, and Contraindications Published outcomes for liver transplantation in children with HCC are shown in Table 33-11.* The following guiding principles have been formulated by centers with particular expertise in pediatric liver transplantation. They are in a greater state of controversy and evolution than are the guidelines for HB. In most centers, the criteria for transplantation of multifocal and unifocal HCC are the same as for HB and do *not* follow adult limitations on size and number of nodules. Unlike HB, however, any history of pulmonary metastatic disease or extrahepatic disease is considered an absolute contraindication. Major vascular involvement, of the portal vein for example, is a relative contraindication depending upon the degree and severity of involvement.[142] It is important that consultation with a transplantation center with special expertise in pediatric liver surgery be considered early in the treatment to prevent delays and unwanted extended courses of chemotherapy while awaiting resection and transplantation.

Response to Chemotherapy HCC tumor progression while on chemotherapy is a relative contraindication to transplantation, because occult extrahepatic micrometastatic disease is increasingly likely in this situation.

Milan Criteria The Milan criteria, introduced by Mazzaferro in 1996, restrict transplantation in adults with HCC as follows: (1) single tumor diameter less than 5 cm; (2) not more than

---

* References 115, 124, 125, 127, 130, 139, 182, 186–194.

TABLE 33-11

Literature, Transplantation for Pediatric Hepatocellular Carcinoma

	No. of Patients	Survival (%)	Tumor Recurrence	Small Incidental*†	Died Comp OLT†
‡Olthoff et al, 1990, Arch Surg, UCLA[186]	16	22	8/16	—	4/16
‡Penn et al, 1991, Surgery, Transplant Registry[187]	429	—	158/429	31/429	—
Tagge et al, 1992, J Pediatr Surg, Pittsburgh, Pa[188]	9	44	3/9	—	1/9
Yandza et al, 1993, Transplant Int, Paris[189]	2	100	—	—	—
Broughan et al, 1994, J Pediatr Surg, multicenter[190]	4	75	¼	0	0
Otte et al, 1996, Transplant Proc, Brussels[191]	5	60	2/5	0	0
Achilleos, et al 1996, J Pediatr Surg, Birmingham, UK[192]	2	0	½	½	½
Superina et al, 1996, J Pediatr Surg, Toronto[139]	3	100	0/3	3/3	0
Reyes et al, 2000, J Pediatr, Pittsburgh, Pa[115]	19	63	6/19	7/19	2/12
Tatekawa et al, 2001, J Pediatr Surg, Kyoto[193]	2	100	0	½	0
Czaudema et al, 2002, J Clin Oncol, SIOPEL 1[182]	2	—	—	½	—
Avila et al, 2006, Eur J Ped Surg, Madrid[124]	1	100	—	—	—
Austin et al, 2006, J Pediatr Surg, UNOS database[125]		41	63%	12/41	—
Beaunoyer et al, 2007, Pediatr Transplant, Stanford, Calif[127]	10	83	1/10	4/10	2/10
Kalicinski et al, 2008, Ann Transplant, Warsaw[130]	8	75	1/8	—	1/8
Ismail et al, 2009, Pediatr Transplant, Warsaw[194]	11	72	1/11	3/11	2/11

*Most are patients with tyrosinemia, other metabolic liver disease, familial intrahepatic cholestasis, hepatitis, or biliary atresia.
†Died as a result of complications of orthoptic liver transplantation.
‡Did not separately analyze pediatric cohort.
Comp, complications; OLT, orthotopic liver transplantation; SIOPEL, International Society of Pediatric Oncology (epithelial) liver tumor study group; UCLA, University of California–Los Angeles; UNOS, United Network for Organ Sharing.

three foci of tumor, each one not exceeding 3 cm; (3) no angioinvasion; (4) no extrahepatic involvement. Since the introduction of these criteria, long-term recurrence-free survival after liver transplantation in adults with HCC improved from 30% to 75%.[195–198] The problem with the Milan criteria in children is that 50% to 70% of children present with large de novo tumors and a large tumor burden in otherwise healthy livers, *and the Milan criteria were developed in adults with small tumors and underlying cirrhotic liver disease.* In children, the number of nodules, as stipulated by the Milan criteria, is usually not considered a contraindication to transplantation as long as the disease is confined to the liver. Furthermore, de novo pediatric HCC often shows features on a continuum with pediatric HB, and these "transitional liver tumors" may have a more favorable biology.[92–200] In view of the lack of improvement in results of conventional treatment of pediatric HCC during the past 2 decades, most clinicians treating pediatric HCC do NOT recommend adherence to Milan criteria in children who present with large de novo tumors, no cirrhosis, and no evidence of extrahepatic disease.[201]

Metastatic Disease Metastatic disease is considered an *absolute* contraindication to liver transplantation in HCC, and a very careful and thorough evaluation to exclude metastatic microdeposits is essential.

Post-transplantation Chemotherapy Guidelines for post-transplantation immunosuppression in HCC are the same as with transplantation for HB with one possible difference. Many centers would consider post-transplantation adjuvant antiangiogenic therapy with sorafenib in HCC. Experience in the transplantation population of patients is limited, but in any patient considered to be at high risk for tumor relapse, options for possible antiangiogenic therapy should be

discussed. Similarly, many centers have begun to experiment with rapamycin (sirolimus) as a post-transplantation immunosuppressant because of its antineoplastic, antiangiogenic properties.[203–205]

New Agents and Treatment Modalities

Antiangiogenesis, Sorafenib New treatment modalities including metronomic chemotherapy,[206] and adjuvant antiangiogenic therapy[207] are the target of investigation based upon some early promising results. Most promising has been the recent adult experience with sorafenib, an antiangiogenic tyrosine kinase inhibitor, where a survival advantage has clearly been shown in prospective trials of sorafenib in the treatment of HCC in adults with unresectable tumors.[202] Interestingly, this seems to be also the case in some preliminary investigation in childhood HCC.[208]

Chemoembolization and Theraspheres Hepatic arterial chemoembolization (HACE) and transarterial chemoembolization (TACE) refers to the intra-arterial administration of chemotherapeutic and vascular occlusive agents (generally gelatin or Lipiodol) along with cytotoxic drugs. The drugs most frequently used for chemoembolization are doxorubicin, mitomycin, and cisplatin. Intra-arterial injection of cytotoxic agents results in higher local concentration of drugs with reduced systemic side effects, while the intra-arterial embolization causes ischemic necrosis of the tumor. This therapeutic strategy has been used in a small number of children and adolescents with recurrent HCC while awaiting the availability of a liver donor, or as adjuvant therapy in an attempt to facilitate tumor resection.[145,209] There are no large trials in children; however, in a study of adult HCC patients without liver failure or cirrhosis, although TACE successfully reduced tumor growth, it frequently caused acute liver failure and did not improve survival.[210] A related approach that combines radiation therapy with angiographic embolization has been the intra-arterial injection of yttrium-90 radioactive microspheres, called Theraspheres.[211]

Portal Venous Embolization   Portal venous embolization has been used in adults with liver disease to induce hypertrophy of the remaining liver remnant[212] and reported experimentally in children.[213] The portal venous branch on the side of the tumor is cannulated percutaneously, and polyvinyl alcohol and coils are inserted to induce portal vein occlusion under fluoroscopic control. This has a dual effect of alcohol thrombosis of the embolized tumor and compensatory hypertrophy of the unharmed opposite liver lobe, increasing the potential hepatic functional reserve in patients with cirrhosis and underlying liver dysfunction in preparation for hepatic resection.

Percutaneous Ablative Therapies   Ablative percutaneous methods of local control may be considered, especially in recurrent tumors. They include percutaneous radiofrequency ablation (RFA), percutaneous ethanol injection (PEI), and cryotherapy. Cryotherapy refers to cold injury produced by cryoprobe delivery of liquid nitrogen, and although once popular in adults, it has now fallen out of favor because of superior results achieved with RFA and PEI. In most cases, these treatment approaches are palliative and are suitable for smaller tumors only, generally below 3 cm to 4 cm maximum diameter. RFA provides slightly better tumor kill than PEI (90% vs. 80% complete tumor necrosis) with fewer sessions (mean of 1.2 vs. 4.8).[199] It is also associated with fewer side effects; thus in many centers, RFA is now preferred versus PEI; however, RFA is contraindicated in lesions located adjacent to the major biliary ducts or to bowel loops. Complications of these ablative techniques occur in about 8% to 9% of cases, mainly in the form of pain, fever, bleeding, tumor seeding, and gastrointestinal perforation.[214] Percutaneous ablation has not been well studied in children.

Hepatic Sarcomas

Primary hepatic sarcomas are rare. Outcome depends primarily on tumor histology, sensitivity to chemotherapy and/or radiotherapy, and the ability to achieve complete tumor resection.[215]

Biliary Rhabdomyosarcoma

The classic presentation of biliary rhabdomyosarcoma is in young children (average age 3½ years) with jaundice and abdominal pain, and it is often associated with distension, vomiting, and fever.[13] Histology is exclusively embryonal or botryoid, both histologic subtypes of rhabdomyosarcoma that are known to have a favorable prognosis. Because the tumor most often involves the central biliary tree and porta hepatis, the ability to achieve gross total resection is rare. Fortunately, the tumor is often sensitive to both chemotherapy and radiation, and long-term survival is seen in 60% to 70% of patients. Surgical intervention has two goals: to establish an accurate diagnosis and to determine the local-regional extent of disease. Although chemotherapy is generally effective at relief of the associated biliary obstruction, patients remain at risk for biliary sepsis until the obstruction abates.

Rhabdoid Tumor

Although pediatric rhabdoid tumors are most common in the kidney and brain, they do occur at other sites, including the mediastinum and liver. When primary to the liver, rhabdoid tumor is difficult to distinguish from the small cell undifferentiated (SCU) variant of hepatoblastoma. Given the aggressive biological behavior and poor prognosis seen with the SCU variant of HB, it has been suggested that some tumors previously classified as HB-SCU may actually have been hepatic rhabdoid tumors. The differentiation of an HB-SCU from a rhabdoid tumor is challenging and is important in terms of research, but possibly clinically irrelevant at present because both are biologically aggressive with poor response to chemotherapy. Malignant rhabdoid tumor of the liver is a rare and aggressive tumor of toddlers and school-age children that may present with spontaneous rupture.[216,217] These rare tumors are often chemoresistant and fatal,[216] although a recent case report documents the potential for cure with multimodal therapy, including ifosfamide, vincristine, and actinomycin D.[217] As with all locally aggressive liver tumors that respond poorly to chemotherapy, the most important treatment goal is complete surgical excision.

Undifferentiated Sarcomas

Undifferentiated (embryonal) sarcoma of the liver is a rare childhood hepatic tumor that has historically been considered an aggressive neoplasm with an unfavorable prognosis. These tumors may arise in a solitary liver cyst.[218] Survival has improved in recent multimodal approaches, designed for patients with soft tissue sarcomas at other sites, including conservative surgery at diagnosis, multiagent chemotherapy, and second-look operation in cases of residual disease. Using these techniques several small series have reported survival in up to 70% of children.[219–221]

Angiosarcoma

Although rare, personal experience and multiple case reports in the literature support the potential for malignant transformation of an infantile hemangioma to angiosarcoma.[222,223] Histologic verification of malignancy may be difficult, and this rare entity must be suspected if the biological behavior of an infantile hemangioma shows unusual progression or recurrence after a period of relative quiescence. Relatively chemoresistant, prognosis is generally poor.

Aggressive Hemangiomatous Tumors

Locally Aggressive Infantile Hepatic Hemangioma   Infantile hemangioma is the most common benign tumor of the liver in infancy[19] with striking variability of the three subtypes of infantile hemangioma: focal, multinodular, and diffuse. Many focal lesions are often discovered incidentally and are localized and small enough to be of little clinical significance. Symptoms seen with larger lesions may include abdominal distention, hepatomegaly, congestive heart failure, vomiting, anemia, thrombocytopenia and consumptive coagulopathy, jaundice secondary to biliary obstruction, and associated cutaneous or visceral hemangiomas.[11] Contrast-enhanced CT scan shows an area of diminished density, and after bolus injection of intravenous contrast, there is contrast enhancement from the periphery toward the center of the lesion. Further, after a short delay, there is complete isodense filling of the lesion and liver. Magnetic resonance angiography (MRA) has been used in complex cases to identify atypical radiographic features that may portend a poor prognosis.[224] Unfavorable radiographic features include central varix with arteriovenous shunt, central necrosis or thrombosis, and diffuse hemangiomatous involvement of the liver with abdominal vascular compression.[224] Arterial angiography may be used in infants with refractory symptoms in whom either hepatic artery ligation or embolization is considered.

If a definitive diagnosis of simple infantile hepatic hemangioma can be made radiographically, management can be noninvasive because spontaneous regression occurs in most cases, especially focal tumors. The terminology is confusing, however, with different authors often using the terms hepatic hemangioma, infantile hepatic hemangioma, hepatic hemangioendothelioma, or kaposiform hemangioendothelioma interchangeably.[225] True kaposiform hemangioendothelioma with Kasabach-Merritt (as opposed to the high-output heart failure from intrahepatic shunts seen in diffuse infantile hemangioma), rarely, if ever, presents as a primary hepatic tumor.[226] Hemangioendotheliomas are occasionally primary to the retroperitoneum, where they can invade the liver and obstruct the porta hepatis, causing portal hypertension. These tumors are discussed in more detail in Chapter 125.

Sometimes a large rapidly growing infantile hepatic hemangioma can be life threatening with intractable high-output cardiac failure from intralesional arteriovenous shunting, intraperitoneal hemorrhage, respiratory distress as a result of pulmonary congestion, and massive hepatomegaly compressing abdominal vasculature and producing abdominal compartment syndrome (Fig. 33-9). Historically, the initial medical intervention for symptomatic tumors has been corticosteroids. Many other medical treatment options exist, although no single treatment has been shown to be universally effective. Congestive heart failure is treated with supportive care, digitalis, and diuretics. Anemia and coagulopathy are treated with corrective blood product replacement therapy. Both success and complete failure have been reported variously with many other treatments, including epsilon-aminocaproic acid, tranexamic acid, low-molecular-weight heparin, vincristine, cyclophosphamide, interferon-2-alpha, AGM-1470, and newer generation antiangiogenic drugs.[227–231] Recent studies have shown that the large tumors may produce

antibodies to thyroid-stimulating hormone (TSH), and screening to rule out secondary hypothyroidism is recommended.[232,233] Most recently, propranolol has been shown to inhibit the growth of infantile hemangioma.[234] Although rare, malignant transformation to angiosarcoma has been reported, and close follow-up is recommended.[223,224,235,236]

In infants who fail medical management, symptomatic solitary tumors may be treated by excision, hepatic arterial ligation, or selective angiographic embolization.[237] Treatment algorithms may stratify treatment based upon whether or not the tumor is solitary, multifocal, or diffuse.[238,239] About 65% of tumors are solitary or unifocal with a survival of 86% and death usually not caused by the tumor but by a comorbidity.[19] Thirty-five percent of tumors are multifocal or diffuse, with a survival somewhere between 60% to 100%, with death usually secondary to cardiorespiratory compromise caused by tumors refractory to medical and interventional management.[19,237,238]

Metastatic and Other Liver Tumors

Metastatic Liver Tumors Unlike the large body of literature concerning liver resection for metastatic colorectal tumors in adults, there is little published data that addresses the treatment of metastatic tumors in the liver following from abdominal solid tumors in childhood. A recent series from a large metropolitan children's cancer center reported only 15 such patients during a 17-year period, including neuroblastoma (7), Wilms' tumor (3), osteogenic sarcoma (2), gastric epithelial (1), and desmoplastic small round cell tumor (2).[240] Eleven of the 15 patients died of progressive disease; 4 had a local recurrence. These results lead the authors to conclude that the overall prognosis in these patients remains poor, and the decision to perform hepatic metastasectomy should be made with caution. The treatment approach should not, however, be uniformly nihilistic, because not all liver lesions in children with abdominal solid tumors turn out to be metastatic disease. Both nodular regenerative hyperplasia and focal nodular hyperplasia have been reported to mimic hepatic metastasis in children[241]; definitive diagnosis requires biopsy and/or resection.

Occasionally, a pancreatoblastoma may present with extensive hepatic metastasis (Fig. 33-10). Despite the alarming radiographic appearance at diagnosis, this tumor was, in fact,

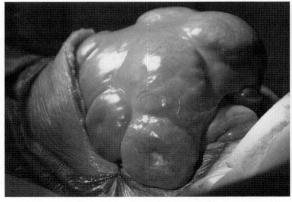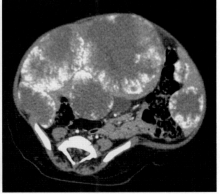

FIGURE 33-9 Symptomatic multifocal/diffuse infantile hepatic hemangioma. These tumors are benign but occasionally will be refractory to aggressive attempts at medical and percutaneous management. This tumor showed progressive growth despite chemotherapy and percutaneous embolization of largest nodules. The baby developed abdominal compartment syndrome and vena cava obstruction. Treated with temporizing abdominal decompressive laparotomy and, definitively, with hepatectomy and live-donor liver transplantation. *(See Expert Consult site for color version.)*

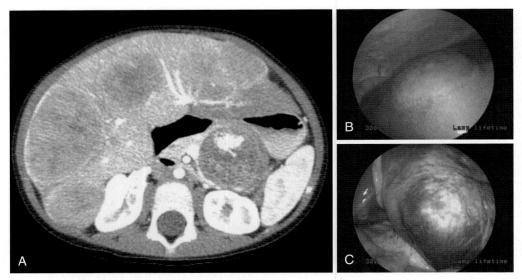

FIGURE 33-10 Metastatic pancreatoblastoma. **A,** Infant with extensive metastatic tumor in the liver at diagnosis. **B** and **C,** Appearance at laparoscopic biopsy. Primary tumor is a pancreatoblastoma involving the body of the pancreas. Although the tumor metastases were extensive at diagnosis, they prove to be exquisitely chemosensitive with cisplatin/doxorubicin chemotherapy. *(See Expert Consult site for color version.)*

exquisitely chemosensitive, and the child did well after neo-adjuvant chemotherapy, subtotal pancreatectomy, hepatectomy, and live-donor liver transplantation. Pancreatoblastomas are treated with multiagent chemotherapy analogous to hepatoblastoma and have a fair prognosis if chemosensitive.

Liver Tumors as Secondary Malignancies

We recently saw a case of multiple lesions of focal nodular hyperplasia in the liver of a 10-year-old boy 9 years after treatment for stage IV neuroblastoma with double autologous stem cell transplantations. Given the history, we initially suspected metastatic neuroblastoma, but diagnostic laparoscopy and laparoscopic biopsy of multiple lesions showed focal nodular hyperplasia (FNH). Another case report of FNH in a child with a history of stage IV neuroblastoma showed foci of small cell undifferentiated hepatoblastoma in the resection specimen; so, very close follow-up is necessary if treatment of the FNH is nonoperative.[242] Liver tumors have been recognized as potential late effects and/or secondary malignancies in children who have previously undergone chemotherapy and radiation as toddlers.

Hemophagocytic Lymphohistiocytosis

Hemophagocytic lymphohistiocytosis (HLH) may occasionally present as an abnormal liver mass in a newborn with coagulopathy. Predisposing factors include familial, herpes simplex virus, and severe combined immunodeficiency.[243] Diagnostic criteria according to HLH-2004 include fever, splenomegaly, bicytopenia, hypotriglyceridemia, hypofibrinogenemia, hemophagocytosis, low natural killer (NK) cell activity, hyperferritinemia, and high interleukin-2 (IL-2) receptor levels.[244] Treatment is with combination chemoimmunotherapy, including etoposide, dexamethasone, cyclosporine A, and anticipated mortality of about 40% is increased if the diagnosis or appropriate therapy is delayed.

Langerhans' Cell Histiocytosis

Morphologic changes and clinical findings in Langerhans' cell histiocytosis (LCH) of the liver may resemble primary sclerosing cholangitis or a chronic nonsuppurative destructive cholangitis.[245] Therefore LCH is an important differential diagnosis of chronic destructive cholangitis with cholestatic liver disease, especially in children and young adults. Other involved organs include bone, pituitary, thyroid, and lungs.[246] The diagnosis can be verified by S-100 and CD-1a (antigen) immunohistochemistry. There have been rare reports of pediatric liver transplantation in toddlers with multisystem LCH, children who developed end-stage liver disease despite intensive chemotherapy.[247,248]

Megakaryoblastic Leukemia

Rarely, congenital acute megakaryoblastic leukemia (AMKL) may present isolated to the liver, with ascites caused by massive infiltration of hepatic sinusoids by leukemic cells.[249] The bone marrow by microscopy and flow cytometry and the peripheral blood smear may not initially show the presence of blasts. Because the marrow fibrosis may not manifest until after the massive hepatic infiltration, it may initially be difficult to diagnose as leukemia. In most children with liver involvement the spleen, lymph nodes, and marrow will also be involved at diagnosis. But even in these cases, the diagnosis may be difficult both clinically and pathologically, and the hepatic and lymph node involvement is not uncommonly misinterpreted as solid tumor.[250]

The complete reference list is available online at www.expertconsult.com.

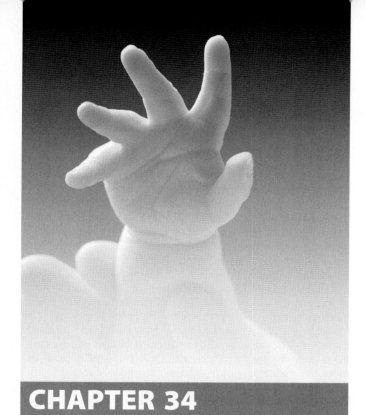

Pediatric Gastrointestinal Tumors

Joseph T. Murphy and Robert P. Foglia

Primary gastrointestinal (GI) tumors are uncommon in infants and children, and GI malignancies account for less than 2% of all cases of pediatric cancer.[1] The presentation and histopathology of pediatric GI tumors differ significantly from those seen in adults. Although rare, GI malignancy should be considered in any child with signs and symptoms of intestinal obstruction, intractable pain, alteration in bowel habits, or GI bleeding that are not attributable to other more common and established diagnosis. Symptoms often persist for several weeks and may progress to intestinal obstruction requiring emergency surgery.[1,2] Children with unexplained gastrointestinal symptoms require a detailed diagnostic evaluation.[3]

Esophageal Smooth Muscle Tumors

Esophageal leiomyomas and leiomyosarcomas are rare in children, with fewer than two dozen patients accounting for all documented pediatric esophageal smooth muscle tumors. Although esophageal smooth muscle tumors are often solitary

in adults, in children they are frequently multifocal, with a third involving the entire esophagus and 70% extending into the proximal stomach. Children typically present with esophageal obstruction and dysphagia, food regurgitation, and chest pain. Barium swallow findings mimic achalasia, and a biopsy is required for definitive diagnosis. Leiomyomas in children are occasionally associated with familial syndromes, such as familial leiomyoma and Alport syndrome. Extensive surgical resection is necessary in the majority of cases.[4,5]

Esophageal and Gastric Adenocarcinoma

Esophageal and gastric cancer in children is extremely rare. Between 1988 and 1996 the Surveillance, Epidemiology, and End Results (SEER) database documented esophageal malignancy in only three patients between 10 and 19 years of age, and none younger than 10 years.[6,7]

The development of Barrett esophagus secondary to chronic gastroesophageal reflux disease (GERD) is a primary risk factor for the development of esophageal adenocarcinoma. Children with severe neurologic deficits, such as cerebral palsy, and those with congenital defects involving the esophagus, such as esophageal atresia and tracheoesophageal fistula, are at increased risk for development of Barrett esophagus.[8] The incidence of Barrett esophagus has been estimated to be 0.02% among children with severe GERD and associated risk factors. Nevertheless, adenocarcinoma of the esophagus has been documented in adolescents with long-standing GERD, and surveillance with upper endoscopy and multiple longitudinal biopsies is appropriate for those children who have the mucosal changes of Barrett esophagus.[9,10]

Barrett changes can also be seen in the retained cervical esophagus following esophageal replacement surgery. Postoperative care of these patients requires control of gastric pH and long-term surveillance endoscopy with biopsy of the retained upper esophageal segment. Esophageal replacement surgery for a patient with esophageal atresia can be performed with retention of the distal esophageal segment. This remnant can develop severe chronic esophagitis and Barrett changes requiring resection. Because Barrett esophagus is a premalignant condition, the distal segment of the esophagus should be removed at the time of esophageal replacement surgery.[11] Esophageal carcinomas may also occur in children after caustic esophageal injuries. Endoscopic evaluation with biopsies should be considered for patients with chemical injuries to monitor for the development of premalignant changes.[12]

Between 1975 and 2007, the SEER database reported a gastric cancer incidence of 9.25 per 100,000 individuals, with an age-adjusted incidence of 0.1% for patients younger than 24 years.[6,13] Despite the rarity of this entity, there are case reports of adenocarcinoma of the stomach in children as young as 2.5 years. The tumors can arise from any anatomic location in the stomach, with nonspecific symptoms including epigastric pain, weight loss, vomiting, anemia, and symptoms associated with esophageal achalasia. Surgical resection is the primary therapeutic modality; however, curative resection is rare and mortality rates are high for children with this tumor.[14–16]

Gastrointestinal Stromal Tumors

EPIDEMIOLOGY

Gastrointestinal stromal tumors (GISTs) are rare mesenchymal tumors whose classification is hindered by anecdotal reports, failure to distinguish between primary and secondary GISTs, and the mixing of benign and malignant tumors in the reports.[17] In addition, GISTs arising from various anatomic sites have been reported together, making prediction of their clinical behavior difficult.[18] The most common site is the stomach (50% to 70%), followed by the small intestine (20% to 30%), colon or rectum (10%), and esophagus (5%).[19]

CLINICAL PRESENTATION

Patients with GIST tumors present with nonspecific symptoms, often generalized abdominal pain, dyspepsia, and occult GI bleeding. Iron-deficiency anemia should prompt an investigation to exclude a GI tract malignancy as the cause.[1] Less commonly, patients present with a palpable abdominal mass or intestinal obstruction.[20] Standard imaging studies may assist in the diagnosis (plain radiographs and computed tomography [CT]). Endoscopy can identify a tumor mass in the stomach, duodenum, or colon.[21]

PATHOLOGY

GISTs are classified as mesenchymal tumors of the GI tract thought to originate from the intestinal cell of Cajal, an intestinal pacemaker cell.[22] Historically, smooth muscle tumors, such as leiomyomas and leiomyosarcomas, and neural tumors, such as nerve sheath tumors, have been categorized as GISTs. GISTs are now defined as cellular spindle cell, epithelioid, or occasional pleomorphic mesenchymal tumors that express the KIT (CD117, stem cell factor receptor) protein, as detected by immunohistochemistry. Additional cell type markers, such as CD34, smooth muscle actin, desmin, and S-100 protein, are also used to establish a diagnosis of GIST. These histologic and immunohistochemical features now distinguish GISTs from leiomyomas, leiomyosarcomas, neural tumors, and other tumors of smooth muscle origin.[23] Prognosis relies on traditional pathologic staging criteria, such as size, extent of tumor invasion into mucosa or surrounding organs, mitotic index, and nuclear pleomorphism. However, no single feature is consistently reliable in predicting outcome.[24]

Determining prognosis of pediatric patients with GIST tumors can be controversial. The usual criteria for assessing risk of malignancy (i.e., tumor size, mitotic activity, anatomic location) are not reliable in pediatric GIST. Children frequently present with multiple gastric nodules, making identification of a dominant mass difficult. Secondly, there exists a wide variation in proliferation index between patients and even among multiple tumors within the same patient. Furthermore, some pediatric patients develop GIST metastasis despite being classified as low risk by adult criteria, and others with low proliferation indices develop recurrent disease in perigastric nodal basins, the peritoneum, or liver.[25] Pediatric GIST is distinguished as a separate clinical, pathologic, and molecular subset with a predisposition for females, multifocal gastric tumors, and wild-type KIT/PDGRA genotype. This is in contrast to older-age, adult GIST and even GIST in young adults. All these factors must be considered when distinguishing benign from malignant pediatric gastric stromal tumors.[18,26]

ASSOCIATED CONDITIONS

The Carney triad consists of a gastric leiomyosarcoma, functioning extraadrenal paraganglioma, and pulmonary chondroma. The gastric stromal tumors are usually located along the lesser curve or antrum and produce few symptoms; however, continued growth leading to mucosal ulceration, GI bleeding, and serosal involvement is common. Despite the possible development of additional gastric tumors in the remaining stomach, if feasible, partial gastrectomy is recommended as the initial operation, to avoid the complications of more extensive gastric resection, particularly in teenaged patients. Because the multifocal nature of the tumor can lead to local recurrence, regular follow-up is mandatory to assess for new gastric tumors. Adjuvant therapy has been unsuccessful in treating metastatic disease. Evaluation for adrenal tumors in patients with gastric stromal sarcomas and pulmonary chondromas should be considered, and a family history should be obtained from patients with the Carney triad. Recently, an autosomal dominant inheritance of paragangliomas and gastric GIST, called the Carney-Stratakis syndrome, has been identified, representing a separate condition affecting both males and females. Succinate dehydrogenase subunit gene mutations, typically associated with familial paragangliomas, have been implicated in the pathogenesis of Carney-Stratakis syndrome.[27–30]

An uncommon, histologically distinct subset of GIST, called a GI autonomic nerve tumor (GANT), has been described in children. Pediatric GANTs have a female prevalence and symptoms that may include anemia, abdominal pain, fullness, emesis, and a palpable abdominal mass. Although adult GANTs are found predominantly in the small intestine, pediatric GANT lesions are primarily gastric tumors. The majority of pediatric patients have localized disease at the time of diagnosis. Younger age, localized disease, gastric location, and small tumor size at diagnosis are associated with favorable prognosis. Immunocytochemical and ultrastructural evaluation is required to differentiate these tumors from GIST. Established pathologic criteria for malignancy are not well defined for the pediatric GANT because of the low incidence of these tumors. Surgical resection of the tumor is the treatment of choice, because there appears to be no definite role for chemotherapy or radiation.[10]

TREATMENT

Complete surgical excision of GISTs, along with the pseudocapsule, is the treatment of choice. Achieving negative pathologic margins is frequently possible, because GISTs tend to hang from and do not diffusely infiltrate the structure from which they arise. Consequently, wedge resection of the stomach or segmental resection of the intestine provides adequate therapy; wide resection is not necessary.[17] In addition, because the status of microscopic margins does not appear to be important for survival, vital structures should not be sacrificed if gross tumor clearance has been attained. GIST rarely metastasizes to lymph nodes; so, lymphadenectomy is seldom warranted.[19]

The high rate of local and distant recurrence underscores the need for adjuvant therapy. GIST has traditionally been resistant to radiotherapy; however, imatinib mesylate, a selective KIT, PDGF-RA, PDGR-RB, and BCR-ABL tyrosine kinase inhibitor, has been successful as a first-line agent in treating advanced and metastatic GIST in adult patients. Imatinib blocks the constitutive activity of KIT receptor in GIST cells.[21] Recently, a mutation in the c-*KIT* gene on exon-11 associated with increased risk of recurrence and higher mortality was identified.[19] The efficacy of imatinib is related to GIST genotype, with *KIT* exon-11–mutated GISTs being more sensitive to imatinib than wild-type (WT) tumors. While imatinib mesylate has been effective adjuvant therapy for adult GISTs, pediatric GIST lesions are frequently less responsive. The lack of efficacy may result from pediatric GISTs being predominantly WT genotype and lacking the *KIT* mutations more commonly detected in adult GIST tumors.[31,32] Second-generation kinase inhibitors (i.e., sunitinib, nilotinib, sorafenib, and dasatinib) have demonstrated in vivo and in vitro efficacy in treatment of malignancy with *KIT* mutations.[33–36] Although investigations of adjuvant and neoadjuvant tyrosine kinase inhibitors are ongoing, surgical excision remains the initial option for pediatric GISTs. Adjuvant chemotherapy with imatinib and other agents may be used in cases of incomplete resection, tumor spillage, or other high-risk factors. For recurrent or metastatic GIST, a trial of a kinase inhibitor, followed by surgical resection, may be effective. Neoadjuvant tyrosine kinase inhibitor chemotherapy may similarly reduce unresectable GIST lesions making surgical resection possible. These therapies may decrease the incidence of postoperative GIST recurrence and spread, and thereby extend survival.[34,35]

SURVIVAL

The long-term survival following surgical resection of pediatric GIST is difficult to determine, because most reports contain small numbers of children or include adults. Moreover, given recent changes in the recognition and pathologic identification of these tumors, many older series contain tumors that are actually not GISTs. Factors associated with long-term survival following surgical resection include small tumor size, low mitotic index, genotype, and gastric primary location.[20] Pediatric GISTs present with a higher incidence of metastasis than comparable adult gastric tumors. However, the biology of pediatric lesions appears more indolent than adult disease with significant long-term survival, despite the presence of metastatic disease and with or without effective adjuvant chemotherapy.[25]

Intestinal Tumors

MYOFIBROMATOSIS

Infantile myofibromatosis is a mesenchymal tumor that can arise in the skin, muscle, bone, subcutaneous tissue, or viscera. It is the most common fibrous tumor of infancy. Myofibromatosis presents with either solitary or generalized lesions, with or without visceral involvement. Most lesions spontaneously regress; however, extensive intestinal myofibromatosis is associated with significant morbidity and mortality.[37,38] Various chemotherapeutic interventions have demonstrated limited efficacy, significant treatment toxicity, and long-term morbidity. However, the combination of low-dose chemotherapy and long-term total parental nutrition for life-threatening infantile myofibromatosis can provide symptomatic relief and inhibit disease progression.[39,40]

LYMPHOMA

Lymphoma is the most common small bowel malignancy in children, with high-grade non-Hodgkin lymphoma comprising 74% of these tumors. Burkitt lymphoma constitutes the most common histologic subtype. The majority of patients (50% to 93%) present with lymphoma localized to the distal small bowel, although tumor may occur anywhere from the stomach to the rectum.[41]

Patients may present with chronic GI distress, occult blood per rectum, hematochezia, and/or an abdominal mass. An acute worsening of symptoms may result in emergency surgery for treatment of ileocolic intussusception, with lymphoma creating the lead point (46%), acute appendicitis (22%), perforation (11%), or obstruction (8%). Higher mortality is associated with advanced disease stage, intestinal perforation, high-grade histology, and T-cell lymphomas.[42]

Surgical management depends on disease presentation, as well as extent of disease at presentation. Bulky disease is usually not completely resectable. Extensive resection of bulky retroperitoneal or mesenteric disease does not enhance survival; nevertheless, complete surgical resection (including bowel resection), if possible, significantly enhances the prognosis of patients with intestinal lymphoma, especially when included in a multimodality treatment approach. Tumor downstaging by complete resection allows for decreased duration and intensity of post-operative chemotherapy. When operating for a complication of intraperitoneal disease, the extent of the procedure should be limited to resolution of the complication and resection of sufficient tissue to ensure an accurate diagnosis. If limited disease is encountered, complete resection and an evaluation of mesenteric, perihepatic, and periaortic nodes should be undertaken to assess for regional metastatic spread. Two-year cumulative survival for intestinal B-cell lymphoma is 94% and 28% for intestinal T-cell lymphoma. The overall 5- and 10-year survival rates for all intestinal lymphoma patients treated with multimodality therapy (surgery, radiation, chemotherapy) are 52% and 44%, respectively. The corresponding disease-free survival rates are 43% and 38%, respectively.[43–48]

Carcinoid Tumors

EPIDEMIOLOGY

Carcinoid tumors originate from neuroendocrine cells within the GI tract. These neoplasms derive from GI epithelial and subepithelial endocrine progenitor cells that function as part of the amine precursor uptake and decarboxylation (APUD) system.[49] Carcinoids can also be found in the lungs, mediastinum, thymus, liver, pancreas, bronchus, ovaries, prostate, testes, and kidneys.[50] Pediatric carcinoid tumors typically occur in the GI tract—stomach, small intestine, appendix (most common), and rectum. Carcinoid tumors of the appendix occur with an estimated incidence of 1 case per million children per year, with a slight female predominance.[51–53]

DIAGNOSIS

Carcinoid tumors are classified according to the location of origin in the primitive gut (foregut, midgut, and hindgut). Foregut tumors include carcinoids of the lung, bronchus, stomach, proximal duodenum, and pancreas. Midgut tumors arise from the distal duodenum, jejunum, ileum, and right colon, including the appendix. These account for 60% to 80% of all carcinoids in adults and children.[54–56] Hindgut tumors arise in the transverse and distal colon and rectum. Tumors can also arise from a Meckel diverticulum, enteric duplications, and the mesentery. Appendiceal carcinoids are the most common, with more than 70% of these tumors developing at the appendiceal tip. Pediatric carcinoid tumors are often discovered incidentally during an operation for presumed appendicitis or another unrelated diagnosis. Although clinical signs of acute appendicitis or gynecologic pathology may prompt exploration, true inflammatory changes of acute appendicitis are not often induced by the carcinoid, possibly because of the distal location of the tumor and absence of proximal luminal obstruction.[51,53,55]

The most serious complication of carcinoid tumors is a carcinoid crisis, which is most often associated with foregut tumors, larger tumors, and high serum/urine 5-hydroxyindoleacetic acid (5-HIAA) levels. Although pediatric carcinoids vary in size, carcinoid syndrome (flushing, diarrhea, abdominal pain, tachycardia, hypertension, hypotension, altered mental status, and coma) has not been typically associated with tumors confined to the appendix.[53,54] In contrast, pediatric patients with extra-appendiceal carcinoid tumors, such as in the lung or liver, are often symptomatic. Biologically active amines (serotonin, catecholamines, histamine) and metabolites (5-HIAA) are characteristically elevated in the plasma and urine of patients with symptomatic carcinoid tumors.[57] Patients with extra-appendiceal carcinoids frequently present with disseminated disease at the time of diagnosis and have a higher incidence of recurrent tumor following the initial diagnosis and resection.[58]

TREATMENT

Tumor size at presentation dictates surgical decision making for carcinoid tumors of the appendix. For appendiceal carcinoid tumors less than 2 cm in diameter, surgical resection of the appendix and mesoappendix is considered curative. Long-term follow-up demonstrates minimal disease recurrence and a rare likelihood of metastatic disease.[51,52,58,59] Carcinoid tumors greater than 2 cm, those with cecal involvement, lymphatic invasion, lymph node involvement, mesoappendix infiltration, positive resection margins, goblet cell malignancy, or cellular pleomorphism with a high mitotic index require a more extensive resection (i.e., a right hemicolectomy with associated resection of the mesocolon).[55,60,61]

SURVIVAL

Complete resection of localized appendiceal carcinoid tumors can result in cure, with greater than a 90% survival rate. Diminished disease-free and overall survival is associated with carcinoids larger than 2 cm, older age, positive lymph nodes, extra-appendiceal spread, distant metastatic disease, and tumors with atypical histologic features.[62]

Colorectal Adenocarcinoma

Adenocarcinoma of the colon and rectum is the most common cancer of the GI tract, with approximately 142,570 new cases and 51,370 deaths in the United Sates in the past year. The lifetime risk of developing colorectal cancer in the general population is 1 in 19.[6] However, colorectal cancer in children is rare, with an estimated incidence of 0.3 to 1.5 cases per million.[63,64] Although reported as early as 9 months of age, the median age at diagnosis for pediatric cases is 15 to 19 years. Pediatric colorectal cancer accounts for 2% of malignancies in adolescents.[65–67]

Colorectal cancer differs greatly between adults and children. These differences include the presenting signs and symptoms, primary site of the tumor, pathologic findings, stage, and prognosis. Carcinoma of the colon is associated with several predisposing factors, including ionizing radiation (e.g., CT scan, therapeutic radiation treatments), polyposis syndromes, urinary diversion with previous ureterosigmoidostomy, and chronic parasitic infection. Various environmental factors, including herbicide exposure, may also be associated with tumor formation.[68]

Polypoid Disease of the Gastrointestinal Tract

Polyps are common, occurring in 1% of all children, and are the most frequent source of rectal bleeding in the young child (2 to 5 years old). Most polyps are benign lesions and are either hamartomas or result from lymphoid hyperplasia. Some hamartomas, however, have the potential for dysplastic, adenomatous or neoplastic transformation because of germline mutations and somatic inactivation of STK11, SMAD4, BMPR1A, and PTEN genes.[68–71]

Isolated juvenile polyps (i.e., retention polyps, inflammatory polyps, cystic polyps) are considered hamartomas. They constitute 80% of polyps in children with 40% to 60% found in the rectosigmoid colon. If multiple (typically two to five polyps) they may be found in the proximal colon as well. They are one of the most common sources of GI bleeding in young children, but are rarely seen in adolescence. Colonoscopy of the entire colon is diagnostic and therapeutic if endoscopic removal is warranted.

Lymphoid polyps (lymphoid nodular hyperplasia) account for 15% of pediatric polyps and are submucosal lymphoid aggregates, specifically localized to distal small bowel, colon, and rectum (Peyer patches). Bleeding results from mucosal erosion and can usually be managed expectantly. Uncontrolled bleeding or irreducible intussusception requires surgical intervention.

Juvenile polyposis coli syndrome is transmitted in an autosomal dominant fashion. Affected individuals are at increased risk for colorectal malignancy with cumulative risk for cancer of nearly 50% to 70% by age 60 years.[63,64,72] A diagnosis of juvenile polyposis coli requires at least 5 polyps throughout the GI tract, or 1 polyp and a family history of juvenile polyposis. Most patients typically have 50 to 100 polyps including gastric and small bowel polyps. Higher numbers of polyps are associated with more severe symptoms, including chronic bleeding, anemia, hypoproteinemia, and failure to thrive.

These patients and their families require long-term endoscopic surveillance (semiannual panendoscopy) with subsequent total abdominal colectomy if mucosal dysplasia, persistent bleeding, or rapid increase in polyp number is detected. Depending on individual circumstance, there also appears to be a role for prophylactic total colectomy and rectal mucosectomy with an endorectal pull-through procedure.

Diffuse juvenile polyposis of infancy is a nearly universally fatal disease typically diagnosed within the first few months of life. Patients present with diarrhea, lower GI bleeding, intussusception, prolapse, obstruction, protein-wasting enteropathy, macrocephaly, and hypotonia. Despite involvement of the entire GI tract, bowel rest and total parenteral nutrition (TPN) permit selective surgical resection. However, survival beyond 2 years of age is rare.

Diffuse juvenile polyposis presents with hematochezia, abdominal pain, and prolapse from hamartomatous polyps in the colon and rectum in infancy to 5 years of age. Although hamartomas typically do not have premalignant potential, chronic polyp inflammation is thought to result in reactive hyperplasia that then progresses to dysplasia or adenomatous changes.

Several genetic disorders carry significant risk for the subsequent development of colon carcinoma and are characterized as polyposis syndromes. They include Gardner syndrome (adenomatous polyposis and soft tissue and bone tumors), Turcot syndrome (familial adenomatous polyps and central nervous system tumors), and familial polyposis coli. Both Gardner syndrome and familial polyposis are autosomal dominant disorders and are associated with adenomatous polyps in the colon and the small intestine. Because the entire surface of the colon can be carpeted with thousands of polyps, the ability to carry out effective surveillance and identify suspicious lesions is low. Recommendations for and the timing of colon resection are based on the likelihood of the development of malignancy. There is little question that colectomy is the appropriate treatment for patients with familial polyposis coli (familial adenomatous polyposis), Gardner syndrome, and Turcot syndrome.

Peutz-Jeghers syndrome is defined by polyposis of the intestinal tract and melanotic skin lesions. It is inherited as an autosomal dominant trait. Germline mutations in *LKB1, STK11,* and *ENG* genes may have a causative role in the pathogenesis of this syndrome.[73,74] Despite equal sex distribution, symptoms appear earlier in males. Brown and black melanotic spots occur in the rectum, around the mouth, lips, buccal mucosa, feet, nasal mucosa, and conjunctivae, typically presenting at puberty. Adolescents characteristically complain of frequent defecation, rectal bleeding, abdominal pain, vomiting, and may present with anemia or recurrent episodes of intussusception. Polyps are found in the small intestine (55%), stomach and duodenum (30%), and the colorectal bowel (15%). The risk of death because of cancer for those with Peutz-Jeghers syndrome is 50% by 60 years of age. There is a 13-fold increased risk of death because of GI cancer and a 9-fold increased risk for all other malignancies. Rapid growth, severe dysplasia, villous changes, or larger polyps (greater than 15 mm) may indicate GI malignancy and necessitate aggressive surgical intervention. However, repeated, extensive intestinal resections may result in short-bowel syndrome resulting from the multifocal and recurrent nature of these polyps.

Gardner syndrome patients present with adenomatous, rather than hamartoma polyposis, and extraintestinal lesions, including bone tumors (80%), sebaceous/inclusion cysts (35%), and desmoid tumors (18%). Bone lesions include cysts of the mandible, fibromas, and osteomas of the skull and face. These patients also may develop hypertrophy of the retinal pigmented epithelium. The syndrome is inherited in an autosomal dominant pattern. Various mutations of the adenomatous polyposis coli (*APC*) gene are associated with Gardner syndrome (*APC* polymorphism in exons 13 and 15), implicating this as a phenotypic variant of familial adenomatous polyposis (FAP). The intestinal polyps that characterize this syndrome have a 100% likelihood of undergoing malignant transformation.[75,76] Desmoids are fibroblastic tumors of the abdominal wall and mesentery that present as dysplasia or a malignant fibrosarcoma. They often become apparent after diagnosis of GI disease and carry a high mortality. Small desmoid tumors, if amenable to excision, have a 10% local recurrence. However, many desmoid lesions are unresectable at presentation. Slow-growing tumors can be treated with sulindac, tamoxifen, vinblastine, and methotrexate, while symptomatic, aggressive tumors require doxorubicin and dacarbazine or high-dose tamoxifen and radiation therapy.

Turcot syndrome, also considered a variant of FAP, is characterized by polyposis and brain tumors (e.g. gliomas, ependymomas). Carcinoma of the colon is prevalent in young adults. Chronic bloody diarrhea, hypoproteinemia, weight loss, anemia, malnutrition, bowel obstruction, and intussusception are common presenting symptoms. Medulloblastoma development is associated with *APC*-related mutations, while microsatellite gene instability (typical of hereditary nonpolyposis colon cancer) is associated with glioblastoma multiforme diagnosis.[77] *Cronkhite-Canada syndrome* is typified by multiple hamartomatous polyps in the stomach and colon. It is a variant of juvenile polyposis and is associated with early-onset skin hyperpigmentation, alopecia, and nail changes. Chronic diarrhea results in malabsorption, hypovitaminosis, hypoproteinemia, and fluid and electrolyte imbalance.

Osler-Weber-Rendu syndrome is characterized by childhood (less than 10 years of age) GI bleeding from cutaneous and hepatic telangiectases and vascular malformations in 50% of affected individuals. Telangiectases are found on the lips, oral and nasopharyngeal membranes, tongue, and perilingual areas. Lesions may also involve the brain, lungs, and liver. Within the GI tract, they occur commonly in the stomach and small bowel, causing significant recurrent GI bleeds throughout childhood. It is inherited in an autosomal dominant manner, and 80% of patients have a family history of the disease. With a high incidence of colon carcinoma or multiple juvenile colonic polyps, all Osler-Weber-Rendu patients with new-onset anemia or GI bleeding require lower GI tract evaluation.[78,79]

Hereditary Associations

Although the majority of childhood colorectal carcinomas are not associated with hereditary factors, approximately 25% of childhood cases have some associated predisposing condition, that is, at least two first-degree relatives with colon cancer, genetic/polyposis syndromes (1%), inflammatory bowel disease (1%), and hereditary nonpolyposis syndromes (5%

to 6%). The progression toward tumor development may occur secondary to tumor suppressor gene mutation, loss of heterozygosity, or a mutational event.[80] Phenotypically normal colonic epithelium may develop hyperplasia as a result, then progress to adenoma formation, dysplasia, and finally, invasive carcinoma. Mutations associated with development of colon cancer may result from exposure to environmental influences or be the result of accumulated DNA transcription errors. Typical of these genetic changes are *APC* inactivation, *K-ras* activation, and *TP53* gene mutations.

Familial adenomatous polyposis (FAP) is inherited as an autosomal dominant trait that accounts for less than 1% of all colorectal cancer. A diagnosis of FAP requires greater than 5 colonic polyps, polyps throughout the GI tract, or polyps associated with a family history of juvenile polyposis. Extensive colonic polyposis (i.e., greater than 100 adenomatous polyps) is common, with some patients having thousands of polyps. Symptomatic patients often present with frequent bloody stools, anemia, and abdominal pain. Long-standing symptoms may signify the presence of a malignant lesion. Patients identified through family history should be assessed in early adolescence prior to the development of symptoms. All patients require early colonoscopic screening to determine the extent of polyposis and the possibility of malignancy. Colorectal carcinoma occurs by age 20 years in 7% of patients and by age 25 years in 15% of patients. Untreated FAP characteristically progresses to colorectal cancer by age 39 years. In contrast, gastric polyps seen with FAP are usually benign hamartomas. FAP patients are also at risk to develop desmoid tumors, congenital hypertrophy of retinal pigment epithelium, duodenal and periampullary adenocarcinomas, thyroid malignancy, and hepatoblastoma.[81,82]

The *APC* gene, a tumor suppressor gene on the long arm of chromosome 5, is known to contain a mutation in 80% to 90% of FAP patients. If a defective *APC* allele is inherited from one parent, a mutation acquired during childhood in the other *APC* gene results in the loss of function of the tumor suppressor gene product.[83] Inactivation of the *APC* alleles results in activation of subsequent signaling pathways leading to uncontrolled cell growth. Malignant progression from adenoma to dysplasia, then to malignancy, may occur. Site-specific *APC* gene mutations correlate with various FAP phenotypes and the development of associated tumors. Classic FAP is associated with central gene mutations, while a less aggressive, attenuated FAP presentation correlates with peripheral *APC* gene mutations. The development of malignancy is also associated with accumulation of other oncogene/tumor suppressor gene mutations, such as *K-ras* activation and *TP53* mutation, in otherwise quiescent adenomas.

Sulindac, a nonsteroidal anti-inflammatory drug (NSAID), and celecoxib, a cyclooxygenase-2 (COX-2) inhibitor, have been used to reduce polyp numbers by induction of epithelial cell apoptosis. Despite the unique mechanism of action of these agents, they have not completely eliminated the risk of colorectal cancer in FAP patients.[84,85] FAP patients with few polyps are still at risk of early colorectal cancer. Resection is indicated even if extensive polyposis does not develop. Surgical options include total proctocolectomy with permanent ileostomy, total abdominal colectomy with ileorectal anastomosis, coloproctectomy with perseveration of the anal sphincter, coloproctectomy with ileoanal pull-through, and total colectomy with rectal mucosectomy and endorectal (J-pouch) pull-through. Each of these procedures has their proponents. Total colectomy with a rectal mucosectomy and endorectal pull-through has gained popularity in recent years. This procedure removes all "at-risk" colonic mucosa and laparoscopic techniques have been demonstrated to be practical, effective, and safe. Endorectal pull-through procedures typically incorporate a distal J-pouch ileal reservoir. Although straight ileal pull-through procedures initially have higher stool frequency, differences in stool frequency between straight pull-through and J-pouch patients have been reported by some authors to be negligible by 24 months. A number of patients treated with a J-pouch may require later treatment for intermittent pouchitis.[86,87] Total proctocolectomy with permanent ileostomy carries significant risk of postoperative urinary bladder atony, impotence, and retrograde ejaculation because of disruption of nervi erigentes during the pelvic dissection. More commonly used for adult colorectal pathology, this technique has limited utility for treatment of pediatric patients because of the psychological and physiologic impact of a permanent stoma.[88] Procedures involving the preservation of the distal rectum can result in the development of colorectal cancer. Forty-four percent of patients undergoing an ileorectal anastomosis require subsequent treatment for rectal polyps that develop in the remaining mucosa. The risk of rectal cancer in these patients is 10% at age 50 years and 29% by age 60 years. Polyps remaining or developing in preserved colorectal segment significantly increases the risk for subsequent cancer. Those with retained rectal mucosa at risk require annual flexible endoscopic surveillance of the pelvic pouch.[89–91] The significant long-term risk of rectal cancer in these patients makes this procedure unacceptable for treatment of FAP in the adolescent population.

Hereditary nonpolyposis colon cancer (HNPCC) has an autosomal dominant inheritance, is the most common hereditary colon cancer syndrome, and accounts for 2% to 3% of all colorectal cancers. It is characterized by early onset, multiple family members affected, and is 5 times more prevalent than familial polyposis–related colon cancer.[92] In contrast to familial adenomatous polyposis, HNPCC malignancy may develop in the absence of adenomatosis of the colon and rectum. Unlike sporadic colorectal tumors, HNPCC colorectal cancer usually develops in a proximal colon lesion and occurs at a younger age (approximately 45 years).

Disease may be limited to the colon in the Lynch syndrome I, where malignancies occur in the cecum and ascending colon more often than in other colorectal sites (70%). These tumors are characterized by poorly differentiated and mucin-producing lesions (i.e., signet cell). Lynch syndrome II is further defined by the development of synchronous and metachronous extracolonic cancers, such as carcinomas of the endometrium, uterus, ovary, stomach, small bowel, pancreas, hepatobiliary tract, brain, genitourinary system, and upper uroepithelial tract. They usually manifest in the second decade of life. HNPCC patients are categorized by the Amsterdam criteria: colorectal cancer in at least three relatives spanning two generations. One of these individuals is a first-degree relative of the other two and one of these individuals must have a diagnosis prior to age 50 years. Patients with the Lynch syndromes have a 50% to 70% lifetime risk of developing cancer and a threefold increased incidence of colorectal cancer compared with the general population.[93–96]

Hereditary nonpolyposis colon cancers, unlike FAP, do not have inherited defects in the *APC* gene. HNPCC tumors are characterized by mutations in genetic loci (*MSH2, MLH1, PMS1, PMS2,* and *GTBP*) resulting in defective DNA nucleotide mismatch recognition and repair. Greater than 90% of these mutations are in *MSH2* and *MLH1* genes on chromosome arms 2p and 3p, respectively. These genes are inherited in a dominant manner with 90% penetrance. Although benign adenomas appear with the same incidence in HNPCC patients as in the general population, DNA-repair–deficient HNPCC adenomas are more likely to grow and progress to invasive cancer than in the general population. As a result, a benign tumor may progress to cancer in as few as 3 to 5 years.[97]

Patients suspected of carrying *MSH2* and *MLH1* mutations may be tested for DNA mismatch-repair gene mutations. A total abdominal colectomy, rather than hemicolectomy or a segmental resection, is recommended, because the risk of recurrent colorectal cancer is 45% spanning 10 years. Patients who have undergone subtotal colectomy must undergo lifelong endoscopic evaluation of their remaining rectal segment. Subtotal colectomy with a rectal mucosectomy and endorectal pull-through has not been studied in this population. Patients who are poorly compliant with colonoscopic surveillance may be candidates for prophylactic colectomy. Asymptomatic HNPCC gene carriers may reduce their risk of invasive cancer through prophylactic colectomy or surveillance colonoscopy and polypectomy, starting with biannual colonoscopy at age 25 to 30 years and annually after age 40 years. All Lynch syndrome patients must undergo lifelong screening for extracolonic malignancies as well.[98,99]

Other Associations

There is a strong association between long-term inflammatory bowel disease and the development of colon carcinoma. After the first 10 years with ulcerative colitis, the likelihood of cancer development increases from 1% to 2% per year.[100] Those with ulcerative colitis–associated carcinoma typically present with malignancy at a young age, have multifocal lesions, and have had a history of colitis involving the entire colon rather than isolated, left-sided disease. Crohn disease is an inflammatory bowel disease in which the risk for colon cancer is significantly greater (more than 20 times) than that in the general population.[101] Crohn-associated colon cancer may develop in an area of colon that appears grossly normal, making the diagnosis of malignancy more difficult than with ulcerative colitis. Routine surveillance contrast enema and colonoscopy are recommended for all patients with either ulcerative colitis or Crohn disease. Biopsies should be performed on suspicious areas as well as on random areas of the colon during the colonoscopy.[102]

Ureterosigmoidostomy performed for urinary diversion predisposes to the subsequent development of malignancy in the colonic segment used as a diversion conduit. Five percent of patients with ureterosigmoidostomy develop colon cancer, often at the site of ureteral implant. Chronic inflammation, possibly resulting from exposure to intermittently infected urine, has been shown to predispose to the development of colon cancer. Close follow-up and annual sigmoidoscopy is warranted for all patients following this type of urinary diversion, which is now infrequently used.

In the United States, approximately 600,000 abdominal and head CT studies are performed annually on children under 15 years of age. The risk of later malignancy related to diagnostic pediatric CT scan is directly proportional to the age of the child at the time of the study. It is estimated 500 of these individuals may ultimately die from a malignancy attributable to the CT irradiation received as a child. Secondary colorectal malignancies may also result from therapeutic radiation, especially if the abdomen was included in the field of primary irradiation. Radiation colitis and adenomatous polyps can develop years after radiation exposure and colonic adenocarcinoma decades later. Immunohistochemical studies suggest a radiation-induced *TP53* mutation may lead to the eventual development of colorectal cancer in these individuals.[67,103–105]

Diagnosis

In children with colorectal tumors, presenting symptoms are nonspecific and include abdominal pain, nausea, and vomiting, and changes in bowel habits with the development of constipation, particularly with left-sided lesions. Physical findings include abdominal distention, tenderness, and a palpable mass. Many will have guaiac-positive stools. Lower GI (rectal) bleeding may be present in a third of patients and, as with adults, is more prevalent in those with cancer of the left colon and rectum. Significant weight loss affects 20% to 30% of patients.

The median length of time from onset of symptoms to presentation is often months; at least one report cited almost a year between the onset of symptoms and the diagnosis.[106] Diagnosis can be delayed if symptoms are repeatedly attributed to common pediatric conditions such as chronic gastroenteritis.[107] Delay in diagnosis may also be related to adolescents' tendency to minimize or hide embarrassing symptoms and the low index of suspicion of pediatricians for this rare entity. Rectal bleeding, commonly a sign of benign pathology, such as polyps or hemorrhoids, should also raise the suspicion of a colorectal malignancy. Delay in diagnosis contributes to the advanced stage of disease in many children. Most colonic lesions in adults are rectosigmoid in location and are identified by sigmoidoscopy. In contrast, childhood colorectal cancer is relatively evenly distributed throughout the colon, with one third of the tumors located in the right colon.[63,107] Colonoscopy, therefore, is required to obtain a biopsy for diagnosis.

Sporadic Colorectal Carcinoma

Sporadic colon cancer in the young is an aggressive disease whose morphology and natural history differ from those of familial adenomatous polyposis, hereditary nonpolyposis colorectal cancer, and adult colon cancer. The location, stage, and histologic type of pediatric colorectal tumors differ markedly than the same disease in adults. Primary colorectal tumors in children occur frequently in the right and transverse colon, as opposed to the predominant rectosigmoid distribution found in adults. Approximately 40% of adults with colon cancer have involvement of regional lymph nodes or have distant metastases (Dukes stage C or D lesions) at diagnosis. In children, more than 80% of tumors are Dukes stage C or

D at diagnosis.[63,64,106,107] In addition, more than half of the colorectal tumors in children are mucinous adenocarcinomas. The mucinous subtype has an aggressive course and is known to metastasize early. Both advanced stage of disease at presentation and the preponderance of mucinous subtype contributes to a poorer prognosis in children.[66] Accumulation of DNA base-pair mistakes resulting from defective mismatch repair processes (microsatellite instability) is an early step in the process leading to malignant transformation. Patients with colorectal cancer and high microsatellite instability are more likely to have multiple synchronous or metachronous colorectal cancers and are diagnosed at a younger age than those without microsatellite instability.[71,108] Microsatellite instability is not, however, associated with a family history of colorectal cancer or of phenotypic features.[81]

The utility of carcinoembryonic antigen (CEA) has been well established in adults with colon cancer; however, there is little evidence of similar utility in pediatric patients. CEA levels correlate with a change in tumor burden in only 60% of children with colorectal tumors. A number of children with Dukes stage C or D lesions have been shown to have normal antigen levels at the time of diagnosis.[107] In addition, CEA levels do not correlate well with long-term response to treatment in children and therefore should not be used as a definitive marker of recurrence.[64]

Treatment

The primary treatment for colon cancer in children is surgical resection consisting of a wide excision of the involved colon, the mesentery, and the lymphatic drainage area. Unfortunately, resection for cure is possible in only 40% to 70% of pediatric patients because of advanced stage at diagnosis; these percentages are much lower than for adults. The ovaries and the omentum are common sites of metastasis. If resection for cure is performed, omentectomy, and in female patients, oophorectomy, is appropriate in patients identified with associated ovarian disease.[109]

No rigorously tested or widely accepted therapeutic protocols are available specifically for children with colorectal carcinoma. The use of adjuvant chemotherapy consisting of irinotecan, oxaliplatin, and leucovorin has been described in conjunction with 5-fluorouracil. The use of adjuvant chemotherapy, combined with second-look surgery in select cases, may improve survival.[3,68,107,110] As in adult rectal cancer, preoperative radiation therapy may convert unresectable rectal carcinoma to resectable tumors in selected patients. Although anecdotal case reports indicate these therapies can be beneficial, no data documents the utility of either chemotherapy or radiation therapy for cure or palliation; hence, prognosis and survival are most directly related to successful complete resection. The overall rate and duration of disease-free survival among children with colon carcinoma are low, with less than 30% of patients surviving 5 years. In patients who have resection for cure, predictors of survival include node involvement and histologic grade.

Summary

The biology of pediatric colorectal carcinoma is different from colorectal malignancy in adults. The presentation, histologic type, stage, and prognosis differ sharply. Most cases of childhood colorectal cancer arise from previous adenomas. Children with syndrome-associated adenomas are at increased risk for colorectal carcinoma. This suggests that genetics play a greater role than previously thought, and fewer cases are truly sporadic. Understanding the molecular basis of colon carcinoma in children should facilitate the identification of patients at high risk and result in prophylactic intervention or earlier diagnosis and reduce mortality.

The complete reference list is available online at www.expertconsult.com.

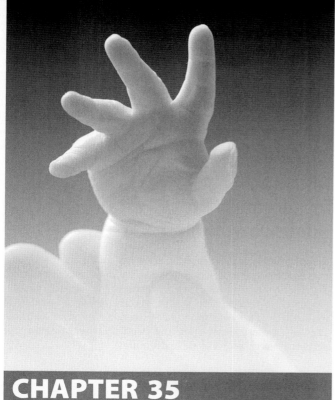

CHAPTER 35

Diagnosis and Treatment of Rhabdomyosarcoma

Kevin P. Mollen and David A. Rodeberg

Historically, the mainstay of therapy for rhabdomyosarcoma (RMS) has been aggressive surgical resection, often including a significant amount of normal tissue along with the tumor.[1] As a result, operations were often disfiguring and outcomes disappointing, with survival rates from 7% to 70% depending on tumor location. It was not until chemotherapy was added to the RMS treatment algorithm in 1961 that outcomes began to improve. The addition of radiotherapy in 1965 to select patients further improved outcomes and decreased the need for aggressive radical operations. Recognition of the crucial contribution of multimodal therapy to the treatment of RMS led to the establishment of the Intergroup Rhabdomyosarcoma Study Group (IRSG) in 1972. The goal of the IRSG was to oversee the development of treatment protocols for RMS. Now called the Soft Tissue Sarcoma Committee of the Children's Oncology Group, this collaborative group has completed a number of cooperative group trials evaluating new drug combinations, chemotherapy dosing, imaging evaluation of tumors, radiotherapy, and surgical strategies for local tumor control and tumor biology.[2] During this time period, the overall 5-year survival rate of RMS has increased from 25% to 70% (Fig. 35-1).[3,4]

Rhabdomyosarcoma Patient Demographics

Rhabdomyosarcoma is the most common type of soft tissue sarcoma diagnosed during the first 2 decades of life, accounting for 4.5% of all cases of childhood cancer.[5] It is the third most common extracranial solid tumor of childhood after Wilms' tumor and neuroblastoma. Age at presentation follows a bimodal distribution, with peak incidences between 2 and 6 years and again between 10 and 18 years of age.[6] This distribution reflects the incidences of the two major histologic subtypes of RMS. The incidence of embryonal RMS is highest at birth and extends through childhood before declining, while alveolar RMS peaks during childhood and adolescence.[7] Approximately 65% of all RMS cases occur in children younger than 6 years of age. Slightly more males (58.4%) are affected than females (41.6%), and whites have a higher incidence than African Americans (rate ratio 1.2).

Rhabdomyosarcoma Tumor Biology

Rhabdomyosarcoma is a malignant tumor of mesenchymal origin.[5] RMS also falls under the greater category of small, blue, round-cell tumors of childhood that includes neuroblastoma, lymphoma, and primitive neuroectodermal tumors (PNET). The two major histologic subtypes of RMS are embryonal and alveolar. Embryonal RMS (ERMS) is the most common type of RMS, affecting two thirds of all patients with disease. ERMS can be further broken down into spindle-cell and botryoid subtypes. ERMS is typically composed of spindle-shaped cells with a rich stroma. In addition to occurring in younger patients, ERMS has a favorable survival rate of 60%. Tumors occur more frequently in the head and neck region as compared with the extremities. Spindle-cell histology is common in paratesticular lesions, whereas botryoid lesions are generally polypoid masses filling the lumen of hollow viscus, such as the vagina, bladder, and extrahepatic bile ducts. Alveolar RMS (ARMS) occurs in older children, and tumors are most commonly located on the trunk or extremities. These lesions are composed of small, round, densely packed cells arranged around spaces resembling pulmonary alveoli. However, this histologic classification of RMS may, in the near future, be supplanted by gene array analysis.[8] Prognosis is worse in ARMS than ERMS, with a 5-year survival rate of 54%. For all histologic types of RMS, outcome is heavily dependent on age at diagnosis, the primary anatomic site, extent of disease (tumor size, invasion, nodal status, metastatic disease), and the completeness of surgical excision. The Soft Tissue Sarcoma Committee is investigating the outcomes of patients by disease characteristics and tumor biology to refine risk-adapted therapy for the treatment of RMS.[2]

The exact nature of the pathogenesis of RMS is unclear; however, many hypotheses exist. It is largely thought that RMS arises as a consequence of regulatory disruption of skeletal muscle progenitor cell growth and differentiation.[9] Pathogenic roles have been suggested for the *MET* proto-oncogene, which is involved in migration of myogenic

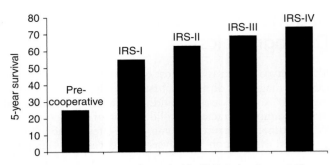

FIGURE 35-1 Improvement in survival for RMS during the past 40 years.

precursor cells, and the *TP53* proto-oncogene, which is responsible for tumor suppression.[10,11] At the chromosomal level, ERMS is characterized by a loss of heterozygosity at the 11p15 locus, with a loss of maternal information and duplication of paternal genetic information. Within this locus lies the insulin growth factor II (IGF-II) gene.[12–14] Both ERMS and ARMS overproduce IGF-II, which has been shown to stimulate RMS tumor growth, suggesting that IGF-II plays a role in unregulated growth of these tumors.[15] Although the significance is unclear, ARMS is frequently tetraploid, whereas ERMS lesions are generally diploid. Translocations of the *FKHR* transcription factor gene from chromosome 13 with either the *PAX3* (chromosome 2) or *PAX7* (chromosome 1) transcription factor genes occur frequently in ARMS.[16–18] In these *PAX/FKHR* fusions, the DNA binding domain of *PAX* is combined with the regulatory domain of *FKHR*. This results in increased PAX activity leading to the de-differentiation and proliferation of myogenic cells. Understanding the role of these fusion proteins in tumor development may provide insight into treatment strategies and potential biomarkers for the diagnosis of RMS.[8] For example, it has been demonstrated that approximately 25% of ARMS tumors are translocation negative. By gene array analysis, these fusion negative ARMS tumors more closely resemble ERMS overall and have a similar prognosis to ERMS. It has therefore been proposed that tumors should be divided into *PAX/FKHR* fusion–positive and –negative tumors rather than the more ambiguous alveolar and embryonal histologies.

Although most cases of RMS occur sporadically, the disease is associated with familial syndromes, including Li-Fraumeni and neurofibromatosis I. Li-Fraumeni is an autosomal dominant disorder and is usually associated with a germline mutation of *TP53*. Patients with this syndrome present with RMS at an early age and have a family history of other carcinomas, especially premenopausal breast carcinoma.[19–22] Neurofibromatosis is an autosomal dominant genetic disorder characterized by optic gliomas, café-au-lait spots, and neurofibromas.[23] The association of RMS with Li-Fraumeni and neurofibromatosis appears to involve malignant transformation through the inactivation of the *TP53* tumor suppressor gene and hyperactivation of the *RAS* oncogene.[24,25] Nevoid basal cell carcinoma (Gorlin syndrome) is an autosomal dominant disorder caused by mutations in the *PTCH* tumor suppressor gene mapping to chromosome 9q22.3.[26] Animals with mutations in the *PTCH* gene have elevated levels of the tumor growth–promoting IGF-II and develop spontaneous RMS.[27,28] The association of mutations in the *PTCH* gene in human disease with spontaneous development of RMS is supported by the finding that up to 30% of sporadic cases of ERMS demonstrate molecular abnormalities at the 9q22.3

locus.[29,30] Autopsy findings suggest that one third of children with RMS also have congenital anomalies, suggesting that prenatal events may also contribute to tumor development.[31] Although no specific carcinogens have been identified, benzenediazonium sulfate has been shown to induce RMS in mice.[32] Maternal marijuana or cocaine use in pregnancy may be an environmental factor that contributes to the development of RMS.[33,34]

Presentation of Rhabdomyosarcoma

Rhabdomyosarcoma typically presents as an asymptomatic mass found by the patient or the parents of younger children.[5] Specific symptoms vary based on the site of occurrence and extent of disease. These symptoms are generally related to mass effect or complications of the tumor. The most common sites of primary disease are the head and neck region, the genitourinary tract, and the extremities.

Preoperative Workup

Patients with suspected RMS require a complete workup prior to surgical intervention.[5] Standard laboratory work, including complete blood counts (CBC), electrolytes, and renal function tests, liver function tests (LFTs), and urinalysis (UA) should be performed. In addition, imaging studies of the primary tumor should be performed with computer tomography (CT) or magnetic resonance imaging (MRI). CT is advantageous for the evaluation of bone erosion and abdominal adenopathy, whereas MRI provides better definition of the tumor and surrounding structures. MRI is preferable for limb, pelvic, and paraspinal lesions. Metastatic workup includes a bone marrow aspirate and bone scan, CT of the brain, lungs, and liver, and lumbar puncture for cerebrospinal fluid collection. Tumor imaging defines the proximity of tumors to vital structures and determines size. Both factors are important when determining if the tumor can be primarily resected or if neoadjuvant therapy is required to decrease tumor size and thereby decrease the morbidity of resection. It has been demonstrated that the size of the primary mass, as determined by pretreatment imaging, carries prognostic significance. Recent evidence would suggest that tumor volume and patient weight may be superior predictors of failure-free survival than tumor diameter and patient age in patients with intermediate-risk RMS.[35,36] Evaluation of regional and distant lymph nodes by clinical and radiographic means should be performed, because this is an important component of pretreatment staging.

Metabolic imaging using ^{18}F-fluorodeoxyglucose positron emission tomography (FDG PET) has become widely used in the adult population to determine the extent of disease in the setting of many cancers; however, there is limited experience in the pediatric population. Recent studies have suggested that FDG PET would be both a sensitive and specific tool in the clinical determination of the extent of disease in childhood sarcomas.[37–40] Further, when combined with CT, it may be more accurate than conventional imaging modalities in staging patients or re-staging patients at the time of recurrence.[41,42]

It is unclear what role FDG PET will have in the clinical evaluation of RMS, although there are several settings in which this imaging modality may improve our pretreatment staging and thus alter treatment for patients. FDG PET may enhance the evaluation of regional adenopathy versus traditional modalities. Similarly, FDG PET may offer improved detection of occult metastases, helping to differentiate them from normal structures. Finally, this modality may offer a guide to the diagnosis and treatment of recurrent disease. The diagnosis of a recurrence in a previously operated field is often difficult to obtain with conventional imaging methods. FDG PET/CT may offer an enhanced diagnostic tool and, more important, may offer tumor viability information which will guide further surgical therapy. One of the goals of ongoing trials will be to investigate the role of FDG PET in RMS.

Pretreatment Clinical Staging

Staging of RMS is determined by the site of the primary tumor, primary tumor size, degree of tumor invasion, nodal status, and the presence or absence of metastases, and it is based solely on the preoperative workup of imaging and physical examination. This is expressed in a tumor-node-metastasis (TNM) classification system modified for the site of tumor origin (Fig. 35-2). Adequate pretreatment clinical staging requires a thorough physical examination and preoperative imaging. Several investigators have validated the modified TNM staging system as a reliable predictor of patient outcome.[43]

Surgical Principles

BIOPSY

Open biopsy of a mass suspected to be RMS should be performed to confirm the diagnosis. Care should be taken to obtain adequate specimens for pathologic, biological, and treatment protocol studies. For small lesions in areas that will be treated with chemotherapy and radiation or for metastatic disease, core needle biopsy may be appropriate for diagnosis.[44,45] Although less invasive than open biopsy, core needle biopsy obtains a smaller tissue sample, which increases sampling error and the number of inconclusive findings. This smaller volume of tissue may prevent the performance of adequate molecular biology studies. Image guidance with ultrasonography may increase the accuracy of sampling while helping to avoid inadvertent puncture of surrounding structures.[46] Clinical and radiographic positive lymph nodes should be confirmed pathologically. Open biopsy is recommended; however, fine-needle aspiration or core needle biopsy of lymph nodes may be performed at the discretion of the surgeon's judgment and pathologist's recommendations.[44,47] Sentinel

Stage	Sites	T	Size	N
1	Orbit Head and neck (excluding parameningeal) GU nonbladder/nonprostate	T_1 or T_2	a or b	N_0 or N_1 or N_x
2	Bladder/prostate, extremity, cranial parameningeal, other (includes trunk, retroperitoneum, etc.)	T_1 or T_2	a	N_0 or N_x
3	Bladder/prostate, extremity, cranial parameningeal, other (includes trunk, retroperitoneum, etc.)	T_1 or T_2	a b	N_1 N_0 or N_1 or N_x
4	All	T_1 or T_2	a or b	N_0 or N_1

Definitions:

Tumor T(site)$_1$– Confirmed to anatomic site of origin
(a) <5 cm in diameter (b) >5 cm in diameter

T(site)$_2$ Extension and/or fixative to surrounding tissue
(a) <5 cm in diameter (b) >5 cm in diameter

Regional nodes–
N_0 Regional nodes not clinically involved
N_1 Regional nodes clinically involved by neoplasm
N_x Clinical status of regional nodes unknown (especially sites that preclude lymph node evaluation)

Metastasis–
M_0 No distant metastasis
M_1 Metastasis present

FIGURE 35-2 TNM Pretreatment Staging Classification. Staging before treatment requires thorough clinical, laboratory, and imaging examinations. Biopsy is required to establish histologic diagnosis. Pretreatment tumor size is determined by external measurement or MRI or CT, depending on anatomic location. For less accessible primary sites, CT also will be used for lymph node assessment. Metastatic sites will require some form of imaging confirmation (but not histologic confirmation, except for bone marrow examination). CT, computed tomography; GU, genitourinary; MRI, magnetic resonance imaging.

node biopsy may offer a safe and less invasive means of lymph node evaluation for extremity and truncal lesions, although its role in RMS is yet to be determined but will soon become the focus of a clinical trial.[48–51]

RESECTION OF THE MASS

Surgical biopsy of a primary lesion is often performed prior to a definitive surgical resection. If this is the case, pretreatment reexcision (PRE) is advisable. PRE is a wide reexcision of the previous operative site with adequate margins of normal tissue prior to the initiation of adjuvant therapy. PRE is most commonly performed on extremity and trunk lesions but should be considered the treatment of choice whenever technically feasible.[52]

The primary goal of surgical intervention is wide and complete resection of the primary tumor with a surrounding rim of normal tissue. A circumferential margin of 0.5 cm is considered adequate; however, there is minimal data to support this recommendation. Such a margin may be unobtainable, however, especially with head and neck tumors. Because of these limitations, adequate margins of uninvolved tissue are required unless excision would compromise adjacent organs, result in loss of function or poor cosmesis, or is not technically feasible. All margins should be marked and oriented at the operative field to enable precise evaluation of margins. If a narrow margin occurs, several separate biopsies of "normal" tissue around the resection margin should be obtained. These specimens should be marked and submitted separately for pathologic review. Communication between the pathologist and surgeon is mandatory to ensure that all margins are accurately examined. The surgeon should not bisect or cut the excised tumor into specimens prior to sending it to the pathologist. Any microscopic or gross tumor should be marked with small titanium clips in the tumor bed to aid radiotherapy simulation and subsequent reexcision. Published outcomes analyses have shown that a clear margin and no residual disease (group I) is superior to residual microscopic margins (group II) or gross residual disease (group III).[2,3,52–54] Tumors that are removed piecemeal are considered group II even if all gross tumor is removed.

LYMPH NODE SAMPLING/DISSECTION

Lymph node status is an important part of pretreatment staging and therefore directly impacts risk-based treatment strategies in RMS. Regional lymph node disease (N-1) has been identified in ARMS as an independent poor prognostic factor in stage 3 patients.[2] Data from IRS-IV would suggest that N-1 disease in patients with ARMS is associated with tumor characteristics that carry a poor prognosis, such as older age, more invasive tumors (T_2), large tumor size (>5 cm), and unfavorable primary sites.[55] In addition, N-1 disease was present in 23% of all RMS patients, predominantly in primary tumor sites, such as perineum, retroperitoneum, extremity, bladder/prostate, parameningeal, and paratesticular. N-1 disease alters both failure-free survival (FFS) and overall survival (OS) for ARMS but not ERMS.[55] For patients with N-1, ARMS outcomes were more similar to patients with single-site metastatic disease than those with only local disease. However, for ERMS other prognostic factors, such as patient age, tumor invasion (T stage), site of primary tumor, and the presence of metastasis at initial presentation, were more

important prognostic factors than N-1 disease. In addition, it has previously been shown that in patients with otherwise localized disease, such as an extremity, N-1 disease may be associated with an inferior outcome.[56,57] Clinical and radiographic positive nodes should therefore be biopsied to confirm tumor involvement, thus ensuring correct assessment of disease risk and assignment of optimal therapy. Lymph node removal has no therapeutic benefit, therefore prophylactic lymph node resection plays no role in therapy.[57] Therefore clinical and/or radiographic negative nodes do not require pathologic evaluation except in extremity tumors and for children older than 10 years of age with paratesticular tumors.[58,59] In both of these sites, the high incidence of nodal disease and false-negative imaging necessitates pathologic evaluation of regional nodal basins.

The use of sentinel node mapping to determine regional node status has proven to be beneficial in adult breast cancer and melanoma. For childhood RMS, sentinel node mapping is not yet the standard of care but may prove to be effective.[48] Sentinel node mapping has proven its utility in determining nodal status in pediatric skin and soft tissue malignancies and will likely become the standard of care for identifying the regional nodes involved with tumor.[60]

If regional nodes are positive then distant nodes should be harvested for pathologic evaluation. Tumor identified in these nodes would be considered metastatic disease and would therefore alter therapy using the current risk-based protocols. For upper extremity lesions, the distant nodes would be the ipsilateral supraclavicular (scalene) nodes. In the lower extremity, the distant nodes would include the iliac and/or paraaortic nodes. For paratesticular RMS, the ipsilateral paraaortic lymph nodes above the renal vein are considered distant nodes.[60]

CLINICAL GROUP

The extent of residual disease after resection is one of the most important prognostic factors in RMS. For this reason, a clinical grouping system was developed in 1972 to stratify patients into groups that would more accurately reflect their prognosis and treatment options. Currently, patients are assigned to a clinical group based on the completeness of tumor excision and the evidence of tumor metastasis to the lymph nodes or distant organs after pathologic examination of surgical specimens (Fig. 35-3). This system differs from TNM staging in that determination of each patient's clinical group is based on the extent of the surgical resection instead of tumor size and site.

Group	Criteria
I	Localized disease, completely resected A. Confined to organ or muscle of origin B. Infiltrating outside organ or muscle of origin: regional nodes not involved
II	Compromised or regional resection including: A. Grossly resected tumors with microscopic residual tumor B. Regional disease, completely resected, with nodes involved and/or tumor extension into an adjacent organ C. Regional disease, with involved nodes, grossly resected, but with evidence of microscopic residual tumor
III	Incomplete resection or biopsy with gross residual disease remaining
IV	Distant metastases present at outset

FIGURE 35-3 Clinical grouping for RMS patients.

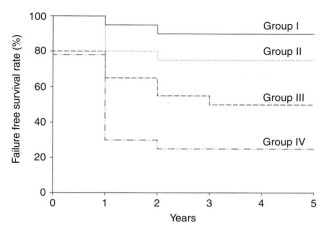

FIGURE 35-4   Rhabdomyosarcoma survival based on completeness of surgical resection (clinical group).

Data from IRS-III and IRS-IV demonstrate that five-year failure-free survival rates vary according to clinical grouping and by histologic type (Fig. 35-4).[2] One criticism of clinical grouping is that variation of surgical techniques make comparisons of clinical grouping between different institutions problematic.[61] Nonetheless, this system offers a tremendous companion to preoperative staging in determining patient risk assessment and prognosis (Fig. 35-5).

SECOND-LOOK OPERATIONS AND AGGRESSIVE RESECTION FOR RECURRENCE

After completing adjuvant therapy, patients with RMS are reimaged with CT or MRI. If residual tumor remains, or if the outcome of therapy remains in doubt, a second-look operation (SLO) may be considered. SLO can be performed to confirm clinical response, to evaluate pathologic response, and to remove residual tumor in order to improve local control.[62] As with the initial operation, the goal of SLO is complete resection of disease. Data from IRS-III suggested that SLO results in the reclassification of 75% of partial responders to complete responders after excision of residual tumors. These operations were most effective in extremity and truncal lesions.

In general, an aggressive surgical approach is used for recurrent RMS. Data would suggest that resection of recurrent RMS confers a 5-year survival of 37% compared with 8% survival in a group of patients without aggressive resection.[63] Given these results, SLO and aggressive resection for recurrence can be important tools for the treatment of RMS.

However, resection of residual masses after completion of adjuvant therapy may not be warranted. Associated morbidity of resection and the inability to achieve complete resection in some cases need to be considered. Further, it is not uncommon to find an absence of viable tumor tissue in resected samples.[63a] This brings into question the utility of aggressive re-resection and suggests that better means of detecting viable tumor is crucial. As discussed, PET/CT may provide the crucial information required to make these decisions.

Chemotherapy

It was not until the 1960s that chemotherapy was recognized as an important adjunct to surgery in the treatment of RMS. Today, all patients with RMS receive some form of chemotherapy. Standard therapeutic regimens consist of a combination of vincristine, actinomycin-D, and cyclophosphamide (VAC). Although tremendous advances have been made in improving the outcomes of patients with isolated local and regional disease, little progress has been made in improving outcomes for advanced RMS tumors. The limiting factor has been an inability to improve significantly upon standard chemotherapeutic regimens. Dose intensification of vincristine and actinomycin-D is not possible because of their neurotoxic and hepatotoxic side effects. Studies evaluating dose intensification of cyclophosphamide found that although patients tolerate higher doses, outcomes of intermediate-risk tumors are not changed.[64] These findings have lead to the evaluation of new drug combinations and the development of risk-based treatment protocols.[65]

The combination of ifosfamide and etoposide was tested in a Phase II therapy window in IRS-IV. When combined with VAC, ifosfamide, and etoposide therapy resulted in a better 3-year survival rate, with less bone marrow toxicity when compared with the use of vincristine and melphalan with standard VAC regimens.[66] Other chemotherapeutic regimens being developed to treat advanced rhabdomyosarcoma have

Risk group	Pretreatment stage*	Clinical group#	Site#	Histology
Low 1	1 or 2	I or II	Favorable or unfavorable	EMB
	1	III	Orbit only	EMB
Low 2	1	III	Favorable	EMB
	3	I or II	Unfavorable	EMB
Intermediate	2 or 3	III	Unfavorable	EMB
	1–3	I–III	Favorable or unfavorable	ALV
High	4	IV	Favorable or unfavorable	EMB
	4	IV	Favorable or unfavorable	ALV

* Pretreatment stage dependent on site of disease
\# Favorable sites: Orbit, genitourinary tract, biliary tract nonparameningeal head and neck

FIGURE 35-5   Risk-based stratification of patients to guide degree of therapy and prognosis for RMS patients. ALV, alveolar; EMB, embryonal.

incorporated doxorubicin and the topoisomerase inhibitor irinotecan. Although used as a single agent, irinotecan is of little value, it may be a useful adjunct to current VAC regimens for the treatment of advanced RMS.[67-69] Another topoisomerase inhibitor, topotecan has shown some promise in patients with stage 4 disease when combined with cyclophosphamide.[70-72] However, alternating these drugs with standard VAC therapy has not shown any benefit in intermediate-risk patients.[73] Multiple drugs are currently being evaluated for the treatment of RMS in Phase I and II trials.

Radiation Therapy

Radiotherapy is an important adjunct to therapy for many children diagnosed with RMS, offering improved local control and outcomes. Candidates for radiotherapy primarily include those with group II (microscopic residual disease) or group III (gross residual disease) disease. The impact of therapy is influenced by the location of the primary tumor and amount of local disease (tumor stage and clinical grouping) at the time radiotherapy is initiated.[74,75] Among patients with group II disease, low-dose radiation (40 Gy at 1.5 to 1.8 Gy/fraction) is associated with local tumor control rates of at least 90%.[76] For patients with group III disease, radiation doses are more commonly 50 Gy.[77] A randomized study within the IRS-IV protocol demonstrated that twice-daily irradiation at 110 cGY per dose, 6 to 8 hours apart (hyperfractionated schedule) for 5 days per week is feasible and safe. This schedule, however, is difficult to accomplish in small children who require twice-daily sedation for treatment. Unfortunately, the hyperfractionated schedule demonstrated no improvement in local control over conventional radiation therapy.[78]

Radiation therapy in very young children with RMS poses a unique therapeutic challenge. Concerns over the technical difficulties associated with external beam radiotherapy in young children and late side effects of therapy have led to the evaluation of strategies that reduce the total burden of therapy without sacrificing local control. Modern techniques, such as intensity modulated radiation therapy (IMRT) and proton beams, may improve outcome without compromising long-term function.[79,80] Ongoing studies continue to evaluate the dose of radiation necessary for local control of the tumor.

Assessment of Response to Treatment

Although European RMS trials have incorporated the use of conventional radiologic modalities to evaluate the response to induction therapy and help tailor subsequent therapy, this has not been employed in the United States. IRS-IV data demonstrated no predictive value of radiographic response after 8 weeks of induction therapy.[81] Further, radiographic evidence of a complete response to therapy in group III RMS was not associated with a reduction in disease recurrence and death.[63a] Clearly, the significance of persistent radiographic masses in patients treated for RMS is unknown. Conventional imaging modalities offer no information about the biology of these masses and are unable to differentiate between active tumors and scar. It is possible that FDG PET may offer useful clinical information in patients treated or partially treated for RMS.

SPECIFIC ANATOMIC SITES

Rhabdomyosarcomas are unique among solid tumors in that they may occur in many different areas of the body. Tumors in different parts of the body may behave differently than those in other areas. In addition, some areas of the body offer unique obstacles to surgical resection. As such, some specific anatomic sites of tumor occurrence will be discussed separately.

Head and Neck (Superficial Nonparameningeal)

Approximately 35% of RMS arises in the head and neck region. Of these tumors, 75% occur in the orbits. Other sites include the buccal, oropharyngeal, laryngeal, or parotid areas.[3] The histologic variant of RMS correlates to some extent with the location of the orbital tumor. ERMS and differentiated types more commonly arise in the superior nasal quadrants, whereas ARMS generally originate within the inferior orbit.[83] For all head and neck RMS, biopsy is required for the confirmation of diagnosis. Resection may be limited by the inability to obtain an adequate margin, and therefore the success of resection is heavily dependent on location.[84-86] Lymph nodes are rarely involved in childhood head and neck RMS; however, clinically or radiographically positive nodes must be biopsied.[87] Outcomes correlate strongly with tumor location. Orbital RMS carries the best prognosis and is least likely to extend to the meninges. These tumors generally present earlier in the course of disease. Tumors arising in nonorbital parameningeal locations have a high likelihood of meningeal extension. If meningeal extension occurs after chemotherapy and radiation therapy, the outcome is often fatal.[88]

Parameningeal Sites

Parameningeal RMS includes tumors arising in the middle ear/mastoid, nasal cavity, parapharyngeal space, paranasal sinuses, or the pterygopalatine/infratemporal fossa region. These tumors are considered high risk because of their propensity to cause cranial nerve palsy, bony erosion of the cranial base, and intracranial extension.[89] Wide local excision is recommended but is often not feasible because of the location of the tumors. Craniofacial resection for tumors of the nasal areas, paranasal sinuses, temporal fossa, and other deep sites are reserved for expert surgical teams. The recognition of poor outcomes associated with meningeal extension has lead to a propensity for early radiation therapy of primary tumors and adjuvant chemotherapy.[87] For patients with unresected tumors and/or lymph node-positive disease, the use of three-drug chemotherapy regimens (including an alkylating agent) plus local or regional radiation may be beneficial. The optimal dosing and timing of radiation are not yet determined.[84]

Trunk

Accounting for only 4% to 7% of tumors, RMS of the trunk is associated with a poor prognosis. Symptoms for RMS of the trunk often occur late in the progression of disease, which leads to late diagnoses. Complete surgical resection is difficult, particularly when the pleura and peritoneum are involved. In addition, resections are frequently morbid and associated with poor cosmetic outcomes. Resection may necessitate major chest wall or abdominal wall reconstruction with prosthetic materials or with flaps.[90,91] Indicators of poor prognosis include advanced stage at presentation, alveolar histology, recurrence disease, tumor size greater than 5 cm, lymph node involvement, and the inability to undergo gross total resection.[92,93]

Abdominal Wall

Abdominal wall RMS generally presents as a painless, firm mass. Many abdominal wall primaries can be removed completely at presentation or following neoadjuvant chemotherapy. However, tumors arising from the interior abdominal wall may not be noticed until significant tumor progression has occurred, thus rendering resection much more challenging. Tumor excision should include full-thickness resection of the abdominal wall, including the skin and peritoneum with a margin of normal tissue. Reconstruction of the abdominal wall can be performed with mesh or myocutaneous muscle flaps in an attempt to preserve function and cosmesis after resection. Data would suggest that localized tumors of the abdominal wall can be resected with good outcomes and that younger children with abdominal wall RMS fare better than adolescents, possibly because of a higher proportion of unfavorable histology in the older group of children.[94] If the size or location prevents adequate excision, neoadjuvant chemotherapy should be initiated to reduce tumor size and facilitate subsequent resection.

Chest Wall

The differential diagnosis for malignant chest wall masses includes Ewing sarcoma, primitive neuroectodermal tumors (PNET), and RMS. Diagnostic biopsies are performed in the long axis of the tumor, parallel to the ribs. Wide local excision of chest wall lesions with a 2-cm margin, including the previous biopsy site, involved chest wall muscles and involved ribs, as well as wedge excision of any involved underlying lung, is recommended. Thoracoscopy performed at the time of resection may be helpful in determining the extent of pleural involvement and tumor extension to the underlying lung. Chest wall reconstruction can be performed using a number of techniques employing prosthetic mesh, myocutaneous flaps, and titanium ribs. Chest wall lesions have a worse prognosis than other trunk lesions, with a 1.8-year survival rate of only 42%.[90] Although radiotherapy may be beneficial for local control of tumor, this option is associated with significant morbidity, including pulmonary fibrosis, decreased lung capacity, restrictive defects from altered development of the thoracic cavity, and scoliosis.[95] There is also no proven survival benefit.

Biliary Tract

Classically, patients with biliary RMS present at a young age (average age 3.5 years) with jaundice and abdominal pain, often associated with abdominal distension, vomiting, and fever. Workup reveals a significant direct hyperbilirubinemia and a mild elevation of hepatic transaminases. Gross total resection of biliary tract RMS is rarely possible and is often unnecessary because of good outcomes with chemotherapy and radiation. Currently, open biopsy is the only definitive role of surgery in the treatment of biliary RMS, although this

is controversial. The histology of these tumors is often the botryoid variant of embryonal RMS, which carries a good overall prognosis.[96] Biliary obstruction can be relieved by stenting, but external biliary drains should be avoided because of infectious complications. Overall, outcomes are good unless distant metastases are present at the time of diagnosis.[97,98]

Paraspinal Sites

Paraspinal RMS is rare (3.3% of all RMS) and carries a poor prognosis. These tumors tend to spread along anatomic structures, such as neurovascular bundles and fascial sheaths, occasionally causing spinal cord compression. Complete excision of paraspinal lesions is often difficult to perform because of large tumor size at presentation and proximity to the vertebral column and spinal canal.[92,99] Recurrence rates for paraspinal RMS are high (55%) with the majority of these occurring at distant locations. The lung is the most common site of distant metastasis followed by the central nervous system.[99]

Retroperitoneum/Pelvis

Like paraspinal tumors, retroperitoneal/pelvic lesions are often discovered at an advanced stage and thus generally carry a poor prognosis. These tumors can envelop vital structures, making complete surgical resection challenging. Neoadjuvant chemotherapy may play a role in tumors that cannot be safely resected at the time of diagnosis. With the exception of group IV metastatic disease, aggressive resection is recommended and has been shown to offer improvement in survival.[100] Group IV patients with embryonal histology and those who present at less than 10 years of age may also undergo surgical debulking.[101] It has been demonstrated that excising greater than half of the tumor before chemotherapy resulted in improved rates of failure-free survival when compared with patients who did not undergo debulking.[102] This is the *only* setting in which surgical debulking of RMS has shown any benefit.

Perineal/Perianal Sites

Perineal tumors are rare and usually present at an advanced stage. Characteristics associated with improved survival include a primary tumor size less than 5 cm, less advanced clinical group and stage, negative lymph node status, and age less than 10 years of age. Interestingly, histology does not affect overall outcome for these tumors. Resection of these tumors can be challenging because of proximity to the urethra and anorectum. At resection, particular care should be taken to preserve continence. If anorectal obstruction exists, a temporary colostomy may be necessary. Patients presenting in clinical group I had 100% overall survival at 5 years compared with 25% for group IV patients.[103]

Extremities

Rhabdomyosarcoma of the extremities accounts for 20% of all new diagnoses. The majority of these tumors have alveolar histology and thus a poor prognosis. The cure rate for children with extremity RMS has, however, improved steadily from 47% in IRS-I to 74% in IRS-III.[104,105] As with many types of RMS, complete gross resection at initial surgical intervention is the most important predictor of failure-free survival. The primary goal of local tumor control in extremity tumors is limb-sparing complete resection. Amputation is rarely necessary for tumor excision. Positive regional lymph nodes are found in 20% to 40% of patients and are associated with decreased overall survival (46% survival rate for node-positive patients compared with 80% survival for node-negative patients). Seventeen percent of IRS-IV patients with clinically negative nodes were found to have microscopic nodal disease on biopsy. In light of this, surgical evaluation of lymph nodes is necessary to accurately stage children with extremity RMS, even in the absence of clinically positive nodes.[60] Currently, axillary sampling is recommended for upper extremity lesions, and femoral triangle sampling is recommended for lower-extremity lesions. Sentinel lymph node mapping may be a useful adjunct in the setting of extremity RMS. If regional nodes are involved, then x-ray therapy (XRT) fields are adjusted to incorporate regional lymph node basins. This approach is associated with decreasing rates of local and regional recurrence.[57] In-transit nodal involvement at the time of diagnosis, present in 4% of IRS-IV patients, has also been identified as a factor contributing to regional treatment failure. This may be evaluated by MRI, or possibly FDG PET, at the time of diagnosis. Radiation therapy (RT) should be used at regional lymph node sites in these patients.[106]

Genitourinary Sites: Bladder/Prostate

Rhabdomyosarcoma of the bladder or prostate typically presents with urinary obstructive symptoms. These lesions are typically of embryonal histology (73%). The major goal of surgery is complete tumor resection with bladder salvage. This can be achieved in 50% to 60% of patients.[107,108] Partial cystectomy has resulted in similar survival rates and improved bladder function compared with more aggressive resections.[109,110] Bladder dome tumors frequently can be completely resected, whereas more distal bladder lesions frequently require ureteral reimplantation or bladder augmentation. Prostatic tumors require prostatectomy, often combined with an attempt at bladder salvage with or without ureteral reconstruction.[53] Continent urinary diversion may be necessary if tumors are unresectable or have a poor response to medical therapy. Lymph nodes are involved in up to 20% of cases. Therefore during biopsy or resection, iliac and para-aortic nodes should be sampled, as well as any other clinically involved nodes. An analysis of patients with bladder or prostate RMS in IRS-IV revealed that 70% of these tumors arose from the bladder with an overall 6-year survival of 82%.[111] Of these patients, 55 retained their bladder without relapse, but only 36 had normal bladder function. Urodynamic studies have been used to evaluate bladder function after treatment.[112]

Genitourinary Sites: Vulva/Vagina/Uterus

Traditionally, females with primary tumors of the genital tract underwent aggressive resection followed by chemotherapy with or without radiation.[113–115] Newer treatment approaches rely more heavily on neoadjuvant chemotherapy to reduce tumor size and minimize the extent of resection in an attempt to preserve organ function. Primary tumors of the vagina are about 5 times more common than cervical tumors. The vast majority of these tumors are classic embryonal or are of the botryoid subtype. This may account for the more favorable prognosis that these tumors display.[116] These tumors respond well to chemotherapy, with impressive tumor regression that often precludes the need for radical operations such as pelvic exenteration. Vaginectomy and hysterectomy are performed only for persistent or

recurrent disease. Primary uterine tumors require resection with preservation of the distal vagina and ovaries if they do not respond to chemotherapy. Oophorectomy is only indicated in the setting of direct tumor involvement. For those patients presenting with nonembryonal RMS of the female genital tract, more intensive chemotherapeutic regimens are recommended to reduce the risk of recurrence. Prognosis for this tumor site with only locoregional disease is excellent, with an estimated 5-year survival of 87%.[117]

Paratesticular Sites

Paratesticular RMS generally presents as a painless scrotal mass. Histology is generally favorable, with most tumors showing the spindle-cell subvariant of embryonal histology. Survival rates are greater than 90% for patients presenting with group I or II disease.[118,119] Radical orchiectomy via an inguinal approach with resection of the spermatic cord to the level of the internal ring is the standard of care. Open biopsy should be avoided, because the flow of lymphatics in this region facilitates spread of the disease. If a transscrotal biopsy/resection has been performed, subsequent resection of the hemiscrotum is required. If unprotected spillage of tumor cells occurs during tumor resection, these patients are considered clinical group IIa regardless of the completeness of resection.[120] The incidence of nodal metastatic disease for paratesticular RMS is 26% to 43%.[121,122] Unfortunately, studies have demonstrated that CT is a poor means of evaluating lymph node positivity in the retroperitoneum.[123] In addition, patients older than 10 years of age or those with enlarged nodes have a much higher incidence of node positivity.[59] Those patients should therefore undergo an ipsilateral retroperitoneal nodal resection. Suprarenal nodes should be evaluated, because positive nodes in this area place a patient in group IV with disseminated metastatic disease.

Metastatic Disease

Rhabdomyosarcoma metastasizes both through hematogenous and lymphatic routes. Children with metastatic RMS have very poor survival rates. For the IRS studies I through III, children with metastatic disease had a 5-year disease-free survival of 20%, 27%, and 32%, respectively, in each of the successive studies. Recently studies have employed the use of upfront "window studies" to address potential chemotherapeutic regimens that would improve the disease-free survival period when given to patients with newly diagnosed metastatic RMS. One such study evaluated the combination of ifosfamide and doxorubicin for the treatment of children with metastatic disease who are less than 10 years of age, have embryonal histology, and lack nodal, bone, or bone marrow involvement. This treatment strategy increased 5-year failure-free survival to 28% and 5-year overall survival to 34%.[68] Despite these improvements, more intensive research into chemotherapeutic regimens for group IV disease should be investigated to improve overall outcome.

Prognosis

The prognosis of patients with RMS is dependent on many factors. Favorable prognostic factors include embryonal/botryoid histology, primary tumor sites in the orbit and nonparameningeal head/neck region and genitourinary nonbladder/prostate regions, a lack of distant metastases at diagnosis, complete gross removal of tumor at the time of diagnosis, tumor size less than or equal to 5 cm, and age less than 10 years at the time of diagnosis.[77] Clinical grouping was identified as one of the most important predictors of failed treatment and tumor relapse.[2,77] These factors become important in the designation of treatment groups for risk-based therapy.

For group II patients, Smith and colleagues performed a retrospective review of patients enrolled in IRS-I through IRS-IV to determine the risk factors for relapse. Those patients in group II at highest risk for treatment failure had alveolar/undifferentiated histology, unfavorable primary sites, regional disease with residual tumor after gross resection and node involvement, or were treated with early therapeutic regimens (IRS-I or IRS-II). Current therapy for patients with group II tumors results in 85% survival long term, indicating that risk-based therapeutic strategies have assisted with failure-free survival.[124]

Patients with group III disease have incomplete resection or biopsy only prior to chemotherapy and irradiation. Wharam and colleagues determined that predictors of failure-free survival in group III include tumor size less than 5 cm, primary sites of orbit and bladder/prostate, and TNM staging equivalent to T_1/N_0N_x tumors in stage I or stage II. Since radiotherapy is important for local control of group III disease, the incidence of local failure was stratified by radiotherapy dosing (<42.5 vs. 42.5 to 47.5 vs. > 47.5 Gy) and was not significantly different among these dose ranges.[125]

Approximately 15% of patients with RMS present with metastases (group IV) at the time of diagnosis.[104] Patients in group IV have poor outcomes despite aggressive multimodality treatments, with only 25% expected to be free of disease 3 years after diagnosis.[104,105] A review of prognostic factors and outcomes for children and adolescents with metastatic RMS in IRS-IV found that 3-year overall survival and failure-free survival was improved if there were two or fewer metastatic sites and the histology of the tumor was embryonal. Compared with patients without metastatic disease, group IV patients in the IRS-IV study were more likely to be older (median age 7 years vs. 5 years), had a higher incidence of alveolar histology (46% vs. 22%), had tumors that were more invasive (T_2: 91% vs. 49%) and larger (>5 cm: 82% vs. 51%), a higher incidence of lymph node involvement (N_1: 57% vs. 16%), and had a greater proportion of extremity and truncal/retroperitoneal primary sites (48% vs. 25%). This study concluded that not all children with metastatic RMS have uniformly poor prognoses, suggesting that therapy should be tailored according to these factors.[126]

Future clinical trials and a better understanding of the molecular biology driving RMS tumor behavior may assist with customized clinical therapies that will improve outcome and failure-free survival in patients diagnosed with RMS.

The complete reference list is available online at www. expertconsult.com.

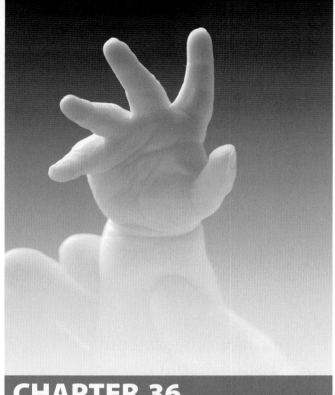

CHAPTER 36

Other Soft Tissue Tumors

Andrea Hayes-Jordan

Nonrhabdomyosarcoma Soft Tissue Sarcoma in Children: Background and Overview

Approximately 8% of childhood malignancies are soft tissue sarcomas. Half of these are nonrhabdomyosarcoma soft tissue sarcomas (NRSTSs). There are more than 50 histologic types, and genetic patterns are poorly understood. When surgical resection is feasible, ≈60% of patients are expected to achieve long-term survival with or without radiation therapy.[1] Patient outcome is largely based on age, the presence of metastasis at diagnosis, and size and depth of the lesion. Here we focus on the most common primary histologic types and differences in presentation and surgical treatment of childhood NRSTS and other common pediatric soft tissue tumors.

The treatment for children and adolescents with NRSTS has not previously been standardized, nor have there been any pediatric cooperative group trials as for rhabdomyosarcoma (RMS). Because there are many histologic subtypes of NRSTS, standardization of treatment is difficult. The first risk-based prospective trial of NRSTS in children and adolescents will complete enrollment soon, with results anticipated in 2013. In this trial, patients with NRSTS are treated as low,

intermediate, or high risk based on criteria previously ascertained in a thorough review of 121 patients by Spunt.[2,3] In patients with surgically resected NRSTS, univariate analysis revealed clear risk factors. Positive surgical margins ($P = 0.004$), tumor size greater than or equal to 5 cm ($P < 0.001$), invasiveness ($P = 0.002$), high grade ($P = 0.028$), and intra-abdominal primary site ($P = 0.055$) had a negative impact on event-free survival (EFS). Multivariate analysis confirmed all of these risk factors, except for invasiveness. Local recurrence was predicted by intra-abdominal primary site ($P = 0.028$), positive surgical margins ($P = 0.003$), and the omission of radiation therapy ($P = 0.043$). As expected, the biology of the tumor, assessed by tumor size greater than 5 cm, invasiveness, and high grade, predicted distant recurrences. Children and adolescents with initially unresectable NRSTSs are a subgroup with pediatric NRSTSs that is particularly high risk. These are large tumors, greater than 5 cm, which involve critical neurovascular structures of the extremity, trunk, abdomen, or pelvis. In these patients, the 5-year estimated overall survival and EFS were 56% and 33%, respectively, and postrelapse survival was poor, 19% despite multimodality therapy.[4]

In addition to the tumor being unresectable, age is a prognostic indicator in pediatric NRSTS. Patients less than 1 year of age have an excellent prognosis, whereas the adolescents and young adults have the worse prognosis compared with younger patients or older adults.[2] A 34-year review of patients treated at St. Jude Children's Research Hospital (SJCRH) revealed the overall 5-year survival estimate for children less than 1 year of age was 92% compared with 36% in those 15 to 21 years of age. Patients between 1 and 15 years of age had an intermediate survival of approximately 60%. Survival after relapse was poor in all age groups less than 18 years, except those less than 1 year of age. The 5-year estimate of postrelapse survival in patients less than 1 year of age was 80% compared with the 15- to 25-years cohort in which survival was 21%. The type of chemotherapy used in these patients was variable; surgical excision was generally completed for lesions less than or equal to 5 cm, and for most patients, incisional biopsy was performed for lesions greater than 5 cm, followed by chemotherapy, reexcision, and radiation therapy or amputation.[5]

INFANTILE FIBROSARCOMA

Patients in the study above who were less than 1 year of age had infantile fibrosarcoma (IF). This is a very rare form of NRSTS that occurs primarily during the first year of life, but can appear up to year 4. IF presents as a rapidly growing mass in the trunk or extremities. It can erode bone and usually reaches a large size.

Most cases of IF have a specific translocation t(12;15) (p13;q25)[6–8] leading to fusion of *ETV6 (TEL)*, a member of the ETS family of transcription factors, on chromosome 12p13, and *NTRK3 (TRKC)*, which encodes a tyrosine kinase receptor for neurotropin-3[9,10] on chromosome 15q25. Other cytogenetic abnormalities include trisomy 11; random gains of chromosomes 8, 11, 17, and 20[11]; deletion of the long arm of chromosome 17[12]; and a t(12;13) translocation.[13] The helix-loop-helix dimerization domain of *ETV6* fuses to the protein tyrosine kinase domain of *NTRK3*. The fusion protein results in ligand-independent chimeric protein tyrosine kinase activity with autophosphorylation. This leads to constitutive activation of Ras-MAPK and P13K-AKT pathways through insulin receptor substrate-1, which is tyrosine-phosphorylated,[14–16] and through the activation of c-Src.[17] The fusion protein also associates with TGF-beta II receptor, which can be oncogenic by leading to inhibition of TGF-beta receptor signals that mediate tumor suppression.[18]

Identical genetic findings have been reported in the cellular variant of congenital mesoblastic nephroma, a microscopically similar tumor of the kidney,[19,20] and in secretory carcinoma of the breast[21] and acute myeloid leukemia,[22] implying oncogenesis by lineage-independent activation of kinase-related signaling pathways.

SYNOVIAL SARCOMA

Synovial sarcoma (SS) and malignant peripheral nerve sheath tumor (MPNST) are the most common pediatric NRSTSs. SS is characterized by a very specific fusion gene 18[t(X;18)(p11.2;g11.2)]. Its etiology is unknown.[23] In evaluating the three largest reviews of pediatric SS, common principles are evident. For children 0 to 16 years old and tumors less than 5 cm in size, overall 5-year survival (OS) is 71% to 88%. In this group, the addition of chemotherapy did not improve survival. In patients 17 to 30 years old, the addition of chemotherapy does improve metastasis-free survival. In patients with SS tumors greater than 5 cm that are deep and invasive and without metastasis, OS is 50% to 75%, and chemotherapy responsiveness is 50% to 60%.[24] It is clear that for SS survival does not depend on surgical margins but depends on size (>5 cm) and local invasiveness. Brecht and colleagues found event-free survival was 92% and 56%, respectively, when SS tumors were less than or equal to 5 cm or greater than 5 cm.[24] Figure 36-1 shows the leg of a child with synovial sarcoma that was not responsive to chemotherapy and required resection down to the periosteum of the tibia. Radiotherapy does have a role in this disease and is recommended after marginal resection or before anticipated marginal resection, such as the one pictured.[23]

MALIGNANT PERIPHERAL NERVE SHEATH TUMOR

Malignant peripheral nerve sheath tumor (MPNST), also called schwannoma or neurofibrosarcoma, usually arises in proximity to nerve sheaths. MPNST develops in a preexisting neurofibroma in approximately 40% of patients, particularly those with neurofibromatosis type 1 (NF-1).[25] In a review of 171 patients the 5-year OS and progression-free survival was 51% and 37%, respectively. Multivariate analysis revealed absence of NF-1 and tumor invasiveness to be poor prognostic variables. The overall response of the patients who received neoadjuvant chemotherapy was 45%. Some partial responses were seen in patients with initial unresectable disease, because of neurovascular involvement.[25] Neoadjuvant radiotherapy failed to maintain or achieve local control in 45% of patients (26 of 58). Neither chemotherapy nor radiotherapy produced any statistically significant difference in outcome. This article concluded by stating "…complete surgical resection is the mainstay of successful treatment."[25] In another much smaller series, the same patterns in outcome were seen.[26]

Surgical Approach and Presentation of Nonrhabdomyosarcoma Soft Tissue Sarcoma

Unlike rhabdomyosarcomas, NRSTSs are relatively chemoinsensitive. In the above pediatric studies and in adult multi-institutional studies, the impact of chemotherapy on outcome is minimal. In large American Joint Commission on Cancer (AJCC) stage 3 tumors, overall survival was no different whether or not chemotherapy was added to surgery and also if neoadjuvant or adjuvant radiation therapy was added.[27] Complete surgical excision provides the best outcome. Patients usually present with a painless mass, sometimes identified after a recent episode of trauma. Pediatric patients who have an extremity or trunk mass that is greater than 5 cm, should have a magnetic resonance imaging (MRI) examination, followed by core needle or open biopsy. If NRSTS is identified and no mutilating limb-sparing surgical excision is feasible, resection should be completed. If margins are microscopically positive, postoperative radiotherapy should be given in high-grade tumors and tumors larger than 5 cm. Low-grade tumors that are less than 5 cm can be reexcised or just watched closely. If surgical excision is not feasible without amputation or severe morbidity, whether less than or greater than 5 cm, preoperative chemotherapy and radiotherapy should be administered. If surgical excision is feasible, but R1 resection is anticipated, the type of radiotherapy, whether

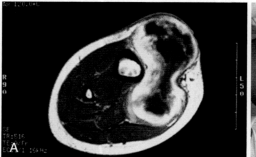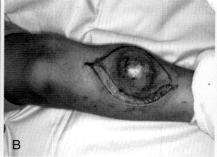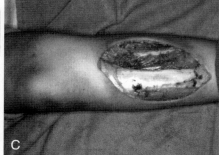

FIGURE 36-1   A-C, Magnetic resonance (MR) image of a child with synovial sarcoma abutting the tibia. Neoadjuvant chemotherapy was not successful in reducing the size of the tumor. Marginal resection with postoperative radiation or brachytherapy is a preferred alternative to amputation.

preoperative or postoperative brachytherapy, proton beam therapy, or external beam therapy, should be discussed with the radiation oncologist, with the goal in pediatric extremity tumors to avoid the growth plate in younger patients who are still growing. In tumors less than 5 cm, complete surgical excision with negative microscopic margins is the goal. In the case of unexpected malignant pathology, primary reexcision is recommended. For all NRSTSs, negative microscopic margins should be achieved; however, there is no consistent reliable evidence to establish the appropriate width of the margins.

NRSTSs are graded histologically to help predict outcome. Grade 1 is any NRSTS with low malignant potential, such as infantile fibrosarcoma, with mitotic activity less than 5 mitoses per high-powered field (HPF). NRSTSs with tumor necrosis less than 15% and mitotic activity of 5 to 10 mitoses per HPF are graded 2, and specific histologic subtypes with known aggressive behavior and/or any sarcoma with tumor necrosis of more than 15% or mitotic activity of more than 10 mitoses per HPF are graded 3.[28]

Cytotoxic chemotherapy (Adriamycin, ifosfamide, vincristine, dactinomycin, etc.), will be effective, at best, in 45% to 50% of patients from the evidence we have to date.[4] (This does not include targeted therapy, because there are not yet sufficient data to analyze at this time.) Very close observation by imaging is warranted if neoadjuvant chemotherapy is chosen, because an increase in tumor size may preclude limb-sparing, nonmutilating surgery, and an abdominal or pelvic tumor may become unresectable.

Sentinel lymph node biopsy, although recommended for rhabdomyosarcoma to evaluate normal-appearing lymph nodes, is only recommended in histologic subtypes of NRSTS that have high risk of lymph node metastasis. These include epithelioid sarcoma and clear cell sarcoma, which have an approximate incidence of lymph node metastasis of up to 30%. Synovial sarcoma metastasizes to the lymph nodes about 15% of the time.

Computed tomography (CT) scan of the chest is a necessary part of the workup to exclude lung metastasis. Lung metastasis occurs in approximately 30% of patients with NRSTS. Because NRSTSs are relatively chemoinsensitive, surgical resection of lung metastasis is recommended. Thoracotomy is the recommended approach in order to palpate the lung for any tumors that may have been missed on imaging.

Desmoplastic Small Round Cell Tumor

Desmoplastic small round cell tumor (DSRCT) is a malignant neoplasm in the soft tissue sarcoma family that arises from the peritoneal surface of the abdomen and pelvis. No more than 200 cases have been reported worldwide since the disease was first described in 1989 by Gerald and Rosai[29] and Ordonez.[30] The tumor is most prevalent in young white males.[29–30] Presenting symptoms include abdominal pain, constipation, and abdominal distension with ascites. Overall survival is approximately 30% to 55% despite chemotherapy, radiotherapy, and aggressive surgical resection.[31,32] Because most DSRCT patients present with multiple abdominal tumor implants (Fig. 36-2), microscopic tumor cells can be left behind, despite the complete resection of dozens to hundreds of tumors. The most widely accepted standard of care for

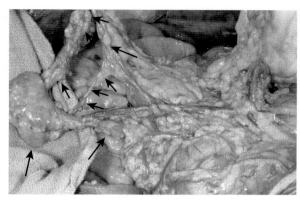

FIGURE 36-2 Desmoplastic small round cell tumor in the omentum of a 5-year-old boy after six cycles of chemotherapy. Peritoneal disease has similar appearance. This child had 402 nodules removed at this operation.

DSRCT was multimodality therapy with the P6 regimen: cyclophosphamide, doxorubicin, and vincristine, alternating with ifosfamide and etoposide for seven total courses,[31] followed by aggressive debulking surgery to remove all visible disease.[32] It is clear that without complete resection of all visible disease survival is poor.[32] Hyperthermic intraperitoneal chemotherapy (HIPEC) is a new therapeutic modality recently used in children; its results are promising, but studies are ongoing. Hyperthermia and chemotherapy have synergistic cytotoxicity that is of value in the treatment of microscopic disease in adult carcinomas. HIPEC has been applied successfully in adults with extensive peritoneal disease, commonly observed with mesothelioma, appendiceal, colon, and gastric carcinoma.[33–37] A recent publication shows that DSRCT can now be treated safely with aggressive cytoreductive surgery followed by (HIPEC) in children.[38] The study included 23 pediatric adolescent and young adult patients with DSRCT. HIPEC was compared with standard chemotherapy, radiation therapy, and surgical debulking. The patients were mostly males (96%). The age of the HIPEC patients ranged from 5 to 25 years of age. Complete resection (CR0) to less than 1.0-cm tumor size was achieved in all 8 patients who underwent HIPEC. Operative times ranged from 7 to 16 hours. Figure 36-3 shows the setup used in the operating room to deliver HIPEC. In the pediatric patients, the estimated 12-month disease-free survival (DFS) rate was 53% for the HIPEC group, compared with 14% for the non-HIPEC group. Median 3-year survival in this small group of patients was 29% with chemotherapy and radiotherapy alone, compared with 71% in the HIPEC with cytoreductive surgery group. The severe morbidities that occurred were partial bowel obstruction managed nonoperatively, prolonged ileus/gastroparesis, transient renal insufficiency, and one patient developed cardiomyopathy secondary to resection of more than 3 kg of tumor, causing release of tumor necrosis factor. HIPEC is an option in treating this rare tumor.[38]

Desmoid Tumors

Desmoid tumors are very different than DSRCT. These are intermediate-grade sarcoma-type tumors that are locally very aggressive and can be fatal, but usually do not metastasize. Desmoid fibromatosis is a mesenchymal neoplasm. It is encountered

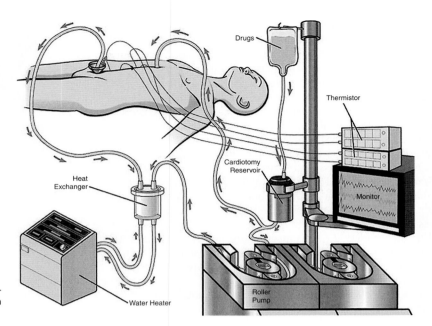

FIGURE 36-3 Setup for hyperthermic intraperitoneal chemotherapy (HIPEC) therapy for children with "sarcomatosis" after cytoreductive surgery.

in two settings—within the context of familial adenomatous polyposis (FAP) and sporadically.[39] Here we focus on the sporadic group. Desmoid tumors can arise in any body site and are much more common in women. Surgery has been the therapeutic mainstay, but radiotherapy plays an important role in treatment as do systemic therapies, such as the tamoxifen and sulindac combination and nonsteriodal anti-inflammatory drugs (NSAIDs).[40–46] Desmoids have a very unique course in that they can recur locally and can be more aggressive or regress spontaneously. However, they have no capacity for metastasis.[39] Resecting recurrent tumors can be potentially mutilating. Some large retrospective studies[42,47,48] demonstrated that microscopically positive (or grossly positive) margins were predictive of increased frequency of local recurrence on retrospective multivariate analysis, although radiation improved outcome in one study. Other studies[40,49–51] have failed to demonstrate an effect of microscopic margin on recurrence. Some of these differences may result from the mixture of disease sites, pattern of application of adjuvant radiotherapy, and selection of patients treated by surgical approach. In the end, surgical therapy must be tailored to what is achievable in terms of margins with preservation of functional status for the individual patient.[39] Incomplete resection or positive microscopic margins in desmoid tumors should be treated with adjuvant radiotherapy. Figure 36-4 provides a helpful algorithm to follow.

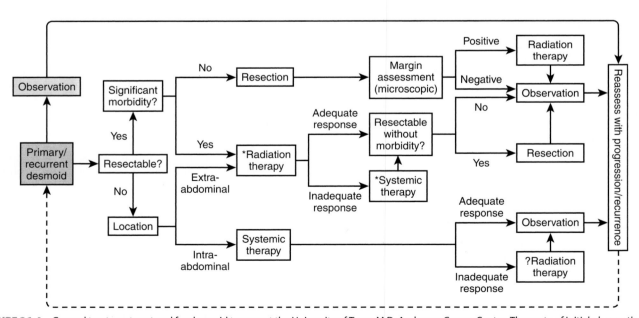

FIGURE 36-4 General treatment protocol for desmoid tumors at the University of Texas M.D. Anderson Cancer Center. The route of initial observation for certain cases, to avoid overtreatment advocated by some, is depicted in *gray*. Given the propensity for progression on treatment and local recurrence, all treatment pathways ultimately end in observation. *Radiation therapy can be preceded, and even precluded, by systemic therapy in certain cases of initially unresectable extraabdominal desmoid tumors.

Dermatofibrosarcoma Protuberans

Dermatofibrosarcoma protuberans (DFSP) is a relatively common soft tissue tumor. Its peak age is in young adulthood, but it is frequently present in children and at birth. DFSP occurs primarily on the trunk and extremities. It can present as a plaque on the skin or in a more diffuse multinodular pattern.[52,53] The latter is more common in children. Pigmented dermatofibrosarcoma, giant cell fibroblastoma, and fibrosarcoma can arise in DFSP.[54,55]

Dermatofibrosarcoma protuberans has a reciprocal translocation, t(17;22)(q22;q13.1), resulting in fusion of the genes *COL1A* (encoding the alpha 1 chain of collagen type 1, a heterotrimer) on 17q21-22 and *PDGFB1* (encoding the beta chain of platelet-derived growth factor, a homodimer) at 22q13.[55,56] The same fusion is also seen in supernumerary ring chromosomes derived from t(17;22),[57] which are found in adult cases of dermatofibrosarcoma. Fusion gene transcripts can be detected by reverse transcriptase–polymerase chain reaction (RT-PCR).[53,58] This is not usually required for diagnosis but might be useful in guiding therapy, especially for superficial fibrosarcomas.

Dermatofibrosarcoma protuberans has a high local recurrence rate, especially if incompletely excised, and can metastasize in 5% of cases, usually after multiple local recurrences. Therefore complete excision with negative margins is crucial, and 2- to 3-cm margins are recommended. However, in areas such as the head and neck, lesser margins are acceptable.

Platelet-derived growth factor receptor (PDGFR) is a receptor tyrosine kinase, which in dermatofibrosarcoma protuberans is constitutively activated by autocrine or paracrine mechanisms as a result of overproduction of its ligand platelet-derived growth factor-beta (PDGFB),[59] leading to cellular proliferation.[60] This has suggested the use of the tyrosine kinase inhibitors imatinib[61] and, more recently, sunitinib or sorafenib in locally advanced or metastatic disease,[62–63] but fibrosarcomatous variants without the translocation do not respond[64,65] so that genetic analysis is indicated before targeted therapy. In the only multicenter Phase 2 study published to date, imatinib was found to be effective preoperative therapy in 36% of patients ($n = 25$) by reducing tumor size by an average of 20%. Response was measured by physical exam, ultrasonography, and MRI. Decrease in average diameter by 1 cm on physical exam, 1 cm by ultrasonography, and 2 cm by MRI were observed, respectively. In 21 of 25 patients, the fusion gene *COL1A1-PDGFB* was detected. Therefore when DFSP is located in places where a decrease in size provides a significant advantage in wound closure, neoadjuvant imatinib is a viable option.

The complete reference list is available online at www. expertconsult.com.

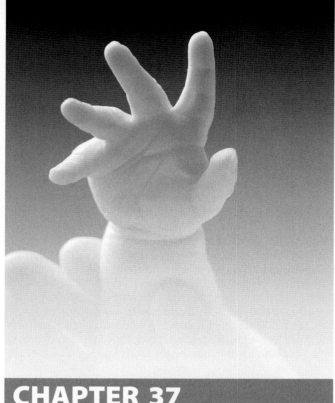

CHAPTER 37

Teratomas and Other Germ Cell Tumors

Frederick J. Rescorla

Pediatric germ cell tumors are rare tumors that are unique due to their varied clinical presentation and locations. Approximately 20% of pediatric germ cell tumors are malignant, and they represent 1% to 3% of all malignant tumors in childhood and adolescence.[1,2] Three features distinguish these childhood tumors from many other malignancies as well as their counterparts: In children, the extragonadal tumor site is more common than the gonadal site, whereas in adults, only 10% are at extragonadal sites; yolk sac tumor is the predominant malignant histology, and a serum marker (alpha fetoprotein, AFP) exists to follow response to therapy and monitor for recurrent disease; and the introduction of modern chemotherapy with cisplatin and bleomycin significantly increased survival for affected children and has allowed neoadjuvant therapy with vital organ preservation in initially unresectable cases.

Abnormal or arrested migration of primordial germ cells results in deposition of cells in the sacrococcygeal region, retroperitoneum, mediastinum, and pineal gland of the brain, resulting in the potential of extragonadal germ cell tumors at these sites. Whereas in adults 90% of germ cell tumors are at gonadal locations, in childhood, the extragonadal site is

more common until puberty, at which time the gonadal sites are more common. The totipotential nature of these cells results in a wide variety of histologic patterns, and in addition, one quarter of pediatric tumors have more than one histologic component.[2] The management of these tumors is dependent upon complete surgical resection at diagnosis or after neoadjuvant therapy, accurate and thorough histologic examination, and selective use of chemotherapy. Prior to the late 1970s, the survival of advanced-stage tumors was dismal; however, Einhorn's introduction of cisplatin, vinblastine, and bleomycin for disseminated testicular cancer in 1977 changed the treatment of all germ cell tumors with dramatic results.[3] Subsequent studies validated the use of chemotherapy in a neoadjuvant fashion, thus allowing vital organ preservation in advanced cases with frequent massive tumor shrinkage. The role of the surgeon in determining resectability and performing a proper staging operation is vital.

Current therapy within the Children's Oncology Group (COG) is risk based: with surgery alone for stage 1 testes and ovary tumors and all immature teratomas, with anticipated survival of 95% to 100%; surgery and chemotherapy for all remaining gonadal tumors (except stage IV ovary) and low-stage (I-II) extragonadal, with anticipated survival of 90% to 100%; and surgery and intensive chemotherapy for high-risk (stage III-IV) extragonadal and stage IV ovary, with survival between 75% and 90%, depending on site and stage.

Embryology and Classification

Primordial germ cells arise near the allantois of the embryonic yolk sac endoderm and are evident at the fourth fetal week. They migrate along the midline dorsal mesentery to the genital ridge, arriving by the end of the sixth fetal week. The migration of the germ cells appears to be mediated by the c-KIT receptor and stem cell factor; the latter is expressed in increasing levels from the yolk sac to the genital ridge.[4,5] Arrested migration is presumed to account for the extragonadal locations in the normal path of the germ cells (retroperitoneum), whereas aberrant migration results in cells at other extragonadal sites (pineal, sacrococcygeal).

CLASSIFICATION

Teilum[6] proposed the germ cell origin of gonadal tumors, and the pathway of differentiation is listed in Figure 37-1. Seminoma (or dysgerminoma) is a primitive germ cell tumor that lacks the ability for further differentiation. It is unusual in childhood and occurs most frequently in the mediastinum, pineal gland, and at the gonadal sites during the adolescent years. Embryonal carcinoma is composed of cells capable of further differentiation into embryonic or extraembryonic tumors. Teratomas are the most common germ cell tumor and are composed of elements from one or more of the embryonic germ layers and contain tissue foreign to the anatomic site of origin.[7,8]

Mature and immature teratomas are considered benign lesions. It is, however, imperative to have a thorough and accurate pathologic review, because 25% of germ cell tumors in childhood are mixed tumors with more than one histologic

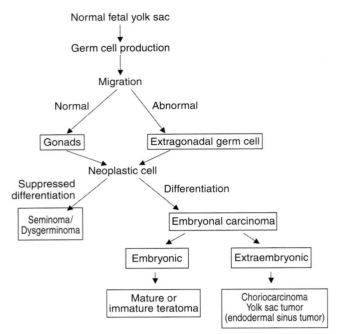

FIGURE 37-1   Classification system for development of germ cell tumors.

component.[2] Certain sites are more likely to have mixed tumor histology, with ovary (46%) and mediastinal (61%) the most common.[9,10] Mature teratomas contain well-differentiated tissue, whereas immature teratomas contain neuroectoderm and are graded between 1 and 3 based on the number of low-power fields of primitive neuroepithelium.[11] There has been debate about the treatment of immature teratomas. Many adult reports of ovarian tumors have considered grade 3 lesions malignant, and these patients have been treated with chemotherapy. A review of childhood immature teratomas demonstrated an association between high-grade immaturity and the presence of microscopic foci of endodermal sinus tumor,[12] with malignant foci observed in 83% of grade 3 immature teratomas as the only risk factor for recurrence.[13]

Yolk sac tumors (endodermal sinus) and choriocarcinoma are well-differentiated, highly malignant tumors. Yolk sac is the more common histology in childhood and occurs primarily in the sacrococcygeal region, ovary, and prepubertal testes.

Genetics and Risk Factors

Germ cell tumors demonstrate a bimodal age distribution with peaks at 2 and 20 years of age. Pediatric germ cell tumors differ in several aspects from their adult counterparts. Pediatric yolk sac tumors are more likely to have DNA ploidy, whereas adolescent and adult germ cell tumors are usually aneuploid.[14] In children younger than 4 years of age, the primary malignant germ cell tumor is yolk sac, and these are diploid or tetraploid; the teratomas are diploid with normal karyotypes and are benign.[15–17] Childhood yolk sac tumors have also demonstrated deletion of chromosomes 1p and 6q in 50% of specimens.[18] In addition, a smaller percentage demonstrates amplification of c-MYC. The isochromosome i (12p), which is identified in most pubertal or postpubertal testes tumors, is not observed in prepubertal tumors. Gains of 12p have been

noted in malignant ovarian germ cell tumors but not in ovarian immature teratomas.[19]

The presence of intersex disorders is a known risk factor for gonadoblastoma, an in-situ germ cell tumor with the ability to differentiate into dysgerminoma, immature teratoma, yolk sac tumor, or choriocarcinoma.[20] One risk group includes testosterone deficiency, androgen insensitivity syndromes, and 5-alpha-reductase deficiency, which are androgen-deficient males. The presence of any portion of a Y chromosome is considered a risk factor in these children.[21] Risk of malignancy in androgen insensitivity is 3.6% at age 20 and 22% at age 30[22]; in view of this, gonadectomy usually in adolescence, is recommended. Gonadal dysgenesis is associated with a risk of malignancy of 10% at age 20 and 19% at age 30.

Undescended testes have an increased risk of malignancy, with the rate highest for intraabdominal testes. Approximately 0.4% of all males have undescended testes, however, it is observed in 3.5 to 12% of the testicular cancer population.[23] One study noted that although intraabdominal testes only account for 14% of undescended testes, they account for nearly 50% of tumors in the undescended testes group. The effect of orchiopexy on the risk of testes cancer is not known, and 20% of the tumors in patients with undescended testis occur in the descended testis.[24] Seminomas occur in a higher percentage of undescended testes (60%) compared with the descended testes tumors (30% to 40%),[25] and one study observed that orchiopexy decreases the incidence of seminoma.[26] The early identification of these children is important, because a recent report noted a 2-year-old boy with a large yolk sac tumor in an intraabdominal testis with lymph node involvement.[27] Surgery and chemotherapy yielded a successful outcome.

Risk-Based Therapy

The survival of patients with advanced-stage germ cell tumors was poor prior to the introduction of modern chemotherapy, with most survivors having had low-stage surgically excised tumors. Surgery and chemotherapy consisting of vincristine, actinomycin, cyclophosphamide, and doxorubicin was the primary therapy in the 1960s and 1970s.[28] In 1975, Samuels and colleagues[29] introduced bleomycin with vinblastine for advanced-stage testicular tumors, and in 1977, Einhorn and Donohue[3] reported success with cisplatin, vinblastine, and bleomycin in disseminated testicular cancer. This therapy dramatically transformed the treatment of germ cell tumors. Even after the introduction of cisplatin-based regimens, the early results in children were poor. A report from the Children's Cancer Group (CCG) of children treated between 1978 and 1984, using cisplatin and bleomycin alternating with other agents (cyclophosphamide, dactinomycin, and doxorubicin), reported 4-year survival and event-free survival (EFS) of 54% and 49%, respectively, with ovarian tumors higher at 67% and 63%, respectively, and extragonadal tumors at 48% and 42%, respectively.[30] The lower survival in the early study may have been due to the inclusion of less effective chemotherapy that lengthened the intervals between the courses of the more effective cisplatin and bleomycin.

The subsequent CCG/Pediatric Oncology Group (POG) intergroup studies conducted between 1990 and 1996 used only cisplatin, etoposide, and bleomycin (PEB). The overall 6-year survival was 95.7% for stage I and II ovarian and testes and 88.9% for stage III-IV gonadal and stage I-IV extragonadal.[31–33] The higher-risk group (stage III-IV gonadal and stage I-IV extragonadal) were stratified to either standard or high-dose cisplatin, and the overall survival was not different between the groups, but the toxicity was higher with the high-dose cisplatin, and it has therefore not been incorporated in the current study.

Based on these past studies, the current COG protocol for malignant germ cell tumors is risk based (Fig. 37-2). The overall goal is to maintain the excellent survival from the past intergroup study while decreasing the toxicity of the chemotherapy. Mature teratoma is considered to be a benign lesion, and these tumors are not entered on the current protocol. Immature teratomas at all sites are treated with surgery and observation. The 3-year survival for immature teratomas on the last study was 93% among 73 patients with immature teratoma, and four of the five recurrences were salvaged with platinum-based chemotherapy.[13,34] Stage I ovarian and testes tumors are treated with surgery and observation, although this portion of the protocol is currently suspended (see Ovary section). Stage II-III ovary and stage II-IV testes currently receive three cycles of PEB administered during 3 days compared with four cycles during 5 days on the prior study, thus resulting in significantly less total chemotherapy. Higher-risk tumors (stage IV ovary and stage III-IV extragonadal), are currently not a part of a protocol but would received PEB.

Testes

CLINICAL PRESENTATION AND INITIAL EVALUATION

Testicular germ cell tumors in children are one of the rarer germ cell tumor types, with an incidence of 0.5 to 2.0 per 100,000.[35] The bimodal age distribution of testes tumors, with a small peak in the first 3 years of life and a much larger peak in young adults, suggests a difference in the tumors of these age groups. The malignant germ cell tumors in the younger group are predominantly yolk sac tumors, whereas most adolescent and adult testes tumors are seminomas and mixed tumors. Several other factors provide evidence of differences between pediatric and adult testes tumors. Intratubular germ cell neoplasia (ITGCN), which is a carcinoma in situ, is commonly identified in adults with malignant germ cell tumors but does not occur in association with prepubertal yolk sac tumor. Adult testes tumors usually have a chromosomal gain of the short arm of chromosome 12p (isochromosome 12p), whereas this is not seen in prepubertal yolk sac tumors.

Testicular tumors are rare in boys prior to puberty, and during this time non–germ cell Sertoli tumors and paratesticular rhabdomyosarcomas are more common, whereas germ cell tumors predominate in pubertal and adult males. Paratesticular neuroblastoma has also been reported arising from an embryonic adrenal rest along the spermatic cord.[36,37] Although it is difficult to determine the incidence of malignancy in prepubertal testes tumors, several reports would suggest that it is less common than in adults. In one large series,[38] 74% of all tumors were benign, with teratoma accounting for 48% and yolk sac tumors only 5%. This has affected the initial surgical evaluation of these children in order to avoid unnecessary radical orchiectomy.

Low risk	
Stage 1 ovary	
Stage 1 testes	Surgery alone
Immature teratoma	COG, AGCT 0132

Intermediate risk	
Stage II–III ovary	
Stage II–IV testes	Surgery and
	Chemo-PEB x 3
Stage I–II extragonadal	COG, AGCT 132

High risk	
Stage III–IV extragonadal	Surgery and
Stage IV ovary	PEB

FIGURE 37-2 Low- and intermediate-risk–based scheme for pediatric germ cell tumors. Children's Oncology Group AGCT 0132, opened November 2003.

Most testicular tumors present as a painless scrotal mass. In the intergroup CCG/POG study (1990 to 1996)[31] of malignant testes tumors, 76% of the stage 1 boys presented with a testicular mass and 17% with generalized scrotal swelling. The preoperative diagnosis was tumor in 79%, hydrocele in 11%, hernia in 3%, and acute scrotum or torsion in 3%.

Preoperative workup includes a thorough physical examination, looking for signs of androgenization as well as metastatic disease. Metastatic disease is relatively uncommon in prepubertal testes cancer, but if present, is usually in the retroperitoneum or chest. Testicular ultrasonography is useful to identify extratesticular lesions and may be useful to identify or raise the suspicion of a teratoma. Benign testes tumors tend to be well circumscribed with sharp borders and decreased blood flow on Doppler studies.[39] Preoperative AFP levels should be obtained, and this level was elevated in 98% of the children with malignant tumors in the most recent study.[31] If the preoperative diagnosis is a testicular malignancy (elevated AFP), it is reasonable to obtain an abdominal computed tomography (CT) scan, because the presence of enlarged nodes after an inguinal exploration can be due to either a reactive or malignant process.

OPERATIVE MANAGEMENT

The standard approach consists of an inguinal incision, with initial control of the vessels at the level of the internal inguinal ring with subsequent mobilization of the testes. A preoperative elevation of AFP indicates the presence of yolk sac tumor and thus precludes consideration of testes-sparing surgery, and a radical orchiectomy is performed with ligation of the cord at the internal ring. If the AFP is normal, there is a much greater chance that the mass represents a benign lesion, and in these instances, the field can be draped off and the tunica opened. Enucleation is often possible, leaving a large amount of residual normal testes.[40] If frozen section analysis reveals a benign lesion, the tunica is closed, and if malignant, an orchiectomy is completed. Unfortunately, this is not always possible, and in a recent review from the U.K. Children's Cancer Group, 48 of 53 boys with mature or immature teratoma had radical orchiectomy.[41] There were no recurrences in the five treated with enucleation. Bilateral testes-sparing surgery

Stage	Extent of disease
I	Limited to testis (testes), completely resected by high inguinal orchiectomy; no clinical, radiographic or histologic evidence of disease beyond the testes.
II	Transscrotal biopsy; microscopic disease in scrotum or high in spermatic cord (<5 cm from proximal end). Tumor markers fail to normalize or decrease with an appropriate half-life.
III	Retroperitoneal lymph node involvement, but no visceral or extraabdominal involvement. Lymph nodes > 4 cm by CT; or > 2 cm and < 4 cm with biopsy proof.
IV	Distant metastases, including liver.

FIGURE 37-3 Current Children's Oncology Group staging system for childhood testes cancer.

TABLE 37-1

Survival for Testes Cancer, POG/CCG 9048/8891; 9049/8882, 1990-1996

Stage	N	Treatment	6-Year EFS (%)	6-Year Survival (%)
I	63 S	78.5	100	
II	17	S + PEB × 4	100	100
III	17	S + HDP/EB vs. PEB	94.1	100
IV	43	S + HDP/EB vs. PEB	88.3	90.6

CCG, Children's Cancer Group; EB, etoposide and bleomycin chemotherapy; EFS, event-free survival; HDP, high-dose platinum chemotherapy; PEB, platinum, etoposide, and bleomycin chemotherapy; POG, Pediatric Oncology Group; S, surgery.

has been reported for testes teratoma.[42] A more recent report noted no atrophy or recurrence with enucleation in a large group of benign testes tumors.[43]

POSTSURGICAL TREATMENT

Testicular teratomas are benign lesions and are treated with enucleation, if possible, and then postoperative observation. Testicular immature teratomas are also benign germ cell tumors, and surgery alone (enucleation if possible) is definitive treatment. Higher-grade immature teratomas are, however, associated with yolk sac tumors. In a (CCG/POG) review, grade 1 and 2 immature teratomas were not associated with yolk sac tumors, whereas 2 of 3 grade 3 lesions were associated with yolk sac tumors.[13]

Yolk sac tumor is the primary malignant prepubertal testes cancer. The current staging is noted in Fig. 37-3. The role of surgery alone for stage I testes tumors was reported in the 1980s[44] and confirmed in an initial small series.[45] The U.K. Children's Cancer Study Group[46] and the Testicular Tumor Registry of the Section of Urology of the American Academy of Pediatrics,[47] in larger series (73 and 181 children, respectively), confirmed the safety of surgery alone for stage I malignant testes tumors.

The intergroup trial of testes cancer (CCG/POG; 1990–1996)[31] confirmed the excellent outcome with stage 1 testes tumors treated with surgery alone (Table 37-1). This study of 63 boys (median age 16 months) reported AFP elevation in 98%. In patients with the preoperative diagnosis of tumor, the surgical guidelines were followed in 84% of boys but were followed in only 27% with a nontumor diagnosis. Although overall adherence to surgical guidelines did not affect outcome, scrotal violation was associated with a 75% recurrence rate compared with 15.5% in those without scrotal violation. All recurrences were successfully treated with surgery and chemotherapy.

Stage 2 boys on the CCG/POG study included only 17 patients, and 11 were stage II because of a transcrotal procedure.[32] Survival was excellent (see Table 37-1) with surgery and chemotherapy. Higher-stage 3 and 4 boys received surgery and were then randomized to standard or high-dose cisplatin, both with etoposide and bleomycin.[33] Sixteen were recurrences from stage 1 disease (median age 3.1 years), and the rest were newly diagnosed and much older (median age 16 years). Despite the advanced disease, outcome was

excellent (see Table 37-1). The toxicity with high-dose cisplatin was significant without added benefit, and it has therefore been eliminated from current protocols.

The current protocol of the Children's Oncology Group is designed to reduce the total dose and days of chemotherapy (Fig. 37-2). As noted in the staging, if the retroperitoneal nodes are greater than 4 cm in size, it is assumed to be due to tumor, whereas nodes between 2 and 4 cm require biopsy to confirm status. There is no role for retroperitoneal lymph node dissection in prepubertal yolk sac tumors at diagnosis and simple biopsy is adequate.

Ovary

CLINICAL PRESENTATION AND EVALUATION

Ovarian tumors are the most common site for germ cell tumors in children and adolescents. Eighty to 90% percent of all ovarian masses are benign (epithelial cyst, mature teratoma), often with predominant cystic components.[10,48] Presenting symptoms often include pain and gradual onset of lower abdominal fullness. Approximately 10% present with an acute abdomen secondary to torsion or tumor rupture.[10] Of all girls presenting with ovarian torsion, only 1.8% to 3% are malignant tumors; however, 33% are benign tumors, including teratoma and cystadenoma.[48]

In nonacute cases, preoperative evaluation should include assessment of AFP and beta-HCG, as well as ultrasonography and usually abdominal and pelvic CT scan. Unfortunately, reliable tumor markers are absent in many tumors. Germinoma is present in one third of malignant tumors, and they have normal markers or mild elevation of beta-HCG, and embryonal carcinomas have normal markers.[2] Benign lesions are primarily cystic, and a 2% risk of malignancy in cystic lesions is frequently quoted based on adult series.[49–51] This, however, is also unreliable, because in the recent intergroup study from the Children's Oncology Group (COG), 57% of malignant tumors had cystic components.[10] A recent study attempting to identify risk factors noted that markers were elevated in only 54% of malignant tumors. The best predictors were a mass with solid characteristics and a mass greater than 8 cm in diameter.[52] They also noted as, in other series, that girls between 1 and 8 years have the greatest incidence of malignancy. In view of these observations, great care should be taken to perform a proper staging operation with lesions with solid components.

1. Collect ascites or peritoneal washings for cytology
2. Examine peritoneal surface and liver; excise suspicious lesions
3. Unilateral oophorectomy
4. Examine contralateral ovary and biopsy if suspicious lesion
5. Examine omentum and remove if adherent or involved
6. Inspection of retroperitoneal lymph nodes, biopsy of enlarged nodes

FIGURE 37-4 Operative procedure for malignant ovarian germ cell tumor.

Stage I: Limited to ovary (ovaries) peritoneal washings negative; tumor markers normal after appropriate half-life decline (AFP 5 days, HCG 16 hours).

Stage II: Microscopic residual; peritoneal washings negative for malignant cells, tumor markers positive or negative.

Stage III: Lymph node involvement; gross residual or biopsy only; contiguous visceral involvement (omentum, intestine, bladder); peritoneal washings positive for malignant cells; tumor markers positive or negative.

Stage IV: Distant metastases, including liver.

FIGURE 37-5 Children's Oncology Group ovarian staging system. AFP, alpha fetoprotein; HCG, human chorionic gonadotropin.

The staging procedure endorsed by COG is listed in Figure 37-4 and the current staging system in Figure 37-5. The importance of an accurate and complete staging procedure and accurate pathologic evaluation cannot be overemphasized. The recent COG intergroup study of 131 girls reported positive ascites/peritoneal fluid in 23 of 100 girls, and 5 of these would have otherwise been stage I tumors.[10] This is particularly relevant, because the current low- and intermediate-risk COG study manages stage I girls with surgery alone.

The survival rates of children in the most recent intergroup study is listed in Table 37-2. The current therapy for ovarian malignant tumors is noted in Figure 37-2. In the most recent study,[33] the results for stage IV ovarian tumors did not allow them to be included in the current low- and intermediate-risk COG study (AGCT 0132) using reduced chemotherapy.

Some tumors are noted with invasion into surrounding structures, and in these cases, recommendations are for initial biopsy, neoadjuvant chemotherapy, and delayed resection. Bilateral ovarian tumors were observed in 8% of girls on the recent study, and 4 of the 11 contralateral tumors were benign teratomas. The current recommendation for bilateral tumors is to attempt ovarian preservation, if possible, on the least involved side, attempting to find a plane of demarcation between the tumor and normal ovarian tissue. The larger tumor should be removed and sent for frozen section. If the first side is malignant and the contralateral side is greater than 10 cm, it should also be removed.

The treatment algorithm for malignant ovarian tumors is surgery and observation for stage I and surgery and chemotherapy for higher-stage tumors (see Fig. 37-2). The surgery-only arm was based on a German and French series of a total of 39 girls with stage I tumors treated with surgery alone who experience a 67% EFS with salvage of 12 of 13 recurrences with chemotherapy for an overall survival of 97.4%.[53,54] The CCG/POG intergroup study noted excellent results in girls with stage I immature teratoma, with microscopic yolk sac tumor

TABLE 37-2

Event-free Survival (EFS) and Survival in Pediatric Ovarian Germ Cell Tumors, POG/COG Intergroup Study 1990-1996

Stage	N	Treatment	6-Year EFS (%)	6-Year Survival (%)
I	41	S + PEB	95	95.1
II	16	S + PEB	87.5	93.8
III	58	S + HDP/EB vs. PEB	96.6	97.3
IV	16	S + HDP/EB vs. PEB	86.7	93.3

CCG, Children's Cancer Group; EB, etoposide and bleomycin chemotherapy; HDP, high-dose cisplatin chemotherapy; PEB, cisplatin, etoposide, and bleomycin chemotherapy; POG, Pediatric Oncology Group; S, surgery.

treated with surgery alone as well as stage I girls treated with surgery and PEB.[55] The current low-risk arm of the study has been closed because of a higher than expected recurrence rate in stage I ovarian tumors. These girls had a less than 70% three-year EFS, thus leading to suspension of the trial; however, with salvage chemotherapy, they have an overall survival of over 95%.[56]

Laparoscopy has been widely used for ovarian cystic disease, and the application of this for malignant procedures has been controversial. The primary concern is adequate completion of the staging procedure (potential understaging) and avoidance of intraperitoneal spill or tumor rupture, which could upstage a stage I to a stage II tumor. The COG germ cell committee and others[10,57] recommend laparotomy for known malignancy; however, this is difficult to determine preoperatively, although preoperative elevated markers and a large solid mass are very suggestive of malignancy. A recent French study suggested that size greater than 7.5 cm or predominately solid components predicted malignancy and thus required laparotomy.[57]

Most primarily cystic lesions, some of which are large, are benign, and a laparoscopic approach is appropriate. One option to avoid spill is to either excise the cyst, as a cystectomy or oophorectomy, and then place it in a retrieval bag, which is then delivered out of the umbilical opening, allowing decompression of the cyst while in the bag without spill and then removal of the bag and cyst. A second option is to glue a bag to the cyst through a small laparotomy, using one of the adhesives, such as cyanoacrylate, as described by Shozu and colleagues.[58] The cyst is incised by cutting through the center of the bag–cyst interface, allowing removal of the fluid without spill, and the decompressed cyst is then delivered from the abdominal cavity. The cyst can then be separated from the normal ovary as a cystectomy, or if not possible or if there is concern for malignancy, an oophorectomy.

Sacrococcygeal Tumors

CLINICAL PRESENTATION AND INITIAL EVALUATION

Tumors of the sacrococcygeal region, referred to as sacrococcygeal teratomas (SCTs) in most reports, generally present in two distinct fashions: neonates with large predominantly external lesions, which are detected in utero or at birth and are rarely malignant (Fig. 37-6); and older infants and children who present with primarily hidden pelvic tumors with a much higher rate of malignancy (Fig. 37-7). Sacrococcygeal teratomas are the most common extragonadal tumor in neonates, accounting for up to 70% of all teratomas in childhood. A 3 to 4:1 female to male ratio is generally reported.[59] Newborns typically present with a mass protruding from the sacral region, and many are detected with prenatal ultrasonography. Abdominal delivery should be considered if the external mass is greater than 5 cm, to avoid dystocia and rupture.[60] In-utero shunting can lead to fetal hydrops, which is associated with high mortality. Adzick and colleagures[61] performed the first successful fetal resection in a fetus that developed placentomegaly and polyhydramnios and, at 25 weeks, underwent

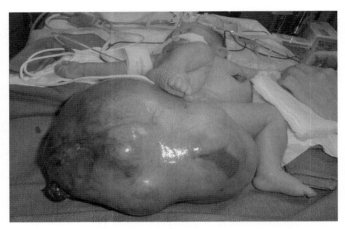

FIGURE 37-6 A newborn with a large ruptured sacrococcygeal teratoma. *(See Expert Consult site for color version.)*

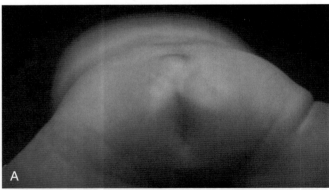

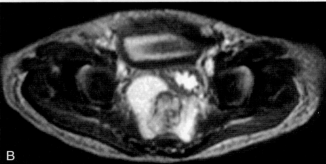

FIGURE 37-7 **A,** Three-month-old boy with a small external mass noted since birth. **B,** Underlying presacral mass noted on magnetic resonance imaging. *(See Expert Consult site for color version.)*

fetal resection of a 400-g immature teratoma. After delivery at 29 weeks, the child underwent exploration, with no residual tumor identified.

Makin and colleagues[62] reported a 77% survival among 41 antenatally diagnosed SCTs but noted survival of 50% in those undergoing fetal interventions and survival of only 14% if the intervention was for hydrops. Intervention included nonresection procedures, such as cyst drainage, laser ablation, or alcohol sclerosis. Another study of prenatally detected lesions noted the highest survival (100%) in lesions less than 10 cm with predominantly cystic tumors, whereas survival was only 48% in tumors greater than 10 cm and in those with increased vascularity, vascular steal syndrome, or rapid growth.[63] This is a difficult group, and the University of California San Francisco experience with fetal resection noted a survival of 20%.[64]

Older infants and children typically present with symptoms related to compression of the bladder or rectum. If a mass has been noted at birth and left in place, an increased rate of malignancy has been noted.[65] AFP levels, which can be normally elevated in newborns, should be obtained and then followed to ensure that they return to normal by 9 months of age. An association of the triad of presacral teratoma, anal stenosis, and sacral defects was first reported by Ashcraft and Holder, who also confirmed the autosomal dominant nature of the condition.[66] Currarino proposed that adhesions between the endoderm and ectoderm form, causing a split notochord that results in this association, and the triad now bears his name.[67]

CLASSIFICATION AND ASSOCIATION WITH MALIGNANCY

Altman and colleagues[68] developed the classification system of SCTs based on a survey of the Surgical Section of the American Academy of Pediatrics (Fig. 37-8). In this study, the malignancy rate increased with the more hidden (type III and IV) lesions. This survey also noted the low rate of malignancy in neonates and young infants (≤2 months of age, 7% girls and 10% boys have malignant tumors) and the higher rates in older infants and children (≥2 months of age, 48% girls and 67% boys have malignant tumors). Several subsequent studies have confirmed this and noted malignancy rates as high as 90%.[65,69]

SURGICAL MANAGEMENT

In neonates presenting with large external masses, the degree of pelvic and abdominal involvement should be assessed preoperatively with either ultrasonography, CT, or magnetic resonance imaging (MRI), and these studies may also offer a clue as to the characteristics of the vascular supply. An open or laparoscopic abdominal exploration may be required to mobilize the pelvic portion and to divide the middle sacral artery.

The neonatal type I and II lesions can usually be approached with the child in the prone position (Fig. 37-9). Removal of the coccyx is an essential step, because Gross and colleagues[70] reported a 37% recurrence rate if it was not removed. In view of the anterior displacement caused by the large mass, the rectum is often brought back to a more posterior location at the time of closure. Fishman and colleagues[71] described a buttocks contouring closure bringing

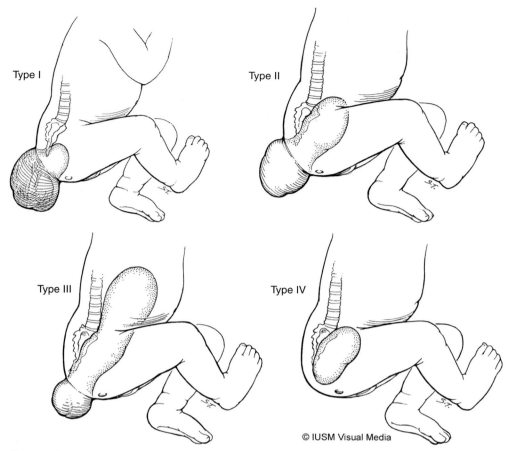

FIGURE 37-8 Classification of sacrococcygeal teratomas based on Altman's study: Type I (46.7% of reported cases) predominantly external, type II (34.7%) external with intrapelvic extension, type III (8.8%) visible externally but predominantly pelvic and abdominal, type IV (9.8%) entirely presacral. (Adapted from Altman RP, Randolph JG, Lilly JR: Sacrococcygeal teratoma: American Academy of Pediatric Surgical Section Survey—1973. J Pediatr Surg 1974;9:389-398.)

the ventral portion of the lateral flaps to a more posterior location, thus resulting in a transverse posterior incision and two vertical incisions in the midportion of each buttock. The operative approach in older infants and children is similar; however, due to the presence of malignancy in many of these cases with invasion of adjacent structures or massive size, initial resection is not possible, and an initial biopsy followed by neoadjuvant chemotherapy is the best mode of management (Fig. 37-10). In the CCG/POG Intergroup study, there was no survival difference between initial and delayed rejections, supporting surgical delay in these cases.[72]

POSTOPERATIVE MANAGEMENT

The staging system for extragonadal tumors is noted in Figure 37-11. Most neonatal tumors are mature or immature teratomas that can be managed by surgery and postoperative observation. Recurrent tumors are noted in 10% to 20% of initially benign tumors, and 50% of these are malignant recurrences.[65,73] The recurrence may be due to a sampling error of the original tumor, incomplete resection of a malignant focus, or transformation of a small benign remnant into a malignant lesion. The large size of the neonatal tumors and frequent cystic components can often result in rupture during resection. Follow-up of these neonates should include

serial AFP levels to ensure return to normal by 9 months of age and rectal examination every 3 months until 3 years of age, because the latest reported recurrence has been at 33 months.[65]

The management of the older infants with malignant tumors has been influenced by the chemosensitive nature of these yolk sac tumors. In the intergroup study of 74 infants and children (median age 21 months; 62 girls, 12 boys), 59% had metastatic disease at diagnosis, and the initial procedure was biopsy in 45 patients and resection in 29 patients.[72] All patients received chemotherapy, and postchemotherapy resection was accomplished in all but three patients. Definitive resection required a sacral approach in 63% and a combined abdominal-sacral approach in 35%. The 4-year EFS and survival was 84 ± 6% and 90 ± 4%, respectively, with no significant difference noted between timing of resection or presence of metastatic disease. In view of these results, it is strongly recommended to avoid resection of normal structures at initial exploration.

Long-term follow-up of the newborns and older children is necessary, because neuropathic bladder or bowel abnormalities have been reported in 35% to 41% of survivors.[74,75] A recent report from the U.K. Children's Cancer Group noted that 10 of 95 survivors of sacrococcygeal tumors had a neuropathic bladder, and two had leg weakness.[41] In a large survey of

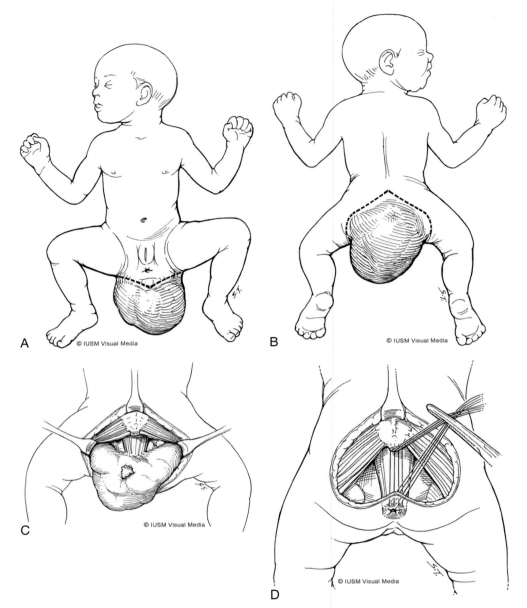

FIGURE 37-9   **A** and **B,** Operative excision of sacrococcygeal teratoma in a neonate with an inverted-V incision. **C** and **D,** The tumor along with the coccyx is excised with careful preservation of the rectum.

79 patients from the Netherlands, 9.2% reported involuntary bowel movements, 13.2% suffered from soiling, 16% had constipation, and 30% reported difficulty with urinary control,[76] with all of these correlating with decline in their quality of life. Interestingly, the Altman classification of the tumor did not correlate with the occurrence of these long-term complications.

Mediastinal Germ Cell Tumors

Mediastinal tumors are relatively common in childhood and adolescence and are more common in boys than girls. Germ cell tumors compromise approximately 6% to 18% of mediastinal tumors,[77] and of these, 86% are benign.[78] Mediastinal germ cell tumors are typically located in the anterior mediastinum. Younger children present predominantly with respiratory symptoms. The most common symptoms during adolescence include chest pain, precocious puberty, or facial fullness related to superior vena caval obstruction. Klinefelter's syndrome is also observed in the adolescent group as are hematologic malignancies. The histology of the malignant mediastinal germ cell tumors is more heterogeneous than other sites. In the intergroup study of 38 children, yolk sac was seen in boys less than 5 years of age and in all girls; the older boys had mixed malignant tumors in greater than 50%.[9] Reflective of this, the AFP was elevated in 29 cases and beta-HCG in 16 cases.

Anterior mediastinal tumors pose significant anesthetic risks because of airway compression and may affect the anesthetic from compression as well as the weight of the tumor,

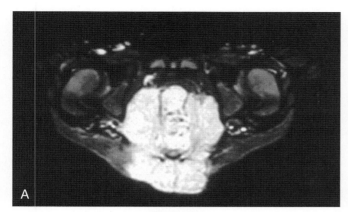

Diagnosis

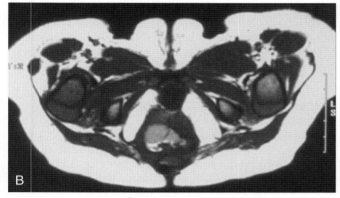

Postchemotherapy

FIGURE 37-10 A, Appearance of a large unresectable malignant yolk sac tumor treated with biopsy and neoadjuvant chemotherapy. **B,** Residual postchemotherapy tumor.

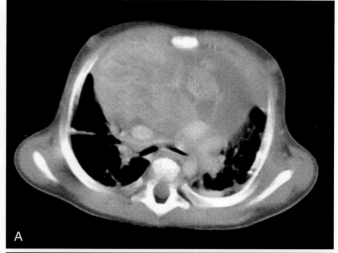

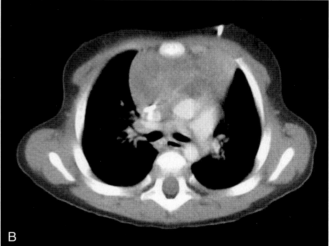

FIGURE 37-12 A, Appearance of a large mediastinal mass causing tracheal compression and cardiac displacement. **B,** Appearance after neoadjuvant chemotherapy.

leading to further compression with loss of spontaneous ventilation. An early report suggested increased risk of respiratory collapse upon induction of anesthesia if the trachea was compressed by one third of the cross-sectional area.[79] Shamberger and colleagues,[80] added pulmonary function tests and observed that general anesthesia was well tolerated if both the tracheal area and the peak expiratory flow rate were greater than 50% of predicted. Alternatives to general anesthesia for diagnostic procedures in children in these situations include aspiration of pleural fluid and needle biopsy or open biopsy

Extragonadal germ cell tumors:

Stage	Extent of disease
I	Complete resection at any site, coccygectomy for sacrococcygeal site, negative tumor margins.
II	Microscopic residual: lymph nodes negative.
III	Lymph node involvement with metastatic disease. Gross residual or biopsy only; retroperitoneal nodes negative or positive.
IV	Distant metastases, including liver.

FIGURE 37-11   Staging system for extragonadal germ cell tumors.

under local anesthesia. Open biopsy can be performed using an anterior thoracotomy (Chamberlin procedure) with excision of a segment of costal cartilage.[81]

In the intergroup study ($N = 38$) 14 children underwent initial resection, with 12 survivors.[9] Twenty-two patients underwent biopsy followed by neoadjuvant chemotherapy and subsequent resection in 18, with 13 survivors. The size of the mass was reduced by a mean of 57% in 12 of the patients and was stable or increased in 6 (Fig. 37-12). Four patients had no further surgery, because of complete radiographic resolution in 1, progressive disease in 1, and death from toxicity in 2. Eight of 10 image-guided biopsies were successful. Of 31 resections, 20 were by median sternotomy and 11 by thoracotomy. Excision was frequently reported as difficult because of adherence to the major arteries and veins as well as the phrenic and vagus nerves and the lung and thymus. The overall survival was 71%, which is higher than the historical series but lower than survivals reported for the other extragonadal sites. The outcome was superior in the patients with yolk sac tumors, and all of the tumor deaths were noted in adolescent boys with mixed germ cell tumors.

Abdominal and Retroperitoneal Germ Cell Tumors

Retroperitoneal and abdominal germ cell tumors account for approximately 4% of germ cell tumors in children. Most present in infancy, although several have been indentified antenatally.[82] Eighty percent were less than 5 years of age in the recent intergroup (CCG/POG) study.[83] Mass and pain are the most common presenting symptoms, but fever, weight loss, constipation, and acute abdomen are also reported. An unusual group within this cohort are the infants with choriocarcinoma, which are thought to be primary placental tumors with metastases to the fetal liver. The beta-HCG production can lead to precocious puberty, and these infants usually present with hepatomegaly and anemia in the first 7 months of life.

Most retroperitoneal germ cell tumors are mature and immature teratomas; reports have noted malignancy rates between 0% and 24%, with the highest percentage occurring in infants.[82,84–87] The histologic pattern of the malignant tumors is most commonly pure yolk sac (63%), but also includes choriocarcinoma and mixed tumors. In the intergroup study,[83] 19 of 24 of the malignant tumors had elevated AFP, indicating yolk sac components were present but also illustrating the difficulty of determining malignancy preoperatively. Prior to attempting resection, a search for metastatic disease is appropriate, because nearly 90% of those with malignancy have stage III or IV disease at presentation.[83]

Primary resection should be attempted if preoperative imaging suggests lack of contiguous organ involvement or metastatic disease. Unfortunately, the benign tumors can also encase blood vessels, and the hazardous nature of these operations was demonstrated by two recent reports about several major vascular, biliary, and intestinal injuries.[82,86] In the intergroup study of 25 children, only 5 underwent initial resection, 13 had resection after chemotherapy and biopsy, or there was partial resection in 7.[83] Of note, 4 had no residual tumor after chemotherapy. The outcome with modern chemotherapy has dramatically improved the outcomes of children with these lesions from a historical survival of less than 20%[59] to current 6-year EFS of 82.8 ± 10.9% and overall survival of 87.6 ± 9.3%.[83] There are other rare abdominal sites that may present later in life, and yolk sac tumors of the pelvis and uterus have been reported in adult patients.[88–90]

Genital (Vaginal) Germ Cell Tumors

Genital lesions are rare and most commonly involve the vagina in girls. Although early reports of surgery alone reported survival rates of 50%, survival has improved with the addition of platinum-based adjuvant chemotherapy.[91,92] Vaginal lesions generally occur in girls less than 3 years of age who usually present with vaginal bleeding. A mass is typically identified within and often protruding from the vagina and uterus, and the actual site of origin may be difficult to ascertain. The CCG/POG report of 13 genital lesions (12 vaginal, 1 penile) confirmed the efficacy of platinum-based chemotherapy administered in a neoadjuvant fashion, with ultimate preservation of the vagina in 10 of 12 girls.[93] This is best accomplished by initial biopsy, followed by chemotherapy, and subsequent excision of the residual tumor, with the goal of partial vaginectomy. Although there is no role for initial total vaginectomy or hysterectomy, this rarely may be required in chemoresistant cases.

Cervicofacial Teratomas

This rare site accounts for 5% to 6% of teratomas, which generally present in the neonatal period with large tumors. Most are mature or immature teratomas, but up to 20% are malignant.[94] A review of 20 neonates noted that 35% presented with airway obstruction.[94] A more recent report of seven giant fetal cervical teratomas observed that four developed hydrops (two died, one aborted), with one undergoing fetal resection.[95] Three neonates without hydrops underwent ex utero intrapartum treatment (EXIT) with intubation, tracheostomy, and resection on placental support in one each. If there is no evidence of hydrops, these can be followed to term. If the fetus is sufficiently mature (≥28 weeks) and hydrops is present, the fetus can undergo delivery; however, if the gestational age is less than 28 weeks, fetal resection should be considered.[95]

Gastric Teratomas

Tumors at this location generally present within the first few months of life with abdominal distention, bleeding, or symptoms of gastric outlet obstruction because of the gastric mass.[96] We have seen older children present with pain and obstructive symptoms as a primary cystic component has enlarged. These tumors occur primarily in males, and there are no reported malignancies at this site. Resection with primary closure of the stomach is the treatment of choice.

The complete reference list is available online at www.expertconsult.com.

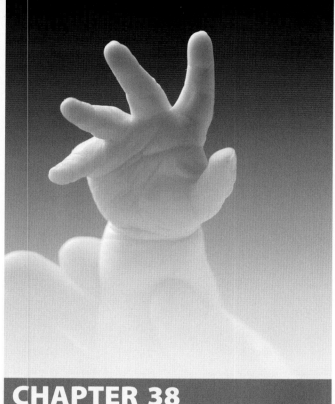

CHAPTER 38

Hodgkin Lymphoma and Non-Hodgkin Lymphoma

Peter F. Ehrlich

Hodgkin Lymphoma

Hodgkin lymphoma (HL) is one of the few cancers that affect both adults and children with a wide spectrum of histopathologic and clinical presentations. Unlike many other cancers, the adult and pediatric forms have similar biology and natural history. Pediatric HL accounts for 12% of all HL cases and represents 6% of all childhood cancers. Cure rates for pediatric HL are excellent, approaching 90% to 95% (Fig. 38-1).[1,2] Despite these excellent rates of cure, treatment can result in significant short-term and long-term morbidity. The aims of current therapeutic trials are to maintain or improve on outcomes while reducing short-term and long-term complications of therapy.[3]

Hodgkin lymphoma is named after Thomas Hodgkin, a British pathologist, who in 1832 described the disease in a paper titled *On Some Morbid Appearances of the Absorbent Glands and Spleen.*[4] One hundred and fifty years later, with the advent of microscopic histology, Sternberg (1898) and Reed (1902) described the distinctive multinucleated giant cell with the prominent nucleoli that are characteristic of Hodgkin disease (HD) (Fig. 38-2). They showed that these cells, now referred to as Reed-Sternberg cells, are derived from germinal center B cells.[5,6] Radiotherapy was the first reported "curative" treatment for HL in the 1930s.[7] In 1950, Peters published the first long-term series of survivors (20 years) treated with radiotherapy.[8] Single-agent chemotherapy (nitrogen mustard) was used to treat HL in 1946, and multiagent treatment with MOPP (Mustargen [mechlorethamine], Oncovin [vincristine], procarbazine, prednisone) was reported in 1967.[9,10] In the 1960s, the staging laparotomy was increasingly used to identify sites of involvement and for research purposes.[11] In the 1980s, oncologists began to appreciate the long-term morbidity of the chemotherapy and radiotherapy regimens used to treat patients with HL. Thus multimodality therapy designed to maintain outcomes while reducing toxicity were initiated. Currently, biologically based therapies, both immunotherapy and small molecules, are being investigated for use as primary and relapse therapy.

INCIDENCE AND EPIDEMIOLOGY

Hodgkin lymphoma accounts for 6% of all pediatric malignancies, with an incidence of about 6 cases per 1 million, with a bimodal distribution with peaks in adolescence (15 to 19 years) and after age 55 years. HL is exceedingly rare in children less than 5 years of age.[12] Epidemiologic studies identify three forms of HL: two that involve the pediatric population and one in adults. Childhood HL is found in children less than 14 years old and accounts for 10% to 12% of cases; adolescent young adults (AYA) HL is defined as occurring in those 15 to 35 years of age and accounts for greater than 50% of the cases. It is the most commonly diagnosed cancer among adolescents 15 to 19 years of age. Older adults HL occurs in those older than 55 years of age and comprises 35% of the cases.[13]

Childhood HL is more common in males, and the histology is more likely to be mixed cellularity or nodular lymphocyte predominant. Risk factors include increasing family size, lower socioeconomic status, and exposure to the Epstein-Barr virus (EBV).[14–17] The EBV viral infection appears to precede tumor cell expansion, and EBV may act alone or in conjunction with other carcinogens.

The AYA form has no gender predilection, and the most common form is nodular sclerosis. Risk factors include higher socioeconomic status, early birth order, smaller family size, and EBV. In the AYA forms, it is hypothesized that EBV exposure is delayed (as opposed to the childhood form), suggesting that delayed exposure to EBV or some other unidentified common infectious agent may be a risk factor for AYA HL.[16–19]

Hodgkin lymphoma is derived from a single transformed B cell that has undergone monoclonal expansion. Classic cells include Reed-Sternberg, lymphocytic, and histiocytic cells. There are also many cytokine-producing and cytokine-responding cells that are responsible for the nonspecific signs and symptoms seen with this tumor. Immune system dysfunction is hypothesized to be one of the primary causes for Hodgkin lymphoma. In the childhood form, it is thought to result from immune immaturity, whereas in the adult form, it is thought to result from immune dysregulation. Support for this hypothesis is found in diseases with altered immune states in which an increased incidence of HL is seen, including

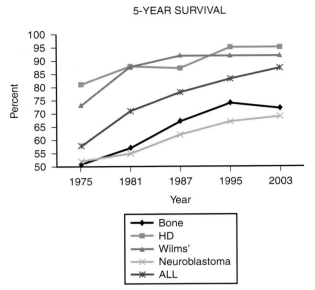

5-YEAR SURVIVAL

FIGURE 38-1 Graph shows survival statistics of different pediatric cancers from 1975 to 2003.

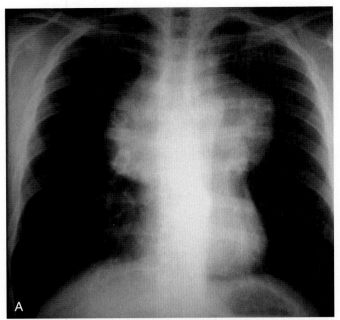

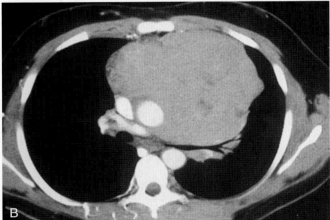

FIGURE 38-3 **A,** Chest radiograph demonstrating a large anterior mediastinal mass. **B,** Computed tomography scan demonstrating a large anterior mediastinal mass.

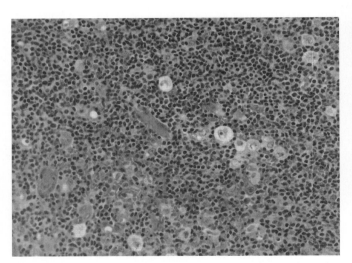

FIGURE 38-2 High-power hematoxylin and eosin–stained slide of a patient with nodular sclerosis Hodgkin lymphoma with typical Reed-Sternberg cells. *(See Expert Consult site for color version.)*

patients with human immunodeficiency viral infection, other acquired immunodeficiency states (post–solid organ or hematopoietic stem cell transplantation), and autoimmune disorders or a family history of autoimmune disorders.[20–24]

CLINICAL PRESENTATION

Hodgkin lymphoma must be considered in any child with lymphadenopathy. Involved nodes are described as firm, nodular, and painless. Children and adolescents most frequently present with cervical and or supraclavicular lymphadenopathy (80%). Patients presenting primarily with enlarged axillary nodes (25% of all cases) or inguinal nodes (5%) are far less common. Associated mediastinal disease is found in up to 75% of adolescents and 33% of children.[13,25–27] Mediastinal

involvement must be assessed prior to any operative intervention; involvement may be extensive and produce major complications upon the induction of anesthesia (Fig. 38-3) Patient's may also present with B symptoms, including fever greater than 38° C, soaking night sweats, and weight loss of 10% or more. These symptoms are not specific to HL and can occur in non-Hodgkin lymphoma. The presence or absence of B symptoms, which occur in up to a third of children, has prognostic significance and is reflected in the staging of HL.[13,25] Respiratory symptoms may also result from large mediastinal masses, including dyspnea on exertion or orthopnea. Itching or pruritus is a frequent finding but is nonspecific.[28]

DIAGNOSIS

A full history and physical examination focusing on nodal areas and the abdomen should be performed. At present there is no specific laboratory test for HL. An excisional biopsy of a suspicious lymph node should be the initial step to diagnosis

TABLE 38-1

Hodgkin Lymphoma Staging: Ann Arbor Classification with Cotswolds Modification

Stage 1	Involvement of a single lymph node region or lymphoid structure (e.g., spleen, thymus, Waldeyer ring) or involvement of a single extralymphatic site
Stage II	Involvement of two or more lymph node regions on the same side of the diaphragm
Stage III III1 III2	Indicates that the cancer has spread to both sides of the diaphragm, including one organ or area near the lymph nodes or the spleen With or without involvement of splenic, hilar, celiac, or portal nodes With involvement of paraaortic, iliac, and mesenteric nodes
Stage IV	Indicates that the cancer has spread to both sides of the diaphragm, including one organ or area near the lymph nodes or the spleen

Modifiers:

A or B: The absence of constitutional (B-type) symptoms is denoted by adding an "A" to the stage; the presence is denoted by adding a "B" to the stage.

E: Used if the disease is "extranodal" (not in the lymph nodes) or has spread from lymph nodes to adjacent tissue.

X: Used if the largest deposit is greater than 10 cm large (bulky disease), or whether the mediastinum is wider than one third of the chest on a chest x-ray.

S: Used if the disease has spread to the spleen.

The nature of the staging is (occasionally) expressed with:

CS: Clinical stage as obtained by doctor's examinations and tests.

PS: Pathologic stage as obtained by exploratory laparotomy (surgery performed through an abdominal incision) with splenectomy (surgical removal of the spleen). Note: Exploratory laparotomy has fallen out of favor for lymphoma staging.

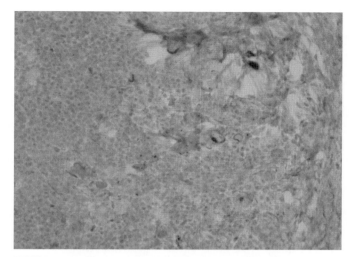

FIGURE 38-4 CD30-positive staining for Reed-Sternberg cells in a patient with Hodgkin lymphoma. *(See Expert Consult site for color version.)*

of Hodgkin lymphoma. Prior to surgery, a chest radiograph must be obtained to assess the presence of mediastinal disease. If a mediastinal mass is detected, a computed tomography (CT) scan of the chest is mandated to assess the tracheal area, and pulmonary function tests further define the extent of respiratory impairment. In some cases, the procedure may need to be performed under local anesthesia because of the size of the mediastinal mass and the resultant respiratory compromise (see Fig. 38-3). Minimally invasive techniques have been used to biopsy mediastinal masses, if no suspicious extrathoracic lymph nodes are available for biopsy. Care must be taken when using a thoracoscopic or laparoscopic technique to ensure that adequate specimens are obtained. A report from the Children's Oncology Group Hodgkin's Lymphoma Committee demonstrated that up to 50% of mediastinal cases required a second diagnostic biopsy when a thoracoscopic biopsy was performed.[29] thoracoscopic biopsy should also be avoided in children with respiratory compromise.

HISTOPATHOLOGY

Reed-Sternberg cells are the pathognomonic cells of HD (see Fig. 38-2). The classification systems for HL have evolved over time from the Rye classification to the Ann Arbor Classification and the Cotswolds modification (Table 38-1).[30-32] The current World Health Organization classification system separates HL into two broad categories: classical and lymphocyte predominant. Classical has four subtypes: lymphocyte depleted, nodular sclerosing, mixed cellularity, and classical lymphocyte rich. Classical HL accounts for 90% of all cases. For children, nodular sclerosis is the most common subtype, accounting for 65% of cases. Immunohistochemical studies

define a common immunophenotype for classical Hodgkin, characterized by CD15-positive and CD30-positive Reed-Sternberg cells (Fig. 38-4). Classical HL expresses CD30, a marker of activated B-lymphoid and T-lymphoid cells, in almost all cases.[25,28,30] About 87% of classical Hodgkin lymphomas express CD15, the carbohydrate X hapten. Classical Hodgkin lymphoma rarely expresses CD45, also known as common leukocyte antigen, which is expressed by nearly all non-Hodgkin lymphomas and can serve as a useful differential marker between HL and non-Hodgkin lymphoma.

The lymphocyte predominant (LPHD) subtype accounts for 10% of all cases and is characterized by lymphocytic and histiocytic (L&H) cells that express markers not typically seen in the classical subtype (Fig. 38-5). These cells are also known as "popcorn cells" and are CD20 positive. Other B-cell immunomarkers found in LPHD include CD79a, CD75, epithelial membrane antigen, and CD45. The lymphocyte predominant subtype historically carries the best prognosis. However, since the development of highly effective multiagent and multidisciplinary treatment regimens, all histologic subtypes have become responsive to therapy.

STAGING

Staging has both clinical and pathologic features. The Ann Arbor staging system and its Cotswolds modification remain the standard for adult and pediatric HL (see Table 38-1).[30,33,34] The original Ann Arbor staging system developed in 1974 was based principally upon the use of staging laparotomy and lymphangiogram, both of which have been abandoned.

Clinical staging requires a complete history and physical examination. Basic tests should include a complete blood cell count with differential, lactate dehydrogenase, alkaline phosphatase, erythrocyte sedimentation rate, or C-reactive protein (CRP), baseline hepatic and renal function tests, and electrolytes. Radiographic studies include a chest radiograph and a computed tomography (CT) scan of the neck, chest, abdomen, and pelvis. Chest radiographs often reveal the presence of a mediastinal mass, and the ratio of its maximal diameter to that of the thoracic cavity on a posteroanterior view is important prognostically. A mass with a ratio greater than 1:3 places

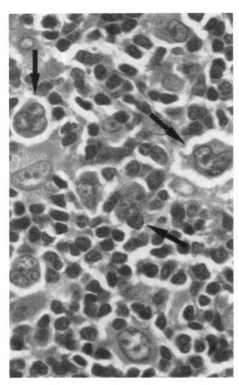

FIGURE 38-5 High-power hematoxylin and eosin–stained slide of a patient with lymphocyte predominant Hodgkin lymphoma demonstrating classical "popcorn" cells as defined by the arrows. *(See Expert Consult site for color version.)*

the patient in the subcategory of bulky mediastinal disease associated with a worse prognosis. Bone marrow biopsy is reserved for those patients with B symptoms or stage III-IV disease. (18F)-2 fluoro-D-2-deoxyglucose positron emission tomography (FDG PET) is replacing gallium scans, and recent studies have assessed the ability of PET scans to replace CT scans and as possible prognostic indicators for response to therapy.[25,28,35–37] Magnetic resonance imaging (MRI) provides a more accurate evaluation of disease in the abdomen compared with CT, with better visualization of fat-encased retroperitoneal nodes, but whether or not this provides clinically significant information has yet to be established.

TREATMENT

Risk Classification

Children and adolescents with HL are divided into three risk categories—low-, intermediate-, and high-risk disease—based on clinical and pathologic staging data, histology, stage at presentation, presence or absence of B symptoms, number of involved sites, and/or presence of bulky disease (>10 cm). The exact definitions of each stage will often change between studies and clinical trial consortiums, such as the Children's Oncology Group (COG).[34] In general, *low-risk* disease is defined as classical Hodgkin lymphoma patients, with clinical stage I or II disease showing no B symptoms or bulky nodal involvement and disease in fewer than three nodal regions. *Intermediate-risk* disease includes stage I, II, and sometimes IIIA disease with criteria that vary from trial to trial.[26,30] Some trials have included B symptoms, bulky disease, a large

number of involved nodal regions, and extranodal involvement of disease. *High-risk* patients are those with stage IIIB and IVA/B disease.[38–40] LPHD is considered a low-risk disease but is often separated from the classical HL studies.

Surgery

The role of surgery in the initial diagnosis and staging for HL has been reduced. With the wide application of chemotherapy in all stages of HL, surgical staging has become irrelevant, because the additional information it provides does not alter treatment.[41,42] The surgeon's primary role is to obtain tissue for diagnosis. Biopsies should be taken from the most easily accessible site, and adequate tissue must be obtained and sent fresh to pathology for immunohistochemistry, immunophenotyping, cytogenetics, and flow cytometry. Fine-needle aspiration is generally discouraged, because it is inaccurate and inadequate tissue is obtained to properly stage and classify the patient. Thoracoscopic biopsy or a Chamberlain procedure can be used for diagnosis in patients with only mediastinal involvement. Retroperitoneal lymphadenopathy is often accessible through laparoscopic biopsy. However, thoracoscopic and laparoscopic, as well as core needle biopsies, have a higher incidence of misdiagnosis and can require multiple procedures to obtain an adequate sample.[29] The second role for surgery is to provide central venous access for chemotherapy. Bilateral oophoropexies are also performed in girls who will receive abdominal radiotherapy.

Chemotherapy and Radiation Therapy

Chemotherapy and radiotherapy (RT) are the mainstay treatments of HL. Although the outcomes for children with HL have improved dramatically, the short-term and long-term toxicity of therapy has been substanial.[43,44] Therefore recent and current therapeutic protocols for HL have focused on maintaining excellent outcomes but reducing toxicity. Ideal chemotherapy regimens use drugs that are individually effective with different mechanisms of action and toxicities, to allow for a maximal dose. The first widespread successful regimen was MOPP (Mustargen, oncovin, procarbazine, and prednisone). In a long-term study of 188 patients from the National Cancer Institute, who were treated with MOPP, the complete remission rate was 89%, and 54% of patients remained disease free at 10 years.[45] In this study, 95% of patients had stage III or IV disease, and 89% had B symptoms. ABVD (Adriamycin [doxorubicin], bleomycin, vinblastine, and dacarbazine) was the second regimen used in the treatment of HD.[46] It was developed for the treatment of patients failing MOPP therapy and contains individually effective drugs with nonoverlapping toxicities.

Historically, radiation therapy was based on the concept of contiguous lymph node basin involvement.[47] The whole nodal region was included as defined by Kaplan and Rosenberg, sometimes additionally covering uninvolved adjacent lymph node region(s), extended field radiotherapy (EFRT).[47] However, radiation therapy is one of the major contributors to early and late toxicity in children with HL. Similar to chemotherapy, treatment has evolved, however, to reduce the radiation necessary. EFRT has been supplanted by involved field radiation therapy (IFRT). Over time, improvements in equipment and targeting have reduced the exposure of uninvolved areas. These practices aim to reduce salivary gland and oral cavity morbidity and to optimally spare the heart from irradiation. A further reduction of RT volume to cover just the nodal tissue involved by disease, without any attempt to include whole nodal region(s), is termed involved node radiation therapy (INRT).[48] Relapses in patients treated with chemotherapy alone occur primarily in the initially involved lymph nodes.[49] Using FDG PET analysis of residual disease and advances in radiation planning, it is possible now to confine the radiation to the initially involved nodal tissues rather than the whole nodal chain. The hope is that a reduction in irradiation volume will result in a lower incidence of late complications. This goal may be particularly important in young females with anterior mediastinal disease, where exclusion of the hilar and subcarinal nodes from the radiation field would lead to significant reductions in radiation dose to the breasts. This is important because the most common malignancy following treatment for HL is breast cancer. In addition, children have been shown to be particularly susceptible to thyroid toxicity following RT, and the transition to INRT may potentially exclude the thyroid from the treated volume for many patients with supradiaphragmatic HL. Preliminary data reported from British Columbia in Canada indicated no increase in relapses with INRT compared with IFRT or EFRT using a current multiagent chemotherapy regimen.[50]

Therapy for Low-Risk Disease

Optimal therapy for low-risk Hodgkin disease in children and adolescents continues to evolve. Protocols using chemotherapy followed by low-dose radiation therapy have achieved cure rates of greater than 90% for patients with low-risk Hodgkin disease and represent the standard of care for children and adolescents with Hodgkin disease. Several multi-institutional trials demonstrate that children and adolescents with low-risk HL can be effectively treated with two to four cycles of chemotherapy followed by 15- to 25-Gy IFRT, with series reporting 90% or better event-free survival (EFS), with overall survival (OS) greater than 95%.[51–54] The most recent COG low-risk HL study used a response-based chemotherapy regimen of AP-PC (Adriamycin [doxorubicin], vincristine, prednisone, and cyclophosphamide) with or without IFRT. After three cycles, those with complete response do not receive IFRT. IFRT consists of 21 GY in 14 fractions of 1.50 Gy per day for 14 sessions.[37] This study closed in the fall of 2010.

Therapy for Intermediate-Risk Disease

Intermediate-risk trials for HL have documented the need for adjuvant radiotherapy in most patients.[54–56] In a German trial, patients who completely responded to induction therapy had radiation therapy omitted, but their event-free survival was lower than expected.[40] In the CCG 5942 trial, intermediate-risk children with complete response were randomized to receive either IFRT or no further treatment.[54] Three-year EFS was 82% with OS of 93%, but the patients who received IFRT had three-year EFS of 88%. Both these studies support the need for IFRT with most intermediate HL patients. The current intermediate-risk COG trial is a randomized trial to see if early complete responders can have a dose reduction of both chemotherapy and radiation therapy without a decrease in their EFS. Induction chemotherapy consists of ABVE-PC (Adriamycin [doxorubicin], bleomycin, vincristine, etoposide, prednisone, and cyclophosphamide) for two cycles. It is a double randomized response–based protocol with both IFRT and chemotherapy intensifications following induction.[36] This study closed in the fall of 2010.

Therapy for High-Risk Disease

Patients with high-risk tumors require both intensification of chemotherapy and radiation therapy. The German (GPOH) HD-DAL 90 protocol treated high-risk patients with two or four cycles of COPP (cyclophosphamide, vincristine, procarbazine, and prednisone) plus 20- to 35-Gy IFRT. Five-year EFS in high-risk groups was 93% and 86%, respectively.[53] The EFS in the high-risk groups was comparable to that seen in the low-risk group. The Children's Cancer Group (CCG) 5942 protocol treated those with high-risk disease with two courses of intensive multiagent chemotherapy with cytarabine/etoposide, COPP/ABV, and cyclophosphamide, vincristine, doxorubicin, and methylprednisolone/prednisone with granulocyte colony–stimulating factor support. Complete responders were randomly assigned to 21-Gy IFRT or no further therapy. Three-year EFS rates in intermediate- and high-risk patients receiving IFRT were 88% and 91%, respectively.[54] In both the GOPH HD-95 and CCG 5942 trials, the benefit of IFRT in reducing relapse rates was most pronounced among high-risk patients. The most recent studies suggest that outcome of patients with high-risk factors can be improved with intensification of chemotherapy and lowering RT based on response. Pediatric Oncology Group (POG) 9425 study reported 2-year EFS for intermediate- and high-risk disease in a response-based paradigm. In this study, 63% of patients received 9 weeks of chemotherapy and 21 Gy of IFRT because of good response, whereas the others received more intensive therapy.[56] The most current COG high-risk study recently opened. This is a nonrandomized response-based protocol. Induction therapy is with ABVE-PC, and patients will be divided into rapid early responders and slow early responders. Response will be determined by PET scan, and further chemotherapy and radiotherapy targets are based on the PET scan.[57]

Therapy for Lymphocyte-Predominant Hodgkin Disease

Lymphocyte-predominant Hodgkin disease (LPHD) is recognized as a distinct clinical-pathologic entity, with a favorable outcome, but also associated with a higher risk of late relapse and subsequent development of non-Hodgkin lymphoma (NHL). LPHD comprises up to 10% of cases in adult and pediatric series. Most patients with LPHD reported in the literature have been treated similarly to patients with classical HD, using chemotherapy, RT, or combined modality treatment.[3,58] However, treatment by surgical resection alone has been reported in adult and pediatric patients. The outcomes suggest that patients with low-stage disease may be effectively treated with surgery alone, particularly considering the toxicity of treatment.[59–61] In 2007, European researchers reported 100% survival in 58 LPHD patients treated initially with surgery alone; 50 had a complete response (CR) and received no adjuvant therapy.[62] In this group, 14 (28%) recurred, but 73% required no other therapy at 43 months follow-up. A recently completed COG protocol treated patients with stage I single node disease with surgery only. Results have not been published.[35]

Novel Therapy

Novel therapies are being investigated for children with HD at diagnosis and relapse. These include rituximab (an anti-CD20 monoclonal antibody) and small molecule agents, such as bortezomib, a reversible proteosome inhibitor that leads to the blockage of NF-kappa beta being explored in HD. Other agents include histone deacetylase inhibitors, such as MGCD0103; however, none of these agents are being incorporated in standard therapies.[3]

Treatment Toxicities

Toxicities of treatment include decreased stature, cardiopulmonary dysfunction, thyroid disease, infertility, second malignancies, impaired psychosocial functioning, and decreases in health-related quality of life.[28]

Growth Problems Full-dose (35- to 44-Gy) RT produces bone and soft tissue hypoplasia in prepubertal children. For patients treated with mantle fields, this manifests as spinal and clavicular shortening and underdevelopment of the soft tissues in the neck.

Cardiopulmonary Dysfunction Long-term survivors of HL treated with full-dose RT have an increased risk of atherosclerotic heart disease, valvular dysfunction, and pericardial disease.[62–64] A study reported a 45-fold mortality risk from acute myocardial infarction in children treated before the age of 20 years with more than 30 Gy of mediastinal radiation.[65] Heart disease and valvular disease tends to occur late—8 to 10 years after therapy. Lower doses and cardiac shielding reduce this risk. Pericarditis can occur, especially if the tumor involved the pericardium. Anthracyclines, such as doxorubicin, cause dose-dependent myocardial heart failure and coronary artery disease.[66] In children, a cumulative dose of 300 mg/m^2 of doxorubicin increases heart failure rate by 11-fold at 15 years after therapy.[67,68] Contemporary chemotherapy regimens delivering 250 mg/m^2 doxorubicin with low-dose IFRT appear to be associated with minimal early cardiac toxicity.[69] Bleomycin results in both short-term and long-term lung toxicity with impaired diffusion capacity and restrictive lung disease.[70] RT can also produce breast hypoplasia and contribute to the pulmonary fibrosis.

Thyroid Hypothyroidism, hyperthyroidism, as well as benign and malignant thyroid nodules have been recognized as problems occurring in long-term survivors of HL.[71,72] In the Childhood Cancer Survivor Study, 34% of 1,791 5-year survivors of HL treated between 1970 and 1986 reported thyroid abnormalities.[72] Thyroid nodules appear late in the follow-up, often 10 or more years after completion of therapy. The relative risk (RR) is 18.3 (confidence interval, 11.4 to 27.6) compared with the general population. Children receiving neck RT also appear to be at greater risk of hypothyroidism than adults.[71]

Infertility Sterility/infertility is a significant risk of alkylating agents, most commonly cyclophosphamide and/or procarbazine.[73] Males in the German GPOH studies receive etoposide in place of procarbazine, because testicular germinal function is more sensitive to alkylating agents than is ovarian function, and current COG protocols limit alkylating agents to doses compatible with preservation of fertility.[35–37,57] Gonadal failure is also a result of pelvic RT. In boys, doses greater than 3 Gy can produce irreversible azospermia.[74] Low-dose IFRT to iliac or inguinal lymph nodes may impair fertility among females if the direct or scattered dose to the ovaries exceeds 2 to 3 Gy. Oophoropexy can help limit the adverse effects of radiation therapy. Also reported in females is a high risk of prematurity and premature menopause.[75]

Second Cancers (SC) The risk of second cancers is significantly increased in the long-term survivors of HL treated with full-dose RT.[76–80] The Late Effects Study Group estimated the 30-year cumulative incidence of SC to be 26.3% among survivors diagnosed before age 16. The two most frequent cancers are breast cancer (20% risk at 45 years of age), followed by thyroid carcinoma (36-fold increased rate).[80] Exposure to alkylating agents, particularly in conjunction with extended-field RT, is associated with an increased risk of leukemia. Leukemias tend to arise 2 to 10 years after therapy. The risk of SC after modern treatment is not yet known, because reduction in exposure to alkylating agents and the use of low-dose IFRT became standard practice within the last 15 to 20 years. The transition from extended-field RT to IFRT significantly reduces the radiation dose to breast and lung tissue.[81] It is thought that modern IFRT should lead to lower SC rates than have been documented in the past.

Non-Hodgkin Lymphoma

Non-Hodgkin lymphomas (NHLs) comprise a heterogeneous group of tumors that has a constantly evolving classification system. The current World Health Organization (WHO) pathologic classification identifies almost 60 unique subtypes based on morphologic, immunophenotypic, and genetic differences, as well as clinical behavior (Table 38-2). NHL can be broadly divided based on the cell of origin (B cell or T cell) or on clinical behavior (indolent, aggressive, or highly aggressive). There are distinct differences between adult and pediatric NHL, with a strong bias toward precursor B-lymphoblastic and T-lymphoblastic lymphoma, anaplastic large cell lymphoma, and Burkitt lymphoma in childhood.

Indolent lymphomas are slowly progressive but incurable diseases, with a median survival time of 8 to 10 years. Aggressive lymphomas, such as Burkitt and Burkitt-like lymphomas, are rapidly progressive at presentation but curable in 70% to 90% of patients, with outcome strongly dependent on clinical and biological features (as identified by current molecular and immunologic approaches) at presentation.

INCIDENCE EPIDEMIOLOGY AND CLASSIFICATION

There are 750 to 800 new cases of non-Hodgkin lymphoma each year in the United States.[82] Non-Hodgkin lymphoma (NHL) accounts for 7% of cancer in children and adolescents, with an incidence of 10 per 1 million population annually in the United States.[83] NHL is rare at less than 5 years of age, with an incidence of 2.8 per million cases but increases dramatically after age 20. NHL is more common in males (1.1 to 1.4:1), with a higher frequency in whites than in blacks or Asians. Certain NHL types cluster according to race, for example, the natural killer (NK) T-cell lymphomas are most frequently encountered in Asian populations. A family history of a hematologic malignancy produces an increased risk, but it is not NHL-disease specific.[82]

DNA and RNA viruses are thought to play an important role in the pathogenesis of NHL.[17,82] The Epstein-Barr virus (EBV)

TABLE 38-2

World Health Organization and Clinical Classification of Selected Subtypes of Non-Hodgkin Lymphoma

WHO Pathologic Category	Clinical Behavior		
	Indolent	Aggressive	Highly Aggressive
Mature B-cell neoplasms	Follicular lymphoma	Diffuse large B-cell lymphoma, NOS	Burkitt lymphoma
	Chronic lymphocytic leukemia/small lymphocytic lymphoma	Primary mediastinal large B-cell lymphoma	
	Hairy cell leukemia	Mantle cell lymphoma	
	Extranodal marginal zone lymphoma		
	Lymphoplasmacytic lymphoma/Waldenstrom macroglobulinemia		
	Splenic B-cell marginal zone lymphoma		
Mature T-cell and NK-cell neoplasms	Mycosis fungoides	Hepatosplenic T-cell lymphoma	
	Sézary syndrome	Peripheral T-cell lymphoma, NOS	
		Angioimmunoblastic T-cell lymphoma	
		Anaplastic large cell lymphoma, ALK+ type	
		Anaplastic large cell lymphoma, ALK− type	

Adapted from Jaffe E, Harris NL, Stein H, et al: Introduction and overview of the classification of lymphoid neoplasms. In Swerdlow SH, Campo E, Harris NL, et al (eds): WHO Classification of Tumours of Haematopoietic and Lymphoid Tissues. Lyon, France, IARC Press, 2008, p 158-166.
ALK, anaplastic lymphoma kinase; NK, natural killer; NOS, not otherwise specified; WHO, World Health Organization.

is the most prominent. EBV was first detected in cultured African Burkitt lymphoma cells and is known to be present in greater than 90% of such cases. EBV is important as a trigger for lymphoproliferations/lymphomas occurring in congenital immunodeficiencies, iatrogenically immunosuppressed organ transplant recipients, patients receiving maintenance chemotherapy, and patients receiving combined immunosuppressive therapy for collagen disorders.[84] EBV is also found in HL (mostly the mixed cellularity type), and patients who have had infectious mononucleosis are at increased risk of HL. Other viruses implicated in the pathogenesis of NHL include the retrovirus human lymphotropic virus type 1 (HTLV-1), with adult T-cell lymphoma and human herpesvirus 8 (HHV-8) as a cause of primary effusion lymphoma, a rare type of large cell lymphoma confined to serous-lined body cavities, which occurs with highest frequency in the HIV-positive population. Bacterial overgrowth can also promote the occurrence of a lymphoma. In gastric lymphoma of mucosa-associated lymphoid tissue (MALT) type, *Helicobacter pylori* infection has been shown to be necessary for the development and early proliferation of the lymphoma.[85]

NHLs in children are typically high grade.[86] Ninety percent are from three main groups. These are (1) mature B-cell NHL, which includes Burkitt lymphoma (BL), Burkitt-like lymphoma (BLL), or diffuse large B-cell lymphoma (DLBCL); (2) lymphoblastic lymphoma (LL); or (3) anaplastic large T-cell lymphoma (ALCL). The other 10% are similar to types seen in adults, such as MALT and mature T-cell natural killer (NK) cell lymphoma (see Table 38-2). NHL subtypes have different cell lineages and cell cycle kinetics with different propensities to invade the bone marrow and central nervous system.[87]

CLINICAL PRESENTATION AND STAGING

Similar to HL, NHL must be considered in any child with lymphadenopathy. However, most children with B-cell lymphoma present with a palpable abdominal tumor or a mediastinal tumor.[88,89] Frequently, the lymphoma presents as a mass in the right iliac fossa and can be confused with appendicitis or an appendiceal abscess. Children may also present with intussusception bleeding, ascites, or a bowel perforation.

As with HL, the presence of mediastinal disease must be assessed, because these masses can be exceedingly large and result in significant morbidity or mortality (see Fig. 38-3). Superior vena cava syndrome and respiratory distress are more common in patients with NHL. In these cases, immediate treatment with corticosteroids with or without cyclophosphamide or radiation may be required. The concern in these situations is that the treatment will make it difficult to establish the pathologic diagnosis. However, there is some thought that treatment for up to 48 hours is beneficial and unlikely to obscure subsequent pathologic diagnosis, but if there is significant resolution of the mass, the tissue may be necrotic.[90] Many children with NHL will present with advanced-stage disease, including bone marrow involvement and malignant pleural or pericardial effusions. Pleural fluid and pericardial fluid often require drainage; cytologic examination of the fluid can be diagnostic.[90] Patients may also present with B symptoms. The presence or absence of B symptoms has prognostic significance and is reflected in the staging of these lymphomas. B symptoms occur in up to one third of children with NHL.[13,25] In NHL, the proper diagnosis allows for classification to the distinct biological subgroups. Specimens should be sent fresh to pathology. Regular histopathology, cytology, immunopathology, cytogenetics using fluorescence in situ hybridization (FISH, to look for chromosomal translocation), polymerase chain reaction (PCR), and growth patterns all are needed to properly classify a case of NHL.[91,92]

Staging

Staging laparotomy is not performed in non-Hodgkin lymphoma, because all patients require systemic chemotherapy. However, patients may require surgical intervention because of abdominal complications, such as intussusception or bleeding or to obtain diagnostic tissue. In some cases, the disease is localized and a total resection can be performed, in others the

TABLE 38-3	
St. Jude's Murphy Staging System for Non-Hodgkin Lymphoma	
Stage	**Description**
I	A single extranodal tumor or single anatomic nodal area with exclusion of mediastinum and abdomen
II	A single extranodal tumor with regional nodal Involvement greater than or equal to two involved nodal regions or localized involvement of extranodal disease on the same side of diaphragm A primary gastrointestinal tract tumor that is completely resected
III	Greater than or equal to two nodal or extranodal tumors on opposite sides of the diaphragm Any primary intrathoracic tumor Unresectable primary intraabdominal disease Any paraspinal or epidural disease
IV	Involvement of central nervous system and/or bone marrow

disease is extensive with involvement of the mesenteric root and retroperitoneum.

Although no staging system is entirely satisfactory, the most widely used staging system for NHL is the St. Jude's Murphy system (Table 38-3).[93] The Children's Oncology Group divides NHL into two categories: limited and extensive. Limited disease corresponds to stages I and II in the St. Jude's system, and extensive correlates with stages III and IV.

NHL SUBTYPES IN CHILDREN AND ADOLESCENTS

A detailed review of all the different types of NHL is beyond the scope of this chapter. The most common subtypes of NHL, accounting for 90% of cases found in children, are presented.

Mature B-cell NHL: Burkitt Lymphoma, Burkitt-Like Lymphoma, and Diffuse Large B-Cell Lymphoma

B cells originate in the bone marrow from totipotential stem cells that differentiate through many intermediate cell types to eventually become antibody-producing plasma cells (Fig. 38-6). Malignant transformation can occur at any point along the path of differentiation. The clinicopathologic subtypes of NHL are determined by the stage of differentiation at which malignant transformation occurs. Because of their appearance by light microscopy, tumors in this category are also called small, noncleaved cell lymphomas. Because B cells develop in the bone marrow and then migrate to secondary lymphoid organs (lymph nodes, spleen, Peyer patches, liver), one would expect clinical localization of the developing neoplasm in those anatomic sites. Alternatively, B-cell lymphoma should not occur in the anterior mediastinum in the region of the thymus, because normal B cells are not thymic dependent. Usually, but not always, this anatomic distribution is consistent with clinical observations.

Burkitt Lymphoma and Burkitt-Like Lymphoma BL was first described in 1958 in Uganda by a surgeon who observed rapidly enlarging tumors involving the jaw in children.[94] BL and BLL account for about 40% of childhood NHLs (Fig. 38-7).[86] There are three variants of BL: endemic, sporadic, and immunodeficiency related. In the United States, BL most frequently occurs in the abdomen; in western

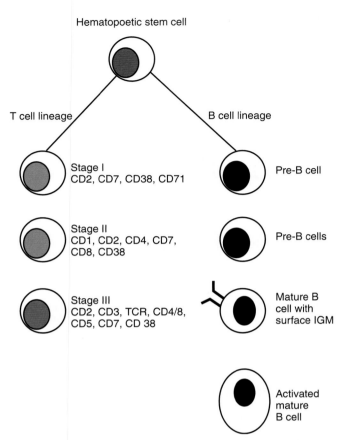

FIGURE 38-6 A schematic of B-cell and T-cell lineages. *(See Expert Consult site for color version.)*

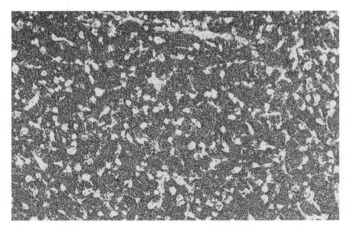

FIGURE 38-7 A low-power hematoxylin and eosin–stained slide of a patient with Burkitt lymphoma. Shows the typical "starry sky" appearance of the tumor. *(See Expert Consult site for color version.)*

equatorial Africa, it usually arises in the mandible, but abdominal lymphoma is also noted in up to 20% of these patients. BL can also be found in the central nervous system and bone marrow. BL of the anterior mediastinum is extremely rare.[95,96] The gold standard for the diagnosis of BL is c-*MYC* rearrangement.[97] This is based on a characteristic chromosomal translocation, usually involving chromosomes 8 and 14, that was discovered in BL in 1976.[98] In 80% of the translocations, this involves the locus at 14q32, in 15% of cases it is 2p11, and in 5% it is 22q11. BL is the most rapidly growing tumor in children, with a doubling time of approximately 24 hours. The rate of cell death or apoptosis is also high, with the dead cells being taken up by pale histiocytic cells within the tumor that punctuate the low-power view, giving a "starry sky" appearance (see Fig. 38-7).[97] BL cells are mature B-cells that are positive for CD19, CD20, CD22, and CD79a and have a monotypic surface IgM.[99] BLL is an aggressive highly proliferative variant with features that overlap classical BL and DLBCL; BLL is treated by BL regimens.[97] The distinction between BL and BLL is controversial. Because of the rapid growth seen in BL and BLL, when the disease is suspected, the pediatric surgeons are often asked to intervene immediately so that treatment can begin.

Diffuse Large B-Cell Lymphoma   DLBCL accounts for 10% of pediatric lymphomas. It is less common in young children and becomes frequent in adolescents. DLBCL is derived from transformed mature B cells of the peripheral lymphoid organs.[100] DLBCL tumors have cells that are 4 to 5 times the size of small lymphocytes. In adults, there is a genetic signature; however, in children this is not the case. The tumors do express c-*MYC*–like BL as well as genes from the NF kappa-beta pathway, but there is no specific marker of DLBCL.[101] The tumors express CD19, CD20, CD22, and CD79a. The three most common morphologic variants are centroblastic, immunoblastic, and anaplastic. Gene expression profiling has identified two subtypes: germinal center B-cell–like (GC) and activated B-cell (ABC). The most common subtype, GC, has a more favorable outcome. A progressively enlarging mass is the most common mode of presentation. Symptoms are based on tumor location. About 20% of pediatric DLBCL present as a mediastinal mass, but the tumors can occur anywhere. Increased lactate dehydrogenase (LDH), pleura effusions, and ascites are less frequently observed than in other NHL. The bone marrow (BM) and the central nervous system (CNS) are rarely involved.[87]

T-Cell Tumors

Lymphoblastic Lymphoma   Lymphoblastic lymphomas (LL) make up approximately 30% of childhood NHL.[12,82,83,86] In pediatric patients with LL, 75% will have a T-cell immunophenotype. The remaining LL patients have a precursor B-cell phenotype more commonly presenting as disease localized in skin and bone rather than T-cell LL. Some oncologists and pathologists feel LL is acute lymphoblastic leukemia in an extramedullarly site. Whether the LL is a T cell or B cell does not affect prognosis. LL tumors have a precursor lymphoblast phenotype (TdT [terminal deoxynucleotidyl] positive) and express T-cell markers, including CD7 or CD5.[12,102] Although there is no genetic signature, T-cell rearrangements are common, as well as several cytogenetic and molecular changes.[12,103,104] Because thymic residence is a necessary part of T-cell development, most lymphomas presenting in the anterior mediastinum originate from the T-cell lineage. Fifty percent to 70 percent of patients with lymphoblastic lymphoma (T cell) present with an intrathoracic tumor. Abdominal involvement is uncommon and, when observed, usually includes hepatosplenomegaly. Bone marrow infiltration is common in this situation, making the distinction from acute lymphoblastic leukemia difficult. In these cases, survival may be better after treatment with a lymphoblastic leukemia–type regimen. Pleural effusions are often observed, and

patients may complain of dyspnea, chest pain, or dysphagia. Superior vena cava syndrome with facial, chest, and upper extremity edema and dilated cutaneous veins over the upper torso and shoulders, or airway compression with severe dyspnea or orthopnea (or both) can also occur. The central nervous system is rarely involved at diagnosis.

Anaplastic Large T-Cell Lymphoma   ALCL is a mature T-cell cancer and accounts for 10% of NHL in children. Morphologically, ALCL are characterized by large cells with big cytoplasms and horseshoe- or kidney-shaped nuclei called hallmark cells.[105] More than 90% of ALCL cases are CD30-positive (Ki- antigen) and have the translocation t(2;5) (p23;q35). This results in production of a fusion protein NPM/ALK, although variant *ALK* translocations have been reported.[106] The WHO divides ALCL into systemic (ALK+ and ALK−) and cutaneous lymphomas. ALK− is predominantly found in adults with a poorer prognosis, with OS of 45%. ALK+ prognosis is good, with an 80% OS.[107–109] The cutaneous form is extremely rare in children and only accounts for 1.7% of ALCL; its OS is 90%. Clinically, ALCL has a broad range of presentations, including involvement of lymph nodes and a variety of extranodal sites, particularly skin and bone. Involvement of the CNS and bone marrow is uncommon. As opposed to other pediatric NHL, ALCL is often associated with B symptoms (e.g., fever and weight loss), and a prolonged waxing and waning course can complicate and often delay diagnosis.

Post-Transplant Lymphoproliferative Disorders   The 2% to 4% risk of developing cancer after solid organ transplantation (SOT) is about 5- to 10-fold greater than that of the general population. The risk correlates with the intensity and cumulative exposure to immunosuppression.[110] The lowest frequency seen is in renal transplant recipients (1%), and the highest is in heart-lung or liver-bowel allografts (5%). EBV seronegativity at time of transplant and young age at transplant are the two greatest risk factors for subsequent PTLD. In children, post-transplant lymphoproliferative disorders (PTLDs) may occur early, because of their risk for a primary EBV infection.[111] Many of the tumors exhibit an EBV-induced monoclonal or, more rarely, polyclonal B-cell or T-cell proliferation as a consequence of immune suppression.[112] The diagnosis can be difficult and patients tend to present with nonspecific findings, such as episodic and unexplained fever, weight loss, and fatigue. A high index of suspicion is needed to diagnose PTLD. The tumors can occur both within and outside the allograph, including lymphoid tissue, gastrointestinal (GI) tract, lung, and liver. Involvement of the GI tract may present with vomiting, diarrhea, bleeding, intussusception, or obstruction. Perforation may occur at presentation or immediately following initiation of therapy in the presence of transmural necrosis of the lesion.

TREATMENT AND OUTCOMES

Chemotherapy for Non-Hodgkin Lymphoma

Non-Hodgkin lymphomas in childhood are in most cases disseminated at diagnosis. Chemotherapy is the primary treatment modality. Each regimen is divided into phases of induction, consolidation, reintensification, and maintenance.

Historically, only 20% to 30% of patients with non-Hodgkin lymphoma survived for 5 years until the pioneering work of Wollner and colleagues in 1975, when the LSA_2-L_2 (cyclophosphamide, vincristine, methotrexate, daunorubicin, prednisone, cytarabine, thioguanine, asparaginase, carmustine, hydroxyurea) regimen, adapted from the treatment of acute lymphoblastic leukemia, resulted in a 73% salvage rate.[113,114] At the same time, Ziegler and colleagues reported similar success with treatment of these patients using the COMP (cyclophosphamide, Oncovin [vincristine], methotrexate, prednisone) regimen.[115,116] A third important NHL treatment regimen is the Berlin-Frankfurt-Münster (BFM). This is a similar regimen to LSA_2-L_2. The main difference is the earlier application of L-Asp and high-dose methotrexate (MTX) in the BFM regimen.

The results of the Children's Cancer Group (CCG) randomized trial CCG-551 is considered one of the main studies to alter therapy for NHL in children. It compared LSA_2-L_2 with COMP. This study stratified treatment modalities by biological subgroups. The three main findings were (1) different chemotherapy regimens exert different effects in different NHL subtypes, (2) differences in treatment efficacy are seen mainly in advanced-stage disease, and (3) in advanced-stage disease, the differences in treatment efficacy are more pronounced in patients with LBL (i.e., patients receiving LSA_2-L_2 had fewer relapses) and BL (i.e., patients receiving COMP did better), while event-free survival (EFS) rates were not significantly different between treatment regimens in patients with large cell lymphoma.[117] A Pediatric Oncology Group trial further helped with the stratification issue by demonstrating that even in patients with localized disease, different strategies had different effects in histologic subgroups.[118] Despite the different disease process, stages, and stratification, most treatment regimens are based on one of the three regimens described previously with adjustment made for stage, histology, and phases of therapy. For example, LBL protocols are continual exposure to cytostatic agents over a long period of time; BL/BLL and DLBCL are treated with rapid repeated short, dose-intense chemotherapy courses. ALCL have a completely different strategy.[90]

Surgery

Initial surgical management includes incisional biopsy for diagnosis, followed by intense, multiagent chemotherapy, except for small, easily resectable lesions.[119] Resection of massive retroperitoneal or mediastinal masses is not indicated. In abdominal BL, the extent of disease is a more significant predictive variable than is completeness of surgical resection. The surgical committee of the Children's Cancer Group (CCG) evaluated the role of surgical therapy in 68 patients with non-Hodgkin lymphoma in the CCG-551 study.[60] Tumor burden was the most important prognostic factor. However, in disease that can be completely resected, it may improve EFS and prevent complications such as bowel perforation. In the setting of localized disease, data do support a role for complete resection.[120–122]

Radiation Therapy

In the treatment of localized non-Hodgkin lymphoma, radiation therapy has been shown to add toxicity with no therapeutic benefit. Several studies continue to show that radiotherapy

has a limited role (stage I disease) in the treatment of NHL.[123] Radiation is used for CNS disease with limited effects and is controversial.[124]

Burkitt Lymphoma and Burkitt-Like Lymphoma and Diffuse Large B-Cell Lymphoma

Most BL and BLL regimens are derived from the LSA_2-L_2 or BFM regimens with the use of methotrexate (MTX) for CNS disease. Rituximab is currently being studied in clinical trials, because it has shown good results in adult NHL. Because of its high proliferation rate, BL therapy uses cytotoxic drug concentrations over a period and drugs with different mechanisms of action with nonoverlapping toxicities that is sufficient to affect as many lymphoma cells as possible during the active cell cycle, using either fractionated administration or continuous infusion.[125] Treatments use high-dose intensity and short treatment intervals. Although these regimens are effective, they are toxic even with use of granulocyte colony–stimulating factor (G-CSF), because up to 3% can die from treatment complications.[126,127] One particular threat is acute tumor cell lysis syndrome (ATLS). Depending on the size of the tumor, the acute lysis of many tumor cells places a tremendous metabolic load on the kidneys, composed of phosphates, potassium, purines, and protein. Patients may present with elevated serum uric acid, lactate, and potassium levels. This syndrome may be further aggravated during the initial massive cell lysis caused by chemotherapy. ATLS can result in hyperuricemic nephropathy and renal shutdown. Patients with localized resected tumors have nearly 100% EFS with two 5-day therapy courses. Recent trials report overall survival rates of 98%, 90%, and 86% in stage I/II, III, and IV disease, respectively.[128] DCLC also has excellent outcomes when treated on BL and BLL protocols with event-free survival reaching 97%.

Lymphoblastic Lymphoma

Event-free survival for children with LL ranges from 60% to 90%, with 5-year survival, with lower stages reaching 90%.[129–132] Most current treatments are based on one of two protocols: the LSA_2-L_2 protocol (cyclophosphamide, vincristine, methotrexate, daunorubicin, prednisone, cytarabine, thioguanine, asparaginase, carmustine, hydroxyurea) or the BFM group strategy. Each uses similar drugs divided into phases of induction, consolidation, reintensification, and maintenance. The main differences between the protocols are earlier application of L-Asp and high-dose MTX in the BFM regimen. Treatment intensity is stratified according to stages I and II versus stages III and IV. Children with stage I/II are rare and achieve EFS rates higher than 90% with reduced-intensity (omission of reintensification in the BFM protocol) and full-length maintenance therapy. Most relapses occur early. Radiation is used for CNS disease with limited effects and is controversial.[124]

A current COG study is looking at the benefit of high-dose MTX with added cyclophosphamide and anthracycline during induction with the regimen from the BFM-95. The study is still open and accruing patients.

Anaplastic Large Cell Lymphoma

ALCL uses different treatment for local and systemic disease. Patients with localized disease show the best results with pulsed multiagent chemotherapy similar to the regimen used in mature B-cell NHL reporting overall survival of 93%. Children and adolescents with disseminated ALCL have a poorer survival of 60% to 75%. It is unclear which strategy is best for the treatment of disseminated ALCL. COG is testing the replacement of vincristine with vinblastine in the maintenance phase of the APO regimen (doxorubicin, vincristine, and prednisone.)

TOXICITIES

The long-term toxicity profile for patients with NHL is very similar to HL. Acutely, the NHL regimens, because of their intensity, tend to be more toxic as described previously.

The complete reference list is available online at www. expertconsult.com.

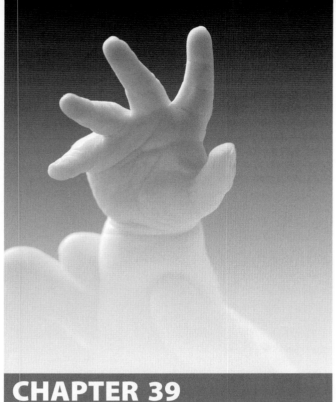

CHAPTER 39

Ovarian Tumors

Daniel Von Allmen and Mary E. Fallat

Ovarian Tumors Incidence

Primary cysts and tumors of the ovaries are uncommon in children. The majority of these masses are not malignant.[1] Gynecologic malignant conditions account for approximately 2% of all types of cancer in children, and 60% to 70% of these lesions arise in the ovary.[2] The North American Association of Central Cancer Registries released data from 1992 to 1997 regarding more than 1.6 million women and children diagnosed with cancer.[3] This report revealed that 1.2% of ovarian cancer cases occurred in females between birth and age 19 years.[3] Lindfors[4] analyzed several large series of ovarian tumors in children and estimated that the annual incidence of combined benign and malignant lesions was 2.6 cases per 100,000 girls younger than 15 years. Using the Surveillance, Epidemiology, and End Results (SEER) registry, 1,037 pediatric patients with malignant ovarian tumors were identified.[5] The age-adjusted incidence of malignant ovarian tumors in those less than 9 years was 0.102 versus 1.072 per 100,000 in those aged 10 to 19 years old. Malignancy is very rare in children less than 5 years old. The predominant pathology was germ cell tumors in all age groups (77.4%) and 61.7% of tumors occurred in patients 15 to 19 years old. The concept that the highest incidence of malignant conditions occurs in the youngest patients has been reassessed. Newer diagnostic imaging techniques have increased the detection of all gonadal masses, and the frequency of ovarian cancer has decreased.

Epidemiology

A few syndromes or diseases are associated with ovarian pathology. The Peutz-Jeghers syndrome is associated with granulosa cell tumors, ovarian cystadenomas, and sex cord–stromal tumors with annular tubules.[6] Juvenile granulosa and Sertoli-Leydig cell tumors are detected with Ollier disease (multiple enchondromatosis)[7] and juvenile granulosa cell tumors and fibrosarcoma with Maffucci syndrome (enchondromatosis and hemangiomas).[8,9] Sclerosing stromal tumors are associated with the Chédiak-Higashi syndrome (oculocutaneous albinism, pyogenic infections, and leukocyte granule abnormalities that result in deficient phagocytosis).[10] The presence of ovarian cysts had been noted in various dysmorphic syndromes, including those with craniofacial, laryngeal, and digital malformations.[11] The McCune-Albright syndrome (triad of café-au-lait macules, polyostotic fibrous dysplasia, and autonomous endocrine hyperactivity) is generally characterized by gonadotropin-independent sexual precocity resulting from recurrent ovarian follicle formation and cyclic estradiol secretion.[12] Fibromas are associated with the basal cell nevus syndrome.[13]

Nulliparity and increased education are associated with a greater risk of the development of ovarian cancer.[14] Women who have never used oral contraceptives have a greater risk than women who have used them, and hormone replacement therapy slightly increases the risk.[15] Other potential but more controversial risk factors include exposure to ovulation-inducing drugs without successful pregnancy and diets high in meat and animal fats, dairy products, and lactose. The risk is not uniform across histotypes for most of these factors. Prior tubal ligation and hysterectomy may reduce the risk of epithelial ovarian cancer.[16–18] More recent reports suggest that higher body mass index (BMI) may predict a higher risk of ovarian malignancy in women presenting with adnexal masses, and avoidance of obesity and smoking seem protective against development of benign serous and mucinous epithelial ovarian tumors.[19,20] Late age at menarche, earlier age at menopause, the use of vitamin E supplements, and fish consumption tend to be associated with a decreased risk of some histologic subtypes. Occupational physical activity seems protective against all histotypes.[16]

Approximately 5% to 10% of women with breast and ovarian cancer have a genetic predisposition. High percentages of hereditary breast and ovarian cancers arise from mutations in the tumor suppressor genes BRCA1 and BRCA2. Approximately 70% of familial ovarian cancer cases are caused by BRCA1 mutations and 20% by BRCA2. These mutations are inherited in an autosomal dominant fashion. If a woman is a carrier of one of these gene mutations, she has a lifetime risk of developing ovarian cancer as high as 60%.[21,17] Genetic testing of adolescents is controversial.[22] Kodish[23] formulated the argument that physicians should respect the "rule of earliest onset" and defer testing until the age when the onset of disease becomes possible. An alternative view proposed by Elger and Harding[24] is that some mature adolescents may obtain significant psychological relief from knowing their mutation status and may be capable of using this information for reproductive and health decisions. In most cases, surgical intervention is not indicated until age 35 years or older or completion of childbearing. The use of oral contraceptives has been shown to reduce the risk of ovarian cancer in the general population. Whether the use of these agents in young women with *BRCA* mutations is beneficial remains to be determined.[17]

Clinical Presentation

The clinical presentation is variable and does not differentiate a benign from a malignant tumor. Abdominal pain is the most common symptom.[22,25] With cysts and other nonneoplastic conditions, the pain can be acute in onset, with a crescendo pattern of severity because of torsion, rupture, or hemorrhage. The clinical picture may mimic appendicitis. A more chronic, insidious pattern of pain, increasing girth, and marked distention over several weeks to months may occur. Secondary symptoms include anorexia, nausea, vomiting, and urinary frequency and urgency. A palpable abdominal mass with or without tenderness is the most frequent finding on physical examination and is detected in more than half of patients with ovarian tumors.[22] These tumors are usually mobile and palpable above the pelvic brim. Bimanual palpation between the lower abdomen and rectum may be helpful in detecting smaller lesions. Vaginal examination is usually reserved for sexually active patients, although vaginal inspection is of value in all patients. An increasing number of ovarian lesions are discovered incidentally by abdominal radiographs or ultrasonography (US) done for other reasons.

Both neoplastic and nonneoplastic ovarian lesions demonstrate endocrine activity in approximately 10% of cases.[13] Ovarian cysts of the simple, follicular, or luteal type may secrete estrogen and can cause precocious isosexual development. The lesions usually function autonomously, and the girls have suppressed gonadotropin concentrations. As a result, they can be distinguished from patients with central precocious puberty (with accelerated skeletal maturation) or premature thelarche (isolated breast development) by estrogen withdrawal and vaginal bleeding after cyst involution or removal. Precocious pseudopuberty may occur because of the production of human chorionic gonadotropin in girls with germ cell tumors, including dysgerminomas, yolk sac tumors (YSTs), and choriocarcinomas. Ovarian tumors most commonly associated with precocious puberty include the sex cord–stromal tumors, such as juvenile granulosa cell tumors or some Sertoli-Leydig cell tumors, which cause elevated levels of circulating estrogen. In the Grumbach syndrome, hypothyroidism presents with precocious puberty and bilateral ovarian cystic masses that resolve with thyroid replacement therapy.

Virilization resulting from androgen excess can occur with Sertoli-Leydig cell tumors, and masculinization is occasionally seen in older girls with dysgerminomas that contain syncytial trophoblastic giant cells. Yolk sac tumors, steroid cell tumors, and polycystic ovaries can be associated with virilization.

Diagnosis

LABORATORY TESTS

Many ovarian neoplasms are associated with the secretion of specific tumor markers or hormones. These are outlined in Tables 39-1 and 39-2 and are discussed further in the sections on individual tumors.

TABLE 39-1

Ovarian Tumor Markers

	CA 125	AFP	hCG	Inhibin
Germ Cell Tumors				
Dysgerminoma	+/−	−	+/−	−
Yolk sac tumor*	+/−	+	−	−
Choriocarcinoma	+/−	−	+	−
Embryonal carcinoma	+/−	+/−	+/−	−
Immature teratoma	+/−	+/−	−	−
Mixed germ cell tumor	+/−	+/−	+/−	−
Epithelial-Stromal Tumors				
Serous carcinoma	+	−	−	−
Mucinous carcinoma	+/−	−	−	+
Endometrioid carcinoma	+	−	−	+
Sex Cord–Stromal Tumors				
Granulosa cell tumor	+/−	−	−	+
Thecoma-fibroma	+/−	−	−	+
Sertoli-Leydig cell tumor	+/−	+/−	−	+

*Endodermal sinus tumor

Comments: CA 125 levels may be slightly elevated in any of the ovarian tumors. LDH levels are useful for staging and risk assessment in germ cell tumors.

AFP, alpha fetoprotein; CA 125, cancer antigen; hCG, human chorionic gonadotropin; LDH, lactate dehydrogenase.

Table courtesy Dr. Robert Debski, Assistant Professor of Pediatrics and Pathology, University of Louisville.

Tumor Markers

Germ cell tumors are associated with various biologic markers that are useful in identifying and managing this group of tumors.[26] Protein markers, including alpha fetoprotein (AFP), beta-human chorionic gonadotropin (beta-hCG), and lactate dehydrogenase (LDH), are the most readily available. They are measured with serum assays or immunohistochemical staining of paraffin-fixed or frozen tumor.

Alpha Fetoprotein

Because the fetal yolk sac is the source of AFP early in human embryogenesis, elevations of the marker occur with yolk sac tumors.[27] This is also true with hepatoblastoma, hepatocellular carcinoma, and teratocarcinoma.[28] The elevation reflects the presence of fetal tissue from which normal progenitor cells arise. There is wide variability in normal levels of AFP from birth through the first year of life,[29] and AFP is significantly elevated in premature and normal newborns. Its usefulness in the diagnosis of yolk sac tumor or embryonal carcinoma in the first month of life is limited. Its value in tumor identification begins when the AFP level is significantly elevated over the normal range at any particular age. The normal serum half-life of AFP is 5 to 7 days. Its decline after removal of an AFP-producing tumor signifies a response to treatment. The goal of any treatment is to return AFP to normal levels. Tumor recurrence is marked by a sudden elevation of the AFP level.

Beta-Human Chorionic Gonadotropin

Beta-hCG is a glycoprotein produced by placental syncytiotrophoblasts. It comprises two subunits, alpha and beta; the latter can be reliably assayed.[30] Beta-hCG elevation in a patient with a germ cell tumor suggests the presence of syncytiotrophoblasts, as seen in seminoma, dysgerminoma, choriocarcinoma,

TABLE 39-2

Ovarian Tumors and Hormones

Histologic Subtype	Estradiol	Testosterone	Urinary 17-ketosteroid	Gonadotropin	MIS
Ovarian cyst					
Simple	↑				
Follicular	↑				
Luteal	↑				
Sex cord–stromal					
Juvenile granulosa	↑	↑‡		↓	↑§
Sertoli-Leydig	↑*	↑†		↓	
Luteinized thecomas	↑	↑‡			
Sex cord tumors with annular tubules	↑				
Steroid cell tumor		↑	↑	↓	
Gonadoblastoma	↑‡	↑	↑	↓	
Choriocarcinoma	↑				↑

*Functioning Sertoli cells predominate.
†Functioning Leydig cells predominate, biologic marker for disease behavior.
‡Indicates rarer variants of the tumor.
§May be useful tumor marker for diagnosis and follow-up.
MIS, Müllerian inhibiting substance.

and, occasionally, embryonal carcinoma.[31] Elevations greater than 100 ng/mL are unusual and suggest the diagnosis of choriocarcinoma.[32] Unlike the much longer half-life of AFP, the beta subunit has a half-life of 20 to 30 hours.[32] Its rapid disappearance implies complete removal of a tumor.

Serum Lactate Dehydrogenase

Serum LDH is a nonspecific marker that is widely distributed in human tissues and is therefore of limited value in establishing tumor type or response to treatment. However, elevated LDH may indicate increased cell turnover and has been used as a nonspecific indicator of malignancy.[33] It is most useful as a prognostic marker for lymphoid tumors and neuroblastoma. The gene for this isoenzyme is located on 12p, and nonrandom structural changes in chromosome 12 have been seen in all histologic subtypes of germ cell tumors, particularly dysgerminoma.

CA 125

CA 125 is the best available marker for epithelial ovarian cancer, although it lacks sensitivity for stage I disease and specificity for early ovarian cancer. Levels greater than 35 U/mL may indicate malignant or borderline ovarian tumors. However, levels are also occasionally raised in some benign conditions, including endometriosis, uterine myomas, acute and chronic salpingitis, and pelvic inflammatory disease.[34] One small series showed a low sensitivity and specificity of CA 125 for detection of epithelial ovarian malignancy in premenarchal girls.[35]

VALUE OF FROZEN SECTION FOR INTRAOPERATIVE DIAGNOSIS

Benign, borderline, and malignant lesions have been identified within the same surgical specimen, suggesting evolution from dysplasia to cancer in some cases, although frequency and speed of this process remain unknown. A quantitative systematic review performed to estimate the diagnostic accuracy of frozen sections compared with paraffin sections, including specimens from 3,659 women aged 1 to 95 years concluded that diagnostic accuracy rates were high for both malignant and benign tumors but low in borderline tumors.[36] This has relevance because a fertility-sparing approach can be used in borderline tumors, but surgeons confronted with this potential diagnosis during surgery should also use a standard approach for staging (discussed later in this chapter), because determination of extent of disease has implications for future treatment and prognosis.[36]

IMMUNOHISTOCHEMISTRY

Immunohistochemistry (IHC) has had a major impact in recent years as an aid to diagnosis in ovarian neoplasia. From a practical standpoint, the time-honored approaches, including gross and microscopic features, thorough sampling, and consideration of patient age and presence or absence of coexisting endometriosis, still take precedence. In general, IHC panels should include markers which are expected to be positive (and negative) in the various tumors in the differential diagnosis. Virtually no antibody is specific for any given tumor, and unexpected positive and negative immunoreactions may occasionally occur. In ovarian pathology, IHC seems to be most valuable in the evaluation of tumors with follicles or other patterns that bring a sex cord–stromal tumor into the differential. The two most useful markers are alpha inhibin and calretinin. Calretinin is a slightly more sensitive marker of ovarian sex cord–stromal tumors as a group, but alpha inhibin, produced by granulosa cells, is a more specific marker, because most other ovarian neoplasms are negative.[37,38]

CANCER GENETICS

Ovarian germ cell tumors are associated with sex chromosome abnormalities. Although a few case studies suggest otherwise, a large study examining 456 first- or second-degree female relatives of 78 patients with ovarian germ cell tumors did not identify an increased risk for occurrence.[39] Some abnormal karyotypes are associated with abnormal gonads that are predisposed to the development of germ cell tumors.

The application of new cytogenetic technologies has increased our understanding of the genetics and molecular mechanisms involved in the development of germ cell tumors. Nonrandom changes in molecular structure have commonly been reported in chromosomes 1 and 12, as well as in others.[40-42] For example, the chromosomal aberration of trisomy 12 has been identified in many stromal tumors.[43] An isochromosome is a chromosome in which both arms are derived from one of the two arms by breakage at the centromere and subsequent duplication. Isochromosome 12p [i(12p)] has been identified in all types of germ cell tumors,[44-47] including testicular germ cell tumors in men.[46] The presence of three or more copies of i(12p) has been associated with treatment failure.[41] Nonrandom endodermal sinus tumors in children involve the deletion of segments of chromosome 1p and 6q. Deletion of the terminal portion of 1p has been identified in other tumors, indicating that it may be a locus of one or more tumor suppressor genes not yet characterized. Endodermal sinus tumors in children may show cytogenetic differences from adults with no evidence of i(12p), but with deletions involving 1p, 3q, and 6q.[48] The c-MYC oncogene has been found in a few endodermal sinus tumors, and the current Children's Oncology Group protocol will begin to correlate amplification with survival and response to therapy.[49] Further studies are required to determine the significance of these findings. Many germ cell tumors in children express P-glycoprotein, a membrane-bound protein that can decrease the response to chemotherapy; this may explain why these tumors are frequently resistant to treatment.[50]

Role of Tumor Markers in the Incidentally Identified Ovarian Mass

If a mixed cystic and solid ovarian mass is discovered incidentally on an imaging study, a preoperative AFP, beta-HCG, and CA-125 assay should be done. If normal, the mass should be removed with ovarian sparing, if possible. If any of these are elevated, a chest CT should be included in the evaluation to look for metastatic disease. Follicle-stimulating hormone (FSH), luteinizing hormone (LH), thyroid-stimulating hormone (TSH), estradiol and lactate dehydrogenase (LDH) serum levels should be added to the preoperative testing if there are signs of precocious puberty.[51]

IMAGING TECHNIQUES

Various radiographic studies play an important role in the clinical evaluation of pediatric ovarian lesions. Prenatal US can usually differentiate ovarian lesions from intestinal duplication, hydronephrosis, duodenal atresia, choledochal cyst, urachal remnants, hydrometrocolpos, and intestinal obstruction (Fig. 39-1). Mesenteric and omental cysts are more difficult to distinguish from simple ovarian cysts, because the ovary is an abdominal rather than a pelvic organ in an infant.

US is the diagnostic study of choice for the initial evaluation of potential ovarian pathology in all age groups. Adequate urinary bladder distention is mandatory to displace gas-filled intestinal loops out of the pelvis and to ensure adequate sound wave transmission through the ovaries. Ovarian volume changes with age from less than 0.7 cm^3 in girls younger than 2 years to 1.8 to 5.7 cm^3 in postpubertal patients.[52] Morphologic characteristics also change. In children younger than 8 years, the ovaries are generally solid, ovoid structures with a homogeneous echogenic texture. During and after puberty, the ultrasonographic spectrum of the gonad undergoes cystic changes that parallel ovulatory follicle activity in the organ. Ovarian cysts are generally anechoic, thin-walled masses with through transmission. With torsion, fluid debris or septation may be present.[53] Most benign tumors are complex masses that are hypoechoic with peripheral echogenic mural nodules, which may exhibit acoustic shadowing. Malignant tumors are

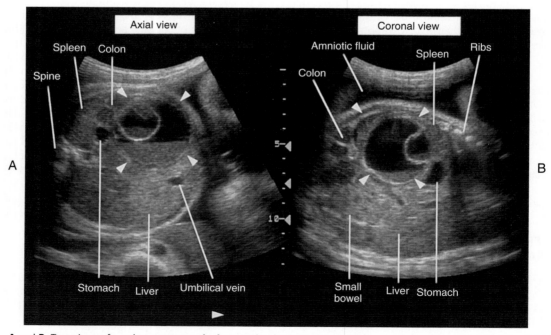

FIGURE 39-1 **A** and **B**, Two views of an ultrasonogram of a fetus in the third trimester. A large, complex ovarian cyst containing fluid debris, internal septation, and solid components can be seen (*arrowheads*). An ovarian neoplasm was identified during surgery after birth. (Courtesy Gary A. Thieme, MD, Prenatal Diagnosis Center, University of Colorado School of Medicine.)

often larger in diameter and appear as complex soft tissue masses with ill-defined, irregular borders and central necrosis, thick septations, or papillary projections on US. Doppler color-flow imaging and transvaginal US are also valuable in postpubertal patients to determine morphologic characteristics of ovarian lesions.[54,55] When vessels are located in the central, septal, or papillary projections, together with a diffuse vascular arrangement, the tumors are likely to be malignant.[56] Other discriminating factors include the presence and nature of solid components and free intraperitoneal fluid. Based on the premise that angiogenesis is a neoplastic marker for malignancy, newer methods of ultrasonography using high-resolution color Doppler with extended flow (e-flow) have resulted in better discrimination of malignancy because of higher sensitivity in detection of blood flow in minute vessels.[57]

Computed tomography (CT) and magnetic resonance imaging (MRI) are useful when the origin of the pelvic mass cannot be established by US or when assessment of the full extent of a noncystic lesion is necessary. The characteristic finding of a benign tumor on CT is a fluid-filled mass with fat and calcifications.[58] Focal solid components arising from the tumor wall are common (Fig. 39-2). Malignant lesions are large and predominantly solid with occasional cystic areas as well as fine or coarse calcifications. Direct extension of tumors to adjacent pelvic structures or to the liver and lungs can also be demonstrated by CT, which provides more accurate staging of disease than US. Adnexal torsion in association with any tumor has a distinct appearance on CT, which is demonstrated by dynamic scanning after the administration of contrast medium. The appearance is generally characterized by lack of enhancement of mural nodules, which indicates interruption of blood flow, and demonstration of thick, engorged blood vessels that drape around the tumor and indicate markedly congested veins distal to the site of torsion.

MRI is well suited for imaging pelvic lesions, because it is not influenced by extensive subcutaneous fat and offers superb soft tissue contrast resolution.[59] The technique is especially valuable in determining whether a mass is ovarian or uterine in origin, and it contributes to the characterization of adnexal masses based on criteria suggestive of benignity (fatty components, shading on T2-weighted images) or malignancy (vegetations or solid portions within cystic masses).[60] MRI accuracy can reach 91%. The long imaging times required may cause peristalsis and respiratory motion to obscure peritoneal and intestinal surfaces, and sedation may be needed in small children. Ovarian torsion with hemorrhagic infarction can be detected on MRI by the finding of a high-intensity rim at the periphery of the mass on the T1-weighted image.[61]

Positron-emission tomography (PET) scanning is a newer modality that may play a role in the differentiation of malignant from borderline ovarian tumors.[62] PET and PET-CT have a potential role in evaluating patients for recurrent ovarian cancer, particularly those with negative CT or MRI findings and rising tumor marker levels. Fused PET-CT scans obtained with combined scanners can help localize pathologic activity and differentiate this activity from physiologic radiotracer uptake.[63]

Disease Classification and Staging

Ovarian lesions are generally divided into nonneoplastic and neoplastic entities; the former category includes functioning cysts, and the latter includes benign and malignant tumors. The clinical system presented here is modified from the most recent version of the World Health Organization's proposal for

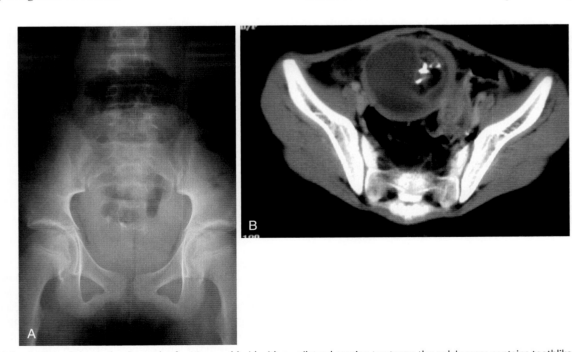

FIGURE 39-2   A, Plain abdominal radiograph of a 16-year-old girl with a unilateral ovarian teratoma; the pelvic mass contains toothlike calcifications. **B,** Computed tomography scan of a large, calcified abdominal mass. The mass has a large cystic component, with solid, thickened walls that are eccentric in appearance. The tumor was a thin-walled fibrous cyst with extensive hemorrhagic infarction throughout the entire cyst wall. Histology was consistent with a benign cystic teratoma.

TABLE 39-3

World Health Organization Histologic Classification of Nonneoplastic Ovarian Lesions

000 Ectopic pregnancy

D27 Benign neoplasm of ovary

E28 Ovarian dysfunction

    E28.2 Polycystic ovarian syndrome

N70-77 Pelvic inflammatory disease

N80 Endometriosis

N83 Noninflammatory disorders of ovary, fallopian tube, and broad ligament

    N83.0 Follicular cyst of ovary

    N83.1 Corpus luteum cyst

    N83.2 Other and unspecified ovarian cysts (simple cyst)

    N83.8 Other noninflammatory disorders of ovary, fallopian tube and broad ligament

From WHO International Classification of Diseases (ICD), 2007. Available at http://www.who.int/classifications/icd/en/. Accessed June 6, 2010. WHO International Statistical Classification of Diseases and Related Health Problems, revision 10, 2007.

TABLE 39-4

World Health Organization Classification of Tumors of the Ovary

1. Surface epithelial–stromal tumors
  1.1. Serous tumors
  1.2. Mucinous tumors
  1.3. Endometrioid tumors
  1.4. Clear cell tumors
  1.5. Transitional cell tumors
  1.6. Squamous cell tumors
  1.7. Mixed epithelial tumors
  1.8. Undifferentiated and unclassified tumors
2. Sex cord–stromal tumors
  2.1. Granulosa–stromal cell tumors
    2.1.1. Granulosa cell tumor group
      2.1.1.1. Adult
      2.1.1.2. Juvenile
    2.1.2. Tumors in thecoma-fibroma group
  2.2. Sertoli–stromal cell tumors
  2.3. Sex cord–stromal tumors of mixed or unclassified cell types
    2.3.1. Sex cord tumor with annular tubules
    2.3.2. Gynandroblastoma
  2.4. Steroid cell tumors
3. Germ cell tumors
  3.1. Primitive germ cell tumors
    3.1.1. Dysgerminoma
    3.1.2. Yolk sac tumor (endodermal sinus tumor)
    3.1.3. Embryonal carcinoma
    3.1.4. Polyembryoma
    3.1.5. Nongestational choriocarcinoma
    3.1.6. Mixed germ cell tumors (specify components)
  3.2. Biphasic or triphasic teratomas
    3.2.1. Immature
    3.2.2. Mature
  3.3. Monodermal teratomas
4. Germ cell sex cord–stromal tumors
  4.1. Gonadoblastoma
  4.2. Mixed germ cell–sex cord–stromal tumor of nongonadoblastoma type
5. Tumors of rete ovarii
6. Miscellaneous tumors
  6.1. Small cell carcinomas, hypercalcemic type
  6.2. Gestational choriocarcinomas
  6.3. Soft tissue tumors not specific to ovary
7. Tumorlike conditions
8. Lymphoid and hematopoietic tumors
9. Secondary tumors

(From International Classification of Diseases for Oncology, ed 3 (ICD-O-3). Creation date: 1976; last date change: 2000.

the international histologic classification of diseases and its adaptation for oncology (Tables 39-3 and 39-4).[64–66] Nonneoplastic and neoplastic lesions may arise from surface epithelium, germ cell components, or support stroma. Neoplastic lesions are listed based on the tissue of origin.

Proper management of ovarian neoplasms requires accurate staging of the initial extent of disease. In malignant cases, recent advances in therapy have resulted in increased survival rates and preservation of fertility. Surgical staging with histologic confirmation must be done to supplement the clinical assessment of disease status. Precise staging is based on clinical examination, surgical exploration, tissue histology, and fluid cytology. In the United States, staging of epithelial ovarian cancer is performed at the time of surgery using the International Federation of Gynecology and Obstetrics (FIGO) staging system of 1988 (which was evaluated and not changed in 2009) (Table 39-5).[67,68] This system is ideal, because it accurately correlates clinical findings with survival in a continuum. However, the FIGO staging protocol does not describe the thoroughness of the lymphadenectomy required for ovarian cancer staging, and it has been suggested that the number of lymph nodes obtained at surgery has prognostic and clinical significance.[68]

Because ovarian neoplasms are relatively uncommon, evaluation and treatment protocols developed from multiinstitutional collaborative studies have been valuable. Stromal and germ cell tumors have been assessed in studies from the Children's Cancer Group (CCG), the Pediatric Oncology Group (POG), and the Gynecologic Oncology Group (GOG).[49,69–71] In children, the intergroup POG 9048/9049 and CCG 8882/8891 studies used a system that incorporated both surgical and pathologic findings.[70] This concept has been preserved by the Children's Oncology Group (COG) (Table 39-6). Uniform surgical guidelines that incorporate standard approaches to these lesions have been formulated, although the approach to ovarian neoplasms has become more conservative with time.[72,73] Preoperative assessment should try to exclude obvious malignancy by the collection of serum tumor markers and carefully performed pelvic US to determine whether the ovarian mass is complex in nature.

Elevated tumor markers and a complex mass on US strongly suggest a malignancy, and an abdominal and pelvic CT scan should be obtained. For potentially malignant lesions, an adequate abdominal incision is used, and violation of the tumor capsule is avoided. Alternatively, if tumor markers are negative and the mass is thought to be benign (e.g., a mature cystic teratoma) a laparoscopic approach can be considered.

Initial resection in pediatric patients should virtually always be conservative. Pelvic washings, unilateral ovarian cystectomy, intraoperative frozen section, and careful visual

TABLE 39-5

Staging of Carcinoma of the Ovary: International Federation of Gynecology and Obstetrics (FIGO)

Stage	Extent of Disease
	Primary tumor cannot be assessed
0	No evidence of primary tumor
I	Tumor confined to ovaries
IA	Tumor limited to one ovary, capsule intact
	No tumor on ovarian surface
	No malignant cells in ascites or peritoneal washings
IB	Tumor limited to both ovaries, capsule intact
	No tumor on ovarian surface
	No malignant cells in ascites or peritoneal washings
IC	Tumor limited to one or both ovaries, with any of the following:
	capsule ruptured, tumor on ovarian surface, malignant cells in ascites or peritoneal washings
II	Tumor involves one or both ovaries with pelvic extension
IIA	Extension to or implants on uterus or tubes or both
	No malignant cells in ascites or peritoneal washings
IIB	Extension to other pelvic organs
	No malignant cells in ascites or peritoneal washings
IIC	IIA or IIB with positive malignant cells in ascites or peritoneal washings
III	Tumor involves one or both ovaries with microscopically confirmed peritoneal metastasis outside the pelvis or regional lymph nodes metastasis
IIIA	Microscopic peritoneal metastasis beyond the pelvis
IIIB	Macroscopic peritoneal metastasis beyond the pelvis 2 cm or less in greatest dimension
IIIC	Peritoneal metastasis beyond the pelvis more than 2 cm in greatest dimension or regional lymph nodes metastasis
IV	Distant metastasis beyond the peritoneal cavity

TABLE 39-6

Clinicopathologic Staging of Ovarian Germ Cell Tumors: Children's Oncology Group (COG)

Stage	Extent of Disease
I	Limited to ovary (peritoneal evaluation should be negative); no clinical, radiographic, or histologic evidence of disease beyond the ovaries (Note: The presence of gliomatosis peritonei does not change stage I disease to a higher stage.)
II	Microscopic residual; peritoneal evaluation negative (Note: The presence of gliomatosis peritonei does not change stage II disease to a higher stage.)
III	Lymph node involvement (metastatic nodule); gross residual or biopsy only; contiguous visceral involvement (omentum, intestine, bladder); peritoneal evaluation positive for malignancy
IV	Distant metastases, including liver

inspection of the contralateral ovary are appropriate in the initial management of benign lesions or tumors of low malignant potential. Pelvic washings are part of the staging system for ovarian tumors and should be performed immediately on entry into the abdomen (by either laparoscopy or laparotomy) in an attempt to avoid contamination in the event of intraoperative tumor rupture. Because the final pathology will not be known until either frozen section or histologic evaluation of paraffin-embedded tissue, peritoneal washings should be performed in all patients with complex adnexal masses in case of an unsuspected malignancy. If there is no evidence of free fluid upon entering the abdomen, lactated Ringer solution can be used to irrigate the pelvis and paracolic gutters, then aspirated and sent as washings.

Malignant germ cell and stromal tumors are almost never bilateral in early-stage disease; so, unilateral salpingo-oophorectomy with a staging procedure is adequate first-line management. Excellent responses have been reported with chemotherapy, even in children with extensive tumors, and maintenance of childbearing capability is possible with this approach. In bilateral or more advanced disease, the current success of in vitro fertilization techniques has prompted the consideration of uterus-sparing procedures during the initial operation.[74,75] The expected biologic behavior of the tumor and its response to adjuvant therapy generally dictate the ultimate extent of surgery required. The value of laparoscopic examination in the assessment of pelvic disease is well established, because it will allow identification and management of ovarian masses as well as identification of nonovarian lesions.[76,77] The American Association of Gynecologic Laparoscopists reviewed more than 13,000 procedures performed for persistent ovarian masses.[78] Stage I ovarian cancer was detected in 0.4% of cases. Although these results are encouraging in adult women, there is concern about the difficulty of establishing the true nature of an ovarian tumor by gross examination in children, because experience with such an evaluation is so infrequent. Nevertheless, techniques are being established to avoid tumor spillage that may expand the use of this method. Experienced surgeons have performed more extensive staging procedures and lymph node dissections using the laparoscope.[79] Studies evaluating the laparoscopic approach have been retrospective and suggested that staging is safe, feasible, and a valid alternative, but there has been no prospective trial to date comparing the laparoscopic to open approach.[68]

Treatment

NONNEOPLASTIC OVARIAN TUMORS

Ovarian cysts are known to arise from mature follicles. Fetal FSH, LH, estrogens (maternal, placental, and fetal), and placental hCG all stimulate the ovarian follicle, and mature follicles can be found in more than half of newborn ovaries.[80] A postnatal decrease in hormonal stimulation often leads to a self-limited process. Autopsy studies of prepubertal girls have documented active follicular growth at all ages and in normal oocytes, granulosa cells, and cysts in various stages of involution.[81,82] By convention, physiologic follicles are differentiated from pathologic ovarian cysts on the basis of size, and any lesion larger than 2 cm in diameter is no longer considered a mature follicle.

Nonneoplastic cysts are benign and generally asymptomatic. Although surgical intervention is rarely indicated, these lesions occasionally have clinical manifestations, based on size or associated functional activity, that warrant differentiation from true ovarian neoplasms. When an operation is necessary, a conservative approach should be undertaken with the goal of ovarian preservation.

Follicular Cysts

Follicular cysts represent about half of nonneoplastic ovarian lesions. They are unilateral, unilocular, and histologically benign and often have a thin, yellowish, clear liquid content. Cohen and associates[83] detected cysts in 84% of all imaged ovaries in 77 patients from birth to 24 months of age. The prevalence was similar in each 3-month age bracket. Parallel findings were noted in premenarchal girls between 2 and 12 years of age,[84] with a generally equal distribution across the age spectrum. Occasionally, ovarian cysts persist and enlarge and are capable of secreting estrogen, thereby leading to precocious isosexual development.[85]

The size of an ovarian lesion has been a major factor in determining clinical management.[80] Simple cysts, regardless of size, are more likely to regress. Larger cysts (>5 cm) have a greater risk of torsion. Larger cysts in children have a greater association with sexual precocity. Complex cysts may already have torsed or may be neoplastic. Complex cysts should be resected, rather than observed, in prepubertal children. Complex cysts in adolescents are most often due to hemorrhage into a functional cyst and can be managed conservatively with symptom control. Operation is indicated for persistent cysts or persistent symptoms despite conservative management.

Ovarian cysts noted in the prenatal period can be expected to spontaneously regress during the first year of life, and in utero therapy is seldom justified.[86,87] Cysts that develop in utero are most often lined by luteinized cells, whereas those in older children are more often lined by granulosa cells.[32] These lesions may occasionally be complicated by torsion, intestinal obstruction, or perforation and cyst rupture.[80,88] Bagolan and colleagues[89] and Giorlandino and colleagues[90] confirmed that echogenic cysts with fluid debris, retracting clot, or septation were associated with torsion and hemorrhage. In newborns, torsion is often a prenatal event, and viable ovarian tissue may not be identified, even with the most expeditious neonatal surgical intervention (Fig. 39-3). Most authors now advocate increasingly conservative measures for neonatal ovarian lesions.[80] Small, asymptomatic cysts are generally observed for regression with serial US. Cysts 5 cm in

diameter or larger and those with a long adnexal pedicle are more likely to undergo torsion and may be excised with ovarian preservation or aspirated.[91] However, in one randomized study of postmenarchal patients, cysts greater than 5 cm in diameter and those with a complex appearance on imaging studies were followed for a short time with serial pelvic US. High regression rates were seen with those followed expectantly.[35] Although practitioners often reflexively prescribe oral contraceptive pills (OCPs), hormonal therapy has not been shown to improve the regression rates of ovarian cysts compared with those followed expectently.[92] Exploratory laparotomy or laparoscopy has been recommended for patients with cysts that do not resolve or increase in size within 2 to 3 months[92] and for cysts associated with acute or severe chronic abdominal pain or intra-abdominal complications.

In prepubertal children, the occurrence of acute symptoms and endocrine activity are more problematic. Surgical intervention is recommended for any cyst that increases in size or fails to regress on follow-up US or if there is evidence of a neoplasm on imaging studies.

As many as 75% of girls with juvenile hypothyroidism have large multicystic ovaries and may show varying degrees of sexual precocity and/or galactorrhea resulting from increased secretion of pituitary gonadotropins and prolactin.[93] Multiple follicular cysts should be distinguished from polycystic ovary syndrome, which is the most common cause of delayed puberty and heavy anovulatory bleeding in adolescent females.[94]

In nonneoplastic ovarian cysts, surgical preservation of as much normal ovarian tissue as possible is a high priority.[95] A plane of dissection can usually be established between the normal gonadal tissue and the cyst after injecting saline with a fine-bore needle beneath the visceral peritoneum. If the surgical manipulation necessary to completely remove the lesion would threaten significant viable ovarian tissue, the cyst should be unroofed and debulked, and the cyst wall excised to the extent possible, while protecting the ovary. Unilateral oophorectomy is indicated only if there is a reasonable certainty that no viable gonadal tissue can be salvaged. The ipsilateral fallopian tube should be spared, because fertilization is still possible from the contralateral normal ovary.

Corpus Luteum Cysts

True functioning corpus luteum cysts develop only in adolescents who are actively ovulating. Although these cysts may be bilateral and become quite large, they usually regress spontaneously with the cyclic decline in serum progesterone. The gross appearance of the external surface is often bright yellow, although it may take on a hemorrhagic appearance when filled with bloody fluid. The cyst lining is composed of luteinized granulosa and theca cells and is capable of actively producing estrogen and progesterone. These cysts may cause acute pelvic pain if they rupture or undergo torsion. Failure of the corpus luteum to involute may cause menstrual irregularity and dysfunctional uterine bleeding. Surgical goals for corpus luteum cysts parallel those for other follicular lesions. Surgical intervention is indicated in the presence of cyst accident or persistence, demonstrated by repeat pelvic US performed 4 to 6 weeks after the initial assessment. Hasson[96] was able to treat 17 of 19 patients who had corpus luteum cysts with laparoscopic aspiration, fenestration, or cyst wall excision. Clinical symptoms resolved in all but one patient. Cyst recurrence was rare.

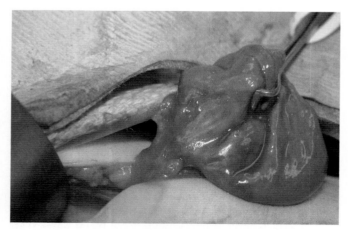

FIGURE 39-3 This newborn female infant had a prenatal diagnosis of an intra-abdominal cystic mass. Postnatal imaging showed a low-attenuation cystic structure with a curvilinear calcification along one wall. Laparotomy disclosed a torsed ovarian cyst and ovary, attached by only a small residual stalk. The fallopian tube was preserved. Pathology showed a thin-walled cyst containing dystrophic calcifications.

Parovarian Cysts

Parovarian cysts are usually small and rarely symptomatic. They do not arise from ovarian tissue but are usually considered with this group of lesions because of their proximity to the gonad. These cysts originate from the epoophoron and are located in the leaves of the mesosalpinx. Parovarian cysts cannot be distinguished from ovarian follicular cysts using any radiographic imaging technique. During an operation, their gross features are virtually identical to those of follicular lesions, but they can usually be accurately distinguished because of their anatomic position. When surgical treatment is required, both standard open and minimally invasive techniques have been used.[96,97] Large parovarian cysts (>3 cm) should be completely enucleated from the mesosalpinx in such a way that the fallopian tube and ovary are not damaged.[98] Those less than 3 cm may be treated with puncture and bipolar coagulation of the cyst wall.[98]

Endometriosis

Endometriosis is a disorder in which the endometrial glands and stroma are implanted on the peritoneal surfaces of extrauterine sites. The proposed mechanisms for the pathogenesis of this disease include menstrual flow obstruction with retrograde menstruation, mechanical transplantation and implantation of endometrial elements, and coelomic metaplasia.[99–101] The interval between the onset of menarche and the diagnosis of endometriosis may be as short as 1 month, and the incidence of disease in teenage girls may be far higher than previously anticipated or described.[102] Extensive disease and the presence of endometriomas is uncommon in children and young adolescents unless it is associated with an obstructive müllerian anomaly.[103] An endometrioma or endometrioid cyst may occur in the ovary and can be diagnosed by ultrasonography. Endometrioid *cysts* are filled with dark, reddish-brown blood and may range in size from 0.75 to 8 inches. Several surgical treatments are available for endometriomas, including simple puncture, ablation, removal of the cyst wall, or drainage and medical therapy, followed by later removal. Complete removal is the procedure of choice to decrease recurrence of disease. The revised American Fertility Society classification of endometriosis is widely accepted as the staging system for the disease and was developed as a prognostic tool for patients with infertility.[104] For patients with pelvic pain and a suspected diagnosis of endometriosis, medical therapy with nonsteroidal antiinflammatory drugs or oral contraceptives should be considered. Both medications act to suppress prostaglandins, which are known to be important in the pathophysiology of dysmenorrhea. These drugs along with gonadotropin hormone antagonists, used for a 6-month period, are the most commonly used medications.

NEOPLASTIC OVARIAN TUMORS

Most neoplastic ovarian tumors develop from cell lines derived from one of three sources: the germinal epithelium covering the urogenital ridge, the underlying stromal elements of the urogenital ridge, or the germ cells that arise from the yolk sac. Cells from each of these lineages may develop into an ovarian neoplasm by de-differentiation, proliferation, and eventually malignant transformation.[105] Malignant ovarian tumors probably arise from their benign counterparts

because of either direct or indirect hormonal stimulation.[106] Histologic and biologically intermediate forms between benign and malignant epithelial lesions have been identified and designate tumors of low malignant potential.

Age influences the relative frequency of the various types of ovarian neoplasms. In adults, most tumors are derived from the epithelial line and adenocarcinomas predominate. In children, germ cell tumors are most common and represent approximately 60% to 77% of cases.[105] Epithelial lesions account for approximately 15% of tumors in the younger age group.[95,107] Although germ cell tumors predominate in each age group, the peak incidence of sex cord–stromal tumors occurs in the first 4 years of life, and epithelial tumors are more common in older teenagers. Neoplasms that are rare in children include endometrioid and clear cell tumors (which are usually malignant); Brenner tumors, which are usually benign; disseminated malignant lymphoma; and metastatic lesions to the ovary.

Surface Epithelial-Stromal Tumors

Epithelial tumors account for 70% of all ovarian neoplasms, but they are much less common in children. In most series, they account for approximately 15% of all surgically resected ovarian masses.[108] Norris and Jensen[109] reported that 67 of 353 ovarian tumors (19%) in children were epithelial in origin and 12% were malignant. The tumors are usually serous or mucinous.[13] Twenty percent of serous tumors are bilateral, and very few are malignant.[13,110] Mucinous tumors are usually unilateral, and 10% are malignant.[13] Deprest and colleagues[111] calculated a 16% malignancy rate for ovarian epithelial neoplasms derived from a collected series that reported more than 1700 pediatric patients with various types of ovarian tumors. Ovarian carcinoma is different in children than in adults. The proportion of mucinous tumors in children was 40% compared with 12% in adults, and 30% were of borderline malignant potential compared with the adult rate of fewer than 10% for these more favorable lesions. As previously discussed, serum CA 125 is a useful tumor marker in malignant epithelial ovarian tumors.[68] However, in premenopausal patients, it may also be raised in several benign gynecologic conditions, including endometriosis, pelvic inflammatory disease, fibroids, and pregnancy.

Proper staging of epithelial tumors is important and differs from the staging algorithm used in pediatric germ cell tumors, which are far more common. Epithelial tumors are staged using the adult FIGO system (see Table 39-5).[67,68] Stage IA tumors may be treated with unilateral salpingo-oophorectomy. The opposite ovary should be examined externally and a biopsy should be taken of any surface abnormalities. Most young patients with stage IB tumors (tumors limited to both ovaries) may be adequately treated by bilateral gonadectomy, but the uterus should be preserved to allow future fertilization.[74,112] In ovarian cancer of a more advanced stage, maximum cytoreduction is important and has been associated with an improved outcome.[113] Total abdominal hysterectomy and bilateral salpingo-oophorectomy with omentectomy and resection of as much gross intraperitoneal disease as possible is necessary. Systemic chemotherapy after appropriate surgery has been beneficial in cases of advanced ovarian carcinoma. Combinations of cisplatin, cyclophosphamide, and paclitaxel are standard agents, while newer biologic therapies hold some promise to improve the overall poor outcome in advanced-stage disease.[114]

Fortunately, advanced-stage disease is uncommon in pediatric patients as tumor stage is the most important prognostic factor.[68]

Tumors of Low Malignant Potential

Ovarian epithelial tumors of low malignant potential or borderline ovarian tumors (BOTs) differ from epithelial cancer in two major ways: They occur in younger patients, and they have a better prognosis than ovarian cancer. They have been described for all subtypes of ovarian cancer.[111] The serous and mucinous tumors are by far the most common and resemble their benign counterparts. These borderline tumors are differentiated from standard adenocarcinoma in that they lack stromal invasion by neoplastic epithelial elements (Fig. 39-4). Up to 50% of these tumors are bilateral, and they demonstrate a characteristic indolent clinical course. However, recurrences may occur as long as 10 to 15 years after surgery for the primary tumor, and they may be in the form of invasive cancer.[115,116]

In adults, 91% of borderline mucinous tumors present with stage I disease and have a 5-year survival rate of 98%. Serous tumors have a similar outcome. The extensive review of Massad and colleagues[117] noted an overall survival of 98% for stage I tumors, 94% for stage II, and 79% for stages III and IV. In children, Morris and colleagues[118] noted that 75% of the cases presented with stage I disease, and overall survival was 100%. The combined 10-year survival rate for all stages was 73%. In a more recent adolescent study, 26/28 cases were stage I, two cases were stage II, and all patients were alive at 5 years.[116]

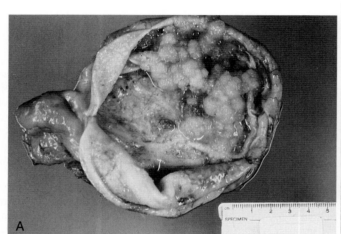

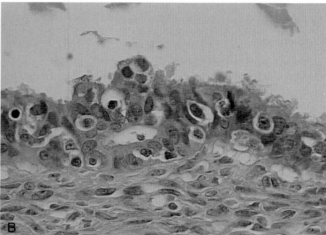

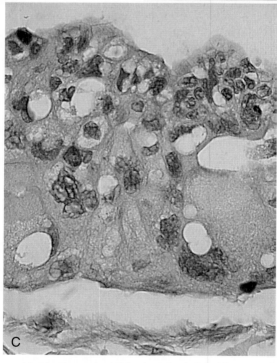

FIGURE 39-4   **A,** Ovarian tumor from a 17-year-old girl with massive bilateral ovarian lesions. The opened specimen shows a cavity filled with clear fluid, and the wall is lined by numerous nodules and papillary protuberances. **B,** Histologic section of the lesion shows serous papillary tumor of low malignant potential (hematoxylin-eosin stain). **C,** Higher-power photomicrograph of a section of the lesion shows mucinous tumor of low malignant potential (hematoxylin-eosin stain).

Surgery is the primary method of therapy. Unilateral salpingo-oophorectomy is adequate for all low-stage tumors and has been standard treatment; however, some studies have shown that ovarian cystectomy can be performed in young patients with careful follow-up.[119] These patients require close follow-up with pelvic exams, CA 125 assay, and ultrasonography every 3 to 6 months, because patients managed with ovarian cystectomy have a higher risk of recurrence than those managed more aggressively.[120] Morice and colleagues have demonstrated this to be 36.3%, 15.1%, and 5.7% after cystectomy, oophorectomy, and hysterectomy/bilateral oophorectomy, respectively.[119] Despite the difference in recurrence risk, there was no demonstrated impact on overall survival, because all patients were salvaged with further surgery. Conservative treatment should therefore be considered in young patients who wish to preserve their fertility and will comply with routine follow-up.[121]

Bilateral tumors will require bilateral oophorocystectomy or salpingo-oophorectomy. Uterine-sparing procedures are probably not appropriate for advanced-stage disease. The pathologic features that identify poor prognosis are being sought,[115] but currently there are no clear candidates. At present, surgery remains the most effective therapy for these patients with the place of adjuvant therapy yet to be established.[122] No individual treatment strategy has led to consistently superior outcomes, but the favorable biology of this tumor minimizes the importance of the limited clinical benefit from adjuvant therapy.

Sex Cord–Stromal Tumors

Sex cord–stromal tumors probably arise from uncommitted mesenchymal stem cells that reside below the surface epithelium of the urogenital ridge.[123,124] This totipotential tissue may differentiate into several different cell lines, including granulosa-theca cells in the ovary and the Leydig-Sertoli cells in the testicular interstitium. Sex cord–stromal tumors are referred to as functioning ovarian tumors, because they produce systemic hormonal effects. They account for 5.7% to 17% of malignant tumors in series of ovarian neoplasms in children.[5] Before 9 years of age, most sex cord–stromal tumors are feminizing, and after 9 years of age, there is a predominance of virilizing neoplasms.[32]

Granulosa-Theca Cell Tumors Granulosa-stromal cell tumors are the most common type of sex cord–stromal neoplasms, and the most common type of functioning ovarian neoplasm. The juvenile granulosa cell tumor is a specific subclassification of these lesions; 44% of these occur in the first decade of life and 97% are seen by 30 years of age.[125] Isosexual pseudoprecocious puberty is the presenting sign in the majority of premenarchal girls who have this tumor (Fig. 39-5).[123] Most patients have elevated serum and urinary estrogen levels, whereas gonadotropin levels are low. This profile assists in differentiating children with these tumors from those with true sexual precocity, gonadotropin-secreting lesions, or feminizing adrenal tumors. The peptide hormones

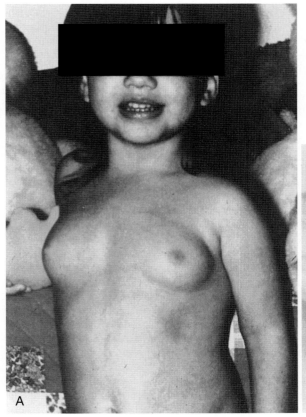
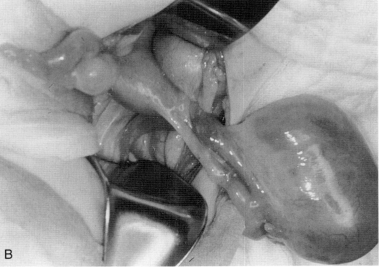

FIGURE 39-5 **A,** Three-year-old girl demonstrating isosexual pseudoprecocious puberty. **B,** Surgery revealed a benign juvenile granulosa cell tumor. Unilateral salpingo-oophorectomy was performed to remove the tumor.

inhibin and antimüllerian hormone are produced by ovarian granulosa cells and may be useful tumor markers for diagnosis and follow-up of granulosa cell tumors.[126]

Clinical findings include premature thelarche, vaginal discharge or bleeding, labial enlargement, development of pubic or axillary hair, increased somatic growth, and advanced bone age. Clitoral enlargement is a rare manifestation of virilization and tumor androgen production. Postpubertal girls may present with an abdominal mass, relatively nonspecific symptoms of abdominal pain, or increased girth. Amenorrhea and other menstrual irregularities may occur.

In addition to differences in clinical presentation, juvenile granulosa cell tumors demonstrate a pattern of histologic features and biologic behavior that are very distinct from the adult counterpart. The juvenile variety is usually a relatively large lesion that averages 12.5 cm in diameter.[127] At laparotomy, it appears as a yellow-tan or gray solid neoplasm with cystic areas that often contain hemorrhagic fluid. In contrast to the adult tumors, the juvenile type has abundant eosinophilic or luteinized cytoplasm with atypical nuclei and a higher mitotic rate. Deoxyribonucleic acid (DNA) content and cell cycle kinetics analyzed by flow cytometry do not necessarily correlate with the prognosis in children as they often do in adults.[128]

Although the adult form is generally an indolent, slow-growing lesion of relatively low malignant potential, the biologic behavior of the juvenile tumor is more aggressive and correlates well with tumor size, disease stage, presence of rupture, and degree of nuclear atypia and mitotic activity. The lesion was unilateral in 122 of 125 cases reviewed by Young and colleagues.[129] If the adult tumor recurs, it is usually more than 5 years after diagnosis. Malignant granulosa cell tumors in young patients tend to recur much more quickly.

Granulosa cell tumors are staged similarly to other ovarian lesions (see Table 39-5). In children, these tumors are associated with a favorable prognosis, because more than 90% of affected children present with stage I disease. In a German series, 69% of patients were less than 10 years of age, and 82% of patients less than 5 years of age presented with endocrine symptoms. Survival of FIGO stage IA patients was 100%, stage IC was 76%, and stage II/III was 67%. Platinum-based chemotherapy is recommended for tumors of stage IC and above.[93]

Fibromas and Thecomas

Fibromas and thecomas account for 14% of sex cord–stromal tumors in pediatric patients.[13] Although they are extremely uncommon in females younger than 20 years of age, fibromas are usually associated with the basal cell nevus syndrome and are frequently bilateral, multicentric, and calcified. Most ovarian thecomas occur in menopausal women; however, two variants of this lesion have been reported in the second decade of life. Calcified thecomas invariably cause amenorrhea or other menstrual irregularities and hirsutism.[130] If these tumors contain a substantial number of lutein cells, they are appropriately called luteinized thecomas and can occur in younger girls associated with androgenic manifestations.

On gross examination, fibromas are firm, solid masses with a whorled, trabeculated appearance on cross section. The lipid content of thecomas imparts a pale yellow to orange color on sectioning the tumor. These lesions are benign, and unilateral oophorectomy is adequate treatment. In the case of bilateral fibromas, all gross tumor tissue should be removed with particular attention to sparing normal-appearing ovarian tissue.[131] Tumor recurrence is rare and managed by reoperation. Virilizing symptoms usually resolve after resection of the tumor.

Sclerosing Stromal Tumors

Sclerosing stromal tumors have recently been recognized as distinct tumors that are separate from fibromas and thecomas. These tumors are seen in girls, with 30% of documented cases occurring in the first 2 decades of life. Estrogen secretion has occasionally been reported, whereas androgen manifestations are quite rare. The typical presentation includes the presence of a pelvic mass and pelvic pain in a young patient with a history of menstrual irregularity. This lesion has also been associated with the Chédiak-Higashi syndrome.[10]

Sclerosing stromal tumors are unilateral, usually larger than 5 cm in diameter, and benign. At laparotomy, these tumors are well-circumscribed, firm, whitish-yellow masses with clearly demarcated areas of edema and cyst formation. Histologically, the tumor is characterized by a pseudolobulated pattern with cellular foci clearly demarcated from the edematous and collagenized areas.[132] Gross tumor removal is generally adequate for treatment.

Sertoli-Stromal Cell Tumors

Sertoli-Leydig cell tumors account for less than 0.5% of all ovarian tumors but represent 10% of the sex cord–stromal neoplasms.[13] Although most of these tumors are masculinizing, some are nonfunctional or even associated with estrogenic effects. Therefore the older terms, *arrhenoblastoma* and *androblastoma* are no longer favored. One third of cases occur in patients younger than 20 years of age. These tumors are almost always unilateral and present as stage IA at diagnosis. Survival is excellent, with tumor-related deaths in only 5% of affected individuals.[32] Similar to granulosa cell tumors, the gross appearance of Sertoli-Leydig cell tumors varies widely, but these lesions are less often filled with hemorrhagic fluid and rarely have a unilocular thin-walled cystic appearance. Current classifications now recognize five histologic patterns based on the degree of differentiation and presence of heterologous, endodermal, or mesenchymal elements. Tumor stage and histologic appearance are important prognostic factors. Sertoli-Leydig cell tumors with heterologous elements are more common in younger patients and may be difficult to distinguish from immature teratomas.[32] There are two phases of the masculinizing effects of androgen overproduction. Initially, defeminization takes place with amenorrhea, breast atrophy, and loss of female body habitus. This may be followed or overlapped by masculinization characterized by hirsutism, clitoral hypertrophy, and deepening of the voice. In prepubertal girls, masculinization and accelerated somatic growth predominate. Postpubertal girls usually have menstrual irregularities, acne, body habitus masculinization, and hirsutism. The virilizing effects are caused by testosterone accumulation resulting from a deficiency in catabolizing enzymes. Gonadotropin levels are low, and excretion of urinary 17-ketosteroids and pregnanetriol is normal. Because the testosterone level is often directly related to tumor tissue volume, this hormone is a biologic marker for monitoring disease behavior.[133] Tumor markers most likely to be elevated are alpha fetoprotein (AFP) and CA 125.[134] LDH may be elevated or normal. The hormonal profile of these lesions assists in differentiating them from exogenous androgen sources, adrenal tumors, true hermaphroditism, and polycystic ovaries. Similar to granulosa cell tumors, the Sertoli-Leydig cell lesions may be associated with multiple enchondromas caused by nonhereditary mesodermal dysplasia (Ollier disease).[124]

Surgical therapy should be conservative for patients with low-stage disease. Unilateral oophorectomy or adnexectomy is adequate for such disease and will preserve later childbearing capacity. If tumors are bilateral, poorly differentiated or have ruptured or demonstrate aggressive behavior, a more aggressive approach similar to that used for granulosa cell tumors is necessary. Oral contraceptives and gonadotropin-releasing hormone agonists may provide some ovarian protection both during and following chemotherapy.[135]

Sex Cord Tumors with Annular Tubules

Sex cord tumors with annular tubules (SCTAT) are rare but distinct variants of sex cord–stromal tumors. They have potential for bidirectional differentiation into granulosa or Sertoli cells.[13] These lesions are observed in patients with Peutz-Jeghers syndrome.[6] When associated with this syndrome, the lesions are small, multifocal, and usually bilateral. The tumors are often calcified and are invariably noted incidentally during autopsy or in an ovary removed for reasons unrelated to neoplasia. Although patients with these tumors occasionally have menstrual irregularities suggesting hyperestrogenism, surgical therapy is rarely indicated. When these tumors occur in the absence of Peutz-Jeghers syndrome, the clinical difference is significant. Such lesions occur in older patients with a mean age of 34 years, although cases have been reported in patients from 6 to 76 years of age. In the younger patients, the tumor is unilateral and almost always larger than 5 cm in diameter; 20% are malignant. Even with aggressive therapy, 50% of patients with these tumors die.[136]

Steroid Cell Tumors

Steroid cell tumor is the now preferred name for lesions previously called lipid cell tumors. This name is more appropriate because of the morphologic features of the tumor, its propensity to secrete steroid hormones, and because many such lesions contain little or no lipids. The group is subclassified into three major categories according to the cells of origin: (1) stromal luteoma is a small steroid cell tumor contained in the ovary arising from the stromal lutein cell; (2) Leydig cell tumor contains the classic intracytoplasmic Reinke crystals and arises from histologically similar precursor cells found in the ovarian hilus; (3) steroid cell tumors not otherwise specified account for approximately 60% of cases and typically occurs in younger patients.

The first and second categories of lesion are usually encountered in postmenopausal women and are only rarely reported in patients in the first 3 decades of life. Most of the cases in the third category and in prepubertal children have been associated with androgenic, heterosexual pseudoprecocity. The tumors are rarely estrogenic, but isosexual pseudoprecocious puberty has been reported.[137] The androgenic tumors show elevated testosterone and androstenedione levels, increased urinary 17-ketosteroid excretion, and decreased gonadotropin levels. In children, these lesions are virtually always benign and of a low stage. Unilateral salpingo-oophorectomy is adequate treatment, but close follow-up is essential. Most of the hormonal symptoms should progressively resolve after removal of the tumor, although younger children may develop true precocious puberty after resection, because chronic androgen exposure appears to induce an early maturation of the hypothalamus.[138]

Germ Cell Tumors

The path of descent of the primordial germ cells is imperfect; as a result, some of the cells may occasionally miss their destination and be deposited anywhere along this migration route. Germ cells have been found in the pineal area of the brain, mediastinum, retroperitoneum, the sacrococcygeal area, and the ovary and testis. If malignant transformation occurs at any of these sites, a gonadal or extragonadal neoplasm will develop. Because these nests of cells are totipotential in nature, a wide variety of tumors are seen. The specific type of tumor depends on the degree of differentiation that has occurred. This has been characterized by Telium.[27] According to this schema, if no differentiation occurs, a germinoma develops; with differentiation, embryonal carcinomas occur; and with extraembryonic differentiation, these lesions become choriocarcinomas or endodermal sinus tumors. If embryonal differentiation occurs, then the teratoma or most mature of these tumors is seen.

Germ cell tumors are rare in children and adolescents, but when they occur, the gonad is the most frequent site. The ovary is the site of origin for 30% of all germ cell tumors in children.[139,140] Epithelial and stromal ovarian tumors prevail in adults; germ cell tumors predominate in children. Several large series of ovarian neoplasms report an incidence of germ cell tumors ranging from 67% to 77%.[5,141] This group of tumors develops from the same totipotential primordial germ cell, but each neoplasm has different behavioral characteristics, and will be presented individually and then as a group relative to overall management decisions.

Germinoma

The term *germinoma* is used to include a group of tumors with common histologic characteristics. It is the primary malignant tumor found in dysgenetic gonads. This tumor may be referred to as a seminoma if found in the testis, a dysgerminoma in the ovary, and a germinoma in an extragonadal site. Germinomas are believed to arise from the totipotential germ cells that were present at the undifferentiated stage of gonadal development.[142] Germinomas represent the most frequent ovarian malignant neoplasm seen both in children and adults.[32] They account for 26% to 31% of malignant ovarian tumors in children.[143,144]

Germinomas are most often seen in prepubertal girls and young women, with 44% of cases occurring before 20 years of age and 87% by 30 years of age.[145] The typical patient is genotypically and phenotypically normal. These often large tumors may reach massive proportions and lead to abdominal pain and symptoms of pelvic pressure, or symptoms related to obstruction of the gastrointestinal or urinary tract. Occasionally, girls with these tumors present with an acute abdomen as a result of torsion, rupture, or hemorrhage into the tumor. Ascites may be present. In pure dysgerminoma, LDH is elevated in 95% of patients, but other markers are negative. In the mixed form of these tumors, other markers may be positive, including neuro-specific enolase, beta-hCG, and CA 125, depending on which germ cell component is present.[146,147] Ovarian dysgerminomas may also be associated with a paraneoplastic syndrome causing hypercalcemia, which typically resolves with removal of the tumor but may persist for several days.[148] On gross examination, these tumors appear bulky, encapsulated, solid, and yellowish in color (Fig. 39-6); they can be bilateral in 5% to 30% of cases.[142,149,150] Germinomas have a rather uniform microscopic appearance consisting of large, round cells that have vesicular nuclei and clear-to-eosinophilic cytoplasm. These cells resemble primordial germ cells. Lymphoid infiltrates may be present.

The management of germ cell tumors begins with surgical excision. Conservative surgery with a unilateral salpingo-oophorectomy, thorough inspection of the contralateral ovary with biopsy of suspicious lesions, and careful staging (as outlined in the section on surgical approach) is mandatory. Although these tumors are very radiosensitive, surgery alone is adequate treatment in stage I disease. In more advanced disease, radiation has been abandoned in favor of effective

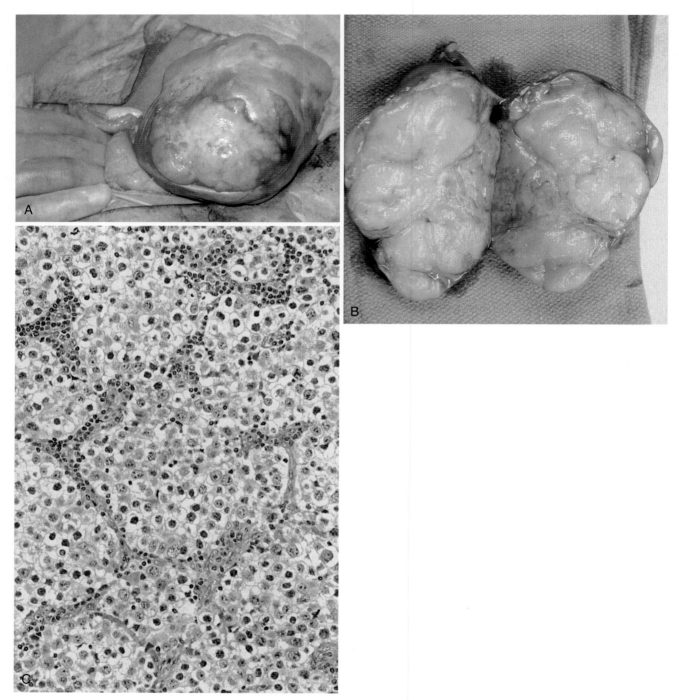

FIGURE 39-6   **A,** This encapsulated mass from a 5-year-old girl with acute abdominal pain proved to be a dysgerminoma. The child's contralateral tube and ovary are seen to the left of the tumor. A small portion of the ipsilateral tube and uterus were in the surgical specimen but uninvolved with tumor. **B,** The cut surface of the tumor is characterized by lobules divided by thin, fibrous septae. **C,** Micrograph of a dysgerminoma demonstrating polygonal, clear tumor cells divided into small lobules by fibrous septae that contain scattered lymphocytes.

multiagent chemotherapeutic programs that include platinum, etoposide, and bleomycin, which is now standard therapy.[146,151,152]

Endodermal Sinus Tumors Endodermal sinus or yolk sac tumors are aggressive malignant neoplasms that, either alone or as a component of a mixed germ cell tumor, are the second most common histologic subtype of malignant ovarian germ cell tumors in children and adolescents.[32,153] In neonates and young children the primary location of these tumors is in the sacrococcygeal area. In older children and adolescents, it is found most frequently in the ovary. The origin of this particular tumor has been debated, and many microscopic patterns of this tumor have now been described. Nogales suggested that this tumor originates from the primary yolk sac, a structure that develops very early in embryogenesis and consists of multipotential primitive endoderm.[154] This tissue is capable of differentiating epithelial somatic tissues as well as secondary yolk sac tissue (a terminal, temporary structure with limited differentiating capacity) and mesenchyme. Yolk sac tumors with pure endodermal sinus subtypes are less mature than the differentiated glandular or hepatoid subtypes.[155] Symptoms are generally present for less than a month and are related to the presence of an intra-abdominal mass. Sixty-three percent of patients present with abdominal pain and/or abdominal distention.[156] Elevation of the biologic marker AFP is the hallmark of this tumor.

The gross appearance of these tumors during surgery is pale yellow-tan and slimy, with foci of cystic areas and necrosis.[157] The tumors are soft and friable when handled. Most tumors show a distinct histologic subtype with differentiation toward vitelline or yolk sac structures.[158] Microscopically, the most common papillary pattern has the so-called endodermal sinus structures (Schiller-Duval bodies) or perivascular sheaths of cells. Most well-differentiated yolk sac tumors also contain extracellular and intracellular droplets that are resistant to periodic acid–Schiff diastase staining and positive for AFP.

Embryonal Carcinomas A relatively uncommon isolated germ cell tumor is embryonal carcinoma, which may resemble an anaplastic carcinoma with extensive necrosis. Embryonal carcinoma is more often found in association with other germ cell tumors and is referred to as a mixed germ cell tumor. One subtype of this tumor, the polyembryoma, is capable of producing both AFP and beta-hCG, resulting in clinical endocrinopathies, including menstrual irregularities and isosexual precocious puberty. The histologic appearance is characterized by bodies that resemble tiny embryos.[159]

The workup and surgical approach to this tumor is similar to that for an endodermal sinus tumor. Isolated, unilateral disease is managed by unilateral salpingo-oophorectomy. Advanced local disease necessitates hysterectomy for local control along with multiagent chemotherapy.[160]

Choriocarcinomas Choriocarcinomas are extremely rare in the pure form but may be present in mixed germ cell tumors as well. They are endocrinologically active, highly malignant germ cell tumors that occur in girls and women. Estrogen is produced both by the tumor and by the ovary itself in response to release of gonadotropin by the neoplastic chorionic tissue. The beta-hCG level is elevated, and AFP is normal. The clinical presentation is influenced by the age of the patient. In a review of 30 cases, Goswami reported a mean age of 13.9 years, with the predominant presenting symptom being abdominal pain. Ten cases occurred in prepubertal girls, three of whom developed isosexual precocious puberty, and in one case a mature teratoma was identified in the contralateral ovary.[161] These usually large, solid tumors generally adhere to surrounding tissues, and distant metastatic disease is associated with this tumor. Operative excision can be a formidable task, because the tumor may be friable, quite vascular, and often invades contiguous structures.[162] If the lesion is localized, surgery is limited to unilateral salpingo-oophorectomy. However, this rarely is the case, and a more extensive extirpative procedure is usually required that involves removing the tumor, the opposite ovary, the uterus, and as much metastatic tissue as possible.

These tumors appear grossly as nodular with a friable consistency. The tumor is purple with variegated areas of dark brown and yellow secondary to hemorrhage and necrosis. Microscopic evaluation of these tumors reveals cytotrophoblasts and syncytiotrophoblasts with evidence of extensive necrosis and hemorrhage. Metastatic implants are friable and have a similar gross and microscopic appearance as the primary lesion. Survival is based on stage at diagnosis and treatment. Platinum-based and methotrexate-based multiagent chemotherapy are described treatment regimens, and platinum-based (bleomycin, etoposide, and cisplatin) chemotherapy has improved survival. Goswami reports an 82% survival in patients treated with chemotherapy versus 28% in those treated with surgery alone.[161]

Teratomas Teratomas are a group of neoplasms composed of tissue elements that are foreign to the organ or anatomic site in which they are found.[163] Classically, these tumors are defined as being composed of tissue derived from the three germ layers: ectoderm, mesoderm, and endoderm. All three germ layers do *not* have to be present in each tumor, but some embryonic tissues must be found in an abnormal location. These tissues show elements of disorganization as well as various levels of maturation. As such, teratomas are histologically classified as mature and immature tumors and those with monodermal components.[164,165] The development of a somatic malignancy within a teratoma is a rare event in childhood, and is thought to occur within differentiated teratomatous elements rather than from totipotent embryonal cells.[32]

Mature Teratomas Most teratomas in children are of the mature type. The majority of mature ovarian teratomas have entered, but have not completed meiosis, suggesting that they arise from germ cells arrested in meiosis I.[32] There is little or no tendency to malignant degeneration of preexisting benign elements or the coexistence of malignant cells in a benign teratoma.[107] In neonates, mature teratomas are found most commonly in the sacrococcygeal area followed by the head and neck.[146,164,166] The ovary becomes an important site later in childhood, especially during adolescence. Ovarian teratomas are predominantly cystic in nature.[107] Overall, benign cystic teratomas are the most common ovarian neoplasms in children[162] and can be bilateral in as many as 10% of patients.[107,165,167]

Symptoms of mature teratomas can be acute or chronic. Acute symptoms that mimic appendicitis are seen when torsion, hemorrhage, or rupture of the mass occurs. Gradual onset of symptoms may be related to the presence of an intra-abdominal adnexal mass, which may cause pressure on adjacent organs.[165] Rarely, a ruptured teratoma may lead to a chronic inflammatory response with the development of a mass of intestine and omentum adhering to the anterior abdominal wall; this condition is associated with pelvic adenopathy, which mimics a malignant tumor.[168] On examination, findings are primarily related to the mass itself. These tumors are located in the abdomen in infants and young children. They are found in the pelvis of adolescents, although large tumors may be palpated in the abdomen, and there may be associated tenderness.

Plain abdominal radiographs demonstrate calcifications in up to 67% of cases.[169] Ultrasonography is a commonly used diagnostic test. The positive predictive ability of ultrasonography approaches 100% when two or more characteristic findings for mature cystic teratoma (MCT), such as shadowing echodensity and regionally bright echodensity, are present.[170] Magnetic resonance imaging has been reported to be more useful than CT scan in the diagnosis of mature cystic teratoma due to its ability to clearly define soft tissue components.[171]

Conservative ovarian surgery in childhood and adolescence is important for the development of normal puberty and future fertility. This must be balanced with complete removal of the mature cystic teratoma. Traditional management of children with mature cystic teratomas has been oophorectomy by laparotomy. However, laparoscopic removal, either by cystectomy or oophorectomy affords a safe alternative option when done by an experienced laparoscopist.[73] Campo and colleagues, in a randomized controlled trial, demonstrated that the use of an endobag in the removal a mature cystic teratoma at the time of laparoscopy decreased spillage from 46% to 3.7% of cases.[172] Aspiration of a giant predominantly cystic lesion in order to facilitate removal through a smaller incision runs the risk of upstaging the patient by spillage of the cyst contents if malignant components are identified. Techniques have been described to minimize this risk while allowing a less invasive approach to large cystic lesions.[173,174] Every effort should be made to spare the ovary when a teratoma is suspected based on radiographic findings and normal tumor markers. Very large or bilateral teratomas can be successfully enucleated in an attempt to preserve hormonal and reproductive functions (Fig. 39-7).[165,175,] If this is not possible, the gonad and tumor alone should be removed, leaving the ipsilateral fallopian tube in place.

Miliary, intraperitoneal glial implants (gliomatosis peritonei) are occasionally encountered in association with mature teratomas.[176] These implants are rarely suspected before surgery. They appear as white or gray nodules, usually 1 to 3 mm in diameter, and are usually confined to the omentum, pelvic peritoneum, or adjacent or adherent to the tumor itself. Several explanations have been offered for the development of these implants.[177] The most recent data using microsatellite DNA analysis suggest that the glial implants arise from subperitoneal cells, presumably pluripotent müllerian stem cells and not from the teratoma.[178,179] Implants can have a disturbing appearance and biopsy is necessary, but no specific treatment is indicated when they are well differentiated, and their presence does not change management of the primary tumor. However, if adjacent components are immature, the lesions may progress and require adjuvant therapy.

Immature Teratomas Immature teratomas are germ cell neoplasms that are composed of tissue derived from the three germ cell layers. These teratomas are clinically distinct from benign or malignant teratomas, because they also contain immature, neuroepithelial elements (see Fig. 39-7). Immature

teratomas can coexist with the more mature solid or cystic benign teratomas or with malignant teratomas, in which case treatment is determined by the malignant component.[180] Immature teratomas are graded based on the relative quantity of immature elements and the presence and quantity of the neuroepithelial components. The grade of the primary tumor is significant and is one of the major determinants of the likelihood of recurrence following resection. Multiple grading systems have been proposed based on the system developed by Thurlbeck and Scully.[181] The criteria outlined by Gonazez-Crussi identified the percentage of incompletely differentiated (embryonal) elements in the tumor as follows: grade 0, 0%; grade I, less than 10%; grade II, 10% to 50%; grade III, greater than 50%.[163,182]

The treatment of immature teratomas has gone through an evolution from aggressive treatment with surgery followed by multidrug chemotherapy to conservative surgical approaches with no adjuvant therapy. In a study of 58 pure immature teratomas published in 1976 by Norris,[180] survival was 82% for patients with grade I tumors, 62% for grade II, and 30% for grade III. Based on this study, along with others, use of multiagent chemotherapy for grade III immature teratomas was advocated. The protocol for extracranial nontesticular germ cell tumors of the German Society for Pediatric Oncology and Hematology (GPOH), which was initiated in 1983, recommended adjuvant chemotherapy for grade II and III immature teratomas of all nontesticular sites.[183] Using this approach, the relapse rate was 13.3% for patients with mature and immature lesions. In a follow-up study from the German registry, immature lesions had a higher rate of recurrence than mature lesions when completely resected (8/78 vs. 3/104), as in the previous study, but the recurrence rate overall dropped from 13.3% to 9.5%. Complete resection was associated with a relapse rate of only 4.2% in both studies, and the malignant relapses were explained by microfoci of yolk sac tumor present in the primary tumor as shown retrospectively in single cases by reevaluation of the primarily resected teratoma.[184] The hypothesis that recurrent tumor stems from microfoci of malignant cells present in the original mass is supported by an intergroup study in the United States in which yolk sac tumor elements were detected in 29% of immature teratoma specimens (73 immature teratoma, 21 with YST-microfoci). It was suggested that the true incidence of such microfoci might be underestimated in these typically large masses, as a result of sampling errors.

The combined report from the Children's Oncology Group and the Pediatric Oncology Group in 1999 included 31 patients with pure immature teratomas of the ovary treated with surgery alone. Eighty-six percent of the tumors were grade I or II and the 3-year event-free survival (EFS) was 97.8%, with only one patient developing recurrent disease. That patient was salvaged with a combination of surgery and platinum, etoposide, and bleomycin. The authors advocate surgical excision alone, with close follow-up as appropriate therapy for all ovarian immature teratomas.[185] Based on the excellent survival and avoidance of the risks of chemotherapy, immature teratomas are treated in the United States with fertility-preserving surgery and observation without adjuvant chemotherapy.[185,186]

Monodermal Teratomas A monodermal teratoma refers to an ovarian tumor composed exclusively or almost exclusively of ectoderm or mesoderm or endoderm, for example, neuroectoderm.[187]

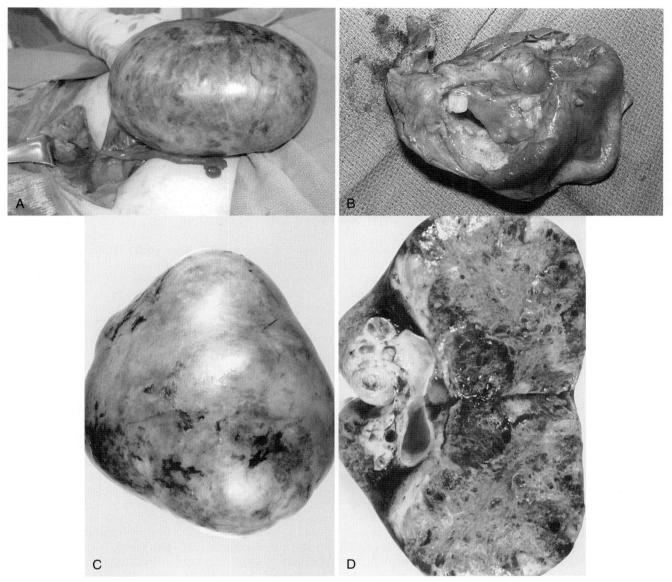

FIGURE 39-7 **A,** Large ovarian dermoid tumor in a 14-year-old girl with acute severe abdominal pain upon awakening. The fallopian tube is seen below the tumor. **B,** Opened gross specimen of ovarian dermoid showing multiple tooth- and jawlike calcifications. **C,** Characteristic gross appearance of an immature teratoma in a 5-year-old girl who presented with a left ovarian mass. The tumor is a solid and cystic globoid mass with a smooth, shiny surface. **D,** Cut section of an immature teratoma shows a variegated, solid, cystic appearance with focal areas of hemorrhage.

Gonadoblastomas

Gonadoblastoma, a tumor first described by Scully[188] in 1953, is relatively rare and occurs most commonly in patients with dysgenetic gonads. Most patients are virilized or nonvirilized phenotypic females. In the only large series reported, Scully[189] reviewed 74 cases and found that 89% were chromatin negative and the most common karyotype was 46XY or 45X/46XY. Troche, in a literature review of 140 cases of neoplasms arising in dysgenetic gonads, found that 80% also had these karyotypes.[190] Patients are usually older adolescents or in the third decade of life with a history of primary amenorrhea. Androgen production by the tumor causes virilization. When a workup for amenorrhea or virilization is undertaken, an abnormal karyotype with a Y chromosome or chromosome fragment can be found in as many as 90% of patients.[190] These often

small tumors may then be identified during examination or exploration. They may also be found incidentally during excision of gonadal streaks or dysgenetic gonads.[191,192] These tumors become invasive early and gonadectomy is recommended as soon as 46XY gonadal dysgenesis is diagnosed.[18,190]

Gonadoblastomas are composed of germ cells and sex-cord derivatives that are similar to granulosa and Sertoli cells, although immunohistochemical and ultrastructural findings are more supportive of Sertoli-like differentiation.[193] Lutein or Leydig-like stromal cells occur in two thirds of cases and probably reflect a stromal reaction to gonadotropin stimulation.[193] These tumors are considered precursors to germ cell tumors in dysgenetic or streak gonads, because they may coexist with dysgerminomas and other germ cell tumors in more than half of the patients.[190] The tumor may be difficult to identify on gross examination because of overgrowth by the malignant component and other changes, including calcification, fibrosis, or both. In fact, calcification may be the only remnant of the gonadoblastoma, and the presence of calcification in a dysgerminoma should raise the suspicion of an underlying gonadoblastoma. The malignant potential of this tumor is determined by the underlying malignant component and should be treated accordingly. The outcome for patients with these tumors may be improved, because abnormal sexual development prompts early evaluation of the patient and subsequent diagnosis of the tumor. The prognosis of nongerminomatous germ cell tumors has improved with the advent of bleomycin, etoposide, and cisplatin protocols, and survival rates of 70% to 90% have been reported.[32]

Mixed Germ Cell Tumors

Germ cell tumors in children are often composed of more than one pure histologic type. Benign but questionably malignant tumors (i.e., immature teratomas) and frankly malignant tumors (germinomas, choriocarcinomas, endodermal sinus tumors, and embryonal carcinomas) may be present. Management of mixed tumors is geared toward the most malignant component of the mass.

Surgical Guidelines for Ovarian Germ Cell Tumors

The goal of surgery is to completely evaluate the extent of disease, safely and completely resect the tumor, and spare all uninvolved reproductive organs. Preservation of reproductive potential is a high priority during surgery for ovarian lesions in children. Laparoscopic procedures are being increasingly performed for evaluation of pelvic masses, and there are now data to demonstrate that the benefits of a faster recovery time and shorter hospital stay seen in adults are also applicable to children.[73,194] If a suspected ovarian malignancy is detected at the time of laparoscopy, complete surgical staging and resection by conventional laparotomy is recommended. Benign lesions require only tumor resection by ovarian cystectomy or unilateral oophorectomy.

Benign tumors, frankly malignant tumors, and those with mixed histologic characteristics often cannot be distinguished based on gross appearance alone. If in doubt, staging is recommended, because treatment and prognosis of malignancies depend on accurate staging. The current intergroup COG protocol includes thorough inspection, palpation, and biopsy of any suspicious peritoneal and liver nodules (including the subphrenic spaces).[49] Both ovaries are inspected. If a tumor is found in an ovary and malignancy is suspected, it should be removed by unilateral oophorectomy if the fallopian tube is not involved. A salpingo-oophorectomy is indicated if the fallopian tube is involved. The contralateral ovary should be inspected, and nodules or suspicious areas should be biopsied. A contralateral salpingo-oophorectomy should be avoided unless malignancy is confirmed.

Staging procedures for malignancies differ somewhat for different cell types, which can result in inadequate staging of unsuspected epithelial tumors. Staging guidelines for germ cell tumors proposed by the Children's Oncology Group (see Table 39-6) include peritoneal fluid aspiration/washings, inspection of the omentum and contralateral ovary with biopsy

of suspicious lesions, biopsy of clinically suspicious lymph nodes, and removal of the primary tumor. Epithelial tumors are staged by the FIGO system (see Table 39-5), which requires peritoneal biopsies, peritoneal washings/aspiration, omentectomy, removal of the primary tumor, and an ipsilateral lymph node dissection. The need for a lymph node dissection is not based on the gross appearance of the nodes, because up to 30% of clinically normal nodes can be positive for metastatic disease.

Chemotherapy for Ovarian Germ Cell Tumors

Forty years ago, no effective therapy for germ cell tumors existed. Based on the early success of management of testicular germ cell tumors using multiagent platinum-based chemotherapy, ovarian tumor treatment evolved along similar lines. The addition of chemotherapy reduced the risk of recurrent disease for adult patients with completely resected ovarian germ cell tumors.[195] Current regimens for ovarian germ cell and sex cord–stromal tumors is platinum-based therapy, and the regimen of cisplatin, etoposide, and bleomycin (PEB) has become the preferred protocol. An 8-year study from the GOG that closed in 1992 evaluated PEB, and 91 of 93 patients were free of recurrent germ cell tumors, with a median follow-up of 38.6 months.[196]

Several chemotherapeutic regimens were also historically tried in children, and the best results were achieved with PEB.[197,198] In a pilot study, Pinkerton and colleagues[199] demonstrated the effectiveness of substituting cisplatin with carboplatin, a less toxic drug; carboplatin was then combined with bleomycin and etoposide. Eight of eight patients with ovarian germ cell tumors survived with this regimen. Using a platinum-based regimen, only 1 of 17 girls with resected ovarian nonseminomatous germ cell tumors in FIGO stage IA relapsed in an analysis of European trials by Gobel and colleagues.[200]

In 1991, the Children's Cancer Group (CCG) experience of 93 children with malignant germ cell tumors included 30 ovarian tumors.[151] By study design, immature teratomas and dysgerminomas were not included. Using a cisplatin-based regimen, the 4-year, event-free survival rate was 63%. Tumor size affected prognosis. If the tumor was larger than 16 cm in diameter, the outcome was worse. Patients in whom complete tumor resection could not be done during the original procedure were more likely to have subsequent adverse events than if the tumor was completely removed ($P = 0.08$). In 1994, Nair and colleagues[201] reported their findings in 107 children with germ cell tumors, including 43 girls with ovarian tumors. Of these, 22 received multiagent chemotherapy. A complete response was seen in 6 of 11 patients treated with platinum, vinblastine, and bleomycin, compared with 10 of 11 patients who completely responded to treatment with PEB (with etoposide replacing vinblastine). The risk for chemotherapy-related complications is low relative to the effectiveness of the PEB regimen and compared with prior regimens that included vinblastine.[202] Others have shown that the PEB regimen is superior to other chemotherapy regimens.[160]

Current efforts in the United States are geared toward reduction of therapy for low- and intermediate-risk tumors. A phase III study undertaken by the Children's Oncology

Group (COG-AGCT0132) stratified malignant germ cell tumors into three risk groups (low, intermediate, and high risk) defined by stage and primary site. Based on data from the POG 9048/CCG 8891 study, demonstrating that patients with stage I ovarian and extragonadal immature teratoma with malignant elements appeared to do well following complete surgical resection,[69] all patients with stage I ovarian tumors were categorized as low risk and were initially treated with surgery, followed by close observation and monitoring. That arm of the study has subsequently been amended to include stage I ovarian tumors in the intermediate-risk group because of a higher-than-expected failure rate with observation alone. Overall survival remains greater than 95%. The intermediate-risk group will consist of patients with stage I to III gonadal tumors. Such patients have been shown to have a 3-year EFS of about 90% with standard-dose PEB.[49,71] These patients will be treated with a modified standard PEB regimen, consisting of three cycles of compressed PEB every 21 days. Saxman and colleagues[203] reported that long-term survival was equivalent for men treated with germ cell cancer for three or four cycles of PEB. Patients who are partial responders (PR) may then have surgical resection of residual tumor. Therapy is discontinued upon pathologic complete response and normal markers, or continued for an additional three cycles in children who remain PR. High-risk patients, defined as those with stage IV disease, showed some improvement in survival with a high-dose platinum regimen that was offset by increased toxicity. Patients with recurring germ cell tumors may be salvaged using high-dose chemotherapy with autologous stem cell transplantation.

Miscellaneous Tumors

Small cell carcinoma of the ovary is an extremely rare condition with a very poor prognosis.[204] These tumors are very aggressive and are the most common undifferentiated ovarian carcinoma in young patients. They have been encountered in patients from 9 to 44 years of age, with a mean age of 23 years.[205] Paraendocrine hypercalcemia occurs in two thirds of cases, but patients rarely have clinical manifestations of this abnormality. Serum parathormone levels are normal. Virtually all tumors are unilateral, although only 40% have been detected at stage 1A. Only one third of patients with stage 1A tumors survive long-term, and survival of patients with more widespread disease is rare.[13] Unilateral salpingo-oophorectomy has been associated with long-term survival in some patients with stage 1A tumors. Asynchronous appearance of tumor in a contralateral conserved ovary has been encountered, and bilateral adnexectomy may be a more appropriate surgical option. Despite various treatment modalities including resection, radiation therapy, and intensive chemotherapy, the average life expectancy remains low at 18 months.[205]

Primary ovarian sarcomas are a heterogenous group of aggressive tumors associated with poor survival. Most cases occur in older women; however, a recent review of 151 cases described 10 of 29 patients with rhabdomyosarcoma who were younger than 20 years of age.[206] These patients presented with nonspecific symptoms of abdominal discomfort or swelling with occasional urinary or gastrointestinal complaints secondary to mass effect. Accurate staging is critical. Hysterectomy with bilateral salpingo-oophorectomy and

debulking of as much diseased intra-abdominal tissue as possible has been done. Radiation therapy was administered for residual pelvic disease, and several chemotherapeutic regimens have been used. In contrast to rhabdomyosarcomas arising at other sites, the outcome for patients with ovarian lesions has generally been poor, perhaps because of the advanced stage of disease at diagnosis. Nevertheless, the most recent chemotherapeutic regimens used in cooperative group studies have been highly effective, and it is reasonable to assume that more conservative surgical resection will provide adequate treatment for these rare tumors.

Stromal sarcomas and low-grade endometrial stromal sarcomas of the ovary have been occasionally reported in the second decade of life. These lesions are believed to arise from ovarian endometriosis, coelomic mesenchyme, or neometaplasia of stromal cells. Lesions are usually discovered because of nonspecific pelvic discomfort, although early infiltration into adjacent tissues may cause intestinal or ureteral obstruction. Tumor infiltration may not be grossly apparent, so initial surgical resection should be aggressive with total hysterectomy and bilateral salpingo-oophorectomy. Progesterone administration may provide effective adjunctive therapy, although this has to be continued indefinitely because stromal sarcomas have been reported to reappear and spread dramatically when the medication is stopped. Radiation therapy has been used for local residual disease, although recurrence is common. The role of chemotherapy for these tumors has not been defined.

Cases of genuine ovarian fibrosarcoma in children are extremely rare. Patients present with pelvic pain and a palpable mass. Fibrosarcoma has been associated with Maffucci syndrome.[8] Although the outcome has been uniformly poor in older patients, survival of younger patients who have undergone aggressive surgical resection, including hysterectomy and bilateral salpingo-oophorectomy, has been reported. Success with subsequent radiation or chemotherapy has not been reported.

Primary leiomyosarcoma of the ovary is extremely rare in children. These tumors may arise de novo from any of the smooth muscle sites in the ovary or may represent malignant degeneration of leiomyoma, a benign counterpart.[207] As with most of these rare tumors, presenting symptoms are nonspecific and discovery may occur in the advanced stage of disease. Aggressive surgical therapy is recommended, because no adjuvant therapy has proven to be effective.

Secondary Tumors

Although secondary ovarian malignancy is rare, the ovaries are a potential metastatic site for a wide variety of childhood malignancies (Table 39-7).[127,208] Distinguishing primary neoplasms from secondary neoplasms is important to prevent inappropriate therapy or adverse sequelae. Metastatic spread to the ovary occurs through four main pathways: (1) hematogenous spread, (2) lymphatic spread, (3) transcoelomic dissemination with surface implantation, and (4) direct spread.[208] Recently described highly malignant tumors that have a predilection for the pelvic region are intra-abdominal desmoplastic small round cell tumors.[209]

Lymphoma can occur in the ovary in children either as a primary tumor or a manifestation of systemic disease. Most

TABLE 39-7

Secondary (Metastatic) Tumors Occurring in the Ovary in Children

Colorectal
Breast
Gastric carcinoma
Carcinoid tumors (liver, lung)
Malignant melanoma
Burkitt lymphoma
Rhabdomyosarcoma
Wilms' tumor
Neuroblastoma
Retinoblastoma
Ewing sarcoma
Rhabdoid tumor of the kidney
Medulloblastoma
Osteogenic sarcoma
Chondrosarcoma
Leukemia

of the reported cases have been of the small, noncleaved cell type (Burkitt or non-Burkitt category), although T-cell non-Hodgkin lymphoma and anaplastic large cell lymphoma have also been reported.[210] Pais and colleagues[211] reviewed 23 cases of ovarian involvement in patients with relapsing leukemia. Abdominal pain was the most common symptom, and a mass could usually be palpated. Although most patients in whom leukemia treatment failed had systemic and not local disease, ultrasonography revealed a characteristic appearance and was effective in detecting ovarian involvement.[212] Survival was based on aggressive systemic multiagent chemotherapy and not on the degree of surgical resection of the ovarian lesion. Routine pelvic radiation therapy was of no benefit.

Reports have noted granulocytic sarcoma of the ovary occurring in patients with acute or relapsed acute myelogenous leukemia.[213] Although aggressive systemic chemotherapy is critical to survival, an ovarian mass should be investigated immediately to determine its nature (i.e., benign or malignant and exact cell type). In this instance, surgical resection of the ovary and any other involved gynecologic organs or pelvic tissue must be done. Radiation therapy has been used for residual disease in the pelvis. Although the ultimate outcome of granulocytic sarcomas is probably more related to effectiveness of chemotherapy, local measures of tumor control cannot be overlooked when this tumor is detected.

Unclassified Benign Tumors

Although the ovary is highly vascularized, hemangiomas are extremely rare; a recent review found only 40 published cases.[214] Their occurrence is relatively evenly distributed between infancy and postmenopausal age groups. The lesions are usually quite small, asymptomatic, and discovered incidentally. Bilateral occurrence is rare, and the tumors are almost always cavernous. Benign-appearing ultrasonographic features have been described.[215] When the tumors are large, associated symptoms include abdominal pain, distention, and bloody ascites. Torsion or rupture may cause an acute surgical emergency. No malignant

tumors of this type have been described, and oophorectomy or adnexectomy is curative if needed.

Primary ovarian leiomyomas are also extremely rare, although they have been reported in teenage girls.[216] Most reported cases are clinically silent; however, the lesion may be large enough to cause increased abdominal girth and pelvic pain. Tumor markers are normal, and imaging studies are generally unable to differentiate this benign solid tumor from a malignant process. Unilateral salpingo-oophorectomy is curative. The ovarian myxoma is a rare benign tumor characterized by conspicuous vascularity and mesenchymal proliferation that requires only a conservative surgical procedure.[217]

Struma ovarii is a benign variant of a germ cell tumor that typically occurs in older women but has been reported in teenagers. It is composed of more than 50% benign thyroid tissue, which is functional in 5% to 12% of cases. Rarely, the tumor contains malignant components and, in some cases, represents the patients' only functioning thyroid tissue. CA 125 levels may be elevated, but other markers are usually normal. Treatment is resection of the mass.[218] In another thyroid-related condition known as the Van Wyk and Grumbach syndrome, long-standing hypothyroidism can lead to large ovarian cysts. TSH levels are extremely high and several theories hypothesize a crossover hormonal effect on FSH or direct stimulation of the ovary by TSH. CA-125 and LDH levels may be elevated. The ovarian cysts resolve with thyroid replacement therapy.[219]

Summary

The diagnosis and management of ovarian lesions in infants and children remains a challenge because of the wide variety of possible pathologies, some of which are extremely rare. Nonneoplastic lesions are being detected more commonly as imaging techniques continue to improve. Neoplastic lesions are more readily diagnosed and completely characterized with advances in biochemical, immunohistologic, and cytogenetic technology.

Because of the relative rarity of ovarian tumors in children, clinical approaches may be based on experience with similar adult lesions. However, it is critical to recognize the differences exhibited by the juvenile forms of many of these entities, which often present at a less advanced stage and have a more favorable natural history and response to therapy. Preservation of reproductive and endocrine function is of paramount importance in the treatment of ovarian lesions in infants and children. Careful observation or nonoperative therapies may be appropriate for many nonneoplastic conditions. Most benign neoplasms are adequately managed with conservative surgical approaches. Even frankly malignant tumors increasingly yield to multimodal therapy, which can include less radically ablative surgery and still result in long-term survival and possible preservation of fertility for young patients.

The complete reference list is available online at www.expertconsult.com.

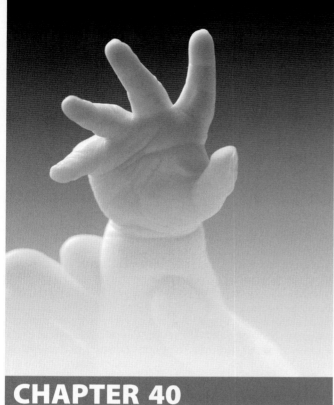

CHAPTER 40

Testicular Tumors

Bryan J. Dicken and Deborah F. Billmire

Historically, prepubertal malignant testicular tumors were managed using the same treatment protocols as their adult counterparts, with radical orchiectomy and retroperitoneal lymph node dissection (RPLND) weighing heavily in the treatment pathway.[1,2] However, with growing clinical evidence, it became clear that prepubertal tumors differed from the postpubertal population not only in presentation but differed in terms of clinical behavior, incidence, histologic diagnosis, and prognosis.[1–6] In recognition of the differences in this population of patients, the Prepubertal Testis Tumor Registry (PTTR) of the urologic section of the American Academy of Pediatrics was established in 1980 to better delineate the natural history of these lesions and to document their response to therapy.[1,2,4] Since its inception, several important features have emerged that have significantly altered the management of testicular tumors in the pediatric population. The management has been further clarified by a series of recent multicenter clinical trials of the most common malignant tumors of the prepubertal testis.[7–12]

The results of the PTTR confirmed that testicular tumors in children are rare, making up approximately 1% to 2% of all pediatric solid tumors, with an incidence of 0.5 to 2/100,000 among whites, while African-American males appear somewhat protected, with an incidence of 0.25/100,000.[1–3,13] Asian/Pacific Island males have a 1.4-fold increased risk of testicular tumors compared with whites.[14] In contrast to adult testicular cancer, which has experienced a marked increase in incidence, pediatric testicular tumor incidence has been stable during the past 30 years.[15] Testicular tumors are 10 times more frequent in the postpubertal cohort compared with boys younger than 12 years of age.[1] Furthermore, epidemiologic data from several sources suggest a bimodal distribution, with a small distinct peak in the first 3 years of life, followed by a large peak in adolescents (15 to 18 years).[2,3] The majority of testicular tumors in the postpubertal age group are malignant, with 90% to 95% demonstrating histologic features of either seminoma or mixed germ cells.[2,6] Initially, the PTTR reported that the yolk sac tumor (62%) was the most common prepubertal testicular tumor, with benign tumors occurring much less commonly.[1,2,13] However, a landmark paper by Metcalfe and colleagues[13] suggested that the PTTR registry and the Armed Forces Institute of Pathology American Tumor registry are subject to reporting bias, with overreporting of malignant tumors and failure to capture the benign tumors. In a series of articles that followed, 74% to 87% of tumors identified were benign, with teratoma making up 43% to 48%, while malignant yolk sac tumors constituted only 15%.[1,5,6,13] Recognition of this fact led to a marked reassessment of the management of testicular tumors in the prepubertal population.

Risk Factors for Testicular Cancer

Although a number of risk factors have been proposed regarding the occurrence of testicular tumors, to date only a few may be considered as "established" based upon a sufficient level of evidence.[16] Other associations that have historically been considered important etiologically have since been refuted. Only four factors have sufficient evidence that links them "highly" with testicular cancer: (1) undescended testis (cryptorchidism), (2) contralateral testicular germ cell tumor (GCT), (3) familial testicular germ cell tumor, and (4) gonadal dysgenesis.[16,17] Associations that may be considered "likely" include infertility, twin-ship, and testicular atrophy. Clinical factors with equivocal/low association include scrotal trauma, inguinal hernia, mumps orchitis, testicular torsion, maternal estrogen exposure, and occupational exposure. Parameters that have historically drawn attention but have since been shown to be irrelevant include obesity, vasectomy, smoking, hydrocele, varicocele, alcohol, and circumcision.[16]

Cryptorchidism occurs in 2% to 5% of term infant males; however, by 12 months of age, this number is reduced to 1%.[18] To date, cryptorchidism is the only factor that has level I evidence linking it with testicular cancer. A meta-analysis of 20 case control studies showed a strong association between undescended testis (UDT) and testicular cancer, with an overall relative risk of 4.8.[16] Similarly, Walsh and colleagues[19] showed boys who underwent orchiopexy after 10 years of age had a 3.5-fold increased risk of testicular cancer, compared with those that had the procedure at an earlier age. In a population-based prospective observational study, Pettersson and colleagues followed 16,983 men treated for UDT for a mean period of 12.4 ± 7.4 years.[20] This study demonstrated two important findings. There was an increased risk of testicular cancer for the entire cohort (relative risk [RR] = 2.23) versus normal population figures, and the incidence of cancer was significantly higher (RR = 5.4) in those who were treated after the age of 13 years.[20] The lowest incidence of cancer was seen in children who underwent orchiopexy before the age of 6 years (RR = 2.02). Orchiopexy before the age of 10 to 12 years results in a twofold to sixfold relative risk decrease in testicular cancer in children with unilateral UDT.[21] Because of the increased risk of malignancy, patients with UDT seen after age 10 may still be candidates for orchiopexy with close surveillance; however, consideration of testicular biopsy may be useful in directing therapy. The decision of timing for orchiopexy should include consideration not only of an effort to reduce the incidence of testicular cancer, but also a consideration of the possibility of spontaneous descent and the evidence regarding preservation of fertility. Canavese and colleagues demonstrated an inverse relationship between age at orchiopexy and total sperm counts and sperm motility, and they recommended orchiopexy during the first year of life.[22] Taking all factors into account, consideration should be given to orchiopexy in all children if complete descent has not occurred by 12 months of age.[21]

Clinical Presentation

The most common presentation of a testicular tumor is a nontender scrotal mass, accounting for 50% to 85% of cases.[5,6,13,23] The presentations of children that were subsequently diagnosed with a prepubertal tumor have included trauma and persistent swelling (3%), hydrocele (10%), epididymitis (13%), incidental discovery during surgical repair of a congenital or acquired disorder (53%), testicular pain/torsion (21%), and bruising.[5,6,13,23] Tumors may also be diagnosed by ultrasonography during investigations for UDT or nonresolving acute hydroceles.

Physical examination should differentiate between those problems arising from the cord (varicocele, spermatocele, epididymitis) and those arising from the testicle (trauma, orchitis, tumor). There may be bruising or a hydrocele present that may confound the diagnosis, because both of these findings may coexist with a tumor. This is particularly true in cases where preceding trauma draws attention to the scrotal area. Careful evaluation of the child's pubertal status relative to their chronologic age is important, because stromal cell tumors may present with precocious puberty (Leydig cell) or gynecomastia (Sertoli cell).

Diagnosis

In addition to a history and physical examination, all boys with testicular masses, and those with a tense hydrocele or with a suspicious examination, should undergo a scrotal ultrasound. Although preoperative ultrasound is highly sensitive for distinguishing intratesticular from extratesticular tumors, it has poor specificity to distinguish between benign and malignant lesions.[5,13,24] Tumor size (volume) on ultrasonography has not been shown to be indicative of benign or malignant tumors.[5] Sonographic features suggestive of benign tumors (epidermoid cyst) include intratesticular cystic lesions with a hypoechoic center, representing central keratinizing debris, and an outer hyperechoic rim. Features of a teratoma may include an entirely intratesticular cystic, septated mass

with intervening solid components with calcifications (bone or psammoma bodies).[13] This contrasts with malignant lesions, which tend to be more solid in appearance. In cases where malignancy is suspected, computed tomography (CT) of the chest, abdomen, and pelvis should be obtained to exclude metastatic disease to the most common sites—lung and retroperitoneum.[2,4]

Tumor Markers

Serum tumor markers are essential in the workup and postoperative monitoring of children with testicular tumors. Human chorionic gonadotropin (HCG) and α-fetoprotein (AFP) are important markers for certain malignant germ cell histologies.[2] AFP is secreted by yolk sac tumors in up to 90% of cases, and β-HCG is secreted by choriocarcinoma. HCG has a half-life of 24 hours, whereas AFP has a half-life of 5 days. In the prepubertal age group yolk sac tumors are the most common malignant histology, and AFP is very important, whereas HCG is rarely elevated. An important consideration is that AFP is normally very high in infancy, and remains elevated for up to 8 months, decreasing to adult levels around 1 year of age.[2,23] Older boys are more likely to have malignant germ cell tumors of mixed histology, and both AFP and HCG may be elevated. For those patients with elevated tumor markers at diagnosis, serial AFP and HCG should be monitored monthly in the first postoperative year, then every other month in the second year to follow current recommendations.[25] Patients presenting with precocious puberty and a testicular mass should prompt assessment of a urinary 17-ketosteroid, serum luteinizing hormone (LH), follicle-stimulating hormone (FSH), and testosterone. Unlike precocious puberty induced by a pituitary lesion, in which the LH, FSH, and testosterone are high, testicular tumors display a low LH and FSH and a high testosterone.

Classification and Stage

Table 40-1 lists the histologic diagnoses for prepubertal testicular tumors from several institutions, and the diagnoses are compared with the 2002 AAP tumor registry.[1,13,26] This table demonstrates the reporting bias of the national tumor registry and the population-based distribution of all testicular tumors. Table 40-2 outlines the Children's Oncology Group (COG) testicular tumor staging system.[7]

PRIMARY TESTICULAR TUMORS

Epithelial-Based Tumors

Epidermoid Cysts The epidermoid cyst is a benign tumor, accounting for 2% to 14% of testicular tumors in the prepubertal population.[1,5,13] They are hormonally inactive and typically present as a smooth, firm intratesticular mass. The tumor consists of a cystic structure filled with keratinizing squamous epithelium, contributing to a characteristic ultrasound appearance: central hypoechoic mass, a surrounding echogenic rim, or a mixed internal echogenicity.[27,28] Epidermoid cysts are rare, making up only 1% of testicular tumors.

TABLE 40-1

Differences in Distribution of Testicular Tumors Based on Tumor Histology among Study Sites

Tumor Type	2002 Registry % (N = 395)	Pohl % (N = 98)	Metcalfe % (N = 51)	Ciftci % (N = 51)
Benign				
Teratoma	23	48	43	18
Epidermoid cyst	3	14	10	6
Leydig cell	1	4	0	6
Sertoli cell	3	3	4	0
Juvenile granulosa cell	3	5	0	N/A
Malignant				
Yolk sac	62	15	8	45
Mixed germ cell	0	0	8	6
Rhabdomyosarcoma	4	Excluded	25	19
Gonadoblastoma	1	2	2	0

N/A, not available.

TABLE 40-2

Staging of Testicular Malignant Germ Cell Tumors

Testicular Stage	
I	Limited to testis, completely resected by high inguinal orchiectomy; no clinical, radiologic, or histologic evidence of disease beyond the testis; tumor markers normal after resection
II	Transscrotal orchiectomy; microscopic disease in scrotum or high in spermatic cord; retroperitoneal node involvement (<2 cm) and/or increased tumor markers after resection
III	Gross residual disease, retroperitoneal lymph node involvement (>2 cm), or malignant cells in pleural or peritoneal fluid
IV	Distant metastases involving lung, liver, brain, bone, distant nodes, or other sites

From Cushing B, Giller R, Cullen JW, et al: Randomized comparison of combination chemotherapy with etoposide, bleomycin, and either high-dose or standard-dose cisplatin in children and adolescents with high-risk malignant germ cell tumors: a pediatric intergroup study—Pediatric Oncology Group 9049 and Children's Cancer Group 8882. J Clin Oncol 2004;22:2691-2700.

These cysts lack atypia and mitotic activity. Although some epidermoid cysts show loss of heterozygosity for certain chromosomal loci, there is currently debate as to whether they represent a true neoplasm.[29]

Stromal Tumors

Sex Cord-Stromal Tumors The stromal tumors consist of three subtypes: Leydig cell, Sertoli cell, and juvenile granulosa cell tumors. This group of tumors accounts for 8% to 11% of pediatric tumors.[1,13] The vast majority of stromal tumors are benign, compared with a 10% rate of malignancy in postpubertal males.

Leydig tumors and granulosa cell tumors are universally benign in children. Leydig cell tumors tend to present in boys 5 to 10 years of age and with precocious puberty.[2] The precocious puberty is a peripherally driven etiology; therefore, the hormone profile consists of a low luteinizing hormone (LH), low follicle-stimulating hormone (FSH), and elevated testosterone. Granulosa cell tumors are rare in children and occur almost exclusively in the first 6 months of life. Chromosomal anomalies of the Y chromosome are common, and granulosa cell tumors have occurred in association with ambiguous genitalia.[2] Because of the benign nature of both Leydig and granulosa cell tumors, both can be treated with either orchiectomy or tumor enucleation in the prepubertal population.[30]

Approximately 10% of adult Sertoli cell tumors are malignant, whereas malignancy is rare in prepubertal males. Review of the PTTR showed a median age of presentation of 6 months, with no cases of malignancy reported in children less than 5 years of age.[31] Therefore complete excision of the tumor is adequate treatment in infants and young children. Presently there are no histologic criteria to predict tumor behavior in older children; however, a full metastatic evaluation should be considered if there is microscopic invasion of the spermatic cord,[31] or worrisome findings, such as a large tumor, necrosis, vascular invasion, cellular atypia, or increased mitotic activity.[2] Large cell calcifying Sertoli cell tumors are histologically distinct tumors occurring in older children and adolescents. One third of these patients have an associated genetic syndrome or endocrinopathy, most commonly, Peutz-Jeghers and Carney syndromes (myxoma of the skin, soft tissue, heart or breast, lentigines of the face and lips, cutaneous nevi, pituitary adenoma, and schwannoma).[2] They have been universally benign in patients less than 25 years of age and may be treated with testis-sparing procedures. Bilateral or multifocal disease is present in 25% of cases, increasing the need for this approach.

Germ Cell Tumors

Teratoma Testicular teratoma is the most common germ cell tumor in prepubertal males according to recent literature.[1,5,6,13] These tumors are invariably benign, unlike the adult population, where 90% to 95%[6] of germ cell tumors are malignant.[32] Teratomas are typically pure; derived from ectoderm, mesoderm, and endoderm; have diploid DNA; and a normal 46 XY karyotype.[29,32] The tissue arrangement is often organized with a gross solid cystic appearance. Dermoid and epidermoid cysts analogous to the prepubertal teratomas occur in the postpubertal testis. The testicular dermoid, like the ovarian dermoid, contains hair within a cystic tumor, and microscopic replication of skin without cellular atypia or widespread mitotic activity. The adjacent testis has normal spermatogenesis.[29] The finding of pilosebaceous units in an epidermal surface, occasionally with a lipoid reaction resulting from leakage of oil from the sebaceous glands, is a prerequisite for diagnosis of a testicular dermoid.

Yolk Sac Tumor The yolk sac tumor comprised approximately 60% of the tumors historically reported in the AAP registry.[2] However, recent population-based studies, including benign testicular tumors, now report the incidence of yolk sac tumors to be 8%[13] to 15%.[1] Most of the yolk sac tumors occur in boys less than 2 years of age, but they are rare in the first 6 months of life. This is important in differentiating this tumor from the juvenile granulosa cell tumor (see previous section).[32] The majority of patients (84.5%) identified in the PTTR presented with localized stage I disease.[33] Prepubertal patients are less likely than adults to have metastasis limited to the retroperitoneum. In a review of the PTTR of the American Academy of Pediatrics, 15.5% of boys with yolk sac tumors presented with metastatic disease. The reported sites included retroperitoneum (27%), retroperitoneal and hematogenous spread (18.8%), chest (24%), lung and an additional hematogenous site (12%), scrotum (3%), and 2% were not documented.[33]

Elevated AFP levels in excess of age-adjusted levels in the context of a testicular mass should raise suspicion of a yolk sac tumor, and the child should be managed with a standard radical inguinal orchiectomy (see later).

Grossly, the tumor is a soft solid, white to grey, or pale yellow mass with cystic degeneration containing areas of necrosis and hemorrhage. Microscopically, the yolk sac tumor characteristically contains solid papillae with a connective tissue core containing a central vessel projecting into cystic spaces; these structures are referred to as Schiller-Duval bodies.[32] The tumor invariably stains positive for AFP and placenta-like alkaline phosphatase.

Embryonal Carcinoma   Embryonal carcinoma is a relatively common testicular germ cell tumor after puberty; 10% are pure embryonal tumors, and a substantial number of tumors will have a mixed embryonal component.[29] This tumor demonstrates distinctive sheets, glands, and papillary structures composed of primitive epithelial cells with crowded pleomorphic nuclei. In poorly differentiated tumors, positive immunostains for CD30 and OCT3 with a c-KIT–negative profile are helpful in confirming an embryonal carcinoma.[32] Embryonal carcinoma is treated with orchiectomy. Tumors composed of more than 80% embryonal cell carcinoma or with elevated preoperative AFP (>10,000 mg/mL), vessel invasion in the primary tumor, and tumors of stage T2 or greater are considered high risk and are treated with postoperative chemotherapy and close follow-up.[34]

Gonadoblastoma   Gonadoblastoma has classically been identified in patients with mixed gonadal dysgenesis (45,X/46,XY), and is likely related to the presence of the testis-specific protein-Y–encoded gene (TSPY).[35] The ectopic location of the testis adds to this risk. The most commonly encountered invasive tumor in the intersex gonad is the seminoma. The development of these invasive tumors is always preceded by the presence of an in situ neoplastic lesion—intratubular germ cell neoplasia unclassified (ITGNU) or gonadoblastoma.[35,36] ITGNU is commonly referred to as carcinoma in situ (CIS). Because gonadectomy is performed prophylactically in early childhood in patients with gonadal dysgenesis, most of the encountered germ cell tumors are benign or CIS lesions. The overall prevalence of germ cell tumors in dysgenetic gonads is 15%, which is much lower than the previously reported prevalence of 33%.[35] The tumor presents with virilization of a phenotypic female harboring an XY karyotype.[37]

Gonadoblastoma typically arises from an intraabdominal testis in a young patient with gonadal dysgenesis. It is usually small, bilateral in 30% of cases, malignant in 10%, and histologically resembles a seminoma. Available data suggest the gonad of origin to include dysgenetic testis in 20%, streak gonad in 26%, and an undifferentiated gonad in 54%.[36] Extension beyond the testis has not been reported. Management has traditionally involved bilateral gonadectomy because

of the risk of degeneration into an invasive seminoma. However, the recognized role of testosterone in gender differentiation has led to a more conservative approach to the contralateral gonad, which may involve a contralateral orchiopexy to allow gender development, followed by annual scrotal examinations and ultrasonography after age 10 years until puberty. At puberty, testicular biopsy should be carried out to evaluate for CIS in the remaining testicle.[38] If no evidence of CIS is identified, annual follow-up with testicular ultrasonography until age 20 is recommended. If CIS is identified at puberty, orchiectomy should be considered.[38]

Choriocarcinoma   Choriocarcinoma is among the rarest of the gonadal germ cell tumors, representing 0.3% of testicular tumors.[29] These tumors elaborate β-HCG, and may be associated with a number of hormonal manifestations. These include precocious puberty from β-HCG–induced Leydig cell stimulation, gynecomastia, and hyperthyroidism because of the similarity of the β-HCG subunits to thyroid-stimulating hormone.[29] Testicular choriocarcinomas frequently have distant metastasis at the time of presentation rather than a scrotal mass. Histologically, they are composed of syncytiotrophoblastic cells with mononucleated cells around foci of hemorrhage. They stain positive for β-HCG and placental lactogen.[32]

Rhabdomyosarcoma

Although technically a paratesticular tumor, rhabdomyosarcoma should be included in the differential diagnosis of scrotal tumors. It is the most frequent tumor of paratesticular origin, accounting for 4% to 25% of scrotal masses.[13] The tumor has a bimodal distribution, peaking between 3 to 4 months of age and 15 to 19 years of age. The infant tumor has a more indolent behavior than the tumor presenting in the adolescent age group (90% vs. 63% failure-free survival).[39] Despite its aggressive behavior, the prognosis of paratesticular rhabdomyosarcoma has improved dramatically from 10% to 77% overall survival with the introduction of vincristine, dactinomycin, and cyclophosphamide (VAC) chemotherapy.[39,40] The most common subtype is embryonal rhabdomyosarcoma, which accounts for 97% of paratesticular tumors.

The tumor consists of small round blue cells and presents as a scrotal mass in 80% of patients. Ultrasonography is highly effective in demonstrating its paratesticular location and distinguishing it from the tumors of testicular origin.[13] CT or MRI of the retroperitoneum should be performed prior to surgery for staging purposes. Thirty to 40 percent of boys will have micrometastasis to the retroperitoneum. The tumor should be resected by a radical inguinal orchiectomy. A retroperitoneal lymph node dissection (RPLND) is recommended for all patients 10 years of age or older for accurate staging, and in patients less than 10 years with radiologic evidence of retroperitoneal involvement.[39] A metastatic workup should include a chest CT, liver function tests, bone scan, and bone marrow biopsy.

SECONDARY TESTICULAR TUMORS

Lymphoma and leukemia are the dominant secondary tumors of the testis. Acute lymphoblastic leukemia (ALL) is a common cause of a prepubertal testicular mass. Microscopic involvement of the testis has been found at autopsy in 66% of patients with ALL.[32] Malignant lymphomas account for 5% of testicular tumors; 10% to 15% are bilateral at presentation.[32]

The management of leukemia and lymphoma are the same. The presence of a palpable mass in a patient with newly diagnosed leukemia/lymphoma should prompt a scrotal ultrasonography. This usually demonstrates a homogeneous hypoechoic mass. Current literature discourages testicular biopsy in patients prior to initiating chemotherapy, because there is no survival advantage.[41] In contrast, a patient with persistent or newly enlarged testis undergoing chemotherapy, particularly in leukemia, implies a relapse while on therapy. This should prompt a biopsy to direct subsequent therapy. This typically involves additional chemotherapy to eradicate residual disease in sanctuary sites and possible systemic residual disease and radiation to the affected testis.

In 25% of cases, testicular lymphoma is a manifestation of widespread systemic involvement, another 25% present with Ann Arbor stage II disease (involvement of lymph nodes below the diaphragm), and the remaining 50% have disease confined to the testis (Ann Arbor stage I).[32]

Metastasis to the testis in children is rare. The most frequent metastasis has been carcinoma from the prostate, colon, kidney, stomach, pancreas, and malignant melanoma in adults, while neuroblastoma and Wilms tumor predominate in children.[32] Most of these tumors have distinctive features that allow easy identification.

Surgical Management

TESTIS-SPARING SURGERY

In the last 2 decades, multiple reports have confirmed that many testicular tumors in the prepubertal population can be managed more conservatively than in adults, because the distribution of prepubertal tumors favors a benign histology. This realization has confirmed the safety and feasibility of testis-sparing surgery, especially when the lesion is evaluated preoperatively by ultrasonography and serum AFP and intraoperatively by frozen section analysis. Metcalfe and colleagues[13] have provided a practical treatment algorithm incorporating the common benign tumors for nonradical surgery (Fig. 40-1).

In general, before puberty, teratoma, gonadal stromal tumors (Leydig cell and Sertoli cell) and epidermoid cyst can be managed with a testis-sparing approach (Fig. 40-2). Postpubertal patients with teratoma or stromal tumors should be treated as adults, with radical orchiectomy because of their more malignant behavior.

Testis-sparing surgery is carried out through an inguinal incision. The cord is mobilized after opening the external oblique aponeurosis to the level of the internal ring. The cremasteric fibers are dissected from the cord structures to allow circumferential control of the cord. The cord should be occluded at the level of the internal ring with a noncrushing clamp. The testis is then delivered through the inguinal incision, and the wound is protected. The tunica vaginalis is opened directly over the mass, and an excisional biopsy of

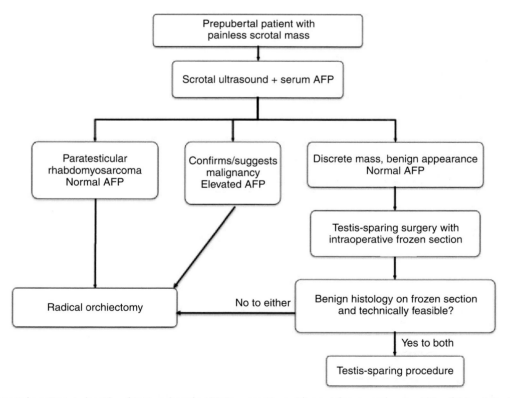

FIGURE 40-1 Proposed treatment algorithm for prepubertal patients presenting with a painless scrotal mass. AFP, α-fetoprotein. (From Metcalfe PD, Farivar-Mohseni H, Farhat W, et al: Pediatric testicular tumors: Contemporary incidence and efficacy of testicular preserving surgery. J Urol 2003;170:2412-2415; discussion 2415-2416.)

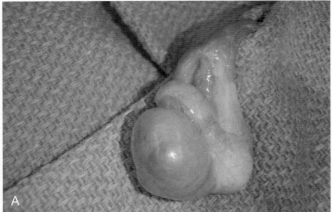

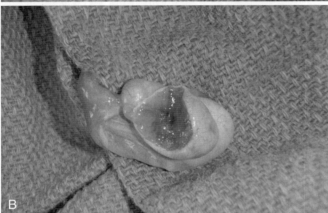

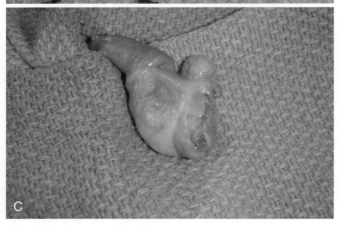

FIGURE 40-2 A, Intraoperative photograph of a child with painless swelling of testicle. **B,** Wedge resection of epidermoid cyst. **C,** Suture closure of testicular capsule. (Courtesy Dr. P. Metcalfe, personal file.) *(See Expert Consult site for color version.)*

the mass is performed without violating the tumor capsule. Frozen section evaluation is obtained. Hemostasis is achieved with electrocautery. If a benign testicular tumor is diagnosed, the tunica vaginalis is closed with fine absorbable sutures (see Fig. 40-2), and the testis is replaced in the scrotum. Normal tissue adjacent to the tumor must be assessed by a pathologist to exclude pubertal changes. It is commonly assumed that the postpubertal testis with a tumor will behave in a similar fashion to the adult testis, although specific data are lacking. Adult testicular tumors are associated with intratubular germ cell neoplasia (ITGCN) in the surrounding parenchyma in more

than 90% of cases. These cells are the precursors for germ cell tumors and are felt to represent a risk for recurrent neoplasia if the residual testicular parenchyma is left in situ. The progression through puberty evolves over a period of time and sequential histologic changes. The testes go through a maturation process starting from simple tubules without lumen and with interstitial Leydig cells in the neonate. The Leydig cells then regress and the tubules become more tortuous. As puberty begins, the Leydig cells become more prominent, and the basal germ cells begin to divide. There are multiple layers of spermatocytes and the tubule lumens form, followed by the appearance of mature sperm. The appearance of mature sperm or ITGCN would be indicative of completion of pubertal changes.

RADICAL INGUINAL ORCHIECTOMY AND RETROPERITONEAL LYMPH NODE DISSECTION

A radical inguinal orchiectomy is performed through a standard inguinal incision, with clear demarcation of the external oblique aponeurosis and external ring and opening of the external ring back to the level of the internal ring. The cremasteric fibers are once again dissected from the cord, and the cord is fully mobilized from the inguinal canal, followed by vascular control at the internal ring. The cord is then clamped and divided at the level of the internal ring, after which the stump is suture ligated. After ligation, dissection proceeds distally with mobilization of the testis from the scrotum and division of the gubernaculum. If the tumor is too large to deliver through the scrotal canal, the incision may be carried onto the superior aspect of the scrotum.[42,43] Once the tumor is excised, the wound is closed in standard fashion.

Current pediatric testicular tumor protocols do not include a RPLND. Postchemotherapy masses are treated with local resection. Postpubertal patients will often be managed with adult protocols, although data regarding adolescents is lacking. The indications for and the extent of RPLND are a matter of some controversy even in adults. Prechemotherapy RPLND is no longer employed, and postchemotherapy RPLND is eliminated in some centers if residual disease is less than 1 cm in dimension by imaging.[44] In the event that a RPLND is required, a midline abdominal incision is made and a thorough laparotomy performed to identify retroperitoneal low-volume metastasis not appreciated on preoperative imaging. There is also controversy regarding the extent of dissection. Because of the morbidity of bilateral RPLND (40%), a variety of unilateral templates have been developed in addition to the concept of nerve-sparing dissection.[45,46] In low-stage disease, lymphatic spread is typically unilateral, and therefore a full bilateral RPLND is not used in some centers.[47] For the unilateral template, dissection for patients with right-sided disease involves removal of the lymphatics in the interaortocaval, precaval, and right paracaval distribution (Fig. 40-3, *A*).[43] For left-sided lesions, this includes the left paraortic and preaortic lymphatics (Fig. 40-3, *B*). This dissection strategy is important, because it preserves the contralateral sympathetics important for emission and ejaculation.[48] Preservation of efferent sympathetic fibers maintains emission and ejaculation rates at 99%.[48] The finding of viable tumor outside of the template distribution has led to the recommendation for bilateral dissection

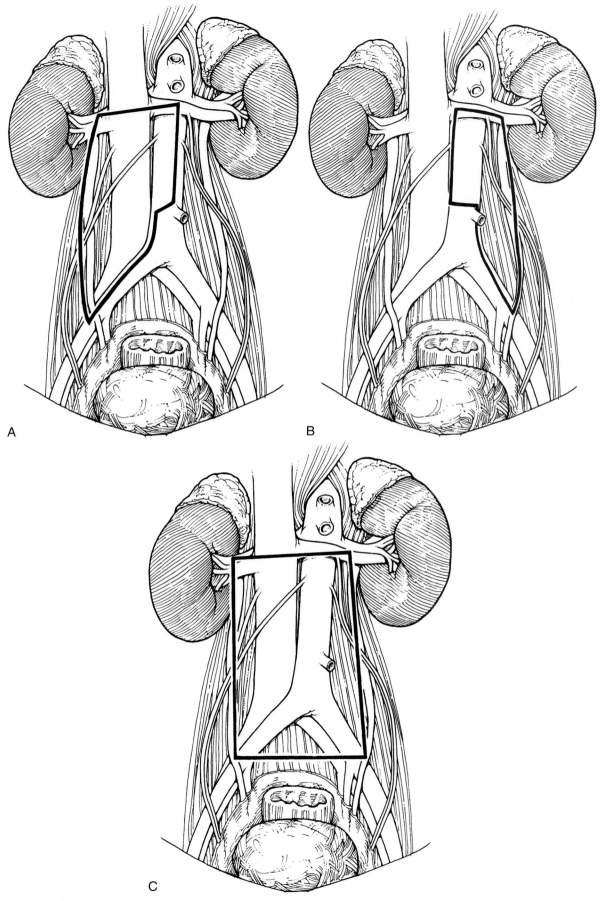

FIGURE 40-3 **A,** Right modified nerve-sparing retroperitoneal lymph node dissection. **B,** Left modified nerve-sparing retroperitoneal lymph node dissection. **C,** A full retroperitoneal dissection involves left and right combined. (From Marshall FF [ed]: Operative Urology. Philadelphia, WB Saunders, 1996, p 368-369.)

in all patients undergoing RPLND in other centers.[46] In advanced-stage/high-volume disease bilateral RPLND is always used, as shown in Figure 40-3, *C*.[45] With either technique, the nodal packets are split at the 12 o'clock position over the vessels and rolled laterally away. The sympathetic fibers are carefully identified and preserved as they cross the iliac bifurcation.

CHEMOTHERAPEUTIC STRATEGIES AND SURVIVAL IN CHILDREN WITH MALIGNANT GERM CELL TUMORS

Prior to effective chemotherapy, children with malignant germ cell tumors (MGCT) had 3-year survival rates of 15% to 20% with surgery and radiation.[7,49] The introduction of cisplatin-based regimens has dramatically improved outcomes (Table 40-3).[11] In patients with low- and intermediate-risk (<15 years of age) MGCT, the 6-year overall survival rates for advanced gonadal tumors (stages III and IV) are now greater than 94%.[7] Standard chemotherapy for children with MGCT of the testes includes standard-dose cisplatin, etoposide, and bleomycin (PEB) for 4 to 6 courses.[2] The current protocol under investigation examines stages II to IV with three courses of chemotherapy. Management of patients is based upon risk groups as proposed by the Children's Oncology Group (COG) as follows (see Table 40-3)[11]:

1. **Low risk:** Stage I immature teratoma and MGCT of the testis. Recommend surgery and close follow-up observation to document normalization of tumor markers following resection

TABLE 40-3

Standard Treatment for Children Younger Than 15 Years with Testicular Germ Cell Tumors by Histology and Stage

Histology	Stage	Treatment	Overall Survival (6-Year)
Mature teratoma	Localized	Surgery + observation	100%
Immature teratoma	Localized	Surgery + observation	100%
MGCT	Stage I	Surgery + observation	100%
	Stage II-IV*	Surgery + PEB	94%

From Cushing B, Giller R, Cullen JW, et al: Randomized comparison of combination chemotherapy with etoposide, bleomycin, and either high-dose or standard-dose cisplatin in children and adolescents with high-risk malignant germ cell tumors: a pediatric intergroup study—Pediatric Oncology Group 9049 and Children's Cancer Group 8882. J Clin Oncol 2004;22:2691-2700; Rogers PC, Olson TA, Cullen JW, et al: Treatment of children and adolescents with stage II testicular and stages I and II ovarian malignant germ cell tumors: A Pediatric Intergroup Study-Pediatric Oncology Group 9048 and Children's Cancer Group 8891. J Clin Oncol 2004;22:3563-3569.

*Patients greater than 15 years old with stage IV testicular tumors should be discussed in a multidisciplinary oncology group for more intensive therapy.

MGCT, malignant germ cell tumors; PEB, cisplatin, etoposide, and bleomycin.

2. **Intermediate risk:** Stages II-IV gonadal tumors (excluding patients >15 years with stage IV testicular tumors).

The complete reference list is available online at www. expertconsult.com.

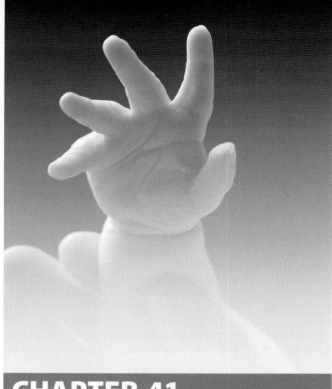

CHAPTER 41

Adrenal Tumors

Michael G. Caty and Mauricio A. Escobar, Jr.

Anatomy

The adrenal glands are found anteromedially to the superior pole of the kidneys, are covered by perirenal fat, and enclosed by Gerota fascia. In adults, the glands weigh approximately 5 g each. The right gland abuts the inferior vena cava and liver and lies on the posterior extension of the diaphragm. The left gland lies next to the splenic vessels and the tail of the pancreas.

Although the blood supply to the adrenal glands is variable, it generally comes from three sources: the inferior phrenic artery superiorly, the aorta medially, and the renal arteries inferiorly. The venous drainage does not parallel the arterial supply; instead, a single large adrenal vein provides the majority of the venous drainage for each gland. The right adrenal vein empties into the inferior vena cava, and the left adrenal vein joins the left renal vein.

The adrenal lymphatics arise from one plexus beneath the capsule and from a second plexus in the medulla. The right adrenal lymph vessels drain into the periaortic lymph nodes near the diaphragmatic crus, and the left adrenal lymphatics empty into lymph nodes near the origin of the left renal artery.

The innervation of the adrenal glands arises from the celiac plexus and the greater thoracic splanchnic nerves. The preganglionic sympathetic fibers enter the hilum and end in ganglia within the medulla.

The cortex and medulla form two distinct regions of the adrenal gland. These regions are distinct on gross examination as well as embryologically, structurally, and functionally. The adrenal medulla is derived from ectodermal cells from the neural crest. These precursors form the chromocell system and the neuronal system, accounting for the potential development of two distinct medullary neoplasms: pheochromocytoma and neuroblastoma. Preganglionic sympathetic neural cells innervate the secretory chromaffin cells, which synthesize norepinephrine and epinephrine.

The cortex comprises the outer portion of the adrenal gland and secretes sex hormones, mineralocorticoids, and glucocorticoids. It is divided into three separate zones that have distinct synthetic functions. The zona glomerulosa is the outermost cortical zone and produces aldosterone and related mineralocorticoids. The zona fasciculata lies beneath the zona glomerulosa and secretes cortisol and the adrenal sex hormones. The inner zona reticularis maintains cholesterol stores as a precursor for steroidogenesis and secretes cortisol, androgens, and estrogens.

Embryology

The primordium of the adrenal cortex becomes visible as early as the fourth week of gestation and is clearly seen by the sixth week. On prenatal ultrasonography (US), the adrenal glands may be visible as early as 20 weeks' gestation and are identifiable in the majority of fetuses by 30 weeks' gestation.[1] During the fourth to sixth weeks of gestation, the mesodermal cells of the posterior abdominal wall at the adrenogenital ridge become more columnar and invade the mesenchyma beneath the epithelial surface, ultimately forming the fetal adrenal cortex. Another proliferation of epithelial cells subsequently forms a cap over these primitive cortical cells, becoming the zona glomerulosa of the definitive cortex. The ectodermal chromaffin cells of the adrenal medulla arise from the neural crest as early as the fifth week, with primitive cells from the thoracic ganglia from the 6th to 12th segments invading the gland and forming the medulla. Differentiation of these primitive medullary cells into chromaffin cells begins at the third month of gestation, ultimately leading to the cells' production of epinephrine and norepinephrine.

The fetal zone of the adrenal cortex begins to appear around the sixth week of gestation. This zone continues to enlarge and occupy the majority of the gland. In fact, because of the large size of the fetal cortical zone, the fetal adrenal gland is 4 times the size of the kidney during the fourth month of gestation. This fetal cortex subsequently decreases in size, disappearing in the first year of life.

During fetal development, ectopic rests of medullary and cortical tissue may remain and persist after birth. Extraadrenal medullary rests are usually found along the aorta and its branches. The organ of Zuckerkandl is an example of a chromaffin mass at the origin of the inferior mesenteric artery. Most extraadrenal chromaffin rests involute after birth; the chromaffin cells in the medulla differentiate.

Extraadrenal cortical rests are common in children and are found in the kidney or liver or along the migratory path of the gonads, in hernia sacs, or in the gonads themselves. Approximately 50% of newborns have adrenocortical rests, but these rests typically atrophy and disappear within a few weeks after birth.[1]

Physiology

ADRENAL MEDULLARY FUNCTION

The adrenal medulla synthesizes and releases catecholamines: dopamine, epinephrine, and norepinephrine. Catecholamine synthesis begins with tyrosine, a nonessential amino acid. Tyrosine hydroxylase converts tyrosine into dihydroxyphenylalanine (DOPA) and is the rate-limiting step in the synthetic pathway. DOPA decarboxylase converts DOPA into dopamine. Phenylamine beta-hydroxylase converts dopamine into norepinephrine. Finally, phenylethylamine *N*-methyltransferase converts norepinephrine into epinephrine.

The chromaffin cells within the medulla contain cytoplasmic granules that store the catecholamines. Preganglionic sympathetic nerve endings release acetylcholine, which causes calcium-dependent exocytosis of these cytoplasmic storage granules and release of the catecholamines. Regulation of adrenal medullary catecholamine release is accomplished through inhibitory feedback mechanisms involving norepinephrine. Norepinephrine inhibits acetylcholine release from the presynaptic alpha$_2$ receptors and also inhibits tyrosine hydroxylase activity when present in high concentrations.

ADRENAL CORTICAL FUNCTION

The adrenal cortex synthesizes three types of hormones: glucocorticoids, mineralocorticoids, and sex hormones. Regulation of these is accomplished by the hypothalamic-pituitary-adrenal axis. The hypothalamus produces corticotropin-releasing hormone (CRH); this is transported to the anterior pituitary gland where it stimulates the release of adrenocorticotropic hormone (ACTH). ACTH then stimulates the production of hormones (glucocorticoids, mineralocorticoids, and sex hormones) from the adrenal cortex.

The physiologic diurnal variation in CRH release leads to a cyclic variation in ACTH and the hormones regulated by it. Serum concentrations peak shortly before or at the time of awakening and decline throughout the remainder of the day. Both cortisol and ACTH inhibit CRH release, creating a negative feedback loop.

Adrenocortical production of glucocorticoids begins with a cholesterol substrate and is regulated by ACTH. The majority of serum cortisol is bound by cortisol-binding protein (90%) and albumin (6%), leaving only a small percentage (4%) free and physiologically active. As with most steroids, the unbound cortisol fraction is lipophilic and therefore readily crosses the plasma membrane of target cells. Specific receptors then bind with cortisol and act in the cell nucleus to regulate messenger RNA synthesis.

Cortisol affects metabolism primarily by opposing insulin. It causes hyperglycemia by increasing the proteolysis necessary for gluconeogenesis and inducing hepatic gluconeogenic enzymes. Cortisol also decreases the use of glucose by peripheral tissues; it inhibits glucose uptake into fat cells and decreases the amount of insulin bound by insulin-sensitive tissues.

Cortisol also decreases inflammation and immune function, affecting wound healing. Cortisol lowers both the lymphocytic and the granulocytic cellular immune response by decreasing the lymphocyte response to antigenic stimulation and impairing chemotaxis and phagocytosis of leukocytes.

These two immune functions are an important part of early wound healing; thus wounds have decreased tensile strength and impaired healing in the setting of excess cortisol.

Aldosterone, a mineralocorticoid, is synthesized in the zona glomerulosa and metabolized primarily by the liver. The renin-angiotensin system controls the majority of aldosterone regulation, with ACTH playing only a small role. The macula densa of the renal juxtaglomerular apparatus releases renin in response to a drop in renal perfusion or hyponatremia. Renin converts angiotensinogen, which is produced by the liver, to angiotensin I. Angiotensin-converting enzyme, found in the lung, converts angiotensin I to angiotensin II. Angiotensin II stimulates the synthesis of aldosterone by directly acting on the cells of the adrenal zona glomerulosa; it also acts as a vasoconstrictor. By increasing the renal retention of sodium, aldosterone increases blood pressure and corrects hyponatremia, thus reducing the release of renin.

The serum potassium concentration also provides a small amount of aldosterone regulation. Hyperkalemia leads to increased aldosterone production by directly acting on the zona glomerulosa cells, as well as increasing renin release from the juxtaglomerular cells. Aldosterone promotes an increased renal excretion of potassium, thus lowering aldosterone production and providing another feedback mechanism.

Adrenal androgens are synthesized in the zona reticularis and are regulated primarily by ACTH. These hormones are released in a cyclic manner, correlating with the release of cortisol and ACTH. The adrenal androgens are only weakly active but are converted by peripheral tissues into more active forms such as testosterone and dihydrotestosterone. Metabolism of these hormones occurs in the liver.

Lesions of the Adrenal Medulla

PHEOCHROMOCYTOMA

In 1886, Frankel of Freiburg, Germany, published the first description of bilateral pheochromocytomas found during the postmortem examination of an 18-year-old woman who had presented with symptoms of anxiety, palpitations, and headache.[2] In 1912, Pick named the tumor for its predominant cell type, the pheochromocyte, but it was not until 1922 that Labbe and colleagues first described a clear relationship between pheochromocytoma and paroxysmal hypertension. In 1927, Mayo performed the first successful removal of a pheochromocytoma in a patient with paroxysmal hypertension who underwent surgical exploration without a preoperative diagnosis. In 1929, Pincoffs made the first correct preoperative diagnosis, and the successful operation was performed by Shipley.[3] Since that time, the behavior of pheochromocytomas has become better understood, particularly with respect to children.

Pheochromocytoma is an uncommon tumor of childhood, and there are several characteristics that distinguish its presentation between adults and children. The incidence of pheochromocytoma in childhood is 10% of the adult incidence, occurring in approximately 1 in 500,000 children compared with 1 in 50,000 adults.[4] Approximately 10% of childhood pheochromocytomas are familial, which is about 4 times the frequency in adults. Whereas only 7% of pheochromocytomas are bilateral in adults, the reported incidence of

TABLE 41-1

Comparison of Pheochromocytoma in Children and Adults

	Pediatric	Adult
Incidence	1:500,000	1:50,000
Familial pattern (%)	10	2-3
Bilateral (%)	24-70	10
Extraadrenal site (%)	30	10
Malignant (%)	3	10

bilateral pheochromocytomas in children ranges from 24% to as high as 70%. Extraadrenal pheochromocytomas are approximately twice as prevalent in children as in adults (Table 41-1).[5,6]

Pheochromocytomas originate from medullary chromaffin cells, which produce the catecholamines that cause the associated symptoms. These cells migrate along the aorta, usually remaining near the branches of the aorta.

SYMPTOMS

In children with pheochromocytoma, the average age at presentation is 11 years, although the tumor can occur at any age. Over half the children present with headaches, fever, palpitations, thirst, polyuria, sweating, nausea, and weight loss, but the most common presentation is sustained hypertension.[4,6,7] In children, most causes of hypertension are secondary, with renal abnormalities being most common (78%), followed by renal artery disease (12%), and coarctation of the aorta (2%).[8] Pheochromocytoma accounts for 0.5% of children with hypertension and must be considered once other causes are eliminated. In children with pheochromocytoma, hypertension is sustained in up to 70% to 90% of cases, with only a small minority presenting with paroxysmal hypertension. In contrast, up to 50% of adults with pheochromocytoma have paroxysmal hypertension.[6]

DIAGNOSIS

The diagnosis of pheochromocytoma relies on the demonstration of elevated levels of blood and urinary catecholamines and their metabolites. A 24-hour urine measurement of catecholamines, metanephrine, and vanillylmandelic acid is the best diagnostic test.[9,10] Urinary metanephrine levels are increased in about 95% of patients, and urinary vanillylmandelic acid and catecholamine levels are increased in approximately 90% of patients.[10] There is also a linear relationship between the amount of vanillylmandelic acid and the size of the pheochromocytoma.[11] The normal 24-hour urinary secretion is less than 100 mg for free catecholamines, less than 7 mg for vanillylmandelic acid, and less than 1.3 mg for metanephrine. Plasma catecholamines can also be measured by radioenzyme assay. However, patients must remain supine and calm during the blood draws, which can be difficult in children. Patients with normal plasma catecholamine levels during a hypertensive episode probably do not have pheochromocytoma, but levels greater than 2000 pg/mL are diagnostic of pheochromocytoma. Plasma catecholamine levels between 500 and 1000 pg/mL are suspicious for a pheochromocytoma, and further testing is indicated.[6] It must be remembered, however, that neuroblastoma can in some cases secrete significant levels of catecholamines.

After establishing the chemical diagnosis of pheochromocytoma, the tumor must be localized. Although large masses such as a neuroblastoma can be seen on plain abdominal films, most adrenal masses cannot be visualized without the use of other imaging methods. Almost all pheochromocytomas occur in the abdomen or pelvis, and although the adrenal gland is the most common site, up to 43% of children may have multifocal disease.[6] The initial study in infants and children is often US, which can be useful in distinguishing between solid and cystic masses while determining their vascularity and avoiding ionizing radiation, but it may not visualize small adrenal lesions. Additionally, it may be difficult to identify the adrenal gland as the organ of origin for large masses, because of compression from adjacent organs such as the kidney. Computed tomography (CT) and magnetic resonance imaging (MRI) offer the advantage of much better resolution and sensitivity (Fig. 41-1). Although CT is an accurate method of diagnosing adrenal lesions, it is less accurate in younger children because of the absence of retroperitoneal fat. Other disadvantages of CT are the need for intravenous contrast material and exposure to ionizing radiation. Simultaneous scanning of the chest to rule out pulmonary metastases in patients suspected of having adrenal carcinoma is a benefit of CT. Currently, both CT and MRI offer multiplanar imaging. Coronal imaging is a useful modality to distinguish

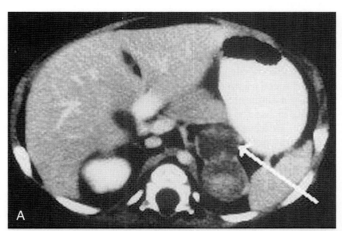

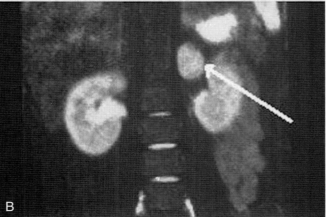

FIGURE 41-1 A, Computed tomography of the abdomen in a 10-year-old girl with a left adrenal mass associated with hypertension. **B,** Magnetic resonance image demonstrates a left adrenal pheochromocytoma. No other masses were noted. No contrast agent was required.

adrenal masses from the adjacent kidney and vice versa.[12–14] Pheochromocytomas demonstrate low or intermediate signal intensity on T1-weighted images and enhance with gadolinium-diethylenetriaminepentaacetic acid (DTPA).[15] One significant disadvantage to MRI is that children often require sedation or general anesthesia, given the length of time the study requires, which may be a risk if children have not been treated with blocking agents.

Another useful imaging technique is ^{131}I-labeled metaiodobenzylguanidine (MIBG) scanning; this radioisotope accumulates where norepinephrine is taken up and allows detection of the tumor. MIBG, which is structurally similar to norepinephrine, is taken up by the norepinephrine transporter system into intracytoplasmic vesicles. Radionuclide imaging is achieved by labeling MIBG with one of two iodine isotopes at the meta position of the benzoic ring. The iodine isotope ^{131}I has a half-life of 8.2 days and emits high-energy radiation. The iodine isotope ^{123}I has a shorter half-life and emits lower-energy radiation.[16] Patients undergoing MIBG scanning should be given a saturated solution of potassium iodide to block thyroid uptake of the free iodine isotope. Scintigraphy is performed at 24 and 48 hours. This technique can be particularly useful in localizing extraadrenal tumors or sites of metastasis. It also confirms the adrenal location of a pheochromocytoma in patients with positive urine or serum catecholamine tests. The head and neck may be a more common site of these tumors in children compared with adults, followed by the retroperitoneum.[17]

Positron emission tomography (PET) may be a useful imaging study for pheochromocytoma in the near future. PET scanning uses short-lived positron-emitting agents to identify specific areas of uptake in the body. Because of the increased metabolism of tumors, labeled glucose can be used to identify malignant tissue. The most common form of labeled glucose in use for PET scanning is (^{18}F)-fluorodeoxyglucose (FDG). However, resolution of pheochromocytoma and distinction between benign and malignant pheochromocytoma are not optimal with FDG PET. A more useful agent may be 6-(^{18}F)-fluorodopamine (DA). The similarity between norepinephrine and DA allows selective uptake by sympathoadrenal tissue.[18] One study found that FDG PET demonstrated metastases better than MIBG scanning did in adults (one patient was 16 years old in this cohort of 29 patients).[19] PET scanning results in lower radiation exposure than standard scintigraphy. When specific agents, such as DA, become generally available, PET scanning may prove to be the imaging method of choice.

TREATMENT

The treatment of pheochromocytoma is surgical excision, although medical management of the hypertension is an essential part of the preoperative preparation. The high levels of catecholamines increase the risk of sudden and severe intraoperative hypertension, as well as profound hypotension once the tumor is removed and catecholamine release has ceased. In fact, these complications accounted for the high mortality rate associated with surgical resection in the past.[6] Improvements in preoperative and intraoperative management have reduced the operative mortality of 24% to 45% in the past to less than 10% today.[20] Preoperative use of alpha-adrenergic blockers, such as oral phenoxybenzamine

and phentolamine, reduces the effects of epinephrine and norepinephrine by blocking the alpha-adrenergic receptors. These agents should be started at least 3 to 7 days before the procedure and the dose increased until the pressures are well controlled to minimize the intraoperative risks. Replacement of intravascular volume is often required as alpha blockade is achieved, because patients with pheochromocytomas tend to be hypovolemic at baseline, with an average 15% reduction in plasma volume. This volume re-expansion also helps minimize intraoperative blood pressure fluctuations and cardiac arrhythmias.

Beta-adrenergic blockade with agents such as propranolol and labetalol may be used once an alpha-adrenergic blockade is achieved, particularly if a resting tachycardia develops despite adequate volume replacement. If these agents are used, it is crucial that alpha blockade be established first. Administration of a beta blocker before an alpha blockade can worsen hypertension secondary to unopposed vasoconstriction.

Methyl-para-tyrosine (metyrosine) competitively inhibits tyrosine hydroxylase, the rate-limiting step in catecholamine biosynthesis. Treatment with metyrosine reduces tumor stores of catecholamines, decreases the need for intraoperative antihypertensive drugs, lowers intraoperative fluid requirements, and attenuates blood loss. It has not been tested in children less than 12 years of age. Metyrosine may not be necessary for patients with minimal or no symptoms from a minimally functioning pheochromocytoma.[21]

Despite good preoperative normalization of blood pressure, the anesthesiologist must be prepared for sudden fluctuations. The times of significant intraoperative risk are during anesthetic induction and intubation, during surgical manipulation of the tumor, and immediately following ligation of the tumor's venous drainage.[22] An arterial catheter and a central venous line are crucial for monitoring intraoperative blood pressure and fluid status. The anesthesiologist must also be prepared to use fast-acting agents to raise or lower blood pressure as needed. Sodium nitroprusside and nitroglycerin are useful agents, as are vasopressors and intravenous fluids. Cardiac arrhythmias can be managed with the use of propranolol, esmolol, and lidocaine. Adrenalectomy is described later.

An adrenal pheochromocytoma is typically encapsulated, and although there may be small amounts of normal adrenal tissue, the entire adrenal gland should be removed. It is rarely necessary to perform a nephrectomy, because the tumor is rarely adherent to the kidney.

As previously mentioned, once the adrenal vein is ligated and the tumor is removed, the patient may become hypotensive because of the removal of the catecholamine excess. In fact, it may be several days before the blood pressure normalizes. If hypertension returns postoperatively, one should suspect a second pheochromocytoma. All patients should undergo follow-up to confirm normalization of catecholamine levels. Long-term follow-up is indicated because of the possibility of a metachronous occurrence of a multifocal pheochromocytoma or occult metastasis.[6,22]

ASSOCIATED DISORDERS

Familial pheochromocytomas may occur in the setting of several syndromes. The most common syndromes are multiple endocrine neoplasia type 2 (MEN-2) and von Hippel-Lindau disease. There is a smaller incidence of familial pheochromocytomas in patients with neurofibromatosis type 1 and in patients without any other abnormalities.

Traditionally, a 10% incidence of familial cases of pheochromocytoma was expected. However, a germline mutation has been identified in up to 59% of apparently sporadic pheochromocytomas presenting at 18 years of age or younger and in 70% of those presenting before 10 years of age in one series.[21] The inherited predisposition may be attributable to a germline mutation in the von Hippel-Lindau gene, the genes encoding the subunits B and D of succinate dehydrogenase, the *RET* proto-oncogene predisposing to multiple endocrine neoplasia type 2, or the neurofibromatosis type 1 gene. Of these, the von Hippel-Lindau gene is the most commonly mutated gene in children presenting with a pheochromocytoma. A mutation of the von Hippel-Lindau gene on chromosome 3 leads to von Hippel-Lindau disease. This condition is characterized by retinal angiomas, hemangioblastomas of the central nervous system, renal cysts, renal cell carcinoma, pancreatic cysts, and pheochromocytomas. These pheochromocytomas are often multifocal and are frequently extraadrenal.

Multiple endocrine neoplasia type 2 is an autosomal dominant disorder caused by a mutation of the *RET* proto-oncogene on chromosome 10. These patients are at risk for medullary thyroid carcinoma, and up to 50% will develop adrenal pheochromocytoma. These tumors are almost always bilateral and are almost never malignant. Patients with MEN-2A are also at risk for hyperparathyroidism, and patients with MEN-2B may have a marfanoid habitus or mucosal ganglioneuromas.

Malignancy has been reported to occur in up to 10% of children with pheochromocytoma.[7] The diagnosis of malignancy is generally based on the tumor's clinical behavior, because the histologic examination is not an accurate predictor. A malignant pheochromocytoma may have local infiltration or distant metastasis, which most commonly occurs in bone, liver, lymph nodes, lung, and the central nervous system. Synchronous or metachronous pheochromocytomas may present anywhere along the sympathetic chain. Although surgical resection remains the treatment of choice, long-term palliation may be obtained through a multimodal approach, including local excision, radiation, and chemotherapy.[23]

Lesions of the Adrenal Cortex

Adrenocortical neoplasms are rare in the pediatric population, accounting for less than 0.2% of all pediatric tumors and 6% of all adrenal tumors in children.[24] The incidence of these neoplasms has been reported to be approximately 25 cases per year in the United States, of which about 75% are adrenocortical carcinomas.[25,26] Adrenocortical tumors occur more frequently in girls, with a male to female ratio of approximately 1:2 to 1:3.[27] Like pheochromocytomas, adrenocortical neoplasms behave differently in children than in adults. Approximately 85% to 95% of these tumors are hormonally active in children, compared with less than 50% in adults.[28,29] Further, whereas there are clear pathologic criteria for malignancy in the adult population, these guidelines are not reliable in the pediatric population. Because the clinical behavior of these tumors does not always correlate with the pathologic appearance, the diagnosis of malignancy should be based

on clinical behavior. Age less than 3.5 years at the time of diagnosis and symptom duration of less than 6 months before diagnosis are favorable prognostic indicators in adrenocortical carcinoma. Early detection is essential in these children, because a delay in diagnosis adversely affects clinical outcome.[1]

Adrenocortical tumors are associated with several congenital anomalies, including hemihypertrophy; other tumors associated with hemihypertrophy include nephroblastoma and hepatoblastoma. Patients with Beckwith-Wiedemann syndrome (exomphalos, macroglossia, and gigantism) also have a higher than expected incidence of adrenocortical carcinoma.[30] Most adrenocortical tumors, however, occur sporadically.[1]

CUSHING SYNDROME

In 1932, Cushing first described the syndrome that bears his name in a patient with a pituitary adenoma. Since that time, the understanding of the pathophysiology and cause has expanded considerably. Endogenous Cushing syndrome is a rare condition in the pediatric population. In general, the incidence of spontaneous Cushing syndrome is approximately 5 per million persons; it occurs primarily in young adult women, with a female to male ratio of 9:1. Ten percent of cases occur in children and adolescents.[31]

The typical manifestation of Cushing syndrome in children is generalized obesity and long bone growth retardation.[31] Other symptoms include hypertension, weakness, thin skin with striae and easy bruising, acne, menstrual irregularity, osteoporosis, and glucose intolerance. Unlike in adults with Cushing syndrome, muscle weakness, sleep disturbances, and mental changes, such as emotional lability, irritability, or depression, are rare in children.[31] Cushing syndrome can be divided into ACTH-dependent and ACTH-independent types. In the former condition, the inappropriately high ACTH levels stimulate the adrenal cortex to produce excessive cortisol. In the ACTH-independent type, abnormal adrenal tissue produces excessive cortisol irrespective of ACTH levels.

Cushing disease refers to Cushing syndrome caused by pituitary tumors that lead to excessive ACTH production. Typically, these tumors are microadenomas and are less than 1 cm in diameter; however, large, invasive pituitary adenomas may develop. These tumors lead to bilateral adrenocortical hyperplasia, with a corresponding glucocorticoid excess. As the age of the patient increases, there is a greater likelihood of a pituitary cause of the syndrome. In patients younger than 6 years, the most likely cause of endogenous Cushing syndrome is an adrenal tumor. Although adrenocortical carcinomas represent only 0.2% of all childhood malignancies and 6% of adrenal cancers, approximately 60% to 80% of pediatric Cushing syndrome cases are caused by adrenocortical carcinomas.[28]

The clinical diagnosis of hypercortisolism must be confirmed biochemically to diagnose Cushing syndrome. In addition, the specific source of the syndrome must be localized (Fig. 41-2). Cortisol production is normally suppressed at night, but in Cushing syndrome, this suppression does not occur. The normal circadian rhythm of cortisol secretion is lost in Cushing syndrome. Random serum cortisol levels are of limited value. The three most common tests used to diagnose Cushing syndrome are the 24-hour urinary free cortisol test,

Diagnostic Studies to Localize Hypercortisolism

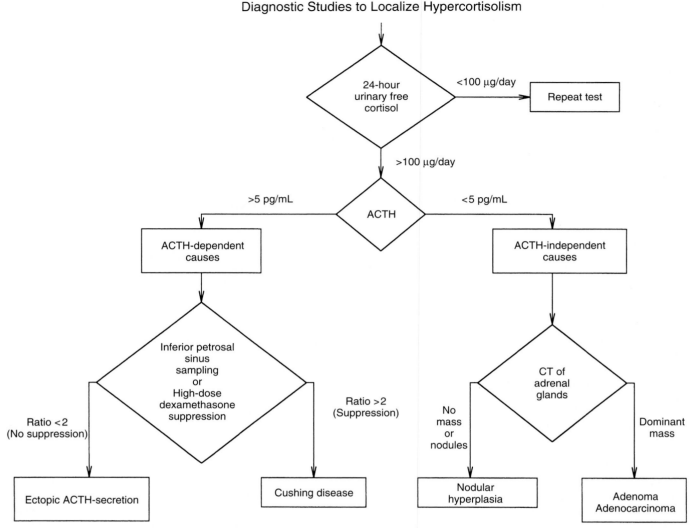

FIGURE 41-2 Algorithm to localize the cause of hypercortisolism in children with suspected Cushing syndrome. ACTH, adrenocorticotropic hormone; CT, computed tomography.

measurement of midnight plasma cortisol or late-night salivary cortisol, and the low-dose dexamethasone suppression test. The dexamethasone-corticotropin-releasing hormone test may be needed to distinguish Cushing syndrome from other causes of excess cortisol. The 24-hour urinary free cortisol level has a sensitivity of approximately 98%.[32] In children, this value must be corrected for size. A normal value is less than 70 $\mu g/m^2$ per day; this is elevated with Cushing syndrome. Another useful test is the 24-hour urinary 17-hydroxysteroid excretion; this is an indirect measure of cortisol secretion and is elevated with hypercortisolism. Once it is corrected for creatinine excretion, the normal value is between 2 and 7 mg per gram of creatinine per day. The overnight dexamethasone suppression test is administered as follows: After the administration of 1 mg (or 0.3 mg/m^2 in children) of dexamethasone, a morning cortisol level greater than 5 $\mu g/dL$ indicates unsuppressed cortisol secretion consistent with Cushing syndrome.

Once the diagnosis of Cushing syndrome has been established, the next step is to determine the underlying cause of the hypercortisolism. As shown in Figure 41-2, measurement of the ACTH level can distinguish between ACTH-dependent

and ACTH-independent causes. If the ACTH level is greater than 5 pg/mL, the source is ACTH dependent; if the level is less than 5 pg/mL, it is ACTH independent.

ACTH-dependent causes of hypercortisolism include both pituitary and ectopic ACTH-secreting neoplasms. Although ectopic production of ACTH is rare in children, Wilms' tumors and tumors of the thymus, pancreas, or neural tissue can produce ACTH. Most patients with ACTH-secreting tumors have Cushing disease (Cushing syndrome caused by a pituitary tumor). Although a high-dose dexamethasone suppression test or an inferior petrosal sinus sampling can distinguish a pituitary source from an ectopic source, MRI can also show a pituitary tumor. An ectopic tumor producing CRH is another ACTH-dependent source of Cushing syndrome, but this condition has not been reported in a child.[32,33]

In both adults and children, the treatment of choice for Cushing disease is a transsphenoidal resection of the pituitary adenoma. In patients with no postoperative improvement or with recurrence, some response may be obtained with pituitary irradiation using cobalt 60.

If an ectopic ACTH-secreting tumor is indicated by the workup, the patient must undergo screening for medullary carcinoma of the thyroid (serum calcitonin levels) and screening for pheochromocytoma (24-hour urine measurement of catecholamines, metanephrine, and vanillylmandelic acid). Other ectopic locations, such as a bronchial, thymic, or intestinal carcinoid tumor, may be seen on CT of the chest and abdomen. Ectopic ACTH-producing tumors should be resected if possible. If resection is not possible, bilateral adrenalectomy can offer an effective treatment of Cushing syndrome.

ACTH-independent causes of Cushing syndrome include adrenal neoplasms and nodular adrenal hyperplasia. ACTH-independent Cushing syndrome is relatively more frequent in children than in adults.[32] In children, an adrenocortical tumor most frequently occurs in the setting of a virilizing syndrome, and the majority of children present with virilizing symptoms. Approximately 33% of these patients have Cushing syndrome; less than 10% present with isolated Cushing syndrome without any virilizing signs.[29,25]

Nodular adrenal hyperplasia is a rare condition that occurs in children and young adults. This disease usually presents in the first 2 decades of life, predominantly in girls. Although this entity can occur sporadically, many cases are familial and appear in an autosomal dominant fashion.[32] The adrenal glands contain multiple nodules approximately 3 to 5 mm in size. Histologic examination reveals lymphocytic infiltration of the cortex, suggesting an autoimmune cause of the disorder. The treatment of this cause of Cushing syndrome is bilateral adrenalectomy.[32] This procedure is associated with significant morbidity and requires permanent postoperative mineralocorticoid and glucocorticoid replacement.

SEX HORMONE–PRODUCING TUMORS

An adrenocortical lesion may lead to either a virilizing or a feminizing tumor. As previously mentioned, most adrenocortical tumors in children are hormonally active. Virilization with or without hypercortisolism is the most common presentation.[26,29,34,35] These virilizing tumors may be more difficult to recognize in boys than in girls. Boys may present with precocious puberty, including penile enlargement, acne, and premature development of pubic, axillary, and facial hair. Girls may develop clitoral hypertrophy, hirsutism, and acne. The treatment of choice is adrenalectomy.

Although feminizing adrenocortical tumors are rare in children, they are usually malignant. In the normal adrenal gland, very small amounts of estrogens may be secreted. With adrenocortical tumors, however, overproduction of estrogens, particularly estradiol, may occur. In girls, these tumors present with precocious isosexual development, including early breast enlargement, accelerated growth, and advanced bone age. In boys, these tumors cause bilateral gynecomastia, accelerated growth rate, and delayed pubertal development; there is also an absence of spermatogenesis.

TREATMENT OF ADRENOCORTICAL TUMORS

Surgical resection is the mainstay of treatment for adrenocortical tumors. The treatment of choice for a benign adrenal adenoma is adrenalectomy. Adrenocortical carcinomas, however, require a wide excision with adequate abdominal exploration for metastatic disease. In either case, postoperative steroid replacement is typically required until the contralateral gland can recover from its suppression.

Computed tomography or magnetic resonance imaging can help distinguish between adrenal hyperplasia and an adrenal tumor. A ^{131}I-iodomethyl-1-19-norcholesterol (NP-59) scintiscan may aid in the evaluation of an adrenal lesion. This cholesterol analogue is taken up as cholesterol into the steroid pathways of the adrenal cortex. Adrenal adenomas usually have an increased uptake of NP-59, whereas adrenocortical carcinomas typically do not take up the isotope. Bilateral uptake of NP-59 indicates bilateral adrenal hyperplasia, which can be the result of ACTH oversecretion.

The most common sites of metastatic adrenocortical carcinomas are the lung, liver, lymph nodes, contralateral adrenal gland, bones, kidneys, and brain. If complete resection is not possible, tumor debulking may be of some benefit to control symptoms. Medical therapy with mitotane may also play a role in treating patients with unresectable disease. Mitotane acts as an adrenolytic agent by altering mitochondrial function, blocking adrenal steroid hydroxylation, and altering the extra-adrenal metabolism of cortisol and androgens. The success of chemotherapy has not been clearly shown, however, and complete surgical resection is the primary determinant of survival.[36]

Hyperaldosteronism

Overproduction of aldosterone, or hyperaldosteronism, may be due to either adrenal dysfunction or overproduction of renin. Primary hyperaldosteronism refers to adrenal dysfunction, such as an aldosterone-secreting tumor or bilateral adrenal hyperplasia. Secondary hyperaldosteronism refers to an overproduction of renin, which can be caused by cirrhosis, congestive heart failure, a renin-producing juxtaglomerular cell tumor, or renovascular abnormalities, such as renal artery stenosis.

The symptoms of hyperaldosteronism include headaches, fatigue, weakness, lethargy, poor weight gain, polyuria, polydipsia, and nocturia. Hypertension develops as a result of increased sodium and water reabsorption. Weakness occurs because of hypokalemia, which is the most common laboratory finding, although metabolic alkalosis may be observed from the loss of hydrogen ions in the urine. The biochemical diagnosis of hyperaldosteronism is demonstrated by excessive aldosterone secretion in the setting of suppressed renin secretion. Once the diagnosis of primary hyperaldosteronism has been established, patients with aldosterone-secreting adrenal tumors must be distinguished from those with the more common condition of bilateral adrenocortical hyperplasia. In patients with bilateral adrenocortical hyperplasia, dexamethasone administration normalizes the abnormally high aldosterone level and low renin level.[10]

In the pediatric population, the incidence of aldosteronoma, or an adrenal adenoma causing primary hyperaldosteronism, is extremely low, with only a handful of reported cases in the literature. As previously mentioned, the more common cause of primary hyperaldosteronism is bilateral cortical hyperplasia.[37] An aldosteronoma is best treated by unilateral adrenalectomy. Patients with bilateral adrenocortical hyperplasia do not respond well to surgical treatment and are best managed with medical therapy using spironolactone and amiloride.[10] Adrenal insufficiency resulting from bilateral adrenalectomy is more difficult to manage than hyperaldosteronism.

Addison Disease

Insufficient production of steroid hormones (either glucocorticoids or mineralocorticoids) can lead to Addison disease. Children with Addison disease present with a variety of symptoms, including weakness, anorexia, weight loss, fatigue, nausea, vomiting, and diarrhea. If the child has an elevated ACTH level, hyperpigmentation will develop, because melanocytes are stimulated by ACTH. Seizures may also occur in the setting of the hypoglycemia, which occurs with adrenal crisis.

There are many causes of adrenal insufficiency in children. Congenital adrenal hypoplasia can result from either an autosomal recessive disorder or an X-linked disorder that occurs in boys. Errors in steroid metabolism can also lead to adrenal insufficiency. The most common group of inborn errors involves defects in glucocorticoid synthesis and is collectively known as congenital adrenal hyperplasia. Acquired lesions involving the hypothalamus or pituitary can also lead to adrenal insufficiency through a reduction in CRH or ACTH secretion.

Destruction of the adrenal glands can also lead to adrenal insufficiency. Conditions causing adrenal demise include hemorrhage, infection, adrenoleukodystrophy, and autoimmune diseases. In older patients, overwhelming infection can lead to adrenal hemorrhage. Tuberculosis used to be a common cause of infectious destruction of the adrenal; however, the incidence of this condition has fallen in modern times. One of the more common causes of acute adrenal insufficiency is cessation of chronic exogenous glucocorticoid administration.

In newborns, adrenal hemorrhage is not an uncommon event. In fact, the adrenal gland is the second most common source of hemoperitoneum in the newborn period.[38] The pathogenesis of adrenal hemorrhage in newborns is not fully understood. Associated factors include traumatic delivery, asphyxia, maternal hypotension, overwhelming infection, or hemorrhagic disorders.[35,39] The incidence of adrenal hemorrhage is almost 2 cases per 1000 live births,[1] but as the sensitivity of imaging technology improves, this number may increase. Adrenal hemorrhage occurs 3 to 4 times more frequently in the right adrenal gland than the left and is bilateral in 8% to 10% of patients.[39] This bias toward the right side may be due to the direct drainage of the right adrenal gland into the inferior vena cava, making the right gland more susceptible to changes in venous pressure. The left gland remains somewhat protected by its drainage into the left renal vein. The fetal cortex contributes to fetal and neonatal adrenal hemorrhage because of both its size and its later involution. The large size of the fetal cortex makes the adrenal glands relatively large, increasing their vulnerability to trauma. The normal adrenal gland is easily visualized by US during the first week of life. The adrenal soon involutes, and the distinction between the cortex and the medulla is lost. The physiologic involution of the fetal cortex may occur quite rapidly, tearing the unsupported central adrenal gland vessels.[38]

On prenatal US, adrenal hemorrhage appears as an echogenic mass. This mass becomes increasingly hypoechoic and usually involutes on subsequent sonograms.[40] The lesion may completely resolve, leaving only residual calcifications. Adrenal hemorrhage may be confused with neuroblastoma. Patients with normal urinary catecholamine levels and the appropriate risk factors for adrenal hemorrhage can be observed and undergo repeat US. Differentiation of adrenal adenoma and carcinoma by US is difficult; in addition, both resemble an adrenal pheochromocytoma. An ultrasonographic characteristic that suggests malignancy is central necrosis from rapid growth. Biochemical testing and the use of CT, MRI, and nuclear medicine studies narrow the diagnostic possibilities.

The treatment of Addison disease is replacement of the deficient steroid hormone. This may be accomplished with a mineralocorticoid, such as fludrocortisone, or a glucocorticoid, such as hydrocortisone or prednisone. During periods of acute stress, such as infection or operation, increased doses of glucocorticoids are needed.

Incidental Adrenal Mass

The incidental discovery of adrenal lesions on imaging studies performed for other reasons has been increasing in both children and adults, perhaps because of the increased frequency of imaging studies being performed and the increased sensitivity of those imaging modalities. In adults, the current recommendation is to remove all hormonally active tumors regardless of size. In the case of nonfunctional adrenal masses, it is considered safe to observe a mass less than 4 cm in size.[41–43] In the pediatric population, however, there are no clear guidelines about incidental, nonfunctional adrenal masses. Because of the higher incidence of both functional tumors and malignant tumors in the pediatric adrenal gland, many surgeons recommend adrenalectomy in this setting.[43]

Adrenalectomy

The objective of adrenal surgery is to attain complete tumor resection, resulting in normalization of endocrine function and cure of malignancy. Perioperative planning includes correction of potential electrolyte abnormalities, establishing alpha and beta blockade in the case of pheochromocytoma, and performing localizing studies to guide the surgical approach. The surgical approach is based on the probable histology of the adrenal mass, the presence of bilaterality, and the surgeon's preference. The introduction of laparoscopic adrenal resection has provided an attractive alternative for the resection of many adrenal masses in children.

Traditional approaches to adrenal resection have included anterior, posterior, and thoracoabdominal approaches. The anterior approach uses a transabdominal incision, usually subcostal, which permits resection of either the left or the right adrenal gland. It also allows bilateral resection through a single incision, as well as visualization of the periaortic sympathetic ganglia, the small bowel mesentery, and the pelvis. More than 95% of pediatric pheochromocytomas are located in the abdomen, and this approach reveals the majority of tumors. The surgeon must make a conscious effort to minimize direct manipulation of the tumor during dissection.

Early control and ligation of the adrenal vein limit the release of catecholamines as the tumor is removed.

During the anterior approach to right adrenalectomy, the duodenum is mobilized by the Kocher maneuver (Fig. 41-3) by reflecting the transverse colon inferiorly and mobilizing the duodenum medially. This exposes the upper portion of the right kidney as well as the right adrenal gland. The Gerota fascia is opened, and the right lobe of the liver is retracted in a cephalad direction. The most important element of the procedure is the dissection between the medial border of the adrenal mass and the lateral wall of the inferior vena cava. This plane is developed in a cephalad direction until the relatively short right adrenal vein is identified entering the vena cava. There is a greater risk of hemorrhage on the right side than on the left, because of the shorter length of

the right adrenal vein and the greater risk of tearing this vessel. Multiple veins may be present and should be identified to prevent accidental avulsion. During the anterior approach to the left adrenal gland, the initial maneuver is to mobilize the splenic flexure of the colon. The pancreas and spleen are retracted superiorly, and the Gerota fascia is opened, exposing the left adrenal gland. Alternatively, the surgeon can divide the gastrocolic ligament, mobilizing the stomach superiorly and the transverse colon inferiorly. The posterior peritoneum along the inferior pancreatic border can then be incised, allowing mobilization of the pancreatic tail and exposure of the adrenal vein. The left adrenal vein enters the renal vein superiorly and can be ligated in this plane. Several arteries enter the medial surface of the adrenal gland from the lateral side of the aorta; these arteries need to be divided before adrenal

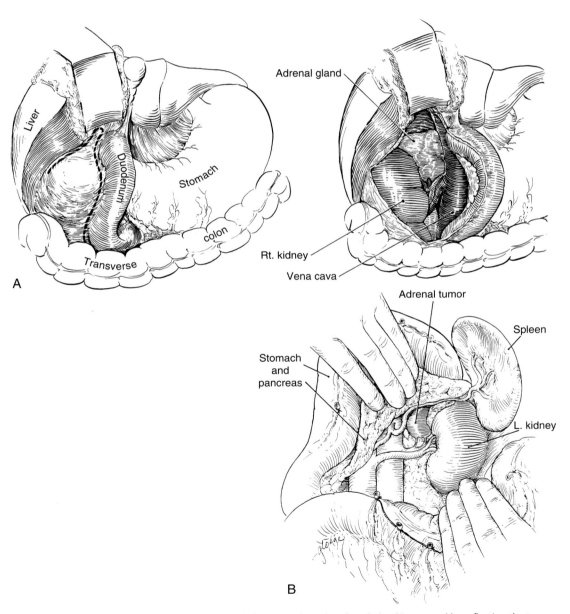

FIGURE 41-3 Transabdominal approach to tumors of the adrenal glands. **A,** The right adrenal gland is exposed by reflecting the transverse mesocolon inferiorly, mobilizing the duodenum medially with a Kocher maneuver, and incising the posterior fascia to expose the diaphragm, adrenal gland, and superior pole of the right kidney. **B,** The left adrenal gland is exposed by dividing the gastrocolic ligament and elevating the stomach. The colon is retracted inferiorly, and the pancreas is elevated, exposing the adrenal gland and left adrenal vein that enters the renal vein.

removal. The posterior approach to the adrenal gland is accomplished most commonly through the bed of the 11th rib. This strategy avoids intraperitoneal dissection, eliminates postoperative adhesions, and decreases postoperative ileus. The posterior approach is not useful for bilateral adrenal lesions, malignancies, or large vascular tumors. The thoracoabdominal approach to adrenalectomy is best applied to very large unilateral lesions. Although this approach provides optimal exposure of large vascular tumors; postoperative pain and impairment of ventilation limit its application.

The first laparoscopic adrenalectomy was reported in an adult in 1991.[44] Since then, a number of studies involving laparoscopic adrenalectomy in children have been published,[45,46] demonstrating the feasibility and safety of this approach. Most commonly, laparoscopic adrenalectomy is performed with the patient in the lateral position. A kidney rest elevates the flank opposite the adrenal lesion. Four or five trocars are placed in a subcostal position on the side of the adrenal gland to be resected. Exposure is improved on the right side by dividing the right triangular ligament of the liver. Division of the lienocolic ligament on the left improves exposure of the left adrenal gland. When possible,

the adrenal vein is ligated with clips at the initial point of dissection. The adrenal specimen should be removed in a specimen bag because of the potential for malignancy. Most adrenal lesions in children are small and benign, making laparoscopic resection an appropriate choice in the majority of cases. Although no absolute contraindications to laparoscopic resection exist, an open approach should be considered in patients with large tumors, malignancies with potential lymph node involvement, and highly vascular pheochromocytomas.

Partial adrenalectomies (termed *cortical-sparing* or *adrenal-sparing*) have been described for bilateral pheochromocytomas, wherein a portion of a single gland or portions of bilateral glands are retained. Preliminary reports indicate few recurrences and maintenance of corticosteroid independence. Children are included in these cohorts but not individually evaluated as a sub-group. Reports are surfacing of successful laparoscopic cortical-sparing adrenalectomies as well.[47] Long-term follow-up and continued surveillance are essential.

The complete reference list is available online at www. expertconsult.com.

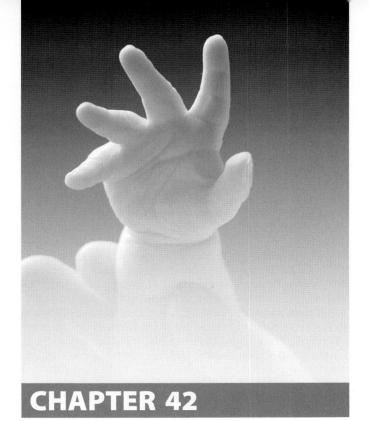

CHAPTER 42

Tumors of the Lung and Chest Wall

Stephen J. Shochat and Christopher B. Weldon

The majority of pulmonary neoplasms in children are due to metastatic disease; however, primary pulmonary tumors of the lung do occur in the pediatric age group. The approximate ratio of primary pulmonary tumors to metastatic neoplasms and non-neoplastic lesions of the lung is 1:5:60.[1] Although primary pulmonary tumors are rare in children, the majority of these tumors are malignant. In a review of 383 primary pulmonary neoplasms in children by Hancock and colleagues,[2] 76% were malignant and 24% were benign. This incidence is similar to that previously reported by Hartman and Shochat.[3] Table 42-1 demonstrates the variety of primary pulmonary neoplasms seen in children. This chapter addresses the more common benign and malignant primary pulmonary tumors in children and discusses the treatment of pulmonary metastatic disease in the pediatric population.

Benign Tumors of the Lung

PLASMA CELL GRANULOMA (INFLAMMATORY PSEUDOTUMOR)

Plasma cell granuloma has also been called inflammatory myofibroblastic tumor, fibroxanthoma, histiocytoma, and fibrohistiocytoma.[4] This lesion, which is seen frequently in adults, occurs rarely in children younger than 10 years (approximately 8% of cases). However, plasma cell granuloma is the most common benign tumor in children and accounts for slightly more than 50% of all benign lesions and approximately 20% of all primary lung tumors.[3] These tumors usually present as peripheral pulmonary masses but occasionally present as polypoid endobronchial tumors.[5,6] The pathogenesis of plasma cell granuloma is not well understood, but an antecedent pulmonary infection has been reported in approximately 30% of cases. The mean age at presentation in children is 7 years of age, and 35% of the children are between 1 and 15 years of age.[5-7] Many children are asymptomatic at the time of presentation, but fever, cough, pain, hemoptysis, pneumonitis, and dysphagia may be present. The natural history is that of a slow-growing mass, starting as a focus of organized pneumonia with a tendency for local invasion. However, rare cases of rapid growth have been reported.[8] Extension of the tumor beyond the confines of the lung is common. At least four deaths have been reported resulting from tracheal obstruction or involvement of the mediastinum by massive lesions.

Treatment consists of a conservative pulmonary resection with removal of all gross disease if possible. Primary hilar adenopathy may be present, and local invasion with disregard for tissue planes mimics malignancy. A frequent problem is identifying the benign nature of these masses. However, the diagnosis can usually be confirmed by frozen section. Malignant fibrous histiocytoma of the lung, an extremely rare tumor in children, can mimic plasma cell granuloma and must be considered in the differential diagnosis.[9] Recurrences following resection are rare but have been reported. Nonsteroidal antiinflammatory drugs have been used to treat large inoperable lesions, with encouraging results.[10]

HAMARTOMA

Pulmonary hamartoma is the second most frequent benign lesion seen in children. These lesions usually present as parenchymal lesions and can be quite large. Approximately one quarter are calcified, and "popcorn-like" calcification is pathognomonic.[11] Two endobronchial lesions have been reported. Four tumors occurring in the neonatal period were quite large and were associated with significant respiratory distress; all were fatal. An interesting triad is the combination of pulmonary hamartoma, extraadrenal paraganglioma, and gastric smooth muscle tumors; the majority of these patients are young women. Carney triad, in addition to its female predilection, is seen in young patients, is associated with multifocal gastrointestinal stromal tumors (GISTs) and has an unpredictable biological behavior.[12] Conservative pulmonary resection is the treatment of choice; however, lobectomy, or even pneumonectomy, may be required, especially for large lesions and endobronchial lesions when sleeve resection is not possible.

Malignant Tumors of the Lung

BRONCHIAL ADENOMA

The most frequently encountered malignant primary pulmonary tumor is bronchial adenoma. These tumors are a heterogeneous group of primary endobronchial lesions. Although adenoma implies a benign process, all varieties of bronchial adenomas occasionally display malignant behavior. There are three histologic types: carcinoid tumor (most common), mucoepidermoid carcinoma, and adenoid cystic carcinoma. Carcinoid tumors account for 80% to 85% of all bronchial adenomas in children.[13] The presenting symptoms are usually due to incomplete bronchial obstruction, with cough, recurrent pneumonitis, and hemoptysis. Because of diagnostic difficulties, symptoms are often present for months; occasionally,

children with wheezing have been treated for asthma, delaying diagnosis for as long as 4 to 5 years. Metastatic lesions are reported in approximately 6% of cases, and recurrences occur in 2%. There is a single report of a child with a carcinoid tumor and metastatic disease who developed the classic carcinoid syndrome.[14] Bronchial adenomas of all histologic types are associated with an excellent prognosis in children, even in the presence of local invasion.[15]

The management of bronchial adenomas is somewhat controversial, because most are visible endoscopically. Biopsy in these lesions may be hazardous because of the risk of hemorrhage, and endoscopic resection is not recommended. Bronchography or computed tomography (CT) may be helpful to determine the degree of bronchiectasis distal to the obstruction, because the degree of pulmonary destruction may influence surgical therapy.[16] However, Tagge and colleagues[17] described a technique for pulmonary salvage despite significant distal atelectasis. Conservative pulmonary resection with removal of the involved lymphatics is the treatment of choice. Sleeve segmental bronchial resection is possible in children and is the treatment of choice when feasible.[18-20] Adenoid cystic carcinomas (cylindroma) have a tendency to spread submucosally, and late local recurrence or dissemination has been reported. In addition to en bloc resection with hilar lymphadenectomy, a frozen section examination of the bronchial margins should be carried out in children with this lesion.

BRONCHOGENIC CARCINOMA

Although bronchogenic carcinoma is rare in children, this tumor was the second most common malignant lesion reported by Hancock and colleagues.[2] Interestingly, squamous cell carcinoma was rare, with the majority of tumors being either undifferentiated carcinoma or adenocarcinomas. The term bronchioalveolar carcinoma has been used in most cases.[21] These tumors are associated with both cystic adenomatoid malformations and intrapulmonary bronchogenic cysts (Table 42-2).[4,11,21-38] Only rare survivors have been reported,

TABLE 42-1
Primary Pulmonary Neoplasms in Children

Type of Tumor	No. of Patients (%)*
Benign (n = 92)	
Plasma cell granuloma	48 (52.2)
Hamartoma	22 (23.9)
Neurogenic tumor	9 (9.8)
Leiomyoma	6 (6.5)
Mucous gland adenoma	3 (3.3)
Myoblastoma	3 (3.3)
Benign teratoma	1 (1.1)
Malignant (n = 291)	
Bronchial "adenoma"	118 (40.5)
Bronchioalveolar carcinoma	49 (16.8)
Pulmonary blastoma	45 (15.5)
Fibrosarcoma	28 (9.6)
Rhabdomyosarcoma	17 (5.8)
Leiomyosarcoma	11 (3.8)
Sarcoma	6 (2.1)
Hemangiopericytoma	4 (1.4)
Plasmacytoma	4 (1.4)
Lymphoma	3 (1.0)
Teratoma	3 (1.0)
Mesenchymoma	2 (1.7)
Myxosarcoma	1 (0.3)

Modified from Hancock BJ, DiLorenzo M, Youssef S, et al: Childhood primary pulmonary neoplasms. J Pediatr Surg 1993;28:1133-1136.
*Percent of benign or malignant tumors.

TABLE 42-2
Bronchioalveolar Carcinoma Associated with Congenital Cystic Lung Malformations

	Year of Publication	Type of Lung Cyst	Age at Diagnosis (Year)	Author Comments
Prichard[22]	1984	CCAM type 1	30	Died of metastatic disease
Hurley[23]	1985	CCAM type 1		
Benjamin[24]	1991	CCAM type 1	19	BAC diagnosed in same lobe with segmental resection 19 years earlier; died at 23 years of age
Morresi[21]	1995	CCAM type 1	20	
Ribet[26]	1995	CCAM type 1	42	
Kaslovsky[27]	1997	CCAM type 1	11	Incomplete resection of CCAM in neonatal period
Granata[28]	1998	CCAM type 1	11	Lobectomy for recurrent infection; BAC was finding
Endo[29]	1982	Bronchogenic (intrapulmonary)	37	Abnormal CXR noted 10 years earlier; presented with dyspnea, BAC was incidental finding
De Perrot[30]	2001	Bronchogenic (intrapulmonary)	79	Long-standing history of cyst infections
MacSweeney[31]	2003	CCAM type 1, 0.5, 13, 18, 30, 36		1 BAC in a recurrent cyst; one other patient with a typical adenomatous hyperplasia (both patients underwent segmental resection)
Sudou[32]	2003	CCAM type 1	17	Abnormality seen on CXR from 10 years earlier

Adapted from LaBerge JM, Puligandla P, Flageole H: Asymptomatic congenital lung malformations. Semin Pediatr Surg 2005;14:16-33.
BAC, bronchioalveolar carcinoma; CCAM, congenital cystic adenomatoid malformation; CXR, chest radiograph.

and mortality exceeds 90%. The majority of children present with disseminated disease, and the average survival is only 7 months. Localized lesions can be treated by complete resection, followed by adjuvant therapy. Mucoepidermoid carcinoma of the bronchus has also been described in children as young as 4 years (Fig. 42-1).[39]

PULMONARY BLASTOMA

Pulmonary blastoma is a rare malignant tumor that occurs primarily in adults and arises from mesenchymal blastema. This tumor is an aggressive lesion, with metastatic disease at presentation in approximately 20% of cases.[40,2] They may arise from the lung, pleura, and mediastinum.[41] These tumors are classified into three types: type I (purely cystic), type II (cystic and solid), and type III (completely solid).[42] Type I tumors may be difficult to distinguish from cystic adenomatoid malformation.[43] Occasionally, these tumors may arise in an extralobar sequestration or in a previous lung cyst (Table 42-3).[22,25,29,36,41,44–73] The majority of cases occur in the right hemithorax (Fig. 42-2). Frequent sites of metastases

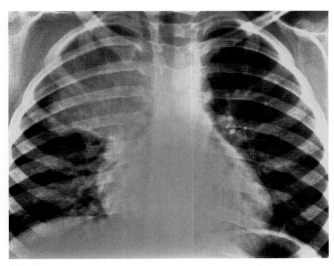

FIGURE 42-1 Anteroposterior view of a right upper lobe lesion in a 4-year-old girl. The tumor was resected by right upper lobectomy and was shown to be a mucoepidermoid carcinoma. (Courtesy Jay L. Grosfeld, MD.)

TABLE 42-3
Mesenchymal Malignancy and Cystic Lung Malformations

Author	Year	Type of Lung Cyst	Type of Malignancy	Age at Diagnosis (Months)
Stephanopoulos[44]	1963	"Cystic hamartoma"	Myxosarcoma	
Ueda[45]	1977	CCAM	RMS	18
Martinez[46]	1978	"Polycystic disease"	Pulmonary blastoma	24
Valderrama[47]	1978	Extralobar sequestration	Pulmonary blastoma	
Sumner[48]	1979	Peripheral cyst	Pulmonary blastoma	48
Weinberg[49]	1980	Congenital lung cyst	Mixed mesenchymal sarcoma	108
Krous[50]	1980	Bronchogenic cyst (intrapulmonary)	Embryonal RMS	30
Weinblatt[51]	1982	"Cystic lung disease"	Pulmonary blastoma	30
Holland-Moritz[36]	1984	"Pneumatocele"	PPB	48
Morales[25]	1986	Congenital cyst	Pulmonary blastoma	
Williams[52]	1986	CCAM	Embryonal RMS	21
Allan[53]	1987	"Congenital origin of cysts not confirmed"	RMS	21, 30
Hedlund[54]	1989	"Cystic hamartoma"	RMS	18, 22
Cairoli[55]	1990	CCAM	RMS	36
Domizio[56]	1990	"Congenital cyst"	Malignant mesenchymoma	48
Senac[57]	1991		PPB	
Murphy[58]	1992	Bronchogenic cyst, CCAM (2)	Embryonal RMS	24, 36, 42
Bogers[59]	1993	Lobar emphysema	RMS	18
Calabria[60]	1993	"Pneumatoceles"	Pulmonary blastoma	
McDermott[61]	1993	Congenital cyst	Embryonal RMS	36
Seballos[62]	1994	CCAM	Pulmonary blastoma	22
Tagge[63]	1996	Bilateral pneumatocele	PPB	45
Adirim[64]	1997	CCAM type 1	Pulmonary blastoma	
D'Agostino[65]	1997	CCAM type 2	Embryonal RMS	22
Federici[66]	2001	CCAM type 1	PPB	36
Ozcan[67]	2001	CCAM	Embryonal RMS	13
Papagiannopoulos[68]	2001	CCAM type 4	PPB	30
Stocker[69]	2002	CCAM type 4	PPB	48

Adapted from LaBerge JM, Puligandla P, Flageole H: Asymptomatic congenital lung malformations. Semin Pediatr Surg 2005;14:16-33.
CCAM, congenital cystic adenomatoid malformation; CPAM congenital pulmonary airway malformation; PPB, pleuropulmonary blastoma; RMS, rhabdomyosarcoma.

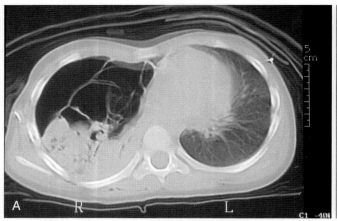
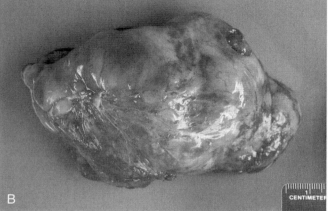

FIGURE 42-2   A, Computed tomography scan of the chest shows a cystic lesion in the right hemithorax. **B,** The tumor was resected (lobectomy), and the histology showed findings consistent with a pleuropulmonary blastoma. (Courtesy Jay L. Grosfeld, MD.)

are the liver, brain, and spinal cord. Local recurrences are frequent, and the mortality rate is approximately 40%.[2,74–76] The majority of children present before 4 years of age, and symptoms include persistent cough, chest pain, episodes of pneumonia that are refractory to antibiotics, and hemoptysis. Diagnosis is achieved by CT of the chest, bronchoscopy, and biopsy. Because most of these tumors are located peripherally, resection is usually possible by segmental or lobar resection. The use of multimodal neoadjuvant chemotherapy and radiation following surgical resection has shown promising results in a few patients with extensive disease and dissemination.[41,75] Chemotherapeutic agents that have been used include actinomycin D, vincristine, cyclophosphamide alternating with courses of doxorubicin, and cisplatin. Histologic evaluation of the tumor shows an exclusive mesenchymal composition, including primitive tubules, immature blastema, and spindle cell stroma. Some demonstrate elements of embryonal rhabdomyosarcoma (RMS) arising within a multicystic lesion.

RHABDOMYOSARCOMA

RMSs of the lung are rare and account for only 0.5% of all childhood RMSs (see Chapter 35).[45,77] Many of the lesions are endobronchial in origin (Fig. 42-3); however, several cases apparently originated in congenital cystic anomalies. (see Table 42-3).* This is an important issue because 4% of benign tumors and 8.6% of malignant tumors enumerated in Table 42-1 were associated with previously documented cystic malformations.[2] Tumors that developed in these malformations included 11 sarcomas, 9 pulmonary blastomas, 3 bronchogenic carcinomas, and 2 mesenchymomas.

COMMENTS

Although children with primary lung tumors represent a heterogeneous group of patients, analysis of the reported cases suggests that evaluation and treatment are similar in the majority of patients. Many children are asymptomatic, especially those with benign tumors; however, cough, recurrent pneumonitis, and

symptoms of atypical bronchial asthma may be the initial presentation. Radiographic findings usually indicate a solitary mass lesion or evidence of airway obstruction with resultant atelectasis and pneumonitis. Because many of these tumors can be visualized by bronchoscopy, a bronchoscopic examination should be performed. Flexible bronchoscopic techniques may be helpful for diagnosis, but the use of rigid bronchoscopy with modern magnification, along with general anesthesia, is necessary if endoscopic biopsy is contemplated. Preparation for emergency thoracotomy should be made at the time of bronchoscopy in the event of life-threatening hemorrhage.

Bronchoscopic removal of some isolated lesions may be attempted, but because of the high incidence of recurrence and the possibility of severe hemorrhage, this technique should be used selectively. Conservative surgical resection is the procedure of choice for benign pulmonary tumors to achieve histologic diagnosis and preserve maximum functioning lung tissue. Thoracoscopic resection is an option in these children.[83] CT and magnetic resonance imaging should be performed in children with large space-occupying lesions to determine resectability. Fine-needle aspiration for cytology or core needle biopsy may be performed as the initial procedure for diagnosis in selected cases. Treatment of malignant lesions varies, depending on location and histology. Sleeve resections should be considered for bronchial adenomas. Resection of involved lymphatics should be considered with malignant lesions. Combined-modality therapy with adjuvant chemotherapy and possibly radiation therapy may be helpful in children with large primary malignancies or dissemination.

An important consideration is the association of primary lung tumors with congenital cystic pulmonary malformations. These lesions may be asymptomatic and are often discovered incidentally. In some instances, the natural history of the lung cyst is unknown, and a few may regress.[80] Although some authors recommend simple observation, most pediatric surgeons argue against prolonged observation of cystic lesions because of an increased risk of infection, pneumothorax, sudden cyst enlargement with potential respiratory compromise, and associated malignancy.* As mentioned previously,

---

* References 3, 23, 25, 26, 31, 36, 44–69, 77–82.

* References 46, 57, 60, 63, 64, 68, 80.

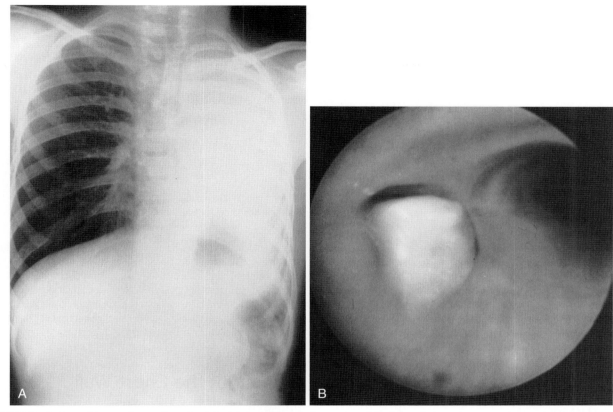

FIGURE 42-3   Patient with complete atelectasis of the left lung **(A)** and obstruction of the left main bronchus secondary to rhabdomyosarcoma **(B)**.

there is evidence suggesting a relationship between type IV cystic adenomatoid malformation and type I pulmonary blastoma. Although complete lobectomy with negative margins is adequate treatment for these patients, close observation is recommended.[31,35,84] If patients with asymptomatic cystic malformations are observed without resection, they should be followed closely and evaluated frequently.

Treatment of Metastatic Disease

Pulmonary metastases occur much more frequently than primary tumors in children, and the surgical approach depends on the histology of the primary tumor and the response of the primary site to combined-modality therapy.[72,85] Pulmonary metastases should not be considered for resection until the primary tumor is eradicated, without evidence of recurrence and other sites of metastatic disease ruled out. Tumors most frequently considered for pulmonary metastasectomy are osteosarcoma (OS), soft tissue sarcoma, and Wilms' tumor.[86]

OSTEOSARCOMA

Children with OS should be considered for resection of pulmonary metastases once the primary lesion is controlled. The overall disease-free survival is approximately 40% in children who develop metachronous pulmonary metastases. Multiple factors, such as number of pulmonary nodules and time of recurrence, play an important role in children with OS and

pulmonary metastases.[87,88] Roth and colleagues[73] showed that patients with fewer than four pulmonary nodules had an improved survival versus those with more than four lesions. According to Goorin and colleagues,[89] a complete resection of all pulmonary lesions is an important determinant of outcome, and penetration through the parietal pleura is associated with an adverse outcome. Although somewhat controversial, the outlook seems to be somewhat improved, even in patients presenting with pulmonary metastases, if complete resection of all metastatic lesions can be accomplished.[90] Harris and colleagues[91] reported a 68% survival rate in 17 patients with fewer than eight pulmonary nodules at presentation following chemotherapy, resection of the primary tumor, and pulmonary metastasectomy. The data in Table 42-4 suggest that an aggressive attempt at surgical resection of pulmonary metastases is indicated in OS, possibly irrespective of the number of lesions or the interval to the development of metastases.* A number of recent studies have shown a survival advantage in patients with repeated metastasectomy, including patients with as many as five recurrences.[74,78,79]

SOFT TISSUE SARCOMA

The usefulness of resecting pulmonary metastases in patients with soft tissue sarcoma depends on the histologic subtype. Rarely is pulmonary resection of metastatic lesions required in RMS, and resection of pulmonary metastasis in Ewing

---

* References 34, 38, 70, 82, 89, 92–95.

TABLE 42-4

Pulmonary Metastasectomy for Osteogenic Sarcoma

	Average Interval to Relapse	No. of Procedures (Months) (Range)	Disease-Free Survival, (No. of Lesions)	Median Follow-up for Survivors/ Author No. (%) (mo)	No. of Patients (Range)
Martini[92]	22	10 (2-25)	59 (113)	7 (32)	33 (15-234)
Spanos[93]	29	15.7 (4-30)	52 (124)	11 (37)	36 (9-234)
Telander[82]	28	9/6 (2-34)	60 (173)	13 (46)	25 (6-48)
Giritsky[34]	12	9 (1-21)	19	6 (50)	17 (9-39)
Rosenberg[94]	18	–	–	7 (39)	–
Marion[70]	12	13 (2-20)	9	5 (42)	(36-72)
Schaller[38]	17	–	34	7 (41)	(12-192)
Goorin[89]	32	12.5 (4-59)	26 (>63)	9 (28)	55 (19-101)
Carter[95]	43	13 (1-83)	–	4 (10)	69 (59-80)

From LaQuaglia MP: The surgical management of metastases in pediatric cancer. Semin Pediatr Surg 1993;2:75-82.

sarcoma has not been found to be efficacious.[71,72] Several European protocols are being developed to better define the role of pulmonary resection in Ewing sarcoma. The remaining sarcomas should be considered for resection if complete excision is possible and the patient's primary tumor is under control. The time to development of pulmonary metastases, number of lesions, and tumor doubling time are all significant prognostic factors in soft tissue sarcomas. Historically, approximately 10% to 20% of these patients can be salvaged by resection of pulmonary metastases.[37]

WILMS' TUMOR

Rarely is pulmonary resection of metastatic disease required in children with Wilms' tumor. In a review of the National Wilms' Tumor Study by Green and colleagues,[96] no advantage of pulmonary resection was found compared with chemotherapy and radiation therapy alone. In an attempt to avoid pulmonary radiation, de Kraker and colleagues[33] suggested a protocol using primary pulmonary resection after chemotherapy for pulmonary metastases. Only 5 of 36 patients ultimately required resection of pulmonary metastases following chemotherapy, because most patients had a complete response with chemotherapy alone. One encouraging finding was that only 4 of 36 children required whole-lung irradiation. Because the results of chemotherapy and whole-lung irradiation are excellent for children with Wilms' tumor and pulmonary metastases, pulmonary resection of metastases should be reserved for selected cases (see Chapter 30).

COMMENTS

Operation for pulmonary metastases in children depends on the histology of the primary tumor, the extent of the metastatic disease, and whether the metastatic disease is responsive to chemotherapy. The surgical approach varies, depending on the disease process and the age of the patient. No difference in survival has been demonstrated with sequential lateral thoracotomy versus sternotomy, but the latter is preferable in older patients with OS. Complete resection of all metastatic disease is an important consideration, and the use of automatic stapling devices can be helpful. Wedge resection is usually possible in children with OS. However, formal lobectomy or segmentectomy may be required to remove all of the tumor completely, especially when the primary tumor

is not responsive to chemotherapy or radiation.[97] Muscle-sparing techniques are available in those children requiring posterolateral thoracotomies, and thoracoscopy may be appropriate in certain cases.[37] New localization techniques are being developed to aid in the thoracoscopic resection of lung lesions.[81] However, port site recurrences have been reported following thoracoscopic resection of pulmonary metastatic disease.[98,99]

Tumors of the Chest Wall

EPIDEMIOLOGY

Tumors of the chest wall are rare entities in the pediatric population with an incidence of no more than 2%,[100,101] and up to two thirds of these lesions are malignant.[102] The majority arise from the bony structures of the chest wall (55%), as opposed to soft tissue (45%).[103] Collectively, a 60% 5-year overall survival rate for all tumors has been reported, with a recurrence rate of 50% (local and distant) and subsequent 5-year survival rate of only 17%.[104]

PRESENTATION

Masses of the chest wall typically present as lumps bulging underneath the skin, and the majority of malignant lesions have pain as a presenting symptom as well. In young children and infants, they are often found incidentally by caregivers, while older children and young adults may present with larger masses that have been present and growing for some time. Incidental discovery on routine chest imaging has been reported to be as high as 20%.[105] They can be found anywhere on the thorax, and the tissue of origin is generally mesenchymal in nature, regardless of whether the tumors are malignant or benign. Hence, sarcomatous variants are the most common malignant tumors, while carcinomas are almost nonexistent. The minority of patients present with nonspecific symptoms of respiratory compromise or dysfunction (tachypnea, hypoxia, cough, dyspnea on exertion), and these symptoms may have been present for quite a while before seeking medical advice. Symptoms stem from parenchymal compression from the mass intruding into the pleural space and onto the lung or from malignant effusions, both of which interfere with normal respiratory mechanics. Regardless of the presentation, a full history and physical exam, including a family history, travel history, injury history, and extensive review of systems, is warranted to document other etiologies or associated conditions. Finally, depending on the degree of respiratory embarrassment, pulmonary function tests may be indicated prior to proceeding with any intervention.

DIAGNOSTIC ADJUNCTS

Once the initial evaluation has been performed in the office, basic laboratory evaluations for complete blood count, coagulation profile, and baseline chemistries are needed. Imaging studies should consist first of erect, posterior-anterior, and lateral chest radiographs to evaluate the location, size, presence of calcifications, osseous involvement, and the presence of pulmonary parenchymal disease. Next, an ultrasound exam to determine the echo features (solid versus cystic, degree of homogeneity) and vascularity of the mass is recommended. Axial imaging (computed tomography or magnetic resonance imaging [MRI]) is performed afterward. The advantages of CT reside in its ability to clearly define the lung parenchyma and pleural space in relation to the osseous, vascular, and soft tissue components of the thorax (and hence mass), and the fact that it is a fast technique requiring minimal to no sedation even in the youngest of patients. The negative aspects of CT are the radiation exposure with subsequent risk of a secondary malignancy.[106] The benefits of MRI include better definition of the soft tissue components versus CT, as well as enhanced evaluation of the osseous and neural structures to determine the extent of central or peripheral nerve involvement and/or the presence of skip lesions or metastases. Unfortunately, this technique is time consuming and generally requires sedation or even general anesthesia to adequately acquire the data. Motion artifact from the heart and lungs can also interfere with this technique, limiting its utility, but this obstacle is being overcome with the use of cardiac-gated, respiratory-triggered protocols.[107,108] Determination of the precise entity from radiology studies alone is impossible, but the accurate construction of a differential diagnosis is readily possible, including the differentiation of malignant versus benign lesions.[107,108] Finally, other imaging studies may also be indicated to determine the presence of metastases (brain and abdominal CT, bone scan, positron emission tomogram [PET] scan) depending on the type of lesion, especially if malignant. Recent reports have suggested that the combination of PET and CT scans yields more accurate data in assessing the primary tumor, local and regional lymph node basins, evidence of recurrence, and for response to ongoing therapies.[109,110] Once initial studies have been performed, retrieval of tissue for histopathologic evaluation and diagnosis is warranted.

DIAGNOSIS

Biopsy options include small or large specimen approaches. If a mass is small (less than 3 centimeters) or thought to be benign, then an upfront excisional biopsy may be warranted. However, the incision should be oriented so that a future reexcision, if needed, can be performed without compromising oncologic principles. Excising a normal rim of tissue circumferentially around the mass is also something for which the surgeon should opt. If the mass is large (greater than 4 to 5 centimeters), fixed to surrounding structures, involving many structures in the thorax, or if it is considered malignant by

imaging, then either an incisional biopsy or core needle biopsy is warranted. Placing the incision in-line with any future resection is of paramount importance, regardless of the technique used, and either approach will yield enough tissue for histopathologic and cytogenetic analyses.[111] Once a diagnosis is confirmed, then disease-specific treatment algorithms may be initiated.

THERAPEUTIC PRINCIPLES

Though treatment regimens are tumor specific, there are certain general principles that apply. For malignant lesions, multimodality therapy is the accepted paradigm for the majority of lesions, while simple extirpation is the rule with benign entities. With surgery, the most important concept to emphasize is that of the need for negative margins to decrease the risk of recurrence and subsequent therapy. Surgical extirpation also mandates wound reconstruction, which must be considered prior to the initiation of operative therapy. Large defects (greater than 5 centimeters, except for posterior and superior lesions where the defect will be buttressed by the scapula) will require the use of prosthetic materials—rigid (silicone, Teflon [DuPont, Wilmington, Del.], methyl methacrylate) or flexible (Prolene mesh [Ethicon, Cincinnati, Ohio], PTFE mesh, Marlex mesh [Chevron Phillips Chemical, Bartlesville, Okla.], Gore-Tex [WL Gore & Associates, Newark, Del.])—and/or autologous tissues (pedicle or free flaps [latissimus dorsi, rectus abdominis, or pectoralis major]) to reconstruct the chest wall and thus ensure normal chest wall mechanics and prevent respiratory embarrassment.

TUMOR TYPES

Chest wall tumors are separated into benign and malignant cohorts (Table 42-5), as well as primary and secondary lesions. Specific tumors and their treatment will be outlined in the subsequent sections, but a discussion concerning secondary tumors is beyond the scope of this work.

Benign Chest Wall Tumors

Aneurysmal Bone Cyst   Aneurysmal bone cysts (ABCs) can be found anywhere on the chest wall, and they generally arise in the ribs. They have characteristic patterns of appearance on both chest radiographs and MRI,[107] and they can grow to be quite large, producing local destruction to the adjacent tissues. Surgical extirpation with complete excision is the treatment of choice, and recurrence is rare. Histologically, the lesions are blood-filled cysts composed of fibrous tissue and giant cells.

Chondroma   Chondromas are slow growing, painless masses that usually arise in the costal cartilages. On imaging studies, they are lytic lesions with sclerotic margins, and unfortunately, they are difficult to distinguish radiographically from their malignant brethren, chondrosarcomas. Hence, complete resection with a wide margin of normal tissue is advocated.[112]

Desmoid   Desmoid tumors are fibrous neoplasms that can be found anywhere in the body. They are thought to be benign, but they have also been reported to undergo malignant degeneration.[112] Desmoid tumors infiltrate adjacent and surrounding tissues, and they are known to travel down fascial planes and to encase neurovascular structures in the mediastinum or

TABLE 42-5
Pediatric Chest Wall Tumors
Benign
Aneurysmal bone cyst
Chondroma
Desmoid
Fibroma
Fibrous dysplasia
Lipoblastoma
Lipoma
Mesenchymal hamartoma
Osteochondroma
Osteoma
Vascular malformations
Malignant
Chondrosarcoma
Ewing sarcoma family
Fibrosarcoma
Langerhans cell histiocytosis
Leiomyosarcoma
Leukemia
Liposarcoma
Lymphoma
Neuroblastoma
Rhabdomyosarcoma
Osteosarcoma

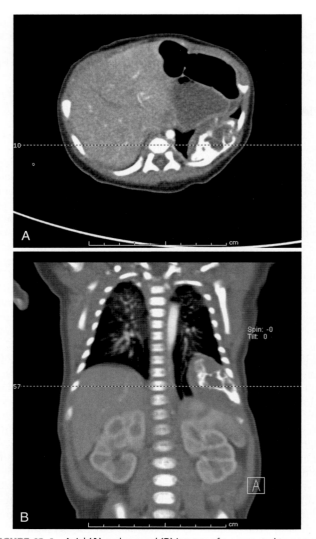

FIGURE 42-4 Axial **(A)** and coronal **(B)** images of a computed tomography scan of the chest in an infant with a mesenchymal hamartoma.

the thoracic inlet. MRI is the radiologic procedure of choice to best define the extent of involvement and the structures involved. Treatment is wide local excision with negative margins, but recurrence rates from 10% (negative margins) to 75% (positive margins) have been described by some authors.[113–115] If a complete resection is not possible, or if vital structures are meant to be sacrificed during operative extirpation, then multimodality therapy consisting of radiation (50 to 60 Gy), and cytotoxic (vinblastine and methotrexate) and cytostatic (tamoxifen and diclofenac) chemotherapy is recommended, though the exact regimen is not well defined.[116–119]

Fibrous Dysplasia Fibrous dysplasia is a benign condition where normal bone is replaced by fibrous tissue. These lesions are generally not large, and patients present with pain, generally from a pathologic fracture. On plain radiographs, these lesions are described as lytic in nature with a characteristic "soap bubble" appearance.[120] Treatment is based on symptoms and concerns for possible fracture secondary to the inherent structural weakness the lesion produces in the bone. Simple excision is the recommended procedure.

Mesenchymal Hamartoma Mesenchymal hamartomas (MH) are masses found in infants or young children that can also be discovered antenatally. The lesions are generally well circumscribed, and though emanating from the chest wall (one or several ribs), they abut or compress, as opposed to invade, thoracic structures (Fig. 42-4). Hence, presenting symptoms are primarily from respiratory embarrassment. These lesions are well defined by radiographic features on cross-sectional imaging, including mineralization and hemorrhagic cystic structures.[121] Histopathologically, these lesions consist of chondroid tissue with blood-filled, endothelial-lined spaces

interspersed with osteoclastic giant cells. Treatment strategies have traditionally consisted of complete resection with subsequent chest wall reconstruction, but considering the large size of these lesions and the small volume of the chest cavity in the infants in which they are discovered, concern over the future complications of scoliosis and respiratory compromise from this approach has been considerable. In light of the fact that they are not known to undergo malignant degeneration,[122] observation[123,124] or other less morbid approaches (radiofrequency ablation[125]) have been described and recommended.

Osteochondroma Osteochondromas are tumors composed of bony and cartilaginous elements more commonly found in males (3:1 ratio).[112] The lesion can present with pain from a pathologic fracture or compression of nearby nerves, or it can be asymptomatic if it grows inward into the thoracic cavity. The lesion is well characterized on plain radiographs, and it arises from the cortex of the rib at the metaphysis and has a "cartilage cap."[120] Malignant degeneration has been documented,[107] and resection is warranted in all postpubertal patients, with symptoms, or if the mass is growing.

Malignant Chest Wall Tumors

The majority of clinically prevalent malignant tumors in the pediatric population are sarcomatous lesions, and a select sampling of these tumors will be addressed individually in the following sections.

Chondrosarcoma Chondrosarcomas (CSs) are derived from cartilaginous elements (costal cartilages) that are the most common primary malignant bone tumor of the chest wall in adults,[126] and they are more common in males.[112] CSs have been associated with a prior history of trauma,[127] as well as being known to form from malignant degeneration of the benign counterpart discussed previously.[126] Some 10% of patients will present with metastatic disease,[103] especially in the lungs and brain. Primary therapeutic intervention is complete surgical extirpation with a margin of normal tissue of at least 4 centimeters[112] secondary to the high risk of local recurrence (up to 75% with positive margins), even with negative margins at the initial operation (10%).[128] These tumors are not chemotherapy responsive, and the role of radiation is only for those lesions that are unresectable or have known positive margins. Five-year survival has been reported to range from 60% to 90%,[128,129] and beneficial prognostic factors are the absence of metastases at presentation and a complete resection.[103,128]

Ewing Sarcoma Family/Primitive Neuroectodermal Tumors Ewing sarcoma family/primitive neuroectodermal tumors (EWS/PNETs) are the most common malignant chest wall lesions in the pediatric population.[123] They are aggressive tumors requiring multimodality therapy, but survival is still poor despite these interventions. The tumors often present as painful masses with frequent metastases (25%) to the lung, bone, or bone marrow.[103] EWS/PNET lesions are characterized by a balanced gene translocation (*EWS/FLI1*) (t11:22 [q24:q12]),[130] and these tumors are defined histologically as sheets of small, round cells with scant cytoplasm. On imaging studies, they have characteristic bony destruction described as lytic or sclerotic lesions.[108] Treatment involves an initial biopsy followed by neoadjuvant chemotherapy (four cycles) with vincristine, actinomycin, cyclophosphamide, and Adriamycin (Adria-VAC) alternating with etoposide and ifosfamide. This regimen has demonstrated a great deal of success in shrinking the tumor to improve survival and facilitate complete resection (Fig. 42-5).[131,132] In fact, with the use of neoadjuvant chemotherapy, complete surgical extirpation with negative margins was possible in 71% of patients versus 37% who underwent primary surgical intervention.[132] The extent of surgery should include all involved structures and a soft tissue or osseous margin. Postoperative adjuvant therapy uses the same preoperative chemotherapy regimens, but not radiotherapy if complete resection is achieved. This should be the goal, despite the known radiosensitivity of this tumor,[133] because of the concern over the late effects (scoliosis, pneumonitis, cardiotoxicity, secondary malignancy, growth retardation, and breast hypoplasia or aplasia) radiotherapy poses.[132] The use of radiotherapy is for residual and unresectable disease and for patients who present with a malignant pleural effusion, where it is an accepted therapeutic intervention. A recent European consensus conference advocated for surgery rather than

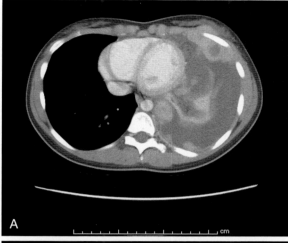

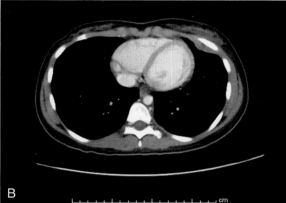

FIGURE 42-5 Axial images of a computed tomography scan of the chest in a child with a Ewing sarcoma family/primitive neuroectodermal tumor (EWS/PNET) of the chest wall before **(A)** and after **(B)** neoadjuvant chemotherapy.

irradiation in all cases.[134] Five-year survival using the previously mentioned protocol was around 70% for nonmetastatic disease,[135] and the 8-year survival was roughly 30% with metastatic disease.[136] In patients presenting with metastatic disease, the European Intergroup Cooperative Ewing's Sarcoma Studies Group demonstrated improved survival with the use of myeloablative chemotherapy followed by stem cell rescue at the conclusion of conventional treatment protocols.[137]

Fibrosarcoma Fibrosarcoma (FS) (also known as infantile or congenital fibrosarcoma) are malignant tumors found throughout the body in infants who present with large masses that often involve, invade, and surround adjacent structures. FS have been found in the chest wall, and several reports have documented the success of multimodality therapy in combating these tumors.[138,139] FS can be distinguished from other myofibrous and sarcomatous lesions by the presence of a unique gene rearrangement between the *TEL* gene (12q13) and *TRKC* gene (15q25).[138] FSs are chemotherapy sensitive, and reports demonstrating the effectiveness of neoadjuvant chemotherapy with vincristine, actinomycin, cyclophosphamide, and Adriamycin, followed by surgical extirpation, are well accepted.[138,139] A recent report[139] from Europe demonstrated that 5-year overall and event-free survival rates were 89% and 81%, respectively. The authors reported that in their series complete surgical extirpation was rarely feasible and that conservative surgical approaches should be adopted. Furthermore, 71% of patients responded to alkylating agent-free and anthracycline agent-free regimens, and hence, this regimen should be started first to limit toxicity.

Osteosarcoma   OS of the chest wall can be primary or secondary tumors (prior sites of irradiation or from preexisting osseous lesions [Paget disease]).[112] Primary lesions are primarily of the ribs, and on imaging, they can be confused with chondrosarcomas.[140] Chest radiographs will demonstrate a "sunburst pattern," and axial imaging concentrating on regional (bony skip lesions) and distant (lung, liver, brain) metastases must be sought.[112] Pretherapy biopsy is the rule, and neoadjuvant therapy precedes extirpative procedures. Overall survival rates are poor (15% to 20%),[103] but in the presence of nonmetastatic disease, 5-year survival rates can exceed 50%.[103] Prognosis is related to the presence of metastases, the degree of tumor burden, and the response to chemotherapy.[141]

Rhabdomyosarcoma   RMS of the chest wall is a rare tumor and encompasses no more than 7% of all RMS in Intergroup Rhabdomyosarcoma Studies (IRS).[142–144] The chest wall site is deemed an unfavorable site, and therefore this is an adverse prognostic factor.[142,143] Other adverse prognostic factors have been reported to be histopathologic findings (alveolar versus embryonal), tumor burden and size, incomplete resection, and presence of metastatic disease (including lymph node metastases).[143,145] Despite advances in the treatment of RMS over the last 40 years, unfavorable sites carry an overall survival of only 55% (versus 90% for favorable sites),[143] and those with truncal RMS have been reported to have a failure-free survival rate of no greater than 67%.[146] These tumors require multimodality therapy, and neoadjuvant chemotherapy followed by surgical extirpation is the norm. Radiation is reserved for lesions with positive margins following surgery, or in unresectable tumors. A report from Saenz and colleagues documented the utility of radiation (median dose of 44 Gy) to salvage some patients with residual disease.[146] However, the necessity for complete surgical resection has been called into question by a recent report from the Children's Oncology Group (COG),[147] where the outcome of patients enrolled in IRS I-IV with chest wall RMS were analyzed. The report documents that regardless of clinical group (I-III) and other tumor-specific factors (histologic subtype, tumor size), the only critical factor to influence failure-free and overall survival was the presence of metastatic disease. In the face of metastases, patients with chest wall RMS had an overall and failure-free survival of 7% and 7% versus 49% and 61%, respectively, in the cohort without metastases ($P < 0.001$). Therefore the authors suggest where gross total surgical resection will produce significant morbidity or physical debilitation, less aggressive operative approaches should be entertained.

The complete reference list is available online at www.expertconsult.com.

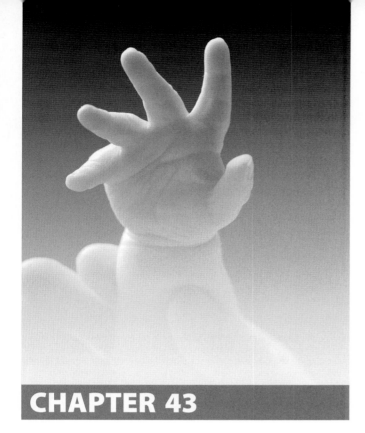

CHAPTER 43

Bone Tumors

Saminathan S. Nathan and John H. Healey

Bone tumors are rare. In the United States, there were 166,487 cases of breast cancer and 164,753 cases[1] of prostate cancer in 2000. By comparison, there were only 2,051 cases of all types of bone sarcomas that year. A large proportion of these tumors, 26.8% in one published database, occur in the pediatric population. There are no population-based benign bone tumor registries; so, it would be impossible to establish their true incidence. Most databases of this nature derive from tertiary referral institutions, and so, benign conditions, which are often asymptomatic, would be grossly underrepresented. Nevertheless, one study has shown that up to 43% of children have a bone lesion that mimics or is a true neoplasm during skeletal development.[2] This implies that the overwhelming majority of lesions are benign.

The pediatric surgeon will often be called into the management of the patient with bone tumors for a number of reasons. The very young child on follow-up for an unrelated condition may manifest with a bone lesion secondary to osteomyelitis or leukemia. The older child with a metastatic osteogenic sarcoma may require the expertise of the pediatric thoracic surgeon for the resection of pulmonary nodules. The teenager with a pathologic fracture through a unicameral bone cyst or nonossifying fibroma may present first to the pediatric surgeon on call in the pediatric emergency department.

The diagnosis of these rare conditions is readily attained through a careful clinical evaluation. In that regard, the utility of plain radiographs can never be overstated. They facilitate the initial workup and allow these patients to be referred to specialized centers with multidisciplinary expertise. Although the subsequent imaging modalities are important, the radiographs form a key part of surgical planning.

It is with the pediatric surgeon in mind that this chapter is written. Lengthy discourse on the pathology is avoided, and several excellent references exist.[3–6] Instead, the format adopted is a practical approach to the management of these conditions. Where prudent, insights and controversies are highlighted to spur interest in specific areas.

General Considerations

PATHOPHYSIOLOGY

The main aim of this section is to illustrate the specific issues of the pathophysiology of bone tumors that distinguish them from tumors of soft tissue. Bone tumors should be approached initially from the standpoint of whether they are benign or malignant. Whereas traditional approaches regarding the treatment of most nonskeletal benign lesions have been ones of benign neglect (if these lesions are not perceived to be causing problems), the management of benign bone lesions is complicated by the potential compromise of skeletal structural integrity. Cortical deficiency weakens bones and can mandate treatment to prevent fracture. The prudent, if rare, consideration is one of syndromic presentation and malignant transformation. Many of these principles are applicable to malignant lesions as well. However, malignant lesions have, as the cornerstone of consideration, their implications on survival, which will be elaborated. Metastatic lesions to bone are uncommon in the pediatric age group. Their pathophysiologic implications tend to be structural or diagnostic.

In the pediatric age group, benign lesions far outnumber primary malignant lesions, which in turn outnumber metastatic lesions. Because of the protean manner in which benign lesions behave, some are not evident in the physician's office. Conclusions about their natural history and malignant potential are therefore difficult to ascertain.[4] This is obviously not the situation with malignant and metastatic lesions. In this section, we discuss pathologic conditions of the bone that occur most commonly in the pediatric age group. In the pediatric population, the commonly occurring benign lesions are the unicameral bone cyst, aneurysmal bone cyst, enchondroma, osteochondroma, nonossifying fibroma, and osteoid osteoma. The common malignant bone tumors are osteogenic sarcomas and Ewing family tumors (Table 43-1). Here we highlight specific features of each tumor. For a more thorough understanding of the pathology, the reader is directed to any of a number of fine books on the subject.[3–6]

Benign Lesions

The typical benign lesion in the pediatric age group (Table 43-2) is identified incidentally, because they rarely cause symptoms. They are often diagnosed when a parent notices a lump or deformity (e.g., osteochondroma) or a radiograph is obtained for an unrelated condition (e.g., nonossifying fibroma). The two main surgical issues are diagnosis

TABLE 43-1

Commonly Occurring Tumors by Age Group

Age	Benign Tumors	Malignant Tumors	Tumor-like Conditions
Birth to 5 years	Eosinophilic granuloma	Leukemia Metastatic neuroblastoma	Osteomyelitis Nonaccidental injury
5 to 15 years	Unicameral bone cyst Osteochondroma Aneurysmal bone cyst Osteoid osteoma Enchondroma Nonossifying fibroma Chondromyxoid fibroma Chondroblastoma	Ewing sarcoma Osteogenic sarcoma	Fibrous dysplasia Osteomyelitis Osteofibrous dysplasia Stress fracture
15 to 20 years	Unicameral bone cyst Osteochondroma Osteoid osteoma Aneurysmal bone cyst Nonossifying fibroma Giant cell tumor Enchondroma Chondroblastoma Chondromyxoid fibroma	Osteogenic sarcoma Ewing sarcoma	Fibrous dysplasia Stress fracture

By considering the factors of age, frequency, and location in the long bones (see Fig. 43-3), a diagnosis can be proposed in the majority of cases. The possibility of trauma should always be borne in mind, and in the noncommunicative child younger than 5 years old, nonaccidental injury may be the cause.

TABLE 43-2

Incidence of the More Commonly Diagnosed Bone Tumors

Bone Tumors	All Bone Tumors (%)	Bone Tumors in the First Two Decades (%)
Benign		
Osteochondroma	7.86	4.69
Aneurysmal bone cyst	2.60	1.96
Osteoid osteoma	2.99	1.94
Nonossifying fibroma	1.13	0.99
Enchondroma	3.02	0.98
Giant cell tumor	5.10	0.80
Chondroblastoma	1.07	0.66
Chondromyxoid fibroma	0.41	0.14
Unicameral bone cyst	Unknown	Unknown
Malignant		
Osteogenic sarcoma	14.9	7.53
Ewing sarcoma	4.6	3.50

In using this table, a number of caveats need to be remembered. Most benign lesions are often asymptomatic, and only symptomatic ones will present. Of these, most will be managed in the primary care setting. Malignant lesions will, however, usually present at a referral center. Hence, in terms of population incidence, these figures are unreliable. In relative terms, however, they have some utility in indicating their prevalence. Unicameral bone cysts are left in this list as a reminder of their frequency.

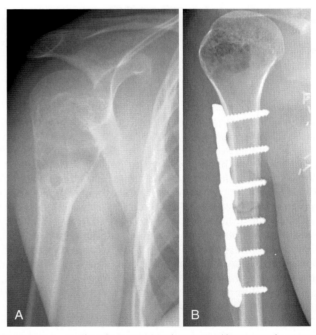

FIGURE 43-1 A, Chondrosarcoma in the proximal humerus of a 13-year-old boy. This is an exceedingly rare diagnosis in this age group. **B,** A proximal humeral resection with allograft reconstruction was performed. In children, the available prostheses may be too large, and hence bulk allografts may be the only choice.

through a biopsy and stabilization of bones that have fractured or are at risk to fracture, especially through a precarious location. For example, a bone cyst in the neck of a femur should be seriously considered for surgical stabilization, because a fracture at this site may result in avascular necrosis of the femoral head. The biopsy itself cannot be undertaken lightly, because it can weaken the bone, mandating surgical or external splinting. The challenge is to use a high-yield biopsy with minimal morbidity.

Size of the Tumor Size is an important consideration for surgical approach. For example, cartilaginous rib tumors larger than 4 cm were found to have increased likelihood of malignant behavior.[3] Hence they should be resected widely despite their relatively bland histologic appearance (Fig. 43-1). Large tumors can also grow into neighboring compartments and cause mechanical compromise to joints. Although this is less critical in joints of the upper limb, it is important in the spine and in the lower limbs, where they cause mechanical impingement and pain. The disruption of a tubular bone by growth of a neoplasm weakens the bone. Lesions that involve more than 50% of the cross section of a bone are at risk of fracture and should be treated from a mechanical standpoint.[7–9] Fracture of a malignant lesion may require amputation rather than a limb-sparing operation.

Fracture Through a Benign Lesion The fractured benign lesion is typified by the unicameral bone cyst. These lesions may appear radiographically to be aggressive, but a careful history and physical examination with appropriate imaging modalities will usually establish their benign nature

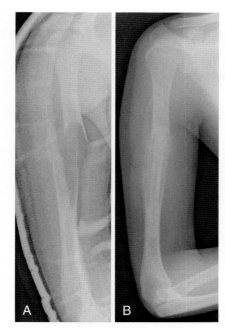

FIGURE 43-2 **A,** Large unicameral bone cyst of the proximal humerus that had fractured. The aggressive appearance may lead one to suspect a malignant process, but a careful evaluation of the margins of this lesion and absence of periosteal reaction reaffirms the management decision of observation before surgery. **B,** This cyst was curetted and packed with an allograft 1 month after the fracture. Treatment with an intramedullary fibular graft provided stabilization, and supplemental bone graft healed the lesion.

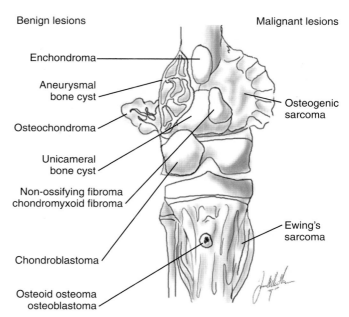

Benign lesions | Malignant lesions

Enchondroma

Aneurysmal bone cyst

Osteochondroma

Osteogenic sarcoma

Unicameral bone cyst

Non-ossifying fibroma chondromyxoid fibroma

Ewing's sarcoma

Chondroblastoma

Osteoid osteoma osteoblastoma

FIGURE 43-3 The location of lesions in relation to the physis gives a clue to the diagnosis. In most cases, the diagnosis can be made on radiographs, leaving further imaging to plan for surgery.

(Fig. 43-2). Unicameral bone cysts that fracture may resolve spontaneously. However, the vast majority continue to fracture throughout a child's lifetime and prove to be disabling.[10] In general, they should be treated surgically, especially if they are symptomatic.

The timing of surgery is critical. An early biopsy after fracture would show callus formation difficult to distinguish from a malignant process. Therefore these lesions should be observed during healing of the fracture for about a month, after which a biopsy and definitive procedure are performed.

Location in Relation to the Physis Location in relation to the physes is an important consideration distinguishing tumor assessment and management of children versus adults (Fig. 43-3). The term diaphyseal aclasis was coined to highlight a condition in which multiple osteochondromas, a condition primarily of the growth plate, caused disordered linear growth of the long bone.[6] These cases are often familial, and children are rarely compromised by their condition. Joints of the upper limb generally have a high tolerance for the resultant deformity. However, occasionally, degenerative arthritis develops, especially in the lower limb, then requiring early surgery.

Multiplicity of Bone Tumors Multiple bone lesions in an individual are often syndromic and may confer a higher incidence of malignant degeneration than when they occur singly.[4–6] Multiple osteochondromas occur in multiple

hereditary exostoses—an autosomal dominant condition caused by abnormalities of the *EXT1, EXT2,* and *EXT3* genes on chromosomes 8, 11, and 19.[11–13] Although each osteochondroma has a low probability of malignant transformation, the cumulative risk is high. Children with this condition have an increased incidence of 10% to 27.6% for malignant degeneration of an osteochondroma into a chondrosarcoma. By comparison, isolated osteochondromas have a malignant degeneration rate of about 1%.[3–5] Because only symptomatic lesions will present to the physician, the true incidence of malignant degeneration in isolated lesions is impossible to ascertain with certainty. Multiple enchondromatoses is a sporadic condition that confers an increased incidence of malignant transformation of up to 50% in the involved bones.[4] Limb-length inequality and malalignment are also common. Ollier disease, as this condition is termed, has another counterpart classically affecting one limb anlage. A variant, Maffucci syndrome, involves widespread enchondromas associated with hemangiomas of the hand. The occurrence of multiple nonossifying fibromas, associated with mental retardation, café-au-lait spots, endocrine disorders, cardiovascular malformations, and ocular abnormalities has been termed Jaffe-Campanacci syndrome, but this entity has no malignant implications.[4,14]

Site of Involvement The site of benign cartilaginous lesions has important implications for malignant potential. Peripheral lesions in the hand rarely turn malignant, while those closer to the axial skeleton have important malignant potential even if they appear benign histologically.[3–6,14,15] Lesions in bones adjacent to weight-bearing joints should be regarded with special concern. In the pediatric group, these lesions are usually chondroblastomas. They grow epiphyseally and in so doing can cause weakening of the subchondral bone and, ultimately, an intraarticular extension or fracture that may even mimic osteochondral defects. In the case of sarcomas, a relatively conservative resection in this context would have to be deferred to an extraarticular resection.

Metastatic Potential A unique feature of benign bone tumors is that there is a small incidence of metastasis in these lesions. Accordingly, 1.7% of chondroblastomas and 3% of giant cell tumors[5,16–18] do metastasize. There is a controversy about whether some of these lesions were, in fact, malignant from the outset.[19] However, the truly benign lesions that do metastasize are atypical lesions that have had surgical manipulation, which may have embolized tumor cells. When followed, some of these metastatic lesions, primarily in the lung, may remain dormant and not progress. The possibility, therefore, is that they represent a transport phenomenon more akin to a mechanical embolism and not a true metastasis.[3,19]

MALIGNANT LESIONS

Epidemiology

The main histologic types of bone tumors are osteogenic sarcoma, Ewing family tumor, chondrosarcoma, and other sarcomas. They affect children at a rate of 6:3:2:1, respectively.[1,5]

Osteogenic sarcomas (also known as osteosarcomas) are malignant bone-forming tumors of the bone. They occur at any age but most frequently present in an extremity in the middle teenage years. There are various subtypes with varying implications for survival. In general, the subtypes behave similarly, except perhaps for telangiectatic osteogenic sarcoma, which bears special mention. In the prechemotherapy era this was regarded as the tumor with the worst prognosis.[20] Presently, however, it has the best prognosis.[21] The lytic nature of these sarcomas weakens bone, resulting in the highest rate of pathologic fracture. Increasingly, rarer forms of osteogenic sarcoma are described. Two variants of note are the small cell sarcoma and giant cell-rich osteogenic sarcoma. The former can be confused with a Ewing family tumor and thus is often treated by similar chemotherapy protocols.[22,23] The latter can be confused, in the appropriate setting, with a giant cell tumor of the bone, which is a benign condition.[24–26]

The Ewing sarcoma occurs at a younger age (see Table 43-1) and may affect any bone, particularly, the femur, pelvis, and humerus. It is the most common cancer in the pelvis, ribs, foot, and fibula. It was once considered to be distinct from peripheral neuroectodermal tumors but has been shown to be genetically identical to this entity. It is presently considered to be in the same family of neoplasms also known as Ewing family tumors.[3,6]

Chondrosarcoma is less prevalent in the pediatric age group. It is more widely distributed in the body compared with its occurrence in adults.

Genetics There have been few consistent genetic or syndromic associations with osteogenic sarcoma. Patients with the Li-Fraumeni syndrome[27] have a *TP53* germline mutation[28,29] on 9p21 and are predisposed to osteogenic sarcoma, breast cancer, and leukemia (Fig. 43-4). Two to 3 percent of patients with osteogenic sarcoma will be the proband for Li-Fraumeni families.[30] Another germline mutation of 13q14, hereditary retinoblastoma (RB), predisposes to osteogenic sarcoma.[31] Children who received radiation therapy for retinoblastoma,

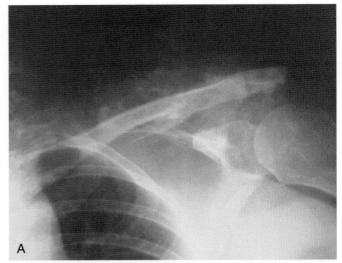

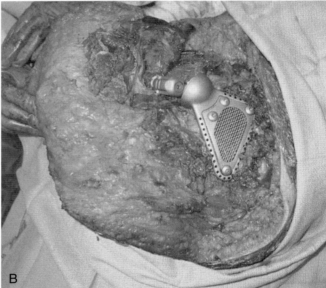

FIGURE 43-4 **A,** Osteogenic sarcoma in the left scapula of a female patient with Li-Fraumeni syndrome. This patient had a family history of osteogenic sarcoma in a first-degree relative. At the time of staging for the osteogenic sarcoma in the scapula, a lesion in the breast was discovered on computed tomography (CT) of the chest. This was subsequently found to be an adenocarcinoma. **B,** The patient underwent a scapular replacement. A latissimus dorsi flap was used for skin cover.

Hodgkin and non-Hodgkin lymphoma, Ewing family tumor, and other cancers are at a 5% to 10% risk of developing osteogenic sarcoma. Patients with an *RB* gene deletion and a history of alkylating agent exposure from a prior malignancy are predisposed to this complication as well. About 5% of all osteogenic sarcomas occur as postradiation sarcomas.

The Ewing family tumor is a malignancy associated with a number of translocations. The 11 to 22 translocation, resulting in an EWS-FLI1 fusion transcript, is the most common variant, and type 1 is associated with the best prognosis.[32] Other translocations include type 2 EWS-FLI1, EWS-ERG from a 21,22 translocation, and EWS-ETV1 from a 7,22 translocation. These rarer variants have not been as well studied but appear to confer a poorer prognosis.[32] Further additive mutations involving cell-cycle genes reduce the prognosis of these tumors still more. The Ewing family tumor is the most common solid tumor to metastasize to the brain.[33]

DIAGNOSIS AND STAGING

Bone tumors are diagnosed based on the well-recognized triad of history, physical examination, and investigation. After a clinical diagnosis, it is imperative that imaging and staging procedures are done before biopsy. Preoperative imaging allows for planning of the definitive procedure and hence placement of the biopsy incision. In addition, changes that would occur in the lesion after biopsy would be difficult to distinguish from changes resulting from tumor growth on imaging. Furthermore, changes in the lung after general anesthesia (e.g., atelectasis) are difficult to distinguish from metastatic deposits.

Clinical Evaluation

Although it is not possible to be comprehensive in this section, the history and physical examination are important parts of the assessment of a patient with a bone tumor. Patient demographics and tumor location narrow the differential diagnosis and focus the workup efficiently.

The patient's age is important (see Table 43-2). Most malignancies occur in the second decade of life.[3-6] Among children, subtle variation occurs in the prevalence of disease with respect to age (see Table 43-1). Demographically, it is exceedingly rare for patients of African descent to have a Ewing family tumor.[6]

Pain at rest is an important sign that occurs in tumors and in other organic conditions, such as infection and bone infarction. It distinguishes these conditions from mechanical pain, which occurs with activity. Most malignant tumors will present with pain. Pain relieved by nonsteroidal antiinflammatory drugs (NSAIDs) is pathognomonic of osteoid osteoma.[34] This lesion can occur at any age and is characterized by painful scoliosis when it occurs in the spine.

A family history of malignancy should be discerned, especially in possible sentinel cases of the Li-Fraumeni syndrome.[27-29] Such patients should have systemic evaluation in the form of radioisotope bone scans or positron emission tomographic scans, to rule out other sites of involvement.

As described earlier, the surgeon should be alert to any dysmorphism that the patient may have. Cutaneous stigmata are evident in patients with neurofibromatosis, fibrous dysplasia, and Jaffe-Campanacci syndrome.[14] Limb length discrepancies are seen in patients with multiple enchondromatoses and multiple hereditary exostoses.[35]

Infection should be considered in the differential diagnosis in almost every case seen. Tumor epidemiology is very telling. For example, childhood leukemia is nearly 10 times as common as Ewing family tumor, and so, rare manifestations of leukemia are more common than routine presentations of Ewing family tumor.

The nature of bony reconstruction also requires that the method chosen be matched with the demands of the patient. As such, an idea of the patient's expectation should be sought at this time.

Radiology

The minimal radiologic assessment at the first visit should be two orthogonal radiographic views of the area in question. A radiograph remains the most specific diagnostic imaging test and is the only one that gives the "gestalt" of overall assessment of skeletal biology and mechanics. By analyzing the location of the tumor (see Fig. 43-3), as well as whether it is benign or malignant, the diagnosis can be made in the majority of cases.[3-6]

Benign lesions are well circumscribed, with a good sclerotic border, and produce no soft tissue edema. Malignant lesions have lucent or variegated matrices and permeative borders. Edema is often apparent with the presence of fat lines.

The often-quoted eponymous phrases are not specific to distinct malignancies. The Codman triangle refers to the lifting and ossification of periosteum at the periphery of an osteogenic sarcoma. The sunburst appearance is due to the ossification of fibers and vessels subperiosteally, as the tumor expands out of the cortex. Onion skinning refers to the periodic ossification and expansion of periosteum from the cortex. Any of these conditions can be seen in tumors or infections that are sufficiently fast growing.

In Figure 43-3, epiphyseal lesions are typical of chondroblastoma or giant cell tumors; physeal lesions are typical of osteochondromas; metaphyseal lesions are typical of osteogenic sarcomas, unicameral bone cysts, aneurysmal bone cysts, and nonossifying fibromas; and diaphyseal lesions are typical of Ewing family tumor, fibrous dysplasia, or enchondromas.

Laboratory Evaluation

The main blood parameters of importance are lactate dehydrogenase and alkaline phosphatase.[36-38] Lactate dehydrogenase levels have been used as a surrogate for tumor load and have been correlated with survival in the case of Ewing family tumor.[36] Serum alkaline phosphatase elevation is characteristic of osteogenic sarcoma and is correlated with poor survival in this condition.[37,38] Glucose intolerance is associated with chondrosarcoma of the bone.[39,40] Erythrocyte sedimentation rates, C-reactive protein, and white blood cell and differential counts should be sought to rule out infection.

Preoperative Planning

Magnetic resonance imaging (MRI) of the lesion offers an assessment of compartmentalization of the tumor. A compartment is an abstract concept and refers to any plane that offers a fascial or cortical bone barrier to contiguous spread. It has implications for the extent of surgery, which by definition must be outside the compartment to be radical (see later).[41] Also, by forming a baseline assessment, one is able to make an assessment of response to chemotherapy in the case of neoadjuvant treatment.[42] It has secondary importance in providing the actual diagnosis. In specific examples it is useful in histologic diagnosis. The aneurysmal bone cyst shows fluid-fluid levels on an MR image. Pigmented villonodular synovitis is hypointense (dark) on T1- and T2-weighted imaging because of hemosiderin deposition. Cartilaginous lesions are hyperintense (light) on T2-weighted imaging. Mineralized and dense fibrous tissues are dark on T1- and T2-weighted imaging.[43,44]

Staging

Staging studies are meant to assess the degree of spread of the disease. In the case of bone tumors two systems are used: the Enneking system or surgical staging system (SSS),[45] as adopted by the Musculoskeletal Tumor Society and the American Joint Committee on Cancer (AJCC) system, which at the time of writing is in its sixth revision.[46] In the case of Ewing family tumor, a different classification than Enneking is used.[47]

In the SSS, tumors are designated G0, G1, and G2 for benign, low-grade, and high-grade lesions, respectively. Benign lesions (G0) are classified as latent, active, or aggressive—designated by Arabic numerals 1, 2, and 3, respectively. Malignant lesions are designated with the Roman numeral I if low grade and II if high grade. The further designation A or B denotes intracompartmental or extracompartmental disease. Stage III disease is metastatic disease. Therefore in this classification, grade, compartmentalization, and metastases are the fundamental prognostic factors.

In the AJCC system, I and II similarly designate low- and high-grade lesions. The letters A and B designate tumors smaller or larger than 8 cm, respectively. The Roman numeral III denotes multicentric disease, and IV denotes metastatic disease. The designation IVA denotes pulmonary metastases, and IVB denotes extrapulmonary metastases. Therefore this classification considers grade, size, multicentricity, and metastases as prognostic factors.

In the Enneking staging system of Ewing family tumor, stage I tumors are solitary intraosseous lesions, stage II are solitary lesions with extraosseous extension, stage III are multicentric lesions, and stage IV are metastatic. It is unclear how to stage patients who have independent sites of bone marrow involvement versus those who have circulating tumor cells identified by light microscopy (i.e., Enneking stage III or IV). Modern pathology analysis extends these concepts to include immunohistochemistry or reverse transcriptase polymerase chain reaction (RT-PCR) of recombinant gene products.

The modalities used for staging are bone scans and computed tomography (CT) of the chest.[45] Positron emission tomography scans are presently being evaluated, but have fundamental utility in the management of recurrent or metastatic disease.[48] In the case of Ewing family tumor, bone marrow biopsies are obtained to try capturing cases that are multicentric at presentation. The utility of this approach is being evaluated.[49]

BIOPSY

The biopsy is a critical procedure that can complicate management severely if not performed appropriately. Misplaced incisions continue to be an important cause of resectable tumors being rendered nonamenable to limb salvage surgery.[41,50] A good pathologist who is comfortable handling bony tissue is critical to this process. In the appropriate case, extra tissue may be needed for cytogenetic studies. Ewing family tumors are particularly fragile, and biopsy specimens should be handled carefully to allow for processing.

Presurgical Considerations

As a general rule, all imaging and staging should be completed before biopsy. The lesion that warrants biopsy should be given consideration for a primary wide excision. This approach is typically applicable to small lesions that are less than 3 cm, lesions in expendable bones (e.g., distal phalanx), distal lesions of the ulna, and proximal lesions of the fibula, where there is a risk of common peroneal nerve contamination (Fig. 43-5).

The lesion should preferably be sampled in the institution where the definitive procedure will be performed and by the same surgeon. It has been shown repeatedly, that when this approach is not used, the results are compromised.[50,51]

Consideration should be given to needle biopsies in the case of lesions in the pelvis or the spine, where the exposure necessary for an open biopsy may be extensive and obliges commitment to a definitive procedure.

A pathologist familiar with processing bone tissue should be on hand to evaluate the biopsy. If tumor tissue can be cut with a knife, then it can be cut with a microtome. Frozen-section analysis is required primarily to ascertain the adequacy and representativeness of the specimen and secondarily for the definitive diagnosis.

Antibiotics should be withheld before the biopsy to improve the yield of cultures. The biopsy may be done with use of a tourniquet, to prevent bleeding and dissemination of the tumor locally. When the tourniquet is applied, simple elevation should be used for exsanguination. Compressive exsanguination should be avoided, because this could rupture the tumor. At all times, the limb should be protected from fracturing, because this would cause extensive local dissemination of disease.

Surgical Considerations

The planned incision for the definitive surgery should be marked. This should generally follow extensile exposures and be longitudinal along the line of the definitive incision. The incision should be placed directly over the lesion. Flaps and dissection should be avoided.

The incision is developed directly into the tumor. If there is a soft tissue component of the tumor, then this alone needs be sampled. If a bone biopsy is necessary, then the edges of the biopsy specimen should be rounded to minimize a stress riser. Frozen-section analysis will confirm the adequacy of the biopsy. In the meantime, a culture is taken, the tourniquet is released, and antibiotics are given. Absolute hemostasis is needed at the conclusion of the procedure to minimize spread of tumor cells in the hematoma.

The wound is closed in layers. If a drain is necessary, this should be brought out in the line of the incision so that it can be excised at the time of definitive surgery.

Postsurgical Considerations

The patient should be limited to protected weight bearing, at least until some healing of the biopsy or ossification of the tumor as a response to neoadjuvant chemotherapy occurs. This typically takes up to 6 weeks.

Fractures through osteogenic sarcomas have traditionally precluded limb salvage surgery. Recent studies have shown that limb salvage may still be possible in selected cases.[52–55] Special surgical consideration is needed in these cases.

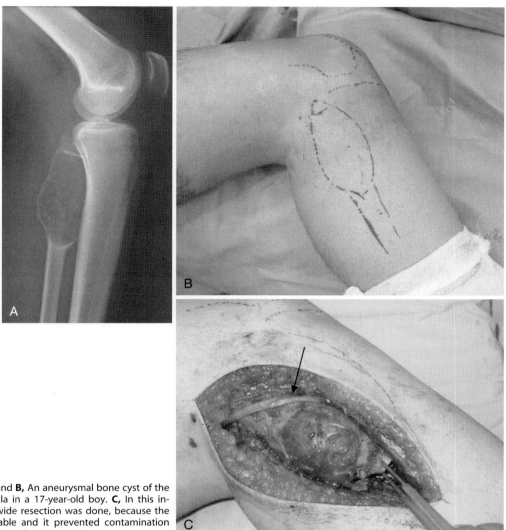

FIGURE 43-5 **A** and **B,** An aneurysmal bone cyst of the right proximal fibula in a 17-year-old boy. **C,** In this instance, a primary wide resection was done, because the bone was expendable and it prevented contamination of the common peroneal nerve (*arrow*).

ADJUVANT THERAPY

This section concentrates on the use of radiation and chemotherapy. In general, these modalities are not used in the treatment of benign conditions. Up to 10% risk of malignant transformation occurs when benign lesions are irradiated.[3–6]

Both chemotherapy and radiation therapy can be used in the neoadjuvant (preoperative) or adjuvant (postoperative) setting in the treatment of malignant conditions. The neoadjuvant approach has the advantage of "shrinking" the tumor and provides a more discernible margin, theoretically improving local control of the disease. In the case of chemotherapy, before the era of modular prostheses, the neoadjuvant route was necessary while the custom prostheses were manufactured. This technique has been shown to be as efficacious as primary surgery. Even so, the one randomized trial of preoperative and postoperative chemotherapy versus only operative and postoperative chemotherapy failed to show any difference in survival. Therefore in selected cases, it is reasonable and may be prudent to perform surgery first.[56]

SURGERY

In bone tumors, resection and reconstruction are two aspects of management that have largely complementary but occasionally conflicting goals (e.g., cryotherapy is good for extending the margins of resection of a tumor but results in weakening of the bone). Therefore, while the goals of resection are generally quite clear (i.e., cure), the goals of reconstruction are often compromised, especially in malignant conditions. In benign conditions, reconstruction usually restores more function. In this section, we present a general list of considerations that will be elaborated further in the section on specific considerations.

Minimally Invasive Options

The minimally invasive option is reserved for benign conditions. It is born of two management philosophies—the desire to effect local control and the hesitation to cause more morbidity than the primary lesion. Whichever modality is chosen, it is imperative that a histologic diagnosis be obtained a priori.

Radiofrequency Ablation   Radiofrequency ablation uses high-intensity heat in proximity to a lesion, to effect thermal necrosis. It has wide utility in the ablation of various solid tumors. In bone tumors, it has been used principally in the ablation of osteoid osteomas. This condition is a painful one, marked by increased night pain and is promptly relieved by the use of NSAIDs. Otherwise, it is relatively benign. It can be found most commonly in the proximal femur. In these locations, surgical ablation in the form of a resection can incur high morbidity. Hence, an option such as radiofrequency ablation is ideal, although it incurs a 10% to 15% recurrence rate[57,58] compared with surgery, which has a near 0% recurrence rate.[59] It has limited utility in the spine because of the indiscriminate high heat generated.

Injection   This technique is principally used in the treatment of unicameral bone cysts. Clinically apparent bone cysts have a tendency to recurrent fracture and need to be treated.[10] However, they have no malignant potential and have been known to regress.[4,10] There is controversy about whether corticosteroid injection is a necessary element of treatment; it has been shown that simple decompression of a cyst is sufficient to induce a regression.[60] Rates of cure up to 50% are reported, with a median injection rate of three and a range of one to nine injections.[61,62] Each of these sessions requires the child to be under anesthesia. Therefore it has not been widely embraced.

As alluded to earlier, various forms of decompression have been advocated in the literature with varying success. One approach involves the injection of bone marrow.[63–67] Rates of cure of up to 50% to 70% may be achieved. However, with this technique, repeated injections may be necessary, incurring multiple episodes of anesthesia and donor-site morbidity.

Curettage, widely regarded to be the gold standard treatment, has a recurrence rate of 5% to 50%.[10] Thus there is no clearly superior modality in the treatment of this condition.

Resection

Surgical decisions are based on the concept of compartments in relation to a tumor (Fig. 43-6). The compartment is bound by a barrier, which naturally limits the expansion of a tumor. When first described, it was useful in teaching the principles of wide resection or a resection with a margin of healthy tissue: If a resection was performed outside a compartment, it resulted in a margin that was free of malignant involvement.[45] This idea was useful in drawing parallels to conventional cancer surgery of that time. We realize now that this theory is flawed at many levels. For example, most osteogenic sarcomas present with tumors that have breached the cortex, and so, their distinction from a "contained" osteogenic sarcoma is moot. In the lower limb, a tumor that has involved the rectus femoris has involved a compartment extending from the anterior inferior iliac spine of the pelvis to the tibial tubercle. Clearly, it would not be practical, in this setting, to perform a hindquarter amputation. Finally, especially in the region

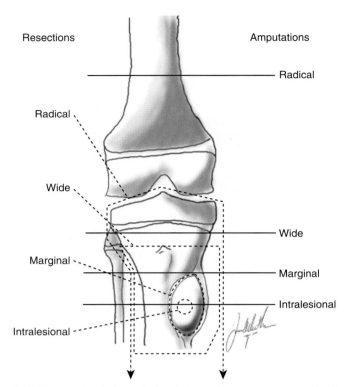

FIGURE 43-6   Surgical margins in relation to the compartments involved. At left are the resections, and at right are the amputations. These classifications are largely academic, because in the strictest terms, most of the resections, except radical resections and only wide or radical amputations, are performed. Radical resections involve the compartment bearing the tumor, and hence, in this case, would amount to removing the tibia (*arrows*). Marginal amputations may be used in the spine and pelvis, whereupon local adjuvants assume significant roles in disease control (see Fig. 43-7). Intralesional amputations are obviously not therapeutic applications in tumor surgery but are included here for completeness. Of interest, intercalary amputations in the pediatric population can be problematic, when the remnant stump elongates through appositional growth. To avoid this complication, it may be necessary to use a through-joint (e.g., through-knee) amputation.

of the linea aspera, there are numerous perforating vessels, which penetrate the lateral intermuscular septum; clearly these do not form a continuous barrier to tumor spread.

Still, the concept of compartmentalization is useful when one describes the surgical procedures as intralesional, marginal, wide, and radical.[41] Although not often used in the context of amputations, the concept of compartmentalization applies here as well. Intralesional procedures, as the name implies, are procedures that leave macroscopic residual tissue. A biopsy or injection of a lesion is an intralesional procedure. A marginal procedure stops at the level of the extent of maximal expansion of a tumor. Curettage is a marginal procedure. A wide procedure goes beyond the reactive zone of the tumor. When first described, the "reactive zone" referred to the zone of reaction around the tumor, marked by inflammatory change (i.e., hyperemia and edema).[41,47] This assessment was made predominantly at the time of surgery. With the advent of more sophisticated imaging modalities, it can now be demonstrated that this "zone" may extend further than previously appreciated. Therefore it appears that the description of a reactive zone is rather more abstract than real. As a general rule, resecting a tumor beyond its capsule, where vessel tortuosity and edema is seen, is a wide resection, and hence this appreciation, while strongly influenced by newer imaging, remains largely surgical. Most malignant tumors are resected widely. A radical resection is an excision of the compartment in which a tumor resides. An above-knee amputation for a tibial lesion is a radical resection.

There are a number of surgical adjuvants that may be used. This can be in the form of heat (e.g., argon beam coagulator) or cold (e.g., liquid nitrogen cryotherapy).[68,69] In addition, chemical measures may be used (e.g., phenol, polymethylmethacrylate cement).[70,71] In the occasional case, specialized forms of radiation (e.g., brachytherapy, intraoperative radiation therapy) may be used, especially in the pelvis (Fig. 43-7). The purpose of these surgical adjuvants is to extend the margins of resection beyond what can be mechanically removed by the surgeon. These improve local control of the tumor.

Benign Lesions   It is useful at this juncture to recall the staging system for benign lesions. These are classified as benign, active, and aggressive. It is evident in these entities that, even within this group, specific nuances of the condition warrant special considerations. In benign bony conditions, the procedures available are curettage, high-speed burring of lesion walls, adjuvant procedures, and wide resection.[68,70] It is helpful to describe these procedures from most to least aggressive.

In benign conditions, wide resection may occasionally be used, when the involved bone is expendable (e.g., rib or terminal phalanx of the little toe) or at the end of a bone (e.g., distal ulna or proximal fibula). In these situations, reconstruction provides little value and can, in fact, be the source of considerable morbidity. Additionally, it may be used in the context of a recalcitrant recurrent benign or aggressive lesion. Typical lesions that are resected in this manner are giant cell tumors, aneurysmal bone cysts, or fibrous dysplasia.

Marginal excision is typified conceptually by the technique used to excise a soft tissue lipoma. Such a procedure is not technically feasible in most bony lesions. Osteochondromas and periosteal chondromas may be removed in such a fashion.

Intralesional procedures are more commonly performed in benign tumors. This typically involves curettage of a lesion with high-speed burring of the wall. In general, this is the typical procedure for most latent or active benign bony conditions (e.g., unicameral bone cyst). The use of heat, cold (Fig. 43-8), or chemical modalities serves to extend this margin of clearance further and is typically used in active or aggressive tumors (e.g., giant cell tumor, chondroblastoma).

Malignant Lesions

The sine qua non of the resection of a malignant bone lesion is that, at minimum, a wide resection must be performed. In certain situations, however, this may not be possible (e.g., a tumor that has expanded into the spinal canal or a tumor that has invaded the pelvic cavity). In these instances, the outcome tends to be suboptimal.

With newer imaging modalities, it is now often possible to perform a physeal-sparing procedure in growing children (Fig. 43-9). Although the physis was thought to be an effective barrier to tumor spread, it has been shown that up to 80% of tumors abutting the physis have, in fact, breached it.[72-75] Physeal-sparing procedures must therefore be carefully balanced with the response to chemotherapy, to determine if this is feasible.

Occasionally, a variation on this theme is to save the epiphysis, and hence the neighboring joint, by performing a distraction procedure through the growth plate. This effectively increases the margin of normal tissue proximal to a tumor. A resection may then be performed through this now-lengthened segment.[76]

Another approach to retaining a joint would be to perform a Van Nes rotationplasty (Fig. 43-10).[77] This procedure, generally undertaken for high-grade tumors near or involving the knee, involves wide extraarticular resections, whereupon the distal leg and foot are joined to the remaining proximal femur. In the process, the sciatic nerve is retained, and a segmental resection of the femoral artery with a true femoral-popliteal arterial anastomosis is performed. The foot is rotated with

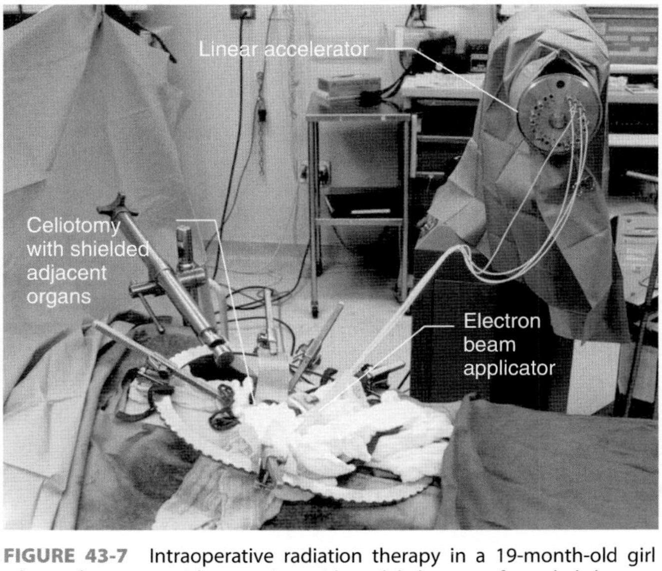

FIGURE 43-7 Intraoperative radiation therapy in a 19-month-old girl who underwent a wide resection with nodal clearance for a rhabdomyosarcoma of the pelvis.

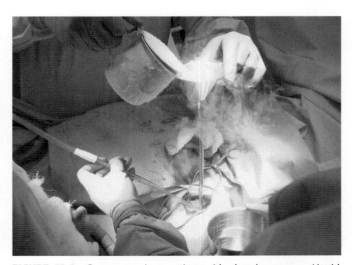

FIGURE 43-8 Cryosurgery in a patient with chondrosarcoma. Liquid nitrogen is poured into a funnel that directs the agent into the lesion, while avoiding contact with the surrounding skin. The effect of freezing extends the margins of necrosis beyond that which can be felt by the surgeon, effectively extending the surgical margins from an intralesional or marginal excision to a wide resection.

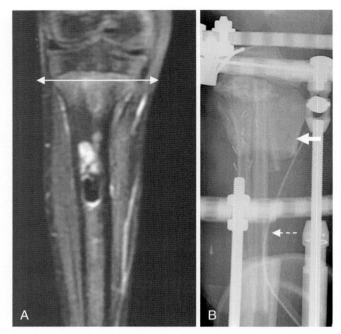

FIGURE 43-9   A, Ewing sarcoma of the tibia in an 11-year-old boy. The lesion extended to 1 cm from the growth plate. It responded well to chemotherapy, with virtually no remaining soft tissue involvement. A physeal-sparing resection was done along a resection plane (*double-headed arrow*), carefully performed under image intensifier guidance. **B,** The use of a pin fixator, in this regard, is extremely advantageous, because it allows stabilization of the small proximal tibial segment that precludes routine pin fixation. The remaining gap was reconstructed with a proximal tibial allograft (*thick arrow*) and vascularized fibular graft (*broken arrow*) harvested with a paddle of skin, which provided skin cover of the construct.

the heel pointing anteriorly. Of practical interest, the distal segment is rotated externally, bringing the sciatic nerve and vessels anteromedial. This should be documented in the surgical note to facilitate further surgical procedures that may be necessary. The ankle, therefore, functions as a knee joint. This procedure has poor acceptance among patients because of their cosmetic abhorrence, but it is highly functional and durable.[78] A similar Winkelmann procedure may be performed, where the proximal tibia is brought to the hip. In children, it is remarkable to note the plasticity and remodeling of these disparate bones, which in time will accommodate each other in a stable fashion.[79,80]

Radical procedures and amputations have received poor support, because they are regarded as being disfiguring. Studies have shown that patients with limb salvage procedures do better in terms of function and cost savings.[81,82] Although this appears true at face value, in-depth analysis shows that these studies are too heterogeneous to allow any firm conclusions. With the aid of modern prostheses, patients with amputations are able to achieve very high levels of activity. Furthermore, complications are 3 to 4 times higher in limb salvage compared with limb ablative surgery. Although most series have not shown a significant survival benefit comparing amputation and limb-sparing surgery, these studies are underpowered or include cases of amputation being used as salvage procedures.[56,83,84] The primary remaining question is whether there is any survival and functional benefit in two-site and stage-controlled groups with respect to amputation or wide resection. This would require a case-controlled study with amputation and wide resection arms, and it is a safe assumption that this will never be performed.

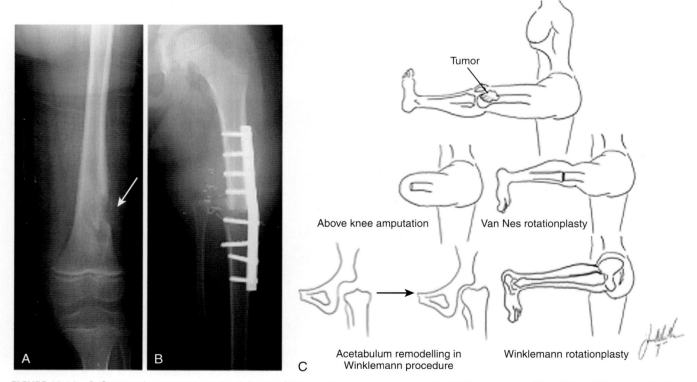

FIGURE 43-10   A, Osteogenic sarcoma (*arrow*) with large soft tissue extension in an 8-year-old child. The small size of the child and high level of activity precluded endoprosthetic reconstruction. **B,** A Van Nes rotationplasty was performed. **C,** Variants of the rotationplasty are compared with the above-knee amputation. The bottom panel illustrates how the proximal tibia remodels and accommodates the acetabulum in the Winkelmann procedure.

There is still a role for amputations, especially when the tumor is in the distal extremity, adjuvant therapies are ineffective, or reconstruction is too problematic because of nerve, vessel, or soft tissue problems.

Local recurrence in malignant lesions is a poor prognostic factor and is associated with a 90% mortality rate. It is generally a reflection of compromised local control, although in one study good chemotherapy response was associated with a low local recurrence rate.[83] Specifically, in this series, when intralesional procedures had been performed for osteogenic sarcoma, standard responders were 3 times as likely to get a local recurrence as good responders. However, even among good responders, local recurrence was 14 times more likely if an intralesional procedure had been done rather than a wide resection. This underscores the need both for good surgical margins and effective chemotherapy.

Reconstruction

In most instances, after the resection of benign lesions, small defects result. These are easily dealt with through the use of various gap fillers. With malignant lesions, large creative solutions are needed. It becomes difficult to determine which lesions are best treated by which technique because of the relative paucity of cases and the high-risk nature of these procedures. In this section, we will highlight the various modalities available and the pertinent qualifiers for each modality.

Benign Lesions Following resection of benign lesions, a small defect usually remains. Thus the aim becomes reconstitution of bone. The modalities that have been used are bone graft and bone graft substitutes. In general, autografts tend to have better rates of incorporation but incur the risk of donor-site morbidity—or worse, donor-site tumor implantation. Allografts have a low risk of disease transmission and immunologic response.[85,86] Synthetic grafts tend not to incorporate as well as allografts or autografts.[87,88]

In the more aggressive lesions, the risk of recurrence increases. In these situations, bone substitutes could be resorbed by the disease process and would increase the delay before subsequent radiologic imaging is able to distinguish between postoperative change and recurrence. In this setting, bone cement becomes a good alternative.[69,71] Furthermore, radiopaque cement acts as a contrast agent. Recurrence at the margin of the cemented defect can be identified readily and treated.

Malignant Lesions The solutions that have been used to solve the complex bone, joint, and soft tissue defects left after tumor resections form a veritable cornucopia of techniques, spanning all of orthopedic and plastic surgery. It is impossible to reiterate all these solutions here. Instead, we present a list of principal solutions pertinent to the specific reconstructive option.

The paramount requirement of all solutions is to provide a space filler and skin closure. Without meeting these two requirements, chemotherapy cannot resume, and the patient will not survive. Most solutions will provide space-filling ability if there is adequate skin for closure. If skin closure is not possible, a local flap or vascularized pedicular graft may be necessary. In some instances, especially with intercalary

resections, the ability to provide intercalary stability with overlying skin closure can be provided by a vascularized fibular graft with a skin paddle. The skin paddle affords the additional advantage of monitoring the viability of the flap. Rotationplasties and their variants are remarkably functional solutions to the problem but have poor acceptance among patients because of their appearance. Similarly, amputations are often an instant solution to the problem, although, even here, the occasional exception exists.[82]

Joint reconstruction is a challenging endeavor. Biologic solutions include the use of bulk allograft (Fig. 43-11). They have the advantage of becoming incorporated by the body. The disadvantages[89] are a high fracture rate of 19%, a nonunion rate of 17%, and an infection rate of 11%. Osteoarticular allografts also become arthritic (16%) with time. Theoretically, however, with good incorporation of the allograft, a conventional, less-constrained joint replacement can be performed (Fig. 43-12). The endoprosthetic solution tends to be easier

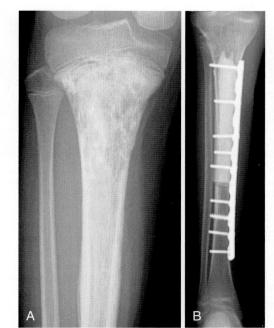

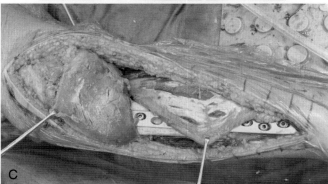

FIGURE 43-11 **A,** Ewing sarcoma of the proximal tibia in an 11-year-old child. **B** and **C,** This was widely resected and reconstructed with an osteoarticular tibial allograft. A gastrocnemius flap was raised to provide soft tissue cover to the construct.

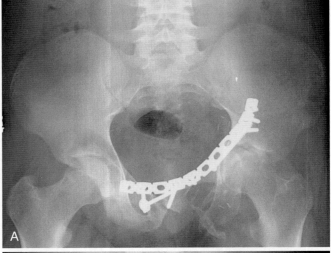

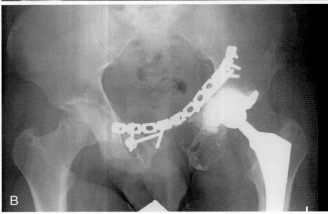

FIGURE 43-12 **A,** Resection and reconstruction of a Ewing sarcoma of the pelvis in a boy. **B,** Two years later, degenerative changes developed in the boy's hip, and he required hip replacement surgery.

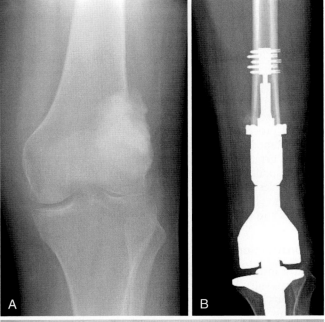

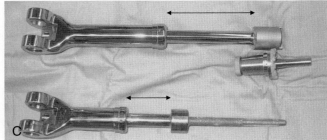

FIGURE 43-13 **A,** Osteogenic sarcoma in a 16-year-old girl. **B,** An endoprosthetic device was placed in the patient after resection of the lesion. **C,** As a child grows, it occasionally becomes necessary to swap implants with devices that can provide further extensibility.

but is less resilient, suffering from wear and loosening with time.[90–92] With advances in technology, better designs will lead to longer-lasting implants (Fig. 43-13). The allograft prosthetic composite is another approach that appears to capitalize on the lasting nature of allografts and their soft tissue capsular attachments and the simplicity of prosthetics (Fig. 43-14). In very young children, the available endoprostheses may be too large, and this may be a relative indication for the use of bulk allografts instead (see Fig. 43-1). Downsized pediatric implants are incapable of holding up in adults and are destined for failure and revision (Fig. 43-15). Prosthetic reconstruction has the distinct advantage of allowing immediate weight bearing, which is very important in patients who may have a reduced life expectancy. In truth, the various modalities are complementary rather than independent.

Growth is a complex issue in the management of patients with bone resection. In the year that patients receive chemotherapy, growth is often stunted. After this, however, the child resumes normal growth. There are various means to predict this growth.[93,94] As a rule of thumb, the distal femur grows 1 cm/year and the proximal tibia grows 7 mm/year. Girls generally stop growing at 14 years of age and boys at 16 years. Therefore a 10-year-old boy who has an extraarticular resection potentially would have 10 cm of growth to accommodate. In general, a 2-cm length discrepancy is considered compensable and does not require treatment. Thus, in this example, an additional 8-cm correction is needed.

The modalities available include contralateral epiphysiodeses. This method ablates the growth plate of the contralateral knee. The procedure needs to be timed accurately and tends to be practical only in the older child approaching the last few centimeters of growth.

Bone transport is another option. This yields good results, but the child must remain in the apparatus for long periods of time. At an elongation rate of 1 mm/day, the child with an 8-cm defect must remain in the apparatus, at minimum, for 3 months for the elongation and a further 3 months for consolidation of the regenerate (Fig. 43-16). This duration is commonly doubled when distraction osteogenesis is done during chemotherapy. Even in healthy individuals, the risk of pin-tract infection during the procedure is greater than

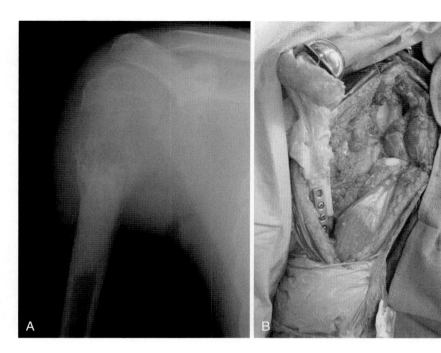

FIGURE 43-14 **A,** Osteogenic sarcoma in proximal humerus of a 16-year-old boy. **B,** A proximal humeral resection with allograft and prosthetic composite was used to reconstruct the defect.

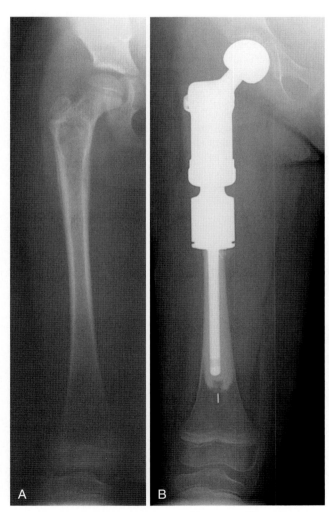

FIGURE 43-15 **A,** Osteogenic sarcoma of the proximal femur in a 14-year-old girl. **B,** A wide resection and bipolar hemiarthroplasty with proximal femoral replacement was performed. Of note, the femoral head matched the acetabulum; so, an additional bipolar component was not added.

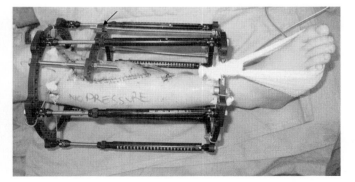

FIGURE 43-16 Ewing sarcoma of the tibia. The patient underwent wide resection and a planned bone transport procedure. The middle ring (*arrow*) is secured to a segment of bone that has been osteotomized. This segment of bone is allowed 5 days for a provisional callus to form. By progressively advancing the ring distally at a rate of 1 mm/day, the segment of bone is transported to fill the defect, while at the same time remaining connected to the proximal tibia. This regenerate is weak and requires an equivalent amount of time to consolidate. For example, an 80-mm defect would require 5 days to form a provisional callus, 80 days to lengthen, and 80 days to consolidate before removal of the frame. This ungainly device needs to be tolerated by the patient for the duration of the limb-lengthening procedure.

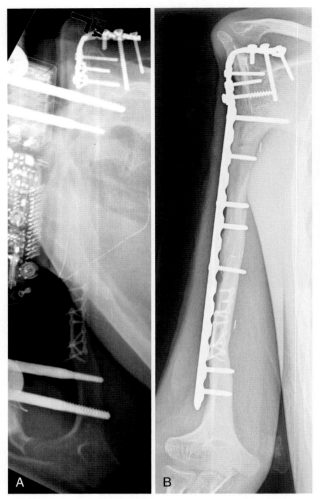

FIGURE 43-17   **A,** A patient presented with osteogenic sarcoma of the proximal humerus that was resected and reconstructed with a vascularized fibular graft shoulder arthrodesis at 6 years of age. He developed a shortened humerus at maturity, which was lengthened. **B,** After lengthening, the regenerate was protected with a plate and hypertrophied with time.

90%.[95] In the patient with malignant disease who is to receive chemotherapy, this would be an important consideration.[96] In addition, the regenerate tends to be weak and is prone to fracture (Fig. 43-17). Patients on chemotherapy are prone to osteoporosis and are already at risk for fracture.

The extensible prosthesis is a marvel of modern science that is presently undergoing "teething" issues.[97–99] The manual expansion designs require repeated surgical procedures to periodically lengthen the limb to keep pace with normal growth (see Fig. 43-13, C). The Stanmore implants (Stanmore Implants Worldwide, Elstree, United Kingdom) have been used for nearly 20 years and have a 23% revision rate.[91] Survivorship analysis, however, shows a near-zero survivorship at 10 years.[100] Self-extending designs work through electromagnetic couplers or heating coils that allow motors or heat-release springs to extend the implant. The Phenix device (Phenix Medical, Paris, France) is presently undergoing evaluation in the United States.[101] Preliminary results show a complication rate of up to 44%, necessitating revision. The Repiphysis system (Wright Medical Technology, Inc., Arlington, TN) uses an external electromagnetic field to provide controlled released of a spring held in place by a locking mechanism. This device is associated with an implant revision rate of 44%.[102] In general, the stems in these devices are too narrow and mechanically insufficient, and fixation techniques remain inadequate. Thus all these designs have poor longevity but reduce immediate surgical complications (e.g., infection). They are well tolerated by patients and families.

There are many solutions to the problem of limb reconstruction in the skeletally immature child, but none is perfect. Therefore it is apparent that the surgeon dealing with potential limb length inequality after tumor resection and subsequent growth must be able to perform, or at least facilitate, the reconstructive procedures previously discussed. Any one of these procedures is applicable to an individual case, and they remain complementary to each other.

The complete reference list is available online at www. expertconsult.com.

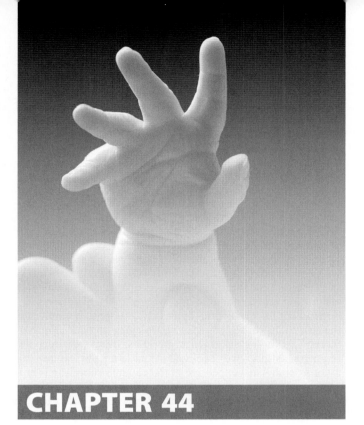

CHAPTER 44

Brain Tumors

Eamon J. McLaughlin, Michael J. Fisher,
Leslie N. Sutton, and Phillip B. Storm

With the exception of trauma, neoplasms are the most common cause of death in children less than 19 years of age. Tumors of the central nervous system are the most common solid neoplasms found in the pediatric population, accounting for 20% of cancer deaths, and are second only to leukemia in overall cancer frequency.[1,2] Approximately 4030 brain tumors are diagnosed each year in the United States, for an overall incidence of 4.71 cases per 100,000 person-years. Of these cases, it is estimated that 2880 will occur in children less than the age 15 years.[1,3]

The important factors in diagnosing brain tumors are location, age, and cell type. Location is probably the most important factor radiographically, followed by the age of the patient. The brain is divided into two compartments by the tentorium. Above the tentorium (supratentorial) are the cerebral hemispheres, basal ganglia, and the thalamus. Below the tentorium (infratentorial) are the pineal gland, the tectum, the pons, the medulla, and the cerebellum. Adult brain tumors tend to be supratentorial; however, pediatric tumors are evenly split between supratentorial and infratentorial. This division of location in the pediatric population is dependent on the age of the patient. In children younger than 2 years of age, the tumors are predominantly supratentorial, whereas children between the ages of 3 and 15 years more often have infratentorial tumors (Table 44-1).[1] The prognosis is usually poor in children with brain tumors younger than the age of 1 year, with choroid plexus papilloma being the main exception.[1,4]

The development of immunohistochemical staining techniques allows pediatric tumors to be classified by histology. Tumors can arise from any of the cell types of the central nervous system. The brain is composed of neurons and glial cells. Glial cells far outnumber the neurons, and provide a nourishing and supportive role. The three main types of glial cells are astrocytes, oligodendrocytes, and ependymal cells, and the neoplasms they give rise to are gliomas. More specifically, they form astrocytomas, oligodendrogliomas, and ependymomas, respectively. Tumors involving both neuronal and glial cells are called ganglion cell tumors and consist of gangliogliomas, desmoplastic infantile gangliogliomas, and gangliocytomas. Another mixed neuronal and glial tumor is a dysembryoplastic neuroepithelial tumor (DNET). Finally, there are embryonal tumors, which include medulloblastoma, primitive neuroectodermal tumors (PNETs), medulloepithelioma, neuroblastomas, melanotic neuroectodermal tumors in infancy, and atypical teratoid/ rhabdoid tumors (ATRTs).[4] Other primary brain tumors include germ cell tumors, choroid plexus tumors, craniopharyngiomas, and meningiomas.

Clinical Features

The signs and symptoms of brain tumors in children vary considerably based on tumor type, location, and age of the patient. In the absence of a seizure or a focal neurologic deficit (e.g., diplopia caused by sixth nerve paresis), the vast majority of the symptoms are nonspecific and easily attributable to many more common and less serious causes. Common symptoms may include headache, nausea, vomiting, lethargy, subtle changes in personality, and worsening school performance. This constellation of symptoms can often be attributed to gastrointestinal problems, depression, school anxiety, migraines, sinusitis, or the need for prescription eyeglasses. Even a long-standing seizure disorder may ultimately be diagnosed as a supratentorial brain tumor. Infants typically present with failure to thrive, decreased intake, macrocephaly, or lethargy. Because of the nonspecific nature of these symptoms, it is common for a patient to present for neurologic evaluation after having visited numerous other specialists without establishing a diagnosis.

Most pediatric patients with brain tumors are between the ages of 2 and 14 years and typically present with a few days to weeks of headache, nausea/vomiting, gait ataxia, and/or diplopia. This constellation of symptoms is caused by hydrocephalus resulting from obstruction of the ventricles by tumor, commonly located in the midline posterior fossa. Headaches are common in children with viral infections, whereas frequent, daily morning headaches should raise the clinical suspicion of an intracranial mass lesion. This is especially true in the absence of a fever or other viral sequelae. Patients with elevated intracranial pressure often have an exacerbation of their symptoms in the morning. Both lying in the recumbent position overnight and sleep-induced hypoventilation (which leads to an increase in Pco_2) cause an increase in intracranial pressure. Elevated intracranial pressure can also cause the cerebellar tonsils to herniate into the foramen magnum and result in occipital headaches and neck pain.

There are two instances in which tumors cause nausea and vomiting. One is the elevation of intracranial pressure, and the other is direct irritation/infiltration of the vomiting center. The

TABLE 44-1

Brain Tumors in Children

Age	Tumor Histology
0 to 2 years	Teratoma
	Primitive neuroectodermal tumor
	Astrocytoma (high grade)
	Choroid plexus papilloma
2 to 15 years	Supratentorial tumors (50%)
	Astrocytoma (low grade)
	Craniopharyngioma
	Hypothalamic glioma
	Primitive neuroectodermal tumor
	Ependymoma
	Choroid plexus papilloma
	Infratentorial (50%)
	Primitive neuroectodermal tumor: medulloblastoma
	Cerebellar astrocytoma
	Ependymoma
	Brainstem glioma

vomiting center (area postrema) is located on the floor of the fourth ventricle and is vulnerable to compression from large posterior fossa tumors or from direct invasion of intrinsic brainstem tumors. Given that an intrinsic tumor in the medulla can cause vomiting in the absence of other neurologic symptoms, persistent vomiting should raise the possibility of a posterior fossa tumor, which could be confirmed through a detailed history and neurologic examination. Ataxia is commonly associated with tumors in the cerebellum and is often described by the parents as clumsiness, "walking like he is drunk," walking with the head tilted to one side, or falling to one side.

The visual complaints associated with posterior fossa tumors are frequently diplopia, difficulty looking up (sunsetting eye or Parinaud syndrome), and occasionally decreased visual acuity. As mentioned before, these symptoms are a result of the hydrocephalus. A decrease in visual acuity can result from papilledema. Loss of vision is a more common symptom of supratentorial tumors, because of optic nerve atrophy from direct compression. Patients with posterior fossa tumors are usually diagnosed with magnetic resonance imaging (MRI), because their other symptoms occur long before any visual defects. Therefore lack of visual signs and symptoms does not exclude a brain tumor. However, patients with poor access to health care can present with posterior fossa tumors and accompanying visual deficits.

Supratentorial tumors are especially common in patients younger than 2 years of age. These children often present with a failure to thrive, hemiparesis, seizures, or a full bulging anterior fontanelle and a rapid increase in head circumference.[5,6] At more than 2 years of age, supratentorial tumors present similarly in both children and adults, most commonly with headaches and/or seizures. When a patient presents with sudden onset of severe headaches or a rapid decline in mental status, it usually indicates a hemorrhage into their lesion. Rarely, obstructive hydrocephalus can cause such a rapid decline in mental status, but this is unlikely because of the slow growth rate of most tumors.

Less commonly, brain tumors can present with endocrine abnormalities. These can include weight gain or loss, diabetes insipidus, short stature, truncal obesity, galactorrhea, and precocious or delayed puberty. These symptoms result from tumors affecting the hypothalamic-pituitary axis. Because of the proximity of these tumors to the optic nerves and chiasm, they often cause decreased vision and visual field deficits.

Radiographic Evaluation

Patients suspected of having a brain tumor should be evaluated with an MRI with and without gadolinium. Although MRI is the gold standard for evaluating tumors, many patients presenting in the emergency department with progressive clinical signs and symptoms of a brain tumor are evaluated with a head computed tomography (CT) without instillation of a contrast medium. CT is the ideal imaging modality to use during emergent situations for a number of reasons. CT is excellent in evaluating hydrocephalus and hemorrhage, the two main causes of rapid neurological decline. Furthermore, CT can be performed in minutes, frequently does not require sedation, gives excellent detail and information, and is considerably less expensive. If the patient's condition is rapidly deteriorating, a contrast agent–enhanced head CT is occasionally performed to better characterize the lesion for the radiologist and neurosurgeon when the patient requires emergent surgical intervention. If the patient's condition is stable, the contrast agent may be omitted, and MRI with and without gadolinium should be performed, the timing of which is dictated by the clinical signs and symptoms.

Magnetic resonance imaging provides much better resolution of the brain and provides images in the sagittal, axial, and coronal planes. Standard MR imaging combined with newer imaging sequences and spectroscopy can even point to a specific histologic diagnosis.[7] Furthermore, it is difficult to evaluate the lower brainstem with CT, because of the bony artifact from the skull base. One limitation of MRI is that it does not show intratumoral calcifications very well, and occasionally, patients require both studies to aid in establishing the proper diagnosis.

Magnetic resonance imaging with and without gadolinium can provide significantly more information about the patient's tumor. The blood–brain barrier is made up of tight junctions in the endothelial cells lining the capillaries in the brain, which prevent most blood contents from entering the brain, including gadolinium. However, certain brain tumors cause breakdown of the blood–brain barrier and permit the gadolinium to enter the tumor and then enhance the tissues (appear bright on T1-weighted images). In general, in the adult population, enhancement in an intra-axial lesion means a more aggressive brain tumor and a poorer prognosis. This is not as consistent in pediatric tumors. There are many enhancing pediatric brain tumors that are not aggressive and are curable with total resection.

When viewing an MRI, the important factors to consider are (1) the location of the tumor (e.g., supratentorial, infratentorial, pineal region, suprasellar), (2) whether the tumor is intra-axial (within the brain tissue) or extra-axial (outside the brain tissue), (3) the age of the patient, (4) whether the tumor enhances, and (5) if there are single or multiple lesions. By systematically assessing the scans and considering these factors, the differential diagnosis can be narrowed considerably, which can be extremely helpful in preoperative planning.

If there are multiple lesions in the brain, or the location and enhancement suggest a tumor type associated with leptomeningeal metastases or "drop mets" to the spine, then a spinal MRI with and without gadolinium is performed. It is preferable to obtain the spinal MRI preoperatively, but this is often dictated by the patient's clinical examination. Postoperatively, brain tumor patients should have an MRI within 36 to 48 hours to evaluate the extent of the resection and rule out hydrocephalus, bleeding, or ischemia. The timing is important, because after 36 to 48 hours, expected postoperative changes can enhance and make it difficult to distinguish scarring from residual tumor. If the patient did not get a preoperative MRI evaluation of the spine and the histologic diagnosis is consistent with tumors that can metastasize to the spine, then the study should be done 2 weeks after surgery, because postoperative debris and blood can be mistaken for metastatic disease

Surgical Intervention

The goal of a surgical intervention for brain tumors is to safely debulk as much tumor as possible, to obtain a histologic diagnosis, to reestablish normal cerebrospinal fluid (CSF) pathways, or to divert CSF. The location of the tumor is often the determining factor as to how aggressively the tumor is debulked. In fact, some tumors, because of their location and their ability to be diagnosed with MRI, are not biopsied. For example, an intrinsic pontine glioma, which is an astrocytoma of the brainstem, cannot be debulked safely and has a characteristic appearance on MRI. Therefore these patients are referred to a neuro-oncologist for management without a tissue diagnosis. Pineal region tumors are another example of a lesion that may be diagnosed without surgical intervention. Patients with pineal region masses should have serum β-human chorionic gonadotropin (β-HCG) and alpha fetoprotein (AFP) levels obtained. If these are negative, then CSF markers are needed. If the serum or CSF markers are positive, then a diagnosis of a germ cell tumor can be made without the need for a biopsy.

However, most tumors require surgical intervention, consisting of either a stereotactic biopsy or an open craniotomy to obtain tissue for a definitive diagnosis. The most important tool for preoperative planning is MRI. Diffuse intrinsic tumors of the thalamus or basal ganglia typically undergo stereotactic biopsy. This procedure involves rigidly fixing an MRI-compatible frame to the patient's skull. The patient then has an MRI, and the x, y, and z coordinates are determined. These coordinates are then used to position the frame and the arc so that the tip of the needle is exactly where these three points intersect in the brain. Given the improvements in frameless stereotaxy, all but the smallest lesions can be biopsied without a rigid frame.[8] The advantages of a stereotactic biopsy include a short procedure time, the possibility of diagnosis in areas of the brain that carry an unacceptable morbidity and mortality with an open craniotomy, and the patient is discharged on postoperative day 1. The disadvantages are that only a small amount of tissue is obtained, which may be nondiagnostic or result in the wrong diagnosis, and if bleeding occurs it is difficult to treat, or it may not be recognized until the patient deteriorates neurologically after the procedure. Lastly, if the diagnosis

cannot be made with a stereotactic biopsy or the diagnosis requires aggressive debulking, the patient will require a second operative procedure.

Because of the fact that the prognosis of many pediatric tumors is strongly influenced by the amount of postsurgical residual tumor,[9] the majority are approached with a craniotomy/craniectomy for open biopsy, with an attempt at maximal microsurgical tumor resection. Cerebral hemispheric tumors are approached through a craniotomy. Preoperative planning consists of an MRI coupled with a frameless stereotactic navigation study. The navigation study allows the neurosurgeon to view the tumor in the operating room in the sagittal, axial, and coronal planes and can be used to find the tumor and plan the incision and approach. However, the main limitation of this technology is that it is not a real-time study, and actions such as retracting the brain or draining cysts or CSF spaces may cause the brain to shift position, thus compromising the accuracy of the intraoperative navigation system. When this occurs, intraoperative ultrasonography is extremely helpful in localizing lesions.

Intraoperative MRI aims to correct the limitations of the navigation system by providing a real-time image. Previous intraoperative MRIs were limited because of poor resolution; however, newer intraoperative suites have 3-tesla magnets and provide excellent resolution. The drawbacks of the intraoperative MRI suites are that they are prohibitively expensive for many institutions, are helpful in only a small number of procedures, and significantly extend the time of the procedure. Nevertheless, this is exciting technology, and as the expense decreases and the efficiency improves, it will be an invaluable tool to surgeons operating upon brain tumors. Functional MRI (fMRI) techniques can localize speech and motor cortex. When tumors involve these areas of eloquent cortex, fMRI can aid in selecting the safest site to incise the cortex.[10] In the pediatric population, fMRI can prove challenging, because it requires a cooperative non-sedated patient. Electrophysiologic recording and stimulation are sometimes helpful in locating the motor strip. Recently, magnetoencephalography (MEG) is being used to help localize motor, sensory, and language cortex for both tumor surgery and epilepsy surgery.[11]

Such advances undoubtedly aid the neurosurgeon throughout the surgical procedure; however, there is still no substitute for an outstanding understanding of the three-dimensional anatomy of the brain. When choosing an approach, anatomic planes, such as the interhemispheric fissure, the sylvian fissure, and the cranial base are used, if possible, to avoid resecting normal brain. If there is no plane available, the approach is usually through the least amount of tissue, while avoiding areas of eloquent language, motor, and visual cortex.

Tumors of the midline (hypothalamus, thalamus, basal ganglia, and brainstem) were once considered inoperable. However, advances in microsurgical techniques and innovative instrumentation now make these tumors approachable. At the same time, advances in chemotherapy and single-dose and fractionated radiosurgery offer alternatives, and it is currently unclear which strategy or combination of strategies is best for a particular tumor. Advances in surgical techniques now allow for multiple options for the approach to tumors. For example, pineal region tumors may be approached through a posterior fossa route (retracting the cerebellum from the underside of the tentorium), by a supratentorial route between the hemispheres and through the posterior corpus callosum, or through the tentorium itself. The relationship of the pineal tumor to the tentorium dictates the approach.

Tumors of the cerebellum and the lower brainstem are approached through a posterior fossa craniotomy or craniectomy.[12] Midline tumors of the fourth ventricle usually present with obstructive hydrocephalus. Some neurosurgeons prefer to place a shunt before tumor resection; however, most now favor giving the child corticosteroids and placing a ventriculostomy at the time of the craniectomy. The ventriculostomy is either removed or converted to a shunt if needed in the postoperative period. Between 20% and 40% of children will ultimately require a shunt.[13] Many neurosurgeons are performing an endoscopic third ventriculostomy (ETV) at the time of the resection. This procedure involves inserting an endoscope into the lateral ventricle, passing it through the foramen of Monro and making a small hole in the floor of the third ventricle. This allows the CSF to bypass the distal obstruction and enter directly into the cisternal system.[14] One series of patients with posterior fossa tumors showed a reduction in the postoperative shunt rate of 26.8% to 6% in patients treated with EVT and tumor removal versus tumor removal alone.[15]

To access the fourth ventricle, the patient is placed in the prone position, and the bone overlying the cerebellum is removed, occasionally including the posterior ring of the C1 vertebrae. After opening the dura, the cerebellar vermis is vertically incised, providing access to the tumor and the fourth ventricle. The tumor is removed with bipolar cautery, suction, or an ultrasonic aspirator. Laterally placed tumors of the cerebellopontine angle are reached by retracting the cerebellum medially. Electrophysiologic monitoring of cranial nerves V, VII, VIII, IX, X, XI, and XII is often required throughout this approach. Tumors of the brainstem may be debulked, if they are dorsally exophytic. The dura is closed and covered with DuraGen (Integra LifeSciences, Plainsboro, NJ), a collagen product that augments dura integrity. Replacement of the bone is not required, but we prefer to whenever possible. Postoperative problems include acute hydrocephalus, pseudomeningoceles, aseptic meningitis, mutism, pseudobulbar palsy,[16] cranial nerve or brainstem dysfunction, and gastrointestinal hemorrhage.[17] Patients with swallowing dysfunction and aspiration may require tracheostomy and feeding gastrostomy.

Tumor Types

CEREBELLAR ASTROCYTOMAS

These tumors are usually low-grade and curable with total surgical resection. The average age at presentation is 9 years, and the patient normally presents with pernicious vomiting, intermittent morning headaches, and disturbances of balance, usually spanning a period of months. The classical CT appearance of these tumors is a hypodense, cystic cerebellar mass (usually around the vermis) with a brilliantly enhancing "mural nodule."[18] However, about one fourth will be entirely solid tumors. MRI is helpful in defining the surgical anatomy, such as the relationship of the tumor to the brainstem, and the nature of the cyst wall. Cerebellar astrocytomas are typically of low signal intensity on T1-weighted MRI sequences, demonstrate increased intensity on T2-weighted sequences, and show enhancement of the solid component with gadolinium (Fig. 44-1). Because of their location and size, they cause

effacement of the fourth ventricle, resulting in obstructive hydrocephalus.

Histologically, they consist of benign-appearing astrocytes.[19] Subtypes are the juvenile pilocytic form (80% to 85%) and the fibrillary form.[4] Detailed examination may reveal cellular pleomorphism and tumor extension to the subarachnoid space, but these tumors rarely disseminate. High-grade astrocytomas in this location are rare and usually follow radiation therapy given for a previous low-grade tumor.[20]

Treatment for cerebellar astrocytomas is complete surgical resection. In tumors with no brainstem involvement, this can be accomplished in a high percentage of cases. If complete surgical excision can be demonstrated radiographically, these tumors rarely recur, and no adjuvant therapy is indicated.[21] Therefore if there is residual tumor on the postoperative scan, reoperation for total excision is recommended. Radiation therapy can be considered for multiple recurrent lesions or in cases in which brainstem involvement precludes complete removal. However, even in these cases, residual tumor may remain indolent for years without additional therapy. Regular postoperative surveillance scanning is appropriate, especially when there is suspicion for residual tumor. Recurrence is treated with reoperation if this is feasible.

PRIMITIVE NEUROECTODERMAL TUMOR AND MEDULLOBLASTOMA

Primitive neuroectodermal tumor and medulloblastoma are related tumors; and, in fact, the term medulloblastoma and posterior fossa PNET are often used interchangeably. Medulloblastoma is the most common malignant brain tumor of childhood. Histologically, the classical medulloblastoma is composed of densely packed cells with hyperchromatic nuclei and little cytoplasm, giving the histologic slides a blue color when stained with hematoxylin and eosin. Tumors with identical histology can occur in the cerebral hemispheres and are termed supratentorial PNETs. Children with medulloblastoma typically present with headache, vomiting, and lethargy of relatively short duration, and the mean age (3 to 4 years) is typically younger than that seen with cerebellar astrocytomas. Infants typically present with failure to thrive. Supratentorial PNETs present with increased intracranial pressure and focal neurologic deficits, depending on the location of the tumor.

On a CT scan, medulloblastomas typically appear as well-marginated homogeneously dense masses filling the fourth ventricle, causing obstructive hydrocephalus. They usually enhance brilliantly with contrast. However, unlike ependymomas, they lack calcifications. On MRI, they can show variable signal characteristics. The images are often slightly hypointense on T1 weighting, becoming brighter on fluid-attenuated inversion recovery (FLAIR) sequences, and may be bright or dark on T2-weighted studies. They usually enhance on MRI (Fig. 44-2) and show restricted diffusion on diffusion-weighted imaging (DWI). MRI of the spine is indicated 2 weeks postoperatively to evaluate for spinal metastases ("drop mets"; Fig. 44-3).[22]

Treatment begins with biopsy and surgical excision. Medulloblastoma and PNET tumors are not curable with surgery alone; and in cases with metastases at diagnosis or extensive brainstem involvement, the major mass should be debulked,

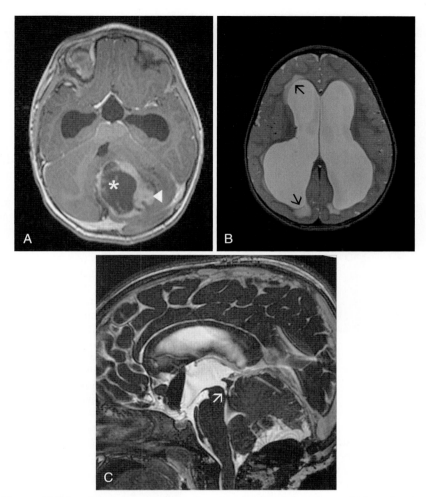

FIGURE 44-1   A, Axial T1WI postgadolinium image of a cerebellar pilocytic astrocytoma, in a 3-year-old boy, showing a large cyst *(white asterisk)* and enhancing mural nodule *(white arrowhead)*. **B,** Axial T2WI image showing markedly dilated lateral ventricles and transependymal flow of cerebral spinal fluid (CSF) out of the ventricles into the surrounding brain parenchyma *(black arrows)*. The obstructive hydrocephalus is a result of the cerebellar astrocytoma. **C,** Sagittal T2WI postoperative image showing resection of tumor and flow through the floor of the third ventricle *(white arrow)* after the endoscopic third ventriculostomy done at the time of tumor resection.

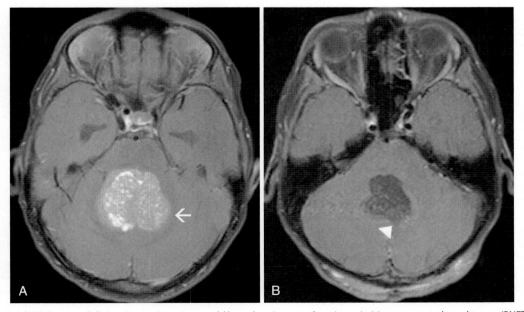

FIGURE 44-2   A, Axial T1WI postgadolinium image, in an 8-year-old boy, showing an enhancing primitive neuroectodermal tumor (PNET) arising from the roof of the fourth ventricle and involving the cerebellar vermis *(white arrow)*. **B,** Axial T1WI postoperative image showing resection of tumor and partial splitting of the vermis *(white arrowhead)*. The patient suffered severe postoperative mutism.

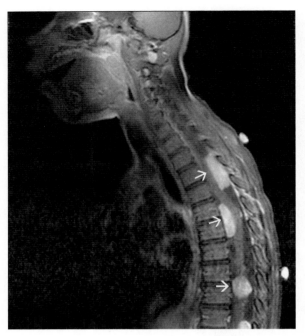

FIGURE 44-3 Sagittal T1WI postgadolinium image of a 4-year-old with metastatic primitive neuroectodermal tumor (PNET) to the spine *(white arrows)* from her fourth ventricular tumor. The "drop mets" were present at the time of her diagnosis.

but no attempt should be made to resect tumor in vital areas.[23] After the operation, radiation therapy is usually administered to the entire brain and spinal canal, with a boost to the tumor bed. Younger children (less than 9 years old) suffer significant, global cognitive problems as a result of whole-brain radiation in an age- and dose-dependent fashion.[24] They are chemotherapy sensitive, and various chemotherapy combinations have been used to improve outcomes and allow for a reduction in craniospinal radiation dose.[25–28] Chemotherapy alone has been shown to have some success in treating these tumors and can be used in the treatment of infants (for whom craniospinal radiation is contraindicated); however, the long-term survival of a chemotherapy-only approach is not as good as combined modality treatment.[29–32] In determining the best treatment, staging criteria are important to define risk groups. In the past, the Chang system was used, which incorporated the surgeon's estimate of the tumor size at operation and the extent of metastatic disease based on postoperative imaging.[33] In most centers today, patients are assigned to a high-risk group based on younger age (<3 years old), supratentorial tumor location, postoperative residual disease greater than a volume of 1.5 cubic centimeters, or presence of disseminated disease.[28,34] Molecular markers have been identified that have prognostic significance, but are not yet being used to dictate therapy.[35–39] The rate of progression-free survival at 5 years ranges from more than 80% in groups with standard-risk factors[40,41] to less than 70% in high-risk groups.[28,42–44] Infants treated with chemotherapy alone historically have progression-free survival rates in the range of 20% to 40%,[29–31] although recent studies suggest that intensification of therapy may improve survival rates.[32,45]

Patients require long-term supportive care, preferably in the setting of a multidisciplinary pediatric neuro-oncology clinic. Surveillance scanning is standard practice, and although rates

of cure for recurrent tumors are low, high-dose chemotherapy and stem cell rescue can salvage some patients at relapse.[46,47] Late sequelae of therapy include pituitary dysfunction, hearing loss, growth delay, cardiomyopathy,[48] cognitive delay,[49] psychosocial adjustment and family problems, and radiation-induced meningiomas, astrocytomas, and sarcomas.[50]

EPENDYMOMAS

Ependymomas occur in the region of the fourth ventricle or cerebellopontine angle, spinal cord, or supratentorial compartment. Most are histologically benign, but despite this, they have a tendency to recur in the local tumor bed and disseminate throughout the neuraxis. The median age at diagnosis is between 3 and 5 years, although tumors in infants and adults are not uncommon.[51] Tumors typically arise in the posterior fossa (60% of cases), and symptoms are similar to those of other tumors in this region. Cranial nerve and brainstem involvement can occur. Vomiting may arise without hydrocephalus, which suggests infiltration of the region of obex, which is characteristic of ependymomas. When the tumors do arise in the supratentorial compartment in children, they are often extremely large, and despite their presumed ependymal origin, may demonstrate no connection with the ventricle.

Computed tomography typically shows an isodense mass with flecks of calcification and an inhomogeneous pattern of enhancement. Posterior fossa lesions may extend through the foramina of Luschka into the cerebellopontine angle (Fig. 44-4). On MRI, ependymomas are usually isointense to hypointense on T1-weighted images, hyperintense on T2/FLAIR images, do NOT show restricted diffusion on DWI, and often enhance inhomogeneously with gadolinium.[52]

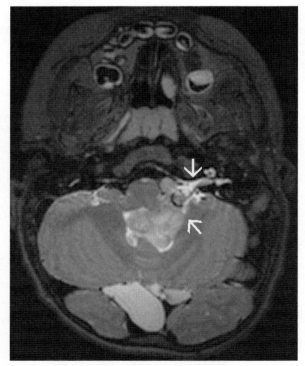

FIGURE 44-4 Axial T2WI image of a fourth ventricular ependymoma, in a 5-year-old boy, growing out of the foramen of Luschka into the cerebellopontine angle *(white arrows).*

Treatment for ependymomas primarily consists of surgery and radiation. Prognosis is highly dependent on the extent of surgical resection as determined by postoperative imaging. The 5-year progression-free survival after complete resection is 60% to 80%, compared with less than 30% after incomplete resection.[53] However, radical surgical resection may result in permanent neurologic damage and may not be possible in some cases. Unless the tumor has disseminated at diagnosis, postoperative radiation is confined to the operative bed. Trials of radiosurgery for unresectable tumors are ongoing at several centers. Ependymomas are now being treated with proton beam therapy because of the decreased radiation exposure to the adjacent, normal uninvolved structures. Adjuvant chemotherapy has minimal impact on survival[54]; however, several chemotherapy agents have activity in this tumor,[30,55] and chemotherapy is being evaluated in a neoadjuvant setting to see whether giving chemotherapy after a subtotal resection may shrink the tumor in such a way that a complete resection can be achieved at a second surgery.

BRAINSTEM GLIOMAS

It is now recognized that there are several types of brainstem gliomas, each associated with very different outcomes.[56] The most common variety is the diffuse intrinsic brainstem glioma, which is not amenable to surgical resection. These tumors are often centered in the pons and typically present with cranial neuropathies rather than hydrocephalus. Patients tend to be less than the age of 4 years, with sixth nerve palsies, facial weakness, and ataxia. The diagnosis is established by MRI, which shows a swollen pons with diffuse signal abnormalities (Fig. 44-5). Surgery is not indicated. Radiation therapy can provide symptomatic relief and prolong survival, but most children die within a year.[57] Chemotherapy has not been shown to be effective.

Cervicomedullary astrocytomas are considered to be rostral extensions of intrinsic spinal cord tumors and carry a better prognosis. Signs and symptoms may include vomiting, torticollis, and slowly evolving motor weakness. MRI shows an enlarged upper cervical spinal cord, with a rostral extension presenting in the cisterna magna. They are often amenable to aggressive surgical resection, and if the histology is benign, adjuvant radiation therapy is usually deferred.

Dorsally exophytic brainstem tumors arise from the floor of the fourth ventricle and present with symptoms of hydrocephalus. These tend to be pilocytic astrocytomas.[58] Treatment is primarily surgical. Gross total resection is difficult to achieve without unacceptable neurologic risk; however, most patients remain progression-free after resection because of the indolent nature of the tumor. Radiotherapy is reserved for recurrence or progression.[59]

Tectal gliomas are now recognized to be a not infrequent cause of hydrocephalus.[60] They typically present with symptoms referable to ventricular obstruction and are usually treated with either a ventriculoperitoneal shunt or endoscopic third ventriculostomy. Biopsy is not required. They are usually extremely indolent, and treatment of the tumor itself is required only if it progressively enlarges.

HYPOTHALAMIC/CHIASMATIC ASTROCYTOMAS

Suprasellar astrocytomas are usually low-grade neoplasms, which may occur in association with neurofibromatosis type 1 or as isolated tumors. The etiology of these tumors is not well described, but the association with neurofibromatosis type 1, which is localized to chromosome 17q, suggests a molecular genetic basis. They may present primarily with vision abnormalities (visual field cuts, asymmetric loss of visual acuity in association with optic atrophy, or nystagmus) or as hypothalamic dysfunction (precocious puberty, diabetes insipidus, other endocrine dysfunction, growth failure, obesity, or diencephalic syndrome, which consists of failure to thrive and vomiting). Often both visual and hypothalamic complaints coexist.[61]

Imaging studies usually cannot distinguish hypothalamic tumors from those arising from the visual apparatus. The tumors typically do not calcify, which helps distinguish them from craniopharyngiomas, and appear as solid hypodense lesions on CT or T1-weighted MRI sequences and enhance

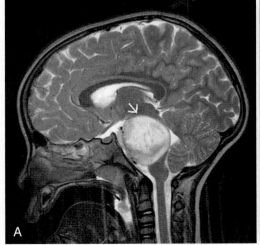
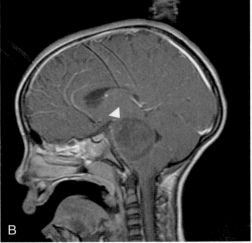

FIGURE 44-5   A, Sagittal T2WI image in a 4-year-old girl showing an infiltrative, hyperintense tumor in the pons *(white arrow)*. **B,** Sagittal T1WI postgadolinium image showing that the tumor does not enhance *(white arrowhead)*. This tumor is an intrinsic pontine glioma, and the diagnosis is made by MRI alone, a biopsy is not required.

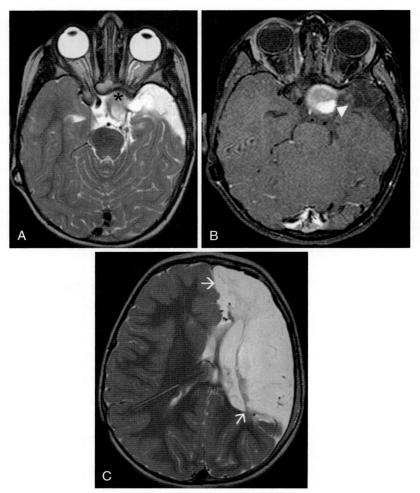

FIGURE 44-6 **A,** Axial T2WI image in a 3-month-old girl who has a hyperintense lesion *(black asterisk)* in the left optic nerve and into the optic chiasm. **B,** Axial T1WI postgadolinium image showing an enhancing tumor *(white arrowhead)*. The tumor causes stretch on the internal carotid artery and middle cerebral artery, putting the patient at risk of a postoperative stroke when this chiasmatic/hypothalamic glioma is resected. **C,** Axial T2WI postoperative image showing a large left internal carotid stroke *(white arrows)* that occurred on postoperative day 4 and was a result of vasospasm in the stretched arteries.

after administering contrast. Extension to the intraorbital optic nerves or along the optic radiations is diagnostic and rules out craniopharyngiomas, germinomas, or other tumors in this location (Fig. 44-6).

Because most of these tumors will not progress significantly (especially in the setting of neurofibromatosis type 1), initial management is usually observation with serial imaging and ophthalmologic screening. Tumors that progress significantly and/or cause worsening vision are treated with chemotherapy. The most common regimen used is vincristine and carboplatin[62,63]; however, thioguanine, procarbazine, lomustine (CCNU), and vincristine (TPCV) are also effective.[64] Radiotherapy is avoided if possible because of the high risk of secondary effects, such as endocrine dysfunction, stroke, secondary malignant neoplasms, and neurocognitive deficits. Although radical surgical resection results in prolonged disease stability in the majority of patients, it carries a higher risk of stroke and injury to the optic pathways and the hypothalamic/pituitary axis.[65,66] Surgery is reserved for cases when the diagnosis is unclear, there is a unilateral optic nerve tumor with severe visual impairment or painful proptosis, and tumors are causing obstruction of the third ventricle or exerting mass effect on surrounding areas of the brain.

CRANIOPHARYNGIOMA

Craniopharyngiomas are histologically benign masses believed to arise from embryonic rests derived from the hypophyseal-pharyngeal duct. Symptoms result from optic chiasm or nerve compression, hypopituitarism, hypothalamic dysfunction, or increased intracranial pressure in association with hydrocephalus.[67] They also occur in adults, but the childhood form represents a distinct entity characterized by large size and extensive calcification. There are two varieties of craniopharyngiomas, the papillary and adamantinomatous types, the latter being the most common in the pediatric population. Histologically, they typically are composed of a squamous epithelial cyst wall, with cystic fluid composed of cholesterol crystals, and calcifications. They tend to be inseparable from the pituitary stalk and may have an interdigitating gliotic interface with the hypothalamus above. This makes complete surgical removal challenging, because small rests of tumor may reside in the brain. This is also the reason for hypothalamic dysfunction that may be seen after surgical excision.[68]

Computed tomography can reveal either a cystic mass with basal calcifications or an entirely solid tumor. MRI shows

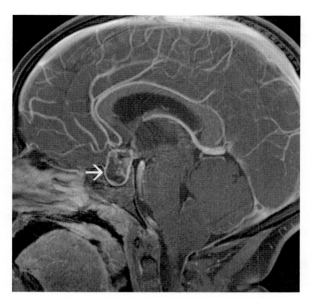

FIGURE 44-7 Sagittal T1WI postgadolinium image, in a 6-year-old boy, showing a sellar/suprasellar craniopharyngioma growing down into the sella turcica and up into the third ventricle *(white arrow)*.

employed with cortical tumors, but simple removal of the tumor usually provides good seizure control, and the value of these strategies is uncertain.[9,80]

The outcome of low-grade astrocytomas,[9] gangliogliomas,[81] (Fig. 44-8), and DNETs (Fig. 44-9) that are completely resected is favorable, although surveillance scanning is

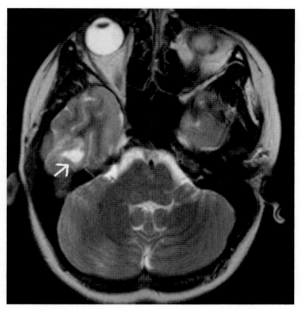

FIGURE 44-8 Axial T2WI image, in a 15-year-old girl, showing a small hyperintense right temporal tumor *(white arrow)*. The patient presented with seizures and the tumor was a ganglioglioma.

the sagittal anatomy well, but may miss the calcifications[69] (Fig. 44-7). In some instances, imaging cannot distinguish a craniopharyngioma from a hypothalamic glioma.

Controversy persists regarding the best treatment approach for patients with this tumor. Gross total resection and subtotal resection with adjuvant radiation have similar local control rates.[70–72] Both are associated with potential post-treatment problems, including panhypopituitarism, diabetes insipidus, obesity, visual problems, stroke, behavioral difficulties, poor school performance, and pseudoaneurysms of the carotid artery.[73–75] Although aggressive resection of very large craniopharyngiomas is often associated with more significant post-treatment complications, gross total resection of smaller tumors in high-volume centers are more likely to be achieved safely. Long-term survival is in the range of 90% at 10 years, but local recurrences are not uncommon.[76] Recurrences are treated by reoperation,[77] instillation of colloidal ^{32}P into cysts, or radiosurgery.

LOW-GRADE SUPRATENTORIAL ASTROCYTOMAS

Low-grade astrocytomas and gangliogliomas involving the cortical regions and temporal lobes can often present with intractable seizures. CT may show masses of low density. MRI usually shows a mass of decreased signal on T1-weighted images and increased signal on T2-weighted images that may or may not enhance with gadolinium.

Complete resection is the goal of surgery, but this may prove difficult because of problems in defining the tumor margins and its proximity to eloquent areas. Adjuncts to aid in this include language and motor mapping using implantable grids or intraoperative electrophysiologic monitoring techniques,[78] functional MRI techniques, and image-directed tumor resection.[79] Tumors of the temporal lobe are often treated by formal temporal lobectomy to decrease the incidence of seizures. Seizure mapping techniques have also been

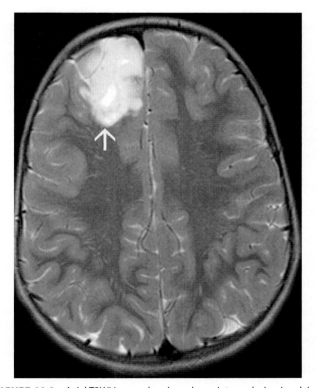

FIGURE 44-9 Axial T2WI image showing a hyperintense lesion involving the white matter and overlying grey matter *(white arrow)*. This 5-year-old boy presented with a seizure, and the tumor was a dysembryoplastic neuroepithelial tumor (DNET).

warranted. About 70% of children will remain recurrence free. Recurrent tumors can be treated by reoperation alone or reoperation followed by radiation therapy.[82]

PINEAL REGION TUMORS

Tumors of the pineal region encompass a wide range of histologic types. They can be divided into germ cell tumors (teratoma, germinoma, choriocarcinoma, embryonal carcinoma, yolk sac tumor), pineal parenchymal tumors (pineocytoma, pineoblastoma), tumors of surrounding structures (astrocytomas, meningiomas), and other benign conditions (cysts, vascular malformations). The older term pinealoma is no longer used.

Patients typically present with signs and symptoms of hydrocephalus and Parinaud syndrome (upgaze paresis, convergence nystagmus, and light-near dissociation). MRI confirms the presence of a tumor, but is nonspecific regarding histologic type. Specific germ cell tumors may secrete "tumor markers," which may be measured in CSF (obtained from a lumbar puncture or ventriculostomy) or blood. Elevated β-HCG is seen in choriocarcinomas, and elevated AFP is seen in yolk sac tumors and embryonal cell carcinomas.

In the past, surgery in the pineal region was considered prohibitively dangerous, and tumors were often treated without histologic confirmation. Today, this region is now readily approachable using supracerebellar/infratentorial or interhemispheric-transcallosal routes with minimal morbidity, and in most centers, biopsy is performed if germ cell markers are negative. As in the suprasellar region, pure germinomas of the pineal gland carry an excellent prognosis after radiation therapy. For focal disease, the radiation field usually includes the whole ventricular volume with a boost to the tumor bed. For disseminated disease, craniospinal radiation is required.[83] Initial treatment with chemotherapy, followed by response-based radiation field and dose, is advocated in some centers. The nongerminomatous germ cell tumors have a worse prognosis and require more intensive chemotherapy along with radiotherapy.[84] Pineoblastomas are treated like PNETs in other regions of the brain. Pineocytomas may be simply observed if totally resected or given focal radiation for residual tumor.

ATYPICAL TERATOID/RHABDOID TUMORS

Atypical teratoid/rhabdoid tumors (AT/RTs) were previously misclassified as PNET tumors, but have been shown to be a distinct entity. They are highly malignant tumors with histologic resemblance to rhabdoid tumors of the kidney. Histologically, they can be distinguished from PNETs by larger cells with pink cytoplasm that show immunohistochemical staining for smooth muscle actin, vimentin, and epithelial membrane antigen. AT/RTs typically occur in young children and most commonly occur in the posterior fossa, but they may be located in the spine or supratentorial space. Fluorescence in situ hybridization (FISH) shows a deletion of the tumor suppressor gene *INI-1* in most cases.[85] The prognosis of these tumors is historically poor; however, treatment consisting of surgical excision, intensive chemotherapy, and radiation in older children has resulted in long-term survival in some patients with localized disease.

MALIGNANT SUPRATENTORIAL ASTROCYTOMAS

Anaplastic astrocytomas and glioblastoma multiforme account for roughly 9% of pediatric tumors, which is a smaller incidence than in the adult population. Clinical signs and symptoms are reflective of their location. Imaging features are similar to those seen in adults, and the masses are often large, with enhancing rings and necrotic centers (Fig. 44-10). Dissemination occurs in about 10% of cases.[86]

Treatment includes maximal resection followed by radiation therapy. Unfortunately, the prognosis is still poor. Although more extensive resection confers better outcome, this may be due to the fact that more favorable tumors are more amenable to aggressive surgery. Chemotherapy has a modest impact on survival.[87,88]

CHOROID PLEXUS TUMORS

Tumors of the choroids plexus are divided into the benign choroid plexus papilloma (CPP) and the malignant choroid plexus carcinoma (CPC). In children, they tend to arise in the trigone of the left lateral ventricle, and the patients often present with hydrocephalus during infancy. On imaging, the appearance is an intraventricular, homogenously enhancing, lobulated mass (Fig. 44-11). Carcinomas are typically larger and may disseminate. The vascular supply is from the choroidal arteries, which may be seen on high-resolution MRI.

Treatment is surgical excision, which is curative for papillomas. The procedure is hazardous, because of the highly vascular tumors and the small size of the patients. Carcinomas are particularly difficult to remove, because of extreme vascularity. This has led some surgeons to biopsy CPCs, followed by chemotherapy and then second-look surgery.[89] Otherwise,

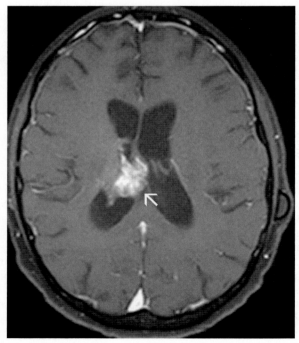

FIGURE 44-10 Axial T1WI postgadolinium image showing a thalamic enhancing tumor in a 14-year-old girl with headaches *(white arrow)*. The tumor was a glioblastoma multiforme (GBM).

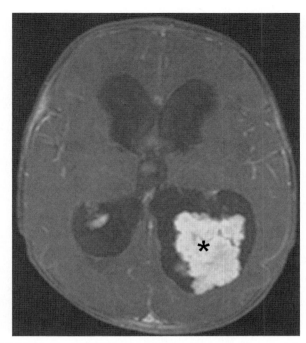

FIGURE 44-11 Axial T1WI postgadolinium image showing an avidly enhancing tumor in the atrium of the left ventricle in a 6-month-old girl with a rapidly growing head circumference *(black asterisk)*. The tumor was a choroid plexus papilloma.

the benefit of chemotherapy and radiotherapy is unproven. With complete tumor removal, prolonged survival and even cure are possible even in the case of CPCs.

MENINGIOMAS

Meningeal tumors are uncommon in childhood, accounting for about 2% of intracranial tumors. Meningiomas can occur in the orbit, sphenoid wing, or virtually any portion of the intracranial compartment, and do not necessarily need a dural attachment. Radiographically, they typically enhance and may be extremely large. Treatment is surgical resection. In adults, a gross total resection is curative; however, in the pediatric population, it is less common to have a meningioma with the typical benign histology seen in adults. Meningiomas in pediatric patients are usually much more aggressive and carry a worse prognosis than in adults.[90]

METASTASES AND DURAL-BASED MASSES

Sarcomas, particularly rhabdomyosarcoma and Ewing sarcoma, are the most common, primary, dural-based non-CNS tumors in children. Metastatic brain tumors are extremely uncommon in the pediatric population and have been reported with most tumor types, including neuroblastoma, Wilms' tumor, osteogenic sarcoma, and hepatoblastoma. Presentation is often abrupt, with potential catastrophic neurologic symptoms resulting from hemorrhage.

Tumor Genetics

In the past 2 decades, there has been a rapid development in imaging, navigational systems, and surgical instruments and techniques. However, despite this rapid increase in surgical technologies, many tumors, especially high-grade lesions, are still incurable with either surgery alone or in conjunction with chemotherapy and radiation therapy. Like much of medicine, the future in treating brain tumors lies in better biological, molecular, and genetic understanding. For example, such techniques have given physicians a better understanding of neurofibromatosis type 2, which is associated with the development of meningiomas and acoustic neuromas in the pediatric population. The gene locus was identified on chromosome 22,[91] the same chromosome that has been identified in pediatric meningiomas in patients without neurofibromatosis type 2.[92] These tumors have been shown to arise from a loss of a tumor suppressor gene.

In contrast, neurofibromatosis type 1 is associated with childhood gliomas, particularly of the optic pathway, hypothalamus, and brainstem. The affected gene locus, located at 17q11.2, encodes for the protein neurofibromin. This protein acts as a negative regulator of the RAS signaling pathway; therefore, a mutation in neurofibromin results in dysregulated RAS signaling, leading to cell growth and differentiation.[93]

Although molecular markers with prognostic significance have previously been identified for medulloblastoma, only recently have pathways been identified that may be implicated in the pathogenesis of certain medulloblastoma subtypes.[35-37,94] Approximately one third of medulloblastoma samples show increased signaling of the Sonic Hedgehog (SHH) pathway, and constitutive activation of SHH pathway promotes medulloblastoma formation in mice. Based on the work implicating this pathway and the preclinical efficacy of inhibition of this pathway on medulloblastoma formation in mice, clinical trials of SHH pathway inhibitors are underway.[84,85]

It has also recently been demonstrated that DNA from sporadic (non–NF1-associated) pediatric low-grade astrocytomas contain a novel duplication at chromosome band 7q34.[95] This duplication was identified in both juvenile pilocytic astrocytomas and fibrillary astrocytomas. This area of duplication contained approximately 20 genes, one of which was shown to be *BRAF*, which plays a regulatory role in the mitogen-activated protein kinase (MAPK) pathway. Reverse transcription polymerase chain reaction–based sequencing reveals that this duplication results in a fusion product between *KIAA1549* and *BRAF*. It is predicted that this fusion gene would lack the N-terminal regulatory domains and could result in constitutive BRAF kinase activity and subsequent unregulated activation of the MAPK pathway. Western blot analysis revealed phosphorylated MAPK protein in tumor cells with this duplication.[95] Further studies are required to determine the actual expression and function of this KIAA1549-BRAF fusion protein. However, neuroscientists are already exploring *BRAF* as a potential tumor marker or even a potential therapeutic target.

This discovery of a novel tumor pathway represents the ongoing trend in how the medical community is approaching the treatment of brain tumors. The future will require continued collaboration between neurosurgeons, oncologists, radiologists, and molecular neuroscientists to continue improving outcomes and diagnosis of patients with pediatric brain tumors.

The complete reference list is available online at www. expertconsult.com.

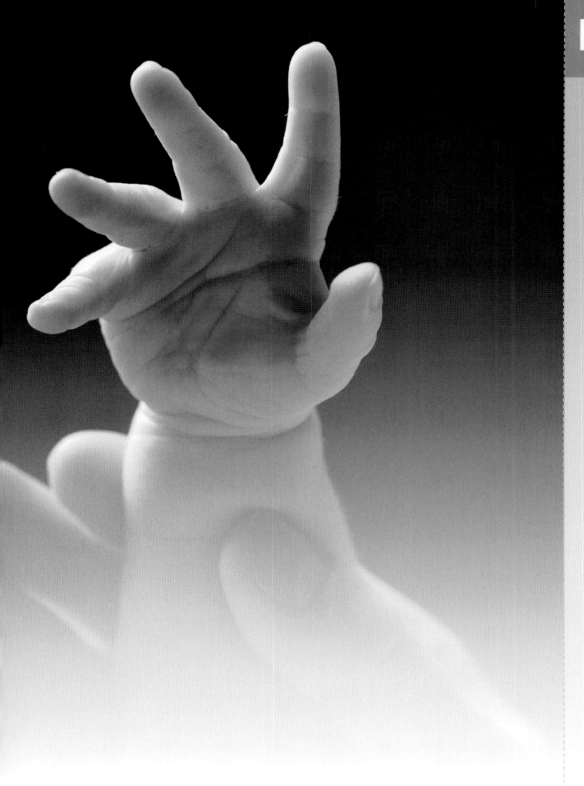

Part IV

TRANSPLANTATION

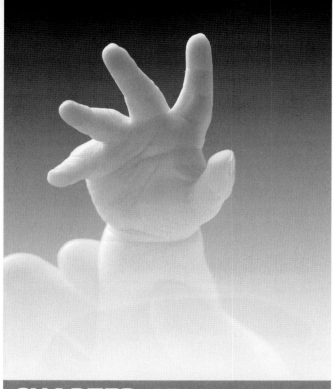

CHAPTER 45

Principles of Transplantation

Jorge Reyes, Noriko Murase, and Thomas E. Starzl

The replacement of failing body parts with the transplantation of organs, cells, and tissues has been a centuries-old dream, fulfilled in the last 50 years. This success with both solid organ and bone marrow cell transplantation has been established on the following principles: histocompatibility matching, immunosuppression, tissue preservation, and techniques of implantation. However, neither kind of transplantation could have emerged as a clinical service if not for the induction by the graft itself of various degrees of donor-specific nonreactivity (tolerance). Without this fifth factor, no transplant recipient could survive for long, if the amount of immunosuppression given to obtain initial engraftment had to be continued.

Enigma of Acquired Tolerance

The variable acquired tolerance on which transplantation depends has been one of the most enigmatic and controversial issues in all of biology. This was caused, in part, by the unexpected achievement of organ engraftment (the kidney) at an early time (a decade before successful bone marrow transplantation) and in ostensible violation of the very principles that would shape the impending revolution in general immunology. As a consequence, clinical organ transplantation was developed empirically rather than as a branch of classic immunology. This occurred in four distinct phases, each lasting more than a decade. Only at the end was it possible to explain organ engraftment and thereby eliminate the mystique of transplantation.

PHASE 1: 1953 TO 1968

The modern era of transplantation began between 1953 and 1956 with the demonstration that neonatal mice[1,2] (with an immature immune system) and irradiated adult mice[3] (with an immune system weakened by total-body irradiation) develop donor-specific tolerance after successful engraftment of donor hematolymphopoietic cells. The key observation was that the mice bearing donor cells (donor leukocyte chimerism) could now accept skin grafts from the original donor strain but from no other strain (Fig. 45-1). The chimeric neonatal mice and the irradiated adult mice were analogues of today's bone marrow transplantation into immune-deficient and cytoablated humans, respectively. But because a good histocompatibility match was required for avoidance of graft-versus-host disease (GVHD) and of rejection,[4] clinical application of bone marrow transplantation had to await discovery of the human leukocyte antigens (HLAs). When this was accomplished,[5–7] the successfully treated human bone marrow recipients of 1968 were oversized versions of the tolerant chimeric mice.

By the time of the clinical bone marrow transplant breakthrough of 1968, kidney transplantation[8–14] already was an established clinical service, albeit a flawed one.[15] In addition, the first long-term survivals had been recorded after liver[16] and heart transplantation[17]; these were followed between 1968 to 1969 by the first prolonged survival of a lung[18] and a pancreas recipient[19] (Table 45-1). All of the organ transplant successes had been accomplished in the ostensible absence of leukocyte chimerism, without HLA matching, and with no evidence of GVHD. By going beyond the leukocyte chimerism boundaries established by the mouse tolerance models, organ transplantation had entered unmapped territory.

"Pseudotolerant" Organ Recipients

Two unexplained features of the alloimmune response had made it feasible to forge ahead precociously with organ transplantation.[14] The first was that organ rejection is highly reversible. The second was that an organ allograft, if protected by nonspecific immunosuppression, could induce its own acceptance. "Self-induced engraftment" was observed for the first time in 1959 in two fraternal twin kidney recipients, first in Boston by Joseph Murray[12] and then in Paris by Jean Hamburger.[8] These were the first successful transplantations in the world of an organ allograft, in any species. Both patients had been conditioned with 450-rad sublethal total-body irradiation before transplantation. The renal allografts functioned for more than 2 decades without a need for maintenance drug therapy, which was, in fact, not yet available.

A similar drug-free state was next occasionally observed after kidney transplantation (and more frequently after liver replacement) in mongrel dogs who were treated with a single immunosuppressive agent: 6-mercaptopurine (6-MP),[20,21] azathioprine,[22,23] prednisone,[24] or antilymphocyte globulin (ALG).[25] After treatment was stopped, rejection in some

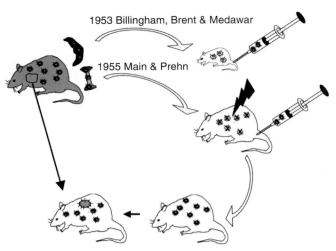

FIGURE 45-1 The mouse models of acquired tolerance described between 1953 and 1956. White cells (leukocytes) were isolated from the spleen or bone marrow of adult donor mice *(upper left)* and injected into the bloodstream of newborn mice *(upper right)* or of irradiated adult mice *(middle right)*. Under both circumstances, the recipient immune system was too weak to reject the foreign cells *(dark shaded)*. With engraftment of the injected cells (i.e., donor leukocyte chimerism), the recipient mice now could freely accept tissues and organs from the leukocyte donor but from no other donor *(bottom left)*.

TABLE 45-1

First Successful Transplantation of Human Allografts (Survival >1 Year)

Physician/ Organ	City	Date	Surgeon	Reference
Kidney	Boston	Jan. 24, 1959	Merrill/ Murray	42, 48
Liver	Denver	July 23, 1967	Starzl	72
Heart	Cape Town	Jan. 2, 1968	Barnard	5
Lung	Ghent	Nov. 14, 1968	Derom	18
Pancreas	Minneapolis	June 3, 1969	Lillehei	34

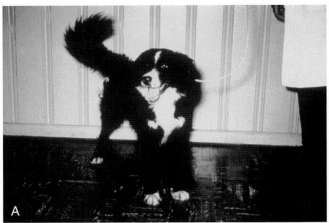

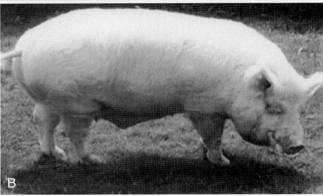

FIGURE 45-2 **A,** Canine recipient of an orthotopic liver homograft, 5 years later. The operation was on March 23, 1964. The dog was treated for only 120 days with azathioprine and died of old age after 13 years. **B,** A spontaneously tolerant pig recipient described by Calne.[29]

animals never developed (Fig. 45-2, *A*). Such results were exceedingly rare, less than 1% of the canine kidney experiments done under 6-MP and azathioprine up to the summer of 1962. However, the possibility that an organ could be inherently tolerogenic was crystallized by the human experience summarized in the title of a report in 1963 of a series of live-donor kidney recipients treated in Denver, "The Reversal of Rejection in Human Renal Homografts with Subsequent Development of Homograft Tolerance."[14] The recipients had been given azathioprine before as well as after renal transplantation, adding large doses of prednisone to treat rejections that were monitored by serial testing of serum creatinine (Fig. 45-3, *A*). Rejection occurred in almost every case, and 25% of the grafts were lost to uncontrolled acute rejection. However, the 1-year survival of 46 allografts, obtained from familial donors during a 16-month period from 1962 to 1963, was an unprecedented 75%.

The development of partial tolerance in many of the survivors was inferred from the rapidly declining need for treatment after rejection reversal (see Fig. 45-3, *A*). Nine (19%) of the 46 allografts functioned for the next 4 decades, each depicted in Figure 45-4 as a horizontal bar. Moreover, all

immunosuppression eventually was stopped in seven of the nine patients without rejection for periods ranging from 6 to 40 years (the solid portion of the bars). Eight of the nine patients are still alive and bear the longest surviving organ allografts in the world.[26]

What was the connection between the tolerant mouse models, the irradiated fraternal twin kidney recipients in Boston and Paris, the ultimate drug-free canine organ recipients (see Fig. 45-2, *A*), and the unique cluster of "pseudotolerant" human kidney recipients in Denver (Fig. 45-4)? What were the mechanisms of engraftment and what was the relationship of engraftment to tolerance? The mystery deepened with the demonstration in 1966 in France,[27] England,[28–31] and the United States[32] that the liver can be transplanted in about 20% of outbred pigs without any treatment at all (see Fig. 45-2, *B*). Because graft-versus-host disease had yet to be seen (despite the use of organs from HLA-mismatched donors) none of the animal or human organ recipients, whether off or on maintenance immunosuppression, was thought to have donor leukocyte chimerism to explain organ engraftment.

False Premises of Phase 1

Organ transplantation became disconnected at a very early time from the scientific anchor of leukocyte chimerism that had been established by the mouse models and was soon to

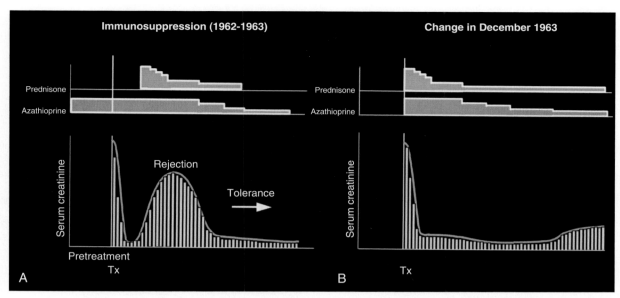

FIGURE 45-3 **A,** Empirically developed immunosuppression used for kidney transplant recipients from 1962 to 1963. Note the reversal of rejection with the addition of prednisone to azathioprine. More than a third of a century later, it was realized that the timing of drug administration had been in accord with the tolerogenic principles of immunosuppression (see text). **B,** Treatment revisions in immunosuppression made at the University of Colorado in December 1963, which unwittingly violated principles of tolerogenic immunosuppression. Pretreatment was de-emphasized or eliminated, and high doses of prednisone were given prophylactically instead of as needed. Although the frequency of acute rejection was reduced, the drug-free tolerance shown in Figure 45-4 was no longer seen. Tx, treatment.

be exemplified by human bone marrow transplantation. The resulting intellectual separation of the two kinds of transplantation (Fig. 45-5) was an unchallenged legacy of phase 1, passed from generation to generation.

There was another dark legacy of phase 1 that began in 1964. This was a modified version of the treatment strategy that had been developed with azathioprine and prednisone (see Fig. 45-3, *B*). The principal change was the use of large prophylactic doses of prednisone from the time of operation, instead of the administration of corticosteroids only when needed. In a second modification, the pretreatment was de-emphasized (see Fig. 45-3, *B*). The incidence of acute rejection was greatly reduced after these changes. However, no cluster of drug-free kidney recipients, such as shown in Figure 45-4, was ever seen again, anywhere in the world. More than

35 years passed before the long-term immunologic consequences of the modifications were realized.

PHASE 2: 1969 TO 1979

Throughout the succeeding phase 2 that began in 1969, immunosuppression for organ transplantation was based on azathioprine and prophylactic high-dose prednisone to which ALG was added after 1966[25,33] in about 15% of centers. Phase 2 was a bleak period. In the view of critics, the heavy mortality, and particularly the devastating morbidity caused by corticosteroid dependence, made organ transplantation (even of kidneys) as much a disease as a treatment. Most of the liver and heart transplant programs that had been established in an initial burst of optimism after the first successful cases closed down.

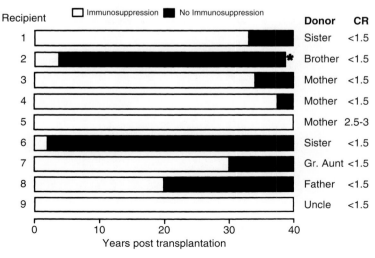

Recipient		Donor	CR
1		Sister	<1.5
2		Brother	<1.5
3		Mother	<1.5
4		Mother	<1.5
5		Mother	2.5-3
6		Sister	<1.5
7		Gr. Aunt	<1.5
8		Father	<1.5
9		Uncle	<1.5

□ Immunosuppression ■ No Immunosuppression

Years post transplantation

FIGURE 45-4 Nine (19%) of the 46 live-donor kidney recipients treated at the University of Colorado during an 18-month period beginning in the autumn of 1962. The solid portion of the horizontal bars depicts the time off immunosuppression. Note that the current serum creatinine concentration (CR) is normal in all but one patient. *Murdered: kidney allograft normal at autopsy.

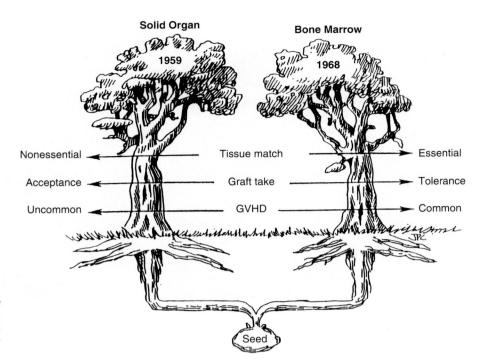

Nonessential ←	Tissue match	→ Essential
Acceptance ←	Graft take	→ Tolerance
Uncommon ←	GVHD	→ Common

Seed

FIGURE 45-5 The developmental tree of bone marrow *(right)* and organ transplantation *(left)* after it was demonstrated that rejection is an immunologic response. GVHD, graft-versus-host disease.

But in the few remaining centers, patients, such as the one shown in Figure 45-6, bore witness to what some day would be accomplished on a grand scale. Four years old at the time of her liver replacement for biliary atresia and a hepatoma in 1969, the patient depicted is the longest surviving recipient of an extrarenal organ.

PHASE 3: 1980 TO 1991

In fact, what had appeared to be the sunset of extrarenal organ transplantation was only the dawn of phase 3, which began with the clinical introduction of cyclosporine,[34–37] followed a decade later by that of tacrolimus.[38–41] The use of these drugs was associated with stepwise improvements with all organs, but their impact was most conclusively demonstrated with liver and heart transplantation. The results with liver transplantation shown in Figure 45-7 using azathioprine-, cyclosporine-, and tacrolimus-based immunosuppression were presented at the meeting of the American Surgical Association in April 1994.[42] By then, intestinal transplantation under tacrolimus-based immunosuppression had become a service.[43,44]

As the new agents became available, they were simply incorporated into the modified formula of heavy prophylactic immunosuppression that had been inherited from phases 1 and 2. Used in a variety of multiple-agent combinations from

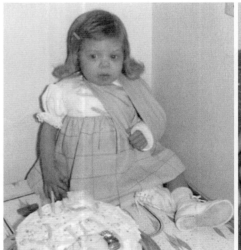
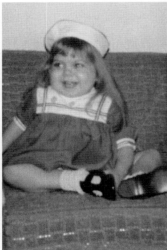
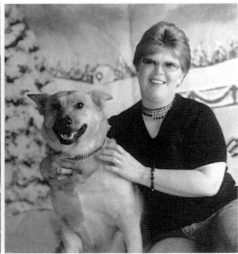

FIGURE 45-6 Four years old at the time of liver replacement for biliary atresia and a hepatoma, but now in her 40th post-transplant year (shown here at 35 years post-transplant), the (former) patient is the longest-surviving recipient of an extrarenal organ.

the time of surgery, the better drugs fueled the golden age of transplantation of the 1980s and early 1990s. Acute rejection had become almost a "nonproblem." However, the unresolved issues now were chronic rejection, risks of long-term immunosuppression (e.g., infections and de novo malignancies),

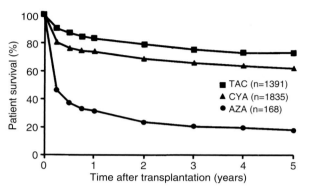

FIGURE 45-7 Patient survival: results with orthotopic liver transplantation at the Universities of Colorado (1963 to 1980) and Pittsburgh (1981 to 1993), in periods defined by azathioprine (AZA)-, cyclosporine (CYA)-, and tacrolimus (TAC)-based immune suppression. Stepwise improvements associated with the advent of these drugs also were made with other organs.

and drug toxicity (e.g., the nephrotoxicity of cyclosporine and tacrolimus).

PHASE 4: 1992 TO PRESENT

It was clear that relief from the burden of lifetime immunosuppression would require elucidation of the mechanisms of alloengraftment and of acquired tolerance. An intensified search for the engraftment mechanisms has dominated the current phase 4, which began in the early 1990s. There was a growing realization (particularly with recipients of liver allografts), that immunosuppression could be withdrawn successfully in selected cases, which sparked various prospective trials of immunosuppression withdrawal.[45]

Historical Dogma

Until this time, organ engraftment had been attributed to mechanisms that did not involve either the presence or a role of leukocyte chimerism. Although it was known that organs contain large numbers of passenger leukocytes, these donor cells were largely replaced in the successfully transplanted allograft by recipient leukocytes as shown in Figure 45-8, *A*. The missing donor cells were thought to have undergone

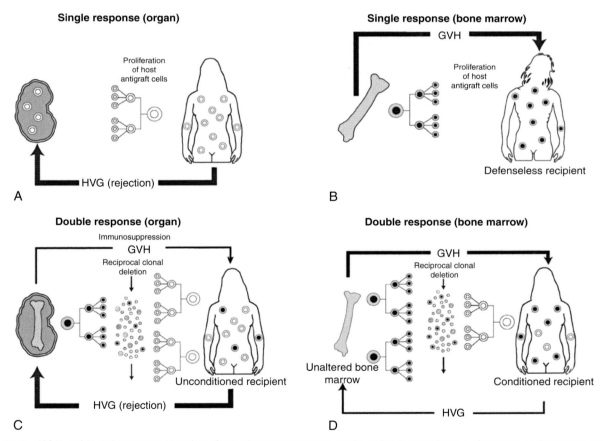

FIGURE 45-8 Old (**A** and **B**) and new views (**C** and **D**) of transplantation recipients. **A,** The early conceptualization of immune mechanisms in organ transplantation in terms of a unidirectional host-versus-graft (HVG) response. Although this readily explained organ rejection, it limited possible explanations of organ engraftment. **B,** Mirror image of **A** depicting the early understanding of successful bone marrow transplantation as a complete replacement of the recipient immune system by that of the donor, with the potential complication of an unopposed lethal unidirectional graft-versus-host (GVH) response, that is, rejection of the recipient by the graft. **C,** Our current view of bidirectional and reciprocally modulating immune responses of coexisting immune-competent cell populations. Because of variable reciprocal induction of deletional tolerance, organ engraftment was feasible despite a usually dominant HVG reaction. The bone silhouette in the graft represents passenger leukocytes of bone marrow origin. **D,** Our currently conceived mirror image of **C** after successful bone marrow transplantation. Recipient's cytoablation has caused a reversal of the size proportions of the donor and recipient populations of immune cells.

immune destruction with selective sparing of the specialized parenchymal cells. As for bone marrow transplantation (see Fig. 45-8, *B*), the ideal result had been perceived as complete replacement of recipient immune cells (i.e., total hematolymphopoietic chimerism).

Discovery of Microchimerism

A flaw in this historical dogma began to be exposed in the early 1990s. The first puzzling observation in Seattle[46] and Helsinki[47] was the invariable presence of a small residual population of recipient hematolymphopoietic cells in patients previously thought to have complete bone marrow replacement (see Fig. 45-8, *D*). This was followed in 1992 by the discovery of donor leukocyte microchimerism in long-surviving human organ recipients. Now it was evident that organ engraftment (see Figure 45-8, *C*) and bone marrow cell engraftment (see Fig. 45-8, *D*) were mirror-image versions of leukocyte chimerism, differing in the reversed proportion of donor and recipient cells.

The discovery of microchimerism in organ recipients was made with a very simple clinical study.[48–52] With the use of sensitive detection techniques, donor hematolymphopoietic cells of different lineages (including dendritic cells) were found in the blood, lymph nodes, skin, or other tissues of 30 of 30 liver or kidney recipients who had borne functioning allografts for up to 30 years. The donor leukocytes obviously were progeny of donor precursor or pluripotent hematolymphopoietic stem cells that had migrated from the graft into the recipient after surviving a double immune reaction that presumably had occurred just after transplantation, years or decades earlier.[53–56]

It was concluded that organ engraftment had been the result of "responses of coexisting donor and recipient cells, each to the other, causing reciprocal clonal exhaustion, followed by peripheral clonal deletion."[48,50] The host response (the upright curve in Fig. 45-9) was the dominant one in most cases of organ transplantation but with the occasional exception of GVHD. In the conventionally treated bone marrow recipient, host cytoablation simply transferred immune dominance from the host to the graft (the inverted curve in Fig. 45-9), explaining the high risk of GVHD. All of the major differences between the two kinds of transplantation were caused by the recipient cytoablation. After an estrangement of more than a third of a century, the intellectual separation of bone marrow and organ transplantation was ended (Fig. 45-10).

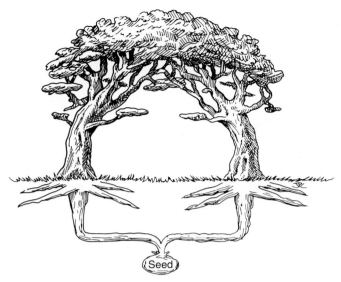

FIGURE 45-10 Unification of organ and bone marrow transplantation (see text).

Immune Regulation by Antigen Migration and Localization

But how was the exhaustion-deletion of the double immune reaction shown in Figure 45-9 maintained after its acute induction by the first wave of migratory leukocytes? Rolf Zinkernagel, in Zurich (Fig. 45-11), had addressed this question during the 1990s in experimental studies of the nonresponsiveness that may develop to intracellular microorganisms, such as tubercle bacillus and noncytopathic viruses.[57–60] The analogies between the syndromes caused by such infectious agents and the events following transplantation were described in 1998 in a joint review with Zinkernagel in the *New England Journal of Medicine*.[61]

The analogies between transplantation and infection had been obscured by the characteristic double immune reaction of transplantation and by the complicating factor of immunosuppression. Now, these analogies were obvious. The antidonor response induced by the initially selective migration of the graft's leukocytes to host lymphoid organs (Fig. 45-12, *left*)[62–65] is comparable to the response induced by a spreading intracellular pathogen. The migration patterns of the donor leukocytes were the same whether these cells emigrated from an organ or were delivered as a bone marrow

FIGURE 45-9 Contemporaneous HVG (*upright curves*) and GVH (*inverted curves*) responses after transplantation. In contrast to the usually dominant HVG reaction of organ transplantation, the GVH reaction usually is dominant after bone marrow cell transplantation to the irradiated or otherwise immunodepressed recipient. Therapeutic failure with either type of transplantation implies the inability to control one, the other, or both of the contemporaneous responses with a protective umbrella of immunosuppression.[61]

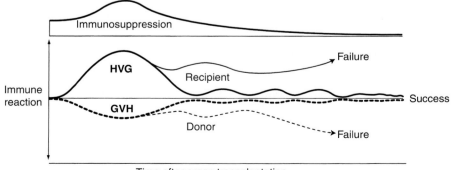

Time after organ transplantation

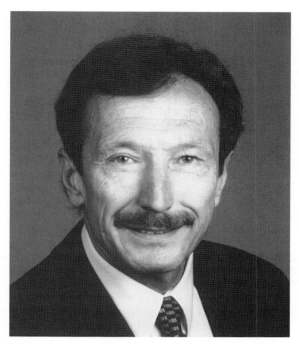

FIGURE 45-11   Rolf Zinkernagel. Swiss physician-immunologist whose discovery, with Peter Doherty, of the mechanisms of the adaptive immune response to noncytopathic microorganisms earned them the Nobel prize in 1996.

cell infusion. Cells that survived the antidonor response that they had induced begin within a few days to move on (see Fig. 45-12, *right*) to protected nonlymphoid niches, where their presence no longer may be detected by the immune system (immune ignorance[61,66–69]). This was a survival tactic of noncytopathic microorganisms.

The migration of donor leukocytes is shown schematically in Figure 45-13, *left* by centrifugal arrows: first by hematogenous routes to lymphoid organs and, after a few weeks, on to nonlymphoid sites (*outer circle*). A subsequent reverse migration of donor cells from protected nonlymphoid niches back to host lymphoid organs is depicted by the inwardly directed *dashed arrows* in Figure 45-13, *right*. The retrograde migration is a two-edged sword. On the one hand, these cells may sustain the clonal exhaustion-deletion induced at the outset, usually requiring an umbrella of maintenance immunosuppression. But on the other hand, these cells can perpetuate alloimmunity in the same way as surviving residual microorganisms perpetuate protective immunity. Not surprisingly, therefore, an alternative consequence of microchimerism may be the high-panel reactive antibody (connoting sensitization to HLA antigens) that commonly develops after unsuccessful transplantation.[70,71]

Therapeutic Implications

How could the new insight be exploited clinically? The window of opportunity for the donor leukocyte-induced clonal deletion that corresponds with collapse of the antigraft response (Fig. 45-14, *left*) is open only for the first few

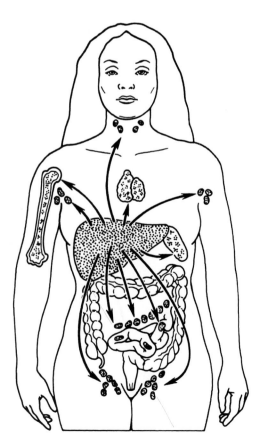
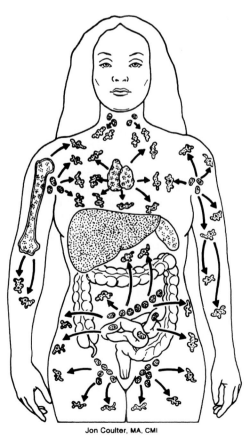

Jon Coulter, MA, CMI

FIGURE 45-12   Initial preferential migration of passenger leukocytes from organ allografts (here a liver) to host lymphoid organs *(left),* where they induce a donor-specific immune response. After about 30 days, many of the surviving cells move on to nonlymphoid sites *(right).*

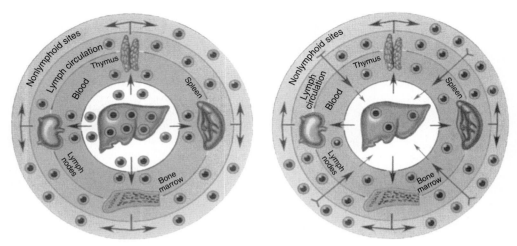

FIGURE 45-13 The migration routes of passenger leukocytes of transplanted organs are similar to those of infused bone marrow cells. *Left,* Selective migration at first to host lymphoid organs. After 15 to 30 days, surviving leukocytes begin to secondarily move to nonlymphoid sites. *Right,* Establishment of reverse traffic by which the exhaustion-deletion induced at the outset can be maintained.

post-transplant weeks.[55,72–74] It was apparent that the window could be closed by excessive postoperative immunosuppression (Fig. 45-14, *middle*). With later reduction of the initial overimmunosuppression, recovery of the inefficiently deleted clone would be expected, leading to the delayed acute rejection, or the chronic rejection, that was being seen in the transplant clinics. Even in the best-case scenario, the patients would be predestined to lifetime dependence on immunosuppression. However, too little immunosuppression would result in uncontrolled rejection (Fig. 45-14, *right*).

The problem faced by clinicians was how to find just the right amount of post-transplant immunosuppression. In 2001, it was suggested that this dilemma could be addressed by successively applying two historically rooted therapeutic principles: recipient pretreatment, followed by minimalistic post-transplant immunosuppression.[75] With pretreatment, the recipient's immune responsiveness would be reduced before exposure to donor antigen, thereby lowering the anticipated donor-specific response to a more readily deletable range (Fig. 45-15). Clonal deletion by the kidneys' passenger leukocytes undoubtedly is what had been accomplished after sublethal irradiation alone in the ground-breaking fraternal twin (i.e., sublethal total-body irradiation or myelotoxic drugs) cases of 1959.[8,12] In fact, radical pretreatment by recipient cytoablation ultimately became the essential therapeutic step for conventional bone marrow transplantation. Because

of the high risk of GVHD, this approach was too dangerous and too restrictive to be practical for organ transplantation.

However, less drastic lymphoid depletion by ALG or other measures (so-called nonmyeloablative conditioning) had been repeatedly shown since the 1960s to be effective without causing GVHD[33] (see Fig. 45-15).

After pretreatment with one of today's potent antilymphoid antibody preparations, the preemptively weakened clonal activation could proceed efficiently to clonal deletion under minimalistic short- and long-term maintenance therapy (Fig. 45-16). In July 2001, we instituted the double-principle strategy in adult organ recipients. The pretreatment was with a single infusion of 5 mg/kg of Thymoglobulin. Beginning in 2002, a single Campath dose of 30 mg was substituted for Thymoglobulin in most adult cases. After either kind of lymphoid depletion, treatment after transplantation was given with a conservative daily dose of a single drug (usually tacrolimus), adding other agents only in the event of breakthrough rejection and for as brief a period as

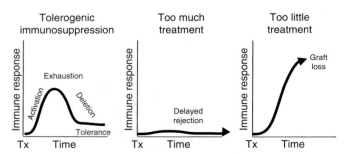

FIGURE 45-14 The effect of post-transplant immunosuppression on the seminal mechanism of clonal exhaustion-deletion. *Left,* Just the right amount. *Middle,* Too much. *Right,* Too little (see text). Tx, treatment.

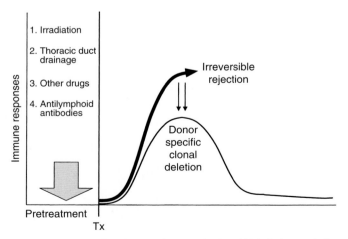

FIGURE 45-15 Rather than producing rejection *(thick dark arrow),* the donor-specific immune response to allografts may be exhausted and deleted, as depicted by the fall of the initially ascending continuous thin line, when recipient immune responsiveness is weakened in advance of transplantation (the pretreatment principle). Tx, treatment.

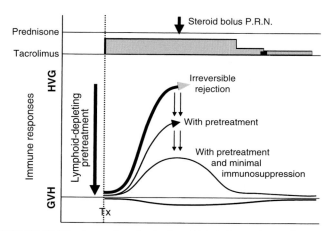

FIGURE 45-16 Conversion of rejection *(thick dark arrow)* to an immune response that can be exhausted and deleted by combination of pretreatment and minimalistic post-transplant immunosuppression. Tx, treatment.

possible. The strategy was extended to infants and children for intestinal transplantation in 2002 and for all kidney transplantations after April 2003.[76]

After 4 to 8 months, weaning from monotherapy to less-than-daily doses was begun in adults whose graft function was stable: every other day, then three times per week, twice a week, and in many cases to once a week by 1 year (Fig. 45-17). The strategy has been used for the treatment of more than 1000 adult kidney, liver, intestine, pancreas, and lung recipients.[77–79] This experience has demonstrated that the quality of life of transplant recipients can be improved. For the first time, children are being considered for spaced weaning.

These and other clinical trials have spawned definitions of clinical or operational tolerance (normal graft function without features of graft rejection and without the need for immunosuppressive drugs), and "prope," or "near" tolerance (the state of normal graft function in the presence of minimal or undetectable levels of immunosuppression).[80,81] However, achieving this on a consistent basis may hinge on the development of standardized clinically applicable markers of immune tolerance that can assess the appropriateness of this clinical strategy on the individual patient. Prospective weaning trials sponsored by the Immune Tolerance Network are currently underway in stable adult and pediatric recipients of liver allografts, incorporating the aforementioned strategies and mechanistic studies.[82]

Organ Preservation

PROCUREMENT

The breakthroughs of the early 1960s that made transplantation clinically practical were so unexpected that almost no formal preparation had been made to preserve the transplanted organs. Cardiac surgeons had used hypothermia for open-heart operations from 1950 onward and knew that ischemic damage below the level of aortic cross-clamping could be reduced by cooling the subdiaphragmatic organs.[83] In an early report, Lillehei and colleagues[84] immersed intestines in iced saline before autotransplantation. In Boston, Sicular and Moore[85] reported greatly slowed enzyme degradation in cold slices of liver.

Despite this awareness, kidneys were routinely transplanted until 1963 with no protection from warm ischemia during organ transfer. The only attempt to cool kidney allografts until then was by the potentially dangerous practice (used by thoracic surgeons for open-heart surgery) of immersing the live donor in a bathtub of ice water (total-body hypothermia).[86] This cumbersome method of cooling was quickly replaced by infusion of chilled solutions into the renal artery after donor nephrectomy,[87] exploiting a principle of core (transvascular) cooling that had been standardized several years earlier for experimental liver transplantation.[88]

Core cooling in situ, the first critical step in the preservation of all cadaveric whole organs, is done today with variations of the technique described in 1963 by Marchioro and coworkers,[89] which permits in situ cooling to be undertaken[90] (Fig. 45-18). Ackermann and Snell[91] and Merkel and associates[92] popularized in situ cooling of cadaveric kidneys with simple infusion of cold electrolyte solutions into the donor femoral artery or distal aorta. Procurement techniques were eventually perfected that allowed removal of all thoracic and abdominal organs, including the liver, without jeopardizing any of the individual organs (Fig. 45-19).[93] Modifications of this flexible procedure have been made for unstable donors and even for donors whose hearts have stopped beating.[94] During the 5 years between 1980 and 1985, such techniques had become interchangeable in all parts of the world, setting the stage for reliable organ sharing. After the chilled organs are removed, subsequent preservation is possible with prototype strategies: simple refrigeration or continuous perfusion (see later).

EXTENDED PRESERVATION

Continuous Vascular Perfusion

Efforts to continuously perfuse isolated organs have proved to be difficult. For renal allografts, Ackermann and Barnard[95] used a normothermic perfusate primed with blood that was oxygenated within a hyperbaric chamber. Brettschneider and colleagues[96] modified the apparatus and were able to preserve canine livers for 2 days, an unprecedented feat at the time. When Belzer and associates[97] eliminated the hemoglobin and hyperbaric chamber components, their asanguineous hypothermic perfusion technique was immediately accepted for clinical renal transplantation but then slowly abandoned

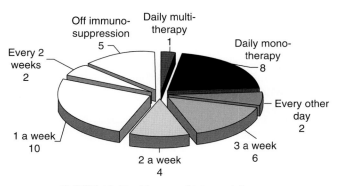

FIGURE 45-17 Diagram of 2.5-year follow-up.

FIGURE 45-18 First technique of in situ cooling by extracorporeal hypothermic perfusion. The catheters were inserted into the aorta and vena cava through the femoral vessels as soon as possible after death. Temperature control was provided with a heat exchanger. Cross-clamping of the thoracic aorta limited perfusion to the lower part of the body. This method of cadaveric organ procurement was used from 1962 to 1969, before the acceptance of brain death criteria. The preliminary stages of this approach provided the basis for subsequent in situ infusion techniques.

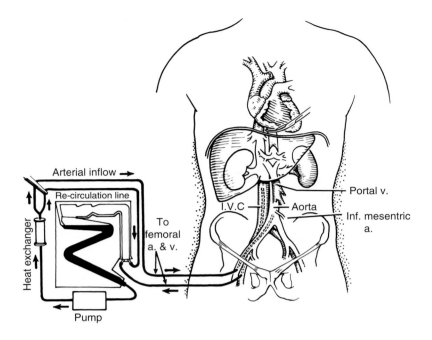

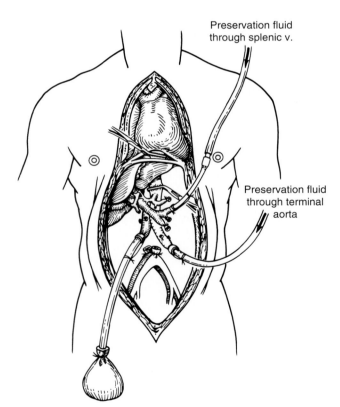

FIGURE 45-19 Principle of in situ cooling used for multiple organ procurement. With limited preliminary dissection of the aorta and of the great splanchnic veins (in this case, the splenic vein), cold infusates can be used to chill organs in situ. In this case, the kidneys and liver were being removed. Note the aortic cross-clamp above the celiac axis.

in most centers when it was learned that the quality of 2-day preservation was not markedly better than that of simpler and less expensive infusion and slush methods (see later). However, refinement of perfusion techniques may someday permit true organ banking.

Static Preservation

With these "slush techniques," special solutions, such as those described by Collins and coworkers,[98] were instilled into the renal vascular system of kidneys or the vascular system of other organs after their preliminary chilling and separation. The original Collins solution or modifications of it were used for nearly 2 decades before they were replaced with the University of Wisconsin (UW) solution that was developed by the team of Folkert Belzer. Although it was first used for the liver,[99–101] the UW solution provides superior preservation of kidneys and other organs.[102,103] The UW preservation permitted longer and safer preservation of kidneys (2 days) and livers (18 hours), a higher rate of graft survival, and a lower rate of primary nonfunction. With the UW solution, national organ sharing was made economical and practical. This success has refocused efforts on understanding the mechanisms involved in the ischemia/reperfusion injury (deprivation and then restoration of tissue oxygen) that impacts organ function, and has resulted in the development of other preservation solutions (Celsior, HTK: histidine-tryptophan-ketoglutarate) and the inclusion of drugs that act on the mediators of injury.[104]

Tissue Typing

ANTIGEN MATCHING

The human leukocyte antigen (HLA) system has an important role in immune regulation and is thus a barrier that must be avoided (with better matching) or modified (with immunosuppressive strategies). HLA class I A, B, and C, and HLA class II DR, DQ, and DP molecules are expressed on various cell types that, when bound to a specific repertoire of peptides, present to CD8+ or CD4+ T cells. Patient and donor matching is of significant importance in bone marrow transplantation in order to prevent lethal GVHD but of variable importance in solid organ transplantation.[105]

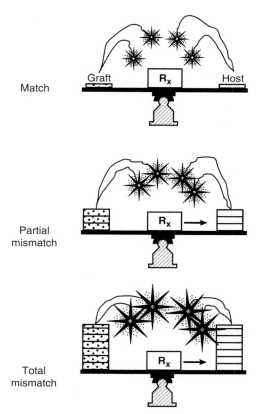

FIGURE 45-20 The nullification effect of simultaneous host-versus-graft (HVG) and graft-versus-host (GVH) reactions when organs are transplanted to recipients whose immune system has not been cytoablated. The reciprocal induction of tolerance, each to the other, of the coexisting cell populations is the explanation for the poor correlation of human leukocyte antigen (HLA) matching with outcome after organ transplantation.

The first prospective antigen matching trials were begun in 1964 by Terasaki and associates[106] in collaboration with the University of Colorado kidney transplantation team. Although the value of this serologic technology was demonstrable when the kidney donor was a highly compatible family member (the "perfect match"),[107] lesser degrees of matching correlated poorly with renal transplantation outcome.[108] The reasons for this paradox were inexplicable until the discovery of recipient chimerism (Fig. 45-20). However, the belief that matching should be a prime determinant of success resulted in its use as an overriding factor for the allocation of cadaver kidneys in the United States.

The propriety of this kidney allocation policy has been repeatedly challenged on ethical as well as scientific grounds for nearly a third of a century. Those in favor of perpetuating the role of graded HLA matches cite multicenter case compilations in the United States and Europe showing a small gain in allograft survival with histocompatible kidneys, whereas many of the individual contributing centers see no such trend in their own experience.[83,109-111] In a compelling study, Terasaki and associates[112] reported that early survival and the subsequent half-life of kidneys from randomly matched, living unrelated donors was identical to that of parent–offspring (one haplotype–matched) grafts. The inescapable conclusion is that more effective timing and dosage of immunosuppressive therapy, rather than refinements in tissue matching and organ sharing, will be the primary method of improving the results of whole organ transplantation.

CROSSMATCHING

None of the immunosuppressive measures available today can prevent immediate destruction of kidneys and other kinds of organ grafts in what has been called hyperacute rejection. This complication was first seen with the transplantation of kidneys from ABO-incompatible donors when they were placed in recipients with antidonor isoagglutinins.[113] After the description by Terasaki and associates[114] of hyperacute kidney rejection by a recipient with antidonor lymphocytotoxic antibodies, Kissmeyer-Nielsen and colleagues[115] and others[116-119] confirmed the association of hyperacute rejection with these antigraft antibodies. Although hyperacute rejection can usually be avoided with the lymphocytotoxic crossmatch originally recommended by Terasaki and associates, the precise pathogenesis of such rejection remains poorly understood more than 30 years after its recognition as a complement activation syndrome.[116,117]

Future Prospects

The revisions in timing and dose control that encourage the seminal mechanisms of clonal exhaustion-deletion and immune ignorance should make it possible to systematically reduce exposure to the risks of chronic immunosuppression. Our prediction is that completely drug-free tolerance will be largely, but not exclusively, limited to recipients of HLA-matched organs. But variable partial tolerance will be more regularly attainable in most of the others, not so much by developing better drugs but by the mechanism-based use of drugs we already have in hand. Xenotransplantation will have to be developed within the same immunologic framework. Here, the problem, in principle, is to create a better interspecies tissue match by transgenic modification. Although the α-1,3GT gene responsible for hyperacute rejection of pig organs by higher primates has been knocked out in pigs,[120] it is not yet known what further changes have to be made before porcine organs can be used clinically. Where stem cell biology will fit remains unknown, but it also will have to conform to the same immunologic rules.

The complete reference list is available online at www. expertconsult.com.

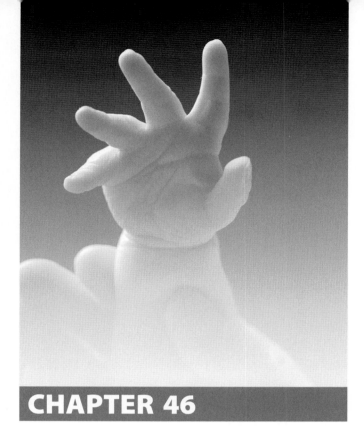

CHAPTER 46

Renal Transplantation

John C. Magee

Transplantation is the preferred treatment for children with end-stage renal disease (ESRD), because it provides the best opportunity for health, growth, and development. Progress continues in pediatric transplantation, and current patient and graft survival is excellent.

Although single-center reports provide insight into many issues, larger registry data provide a more substantive overview of the state of transplantation. The leading registry is the North American Pediatric Renal Trials and Collaborative Studies (NAPRTCS).[1,2] In addition, data for all transplantations performed in the United States are collected through the Organ Procurement Transplant Network (OPTN), and they are regularly analyzed by the Scientific Registry of Transplant Recipients (SRTR).[3,4]

End-Stage Renal Disease in Children

According to the United States Renal Data System (USRDS), 1343 individuals aged 19 years or younger began treatment for ESRD in 2008.[5] The incidence of ESRD in this age group is 15.5 per million per year. Because ESRD is much more

uncommon in children, this rate is well below the overall national incidence of ESRD of 362 per million per year.

The etiology of renal disease in the pediatric transplantation population is summarized in Table 46-1. According to these NAPRTCS data, the five most common diagnoses are renal aplasia/hypoplasia/dysplasia, obstructive uropathy, focal segmental glomerulosclerosis (FSGS), reflux nephropathy, and chronic glomerulonephritis.[1] These diagnoses account for just over half the transplantations performed. The causes of renal failure are distinctly different from those in adults; specifically, congenital abnormalities and obstructive uropathy are the leading causes for transplantation. In addition, FSGS is the most common acquired renal disease and is much more common in children compared with adults.

Within the pediatric population, the prevalence of causes varies by age, sex, and race.[1] Congenital causes are more prevalent in younger children, whereas acquired diseases tend to become manifest in older children. Overall, 59.4% of the recipients are male, and males represent the majority of the recipients with obstructive uropathy (85.2%), aplasia/ hypoplasia/dysplasia (61.8%), and FSGS (57.8%). Reflux nephropathy, chronic glomerulonephritis, and lupus nephritis are more prevalent in females, with females accounting for 56.7%, 57.0%, and 83.3%, respectively. Regarding race, for black children, FSGS was the most prevalent diagnosis (23.1%), followed by obstructive uropathy (15%) and aplasia/hypoplasia/dysplasia (13.5%). In white recipients, obstructive uropathy was the most prevalent etiology (17.0%), followed by aplasia/hypoplasia/dysplasia (16.9%) and FSGS (9.0%).

Recipient Evaluation

Any child with ESRD should be considered for transplantation. Absolute contraindications are rare and include untreated malignancy or systemic sepsis. Relative contraindications include severe systemic disease that profoundly limits the patient's life span or a social situation that makes follow-up with post-transplantation care and immunosuppression regimen absolutely impossible. At times, the decision whether to transplant a child with a poor quality of life or significant impairment can be extremely difficult. In such situations, a thorough discussion focused on the expectations and goals for that child is helpful.

All children with progressive chronic renal insufficiency should be evaluated by a multidisciplinary pediatric transplantation team, including a pediatric nephrologist, a transplantation surgeon, social worker, and nutritionist. In addition, many teams include pediatric urologists and clinical psychologists, with other experts included as indicated. Ideally, the child would be fully evaluated before initiating dialysis. This can facilitate evaluation of potential living donors and permit preemptive transplantation, obviating the need for dialysis. Regarding infant size, although it is often stated that approaching 10.0 kg is ideal, it is clear that transplantation can be performed successfully in smaller infants at experienced centers.[6–8] The guiding principle should be to optimize the situation as much as possible but not let an arbitrary weight target compromise the health of the child.

Our standard evaluation process is summarized in Table 46-2. Every effort should be made to optimize the

TABLE 46-1

Primary Diagnosis for Renal Transplantation Recipients (N = 9854) Age 20 Years and Younger

Disease	%
Aplasia/hypoplasia/dysplasia	15.9
Obstructive uropathy	15.6
Focal segmental glomerulosclerosis	11.7
Reflux nephropathy	5.2
Chronic glomerulonephritis	3.3
Polycystic disease	2.9
Medullary cystic disease	2.8
Hemolytic-uremic syndrome	2.6
Prune-belly syndrome	2.6
Congenital nephrotic syndrome	2.6
Familial nephritis	2.3
Cystinosis	2.0
Pyelointerstitial nephritis	1.8
Membranoproliferative glomerulonephritis type I	1.7
Idiopathic crescentic glomerulonephritis	1.7
Systemic lupus erythematosus nephritis	1.5
Renal infarct	1.4
Berger (IgA) nephritis	1.3
Henoch-Schönlein nephritis	1.1
Membranoproliferative glomerulonephritis type II	0.8
Wegener granulomatosis	0.6
Wilms' tumor	0.5
Drash syndrome	0.5
Oxalosis	0.5
Membranous nephropathy	0.4
Other systemic immunologic disease	0.3
Sickle cell nephropathy	0.2
Diabetic glomerulonephritis	0.1
Other	9.8
Unknown	6.2

From North American Pediatric Renal Trials and Collaborative Study (NAPRTCS) 2008 Annual Report. Available at www.naprtcs.org. Accessed March 20, 2010.

TABLE 46-2

Evaluation of Pediatric Kidney Transplantation Candidate

History and physical examination
Laboratory tests:
   Hematologic (complete blood cell count with platelets; prothrombin time/partial thromboplastin time)
   Biochemistry (renal function, electrolytes, liver function)
   Serologic studies (hepatitis herpesvirus B and C, cytomegalovirus, Epstein-Barr virus, varicella-zoster virus, human immunodeficiency virus)
   ABO blood typing
   Tissue typing (human leukocyte antigen typing; alloantibody screening)
Urinalysis
Chest radiograph
Electrocardiogram
Psychosocial assessment
As indicated evaluations:
   Voiding cystourethrogram/urodynamic studies
   Vascular imaging
   Hypercoagulable workup

medical management of the child with ESRD, including management of bone disease, optimization of nutrition, and completing childhood immunizations. Several aspects of the evaluation of the pediatric recipient are unique and deserve special attention. One is the evaluation and management of bladder function. Urologic anomalies are common, and many will have also undergone previous urologic procedures. Rarely, the bladder may be inadequate for transplantation. Expertise in such issues, or a close working collaboration with pediatric urology, is essential. Nutrition is also of paramount importance to optimize growth and development. Finally, it is important to evaluate and optimize issues related to the psychological state of the child and caregivers.[9] Adequate social support is vital for all involved. The stress of a chronically ill child undergoing a complex procedure places a great strain on all, and the need for ongoing education and reassurance is significant. In older children, it is important to ensure they are actively involved. Adolescents can be particularly challenging, because the risk of noncompliance appears to be greatest in this group.

In addition to these factors, several other issues require special attention. One is the potential need to evaluate the patient's vasculature. As renal replacement therapy has improved, it is now possible to successfully hemodialyze smaller children, including neonates. These therapies require indwelling catheters, leading to increased rates of iliac and vena cava thrombosis. The lack of adequate venous outflow can make transplantation difficult and limit the standard options.[10] Thomas and coworkers proposed a screening algorithm for patients at risk, focusing on young children with a history of femoral vein catheterization or history of any intra-abdominal process associated with inflammation.[11] In addition, patients with a history of venous thrombosis, early graft loss, or recurrent vascular access thrombosis should be under evaluation for a hypercoagulable state. Good results can be obtained in such patients with anticoagulation prophylaxis.[12]

The potential need for native nephrectomy should be addressed. Native nephrectomy is much more common in children compared with adults. Nationally, 22% of children have had all native renal tissue removed before transplantation.[1] Potential indications for native nephrectomy include recurrent severe infections because of reflux nephropathy, uncontrolled hypertension, and congenital nephrotic syndrome. In the case of nephrotic syndrome, the concern centers on these children being hypercoagulable because of the significant proteinuria. Children with polycystic kidney disease may require native nephrectomies if there is recurrent bleeding, infections, or pain. In select cases, nephrectomy may be warranted if the kidneys are so enlarged that the transplanted kidney would be compromised. Some contend that massive polyuria in small infants is an indication for nephrectomy, arguing that postoperative fluid management is made easier, thus decreasing the risk of graft hypoperfusion. Although this may have appeal, careful attention to postoperative management can often avoid this as the sole indication for nephrectomy. In addition, some believe that children with FSGS should undergo native nephrectomy, suggesting it simplifies the diagnosis of recurrent disease, because any proteinuria reflects disease in the graft rather than persistent proteinuria from the native kidneys. In such situations, an attempt at "medical nephrectomy" with nonsteroidal therapy is worth consideration.

In addition to a rational consideration of the risks and benefits of native nephrectomy, the timing of the nephrectomy is important. In children on renal replacement therapy, bilateral native nephrectomies may be safer and easier to accomplish in the weeks before transplantation. In children not on renal replacement therapy, the issue is more complex. We prefer not to perform bilateral nephrectomies at transplantation because this combines two major procedures. We also perform the transplant through a retroperitoneal approach even in small infants, which does not provide access to the contralateral native kidney. For children requiring bilateral native nephrectomy, and who are not yet on dialysis, some will have sufficient renal reserve to tolerate a unilateral left nephrectomy before transplantation and still not require dialysis. In this situation, at transplantation we extend the standard right retroperitoneal incision slightly cephalad and perform a right native nephrectomy. In cases where unilateral native nephrectomy prior to transplantation would require initiation of renal replacement therapy, we typically remove the ipsilateral native kidney during the transplantation procedure. The remaining contralateral native kidney can be removed several months after transplantation if still indicated.

In considering when to perform the transplantation, any child currently on renal replacement therapy should undergo transplantation as soon as a suitable living donor is identified or a deceased donor organ becomes available. In children not yet on dialysis, transplantation should be performed before the onset of symptoms of uremia. It is important to be aware of the impact of ESRD on growth and development. In patients with FSGS or lupus nephritis, transplantation is typically delayed until the disease is quiescent, which may preclude preemptive transplantation. In most other situations, preemptive transplantation provides significant benefit by obviating the need for dialysis. Unfortunately, only 33% of children who receive a living donor transplant and only 13% of deceased donor recipients are transplanted before initiation of dialysis.[13]

Urologic Issues

The high incidence of urologic issues in children requires careful evaluation of bladder function before transplantation.[14] In addition to dysplasia and bladder outlet obstruction, bladder function may be abnormal because of neuropathy, acquired voiding dysfunction, or acquired bladder pathology. Any previous surgical bladder augmentation will impair normal bladder function. A history of urinary incontinence, frequent urinary tract infections, previous urologic procedures, and the need for bladder catheterization should prompt further investigation. In patients with suspected bladder dysfunction, a voiding cystourethrogram (VCUG) should be obtained with urodynamic measurements. A pressure of less than 30 cm H_2O during the filling portion of the VCUG generally indicates the bladder will be suitable.

The timing of any surgical intervention warrants careful consideration. In some patients with anuria/oliguria, the bladder may not be functional, although it is often too early to tell if it will eventually become suitable. Once bladder augmentation is performed, the patient will need to continue catheterizing long term, because the bladder will not have normal function. Urologic procedures that preserve native renal function for many years are clearly prudent, but interventions before transplantation should be planned by carefully considering the risks and benefits of the procedure and being mindful of the impact on subsequent transplantation and long-term management.

Dialysis Access

For children who do not undergo preemptive transplantation or who initially present with ESRD, establishment of adequate dialysis access is of paramount importance. Proper dialysis access is necessary for adequate dialysis, which is directly linked to the quality of life and health of the patient. According to USRDS data, at the end of 2008, 60% of patients aged 19 years and younger were on hemodialysis, whereas 40% were on peritoneal dialysis.[5] Both are suitable options, and the choice is best made on an individual basis, considering the patient's and family's preferences and skill levels, as well as the treatment options available at the local site.

Regarding hemodialysis, all attempts should be made to create a primary arterial venous fistula. For patients without adequate veins, a polytetrafluoroethylene graft is required. A native fistula is preferred because of superior patency rates, but they require several weeks to mature before being accessed. For patients in need of urgent hemodialysis, the only option is a temporary catheter. Approximately three fourths of pediatric patients have a temporary catheter at the time of initiation of dialysis.[15] The use of these catheters is associated with increased risks of infection and poor clearance with dialysis. In addition, catheters can lead to central venous stenosis and thrombosis, making future vascular access efforts more difficult. Accordingly, the jugular vein is preferred rather than the subclavian vein for catheter placement.

Peritoneal dialysis requires placement of a Tenckhoff catheter. A double-cuffed peritoneal dialysis catheter is inserted with the loop of the catheter placed in the pelvis. During the procedure, it is important to ascertain that fluid can instill and drain easily. The use of double-cuffed catheters and orienting the catheter so that it exits the skin pointing downward are associated with a lower incidence of infection.[15]

Donor Selection

Living donor transplantation is the preferred option for all patients with ESRD. Living donor transplantation offers the best outcomes, compared with deceased donor transplantation.[4,16] In addition, living donor transplantation can be performed as soon as a suitable donor is identified, minimizing exposure to ESRD. Living donors may be either genetically related or unrelated to the potential recipient. The results from both types of living donors are equivalent, and both are superior to outcomes from deceased donors. Potential living donors should undergo a full evaluation by a transplant center experienced in this process. The donor must be willing, be in good health, and have two normal kidneys. In addition, the donor and recipient must be ABO compatible. Although there is a growing interest in strategies to cross this barrier, efforts are relatively limited in the pediatric population.[17]

The recipient should also have a negative lymphocytotoxic crossmatch with the potential donor. Crossmatching is done to determine that the recipient does not have preformed antibodies directed against the donor's human leukocyte antigens (HLA), which would likely cause hyperacute rejection and rapid graft loss. The most common causes of anti-HLA antibodies are blood transfusions, previous transplantation, and pregnancy. Strategies to manipulate antidonor antibodies are being investigated and include intravenous immunoglobulin, plasmapheresis, and other agents designed to alter B-cell responses and/or complement.[18–21] Transplanting recipients who are either ABO or anti-HLA antibody incompatible with their donors requires additional immunologic manipulation, with its attendant risks, and the long-term results appear inferior compared with compatible transplantations. Accordingly, there is growing interest in paired kidney exchange programs, which offer a larger living donor pool and the possibility of finding a more compatible donor.[22]

EVALUATION OF THE POTENTIAL LIVING DONOR

Evaluation of potential living donors should occur independent of the recipient's evaluation, giving donor safety the highest priority. Our standard evaluation process is summarized in Table 46-3. Although HLA matching has traditionally played an important role in choosing which living donor to evaluate, current immunosuppression has minimized the impact of matching, and we believe the best potential living donor is the individual who is most motivated. Lacking that distinction, and all other factors being equal, we would choose the donor with the best HLA match. It is also important to consider other issues unique to each donor, including psychosocial concerns (such as the need to care for other children), the need to care for the recipient, and what options would be least disruptive to the family unit. When discussing the situation with the family, it is important to consider other siblings who may also need renal transplantation in the future, because this can play a role in deciding which donor donates to which recipient.

Living-kidney donation appears to be safe and has been practiced for more than 50 years. The risk of operative mortality appears to be 3 in 10,000.[23,24] After the procedure, living kidney donors appear to do well over the long term as well. The introduction of laparoscopic donor nephrectomy has been a significant step forward for the individuals who consider kidney donation. For the donor, the laparoscopic procedure is associated with quicker recovery and appears as safe as open-donor nephrectomy. Although there was some concern that laparoscopic donation might result in inferior outcomes compared with open-donor nephrectomy, particularly in small infants, this concern has not been substantiated.[25–27]

EVALUATION OF THE DECEASED DONOR

For children who do not have a living donor, deceased donor transplantation is the only option. Deceased donors are individuals who have either suffered brain death or whose heart has irreversibly stopped beating. The latter group has often been referred to as "DCD" for donation after cardiac death. In the United States, deceased donor organ allocation is governed by policies established by the OPTN. These policies undergo constant refinement as data support more rational and fair allocation strategies. After a potential deceased donor is identified, the blood type, HLA type, and other relevant donor factors are entered into the national database maintained by the United Network for Organ Sharing (UNOS). Kidney allocation is driven by a point system based on HLA matching, the level of anti-HLA antibodies in the candidate, and waiting time. Waiting times in many areas of the country for adults are 5 or more years.

The OPTN has recognized the special needs of children with end-stage organ disease and continuously reviews policy in an effort to provide them optimal access to deceased donors. In 2005, the kidney allocation system was changed from a system that provided pediatric priority points based on age and waiting time to a system that provides relative priority to donors less than 35 years of age. At present, candidates who are listed at less than 18 years of age are offered kidneys from donors less than age 35 after any zero mismatch candidates, candidates with a panel reactive antibody greater than 80%, or candidates receiving a kidney with a nonrenal organ. The rationale for this modification was based on the observation that pediatric waiting times remained substantial despite the efforts to provide priority. In addition, in an effort to optimize outcomes, centers were waiting for the best donors. The donor age threshold was based on an analysis demonstrating donor age between 5 and 35 years had the lowest relative risk of graft failure.[28,29]

The new policy has decreased pediatric waiting time while maintaining access to the best deceased donors. As was expected, the shorter waiting time has been associated with lower HLA matching, reflecting the greater priority for transplantation compared with HLA matching. The decrease in HLA matching is small, and there appears to be no adverse impact on outcomes.[28] Waiting for a better-matched kidney is not prudent, because there is no advantage, and it only delays the benefit of transplantation. In addition, because of the relatively good access to the best deceased donors, the need to use expanded criteria kidneys,[30] DCD kidneys,[31] and en-bloc kidneys from small pediatric donors[32] is less than in the adult population. An important exception might be the highly sensitized recipient who has waited for a long period of time. In such situations, the decision needs to consider the risks and benefits of the options available.

TABLE 46-3

Evaluation of Living Kidney Donor

History and physical examination
Laboratory tests:
　　Hematologic (complete blood cell count with platelets; prothrombin time/partial thromboplastin time)
　　Biochemistry (renal function, electrolytes, liver function)
　　Serologic studies (hepatitis herpesvirus B and C, cytomegalovirus, Epstein-Barr virus, human immunodeficiency virus)
　　ABO blood typing
　　Tissue typing (human leukocyte antigen typing)
Urinalysis
Chest radiograph
Electrocardiogram
Psychosocial assessment
Helical computed tomography scan

The improved access to deceased donors has been associated with a decrease in the number of living donor transplantations performed in children. Prior to 2005, living donors accounted for more than half of the pediatric transplantations. This proportion has fallen to less than 40% in recent years and is a source of concern. Although greater access to the best deceased donors is appealing, it is important to note that outcomes are significantly better with living donors compared with deceased donors. Specifically, living donors up to 55 years of age provide greater long-term survival compared with even the ideal deceased donor.[16]

Transplantation

PREOPERATIVE PREPARATION

Deceased donor recipients are admitted once a kidney is accepted. We typically also admit our living donor recipients, although they can be admitted on the day of surgery if their dialysis regimen is stable or if they are not on dialysis. On admission, the need for dialysis is assessed. It is important to ask about intervening health issues since the last visit, as well as examining for any evidence of ongoing infection.

ANESTHESIA

Close coordination with the anesthesia team is vital to the conduct of any operation, and it is particularly important in kidney transplantation in small infants. Maintaining adequate volume status is critical. Because a kidney from an adult donor is typically used, blood flow to the graft often equals the entire cardiac output of the recipient. Hypotension can be particularly problematic. Many children have an obligate polyuria that can cause hypovolemia if not carefully monitored. After reperfusion, the new kidney can also sequester several hundred milliliters of blood, further aggravating hypovolemia.

OPERATIVE PROCEDURE

After induction of general anesthesia, adequate intravenous access is established. In children larger than 20 kg, we do not place a central venous line if adequate peripheral access can be established. For smaller children, we find central venous access useful, both for fluid administration as well as for monitoring central venous pressure. In these smaller children, we also place an arterial line to permit constant blood pressure monitoring. The child is positioned supine. A Foley catheter is inserted and connected to a three-way irrigation system, using dilute providone-iodine (Betadine) in saline. In other centers, an antibiotic solution may be preferred. This arrangement allows the bladder to be filled and drained outside of the operative field as necessary. The child's temperature should be monitored closely, especially with small children who may become hypothermic with either fluid resuscitation or the perfusion of the cold kidney. In addition to routine monitoring, ongoing attention must be directed to volume status. It is vital that the arterial blood pressure and central venous pressure are adequate when the kidney is reperfused. For infants and small children, the central venous pressure is usually maintained in the range of 12 to 18 cm H_2O by administration of crystalloid and/or colloid as necessary. Near completion of the vascular anastomoses, we typically give 0.5 mg/kg of mannitol intravenously. We do not routinely employ a loop diuretic.

OPERATIVE TECHNIQUES

Small Children (<20.0 kg)

Historically, many have performed kidney transplantations intra-abdominally in infants and small children using a midline incision. Since 1998, we have used a retroperitoneal approach similar to that used in adults, even in infants. Placing the kidney on the right side is preferable, because this gives the easiest access to the vena cava. A curvilinear skin incision is made in the lower quadrant. The abdominal wall musculature is divided, and the preperitoneal space is entered. Attempts are made to stay extraperitoneal. The spermatic cord is mobilized and preserved in males, whereas the round ligament is routinely divided in females. The dissection is carried medially until the common iliac vessels, the distal aorta, and vena cava are visualized. If a right native nephrectomy is necessary, this is performed at this point.

The site of the vascular anastomosis depends on kidney size as well as the size of the child. In general, in small children, the renal vein is anastomosed to the vena cava, and the renal artery is anastomosed to either the distal aorta or the common iliac artery. The lymphatics overlying these vessels are divided between ties in an effort to minimize the risk of a lymphocele. When an aortic anastomosis is planned, the aorta is mobilized from below the inferior mesenteric artery to the bifurcation. Lumbar branches are controlled with Pott ties rather than ligated. The common iliac arteries are controlled just distal to the aortic bifurcation. The vena cava is mobilized to allow placement of a side-biting vascular clamp, which can require ligation of several lumbar veins. Once the recipient's vessels have been exposed, the donor kidney is brought into the operative field. The kidney should be inspected for any evidence of unsuspected pathology. The renal vessels are examined. After preparing the kidney, thoughtful consideration needs to be given for the fit of the kidney in the recipient's body cavity. Particular attention must be focused on the length of the renal vessels as well as their orientation. It is important to consider the final resting position of the kidney after it is perfused, the retractor is removed, and the fascia closed.

The venous anastomosis is performed first. The vena cava or iliac vein is controlled with a side-biting clamp. A longitudinal venotomy is made along the anterolateral or lateral aspect of the vein. The renal vein is cut to length, again after considering the ultimate lie of the kidney, and mindful that a redundant renal vein may predispose to thrombosis. We place two corner sutures of 5-0 Prolene. The anastomosis is performed in a running manner. An end-to-side arterial anastomosis is then performed to the recipient's distal aorta or common iliac artery. The recipient vessels are controlled using vessel loops or gentle spring clips. A longitudinal arteriotomy is made, mindful of the final orientation of the renal artery. We enlarge the arteriotomy using a 4.0-mm aortic punch. The renal artery is then sewn end-to-side using a running 6-0 Prolene suture. We typically perform the procedure with loupe magnification.

If multiple renal arteries are present, they can either be implanted separately or syndactylized before reimplantation. When the vessels are syndactylized, it is important to consider if this will allow the vessels to lie in good position, because syndactylization will fix the vessels relatively firmly in two dimensions. This can limit the options of where the anastomosis can be suitably performed or lead to kinking of one or both of the donor arteries if the final position of the kidney is not anticipated.

Before completion of the arterial anastomosis, the hemodynamic state of the patient should be considered. Intraoperative assessment of the vascular volume by direct assessment of the vena cava is possible. Mannitol is also given at this time. Because of the size of the adult kidney, it can be both slow to perfuse as well as sequester a significant volume of blood. The anesthesiologist must be ready to give volume replacement promptly as indicated. At this point, the clamp is removed from the vein and bleeding assessed. Next, while the renal artery is gently compressed with vascular pickups, the arterial clamps are removed, restoring distal blood flow. After a few seconds, flow is established to the kidney. In small children, we occasionally will briefly reclamp the recipient's vessels distal to the arterial anastomosis to provide preferential flow to the kidney. The field is carefully examined for bleeding. The color and turgor of the graft are assessed. The renal artery should have a good pulse, and a thrill can usually be appreciated as well. Both the lower and upper poles should be assessed for perfusion. The renal vein should be full but not tense, with a turgor similar to the vena cava. The lie of the kidney is again examined.

Attention is then directed to the ureteroneocystostomy. We generally perform the ureteral anastomosis as an extravesical ureteroneocystostomy,[33-35] although others routinely prefer the transvesical Politano-Leadbetter approach.[7,36] The Foley catheter is clamped and the bladder is filled. A site on the dome of the bladder is selected where the ureter will sit without any angulation. The muscle wall of the bladder is divided, exposing the bladder mucosa. An opening is then made in the mucosa. The donor ureter is trimmed to length. Care should be taken to make sure it is sufficient to allow a tension-free anastomosis, but excessive length should be avoided because of the risk of ureteral obstruction or stricture resulting from inadequate perfusion of the distal ureter. The end of the ureter is spatulated, and a mucosa to mucosa anastomosis is performed using running 5-0 polydioxanone (PDS) suture. The caveat with running suture is that care must be taken to avoid cinching on the suture line, because this results in a purse-string effect causing stenosis. To prevent vesicoureteral reflux, the bladder muscle wall is approximated over the anastomosis using interrupted 4-0 PDS suture. This allows the ureter to take a tangential course under the bladder wall so that during micturition, the transvesical portion of the ureter is compressed by the overlying bladder wall. An adequate length for this tunnel is essential to prevent vesicoureteral reflux. In patients with a normal bladder and a good blood supply to the distal ureter, we do not routinely place a stent. If there is any concern regarding the ureteral anastomosis, either because of the donor ureter or the quality of the recipient's bladder, we place a double-J ureteral stent, which is removed after a few weeks as an outpatient procedure.

After completing the ureteral anastomosis, the kidney is again inspected with attention to the renal vessels and the lie of the kidney once the retractor is removed. Careful planning and attention to detail before performing the anastomosis is usually rewarded at this point. The fascia is closed in one layer with a running suture. The skin is closed using a running absorbable suture. The urinary catheter is flushed with saline to remove any clots that might obstruct the catheter. For small infants, the volume resuscitation required to ensure excellent renal perfusion, combined with the size of the kidney decreasing respiratory excursion, may make ventilatory support in the immediate postoperative period necessary. If the patient's oxygen saturation and pulmonary mechanics are satisfactory, the patient can be extubated in the operating room.

Larger Children (≥20.0 kg)

The technique for transplantation in larger children is similar to that in adults. We prefer to put the kidney on the right side when possible. An incision is made in the right lower quadrant, extending from one to two fingerbreadths above the pubis to just lateral of the rectus sheath. As in smaller children, the placement of the arterial and venous anastomoses depends on the size of the child and the renal vessels. The venous anastomosis can be done to the vena cava, the common iliac, or the external iliac vein. The arterial anastomosis is performed to the distal aorta, the common iliac, or the external iliac artery. After revascularizing the kidney, the ureteroneocystostomy is performed using an extravesicular technique. At the completion of the operation, these larger children are extubated.

Ureteral Reconstruction in Patients with Previous Urologic Procedures

The ideal urinary reservoir stores a reasonable volume at a low pressure, does not leak, and empties nearly completely with voiding.[14] In the majority of cases, the ideal reservoir is the patient's bladder. If the bladder functioned normally before development of oliguria, it is likely to function adequately after transplantation. Nonetheless, up to 30% of pediatric recipients will not have normal bladder function, and frequently a surgical augmentation or other urologic procedure has been performed before referral for transplantation.

Drainage into an augmented bladder or urinary conduit is an appropriate management strategy when the native bladder is unsuitable or absent.[37,38] When indicated, we prefer to have the intended urinary reservoir created and suitable for use before the transplant procedure. Intraoperatively, when planning the ureteroneocystostomy to an augmented bladder, it is important to consider the blood supply to the augmented section so as not to compromise it during the transplant. It is preferable to perform the ureteroneocystostomy to the native bladder, and this can be accomplished in most situations. An antireflux ureteroneocystostomy is essential, and it is most readily performed with the bladder wall.

Patients with an augmented bladder or urinary conduit are at increased risk for urine infection, but compared with historical controls, graft survival is not adversely affected.[39] The rate of surgical complications related to the ureteral anastomosis is higher in these patients, approximately 20%.[39-41] Regardless of the etiology of the bladder dysfunction, these patients require regular clean intermittent straight catheterization after transplantation.

Children with obstructive uropathy from posterior urethral valves will not have normal bladder function, and this can contribute to renal dysfunction after transplantation.[37]

Awareness of these issues is vital, and evaluation with follow-up urodynamic studies is frequently indicated in children with voiding disorders. Bladder dysfunction, such as hypo-compliance and/or hyper-reflexia, requires medical or surgical treatment.

Postoperative Care

Attention to detail in the postoperative period is essential. Special care must be directed to the fluid and electrolyte status. Many children are polyuric before transplant, and this obligate urine loss will continue in the immediate postoperative period. Intravenous fluids are administered, taking into account urine output as well as insensible losses. The composition of these solutions is adjusted as needed, depending on regular measurement of serum electrolytes. Serum sodium, potassium, and calcium levels are followed closely and replaced as necessary. Heart rate, blood pressure, and central venous pressure are carefully monitored. No single factor alone is entirely reliable in assessing intravascular volume.

For patients who were oliguric or who had native nephrectomies before transplantation, monitoring urine output is an excellent monitor of graft function. For patients who made significant urine before transplantation, evaluation of graft function is more difficult. The volume of urine production may be suggestive. In addition, the serum creatinine concentration should fall with time. Recipients with oliguria should be rapidly evaluated. The urinary catheter should be flushed with small volumes of sterile saline. The volume status of the patient should be carefully assessed. A fluid bolus is usually warranted, both as a diagnostic test and as therapeutic intervention. Doppler ultrasonography will confirm adequate arterial flow and venous outflow. Ultrasonography will also show evidence of fluid or blood around the kidney, as well as assess for possible ureteral obstruction. In patients who appear to be adequately volume loaded and hemodynamically stable, a dose of diuretic can be given. It is important to do this carefully, because sudden massive urine output can cause significant intravascular volume depletion, which can then lead to problems with renal perfusion. In patients who are massively volume overloaded or have significant electrolyte abnormalities, dialysis may be indicated.

If ventilated postoperatively, the smaller children are weaned from the ventilator generally within the first 24 hours. Enteral feedings can be started at a slow rate almost immediately after the extraperitoneal approach. Infants who were on tube feedings before transplantation should resume these tube feedings, because they usually will not feed orally in the immediate post-transplantation period. Hypertension can be problematic. The volume loading associated with the procedure as well as the use of calcineurin inhibitors (CNIs) for immunosuppression can result in significant hypertension, which can be severe and require aggressive therapy to prevent seizures and other sequelae.

To monitor and replace urine output on an hourly basis, we admit our children to the intensive care unit (ICU). If this can be accomplished on a surgical floor unit, larger children could be admitted to an area specializing in the care of renal transplant patients. Children who are admitted into the ICU are typically transferred to the floor unit within 1 to 2 days. Most children leave the hospital 5 to 7 days after transplantation, assuming the family is comfortable with the immunosuppression regimen.

Evaluation of Early Allograft Dysfunction

Ideally, the donor kidney should begin to make urine shortly after revascularization. The likelihood of this occurring depends on multiple factors, beginning with the quality of the donor organ. Living donor kidneys will generally function immediately because of the healthy state of the donor as well as the shorter cold ischemic time for the kidney. For deceased donor kidneys, the cold ischemic time is generally longer. In addition and more important, there are multiple factors associated with the donor death, including hypotension, the potential need for high doses of vasopressors, and other issues related to the overall health of the donor.

Regardless of the donor source, the assessment of the graft begins in the operating room, evaluating the graft for color and turgor as well as vascular anastomoses. Particular attention should be directed to considering how the kidney is positioned once the abdomen is closed and how this could impact the vasculature. The renal artery will often have a thrill suggestive of excellent flow and low intrarenal resistance. Assuming the technical aspects of the procedure appear satisfactory, additional volume for the kidney not making urine is the best option. Once the patient is adequately volume loaded, loop diuretics may be used to gently encourage a diuresis. In patients who were anuric before the procedure, continued failure to make urine in the postoperative period should prompt a bedside Doppler ultrasound examination. For patients who made urine before the transplantation, determining whether the transplanted kidney is making urine is more difficult, although sometimes the amount of volume being produced will give a sign that the kidney is working. During the first 24 hours, the serum creatinine level should fall as well. If there is still concern about function, a Doppler ultrasound study should be obtained, and any suggestion of problems with the arteriovenous signal should initiate a prompt return to the operating room. In general, the ultrasound evaluation will be fine, or, occasionally, there will be a modest reduction in flow suggestive of increased intrarenal resistance, most commonly because of acute tubular necrosis. This condition resolves without any specific intervention. Other diagnostic studies are less frequently required. Renal arteriography is rarely indicated. Radionucleotide scans are used by some centers, but we find them less helpful than ultrasonography. A radionucleotide scan may be helpful in documenting a suspected urinary leak.

Complications related to the ureteral anastomosis include leaks and obstruction. The risk of ureteral complications is approximately 7% to 9%.[7,42,43] A leak at the ureteral anastomosis generally manifests in the first few days after the transplant. Leaks detected in the first 2 to 3 days may be repaired operatively. Leaks detected later can generally be managed nonoperatively with a percutaneous nephrostomy. This stent is subsequently advanced across the anastomosis into the bladder. The stent is usually left to external drainage for several days and is then capped. If a large urinoma is present, separate drainage of this collection may be required.

Obstruction of the urinary system can occur at any time. An early obstruction is usually related to technical problems with the anastomosis or other mechanical issues, such as torsion of the ureter, while later obstruction often reflects ischemic stricture. Because the ureter relies on small arterial vessels from the lower pole of the kidney, it should be no longer than necessary. Late ureteral stenoses generally require operative intervention, with resection of the stenotic segment and reconstruction. Vesicoureteral reflux may cause recurrent urinary tract infections or graft dysfunction, and require operative intervention in up to 5% of patients.[44]

Another complication after retroperitoneal kidney transplantation is lymphocele. Lymphoceles may produce discomfort or allograft dysfunction. The diagnosis is established by ultrasound-guided percutaneous aspiration of clear fluid with a creatinine concentration equivalent to serum. Percutaneous drainage is associated with a very high incidence of recurrence, and the preferred treatment is creation of a peritoneal window. This can be accomplished laparoscopically or through a small open incision, with drainage of the lymphocele into the peritoneal cavity.

In instances of renal vein thrombosis, the graft is usually not salvageable. The causes of renal vein thrombosis are several, and the exact mechanism may be difficult to ascertain but include immunologic factors, a hypercoagulable state, and technical issues.

Immunosuppression

Significant advances have been made in understanding the immune response and several new immunosuppressive agents have been developed. The introduction of new agents has permitted consideration of avoidance, conversion, and minimization strategies in an effort to minimize toxicities associated with specific agents. There are several potential regimens, but all require a balance between prevention of rejection and unwanted side effects of immunosuppression. Most centers use standardized protocols for recipients based on immunologic risk. Immunosuppressive agents are used for induction, maintenance, and treatment of rejection episodes.

ANTIBODY PREPARATIONS

Antilymphocyte Antibodies

Antilymphocyte antibodies include polyclonal preparations, such as equine antithymocyte globulin (ATGAM) and rabbit antithymocyte globulin (Thymoglobulin), and the monoclonal antibody preparations muromonab-CD3 (OKT3) and anti-CD52 (Alemtuzumab). Of these antilymphocyte agents, Thymoglobulin is currently predominant, and the use of the others is either rare or of historic interest. Antilymphocyte antibodies act by lymphodepletion, as well as by interactions with cellular receptors. The use of antilymphocyte induction regimens has declined precipitously with time.[1,2] We currently restrict the use of Thymoglobulin to recipients at higher risk for immunologic graft loss, such as patients requiring retransplantation, highly sensitized patients, or black recipients. These agents are also effective in the treatment of acute cellular rejection.

Anti–interleukin-2 Receptor Monoclonal Antibodies

Two monoclonal antibodies have been developed that bind to the alpha subunit of interleukin (IL)-2 receptor (CD25) and inhibit IL-2–mediated lymphocyte proliferation. Basiliximab (Simulect) and daclizumab (Zenapax), received approval by the U.S. Food and Drug Administration (FDA) in 1998, though only basiliximab is currently marketed. Basiliximab is a chimeric human/mouse monoclonal antibody that is effective in reducing the incidence of acute cellular rejection, with good long-term results and no evidence of increased risk of infection or malignancy.[45–47] The IL-2 receptor antibody is used in induction regimens but is not effective in treating rejection.

CALCINEURIN INHIBITORS

The introduction of cyclosporine after its FDA approval in 1983 was one of the most significant advances in transplantation. Tacrolimus received FDA approval in 1994. Both agents act through inhibition of calcineurin activity. They first bind to specific cytoplasmic proteins; cyclosporine binds to cyclophilin, and tacrolimus binds to tacrolimus binding protein (also known as FK-binding protein). Both drug-protein complexes then bind to calcineurin, a phosphatase that controls the transport of transcriptional regulator factors across the nuclear membrane. By inhibiting the translocation of these factors into the nucleus, both drugs inhibit transcription of several early T-cell activation genes, most significantly IL-2.

Both cyclosporine and tacrolimus are effective at preventing rejection. A randomized prospective open-label trial performed in Europe in pediatric renal recipients compared tacrolimus with cyclosporine, along with azathioprine and steroids. There was a significantly lower incidence of acute rejection in the tacrolimus group (36.9%) compared with cyclosporine therapy (59.1%).[48] In contrast with this observation, a retrospective analysis of NAPRTCS data comparing cyclosporine with tacrolimus, along with mycophenolate mofetil and corticosteroids, showed equal rates of rejection and graft survival. Although rejection rates were similar, tacrolimus therapy was associated with improved graft function at 1 and 2 years after transplant.[49] Currently, approximately 70% of pediatric recipients are reported as being discharged on tacrolimus compared with 10% on cyclosporine.[1,2]

Cyclosporine side effects include hirsutism and gingival hyperplasia, whereas tacrolimus is associated with increased incidence of post-transplantation diabetes and neurotoxicity. In children who develop a problematic side effect from one agent, conversion to the other agent is appropriate. Both calcineurin inhibitors have significant nephrotoxicity that impact graft function with time.

MYCOPHENOLATE

Mycophenolate mofetil (MMF) (CellCept) and mycophenolic acid (MPA) (Myfortic) inhibit purine synthesis. MMF is converted in vivo to mycophenolic acid, a noncompetitive inhibitor of inosine monophosphate dehydrogenase (IMPDH), which is a key enzyme in de novo purine biosynthesis. Although most cells can synthesize purines by either the de novo or the salvage pathway, B and T lymphocytes lack the salvage pathway. Mycophenolate is thus a selective inhibitor of lymphocyte proliferation, and it has replaced azathioprine (Imuran) as the primary antiproliferative agent.[50] MMF has been demonstrated to be safe and effective in pediatric patients.[51] Experience with MPA in children is more limited, though it appears equivalent.[52,53] The primary side effects are related to leukopenia and gastrointestinal intolerance.

PREDNISONE

Glucocorticoids have played an integral role in immunosuppression regimens since the earliest days of transplantation. They act primarily through transcriptional regulation, diffusing across the plasma membrane and binding to cytoplasmic steroid receptors. This complex is translocated to the nucleus, where it binds to specific gene promoters and other regulatory regions, inhibiting cytokine synthesis. Corticosteroids are also lymphocytotoxic and possess significant anti-inflammatory activity, inhibiting macrophage function and other nonspecific aspects of the inflammatory response.

Long-term corticosteroid therapy is associated with increased risk of hypertension, hyperlipidemia, diabetes, bone loss, cosmetic disfigurement, and cataracts. Attempts at minimizing corticosteroids have not had a significant effect on these side effects, and efforts are being directed to corticosteroid avoidance. Although it is appealing to consider withdrawal of corticosteroids with time, late corticosteroid withdrawal appears associated with increased risk of acute and chronic rejection. Early corticosteroid withdrawal and corticosteroid-free regimens, with and without antibody induction, have shown promise. Sarwal and associates, at Stanford University, have reported excellent results in a corticosteroid-free protocol using an extended induction with daclizumab, tacrolimus, and MMF.[54] In their recent report, 129 recipients have been treated with a mean follow-up of 5 years. One-year graft and patient survival were 93% and 96%, respectively. The rate of acute rejection was 12% during the first year. Significant improvements in post-transplantation growth and avoidance of steroid side effects were noted. This experience led to a prospective, multicenter randomized study that has been completed, though the results have not yet been published. Similar results have also been reported by the Stanford group in 13 recipients using Thymoglobulin induction in place of daclizumab.[55]

Another large randomized multicenter international trial with 196 pediatric kidney recipients compared rapid steroid withdrawal in children treated with daclizumab, tacrolimus, and MMF with recipients maintained on steroids along with tacrolimus and mycophenolate.[56] Early steroid withdrawal was associated with improved growth and metabolic profiles, with similar acute rejection rates (10.2% vs. 7.1%, respectively) and equivalent graft and patient survival during the first 6 months.

Although encouraging, efforts to withdraw steroids while maintaining acceptable rejection rates have also resulted in regimens with a greater rate of complications of immunosuppression. One multicenter randomized trial of steroid withdrawal after 6 months in recipients treated with basiliximab induction, cyclosporine or tacrolimus, sirolimus, and steroids was halted early because of a high rate of post-transplantation lymphoproliferative disorder (PTLD).[57]

It appears steroid avoidance or early withdrawal is possible in selected patients with good short-term results. Longer-term data are needed, and striking the correct balance of immunosuppression and other side effects remains critical.

PROLIFERATION SIGNAL INHIBITORS

Proliferation signal inhibitors are a relatively new class of immunosuppressants. Sirolimus (rapamycin) and everolimus are macrolide agents that inhibit a protein, mammalian target of rapamycin (mTOR), which is a critical regulatory kinase controlling cytokine-mediated proliferation. A potential role for sirolimus in renal transplantation has been established.[58] Everolimus also appears effective.[59] There is interest in using mTOR inhibitors to avoid or minimize calcineurin inhibitors and/or corticosteroids, though the optimal strategy remains elusive. Experience to date suggests that complete CNI avoidance is often associated with higher rejection rates, while late CNI replacement or minimization may not offer any benefit with respect to reversing CNI nephrotoxicity.

Sirolimus interacts with calcineurin inhibitors, particularly cyclosporine, and careful monitoring is essential. Like many other immunosuppressive agents, there is evidence to suggest more rapid metabolism of sirolimus in children compared with adults.[60]

TREATMENT OF REJECTION

Suspected rejection should be confirmed by biopsy. The first-line therapy for acute cellular rejection is pulse corticosteroids. Typically, intravenous methylprednisolone is administered for 3 days, with doses ranging from 5.0 to 25.0 mg/kg/day (maximum dose, 1.0 g). We use 10.0 mg/kg for children younger than aged 6 years and 5.0 mg/kg for children aged 6 years and older, with a maximum dose of 500 mg/day. Severe rejection or rejection refractory to corticosteroids is treated with Thymoglobulin. Treatment of acute rejection is nearly always successful, although late episodes of rejection are less likely to respond. After successful treatment, many consider altering maintenance immunosuppression, including changing to the other calcineurin inhibitor, or substituting sirolimus for MMF; however, there is little evidence to support this approach. An assessment of adherence to the immunosuppression regimen should also be initiated. If the patient's creatinine level does not return to baseline, a follow-up biopsy should be strongly considered. Although most acute rejection episodes reflect primarily T-cell–mediated processes, there is growing recognition of the role of B cells and alloantibodies in immunologically mediated graft injury.

Outcomes

GRAFT AND PATIENT SURVIVAL

There are approximately 800 pediatric kidney transplantations performed annually in the United States. In 2009, there were 866 transplantations, with 38.8% living donor and 61.2% deceased donor kidneys. Short-term graft and patient survival after transplantation is excellent. Current graft survival for living donor and deceased donor kidney transplantations in children, stratified by recipient age, is summarized in

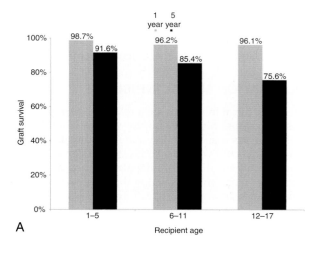

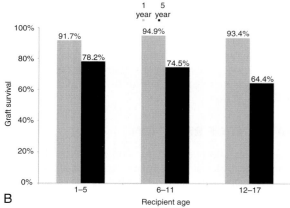

FIGURE 46-1 **A,** One- and 5-year graft survival of living donor kidney transplantations by recipient age. **B,** One- and 5-year graft survival of deceased donor kidney transplantations by recipient age. (From Organ Procurement Transplant Network/Scientific Registry of Transplant Recipients: 2009 Organ Procurement Transplant Network/Scientific Registry of Transplant Recipients Annual Report: Transplant data 1999-2008. Health and Human Services/Health Resources and Service Administration/Special Pathogens Branch/Department of Transportation. Available at www.ustransplant.org. Accessed September 29, 2010.)

Figure 46-1. Recipient survival stratified by age range is summarized in Figure 46-2. The leading causes of death are infection (28.9%), cardiopulmonary (15.7%), and malignancy (11.0%).[2] Although patient survival is good, it is important to realize that even with transplantation, these children face a significantly increased risk of mortality compared with the general population.[61]

With time there has been improvement in outcomes for all pediatric age ranges. This improvement is particularly noteworthy in children younger than 2 years of age who previously had the worst graft survival but now have outcomes that equal the outcomes of any age group.[13,50] In fact, the longest transplant half-lives of all recipients are now the youngest recipients, especially if the pediatric recipient receives an adult kidney that functions immediately.[62] These improvements likely reflect better donor selection, improvement in surgical techniques, better immunosuppression agents, and a better understanding of immunosuppression management in children.

Although short-term graft survival in children is excellent, it is important to appreciate that long-term graft survival in the

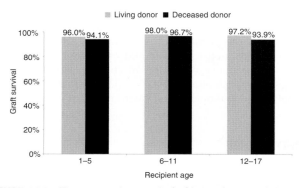

FIGURE 46-2 Five-year patient survival of living donor and deceased donor kidney transplantations by recipient age. (From Organ Procurement Transplant Network/Scientific Registry of Transplant Recipients: 2009 Organ Procurement Transplant Network/Scientific Registry of Transplant Recipients Annual Report: Transplant data 1999-2008. Health and Human Services/Health Resources and Service Administration/Special Pathogens Branch/Department of Transportation. Available at www.ustransplant.org. Accessed September 29, 2010.)

adolescent group (ages 11 to 17 years) is poor (see Fig. 46-2). Adolescent graft survival is less than in all recipient age groups except adults older than 65 years.[4] The reasons behind this significant rate of graft loss are speculative, but noncompliance likely plays a significant role.[63] The higher incidence of recurrent FSGS in this age group may also contribute to graft loss. Regardless of the cause, improving the long-term outcomes in this patient population represents an important focus.

POST-TRANSPLANTATION OUTCOMES AND RISK FACTORS ASSOCIATED WITH GRAFT LOSS

Smith and coworkers reported that the most common causes of allograft failure reported to NAPRTCS for transplantations performed between 2000 and 2005 are chronic rejection (41.3%), vascular thrombosis (8.1%), recurrence of the primary disease (7.9%), acute rejection (6.3%), and discontinuation of immunosuppression (6.3%).[2] Analysis of large single-center experiences and registry data has revealed risk factors associated with specific post-transplantation outcomes.[2,13,64] For a given child, some of these risk factors, such as their race, age, or primary disease, are not modifiable. Other factors are potentially modifiable, and efforts should be made to mitigate risk.

The type and timing of the transplant affect outcomes. Living donor transplantation is associated with better graft survival compared with deceased donor transplantation.[2,4] Preemptive transplantation is associated with better graft survival compared with patients on dialysis at the time of transplantation. For children on dialysis, the choice of dialysis therapy does not impact graft survival, although graft loss from vascular thrombosis is more common in children on peritoneal dialysis compared with hemodialysis.[65]

DELAYED GRAFT FUNCTION

Delayed graft function (DGF) is defined as the need for dialysis during the first week after transplantation and is a manifestation of acute tubular necrosis (ATN). DGF is more common in recipients of deceased donor kidneys compared with living donors, because of the impact of cold ischemic time and donor quality. Nationally, the incidence of DGF after deceased donor renal transplantation is 12.5% in pediatric recipients compared with 23.4% in adult recipients,[50] reflecting the differential donor selection made possible by the allocation system. An analysis of more than 5000 pediatric transplantations has demonstrated that DGF is an independent risk factor for subsequent graft loss.[66] DGF is also associated with increased risk for acute and chronic rejection, likely reflecting the impact of renal injury on the subsequent immune response. DGF limits the ability to use renal dysfunction as a sign of acute rejection, potentially delaying the diagnosis of rejection. We believe that all recipients with DGF longer than 5 to 7 days should be biopsied, and even earlier in patients with increased risk of rejection.

VASCULAR THROMBOSIS

Vascular thrombosis is currently the second most common reported cause of graft loss.[2] Risk factors include donor age younger than 6 years, cold ischemic time greater than 24 hours, prior transplantation, and peritoneal dialysis before transplantation.[65] Careful consideration of donor quality, along with efforts to ensure adequate perfusion to the graft, may minimize the risk of thrombosis. Patients with ESRD have a higher incidence of hypercoagulable conditions, and any history of thrombosis, including recurrent or unexplained thrombosis of hemodialysis access, should prompt further evaluation.

ACUTE REJECTION

Acute rejection typically occurs between 1 week and 3 months after transplantation, although it can happen at any time. A rise in the serum creatinine level is frequently the first sign of rejection. Findings such as low-grade fever, graft tenderness, hypertension, or decreased urine output are infrequent. Any renal dysfunction should be promptly investigated. A percutaneous biopsy should be obtained to confirm the diagnosis, because many other processes can lead to allograft dysfunction, including calcineurin inhibitor toxicity, ureteral obstruction, infection, renal artery stenosis, and recurrence of original disease. Acute rejection episodes are treated by either pulse corticosteroids or antilymphocyte antibodies as detailed previously.

Risk factors associated with acute rejection include African-American race, delayed graft function, and a history of allosensitization. Acute rejection, and, in particular, late acute rejection episodes occurring more than 1 year after transplant, are independent risk factors for graft loss because of chronic rejection.[67] One episode of acute rejection increases the risk of graft loss from chronic rejection graft failure threefold, and two episodes of acute rejection increase the risk 12-fold. The incidence of acute rejection is decreasing with time. In the 2003 to 2005 NAPRTCS cohort, 12.2% of living donor recipients and 15.8% of deceased donor recipients had a rejection episode in the first year after transplant.[2]

Acute rejection, even if successfully treated, impacts graft survival and all efforts to minimize this risk are important. Unfortunately, intensifying the immunosuppression regimen is limited by the consequences of nonspecific systemic immunosuppression. Ensuring the patient remains on therapeutic immunosuppression is vital, because noncompliance can

be disastrous. Prompt recognition and treatment of rejection is important. Because serum creatinine is a relatively insensitive indicator, particularly in small children with an adult kidney, many advocate protocol biopsies to detect subclinical rejection that may benefit from treatment.

CHRONIC ALLOGRAFT NEPHROPATHY

Whereas short-term results are excellent, progressive renal dysfunction frequently occurs and is the leading cause of graft failure. This process of chronic allograft nephropathy, often called "chronic rejection," involves both immunologic and nonimmunologic factors. Although acute rejection episodes are a major risk factor for chronic allograft nephropathy, it is clear other processes can contribute as well. Evidence of antibody-mediated injury is also present in 57% of patients with late allograft dysfunction.[68] Efforts to reduce chronic allograft nephropathy are limited by our understanding of the process. Aside from graft loss, the gradual renal dysfunction associated with chronic allograft nephropathy also adversely impacts the recipient's general health.

NONADHERENCE

Adherence with the medical regimen is essential for the success of transplantation. Nonadherence is believed to be largely responsible for the poorer long-term graft survival seen in adolescent recipients. Shaw and coworkers reviewed 112 pediatric renal transplant recipients and found one third had clinically significant periods of medication nonadherence.[69] Nonadherence was significantly more common in adolescents compared with younger recipients. Nonadherence was associated with both acute and chronic rejection, as well as graft loss. The relative lack of reliable measures of adherence and effective interventions has focused research in the field.[70,71] Improved parental involvement and discussion of the child–parent relationship may improve adherence.

RECURRENT DISEASE

The recurrence of the patient's primary disease is variable, and recurrence may or may not lead to graft loss. Recurrent disease is a more significant issue in the pediatric population, because of the diagnoses leading to ESRD and their association with higher rates of graft loss after recurrence. FSGS is the most prevalent and clinically significant disease to recur after renal transplantation. In children, the recurrence rate can be as high as 40% to 50%.[72] It can recur almost immediately after transplant, and most recurrences are within the first month. Patients with FSGS should be followed closely after transplantation with urine protein measurements. Graft survival is often worse in adolescents with recurrent FSGS, with up to a 38% risk of graft loss.[73] A circulating permeability factor is believed to play a critical role in the pathogenesis of FSGS. Plasmapheresis is the most frequently used therapy for recurrence, although controlled trials supporting its efficacy are lacking. Some have proposed a role for preoperative plasmapheresis to decrease the risk of recurrence.[74] Others have suggested a role for intensifying the immunosuppression and potentially rituximab. In addition to FSGS, other primary renal causes associated with recurrent disease include membranoproliferative glomerulonephritis types 1 and 2 and IgA nephropathy.[75]

Again, the risk of graft loss is variable, and none constitute an absolute contraindication to transplantation.

In addition to these primary glomerulopathies, other recurrent diseases disproportionately affect the pediatric population. Hemolytic-uremic syndrome can recur after transplantation. Nearly all the risk of recurrence and subsequent graft loss is in those with atypical nondiarrhea-associated hemolytic-uremic syndrome.[76] The risk of recurrence appears related to specific defects of complement activation, and screening for these defects is recommended pre-transplant.[77] Henoch-Schönlein purpura can also recur. The overall risk of renal recurrence after transplantation is 29%, and the risk for graft loss appears equivalent to that observed in IgA nephropathy.[78]

Oxalosis (primary hyperoxaluria type 1) is a metabolic disease caused by a defect in hepatic peroxisomal alanine:glyoxylate aminotransferase, which leads to increased synthesis and excretion of oxalate. The excessive oxalate load leads to urolithiasis, medullary calcinosis, and eventual ESRD. The primary metabolic defect is not corrected by kidney transplantation, and the persistent oxalate load causes subsequent renal graft loss. Simultaneous liver-kidney transplantation is generally advocated as the primary treatment.[79,80] Kidney transplantation alone is uncommon, but has been advocated in selected patients, most notably those who are pyridoxine sensitive or those with lower oxalate burdens.[81]

MEDICAL COMPLICATIONS

Infection

Infection is a constant risk of immunosuppression and is one clinical representation of the precarious balance between overimmunosuppression and underimmunosuppression. Great vigilance should be maintained during periods of heaviest immunosuppression, as occurs immediately after transplantation or during treatment of rejection. Additional prophylaxis is warranted during these periods of greatest risk.[82]

Post-transplantation infection accounts for more hospitalizations than acute rejection, even in the first 6 months after transplantation.[83] Post-transplantation infections are predominantly bacterial and viral. Fungal infections, although accounting for 0.2% to 2.7% of infection-related hospitalizations, can be particularly dangerous. Pediatric recipients are often at higher risk, reflecting the fact that they are more likely to be naïve to a particular pathogen than the general population. Younger age and the use of antibody induction immunosuppression are significant independent risk factors for infectious complications.[84]

Cytomegalovirus

Cytomegalovirus (CMV) represents the most common viral infection after transplantation. CMV infection can occur in any recipient, although the risk is highest when a seronegative recipient receives a kidney from a seropositive donor. Infection occurs in seropositive recipients as well because of activation of latent virus. The incidence and the severity of CMV have declined with more effective prophylaxis. The severity of CMV infection may range from asymptomatic to organ involvement and death. The typical presentation occurs 1 to 6 months after transplantation, with the patient feeling relatively well but having fevers or sometimes flulike symptoms.

Leukopenia is common. Patients with tissue-invasive CMV disease will appear toxic, and there will be evidence of end-organ dysfunction. The diagnosis is confirmed using either a CMV pp65 antigenemia assay or the CMV polymerase chain reaction (PCR) assay. Both methods allow monitoring of the response to therapy. Valganciclovir is effective for both the prophylaxis and treatment of CMV disease.[85] In more severe cases, treatment with intravenous ganciclovir and CMV hyperimmune globulin may be helpful.

Varicella-Zoster Virus

In pediatric recipients, there is high risk of a primary chickenpox infection. Treatment is with intravenous acyclovir until the lesions crust over, then conversion to oral acyclovir. Primary infections can be severe. We immunize our candidates who are seronegative for varicella-zoster virus (VZV) before transplantation. For seronegative recipients who have a defined exposure, we administer VZV immune globulin.

BK Virus

BK virus is a ubiquitous polyomavirus that is a significant concern in renal transplantation.[86] There is a high incidence of seroconversion by late childhood, and the virus is dormant in the renal epithelium until reactivated. BK virus appears to be an under-recognized cause of allograft dysfunction, with BK interstitial nephritis resulting in a graft loss in 45% to 70% of affected recipients.

The incidence of BK virus-associated transplant nephropathy is estimated to be 4% to 7%.[86] Smith and coworkers evaluated a single-center cohort of 173 pediatric renal recipients and identified BK nephropathy in 6 children (3.5%).[87] The diagnosis was made on biopsy at a median of 15 months after transplantation. There was a strong association between BK nephropathy and recipient seronegativity. In a subsequent analysis of the NAPRTCS database from 2000 to 2004, the incidence of BK nephropathy was 4.6% with a median onset of 10.1 months post-transplantation. Graft failure occurred in 24% of patients at a mean of 24 months after diagnosis. There was an association with polyclonal antibody induction therapy.[88]

BK nephropathy should be considered in the evaluation of renal allograft dysfunction. BK nephropathy can be definitively diagnosed on biopsy using immunohistochemistry, but the histology can be confused with acute rejection. Treatment with additional immunosuppression does not improve renal function and often will cause further deterioration. The initial treatment for BK nephropathy consists of decreasing immunosuppression. The addition of antiviral therapy and intravenous immunoglobulin has been reported, but there are no controlled trials and compelling data are lacking.[89] Measurement of BK virus by PCR helps with diagnosis and subsequent monitoring of the response to treatment. It is hoped that improved awareness, prompt diagnosis, and treatment may reduce the risk of graft loss initially associated with this disease process.

Malignancy

Transplant recipients face an increased risk of de novo malignancy related to their immunosuppression. Lymphomas, specifically post-transplantation lymphoproliferative disorder (PTLD), are the most common, with an incidence of 1% to 4% in renal transplantation.[90–92] PTLD actually represents a spectrum of pathology, and the treatment and prognosis depends on the histology.[90,93] Epstein-Barr virus (EBV) is believed to be the causative agent in the progression to PTLD, especially in B-cell lymphomas. A wide variety of factors have been proposed to be associated with an increased risk, including the use of antilymphocyte induction therapy, EBV-seronegative recipient, EBV infection, and era of transplant. Young white males appear to be at greatest risk.[92] The incidence of PTLD is associated with the overall intensity of immunosuppression.[91,92,94,95]

The second most common cancer in pediatric recipients is skin cancer. Squamous cell carcinoma accounts for the majority, followed by malignant melanoma and basal cell carcinoma. The best strategy combines sunblock and sun avoidance. All recipients should undergo regular dermatologic follow-up, specifically focusing on this risk. Long-term immunosuppression is also associated with increased risks of cervical, vulvar, and anal carcinoma.

Other Medical Issues

In addition to the risks of infection and malignancy, transplant recipients face many other risks secondary to their history of ESRD, their underlying renal disease, and the individual risks associated with all their medications.

Renal transplant recipients are at high risk for cardiovascular disease.[96] Preexisting renal insufficiency, time on dialysis, and immunosuppressive medications after transplantation all contribute to this risk. In addition, the prevalence of hypertension in pediatric kidney recipients is 50% to 80%.[97,98] The incidence of left ventricular hypertrophy at initiation of renal replacement therapy ranges from 54% to 82%, though it generally improves after transplantation.[99–101] Many children and adolescents will have additional cardiovascular risk factors, including hyperlipidemia, hyperhomocysteinemia, anemia, malnutrition, and chronic inflammation.

Although there are few data examining the magnitude of the risk in pediatric patients, young adult patients with ESRD have a 1000-fold higher risk of cardiovascular death compared with the general population. Although the risk of cardiovascular death decreases after successful transplantation compared with dialysis, it does not become normal.[102] In addition to contributing to cardiovascular risk, hypertension is associated with a higher risk of graft dysfunction and graft loss.[98,103]

Transplantation recipients also face significant problems with bone metabolism and growth because of a history of chronic renal insufficiency, malnutrition, graft dysfunction after transplantation, and immunosuppressive medications. Renal osteodystrophy is a substantial problem, but proper calcium and vitamin D supplementation, along with other agents, has improved overall bone health. The risk of osseous complications has decreased with time, and the risk decreases after transplantation compared with dialysis therapy.[104] The impairment in linear growth impacts final adult height, but significant progress has been made.[105,106] Height at transplantation is one of the best predictors of final adult height, and better management prior to transplantation, including nutrition and the use of recombinant human growth hormone, have improved height z-scores at transplantation. Catch-up growth post-transplantation occurs, but appears limited to recipients less than 6 years of age at transplantation. Steroid avoidance protocols are also associated with catch-up growth, adding a potential benefit to consider with respect to immunosuppression regimens.

Cognitive and Psychosocial Development

The negative impact of ESRD on cognitive development has diminished because of significant improvements in medical management and renal replacement therapy. Children with ESRD who undergo transplantation appear to have improvement in their level of cognitive function.[107] Psychosocial development tends to be below the healthy population, though transplantation offers benefit compared with dialysis. Overall quality of life for the child and family appears to be better after transplantation compared with dialysis, although again, when compared with the normative population, there are disparities.[108–111]

The complete reference list is available online at www.expertconsult.com.

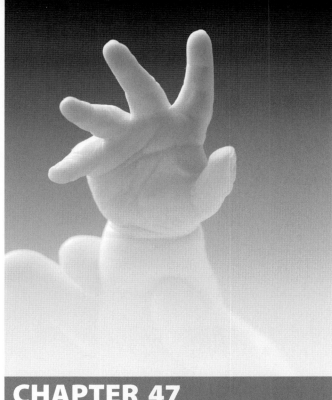

CHAPTER 47

Pancreas and Islet Cell Transplantation

David E. R. Sutherland, Angelika C. Gruessner, Bernhard J. Hering, and Rainer W. G. Gruessner

Type 1 diabetes is an autoimmune disease in which the pancreatic islet insulin-producing beta cells are selectively destroyed.[1] It most commonly presents in childhood and continues to represent a therapeutic challenge. Secondary diabetes complications, observed in 30% to 50% of patients who live more than 20 years after onset of the disease, result in poor quality of life, premature death, and considerable health care costs.[2] The principal determinant of the risk of devastating diabetes complications is the total lifetime exposure to elevated blood glucose levels.[3] Therefore establishing safe and effective methods of achieving and maintaining normoglycemia will have substantial implications for the health and the quality of life of individuals with diabetes.

The Diabetes Control and Complications Trial (DCCT) demonstrated that, given a qualified diabetes care team and intensive insulin treatment control, near-normalization of glycemia could be achieved and sustained for several years.[4] However, such a near-perfect level of treatment would increase a patient's burden of day-to-day diabetes management, be difficult to implement for many patients, require more attention and medical services than are routinely

available in clinical practice,[5] and be accompanied by an increased frequency of severe hypoglycemia.[4] Currently, the only way to restore sustained normoglycemia without the associated risk of hypoglycemia is to replace the patient's glucose-sensing and insulin-secreting pancreatic islet beta cells[6,7] either by the transplantation of a vascularized pancreas[8,9] or by the infusion of isolated pancreatic islets.[10–12] The trade-off is the need for immunosuppression to prevent rejection of allogenic tissue, and for this reason, most pancreas or islet transplant recipients have been adults. However, the potential for application earlier in the course of the disease exists, particularly in diabetic children already on immunosuppression for other indications.[13] Of the nearly 24 million people estimated to have diabetes mellitus in the United States, 5% to 10% have type 1 diabetes mellitus,[14] and the prevalence in children is increasing.[15]

Pancreas Transplantation

HISTORY

The first clinical pancreas transplantation was performed in 1966 by Drs. William Kelly and Richard Lillehei, simultaneous with a kidney transplantation, in a uremic diabetic patient at the University of Minnesota.[16] Shortly thereafter, a few institutions around the world began to perform pancreas transplantations, as detailed in a comprehensive history in another book.[17]

The success rate (long-term insulin independence) with pancreas transplantation was initially low but increased considerably in the 1980s, leading to increased application (Fig. 47-1). Innovations in both surgical techniques and immunosuppression were responsible for the improvements.

The first pancreas transplantation was a duct-ligated segmental (body and tail) graft,[16] but this approach was associated with multiple complications. In a series of 13 more pancreas transplantations between 1966 and 1973 at the University of Minnesota,[18,19] Lillehei devised the whole pancreas–duodenal transplantation technique to the iliac vessels with enteric drainage through a duodenoenterostomy to native small bowel, which is now routine at most centers. The initial results, however, were not as good as today, and several surgeons devised alternative techniques during the 1970s and early 1980s.[17] Dubernard, in Lyon, France, introduced duct injection of a synthetic polymer as a method to block secretions and cause fibrosis in the exocrine pancreas of a segmental graft, with sparing of the endocrine component,[20] and many pioneering centers adopted this technique, although it is little used today. Gliedman introduced urinary drainage through a ureteroductostomy for segmental grafts,[21] and Sollinger later modified this approach with direct anastomosis of a duodenal patch of a whole pancreas graft to the recipient bladder.[22] Drs. Dai Nghiem and Robert Corry did further modification of urinary drainage,[23] retaining a bubble of duodenum for duodenocystostomy, as Lillehei had done for duodenoenterostomy.[18] From the early 1980s until the mid-1990s, the bladder-drainage technique with duodenocystostomy was the predominant technique for pancreas transplantations. The bladder-drainage technique had a low acute complication rate and was helpful in monitoring for rejection by detection of a decline in urine amylase activity, but chronic complications, such as recurrent urinary tract

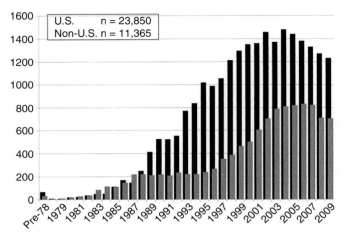

FIGURE 47-1 Annual number of U.S. and non-U.S. pancreas transplantations reported to the International Pancreas Transplant Registry (IPTR), 1978-2009.

infections or dehydration from fluid loss through the exocrine secretions, were common. Thus in the mid-1990s, described by Lillehei and colleagues,[18] a change occurred and enteric drainage, which was never totally out of fashion,[24,25] overtook bladder drainage as the predominant drainage procedure. In addition, portal rather than systemic venous drainage was used by some groups for enteric-drained whole pancreas–duodenal transplantations.[26] Portal venous drainage was originally introduced by Calne in 1984 for segmental pancreas grafts as a more physiologic technique[26] and was applied by several groups sporadically over the years.[17]

With advances in immunosuppression, including the introduction of cyclosporine by Calne and coworkers in 1979,[27] tacrolimus by Starzl and associates in 1989,[28] and mycophenolate mofetil by Sollinger and coworkers in 1995,[29] bladder drainage had become less important for monitoring rejection. Furthermore, in recipients of simultaneous pancreas and kidney transplants from the same donor, the kidney could be monitored for rejection episodes (elevation of serum creatinine) as a surrogate marker for pancreas rejection before there was sufficient pancreatic damage to cause hyperglycemia. However, in solitary pancreas transplants, serum creatinine could not be used as a marker for rejection, and in such cases, bladder drainage is useful and continues to be used.[17]

DETAILS OF SURGICAL TECHNIQUES

As mentioned in the history section, a variety of techniques have been used for management of the exocrine secretions and venous drainage of pancreas transplants.[30,31] The majority of pancreas grafts are procured from multiorgan deceased donors, and because the liver and pancreas share the origins of their arterial blood supply, a whole organ pancreas graft usually requires reconstruction.[32,33] The blood supply to the tail of the pancreas is supplied by the splenic artery, originating from the celiac axis, and the head of the pancreas is supplied by the pancreaticoduodenal arcades, originating from the superior mesenteric artery and the hepatic artery. Because the latter goes with the liver, along with the celiac axis, the usual approach is to attach an arterial Y-graft of the donor iliac vessels, with anastomosis of the hypogastric artery to the graft splenic artery and the external iliac artery to the graft superior mesenteric artery,

leaving the common iliac artery segment of the Y-graft for anastomosis to the recipient arterial system, usually the right common iliac artery. The portal vein of the donor is usually divided midway between the upper border of the pancreas and the liver, leaving adequate length for transplantations of both organs, but if necessary, an extension graft of donor iliac vein can be anastamosed to the pancreatic graft portal vein portion. In the recipient, the pancreas graft portal vein, with or without an extension graft, can be anastomosed to the systemic venous system (usually the iliac vein or vena cava) or to the portal system (usually the superior mesenteric vein).

When venous drainage is to the recipient's iliac vein, the whole pancreas graft can be oriented with the head directed into either the pelvis or the upper abdomen. When directed cephalad, enteric drainage is the only option. When directed caudad, the duodenum can be anastomosed to either the bladder (Fig. 47-2) or bowel (Fig. 47-3). Figure 47-2

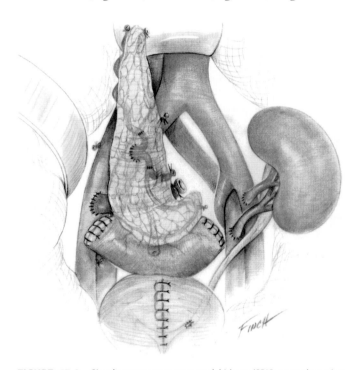

FIGURE 47-2 Simultaneous pancreas and kidney (SPK) transplantation using a whole pancreas/duodenal graft from a deceased donor with systemic venous drainage to the right iliac vein and bladder drainage of the pancreas exocrine secretions through a duodenocystostomy. Both the pancreas and kidney are placed in the peritoneum through a midline incision. The donor splenic artery, supplying the pancreatic tail, and the donor superior mesenteric artery, supplying the pancreatic head, have been joined by a Y-graft constructed from the donor common external/internal iliac artery complex during a bench procedure, and the base of the Y-graft is anastomosed to the recipient common iliac artery. The mid-duodenum is anastomosed to the posterior dome of the bladder, and the duodenal stumps are oversewn. The kidney graft could be from a living donor or the same deceased donor as the pancreas graft, but, in either case, is preferentially placed to the left iliac vessels so that the right side, with its more superficial vessels, can be used for the pancreas transplant. In this particular illustration, the donor ureter was implanted into the bladder using the Politano-Leadbetter technique through an anterior cystotomy, a technique that also allows the duodenocystostomy to be performed with an end-to-end anastomosis (EEA) stapler, with internal oversewing of the anastomotic line using an absorbable suture to cover the staples, followed by closure of the cystotomy. However, when enteric drainage is used for an SPK transplantation, an external ureteroneocystostomy is usually performed. (Reproduced from Gruessner RWG, Sutherland DER [eds]: Transplantation of the Pancreas. New York, Springer-Verlag, 2004.)

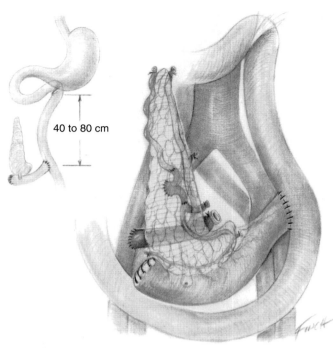

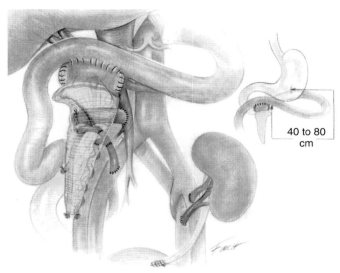

FIGURE 47-3 Pancreas-duodenal transplantation using a deceased donor with systemic venous drainage and enteric drainage of graft exocrine secretions to a proximal loop of recipient jejunum. In this particular case, an end-to-side two-layer duodenojejunostomy, using the distal end of the graft duodenum, is illustrated, and the anastomosis is located 40 to 80 cm distal to the ligament of Treitz (inset). Alternatively, a side-to-side stapled or handsewn duodenojejunostomy, with or without a Roux-en-Y loop, can be done. (Reproduced from Gruessner RWG, Sutherland DER [eds]: Transplantation of the Pancreas. New York, Springer-Verlag, 2004.)

FIGURE 47-4 Whole pancreas/duodenum transplantation using a deceased donor with portal venous drainage with an end-to-side anastomosis to the recipient superior mesenteric vein, accessed below its confluence with the splenic vein. Drainage of exocrine secretions is through a side-to-side duodenojejunostomy, 40 to 80 cm distal to the ligament of Treitz. Note that the cephalad position of the pancreatic head, when portal venous drainage is used, as opposed to the caudal orientation possible with systemic venous drainage, is no different than that needed when bladder drainage is done. In this particular illustration, the pancreas graft overlies the root of the small bowel mesentery, with the duodenal segment below the transverse colon, and the arterial Y-graft is anastomosed to the recipient common iliac artery through a mesenteric tunnel. However, a retroperitoneal approach under the right colon is also possible, in which case the arterial Y-graft can be anastomosed directly to the recipient iliac artery, but the enteric anastomosis must be through a Roux-en-Y limb of recipient bowel brought through the mesentery. If a kidney is simultaneously transplanted to the left iliac vessels, the ureter can be implanted into the bladder using the extravesical ureteroneocystostomy (Lich) technique, as illustrated. (Reproduced from Gruessner RWG, Sutherland DER [eds]: Transplantation of the Pancreas. New York, Springer-Verlag, 2004.)

shows the bladder-drainage technique and also depicts a kidney transplantation to the left iliac vessels, but, as mentioned, with a kidney transplantation, enteric drainage is more common than bladder drainage.

With the bladder-drainage technique, the anastomosis may be handsewn or performed with an end-to-end anastomosis (EEA) stapler brought through the distal duodenum (which is subsequently stapled closed) for connection to the post of the anvil projected through the posterior bladder by an anterior cystotomy (see Fig. 47-2). The inner layer is then reinforced with a running absorbable suture for hemostasis and for burying the staples under the mucosa.

With enteric drainage/systemic venous drainage, the anastomosis may be handsewn in an end-to-side fashion (see Fig. 47-3), or it can be done in a side-to-side fashion by handsewing or by using an EEA stapler.[34] The barrel of the EEA stapler is inserted into the end of the graft duodenum, and the post is projected through the side wall. The anvil is inserted into the recipient bowel through an enterotomy secured around the connecting post by a purse-string suture. The two posts are connected and the stapler is fired, creating the anastomosis. The end of the duodenum is then closed with a simple stapler. The enteric anastomosis can be done directly to the most convenient proximal small bowel loop of the recipient or to a Roux-en-Y segment of recipient bowel that is created at the time. Outcome analyses do not show any statistical advantage of a Roux-en-Y loop.

For portal drainage of the pancreas graft venous effluent (Fig. 47-4), the head and duodenum of the graft is oriented

cephalad, and the graft portal vein is anastomosed directly to the recipient superior mesenteric vein. In the illustration, the pancreas graft is ventral to the recipient small bowel mesentery so that the venous anastomosis is to the ventral side of the vein, and the arterial Y-graft must be brought through a window of mesentery for anastomosis to the recipient's aorta or common iliac artery. The graft duodenum is anastomosed to recipient's small bowel by the same techniques described for systemic venous drainage, with or without (as depicted) a Roux-en-Y loop of recipient bowel.

An alternative approach for portal venous drainage of the pancreas graft effluent is to place the pancreas retroperitoneally by reflecting the right colon to the left and exposing the dorsal surface of the superior mesenteric vein, as described by Boggi and associates.[35,36] The arterial Y-graft can then be anastomosed directly to the right common iliac artery, but this approach does mandate creation of a Roux-en-Y limb of recipient bowel to bring through the small bowel or transverse colon mesentery for a graft duodenoenterostomy.

Other techniques can be used, including duct injection for a segmental graft. Segmental grafts are rarely used, except in the few cases of living donor pancreas transplantations,[37–42] and most of these have the exocrine secretions managed by either a ductoenterostomy to a Roux-en-Y limb of recipient bowel or a ductocystostomy to the recipient's bladder

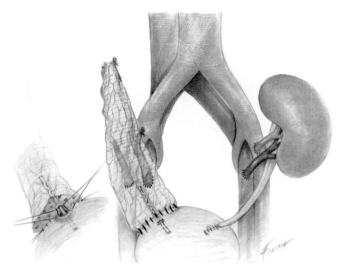

FIGURE 47-5 Living donor segmental (body and tail) pancreas transplantation to right iliac vessels (systemic venous drainage) and bladder drainage of exocrine secretions through a ductocystostomy by means of an intraperitoneal approach. The donor splenic artery and splenic vein are anastomosed end to side to the recipient external iliac artery and vein after ligation and division of all hypogastric veins to bring the main vein as superficial as possible. The splenic artery anastomosis is lateral and proximal to the splenic vein anastomosis. A two-layer ductocystostomy is constructed: The pancreatic duct is approximated to the urothelial layer (inner layer) using interrupted 7-0 absorbable sutures over a stent *(inset)*. If the kidney is transplanted simultaneously, the donor ureter is implanted into the bladder using the extravesical ureteroneocystostomy (Lich) technique. (Reproduced from Gruessner RWG, Sutherland DER [eds]: Transplantation of the Pancreas. New York, Springer-Verlag, 2004.)

(Fig. 47-5). Segmental pancreas transplantations from living donors, with or without a kidney transplantation, are particularly useful in candidates who would otherwise have a long wait for a deceased donor organ, such as those with a high level of human leukocyte antigen (HLA) antibodies but with a negative crossmatch to a living volunteer.[40] However, there are circumstances where a segmental graft from a deceased donor is still appropriate for technical reasons, particularly for retransplantations where conventional sites have been used previously in such a way they cannot be reused and one has to use unconventional sites, even orthotopically.[43] For more details concerning the variety of surgical techniques in pancreas donors (deceased and living) and recipients, the reader is referred to work by Benedetti and colleagues.[44]

GENERAL INFORMATION, PANCREAS TRANSPLANTATION CATEGORIES, AND IMMUNOSUPPRESSION

By the late-1990s, more than 2500 pancreas transplantations were being done annually worldwide (see Fig. 47-1), as reported to the International Pancreas Transplant Registry (IPTR).[45] By 2010, more than 35,000 vascularized pancreas transplantations had been performed, more than half in the United States, with very large series at some centers,[25,46-48] more than 2000 total at the University of Minnesota,[49] and more than 1000 simultaneous pancreas and kidney (SPK) transplantations at the University of Wisconsin.[47] The vast majority were done to establish insulin independence in patients with de novo type 1 diabetes mellitus, but enteric-

drained pancreas transplantations have been used to correct both endocrine and exocrine deficiency after total pancreatectomy in some patients[51-53] and to treat diseases such as cystic fibrosis in others.[54]

Specialists in more than 150 institutions in the United States, and nearly the same number elsewhere, have performed pancreas transplantations.[55] The IPTR was founded in 1980 to analyze the results.[56] In 1987, reporting of U.S. cases became obligatory through the United Network for Organ Sharing (UNOS), and near-annual reports have been made thereafter.[57-60]

There are three categories of pancreas transplantation recipients: (1) uremic diabetic patients who undergo a simultaneous pancreas and kidney transplantation from either a deceased or living donor[61]; (2) nephropathic patients who already have had renal insufficiency corrected, usually by a living donor kidney transplantation, and then undergo a pancreas after kidney (PAK) transplantation[62-64]; and (3) nonuremic diabetic patients who undergo a pancreas transplantation alone (PTA).[65] The Pancreas Transplant Registry has compared outcomes in the three categories spanning several eras of data collection.[57-60,66,67]

The majority of pancreas transplantations have been in the SPK category, but in recent years, there has been an increased emphasis in performing living donor kidney transplantations to preempt the need for dialysis in diabetics with nephropathy.[68] Thus until 2004, the number of PAK transplantations increased, but the number of SPK transplantations did not change (Fig. 47-6). Concomitantly, there has also been an increase in the number of PTA cases to treat diabetics without advanced nephropathy who have diabetic management problems justifying immunosuppression, and to treat patients who would also be candidates for islet transplantation, given the conditions discussed later. Although most pancreas transplantation recipients have type 1 diabetes, insulin-treated type 2 diabetics also become insulin-independent after a pancreas transplantation.[69-71]

Immunosuppression management of pancreas transplantation recipients is similar to that of recipients of other solid organs, including kidneys, which the majority of pancreas recipients also receive.[72] Thus induction immunosuppression

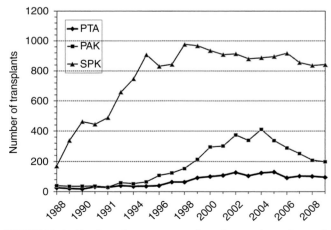

FIGURE 47-6 Number of pancreas transplantations performed annually in the United States from 1988 through 2009 by recipient category. PAK, pancreas after kidney transplantation; PTA, pancreas transplantation alone; SPK, simultaneous pancreas and kidney transplantation.

with anti–T-cell monoclonal or polyclonal depleting or nondepleting agents may be used or reserved for rejection episodes.[73] Maintenance immunosuppression usually consists of a combination of a calcineurin inhibitor (cyclosporine or tacrolimus), with the dose and blood levels adjusted to minimize nephrotoxicity, and an antiproliferative agent (mycophenolate mofetil or sirolimus), with or without prednisone. Corticosteroid-free regimens are now quite common for all organ transplantations, including the pancreas.[74–83] Suspected pancreas allograft rejection episodes, based on transient rise of serum amylase or lipase in enteric-drained grafts or on a decline in urine amylase in bladder-drained grafts, or by a rise in serum creatinine in SPK transplantations, can be confirmed by biopsy of the graft.[84,85]

PANCREAS TRANSPLANTATION OUTCOMES

Current outcomes with deceased donor pancreas transplantations, according to recipient categories, surgical technique, and immunosuppression protocol, for U.S. cases as reported to UNOS from January 2005 to December 2009, are summarized here.[55] During this period, 5567 primary deceased donor pancreas transplantations were reported to UNOS, including 4155 SPK, 947 PAK, and 465 PTA transplantations.

The primary transplantation patient survival rates in the three recipient categories are shown in Figure 47-7. At 1 year, 96% of the SPK, 97% of the PAK, and 97% of the PTA recipients were alive; at 3 years, 92%, 91%, and 92%, respectively, were alive. The highest patient survival rate could be found in PTA subgroups, presumably because this group had less advanced complications before transplantation.

The primary pancreas graft survival rates in the three recipient categories are shown in Figure 47-8. At 1 year, 85% of the SPK, 79% of the PAK, and 78% of the PTA recipients were totally insulin-independent; at 3 years, 79%, 68%, and 62%, respectively, were insulin-independent ($P < 0.001$). The highest pancreas graft survival rates are in the SPK category, presumably because the kidney graft (usually from the same donor as the pancreas) can be used to detect rejection episodes earlier than in the other categories, where only the pancreas can be monitored. Support for this hypothesis comes

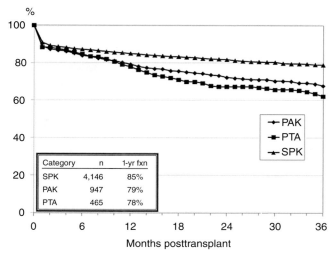

FIGURE 47-8 Pancreas graft functional survival rates (insulin independence) for 2005 to 2009 U.S. deceased donor primary transplantations by recipient category. Fxn, function; PAK, pancreas after kidney transplantation; PTA, pancreas transplantation alone; SPK, simultaneous pancreas and kidney transplantation.

from Registry data showing significantly higher early technical failure rates and also large differences in rejection loss rates for solitary transplants.

Of the 2005 to 2009 primary pancreas grafts, 6% of SPK and 9% of solitary transplants failed for technical reasons, with thrombosis being the highest risk for technical loss (5%); infection, pancreatitis, and anastomotic leak made up the rest. Technical graft loss was significantly higher in solitary transplants than in SPK ($P = 0.0009$).

The primary pancreas graft failure rates from rejection are shown in Figure 47-9. At 1 year, 2% of the SPK, 4% of the PAK, and 6% of the PTA recipients of technically successful grafts had to resume exogenous insulin (significantly lower in the SPK category; $P = 0.0001$).

Regarding management of pancreatic duct exocrine secretions for the 2005 to 2009 cases, enteric drainage predominated

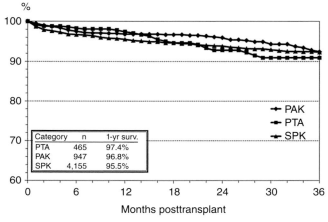

FIGURE 47-7 Patient survival rates for 2005 to 2009 U.S. deceased donor primary transplantations by recipient category. PAK, pancreas after kidney transplant; PTA, pancreas transplant alone; SPK, simultaneous pancreas and kidney transplantation; surv., survival.

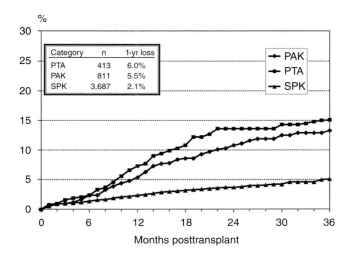

FIGURE 47-9 Technically successful pancreas graft immunologic failure rates (return to exogenous insulin) for 2005 to 2009 U.S. deceased donor primary transplants by recipient category. PAK, pancreas after kidney transplantation; PTA, pancreas transplantation alone; SPK, simultaneous pancreas and kidney transplantation.

for SPK transplants (91%); for PAK and PTA, the proportion that were enteric drained was slightly lower (86% and 79%, respectively). Overall, the technical failure rate was significantly higher with enteric-drained SPK than with bladder-drained SPK (7% vs. 4%) transplants. No difference was found for solitary transplants. Pancreas graft survival rates, however, were not significantly different for enteric-drained versus bladder-drained transplantations in any of the categories: At 1 year, the rates were 85% ($n = 3665$) versus 86% ($n = 366$) for SPK, 79% ($n = 790$) versus 82% ($n = 130$) for PAK, and 80% ($n = 366$) versus 75% ($n = 99$) for PTA cases. No difference in the failure rate from rejection for technically successful grafts for enteric-drained versus bladder-drained transplantations could be found anymore.

In the SPK category, bladder drainage and enteric drainage would be expected to give similar results: In most cases, both grafts come from the same donor, and monitoring of serum creatinine serves as a surrogate marker for rejection in the pancreas transplant, allowing easy detection and reversal by treatment. In contrast, for solitary pancreas transplants (PAK and PTA), serum creatinine cannot be used as a marker of pancreas rejection, hyperglycemia is a late manifestation of rejection, and exocrine markers must be used. Although serum amylase and lipase may elevate during a rejection episode, this does not occur in all cases, but for bladder-drained grafts, a decrease in urine amylase eventually always accompanies rejection (100% sensitive, even though it is not specific) and nearly always precedes hyperglycemia so that a rejection episode is more likely to be diagnosed in a bladder-drained graft and lead to treatment and reversal.

Approximately one quarter of enteric-drained pancreas grafts reported to UNOS were done with a Roux-en-Y loop; in the past, the outcomes were not improved by this procedural addition,[45] and that is still the case.[55]

Another variation in surgical technique is portal drainage of the venous effluent for enteric-drained grafts.[30,86] It establishes normal physiology and a theoretic metabolic advantage versus systemic venous drainage, and some groups have reported that portal venous enteric-drainage grafts are less prone to rejection than systemic venous enteric-drainage grafts,[87,88] although others have not.[89] The latest Registry analysis shows that portal venous drainage was used for one fifth of enteric-drainage transplantations, but there were no significant differences in pancreas graft survival versus systemic venous enteric-drainage transplantations in any of the categories: at 1 year, 84% ($n = 718$) versus 86% ($n = 2896$) for SPK, 79% ($n = 130$) versus 79% ($n = 651$) for PAK, and 78% ($n = 51$) versus 80% ($n = 305$) for PTA cases.

Regarding immunosuppression, according to the latest Registry analysis, anti–T-cell agents were used for induction therapy for more than 80% of the 2005 to 2009 U.S. pancreas recipients in each category.[55] The most frequently used regimen for maintenance immunosuppression (more than two thirds of the recipients in each category) was tacrolimus and mycophenolate mofetil in combination, with or without prednisone. In recipients of primary deceased donor pancreas grafts given anti–T-cell agents for induction and tacrolimus and mycophenolate mofetil for maintenance immunosuppression (Fig. 47-10), the 1-year graft survival rates in the SPK, PAK, and PTA categories were 86% ($n = 2737$), 81% ($n = 544$), and 86% ($n = 271$), respectively. A sirolimus-based regimen was used as a maintenance immunosuppressive drug

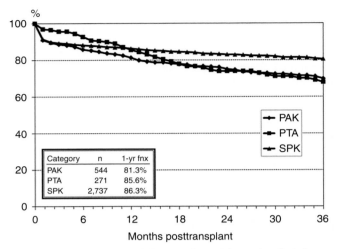

FIGURE 47-10 Pancreas graft functional survival rates (insulin independence) for 2005 to 2009 U.S. deceased donor primary transplantations by category in diabetic recipients given anti–T-cell agents for induction and tacrolimus (TAC) and mycophenolate mofetil (MMF) for maintenance immunosuppression. Fxn, function; PAK, pancreas after kidney transplantation; PTA, pancreas transplantation alone; SPK, simultaneous pancreas and kidney transplantation.

in more than 13% of recipients in each category (Fig. 47-11), with excellent outcomes: The 1-year pancreas graft survival rates in the SPK, PAK, and PTA categories were 90% ($n = 407$), 89% ($n = 94$), and 89% ($n = 84$), respectively. In contrast, the remaining recipients given alternative immunosuppressive regimens had distinctly lower pancreas graft survival rates in each category: at 1 year, 74% in SPK ($n = 153$), 61% in PAK ($n = 71$), and 29% in PTA ($n = 35$) cases. A center effect may play a role in the outcomes of the Registry analysis according to immunosuppressive regimens.

Regarding the logistics of pancreas transplantation, the recent Registry data[55] showed a significant increase in technical

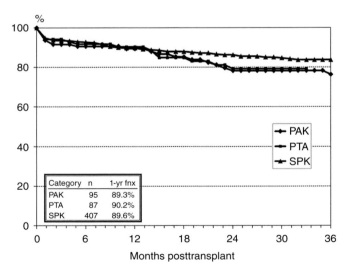

FIGURE 47-11 Pancreas graft functional survival rates (insulin independence) for 2005 to 2009 U.S. deceased donor primary transplantations by category in diabetic recipients given sirolimus-based maintenance immunosuppression. Fxn, function; PAK, pancreas after kidney transplantation; PTA, pancreas transplantation alone; SPK, simultaneous pancreas and kidney transplantation.

failure rates and a decrease in graft survival rates with increasing preservation time. The relative risk (RR) to lose the graft doubled for SPK grafts with a preservation time greater than 24 hours compared with a preservation time of 12 to 24 hours. Shorter SPK preservation time showed a decreased risk of one third. HLA matching had virtually no impact on SPK graft survival rates, but matching at least at the class I loci had a beneficial effect in the PAK and the PTA categories.

Regarding pancreas recipient age, the recent Registry analysis of the 2005 to 2009 cases showed an effect on outcome mainly in solitary recipients, with rejection more likely in younger patients. In the SPK category, only 3 patients were younger than 15 years of age, and 312 recipients (7%) were between 15 and 29 years of age. In PAK, 5% ($n = 60$) were between the age of 15 and 29 years of age, and 15% ($n = 75$) in PTA. The relative risk for graft loss was not significantly increased for younger SPK recipients ($P = 0.21$) but clearly higher for PAK recipients (RR = 1.75, $P = 0.003$) and PTA recipients (RR = 1.99, $P = 0.009$) compared with recipients 30 to 45 years of age. Thus the young nonuremic diabetic is highly immunocompetent and more prone to reject a pancreas graft, consistent with an earlier analysis of outcomes in U.S. pediatric pancreas transplantation recipients from 1988 to 1999.[90] In that analysis, of slightly more than 8000 pancreas transplantations, only 49 were in recipients younger than 21 years of age (<1%), 34 in the SPK, 2 in the PAK, and 13 in the PTA category; all were deceased donor pancreas transplantations, except for two PTA segmental grafts from living donors. Less than half of the pediatric pancreas recipients were younger than 19. In the PTA recipients, the 1-year graft survival rate was only 15%, with all but one loss being from rejection in less than 1 year. The Registry data do not include the indications for a PTA in the pediatric recipients, but presumably they had extremely labile diabetes, justifying placement on immunosuppression in an attempt to gain control. In the pediatric SPK recipients, however, the 1-year patient, pancreas, and kidney graft survival rates were 96%, 78%, and 71%, respectively, which were outcomes comparable to those of adult SPK recipients for the entire period. Of the pediatric SPK recipients, most had a renal disease other than diabetic nephropathy.

Thus pancreas transplantations in the pediatric age group are uncommon, and most are in diabetic children who also have renal failure and thus need a kidney transplantation, obligating them to immunosuppression. At least in this group, the outcomes are such that it seems reasonable to recommend the addition of the pancreas so that the child can become insulin independent as well as dialysis free for the price of immunosuppression.[13] For nonuremic diabetic children with extreme lability, in whom a successful pancreas transplantation would be appropriate treatment, the antirejection strategies need to be optimized to improve the graft survival rates versus what has been achieved in the past.

With respect to outcome measures other than insulin independence, prevention and reversal of secondary complications, improvement in quality of life, extension of life span, and reduction of health care costs per quality-adjusted life-year have all been positively demonstrated in type 1 diabetic pancreas transplant recipients.[91-97] In patients with labile diabetes and hypoglycemic unawareness, a pancreas transplantation can resolve an otherwise intractable and life-threatening course.[98-100]

Whether a pancreas transplantation has an effect on survival probabilities for the diabetic population selected for the procedure is controversial. Two separate analyses of U.S. data from UNOS and the Organ Procurement Transplant Network (OPTN) for pancreas transplantation candidates and recipients between 1995 and 2000 compared the survival probabilities for patients who remained on the waiting list with those receiving a transplant by category.[103,104] In the first analysis,[103] SPK recipients had a significantly higher probability of survival than those remaining on the waiting list for the procedure, but, for solitary (PAK or PTA) recipients, just the opposite was the case. In the second analysis,[104] the higher survival probability for SPK recipients was confirmed, and, in addition, the overall survival probabilities of solitary pancreas transplant recipients compared with those waiting, and even after 1 year, were favorable for transplantation. In the second analysis, patients who listed at multiple centers were identified and were counted only once from the time of first listing, corrections were made for patients who changed categories, and longer follow-up was available. Thus pancreas transplantation does not entail a higher risk than staying on exogenous insulin for those on the waiting list and may improve survival probabilities for solitary as well as SPK recipients.[105]

In regard to secondary complications of diabetes,[106] numerous studies show a beneficial effect on neuropathy,[94,107-113] retinopathy[114-118] and nephropathy[92,119-122] as well as on cardiovascular disease,[123-128] and quality of life.[129,130] In regard to nephropathy, specifically in PTA recipients, even though the diabetic lesions in the native kidneys can improve,[131] this can be offset by the nephrotoxicity of the calcineurin inhibitors given for immunosuppression.[132]

It should be noted that pancreas retransplantation can be done if the first graft fails, with only slightly lower graft survival rates than for primary transplants.[66,67,133,134] Indeed, even third transplants can do well.[134]

Also of note, pancreas allografts are often procured by one center and transplanted at another, and there are studies showing no difference in outcomes compared with locally procured organs.[135]

Surgical complications of pancreas transplantation are numerous and are the subject of an extensive review recently published.[136] The most frequent complication leading to graft loss is venous or arterial thrombosis (5% to 10%). Anastomotic leaks are also common, but if diagnosed early, graft salvage is possible.

Islet Transplantation

Human islet transplantation, the less invasive islet beta cell replacement alternative to transplantation of the vascularized pancreas, has been investigated for more than 3 decades[137-140] after the first clinical islet allograft was performed in 1974.[141] Since then, nearly 1000 islet allotransplantations have been performed worldwide.[142,143]

Islet autotransplantations have had a relatively high success rate in preventing diabetes after total pancreatectomy for more than 2 decades; so, they are briefly described before reviewing the current status of islet allografts for type 1 as well as for surgical diabetes.

ISLET AUTOTRANSPLANTATIONS AFTER PANCREATECTOMY FOR BENIGN DISEASE

Islet autotransplantations to prevent diabetes after a total pancreatectomy for benign disease, primarily painful chronic pancreatitis, have been successful since the first case was performed in the 1970s[144,145] but depend on the number of islets transplanted.[146–151] Children with chronic pancreatitis and intractable pain who require pancreatectomy for relief of the pain and resolution of narcotic dependence nearly always have some beta cell function preserved by an islet autotransplantation, and they are either nondiabetic (more than a third) or can maintain euglycemia with once-daily long-acting insulin or near euglycemia with standard basal-bolus insulin.[152–155] Total pancreatectomy is highly successful in relieving the pain of chronic pancreatitis in both adults and children, particularly if done early before years of narcotic dependence.[148,150,153] The islet yield is also better if the pancreatectomy is not delayed, because the number of islets isolated correlates with the degree of pancreatic damage in both adults[156] and children.[157]

The surgical technique of pylorus-sparing total pancreatectomy and duodenectomy is shown in Figure 47-12. The procedure can be staged, but when the body and tail of the

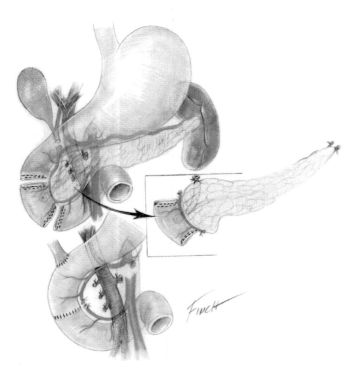

FIGURE 47-12   Pylorus-sparing total pancreatectomy and partial duodenectomy technique for patients with chronic pancreatitis undergoing islet autotransplantations. The bile duct is transected and reimplanted into the duodenum, shown here proximal to a duodenoduodenostomy or duodenojejunostomy, but, more commonly, it is placed distal to the enteric anastomosis, with the site depending on the individual anatomy. When possible, only the second portion of the duodenum is resected, and an end-to-end duodenoduodenostomy is created; but if viability is not maintained, the entire distal duodenum must be resected and an end-to-end or end-to-side duodenojejunostomy performed. The short gastric vessels are preserved, as well as the gastroepiploic artery if possible, and the spleen is not removed if its viability is maintained. (Reproduced from Gruessner RWG, Sutherland DER [eds]: Transplantation of the Pancreas. New York, Springer-Verlag, 2004.)

pancreas are removed, they should always be processed for islet isolation for an intraportal autotransplant (Fig. 47-13, *A*).

If a distal pancreatectomy is the primary procedure and a Whipple (completion) pancreatectomy becomes necessary, diabetes will have been prophylactically prevented by the initial islet autograft. If a Whipple procedure was the primary procedure, but pain persists and a distal (body and tail) completion pancreatectomy is required, it should be done in an institution capable of isolating islets from the excised gland for an autotransplantation.[158]

ISLET ALLOTRANSPLANTATIONS

Islet allotransplantations have been performed for the treatment of surgical and type 1 diabetes. As with autotransplantations, islet allotransplantations are usually done with embolization of the islets to the liver via the portal vein, where at least some islets will survive by nutrient diffusion until revascularization occurs (Fig. 47-13, *B*). A drawback of islet allotransplantations, as compared with pancreas transplantations, is the reduced beta cell mass; much attention has been given to compensating for the attrition that occurs. Islet allografts in patients with surgical diabetes have been associated with a very high success rate,[159,160] possibly because of the avoidance of diabetogenic steroids and the lack of an autoimmunity.

Islet allograft transplantations in patients with autoimmune type 1 diabetes have initially been performed simultaneously with a kidney transplant or in patients with established kidney transplants.[142] Insulin independence in this recipient group, even on an anecdotal basis, was not achieved until the early 1990s.[161–165]

Islet allografts have also been performed in patients in whom type 1 diabetes (T1D) is complicated by hypoglycemia unawareness and defective hormonal glucose counter-regulation resulting in recurrent episodes of severe hypoglycemia.[166] Today, the majority of human islet allografts are performed in this recipient group.[143] Acute complications are frequent in the 12.5% of T1D patients who have become aware of hypoglycemia 20 years after diabetes onset.[167] Iatrogenic hypoglycemia is the most limiting factor in the glycemic management of T1D;[168] it causes recurrent physical and psychological morbidity, including coma, seizures, and significant social embarrassment, and 7% to 10% of all deaths in patients with T1D are the result of hypoglycemia.[169,170] Hypoglycemia-related problems have not abated during the more than 18 years since they were first highlighted by the landmark report of the DCCT in 1993.[168,171] New glucose monitoring technologies are being developed; however, continuous glucose monitoring did not lower the rate of severe hypoglycemia in patients with T1D.[173,174]

A major milestone was reached in 2000 when Dr. Shapiro and colleagues at the University of Alberta in Edmonton achieved diabetes reversal in seven of seven recipients by using islets from more than one donor pancreas and by using corticosteroid-free, less diabetogenic immunosuppression.[175] Since then, several groups around the world have reported restoration of insulin independence after human islet allotransplantation in type 1 diabetic recipients.[11,176–194]

Furthermore, remarkable additional progress has been made in the past decade toward developing islet transplantation into a vital treatment option for T1D. First, new protocols

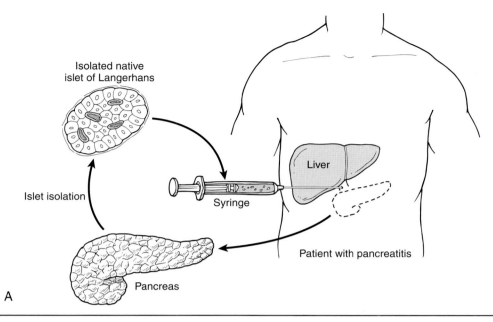

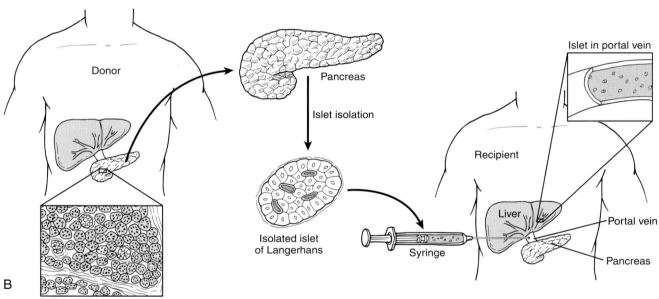

FIGURE 47-13   Islet transplantation using the portal vein for embolization to the liver where revascularization will occur, either as an autograft of islets isolated from the excised specimen after pancreatectomy for benign disease **(A)** or as an allograft of cells isolated from a donor for treatment of a patient with type 1 diabetes **(B)**.

succeeded in achieving insulin independence with islets from a single donor pancreas.[179,180,187–191] Many of these protocols include adjunctive peritransplant anti-inflammatory and/or cytoprotective therapy, likely facilitating improved islet engraftment. Second, recent data indicate that islet allograft survival in T1D can be sustained with calcineurin inhibitor–free protocols.[188–190] Two immunosuppressive regimens, based on the costimulation blocker belatacept or the antileukocyte functional antigen-1 antibody efalizumab, were effective, well tolerated, and involved the first calcineurin inhibitor/steroid-sparing islet protocols resulting in long-term insulin independence. Although efalizumab is no longer available for clinical use, these early results demonstrate that

calcineurin inhibitor–free regimens may be an effective alternative to improve graft function and longevity while minimizing renal and islet beta cell toxicity. Third, Berney and colleagues reported on the first type 1 diabetic patient who remained insulin independent for more than 10 years after islet allotransplantation.[195] Preliminary data now suggest that long-term insulin independence (>5 years) can be achieved in 50% of recipients given T-cell–depleting induction immunotherapy, matching insulin independence rates of solitary pancreas transplantation.[196] Early studies examining long-term islet function suggested a rapid loss of insulin independence beyond 1 year in many patients.[183,197] One possible factor contributing to islet loss is recurrent beta cell autoimmunity.[198,199]

Anti-CD3 antibodies and T-cell–depleting therapies, including anti-Thymoglobulin, have proved promising agents for minimizing autoimmunity in murine models of autoimmune diabetes and in clinical trials for new-onset T1D.[200–204] A recent analysis of University of Minnesota data and data reported to the Collaborative Islet Transplant Registry indicated that patients receiving an induction immunosuppression regimen that includes T-cell–depleting agents, either anti-CD3 antibody alone or either antithymocyte globulin (ATG) or alemtuzumab plus short-term TNF-α inhibition, for alloislet transplantation are more than twice as likely to maintain long-term insulin independence for at least 5 years post-transplant.[196] Three-year and 5-year insulin independence rates in these recipients are comparable with rates previously only attainable in recipients of pancreas transplants alone. Fourth, numerous reports have confirmed that human islet transplants are remarkably effective in protecting recipients with full and even partial islet graft function from severe hypoglycemia.[166,205,206] Finally, a prospective clinical trial demonstrated reduced progression of diabetic microvascular complications after islet transplantation compared with intensive medical therapy.[207] These data extend previous reports by the Milan group[208,209] and highlight the immense potential of cell-based diabetes therapy.

The unlimited and on-demand availability of xenogeneic pig islets would boost access to islet beta cell replacement. The quality of islet products from healthy, young, and living donor pigs would be predictably high and not compromised, as with human islet products, by comorbidity, brain death, age, and cold ischemia. The actual risks of infectious disease transmission from designated pathogen-free (DPF) source pigs are lower compared with risks associated with the use of deceased human donor organs.[210] Finally, genetic modification of source pigs would present opportunities for minimizing recipient immunosuppression not available to recipients of human islet allografts.[211] Thus exploiting the unique possibilities associated with porcine islet products would increase the availability and benefit-risk ratio of islet replacement therapies when compared with human islet products. The impact of such medical products on addressing unmet clinical needs in diabetes would be profound.

During the past few years, prolonged diabetes reversal exceeding 6 months has been demonstrated after porcine islet xenotransplantation in immunosuppressed nonhuman primates (NHPs) and for up to 6 months in nonimmunosuppressed NHPs.[212] Porcine C-peptide has been positive in the plasma of these recipients, and their fasting and, in some studies, also their non-fasting blood glucose levels have been in the normoglycemic to near-normoglycemic range. Perhaps most intriguing is that success has been achieved by five independent groups involving the use of various tissue sources (adult, neonatal, and embryonic pig islet tissue; wild-type and transgenic), implantation sites (portal vein, omental pouch, subcutaneous space), immunosuppressive protocols (with and without anti-CD154 monoclonal antibodies or encapsulation, avoiding immunosuppression), and animal models (streptozotocin-induced and surgical diabetes; in cynomolgus and rhesus monkeys).[213–216] Collectively, the demonstration of prolonged functional islet xenograft survival in nonhuman primates with several distinct xenotransplantation strategies suggests that porcine islet

products could potentially be developed into a more widely available cellular therapeutic for T1D.

Although a transition from pancreas to islet transplantations as the dominant form of beta cell replacement therapy may occur during the next few years, pancreas transplantations will not disappear entirely. Patients with high pretransplantation insulin requirements, in whom diabetes reversal with islet transplantations is less likely, would best be served with a vascularized pancreas transplant, at least as long as other more unlimited sources of beta cells, such as porcine islets, are not available for clinical therapy. Furthermore, diabetic patients with exocrine deficiency would best be served by an enteric-drained pancreas transplant. In addition, in patients who have very high insulin requirements or insulin resistance (type 2 diabetes), an intact organ may be needed to obtain a sufficient islet mass to restore insulin independence from a single donor in the presence of insulin resistance.

Tissue availability will be the limiting factor in determining the magnitude of the impact of beta cell replacement therapy. Six thousand deceased donors are available each year in the United States, but it is estimated that only half have a pancreas suitable for transplantation. Thus the maximal number of pancreas transplantations that could be done in the United States is 12,000 per year, assuming that each deceased pancreas could be split for use in two recipients,[217] and that living donors would be used for segmental pancreas transplantations[61] to the extent that they have been for kidney transplantations (currently about 6000 per year in the United States). This scenario has not yet materialized, but the potential is there to transplant at a rate approaching half of the annual incidence of new-onset cases of type 1 diabetes (30,000/year in the United States). The numbers could be increased further if enough islets could be isolated from one donor for transplantations into more than two recipients. Although the efficacy of islet transplantation protocols will continue to improve, and the procedural and immunosuppressive risks now associated with islet transplantations will continue to diminish, islet transplantations will not be the ultimate approach to diabetes care. Just as pancreas transplantations set the stage for islet transplantations, the real value of islet transplantations will be to create and build momentum for the development of xenogeneic and stem/precursor cell–derived islet beta cell therapy[218] that will then make cell replacement therapy routine and commonplace in diabetes care.

Pancreas transplantations, and eventually islet transplantations, should be in the armamentarium of every transplantation center for the treatment of diabetic patients. Likewise, every endocrinologist should consider beta cell replacement in the treatment of patients in whom type 1 diabetes is complicated by hypoglycemia-associated autonomic failure[219] and/or progressive microvascular complications. Continued clinical research on pancreas and islet transplantations is needed to identify the most appropriate recipient population, the optimal timing in the course of diabetes, and the most suitable donor tissue and transplantation protocol for a given patient. Both pancreas and islet transplants need to be made as economical as possible.[220] Studies such as those done in pancreas-kidney transplant recipients, showing the efficiency in the treatment of complicated diabetes,[221] are needed in islet recipients as well. Currently, beta cell replacement has a well-defined clinical role for adult patients with incapacitating hypoglycemic unawareness and is also appropriate in children and adults who otherwise need immunosuppression, such as for a kidney transplantation. As antirejection strategies become safer and with fewer side effects, the indications for pediatric beta cell replacement therapy can be liberalized.

Acknowledgments

We are indebted to Christine Johnson and Heather Nelson for assistance in preparing the manuscript.

The complete reference list is available online at www. expertconsult.com.

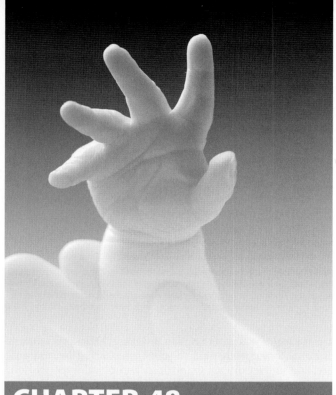

CHAPTER 48

Liver Transplantation

Bob H. Saggi, Douglas G. Farmer,
and Ronald W. Busuttil

The treatment of liver disease in children with transplantation has its roots in the origin of liver transplantation itself, with the initial cases performed by Thomas E. Starzl on two children in 1963 and 1968.[1] Although the initial results were disappointing, during the ensuing 2 decades, liver transplantation developed into the standard therapy for decompensated cirrhosis, certain malignancies of the liver and biliary tract, acute liver failure, and many metabolic derangements. The National Institutes of Health Development Conference designated it as such in 1983, and the National Organ Transplantation Act created a nationally regulated system of organ allocation in 1987. The United Network for Organ Sharing (UNOS) was subsequently created and currently regulates the field through a peer review process. In 2009, 6320 liver transplantation procedures were performed in the United States, and of these, 572 were in the pediatric population.[2] This number of transplantation procedures has remained relatively stable since the late 1990s, although an increasing number of "partial" liver grafts from cadaveric and living donors are now being used. Pediatric liver transplantation offers unique challenges because of size, perhaps enhanced immune responsiveness, and the paucity of donor organs. Although nearly 65% of pediatric liver transplantation recipients are less than 6 years of

age, only 25% of the pediatric cadaveric donor population comes from this same age group (Fig. 48-1).[2] As a consequence, achieving success in this arena requires technical perfection, both from the standpoint of obtaining a suitable graft and performing a meticulous transplantation operation. With reduction in transplantation waiting time and with improvements in immunosuppression, surgical technique, and long-term post-transplantation care, survival has markedly improved and now exceeds 90% at 1 year and 80% at 5 years, with many children surviving into adolescence and adulthood with a good quality of life.[3,4] In this chapter, we review the major indications for liver transplantation in children, the basic pathophysiology and clinical presentation of liver failure, operative strategies with emphasis on the unique surgical options available to children, postoperative management with emphasis on management of surgical complications, and outcome analysis.

Indications and Pretransplant Care

INDICATIONS FOR LIVER TRANSPLANTATION

Liver transplantation is currently indicated for children with decompensated cirrhosis because of cholestatic and noncholestatic causes, acute hepatic failure, some metabolic liver diseases, select tumors, and a variety of miscellaneous indications (Fig. 48-2). The general indication for liver transplantation in children is liver disease that limits long-term survival or quality of life, or markedly impairs normal growth and development. Cirrhosis alone is not an indication for transplantation, because many patients can be medically managed for a prolonged period prior to decompensation. In acute liver failure, the development of clear symptomatology, such as refractory coagulopathy, acidosis, and encephalopathy that correlate with a poor prognosis for spontaneous recovery of liver function, is an indication for transplantation. Otherwise, medical support in those with a better prognosis is provided until liver function returns to normal.[5,6] Finally, metabolic inborn errors of metabolism are a unique and not uncommon indication for transplantation in children, making up 9% of transplantation in children compared with approximately 2% in adults. Parenteral nutrition–associated liver disease accounts for 8% of liver transplantations, and less than 1% of adults are transplanted for this reason. Most of these transplantations are combined with an intestinal graft (Chapter 49).

With long-standing cirrhosis, the development of a constellation of symptoms and signs that represent decompensation of hepatocellular function or portal hypertension herald a need for transplantation. These include progressive jaundice, coagulopathy, protein-calorie malnutrition and growth retardation, impaired cognitive development, encephalopathy, hypersplenism, variceal hemorrhage, and advanced or refractory ascites. The majority of patients undergoing transplantation in this population are deeply jaundiced because of secondary or primary biliary cirrhosis from long-standing intrahepatic and/or extrahepatic biliary obstruction. On physical examination, these patients often have muscle wasting, an enlarged spleen, a hard palpable liver, abdominal distention

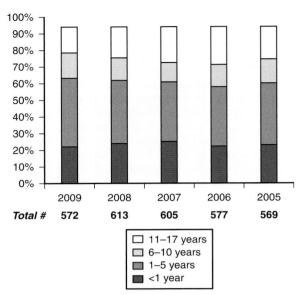

FIGURE 48-1 Distribution of pediatric liver transplantations by age. Data obtained from www.unos.org.

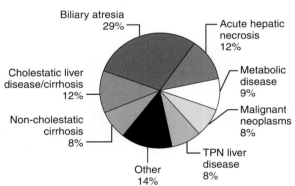

FIGURE 48-2 Indications for pediatric liver transplantation. Data obtained from www.unos.org, based on 2008 transplantations. TPN, total parenteral nutrition.

from ascites, and peripheral edema. With decompensation, long-term survival without liver transplantation is limited, and referral for transplantation must be made prior to decompensation.[3,7–9]

CHOLESTATIC LIVER DISORDERS

The most common indications for liver transplantation are the cholestatic liver disorders, with the most common being biliary atresia (BA). This group accounts for roughly 40% of the transplantation performed on children in 2008, and BA accounts for 70% of this cholestatic group (see Fig. 48-2).[2] The management of BA rests on early diagnosis, using surgical exploration with biopsy as the central confirmatory test in most cases. The diagnostic workup is detailed in Chapter 105. Portoenterostomy (PE) is the preferred treatment if diagnosis precedes the development of cirrhosis, usually before 3 months of age, though long-term results from PE

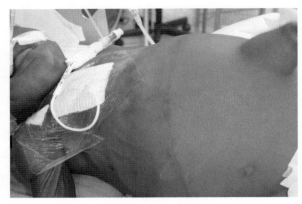

FIGURE 48-3 Decompensated cirrhosis after a Kasai portoenterosotomy. This 6-month-old, 5-kg child presented for liver transplant with the advanced findings of hepatosplenomegaly, extensive abdominal wall venous collaterals, tense ascites, jaundice, and profound malnutrition.

are optimal if it is done prior to 8 weeks.[10] This procedure is essential for slowing, and, in some cases, arresting, the progression of liver disease to cirrhosis and portal hypertension. Unfortunately, despite effective biliary drainage, more than 70% of patients will go on to develop decompensated cirrhosis by the age of 5 years and require transplantation.[10,11] However, in many cases, PE allows reasonable growth so that transplantation is forestalled until the child is older and larger. Primary PE performed late in the course of BA and reexploration for a failing biliary drainage procedure are both usually unsuccessful and only complicate transplantation outcomes. Instead, once a PE has failed, patients should be evaluated for transplantation. Liver transplantation is indicated when the diagnosis is made beyond 3 months of age, when decompensated cirrhosis is clearly present at any age, or after a PE has failed. Patients with BA should be managed by a pediatric hepatologist experienced in transplantation to ensure early referral for transplantation. This should occur prior to severe liver decompensation when signs are obvious on physical examination, especially with an advanced presentation at a late stage (Fig. 48-3).

Other uncommon etiologies of cholestatic liver injury and cirrhosis include familial paucity of intrahepatic bile ducts, which exists in a syndromic (Alagille syndrome) and nonsyndromic form, familial cholestatic syndromes, primary or secondary sclerosing cholangitis, and uncorrectable choledochal cyst disease, including Caroli disease. The cystic diseases have a component of uncorrectable extrahepatic obstruction while the others are the result of malformation or destruction of intrahepatic bile ducts and/or arterial systems. All these share in common a variable and unpredictable progression to advanced fibrosis, cirrhosis, and portal hypertension. These patients typically present with progressive jaundice at an older age than patients with BA. Although their management does not entail a PE, the indications for transplantation in these patients follow the same rationale as that for BA.

NONCHOLESTATIC CIRRHOSIS

Noncholestatic cirrhosis is an uncommon indication for liver replacement in children, accounting for less than 10% of all procedures performed in 2008 (see Fig. 48-2).[2] These children usually present later in life than the cholestatic disorders.

Etiologies of cirrhosis and decompensated cirrhosis in these patients include chronic autoimmune hepatitis, neonatal hepatitis, chronic viral (B or C) hepatitis, and cryptogenic cirrhosis.

ACUTE LIVER FAILURE

Fulminant hepatic failure is usually defined as the onset of encephalopathy within 28 days after the onset of jaundice in a patient with acute liver failure without evidence of chronic liver disease. The hallmarks of acute liver failure include profound coagulopathy, acidosis, hypoglycemia, and progressive hyperbilirubinemia. Acute liver failure patients can develop acute renal failure, systemic inflammatory response with multiorgan failure syndrome, or cerebral edema progressing to herniation. Early referral is essential to avoid progression to a condition that contraindicates transplantation. A variety of criteria to determine the need for transplantation have been devised in European centers, where these patients are managed in a highly structured and centralized manner.[12] The most common established etiology in children is viral hepatitis, followed by acetaminophen and other drug toxicities and Wilson disease. However, in nearly two thirds, an etiology cannot be identified. Liver transplantation is the only acceptable therapy in patients who meet the criteria of fulminant hepatic failure, and early referral of all patients with acute liver failure is essential.[5,6]

METABOLIC LIVER DISEASE

These disorders have in common an enzyme deficiency or some other defect in hepatocellular function. This impairment can result in progressive fibrosis or cirrhosis (e.g., cystic fibrosis, chronic Wilson disease, and neonatal iron storage disease), with a typical presentation of decompensated cirrhosis. In other cases, the liver is structurally normal, but harmful byproducts of metabolism accumulate to cause neurologic injury (e.g., Crigler-Najjar syndrome, ornithine transcarbamylase deficiency, and acute Wilson disease), cardiovascular disease (e.g., familial hypercholesterolemia), or renal injury (familial hyperoxaluria). Some disorders are associated with the development of malignancies (e.g., tyrosinemia), and transplantation should be considered preemptively. Transplant evaluation of all patients with known metabolic disorders of the liver involves a thorough evaluation of extrahepatic function. This will ensure transplantation of only those patients who can benefit from liver transplantation and prevents progression of extrahepatic disease. In some patients, simultaneous or sequential or dual organ transplantation may be necessary (e.g., lung, kidney, heart).

TUMORS

The most common liver malignancy in children is hepatoblastoma.[13,14] Although sporadic cases have been reported, hepatocellular carcinoma (HCC) is primarily seen in children with viral hepatitis, tyrosinemia, some of the glycogen storage diseases, or in association with cirrhosis from other causes. Primary liver malignancies in pediatric patients are managed by surgical resection unless tumor size and/or location preclude resection. The benefit of neoadjuvant and/or adjuvant chemotherapy and radiation for hepatoblastoma has been well documented.[15–17] In HCC, multimodal therapy can be used to prevent further cancer progression or perhaps to improve the outcome of highly selected patients with advanced HCC. Both may benefit from preoperative transarterial chemoembolization and/or radiofrequency ablation.[18] If the lesion is unresectable, transplantation can be considered after excluding extrahepatic disease.[15,17] With multimodal therapy to include liver transplantation, the long-term survival with hepatoblastoma now exceeds 50%, while outcomes from HCC are in excess of 70%.[15,17,19] The major controversy that exists is whether transplantation should be attempted for large hepatoblastomas primarily or as a salvage after recurrence following resection, and whether focal lung metastases contraindicate transplantation if they can be resected The most common benign tumor of the liver is hemangioendothelioma, and although the vast majority regress with growth and medical therapy, occasionally, progression of heart failure or mass effect warrants transplantation.[13,19]

MISCELLANEOUS CONDITIONS

These conditions include diagnoses such as Budd-Chiari syndrome, trauma, biliary cirrhosis secondary to intestinal failure, and long-term total parenteral nutrition (TPN) use. The latter is detailed in Chapter 49.

Organ Allocation and Pretransplant Care

Patients who have evidence of decompensated cirrhosis are candidates for liver transplantation. However, the small size of the pediatric patient combined with a nationwide shortage of organs relative to wait-listed patients makes achieving transplantation in a timely fashion problematic. In 2008, there were 613 pediatric liver transplantations performed. In that same year, there were 773 pediatric-aged cadaveric liver donors. The problem with a discrepancy between donors and recipients is primarily a problem in the less-than-6-year age category, where there were 423 liver recipients but only 274 donors.[2] Another problem is, of course, timing: When a pediatric donor is available, there is not necessarily a size-matched pediatric recipient available. This creates a relative shortage of organs that necessitates a system to allocate these scarce organs to those who will derive the most benefit. Since 2002, the Pediatric End-Stage Liver Disease (PELD) score was implemented to allocate organs based on this "sickest first" paradigm.[9] The PELD score consists of five variables: international normalized ratio (INR), total bilirubin, serum albumin, growth retardation (≥ 2 standard deviations below the median height or weight for age), and young age (<1 or 1 to 2 years). Status I-A is used to designate patients with fulminant hepatic failure, primary graft nonfunction after transplantation, early hepatic artery thrombosis, and miscellaneous acute conditions. Unlike adults, pediatric patients with decompensated cirrhosis requiring intensive care unit (ICU) stay for accepted reasons, and occasional exceptions can be listed as status I-B. This is because their mortality is high despite an often minimal change in PELD score with a decompensation requiring ICU stay. In an effort to ameliorate the shortage of potential organs, the livers of all donors 18 years of age and younger are preferentially allocated to pediatric recipients before being offered to adults.

Also, in 2006, organ allocation policy was changed so that rather than allocating livers from donors less than age 18 years locally, they are allocated at a regional level to children to increase the probability of use of the organ in pediatric patients and to facilitate liver splitting. These changes in organ allocation combined with the widespread use of split-liver transplantation (see later) has markedly reduced waiting times and positively impacted wait list mortality.[3,20]

Donor Procurement and Hepatobiliary Anatomy

HEPATOBILIARY ANATOMY

The performance of a donor hepatectomy or transplant operation requires a thorough understanding of foregut anatomy. In addition, a very detailed understanding of this anatomy is essential to the field of segmental liver transplantation and has impacted hepatobiliary surgery. The blood supply to the liver is based on a highly variable arterial and portal system. Venous drainage is through the right, mid-, and left hepatic veins that join the inferior vena cava, which traverses the dorsal surface of the liver (the retrohepatic cava). The liver is composed of the major right and left lobes that are separated by external landmarks and further subdivided into the right anterior and posterior sectors and left medial and lateral sectors. This nomenclature is still used to describe major anatomic liver resections. However, through the elegant anatomic techniques of the pioneering surgical anatomist Claude Couinaud, hepatic anatomy was found to be much more intricate (Fig. 48-4). The "Couinaud nomenclature" describes nine hepatic segments based on portal vein branching in relationship to the transverse plane (a cross-sectional plane located at "midpoints" of the hepatic veins) and the longitudinal planes of the individual hepatic veins (see Fig. 48-4). Each of the segments is supplied by an independent portal and hepatic arterial branch and drained by an independent biliary radicle. The biliary tree is second only to the arterial system in its variability. The hepatic venous drainage is intersegmental.

Donor Operation

The use of organs from cadaveric donors in pediatric liver transplantation involves selecting an appropriate quality and size-matched donor, organizing an experienced transplantation harvest team, and performing a precise technical operation that recognizes arterial anatomical variants and allows for multiorgan procurement. The advent of segmental liver transplantation has expanded the acceptable donor age to approximately 40 years. Preharvest donor management should focus on maintenance of hemodynamic stability with adequate but not excessive volume loading, the minimization of vasopressors, optimization of oxygenation without excessive use of positive end-expiratory pressure (PEEP), and correction of hypernatremia that results from diabetes insipidus. In the stable donor, once these goals are achieved, the procurement operation can be performed. In the properly selected unstable donor, unnecessary delays are to be avoided, because expedient hypothermic perfusion and cold storage only help minimize the ongoing organ ischemia.

The donor operation begins with midline laparotomy and median sternotomy for wide exposure (Fig. 48-5). The abdominal great vessels are exposed by a medial visceral rotation of the right colon and small intestine, and the aorta and inferior mesenteric vein are cannulated. The liver quality is assessed, and the biliary tree is flushed via the gallbladder. After full systemic heparinization, the supraceliac aorta is cross-clamped, and the intrapericardial inferior vena cava is incised to exsanguinate the donor. Then cold-organ perfusion is begun through the previously placed cannulas, and the abdominal cavity is immersed in ice to attempt achieving a liver core temperature of 4°C. University of Wisconsin (UW) solution has been used as the standard solution in the United States since 1987 when it was developed by Belzer and Southhard. This solution extended the limit of preservation to as long as 12 to 18 hours, after which the incidence of primary

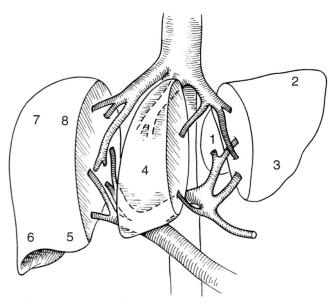

FIGURE 48-4   Segmental liver anatomy. The division of the liver into independently vascularized and drained segments is based on the parallel bifurcation of the portal vein and hepatic artery.

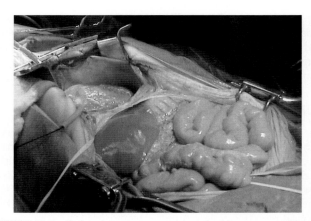

FIGURE 48-5   Cadaveric organ procurement. A wide exposure with median sternotomy extending to midline laparotomy is made for multiorgan procurement. This harvest resulted in the procurement of six organ grafts from a single recipient, benefiting six different recipients.

graft failure increases substantially. However, the acceptable preservation time depends on numerous donor and recipient variables and should still be minimized when possible. This is particularly the case with reduced-size or split-liver transplantation. The UW solution is a hyperkalemic, hyperosmolar solution that prevents cell swelling, maintains stable transmembrane electrical gradients upon reperfusion, by preventing efflux of intracellular potassium during storage, and contains a variety of oxygen free radical scavengers. Many centers are now using a histidine-tryptophan-ketoglutarate solution because of its lower potassium content and viscosity.[21] Once procured, the harvest team typically transports the liver graft to the transplantation center and prepares it for engraftment for a separate recipient team.

Segmental Liver Transplantation: Living Donor, Reduced Size, and Split

The shortage of pediatric organs coupled with a significant wait-list death rate has driven the development of alternative organ sources. Three alternatives to use of a whole organ graft are available to these patients: living donor, reduced-size and split-liver grafts.[7,20,22,23] Living donor transplantation was developed as an alternative to scarce whole organ grafts and typically uses a segment 2 and 3 (left-lateral sector, LLS) graft. Because of the small but real risk of safety in a healthy donor, reduced-size transplantation was simultaneously developed as an alternative and involves resecting the LLS graft prior to or after cold-organ perfusion and discarding the remaining liver. Obviously, this benefits the pediatric recipient but wastes an organ that could be used by an adult recipient. Splitting the whole organ into a right trisegment and LLS graft to use in an adult and pediatric recipient, respectively, was first reported by Pichlmayr in Hanover in 1988. This can be done either prior to cold organ perfusion (in-situ technique) (Fig. 48-6) or after cold-organ perfusion and removal of the liver from the donor (ex-vivo technique).[22] This provides a

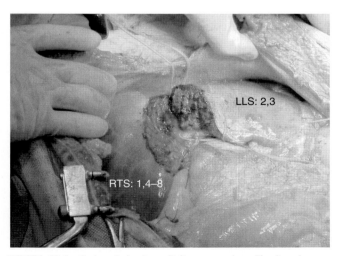

FIGURE 48-6 Cadaveric in-situ split-liver procedure. The liver is separated just to the left of the umbilical fissure into a right trisegment (RTS) graft and a left-lateral segment (LLS) graft.

suitable graft for the pediatric population without worsening the already severe organ shortage in the adult population. Although the initial results were discouraging, with increased experience, the survival rates of patients and grafts are nearly equal to whole organ and living donor transplantation, though the risk of vascular and biliary complications is somewhat higher.[27,23–25] At the University of California in Los Angeles (UCLA), we are only performing living donor transplantations when a whole or split graft is not available in a timely fashion or for special indications. There has been a marked reduction in transplant wait time since the routine use of segmental grafts with this strategy.[3,20,23]

Liver Transplant Operation

The performance of the whole organ cadaveric liver transplant procedure has changed little during the last 2 decades. Although there are tremendous individual and institutional differences in the subtleties and how certain techniques are used or not used, the basic steps in the procedure remain the same. What follows is a description of how the procedure is generally performed at UCLA today and has been applied in more than 3000 cases.[26] The procedure can be roughly divided into four major phases, each with its own anatomic and physiologic challenges: hepatectomy phase, anhepatic phase with engraftment, reperfusion with arterialization, and biliary reconstruction. Perhaps the most challenging step during liver transplantation is the hepatectomy. Coagulopathy, portal hypertension, and poor hepatic and renal function create a surgical environment wherein continuous bleeding is possible. During this phase, the anesthesiologist plays a key role in maintaining volume by rapid transfusion, correcting coagulopathy and fibrinolysis, and maintaining body temperature. The goal of this phase is to devascularize the liver by ligating and dividing the hepatic artery and portal vein as well as to mobilize the suprahepatic and infrahepatic vena cava to enable removal. These goals are achieved while leaving in the recipient adequate lengths of each vessel for later implantation of the donor graft. In the majority of pediatric liver transplant operations, the retrohepatic vena cava is retained as the liver is dissected off the vena cava by dividing the tributaries from the right and caudate lobes, and often only partial occlusion of the vena cava is necessary. Meticulous but expedient surgical technique is essential during the hepatectomy to ensure optimal patient outcome. During the anhepatic phase, the anesthesiologist must support certain aspects of hepatic function to prevent or treat acidosis, hypothermia, coagulopathy, and occasionally fibrinolysis. In addition, they must ensure adequate circulating volume and maintain hemodynamic stability. In children, venovenous bypass is rarely used.

While the patient is anhepatic, the liver graft is taken out of hypothermic storage and engrafted. This begins with the suprahepatic caval, followed by the infrahepatic caval and the portal anastomoses. If the retrohepatic cava was retained, the "piggyback" technique is used, in which the suprahepatic cava of the graft is sewn to the cloacae created from the confluence of the recipient hepatic veins, and the donor infrahepatic cava is ligated (Fig. 48-7). Prior to reperfusion, the liver is flushed with a cold colloid and albumin solution through the donor portal vein to lessen the potential reperfusion-associated complications.

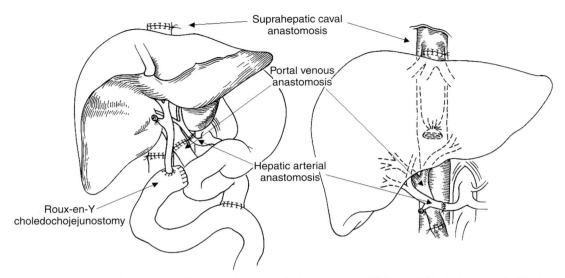

FIGURE 48-7 Whole organ engraftment. Both the standard orthotopic and "piggyback" techniques are depicted.

Reperfusion is then undertaken in a controlled manner. Communication between the surgical and anesthesia teams is essential to allow the anesthesiologist time to institute preparative and preventive measures. Reperfusion is undertaken by first removing the suprahepatic vena cava clamp, then the infrahepatic vena cava clamp and, lastly, the portal venous clamp. As blood is reintroduced into the liver allograft and allowed to drain into the right atria, many serious and life-threatening complications can develop. The major challenges encountered by the anesthesiologist at this point are life-threatening hyperkalemia, acidosis, arrhythmias, and hemodynamic instability with or without surgical or coagulopathic bleeding. Factors that contribute are the return of cold, acidotic, and hyperkalemic blood directly into the right atrium. It is at this point that maintenance of physiologic stability by the surgeon and anesthesiologist in the preceding phases, the preoperative state of the recipient, and the intrinsic quality of the graft converge to determine early graft function as well as the course of the remainder of the operation. Without a doubt, this is one of the most hazardous portions of the liver transplant process.

The hepatic arterial anastomosis is then performed. In general, arterial inflow is obtained from one of the branches of the celiac trunk. However, in some instances, inflow from these vessels is not adequate, thus necessitating the use of aortic conduits. A conduit can be placed either on the supraceliac or infrarenal aorta. In some cases, when the arteries are of very small caliber (<3 mm), the arterial anastomosis is performed prior to reperfusion. The biliary tree is then reconstructed by choledochocholedochostomy or by Roux-en-Y choledochojejunostomy, the latter being more common in small children and used exclusively in partial liver grafts because of the size of the donor duct (Fig. 48-8). After ensuring sufficient hemostasis, drains are placed and the abdominal cavity is closed. The patient is then transferred directly to the ICU. Segmental transplantation, using split, reduced-size, or living donor grafts, involves variations in the manner in which the anastomoses are performed, but the general steps are the same (see Fig. 48-8).

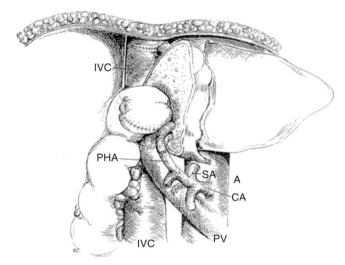

FIGURE 48-8 Left-lateral segment engraftment. A, aorta; CA, celiac artery; IVC, inferior vena cava; PHA, proper hepatic artery; PV, portal vein; SA, splenic artery. (Reprinted with permission from Goss J, Yerziz H, Shackelton H, et al: In situ splitting of the cadaveric liver for transplantation. Transplantation 1997;64:871-877.)

Post-transplant Care

EARLY POSTOPERATIVE CARE

The early and long-term postoperative care of the liver transplant recipient is almost as important as the performance of the operation in ensuring optimal outcomes. The immediate postoperative care is aimed at assessing graft function, providing supportive care for the recipient, and early detection of complications. Graft function can be assessed in many ways. Physiologic and clinical assessment can be done almost immediately with a warm, arousable, hemostatic, and hemodynamically stable patient whose liver is making "golden-brown" bile (in the infrequent case where a biliary drainage tube is placed), characteristics that are the hallmarks of a functional graft. Graft function is then confirmed biochemically by evidence of synthetic and metabolic function (e.g., correcting prothrombin time, reversal of acidosis). The degree of preservation injury, as measured by liver enzyme levels, does not linearly correlate with graft function, but grafts with severe injury are more likely to exhibit delayed function or nonfunction. Failure of a graft without vascular compromise (primary nonfunction [PNF]) is treated by retransplantation in almost all cases, with outcome directly related to the time to retransplantation. The incidence of PNF in pediatric patients is 5% to 10%.[7,8,23,24,27]

Technical Complications

Technical complications can be divided into vascular, biliary, and general surgical complications. In the early postoperative period, infectious and general surgical complications of liver transplantation today are similar to those that occur after any major abdominal operation. However, the incidence of fungal infection is higher, and the incidence of bowel perforation in pediatric recipients is as high as 19% in some series. Also, early exploration or computed tomography (CT) imaging should be considered when sepsis is suspected and no other etiology can be found.

VASCULAR COMPLICATIONS

Major vascular complications include hepatic artery thrombosis (HAT), portal vein thrombosis, and caval thrombosis or stenosis. Intravenous low-dose unfractionated heparin with or without low-molecular-weight dextran is routinely used for prophylaxis against vascular thromboses. Duplex ultrasonography and computerized tomographic or conventional angiography are accepted means of diagnosis. HAT is the most common complication, and its incidence varies from 5% to 18% depending on patient age and type of graft.[7,8,23,24,27,28] Early vascular complications are usually technical in nature, while immunologic and infectious (e.g., cytomegalovirus [CMV]) etiologies have been ascribed to those occurring months after transplantation. HAT occurring in the first week is commonly associated with graft nonfunction and biliary necrosis or leak, while those occurring later do not necessarily affect graft function immediately, but usually produce biliary complications. These include intrahepatic biliary abscesses, biliary anastomotic stricture, and sclerosing cholangitis with sepsis, all of which lead to significant morbidity. If diagnosed early, some patients can be managed by thrombectomy and surgical revision. However, most early HATs require urgent retransplantation. Late HATs with preserved graft function can be managed by radiologic interventional techniques and retransplanted remote from initial transplantation. Thrombosis of the portal vein occurs in 2% to 4% of pediatric liver transplantations and is usually associated with loss of the graft. Prompt retransplantation is required for patient salvage. Late portal vein thrombosis usually presents with recurrent variceal bleeding or ascites and can be managed medically, endoscopically, or surgically with shunting or retransplantation. Vena caval or hepatic vein thrombosis or stenosis occurs in 3% to 6% of

pediatric patients and presents with variceal bleeding and/or ascites and is usually best managed with balloon dilation in interventional radiology[7,8,23,24,27,28]

BILIARY COMPLICATIONS

Biliary complications that are not associated with HAT occur in 3% to 20% of patients depending on the type of graft and whether a choledochojejunostomy was used. These usually result from technical factors, but occasionally warm ischemia or immunologic and infectious factors can be implicated (e.g., CMV). Diagnosis is by cholangiography and treatment can be by endoscopic or radiologic intervention or by surgical revision.[7,23–25,27]

Immunosuppressive Therapy and Rejection

Immunosuppression for liver transplantation in the modern era rests on a class of drugs known as calcineurin inhibitors (CNI), the prototype being cyclosporine (Table 48-1). Cyclosporine, especially its microemulsion formulation, which allows better bioavailability and more consistent therapeutic levels, revolutionized organ transplantation by reducing the incidence of rejection in all solid organs. The second-generation CNI, tacrolimus, was first used clinically in 1990. The greater potency of tacrolimus allowed for a further reduction in the early incidence of rejection following liver transplantation, while also allowing the earlier weaning of steroid therapy. Also, the incidence of chronic rejection has significantly decreased with the use of tacrolimus, which can also effectively treat episodes of acute rejection. Currently, most liver transplant centers use a tacrolimus-based regimen combined with steroid therapy with or without adjunctive agents. Cyclosporine and tacrolimus share certain acute and long-term side effects while having some that are unique to the agent. The most important of these is nephrotoxicity, which occurs in an acute variety from vasoconstriction of the afferent renal arterioles and is reversible, as well as a more chronic variety marked by tubular atrophy, interstitial fibrosis, and glomerulosclerosis. The latter is variably reversible depending on the degree of disease. To minimize acute toxicity and to allow lower early CNI levels, especially with pretransplant renal insufficiency, a purine antimetabolite, mycophenolate mofetil, is sometimes used as an adjunctive agent (see Table 48-1). The newest class of immunosuppressants is the inhibitors of mammalian target of rapamycin, the prototype being sirolimus. This agent has been used sparingly in pediatric liver transplantation, and only preliminary data exist. Although this drug has no nephrotoxicity, it has other long-term sequelae, such as hypercholesterolemia. No perfect immunosuppression (i.e., one with minimal side effects) has been developed yet.

Acute rejection (AR) is common in pediatric liver transplantation, with the peak incidence being within the first 6 months, during which 30% to 50% of patients experience at least one episode.[7,8,23,27] It is less common after the first post-transplant year, occurring in 10% or less of patients. AR is suspected with elevated aspartate or alanine transaminase levels or by elevated alkaline phosphatase levels and gamma-glutamyl transferase levels. AR is an alloantigen specific, T-cell–mediated inflammatory process that targets

TABLE 48-1

Modern Immunosuppressants Used in Liver Transplantation

Name	Mechanism of Action	Principal Use	Common Toxicities
Calcineurin inhibitors (CNI) cyclosporine tacrolimus	Exact and complete mechanism unknown; inhibits IL-2 and other cytokine gene transcription, thus preventing T-helper cell expansion	Induction and maintenance of immunosuppression long term; tacrolimus is the only agent approved for monotherapy, while cyclosporine must generally be used with another agent long term	Shared: nephrotoxicity, hypertension, hyperglycemia, neurotoxicity (seizures, myoclonus, essential tremors) Cyclosporine: hirsutism, gingival hyperplasia, more diabetes Tacrolimus: diarrhea, anorexia, more neurotoxicity, more hypertension
Glucocorticoids methylprednisolone prednisone	Diffuse action on immune system by its anti-inflammatory properties, especially inhibition of IL-1	Induction of immunosuppression and maintenance; may be weaned off long term in some patients	Hyperlipidemia, osteopenia, hypertension, diabetes, impaired wound healing, growth retardation, Cushingoid features, striae, acne
Mycophenolate mofetil	Purine antimetabolite, semiselective for salvage pathway present primarily used in lymphocytes	Used as an adjunctive agent to reduce the dose of CNI or steroid	Myelosuppression, diarrhea, anorexia, nausea, vomiting, GI mucosal ulceration
Mammalian target of rapamycin inhibitors rapamycin	Inhibits cell cycle progression in stimulated cells, thus preventing clonal expansion of stimulated B and T cells	Unclear, use in pediatric patients preliminary; may be useful in minimizing CNI dose when toxicity exists or in refractory AR or chronic allograft rejection	Hyperlipidemia, impaired wound healing, pneumonitis, oral ulceration
OKT3 monoclonal antibody	Clonal deletion of (CD3+) T cells	Severe or refractory acute allograft rejection	SIRS and other infusional reactions, increased risk of viral infections and PTLD
Antilymphocyte globulin (Thymoglobulin)	Exact and complete mechanism unknown, but produces central and peripheral deletion of lymphoid cells	Severe or refractory acute allograft rejection	Increased risk of viral infections and PTLD, lower incidence of infusional reactions than OKT3, thrombocytopenia
IL-2 receptor antagonists basiliximab daclizumab	Competitive inhibition of IL-2 receptors	Induction of immunosuppression as an adjunct to CNI; used to minimize other immunosuppression (CNI, steroids)	Increased risk of viral infections, possible PTLD, rare infusional reactions

AR, acute rejection; GI, gastrointestinal; IL-1, IL-2, interleukin-1, interleukin-2; PTLD, post-transplant lymphoproliferative disorder; SIRS, systemic inflammatory response syndrome.

vascular endothelium and biliary epithelium but not hepatocytes. This is based on the greater expression of donor human leukocyte antigens on the former cell types. The histologic hallmark of AR is a mixed cell inflammatory infiltrate (polymorphonuclear cells, lymphocytes, and eosinophils) in the portal triad, with evidence of inflammation of the endothelium and/or biliary epithelial injury. Rejection can be graded as mild, moderate, and severe depending on the proportion of involved portal triads, the degree of infiltrate and injury, and the presence of central vein endothelial inflammation, which is a sign of severe AR. Treatment of AR is centered on a high-dose methylprednisone bolus, but cases unresponsive to this may require use of antibody therapy (OKT3, antithymocyte globulin [ATG], see Table 48-1). Mild AR can often be treated by simply increasing the tacrolimus level, though steroid bolus should be considered if there is not a prompt response. AR does not influence long-term graft survival in adults or children, unless it occurs in multiple or steroid refractory episodes, or if it occurs beyond the first year post-transplant.[4,7,29] AR accounts for less than 3% of overall patient and graft loss. However, treatment for AR is an important risk factor for the development of cytomegalovirus and Epstein-Barr viral infections in children. The latter is a risk factor for the development of post-transplant lymphoproliferative disorder. Therefore a balance between adequate immunosuppression to prevent AR and over-immunosuppression to avoid toxicity is necessary. Currently, long-term morbidity from immunosuppressive drug therapy is the major challenge facing long-term survival and quality of life in the pediatric population.

Chronic rejection is a common cause of late graft loss in children, because disease recurrence is uncommon. It is not felt to be entirely alloantigen driven, and may be due to a number of factors that share final common pathway of graft injury. Its hallmark is the intrahepatic loss of bile ducts and has been termed "vanishing bile duct syndrome" in the past because of this histologic finding on biopsy. This diagnosis is suspected if progressive jaundice and rising levels of alkaline phosphatase occur. Currently, there is no prophylactic or therapeutic agent for chronic rejection, though progression of graft fibrosis may be forestalled by sirolimus, based on animal and preliminary clinical data.[30] Although maintenance immune suppression is often enhanced, the only definitive treatment when decompensated graft failure occurs is retransplantation.

Infectious Complications

Post-transplant infections are the most common cause of morbidity and mortality after liver transplantation (Table 48-2). The highest incidence of bacterial and fungal infections is in the first month after transplantation. Fungal infections occurring months to years after transplantation are unusual and are more commonly the atypical or endemic organisms, such as *Cryptococcus* spp., *Mucormycosis* spp., *Blastomycosis* spp., or *Coccidiomycosis* spp. Viral infections are the most common infections after the early post-transplant period. Cytomegalovirus (CMV) and Epstein-Barr virus (EBV) infections account for the vast majority of opportunistic viral infections. Overall

TABLE 48-2

Infectious Complications after Liver Transplantation

Organism	Presentation	Diagnosis	Antimicrobials
Cytomegalovirus (CMV)	Infection results from reactivation of virus; blood transfusion; infected transplanted organ Mild viral, "flulike" syndrome Invasive tissue infection (retinitis, pneumonitis, myocarditis, enterocolitis, hepatitis, CNS)	Quantitative CMV-DNA PCR pp65 antigen Tissue cultures Blood or fluid cultures Biopsy with immunostains	Prophylaxis: IV ganciclovir, oral valganciclovir Therapy: IV ganciclovir with or without CMV immunoglobulin
Epstein-Barr virus (EBV)	Spectrum: infectious mononucleosis to lymphoproliferative disease to lymphoma to EBV-associated soft tissue tumors Occurs with EBV and immunosuppression, 10%-15% infant liver transplantation GI tract, neck, thorax, CNS	Quantitative EBV-DNA PCR Blood smear Biopsy with immunostains CT scans of suspected sites	Prophylaxis: IV ganciclovir, oral valganciclovir Therapy: Acyclovir, reduction or withdrawal of immunosuppression; possible use of systemic chemotherapy for lymphoproliferative disorders or lymphoma
Herpes simplex virus (HSV)	Skin lesions, GI tract disseminated herpes—fever, fatigue, abnormal liver functions, hepatitis, pneumonia	HSV-1 and HSV-2 antibodies Biopsy with viral cultures	Acyclovir
Pneumocystis	Atypical pneumonia, can progress to life-threatening pneumonitis	BAL, lung biopsy	Prophylaxis: low-dose oral sulfamethoxazole/trimethoprim, Dapsone, or pentamidine Therapy: high-dose IV sulfamethoxazole/trimethoprim
Candida	Local mucous membrane, invasive tissue infection, fungemia	Blood, fluid, and tissue cultures, fundoscopic exam	Prophylaxis: fluconazole, possibly lipid formulation of amphotericin B in very-high-risk patients Therapy: fluconazole (for sensitive candidal species) or lipid formulation of amphotericin B, caspofungin, or voriconazole (insensitive Candida or Aspergillus)
Aspergillus	Entry via upper or lower respiratory tract with metastatic spread (CNS, intra-abdominal, solid-organ)	Blood, fluid, and tissue cultures, BAL, CT scans	
Bacteria	Gram negative: enterobacteria, E. coli, Pseudomonas Gram positive: Enterococcus, Staphylococcus	Blood, fluid and tissue cultures, BAL, CT scans, surgical exploration	Varies

BAL, bronchoalveolar lavage; CNS, central nervous system; CT, computed tomography; GI, gastrointestinal; IV, intravenous; PCR, polymerase chain reaction.

reduction and more selective immunosuppression and prophylaxis with ganciclovir have reduced the incidence and morbidity of these infections. The other agents responsible for infectious morbidity, their presentation, diagnosis, and treatment are included in Table 48-2. Of particular importance in children is the prophylaxis and effective treatment of EBV. This is associated with the development of numerous malignant consequences. The most common of these is a diffuse proliferation of lymphoid tissue known as post-transplant lymphoproliferative disorder (PTLD). PTLD can present as a mononucleosis-like syndrome with diffuse lymphadenopathy or as lymphoma involving any organ. A variety of other tumors are also associated with EBV infections.[29] The general therapy for PTLD is reduction or elimination of immunosuppression, and, occasionally, surgical intervention and/or chemotherapy. The complete discussion of these disorders is beyond the scope of this chapter but is extensively covered elsewhere.[29]

Outcome and the Future

Numerous factors are known to impact patient and graft survival in this population of liver transplant patients.* Overall, survival has improved with 1-year and 5-year patient survival exceeding 90% and 80%, respectively, in patients less than 18 years of age.[3,4] Age, nutritional status, urgency of transplantation, the indication for transplantation,

and presence of renal dysfunction are all major factors that determine the outcome in any individual patient. Although early data suggested that patients with BA have worse outcomes because of their often-malnourished state, young age, and previous surgical intervention, more recent data suggest that this difference is not significant.[11,31] Patients with metabolic disease do exceedingly well, because they often are older, do not have liver failure and its sequelae, and have not previously undergone abdominal operation. Finally, transplantation for malignancy in children is associated with survival that is substantially less than that of transplantation for other indications but much better than the natural history of the disease. Numerous large series exist in the literature detailing the improvement in outcome with experience.[4,7,8]

Although outcomes have improved, many issues still remain to be resolved. The first and foremost is the organ shortage. The number of listed patients is increasing, while the number of suitable donors (even with segmental liver transplantation and improved organ allocation policies) has plateaued. Strategies aimed at expanding the donor pool and allocating organs to those patients that not only have the greatest survival benefit compared with pretransplant survival, but also the greatest chance of optimal post-transplant outcome are essential. National policies aimed at effectively identifying donors for splitting and development of local, regional, and national sharing of split grafts still await refinement. Finally, the development of gene therapy or optimization of hepatocyte transplantation as alternatives

* References 3, 4, 7, 8, 23, 24, 27, 31.

to transplantation for metabolic diseases may alleviate some of the organ shortage.

Another important challenge for the liver transplant community is the perfection of immunosuppression. Currently, all immunosuppressants have long-term side effects that result in impaired growth and development, infectious morbidity, malignancies, and numerous medical complications such as renal failure. The development of drug therapy that minimizes or eliminates these is essential. Furthermore, a better understanding of the immunology of peripheral T-cell tolerance and chronic rejection is essential. Although the last decade saw improvements in many technical and immunosuppressive aspects of liver transplantation, improvements in survival and quality of life in the next decade will rest firmly on a better understanding of our immune system on a cellular and molecular level.

The complete reference list is available online at www. expertconsult.com.

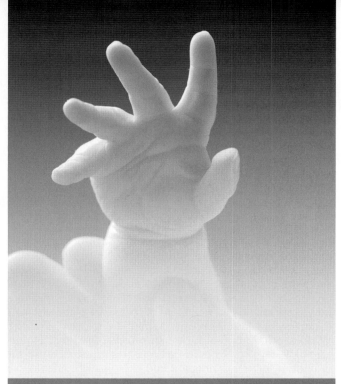

CHAPTER 49

Pediatric Intestinal Transplantation

Yann Révillon and Christophe Chardot

Intestinal failure (IF) is characterized by the inability of the gastrointestinal tract to provide sufficient digestion and absorption capacities to cover the nutritional requirements for maintenance in adults and for growth in children.[1] The first-line treatment for IF is parenteral nutrition (PN). In patients with life-threatening complications of PN, intestinal transplantation (IT)—isolated or combined with the liver and/or other organs—provides children with a second chance for survival. Since the early days of IT in the 1980s (treatment with cyclosporine-based immunosuppressive regimens), significant progress has been made in the medical and surgical management of children requiring IT, with short-term results (1-year patient survival) now approaching those of liver transplantation.

Indications for Intestinal Transplantation

The causes of intestinal failure in children can be divided into five groups[2] (Fig. 49-1): (1) short bowel, mainly resulting from gastroschisis, midgut volvulus, necrotizing enterocolitis, and intestinal atresia; (2) motility disorders: long-segment Hirschsprung disease and chronic intestinal pseudo-obstruction;

(3) epithelial disorders with intractable diarrhea, such as microvillous inclusion disease and tufting enteropathy; (4) children with a failed intestinal transplant; and (5) miscellaneous, including tumors.

Parenteral nutrition, including home PN, is the first-line treatment for children with intestinal failure and allows satisfactory growth and acceptable (although not normal) quality of life in most patients.[1,3] However, life-threatening complications of PN may occur, primarily line sepsis, loss of venous access resulting from thrombosis, and liver disease leading to cirrhosis. In such cases, intestinal transplantation may be the only lifesaving alternative. Depending on the underlying disease and the complications of PN, transplantation of additional organs may be required: liver in patients with cirrhosis, stomach and duodenopancreas in patients with extended motility disorders, and kidney(s) in patients with renal failure.[4]

The management of children with intestinal failure requires a multidisciplinary approach and is a continuous process that may last the whole life of the child. In most patients, the disease starts in the neonatal period and requires initial surgery. The possibility that the child may need other operations in the future should be considered at each surgical intervention. Adequate parenteral nutrition and prevention of line infections have paramount importance for the long-term prognosis of children with intestinal failure.[3,5] If long-term dependence on PN is expected, early contact with a team specializing in the management of children with intestinal failure is recommended before the onset of PN-related complications, to optimize the overall management of the child: adaptation of long-term PN and prevention of its complications, education of parents about home PN, and anticipation and preparation of further steps of the medicosurgical management, which may include nontransplant surgery or transplantation. This early contact with the intestinal failure team is recommended for every child whose requirements for PN are anticipated to be more than 50% at 3 months after initiating PN.[6] In a retrospective study, including 302 children followed for home PN in our center between 1980 and 1999, the median duration of home PN was 1.3 years. By January 2000, 54% had been weaned from PN, 26% were still receiving PN, 16% had died, and 4% had undergone intestinal transplantation. Patient survival rates at 5, 10, and 15 years were 89%, 81%, and 72%, respectively. Nine percent of children with primary digestive disease died versus 38% of children with nonprimary digestive disease.[3] In a multicenter prospective European study, including 688 adults and 166 children on home PN, the candidacy rate for transplantation was estimated at 16% in adults and 34% in children, and it varied greatly among home PN centers.[7,8] The 5-year survival rate on home PN was 87% in noncandidates for transplantation, 73% in candidates with home PN failure, 84% in those with high risk of death attributable to the underlying disease, 100% in those with IF with high morbidity or low acceptance of PN, and 54% in IT recipients ($P < 0.001$). Nontransplant surgery may have a place in the rehabilitation program of such children, especially bowel lengthening procedures in those with a short bowel and limited hepatic or vascular complications.[9,10]

The appropriate timing of intestinal transplantation sometimes is not easy to determine, because it is difficult to predict the ability of the native intestine to adapt, as well as the course of PN-related complications. On the one hand, intestinal adaptation may allow digestive autonomy in some patients with

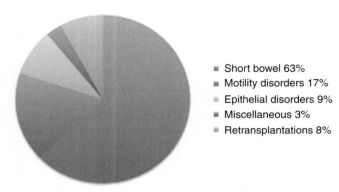

- Short bowel 63%
- Motility disorders 17%
- Epithelial disorders 9%
- Miscellaneous 3%
- Retransplantations 8%

FIGURE 49-1 Indications for intestinal transplantation. From the Intestine Transplant Registry 2003 report[2]: 606 grafts (223 isolated bowel, 306 liver and intestine, 77 multivisceral) in 563 children (age ≤ 18 years). *(See Expert Consult site for color version.)*

a short bowel,[9] and PN-associated liver disease may regress after optimization of PN, especially regarding the quality of lipid intake.[11–13] On the other hand, transplantation results are better in children who are in good general condition, as opposed to children with end-stage disease.[2] However, early referral to a specialized center for intestinal failure does not necessarily result in finding an indication for transplantation. In a series of 118 patients referred to our center for transplantation assessment, 10 could be weaned off PN, 12 patients were unsuitable for transplantation, 65 patients were listed for transplantation, and 31 remained potential candidates.

The two following examples of children treated by our team illustrate how the same condition (short bowel syndrome) may require very different therapies, based on the specifics of the patient.

Yasmine was born in 1971. In 1981, she presented with a midgut volvulus and complete necrosis of the small bowel and right colon. She underwent a duodenocolic anastomosis, and she has been on PN since then. Because of loss of venous access, an arteriovenous fistula was created in 1983. Today, she eats normally and receives home PN 5 nights per week. She has three bowel movements per day. Her general condition is good. She sometimes complains of anal burns or abdominal distension. She has an ovarian cyst and renal stones. She works in business, was married in 2002, and gave birth to two children. She enjoys dancing, skiing, and diving. She does not wish to receive an intestinal transplant.

Virginie was born in 1988, and underwent an extensive intestinal resection at birth after midgut volvulus. Because of complications of PN, she underwent intestinal transplantation, in 1989, with cyclosporine-based immunosuppression. Today, she eats normally and is off PN, with normal intestinal biopsies. Her weight and height are normal. She has mild intellectual retardation and does not work. Her renal function is moderately impaired. She is the world's longest survivor (22 years) with a functional intestinal graft. However, it is still impossible to predict whether this situation will last for a normal lifespan.

Assessment and Preparation for Intestinal Transplantation

Potential candidates for IT usually have a complex medical history and may have undergone several prior operations. A detailed workup is needed to precisely evaluate (1) the level

of IF and its potential reversibility; (2) the history of PN and central-line complications—number of catheters, number of episodes of line sepsis, and bacteria involved (antibiotic resistance profiles); (3) thrombotic complications and current cartography of patent vascular access; (4) intestinal failure–associated liver disease (IFALD)—liver fibrosis or cirrhosis, jaundice, ascites, portal hypertension (esophageal and/or gastric and/or peristomal varices, thrombocytopenia), liver insufficiency; (5) surgical status of the abdomen—previous operations, length and function of remaining bowel, stomas; (6) function of other organs, especially heart, lungs (pulmonary shunts or pulmonary hypertension), and kidneys; (7) neurologic development and potential neurologic impairment; (8) serologic status and immunizations; (9) immunologic status (anti-HLA antibodies); and (10) sociofamilial and psychological assessment and ability of the family to manage the child before and after transplantation. The indications for transplantation as well as all of these issues and alternate therapies are discussed in a multidisciplinary meeting. Whatever the proposal for treatment, the child will require careful follow-up, with further reassessments, because the indication for transplantation and the type of graft needed may change with time.

The general condition of the child has a strong impact on the results of transplant surgery; therefore careful preparation is required, focusing especially on (1) optimization of PN to improve nutritional status and reduce its toxicity; (2) prevention and treatment of infections (optimization of central venous-line management) and immunizations; (3) treatment of the complications of liver disease, primarily ascites and portal hypertension (sclerosis or ligation of esophageal varices, transjugular intrahepatic portosystemic shunt). Education of the child and family about transplantation is done simultaneously.

Transplantation Surgery

The donor is usually a deceased donor, although a few living-related donations have been reported for isolated small bowel transplants.[14] The volume of the graft must correlate with the abdominal cavity of the recipient; this depends on (1) the donor to recipient weight ratio, (2) the native organs removed and the type of graft implanted, and (3) whether the abdominal cavity is small (IT for short bowel) or distended (IT for intestinal motility disorders with chronic intestinal distention).

A wide variety of grafts can be implanted, from isolated small bowel to multivisceral grafts, including stomach, pancreas and duodenum, small bowel, right colon, liver, and kidneys (Fig. 49-2). These grafts can be classified as

1. Isolated intestinal transplantation: small bowel ± right colon. This type of graft is generally indicated for IF with normal motility of the stomach and duodenum, and without significant liver disease. The native stomach, duodenum, pancreas, spleen, and liver are preserved. The superior mesenteric artery of the graft is connected to the recipient infrarenal aorta, and the mesentericoportal axis of the graft is joined to the native infrarenal vena cava. The proximal jejunum of the graft is connected to the native jejunum.

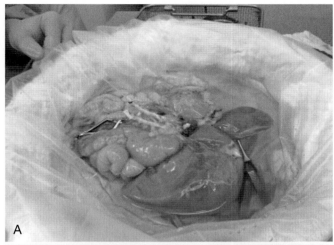

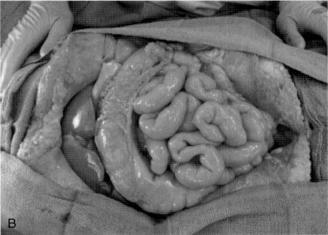

FIGURE 49-2 **A,** Multivisceral transplantation: the graft before implantation. The graft includes stomach, pancreas, duodenum, small bowel, right colon, liver, and two kidneys. **B,** Multivisceral transplantation: the graft after implantation and reperfusion. *(See Expert Consult site for color version.)*

2. Modified multivisceral transplantation: stomach, pancreas and duodenum, small bowel ± right colon. This type of graft is indicated for IF with impaired motility of the native stomach and duodenum (i.e., pan-intestinal Hirschsprung disease and chronic intestinal pseudo-obstruction), without significant liver disease. The upper part of the native stomach, duodenum, pancreas, spleen, and liver are preserved. The arterial axis of the graft (including celiac trunk and superior mesenteric artery) is connected to the recipient infrarenal aorta, and the mesentericoportal axis of the graft is joined to the recipient infrarenal vena cava. The native and transplanted hemistomachs are connected, the native first portion of duodenum is closed, and the native jejunum is connected to the transplanted jejunum as a Roux loop.

3. Combined liver and intestinal transplantation: liver, pancreas and duodenum, small bowel, ± right colon. This type of graft is indicated for IF with normal motility of the stomach and duodenum, and with significant liver disease. The native liver is removed, and a portocaval anastomosis is fashioned between the native portal vein and vena cava. The native stomach, duodenum, pancreas, and spleen are preserved. The arterial axis of the graft (including celiac trunk and superior mesenteric artery) is connected to the recipient infrarenal aorta, and the suprahepatic vena cava of the graft is connected to the native suprahepatic vena cava in a "piggyback" fashion. The first portion of the duodenum of the graft is closed, and the graft jejunum is connected to the native jejunum as a Roux loop.

4. Multivisceral transplantation: liver, stomach, duodenum and pancreas, small bowel, ± right colon, ± kidneys. This type of graft is indicated for (1) IF with impaired motility of the stomach and duodenum (pan-intestinal Hirschsprung disease and chronic intestinal pseudo-obstruction), with significant liver disease; (2) when en-bloc ablation of native organs (liver, pancreas, duodenum, and intestine) is needed,[4] either due to previous surgeries and portal hypertension, making selective dissection of native abdominal organs impossible, or (rarely) because of a tumor. All abdominal organs anterior to the aorta and vena cava are removed. The arterial axis of the graft (including celiac trunk and superior mesenteric artery) is connected to the recipient aorta, and the suprahepatic vena cava of the graft is connected to the native suprahepatic vena cava in a "piggyback" fashion. The native lower esophagus is connected to the transplanted stomach.

In all cases, a distal ileostomy is performed to provide easy access to the graft for intestinal biopsies. When the right colon is transplanted, its distal end is either anastomosed to the remaining native rectum (patients with short gut or mucosal diseases) or a temporary distal colostomy is created (Hirschsprung disease). Cholecystectomy and gastrostomy (for continuous enteral feeding) are generally performed if not done previously.

Abdominal wall closure is an issue after intestinal transplantation, because of the size discrepancy between the graft and the abdominal cavity of the recipient and post-reperfusion edema of the graft. Reduction of the liver and/or intestinal graft is possible.[15,16] Staged abdominal closure, using a temporary Silastic sheet and a vacuum dressing, avoids abdominal compartment syndrome. The final abdominal closure is usually possible after 5 to 7 days (Fig. 49-3).

Postoperative Care

The intestinal transit generally resumes quickly after surgery, and enteral feeding is progressively introduced 2 to 7 days after the operation. Transit time is accelerated because of the graft's denervation, and if dysfunction of the graft (mainly rejection or infection) has been ruled out, antimotility agents, such as loperamide or codeine, can be used to slow down the intestinal motility. In an uncomplicated postoperative course, full enteral feeding can be achieved 1 month after the operation.

Various surgical complications may occur (obstructions, peritonitis, fistulas, and pancreatitis), and may be difficult to detect under steroid therapy. Vascular monitoring of the graft relies on observation of the color of the stoma and, if the graft includes the liver, repeated ultrasonography (US) of the liver.

The intestine is highly immunogenic, and IT requires high-level immunosuppression. As understanding of the mechanisms of rejection progresses and new immunosuppressive

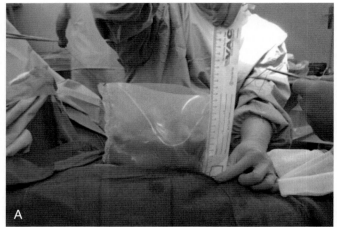

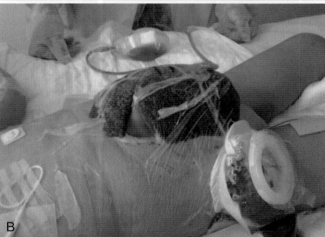

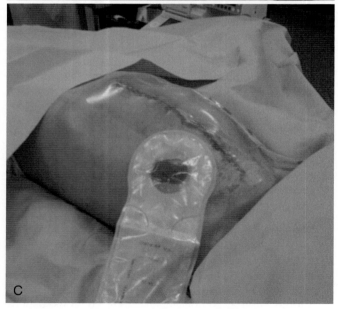

FIGURE 49-3 **A,** Intestinal transplantation, end of operation. The edema of the graft after reperfusion prevents primary abdominal closure. A Silastic silo is performed. **B,** Staged abdominal closure. The Silastic silo is covered with a vacuum dressing. The silo is progressively tightened over the next days at the bedside, as edema progressively resolves and graft reintegrates the abdomen. **C,** Final abdominal closure. After 5 to 7 days, the edema of the graft has diminished, and final abdominal closure can be achieved; the musculoaponeurotic layer can be closed either completely or with a wound prosthesis (for instance, a GORE-TEX sheet). *(See Expert Consult site for color version.)*

drugs become available, immunosuppressive protocols evolve. The current standard immunosuppressive regimen is a combination of tacrolimus, steroids, and basiliximab or daclizumab (anti–IL-2 receptor antibodies). Monitoring of intestinal rejection is based on stoma output, protein concentration in the stools, and repeated intestinal biopsies through the stoma. Other markers, such as stool calprotectin or serum citrulline, have also been used. In case of biopsy-proven rejection, first-line treatment relies on high-dose steroid pulses. Second-line treatments are available but expose the child to complications of overimmunosuppression, primarily opportunistic infections, and post-transplant lymphoproliferative disease (PTLD). In case of uncontrolled rejection, removal of the transplanted intestine may be needed. Recently, humoral rejection has increasingly been studied: Donor-specific anti-HLA antibodies are monitored, and high levels can be treated by high-dose intravenous (IV) immunoglobulins, rituximab (anti-CD20 antibody), and plasmapheresis.

Because of the high level of immunosuppression, opportunistic infections are a constant threat after IT. Various infectious agents can be involved, the most common being cytomegalovirus (CMV) and Epstein Barr virus (EBV). CMV can cause severe graft enteritis and trigger rejection. EBV can trigger lymphoproliferation. Monitoring of the viral loads is currently determined by polymerase chain reaction (PCR), which guides the prophylactic or curative treatments.

Post-transplant lymphoproliferative disease is nowadays detected at earlier stages. First-line treatment relies on reduction of immunosuppression and rituximab.

Drug toxicity is an issue after IT, because these children receive many drugs, some of them at high doses. Impairment of renal function, hypertension, and seizures are the most common side effects, which are usually reversible after dose reduction or a switch to alternate therapies.

Progressively, all treatments are decreased or withdrawn. Stoma closure can be considered when the child has been stable, without rejection, under maintenance immunosuppression for several months.

Results of Intestinal Transplantation

Short-term results of intestinal transplantation have improved with increasing experience.[2] In the United States, current 1-year patient and graft survival is 89% and 79%, respectively, for isolated bowel recipients, and 72% and 69%, respectively, for liver-intestine recipients. However, medium-term results remain unsatisfactory; by 10 years, patient and graft survival falls to 46% and 29%, respectively, for isolated bowel recipients, and 42% and 39%, respectively, for liver-intestine recipients.[17,18] According to the International Intestine Transplant Registry (1985 to 2003 data: 989 grafts in 923 patients),[2] causes of death were sepsis (46.0%), multiorgan failure (2.5%), graft thrombosis (3.2%), graft rejection (11.2%), post-transplant lymphomas (6.2%), respiratory causes (6.6%), technical reasons (6.2%), and other causes (17.3%).

Our team in Paris performed 97 transplants in 90 children, between November 1994 and April 2011, using tacrolimus-based immunosuppression: isolated bowel in 55; stomach, pancreas, duodenum, and bowel (modified multivisceral) in 1; combined liver and bowel in 39; liver, stomach, pancreas,

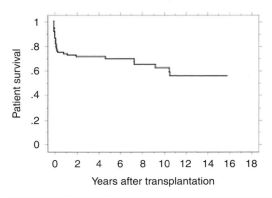

90 patients	1-year	5-year	10-year	15-year
Patient survival	73.0%	61.8%	48.6%	43.7%
Standard error	4.5%	5.2%	6%	6.3%
Number of patients reaching considered follow-up	66	43	21	2

FIGURE 49-4 Patient survival after intestinal transplantation in the tacrolimus era. Paris series from November 1994 to March 2011: 90 patients.

duodenum, and bowel in 1; liver, stomach, pancreas, duodenum, bowel, and two kidneys in 1 (see Fig. 49-2). In 63 of 97 transplants (65%), the graft included the right colon. One-year, 5-year, 10-year, and 15-year patient survival rates are 73.0%, 61.8%, 48.6%, and 43.7%, respectively, and 1-year, 5-year, 10-year, and 15-year graft survival rates are 59.5%, 45.0%, 33.6%, and 31.2%, respectively (Figs. 49-4 and 49-5). Early mortality is higher, but long-term graft survival is better after combined liver and intestine transplantation compared with isolated intestinal transplantation. This is probably due to the protective effect of the liver against intestinal rejection.[19,20]

In a study of 31 children treated by our group, and who are alive with their graft 2 to 18 years after transplantation,[21]

all were weaned from PN after transplantation, and 26 of 31 (84%) remained PN-free at last follow-up. Enteral nutrition was still required for 14 of 31 (45%) patients 2 years after transplantation. All children had high dietary energy intakes. The degree of steatorrhoea was fairly constant, with fat and energy absorption rates of 84% to 89%. After transplantation, two thirds of children had normal growth, whereas in one third, growth remained delayed, concomitant to a delayed puberty. Endoscopy and histology analyses were normal in asymptomatic patients. Five intestinal grafts (16%) were removed 2.5 to 8 years after transplantation for acute or chronic rejection. Late complications also include impairment of renal function and malignancies.

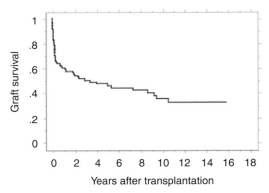

97 grafts	1-year	5-year	10-year	15-year
Graft survival	59.5%	45%	33.6%	31.2%
Standard error	5%	5.3%	5.7%	5.8%
Number of grafts reaching considered follow-up	53	31	14	2

FIGURE 49-5 Graft survival after intestinal transplantation in the tacrolimus era. Paris series from November 1994 to July 2010: 97 grafts.

Results of intestinal transplantation have improved in the recent decades,[2,18] because of better preparation of patients and timing of transplantation, progress in surgical techniques, availability of new immunosuppressive drugs and improved immunosuppressive regimens, and better monitoring and treatments of postoperative complications. The scarcity of grafts remains an important issue, and patients still succumb while waiting for a graft. With expected improvements in the outcomes (especially in the long term), intestinal transplantation may move from a lifesaving procedure to an improving quality-of-life procedure,[22] which may also have economic advantages compared with PN.

Conclusion

Home PN remains the first-line treatment of intestinal failure. Intestinal transplantation and its technical variants are indicated only in case of life-threatening complications of PN. Intestinal failure requires a multidisciplinary approach in specialized centers. Early assessment of the child in such a center, before the onset of complications of PN, is recommended. This does not mean early transplantation, but adequate planning of medicosurgical strategies to provide the child with the best chances of survival and an optimal quality of life.

Acknowledgments

The authors, Yann Révillon and Christophe Chardot, who are part of the surgical team, wish to thank the following pediatric multidisciplinary team members*:

1. Current team members treating intestinal failure and performing transplantations:
   Surgery: Sabine Irtan, Sabine Sarnacki, and Yves Aigrain.
   Gastroenterology, hepatology, and nutrition: Florence Lacaille, Virginie Colomb, Cécile Talbotec, Franck Ruemmele, Muriel Girard, Dominique Debray, Jean-Pierre Hugot, and Olivier Goulet.
   Pathology: Nicole Brousse, Virginie Verkarre, Danièle Canioni, Julie Bruneau, and Jean-Christophe Fournet.
   Intensive care: Fabrice Lesage, Laurent Dupic, Jean Bergounioux, Olivier Bustaret, Sandrine Jean, and Philippe Hubert.
   Radiology: Karen Lambot, Sophie Emond, Laureline Berteloot, and Francis Brunelle.
   Anesthesiology: Nadège Salvi, Nathalie Bourdeau, and Caroline Télion.
   Research laboratory: Nadine Cerf-Bensoussan.
2. Former members of the team: Claude Ricour, Jean-Pierre Cézard, Dominique Jan, Jean-Luc Michel, Frédérique Sauvat, Patrick Jouvet, and Francis Jaubert.

The complete reference list is available online at www.expertconsult.com.

*All members are affiliated with Hôpital Necker-Enfants Malades, Paris, France, except Jean-Pierre Hugot and Jean-Pierre Cézard, who are affiliated with Hôpital Robert Debré, Paris, France.

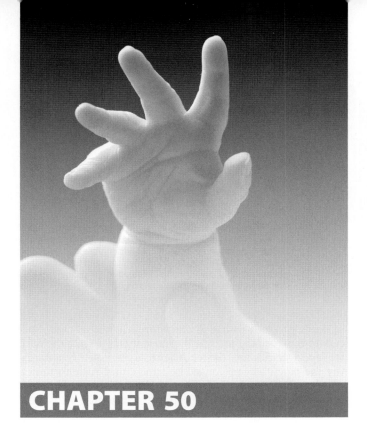

CHAPTER 50

Heart Transplantation

Stephanie M. P. Fuller and Thomas L. Spray

Thoracic organ transplantation has been successfully performed in pediatric patients since the mid-1980s and now serves as an important option in the treatment of both congenital and end-stage heart and lung disease in children. Approximately 400 pediatric heart transplantations are performed annually in the United States, or roughly 16% of all pediatric solid organ transplantations.[1] Despite the clinical success of heart and lung transplantation in children, limited donor availability has prevented broader application of this therapy. Infants awaiting heart transplantation face the highest wait-list mortality among all children and adults listed for a heart transplantation in the United States, with one in four infants dying before a donor heart can be identified.[2] Complications, such as acute and chronic rejection, graft coronary artery disease (CAD), and bronchiolitis obliterans, as well as the infectious and neoplastic complications of current methods of immunosuppression, threaten cardiac transplant longevity. This chapter focuses on the clinical aspects of heart transplantation in infants and children, including indications, preoperative evaluation, operative techniques, postoperative management, complications, and outcomes.

Historical Notes

Kantrowitz and colleagues[2a] performed the first pediatric heart transplant in 1967 when they transplanted the heart of an infant with anencephaly into a 3-week-old infant with tricuspid atresia. The next year, Cooley[2b] transplanted the heart and lungs of a newborn with anencephaly into a 3-month-old with an atrioventricular septal defect and pulmonary hypertension. Although neither of the infants survived for more than a few hours because of allograft rejection, these pioneering procedures emphasized the technical feasibility of thoracic organ transplantation in children. It was only in 1980 with the introduction of cyclosporine as an immunosuppressive agent that meaningful clinical success became possible. In November 1985, Bailey performed the first successful cardiac transplantation on a 4-day-old neonate with hypoplastic left heart syndrome (HLHS) at Loma Linda.[3,4] During the last 2 decades, outcomes have been improved by technical advances, better immunosuppression, including reduced steroid use and the advent of induction therapy, a decreased incidence of rejection, increased attention to viral prophylaxis, and aggressive treatment of post-transplant lymphoma and other post-transplant complications.

Indications

As published by the Registry for the International Society for Heart and Lung Transplantation in the Thirteenth Official Pediatric Report in 2010, the number of pediatric heart transplantations has remained relatively constant during the last 10 years (Fig. 50-1).[5] The most common indications for cardiac transplantation in the pediatric population remain congenital cardiac disease and cardiomyopathy, as demonstrated in Figures 50-2 and 50-3. Congenital heart disease is seen more commonly in infants, whereas cardiomyopathy is more prevalent in older children. As expected, the incidence of retransplantation increases with increasing patient age.

When examining the congenital heart disease population, the most common anomaly treated by transplantation is hypoplastic left heart syndrome (HLHS), a group of defects characterized by aortic or mitral atresia/stenosis with a diminutive left ventricle. Initial poor results with a staged palliative approach to HLHS led some centers to consider orthotopic heart transplantation as the primary treatment of this anomaly. Long transplantation waiting lists have led other institutions to advocate a stage I palliation (Norwood or Sano procedure) to help stabilize the patient and then list the patient for transplantation.[6] However, with improvement in early survival from the Norwood procedure followed by a Fontan repair, the majority of cardiac centers have abandoned primary transplantation as initial therapy for HLHS. Transplantation is an option now reserved for patients with unusually high risk, including aortic atresia with a diminutive ascending aorta and severe tricuspid or atrioventricular valve regurgitation.[7]

Other forms of congenital heart disease that have been treated by cardiac transplantation during infancy include an unbalanced atrioventricular canal, single ventricle, the Ebstein

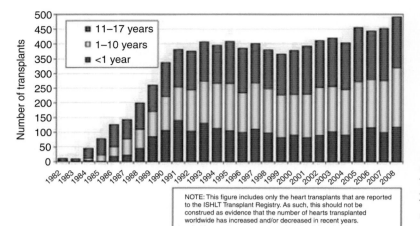

FIGURE 50-1 Age distribution of heart recipients by year of transplantation. (From Kirk K, Edwards LB, Kucheryavaya AY, et al: The Registry of the International Society for Heart and Lung Transplantation: Thirteenth official pediatric heart transplantation report—2010. J Heart Lung Transplant 2010;29:1119-1128.) *(See Expert Consult site for color version.)*

NOTE: This figure includes only the heart transplants that are reported to the ISHLT Transplant Registry. As such, this should not be construed as evidence that the number of hearts transplanted worldwide has increased and/or decreased in recent years.

anomaly, L-transposition of the great arteries, and pulmonary atresia with an intact ventricular septum (Table 50-1).[8,9] Even the most complex forms of congenital heart disease, such as heterotaxy syndromes with anomalies of systemic and venous drainage, are amenable to cardiac transplantation with suitable reconstruction.[10] Other pediatric candidates include infants with congenital heart disease who have undergone previous corrective or palliative procedures, yet who exhibit residual or progressive cardiac dysfunction manifested by left ventricular failure that ultimately requires transplantation. Postoperative cardiac dysfunction is often related to atrioventricular or semilunar valvar insufficiency that eventually results in dilated cardiomyopathy. In some cases, ventricular function may be preserved, but the indication for transplantation is for hemodynamic compromise secondary to anatomic abnormalities not amenable to surgical intervention, intractable arrhythmias, or complications that arise following the Fontan operation, such as protein-losing enteropathy. Of note,

multiple previous palliative procedures do not preclude successful transplantation.[11] In the current era, despite the need for repeat sternotomy, the tendency toward diffuse coagulopathy and potentially prolonged ischemic times, patients undergoing transplantation for congenital heart disease experience no actuarial difference in survival compared with those patients undergoing transplantation for cardiomyopathy who undergo first-time sternotomy and dissection of mediastinal structures.[8,12]

Cardiomyopathy is the other most common indication for heart transplantation in infancy and childhood. Most pediatric heart transplantations outside infancy are performed for dilated, idiopathic cardiomyopathy. Other causes of cardiomyopathy include viral, familial, and hypertrophic. Despite the diverse causes of cardiomyopathy, several variables have been associated with poor outcome, including a very high left ventricular end-diastolic pressure, a left ventricular ejection fraction less than 20%, ventricular arrhythmia, and a family

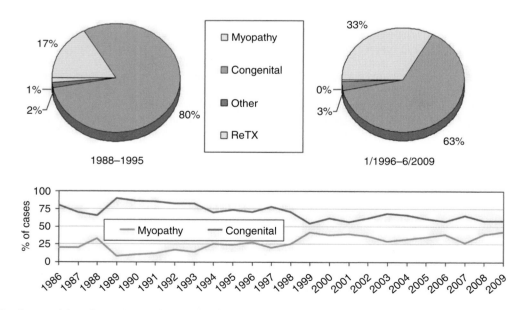

FIGURE 50-2 Infant heart recipient diagnosis according to year of transplantation. ReTx, retransplant. (From Kirk K, Edwards LB, Kucheryavaya AY, et al: The Registry of the International Society for Heart and Lung Transplantation: Thirteenth official pediatric heart transplantation report—2010. J Heart Lung Transplant 2010;29:1119-1128.) *(See Expert Consult site for color version.)*

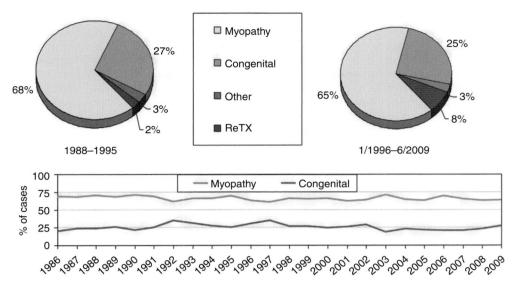

FIGURE 50-3 Diagnosis of heart recipients aged 11 to 17 years according to year of transplantation. ReTx, retransplant. (From Kirk K, Edwards LB, Kucheryavaya AY, et al: The Registry of the International Society for Heart and Lung Transplantation: Thirteenth official pediatric heart transplantation report—2010. J Heart Lung Transplant 2010;29:1119-1128.) *(See Expert Consult site for color version.)*

history of cardiomyopathy.[13,14] Cardiomyopathy attributable to inflammation or arrhythmia tends to have a more favorable outcome, and these patients should be supported as long as possible before transplantation to allow for the possibility of spontaneous recovery. Other less common indications for cardiac transplantation are doxorubicin-induced cardiotoxicity from chemotherapy for malignancy and obstructive cardiac tumors, such as fibromas and rhabdomyomas that are not amenable to surgical resection.

Regardless of the diagnosis, there are several clinical indications for heart transplantation in children, many of which have been borrowed from the adult population. These include the need for ongoing intravenous inotropic support or mechanical circulatory support. Transplantation is indicated in those patients who experience a progressive deterioration of ventricular function despite optimal medical care or those with life-threatening arrhythmias unresponsive to medical treatment, ablation, or automatic implantable defibrillator. Progressive pulmonary hypertension secondary to systemic

ventricular failure is an indication for cardiac transplantation, whereas pulmonary hypertension may otherwise be an indication for lung transplantation. Growth failure secondary to severe heart failure and unacceptably poor quality of life are considered indications as well as certain high-risk conditions following the Fontan procedure, such as protein-losing enteropathy and plastic bronchitis.[15]

Preoperative Evaluation

The pretransplant evaluation is a multidisciplinary screening process that serves as the key to successful organ transplantation (Table 50-2). Potential recipients go through a thorough

TABLE 50-1

Distribution of Anatomic Diagnoses in Children Older Than 6 Months of Age and Adults Undergoing Transplantation for Congenital Heart Disease in the Pediatric Heart Transplant Study and Cardiac Transplant Research Databases

Diagnosis	N	% of Patients
Single ventricle	176	36
Dextrotransposition of the great arteries	58	12
Right ventricular outflow tract lesions	49	10
Ventricular/atrial septal defects	38	8
Left ventricular outflow tract lesions	38	8
Levotransposition of the great arteries	39	8
Complete atrioventricular canal	37	8
Other	53	11
Total	488	100

Modified from Chen JM, Davies RR, Mital SR, et al: Trends and outcomes in transplantation in complex congenital heart disease: 1984-2004. Ann Thorac Surg 2004;78:1352-1361.

TABLE 50-2

Pretransplant Recipient Evaluation

Cardiac catheterization	Assess pulmonary vascular resistance and reactivity Delineate complex anatomy
Exercise testing	Obtain mVo$_2$
Assessment of end-organ function	Pulmonary function tests to evaluate lung function Liver and kidney function
HLA sensitization	Panel reactive antibody
Psychosocial evaluation	Social work assessment of family dynamic Psychiatric evaluation
Financial evaluation	Insurance evaluation
Blood work	Complete blood count with differential chemistry Lipid profile Thyroid function Hepatic function test Blood type Urinalysis Viral testing for cytomegalovirus, Epstein-Barr virus, herpesvirus, HIV, varicella, toxoplasmosis, hepatitis virus, tuberculosis

HIV, human immunodeficiency virus; HLA, human leukocyte antigen; mVo$_2$ myocardial oxygen consumption.

physical and psychosocial evaluation with careful examination of the cardiac, pulmonary, neurologic, renal, infectious, and socioeconomic systems. The presence of an adequate family support system is of paramount importance to survival postoperatively. Parents must demonstrate the ability and resources to comply with the complex medical regimens required and to cope with the potential for long or frequent hospitalizations even years after transplantation. As part of this multidisciplinary evaluation, patients undergo screening laboratory tests, including a viral serology panel (e.g., human immunodeficiency virus [HIV], cytomegalovirus [CMV], human Epstein-Barr virus [EBV], hepatitis).

Cardiac evaluation is performed mainly by echocardiography and cardiac catheterization in which the anatomy of the systemic and pulmonary venous connections of the heart and lungs are precisely identified. Important hemodynamic data, including systemic cardiac output and pulmonary vascular resistance (PVR), both indexed to the patient's body area, are obtained at cardiac catheterization and used to screen candidates. These numbers become significant, because the major contraindication to transplantation is fixed pulmonary hypertension unresponsive to pulmonary vasodilators. Patients with elevated PVR (>4 to 6 Wood units) are tested with pulmonary vasodilators, including sodium nitroprusside, oxygen (Fio_2 100%), and inhaled nitric oxide, to establish whether the pulmonary vascular bed is reactive. In general, the presence of a fixed PVR in excess of 6 to 8 Wood units is a contraindication to orthotopic heart transplantation, because the donor heart is unable to tolerate right-sided dilation caused by high pulmonary vascular resistance. Patients who demonstrate improvement with vasodilators may undergo transplantation with a survival rate comparable to that in patients with normal resistance.[11] Although patients with fixed pulmonary hypertension have successfully undergone transplantation, they have a much higher mortality rate, usually because of postoperative right ventricular failure. Other contraindications to cardiac transplantation include multiple noncardiac congenital anomalies, active malignancy, infection, severe metabolic disease (i.e., diabetes mellitus), multiple organ failure, multiple congenital anomalies, and the lack of an adequate family support system, in addition to socioeconomic factors that lead to noncompliance with drug regimen and follow-up care (Table 50-3).

Children suffering from cardiomyopathy and manifesting symptoms of chronic congestive heart failure that limit activity or uncontrollable arrhythmias are often referred for transplantation, particularly if they are unresponsive to medications. The timing for transplantation, especially for those children with hypertrophic cardiomyopathy, is less clear because some patients may improve with medication and conservative therapy. As previously stated, the mortality for idiopathic dilated cardiomyopathy in children is highest in the first year after diagnosis and is mainly determined by the degree of left ventricular failure.

Children listed for heart transplantation should be closely monitored until their transplantation, either as outpatients, if their condition permits, or while hospitalized. Good nutritional status should be maintained, and supplementation, such as tube feedings or total parenteral nutrition, is used as needed. A close watch for infectious complications is important, and any subtle indications of infection should be thoroughly investigated. Major infections require patients to have their transplantation status put on hold until they are treated adequately. Anticongestive therapy should be optimized with digoxin, diuretics, and afterload reduction with captopril or other angiotensin-converting enzyme inhibitors. If heart failure worsens, hospitalization may be required for inotropic support with dobutamine or phosphodiesterase inhibitors such as milrinone. Long-term therapy may require the placement of an intravenous access device such as a Broviac catheter.

The use of mechanical support as a bridge to cardiac transplantation in critically ill children had been limited mostly to those with postcardiotomy ventricular failure. In general, the results have been poor, although several studies show survival rates ranging from 45% to 73% when extracorporeal membrane oxygenation (ECMO) is used as a bridge to cardiac transplantation.[16,17] ECMO is restricted to short-term use. Additional limitations are the inability to ambulate and undergo effective physical therapy while on ECMO, as well as the damage to circulating red blood cells and platelets requiring persistent transfusion. In the current era, children have excellent survival with the use of long-term ventricular assist devices (VADS) as a bridge to transplantation. Although adult systems can be used in adolescent patients, the Berlin Heart VAD (Berlin Heart AG, Berlin, Germany) is a pulsatile, paracorporeal VAD that is suitable in neonates and infants for both single and biventricular support. The North American experience from 2000 to February 2007 details approximately 80 patients supported for more than 200 days, with the smallest patient being 3.0 kg. Overall, approximately 55% of the patients have undergone transplantation, 13% were weaned, and 25% died during device support.[18]

A neonate referred for cardiac transplantation requires several other unique considerations. Infants with complex congenital heart disease, such as HLHS, are commonly confined to a neonatal intensive care unit and are usually maintained on a continuous infusion of prostaglandin E_1 to prevent closure of the ductus arteriosus if there is ductal-dependent physiology. Implantation of expansile stents in the ductus may allow for discontinuation of prostaglandin therapy while waiting. Initial palliative procedures, such as the Norwood procedure for HLHS or a Blalock-Taussig shunt for lesions with ductal-dependent pulmonary blood flow, can be performed in the face of a prolonged wait for a

TABLE 50-3	
Potential Contraindications to Cardiac Transplantation	
General	Presence of any noncardiac condition that significantly shortens life expectancy
Specific	Active infection
	Active ulcer disease
	Active neoplasm
	Morbid obesity (BMI > 32)
	Renal insufficiency with creatinine greater than 2 times normal
	Hepatic dysfunction with elevated transaminases or cirrhosis
	Elevated, nonreactive pulmonary vascular resistance
	Recent pulmonary embolic event with infarction
	Recreational drug use
	Recurrent medical noncompliance

BMI, body mass index.

donor. Balloon atrial septostomy, with or without stenting to improve mixing of saturated and desaturated blood and to decompress the left atrium, can be helpful if there is a restrictive patent foramen ovale. Other important issues are the maintenance of adequate nutritional support, avoidance of renal and metabolic complications, and prompt and thorough treatment of any infectious complications, especially line sepsis, in these fragile infants. Common neonatal problems, such as seizures, necrotizing enterocolitis, and intraventricular hemorrhage are also seen. At the minimum, 10% to 20% of infants die while awaiting a donor heart.

In all cases, important consideration is given toward pretransplantation recipient human leukocyte antigen (HLA) sensitization. Circulating antidonor antibodies may result in either cellular or humoral rejection culminating in early graft failure.[19] The presence of HLA antibodies is reported as a panel reactive antibody (PRA), and a panel percentage of greater than 10% is considered elevated. Patients prone to developing anti-HLA antibodies include those who have received blood and platelet transfusions during prior surgeries, postgravid adolescent girls, children who have undergone implantation of cryopreserved tissue valves or allograft conduits, and patients with previous organ transplants. Strategies for reduction in PRA include the use of intravenous immunoglobulin as well as agents that may inhibit antibody production by B cells. Candidates who are high risk are managed with pretransplantation plasmapheresis that is continued postoperatively, resulting in good short-term outcomes. However, long-term outcomes are unknown. The United Network for Organ Sharing determines organ allocation and, in 2002, revised their classification for pediatric patients awaiting heart transplantation. Status 1A applies to patients requiring ventilatory or mechanical circulatory support (i.e., left ventricular assist device, ECMO, or a balloon pump) or multiple- or high-dose inotropes, infants younger than 6 months with pulmonary pressure greater than 50% of systemic levels, or any patient with a life expectancy of less than 14 days without a heart transplantation. Status 1B applies to patients requiring single-dose inotropic support or infants younger than 6 months who have significant failure to thrive (less than the 5th percentile for weight or height or loss of 1.5 standard deviations [SD] of expected growth). All other patients with less acuity are classified as status 2. A patient's status may change depending on changes in clinical condition, or the patient may be placed on hold (status 7) because of an infectious, malignant, or other complication and then reactivated.

Donor Evaluation and Organ Procurement

The criteria for an ideal organ donor are as follows: meets requirements for brain death, consent from next of kin, ABO compatibility in older children, weight compatibility (1 to 3 times that of the recipient), normal echocardiogram, age younger than 35 years, and normal heart by visual inspection at the time of harvest. A history of cardiopulmonary resuscitation is not an absolute contraindication to cardiac donation for pediatric recipients. All potential donors are evaluated carefully for the cause of death, including the presence of

chest trauma, need for cardiopulmonary resuscitation, and cardiac function before death. For neonates, most donors have suffered sudden infant death syndrome or birth asphyxia, whereas older donors are victims of violence and car accidents.

The shortage of suitable organ donors, especially for neonatal recipients, has led to many attempts at expanding the donor pool. Hearts from donors with moderately impaired ventricular function by echocardiography (left ventricular shortening fraction greater than 25% without major wall motion abnormalities) have been successfully transplanted into infant recipients.[10] Donor-to-recipient weight ratios of up to 4:1 have been used in infants. Tamisier and colleagues demonstrated that the higher the PVR, the larger the donor heart needed for successful transplantation and that hearts with PVR values thought to be in excess of normal can also be used.[20] Although ideal donor ischemia time is from 2 to 4 hours, ischemic times have been successfully extended beyond 9 hours. Deviations from the "ideal" donor criteria should be individualized, and even though the use of a marginal donor for a dying infant maintained on ECMO may be justified, use of the same heart for a child who is stable as an outpatient might not.

ABO-incompatible transplantation has been introduced as a method to decrease recipient waiting time and associated waiting list mortality.[19] Because neonates do not have the ability to produce antibodies to T-cell antigens, including major blood group antigens, ABO incompatibility becomes a negligible complication. ABO-incompatible transplantation has been infrequently used in the United States, and the age at which it is no longer feasible is still not clearly defined. Despite ABO-incompatible listing, it has not yielded lower wait-list mortality under the current UNOS allocation algorithm.[21]

Good donor management is a vital part of successful organ transplantation. The main goals are maintenance of normothermia, euvolemia, and adequate tissue perfusion and prevention of infection. Often, donors with poor cardiac function on initial evaluation will respond to volume loading and low-dose inotropic support with a significant improvement in function after heart retrieval, usually as part of a multiorgan retrieval procedure. Similar to recipients, all donors are screened for agents that might cause serious infection in an immunocompromised host, such as CMV, EBV, HIV, hepatitis, and *Toxoplasma*. The presence of antibodies is not a contraindication to transplantation but helps guide post-transplant therapy.

The four major goals in procurement of a donor heart are to (1) work effectively with the other teams to ensure the optimal condition of each recovered organ, (2) evaluate the hemodynamic status of the patient and the gross function of the heart by inspection, (3) use an effective cardioplegia and venting procedure that maximizes preservation of the heart, and (4) expertly remove the heart and adjoining vascular connections to ensure optimal anatomy for implantation. Procurement is performed through a median sternotomy. Donor blood is obtained for viral titers and retrospective HLA typing. The initial dissection involves separating the aorta from the main pulmonary artery to allow cross-clamping. Careful inspection of the heart is performed, and the patient is systemically heparinized. Procurement commences when the aorta is cross-clamped. Cardioplegia solution is infused through the aortic root, and the heart is vented through the right atrial appendage or superior or inferior vena cava for the right side and through the superior pulmonary vein or left atrial appendage for the left side. The superior vena cava is dissected free of its pericardial attachments up to the innominate vein, and the azygous vein is ligated and divided. The pericardial reflections around the right superior pulmonary vein and the inferior vena cava are sharply divided. The cardiectomy begins with inferior vena cava transection at the pericardial reflection. The main pulmonary artery is divided and then the posterior pericardial attachments and the superior vena cava. Last, the aorta is transected at the level of the innominate artery or more distally if the aorta is needed for the recipient. The donor heart is immersed in cold (4° C), sterile saline and then triple-bagged in a sterile manner for transport. In general, the cold ischemia time should be limited to a maximum of 4 to 5 hours.

Recipient Preparation and Techniques of Implantation

The standard technique for orthotopic heart transplantation was first described by Lower and Shumway in 1960 and consists of biatrial anastomoses, thus avoiding individual caval and pulmonary vein connections (Fig. 50-4).[22] Currently, however, the majority of cardiac transplant centers now use the bicaval technique, because it preserves atrial morphology and kinesis and is simpler when reconstruction after previous congenital heart repair is necessary. Once adequate hemodynamic monitoring is in place and the recipient is properly anesthetized, a median sternotomy is performed and the heart is suspended in a pericardial cradle. If previous sternotomies have been performed, appropriate precautions should be taken, including exposing the groins in the sterile field for access for femoral bypass. Once in the chest, the main pulmonary artery is dissected off the aorta past the bifurcation, and the pericardial reflection is mobilized off the aortic arch. Normally, aortic and bicaval cannulation is used.

In the case of a neonatal recipient with HLHS, the aortic arch vessels are mobilized proximally and controlled with snares, and the descending thoracic aorta is dissected to a level 2 to 3 cm below the insertion of the ductus arteriosus. The right and left pulmonary arteries are mobilized and controlled with snares in preparation for cardiopulmonary bypass. After heparinization, the main pulmonary artery is cannulated for arterial inflow, and a single venous cannula is placed in the right atrium, because circulatory arrest will be used. Immediately on instituting cardiopulmonary bypass, the pulmonary arteries are snared tight and the body perfused though a patent ductus arteriosus. The recipient is cooled to 18° C for circulatory arrest.

Once the donor organ is available in the operating room and the patient has been adequately cooled, circulatory arrest is established, the arch vessels are snared tightly, and the patient is exsanguinated into the venous reservoir. The aorta is divided just above the valve and incised longitudinally along the lesser curve of the aortic arch to a level 1 to 2 cm below the ductal insertion site on the descending aorta. The ductus is ligated next to the pulmonary artery and divided, and then the main pulmonary artery is transected just below the bifurcation. The right atrial incision is started superiorly at the base of the appendage. This incision is then carried down into the coronary sinus and across the atrial septum into the left atrium. The superior aspect of the right atrial incision is next carried across the septum to open the roof of the left atrium. The lateral wall of he left atrium is incised above the left pulmonary veins with the left atrial appendage included with the specimen.

The donor organ is prepared on the back table in cold saline solution. The right atrium is incised from the inferior vena

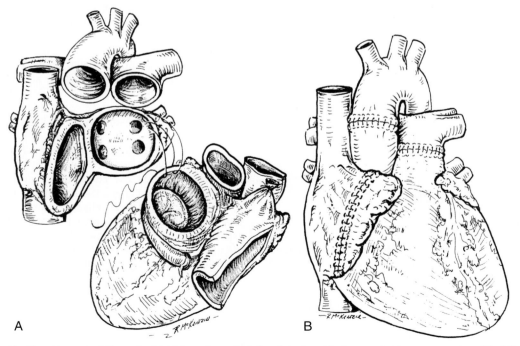

A   B

FIGURE 50-4   Standard heart transplantation using biatrial anastomosis. **A,** A recipient ventricular mass has been removed, and the left atrial anastomosis has been started. **B,** Final appearance after all anastomoses are completed.

cava laterally to the base of the appendage; the area of the sinoatrial node is avoided if atrial anastomoses rather than caval anastomoses are to be performed. The pulmonary vein confluence is excised off the back of the left atrium, leaving an opening comparable in size to the recipient left atrial cuff. The pulmonary artery is transected just below the bifurcation to provide a wide anastomosis. The aorta is trimmed, depending on the level required in the recipient. Care must be taken to check for and adequately close a patent foramen ovale, which is frequently present, especially in infant hearts. Failure to do so may result in significant postoperative right-to-left shunting in the face of pulmonary hypertension.

The implantation is begun by forming an anastomosis between the lateral wall of the left atrium from the level of the left atrial appendage inferiorly. A left ventricular vent is placed through the right superior pulmonary vein, and the left atrial anastomosis is completed by reconstructing the intra-atrial septum. The arch of the aorta is then reconstructed. The right atrial anastomosis is begun at the inferior vena cava orifice and then taken superiorly along the intra-atrial septum. The ascending aorta is then cannulated by a new purse-string suture, air is evacuated, and cardiopulmonary bypass is resumed. The snares are released from the head vessels and warming is commenced. The pulmonary anastomosis is then performed in an end-to-end fashion. If time permits, this step may be done during circulatory arrest in a drier field. After adequate warming, the patient is weaned from cardiopulmonary bypass and the cannulas removed (Fig. 50-5).[22] Right atrial, left atrial, and, occasionally, pulmonary artery pressure catheters are placed before discontinuing bypass and brought out through the skin below the incision.

In older children with cardiomyopathy or infants without aortic arch abnormalities, the recipient procedure is similar to that performed in adults. The ascending aorta is mobilized to the pericardial reflection and used for arterial cannulation. The child is cooled to 28° C to 34° C, because the implantation is performed under aortic cross-clamp rather than circulatory arrest. After the left atrial anastomosis has been completed, the right atrial connection can be sewn either directly or by using a bicaval technique if a previous cavopulmonary connection has been performed. This may decrease the incidence of tricuspid regurgitation in certain patients. The aortic anastomosis is then completed in an end-to-end fashion in the midascending aorta. The pulmonary artery anastomosis may or may not be performed during aortic cross-clamp, depending on how long the implant procedure takes.

Numerous other variations of the implantation procedure can be used, depending on the recipient anatomy. Modifications accounting for a persistent left superior vena cava, previous cavopulmonary shunt or Fontan procedure, corrected transposition of the great arteries, and situs inversus totalis have been described.

Postoperative Management

The recipient is returned from the operating room to an isolation room in the intensive care unit. Mechanical ventilation is required initially but is weaned as rapidly as possible. Antibiotics are continued until all monitoring lines and chest tubes have been removed.

Some level of inotropic support is required in virtually all heart transplant recipients. Isoproterenol is often an ideal choice because of its pulmonary vasodilatory effects, as well as its inotropic and chronotropic effects, because many patients have a slower than optimal heart rate initially. This transient sinus node dysfunction is rarely permanent. Dobutamine and dopamine, especially at "renal doses," are also frequently used to augment ventricular contractility. Epinephrine and norepinephrine are usually reserved for poor graft function. Sodium nitroprusside infusion or phosphodiesterase inhibitors are used for afterload reduction in the early postoperative period. Right ventricular dysfunction secondary to pulmonary hypertension may respond to phosphodiesterase inhibitors, which are used for afterload reduction in the early postoperative period. Right ventricular dysfunction secondary to pulmonary hypertension may respond to phosphodiesterase inhibitors such as milrinone. Inhaled nitric oxide has been shown to be an effective selective pulmonary vasodilator with few systemic side effects and is useful in cardiac transplant recipients with pulmonary hypertension.

Transplant Immunosuppression

A combination of immunosuppressive agents is used for the prevention and treatment of rejection. Standard triple-drug immunosuppression therapy consisting of prednisone, cyclosporine, and azathioprine has been successfully used in pediatric cardiac transplant recipients and remains the most common regimen.[23] In 2009, more than 70% of transplant recipients received induction immunotherapy. The induction and maintenance doses of medications used for immunosuppression at the Children's Hospital of Philadelphia are listed in Table 50-4. Because of the adverse effects of corticosteroids, withdrawal from prednisone is usually attempted 6 months after transplantation.[24] Up to 80% of recipients may be successfully weaned from steroids; only a quarter of these patients have an episode of rejection in the first 6 months.[25]

Most patients are maintained on an immunosuppressive regimen that is a combination of calcineurin inhibitor and cell-cycle inhibitor. Tacrolimus (formerly called FK-506) has been shown to be an effective immunosuppressive agent in children, and its use has increased over the last 5 years, with approximately 66% of all pediatric cardiac transplant patients receiving it for maintenance immunosuppression 1 year after transplantation in the place of cyclosporine. Overall, patients taking tacrolimus appear to have a lower incidence of rejection. Side effects of azathioprine therapy, such as bone marrow depression, have precipitated the use of mycophenolate mofetil (MMF) in its place. It is estimated that approximately 66% of patients use MMF as a cell-cycle inhibitor. It is well tolerated with few side effects and has been shown in large clinical trials to have benefits in survival and treated rejection episodes.[26]

An increasing number of centers use induction immunosuppression in pediatric cardiac recipients, with nearly 70% of patients now receiving a polyclonal anti–T-cell preparation, OKT3 (a murine monoclonal CD3 antibody), or an interleukin-2 receptor antibody immediately after transplantation. However, there have been no significant

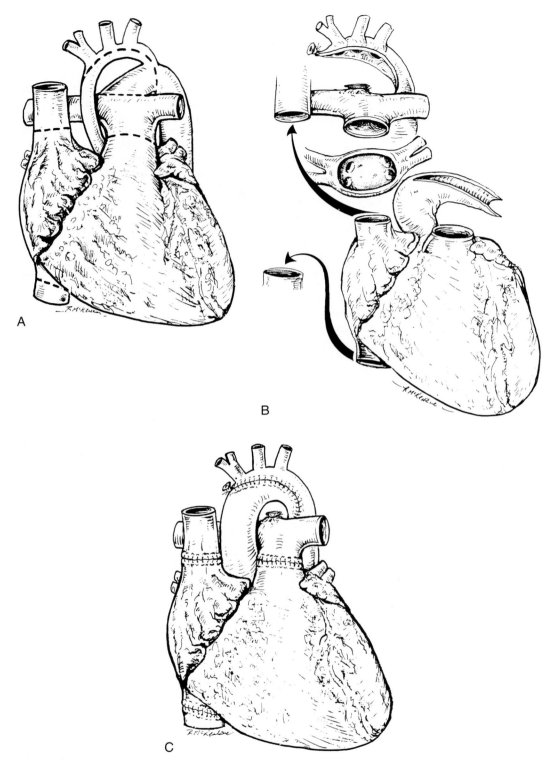

FIGURE 50-5   Technique for transplantation in hypoplastic left heart syndrome (with the use of bicaval anastomosis). **A,** Recipient anatomy before cardiectomy. **B,** Appearance of the recipient after cardiectomy. Note that the aortic incision must be extended into the descending aorta beyond the level of the arterial duct. **C,** Final appearance after all anastomoses are completed.

differences in the average number of rejection episodes in patients treated for rejection regardless of the type of induction used. In addition, there is no significant difference in survival between the induction groups or between use of induction versus no induction. Induction therapy does not increase

the risk of CMV disease or post-transplant lymphoproliferative disease.

Infectious prophylaxis includes oral nystatin for fungal prophylaxis and oral trimethoprim-sulfamethoxazole 3 times per week. Pentamidine inhalation treatment is an effective

TABLE 50-4

Heart Transplantation Immunosuppression Regimen at the Children's Hospital of Philadelphia

Drug	Dosage
Rabbit antithymocyte globulin (ATG)	1.5 mg/kg IV given in operating room before transplantation for sensitized patients and once daily for 5 days; titrated to CD3 count
Azathioprine/mycophenolate mofetil (MMF)	2 mg/kg IV given in the operating room before transplantation Then 2 mg/kg IV given once daily for 5 days (neonates), 7 days (infants), 9 days (adolescents) Change to MMF 600 mg/m² IV given twice daily Change to MMF orally once intestinal function resumes
Tacrolimus	0.05 mg/kg every 12 hours orally
Cyclosporine	0.02 mg/kg/hr IV infusion beginning in the operating room before transplantation Then 0.02 mg/kg/hr IV infusion for 24 hours Change to ATG on postoperative day 3 and give 1.5 mg/kg IV once daily for 3 days (neonates), 5 days (infants), or 7 days (adolescents) Change back to cyclosporine orally once ATG course completed Dosing should be carefully adjusted to maintain levels of 125-150 mg in neonates, 175-200 mg in children, 250 mg in 6- to 12-year-olds, and 250-300 mg in adolescents
Solumedrol	15 mg/kg in operating room before transplantation 3 mg/kg IV twice daily for 3 doses 0.5 mg/kg twice daily for sensitized patients followed by oral prednisone taper

alternative to trimethoprim-sulfamethoxazole for *Pneumocystis carinii* prophylaxis if bone marrow suppression is a problem. Routine CMV prophylaxis is used in cardiac transplant recipients at our institution.

Early Complications

Acute rejection and infection are the most common early complications after cardiac transplantation. Nearly 60% to 75% of patients have at least one episode of rejection, and it should be expected that about a third will have an episode in the first 3 months and 50% within the first year after transplantation.[27] Some studies suggest that infants may be less prone to rejection than older children. Rejection surveillance is based on clinical evaluation, echocardiography, and endomyocardial biopsy. Clinical assessment includes observation of changes in a patient's activity or appetite. Atrial or ventricular ectopy, including tachycardia, is suspicious for rejection and mandates evaluation. Echocardiography is particularly useful in neonates, in whom biopsy is technically difficult and carries significant risk because of patient size. Echocardiographic evaluation is typically performed weekly for the first month and then monthly for the first year after transplantation. Echocardiography-guided transjugular endomyocardial biopsy has been shown to be an effective means of monitoring pediatric transplant recipients for rejection and remains the gold standard for detection of rejection.[28] An aggressive approach, consisting of routine endomyocardial biopsy weekly for the first month after transplantation, every second week for the second month, and then once monthly for the remainder of the first year, has been adopted at the Children's Hospital of Philadelphia for rejection surveillance. Subsequent biopsies are obtained twice annually or whenever rejection is clinically suspected. Most biopsies are performed on an outpatient basis. The international grading system for cardiac transplant rejection is shown in Table 50-5.

Episodes of acute rejection are usually treated with a 3-day course of intravenous methylprednisolone (10 mg/kg). OKT3 and antithymocyte globulin are reserved for an incomplete response or rejection refractory to steroids. Response is confirmed by follow-up biopsy 1 to 2 weeks after treatment.

TABLE 50-5

International Society of Heart and Lung Transplantation Grading System for Evaluation of Cellular Rejection

2005 Classification	
0	No acute rejection
1R	Interstitial and/or perivascular infiltrate with up to 1 focus of myocyte damage
2R	Two or more foci of infiltrate with associated myocyte damage
3R	Diffuse infiltrate with multifocal myocyte damage, edema, hemorrhage, vasculitis

1990 Classification	
0	No acute rejection
1A	Focal, mild acute rejection
1B	Diffuse, mild acute rejection
2	Focal, moderate acute rejection
3A	Multifocal moderate rejection
3B	Diffuse, borderline severe rejection
4	Severe acute rejection

Modified from Billingham ME, Cary NRB, Hammond ME, et al: A working formulation for the standardization of nomenclature in the diagnosis of heart and lung rejection: Heart Rejection Study Group. J Heart Lung Transplant 1990;9:587-593; Stewart S, Winters GL, Fishbein MC, et al: Revision of the 1990 working formulation for the standardization of nomenclature in the diagnosis of heart rejection. J Heart Lung Transplant 2005;24:1710-1720.

Although infectious complications are common in cardiac transplant recipients, infection-related deaths do not appear to be. Bacterial infections are most frequent in the early post-transplant period, but can occur late after transplantation and usually respond to proper antibiotic therapy. Of viral infections, CMV appears to be the most common and is treated with intravenous ganciclovir. Viral respiratory infections usually occur at a frequency similar to that in normal children and appear to be well tolerated by the recipient.

Aside from rejection and infection, the immediate postoperative complications after heart transplantation are hypertension, seizures, renal dysfunction, and diabetes. Nearly 10% of infant heart transplant recipients require perioperative peritoneal dialysis. Among neonates, 10% to 15% require phenobarbital therapy for postoperative seizures.

Late Complications

The primary late complications in pediatric cardiac transplant recipients are chronic rejection, post-transplant lymphoproliferative disease (PTLD), and transplantation CAD. Rejection may account for up to 40% of deaths after cardiac transplantation. Lymphoproliferative disease is associated with EBV infection and is currently treated by a reduction in immunosuppressants, acyclovir, and chemotherapy.[29]

The onset of transplant CAD has a prevalence of 10% to 15% and may be suggested by symptoms of congestive heart failure in recipients. Echocardiograms are performed routinely during follow-up visits of heart transplant recipients, and worsening ventricular function is a sign of graft CAD. A new onset of arrhythmias after transplantation, especially ventricular arrhythmias, may also be an indication of underlying CAD. Additionally, CAD may be found on routine follow-up catheterization or intracoronary ultrasonography, without any previous suggestion of disease. A number of causes have been implicated in the development of graft CAD, including chronic cellular rejection, hyperlipidemia, vascular rejection, and CMV infection. Unlike adult cardiac transplant recipients, CAD appears to develop in pediatric patients relatively early after transplantation, with one series demonstrating an incidence of 35% by 2 years after transplantation. A review of 815 pediatric transplant patients found nearly 8% to have significant CAD by angiogram or autopsy findings. The mean time after transplantation to diagnosis was 2.2 years, with one patient having significant CAD 2 months after transplantation. Only 20% of patients in whom graft CAD was diagnosed were still alive, and most of the deaths were sudden or unexpected. Retransplantation appears to be the only viable option for these patients, although the results in general are not encouraging, with 1- and 3-year survival rates of 71% and 47%, respectively, and CAD developing in the second grafts in 20% of retransplantation patients. However, the Loma Linda group has reported a significantly better retransplantation experience in infants who were first transplanted when younger than 6 months. In this group, a 10-year actuarial survival rate of 91% was observed after retransplantation. Potential medical treatment targeted at cholesterol and lipid-lowering therapies are currently under investigation.

Results

The largest group of infant cardiac transplant recipients reported in the literature is from Loma Linda, where 233 heart transplantations in infants younger than 6 months have been performed. Nearly 65% were for HLHS, and the rest were for other complex congenital anomalies (29%) or cardiomyopathy or tumor (8%). The operative (30-day) survival rate was 89%, with the primary causes of mortality being primary graft failure, technical problems, pneumonia, or acute rejection. The overall 1-year survival rate was 84%, with a 5- and 10-year actuarial survival rate of 73% and 68%, respectively. In addition, patients undergoing transplantation when younger than 30 days had a significantly better outcome than did older infants, with an actuarial survival rate of 80% and 77% at 5 and 10 years, respectively, potentially related to improved immune tolerance in the younger subgroup.

Stanford University reported its series of 72 patients younger than 18 years who have undergone heart transplantation since 1977. Only 25% were younger than 1 year (mean of 9 years), and nearly two thirds had cardiomyopathy unrelated to congenital heart disease. The operative survival rate was 87.5%, with deaths mainly caused by pulmonary hypertension/right ventricular failure and acute rejection. There were 20 late deaths, 24% were due to rejection, and 17% were due to graft CAD. Actuarial survival rates at 1, 5, and 10 years were 75%, 60%, and 50%, respectively.

At St. Louis Children's Hospital, 45 heart transplants were performed from 1983 to 1993, more than half in infants with HLHS. The infant group had a survival rate (92%) similar to that of the Loma Linda series, whereas the pediatric group (older than 1 year) had an 80% early survival rate. Morales and colleagues published results of their experience spanning more 2 decades at Texas Children's Hospital and reported no change in mortality in survivors after the first post-transplant year.[30]

Results from the Registry of the International Society for Heart and Lung Transplantation reveal a perioperative mortality rate higher for infants than for older children (Fig. 50-6). Despite the much greater early mortality, however, the half-life of 18.3 years is longer than that of the childhood or adolescent survivors. For the childhood age group of 1 to 10 years, the half-life was 17.5 years versus 11.3 years for the adolescent age group, thus conferring the younger patients a significant survival advantage. If those patients who died within the first year after transplant were excluded, the median conditional survival was 21.4 years for those who underwent transplantation in the first year of life, 19.3 years for those aged between 1 and 10 years, and 15.2 years for older children (Fig. 50-7). Survival has been improving in relation to the era of transplantation, with the median survival increased

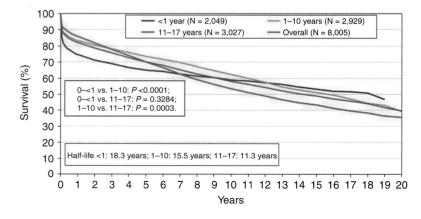

FIGURE 50-6 Survival analysis for transplantations performed January 1982 to June 2008. (From Kirk K, Edwards LB, Kucheryavaya AY, et al: The Registry of the International Society for Heart and Lung Transplantation: Thirteenth official pediatric heart transplantation report—2010. J Heart Lung Transplant 2010;29:1119-1128.) *(See Expert Consult site for color version.)*

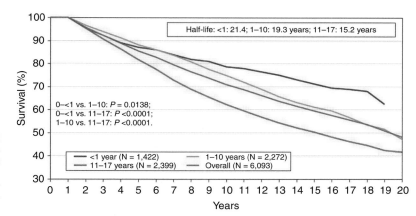

FIGURE 50-7 Survival analysis for transplants performed January 1982 to June 2008 and surviving to 1 year after transplantation. (From Kirk K, Edwards LB, Kucheryavaya AY, et al: The Registry of the International Society for Heart and Lung Transplantation: Thirteenth official pediatric heart transplantation report—2010. J Heart Lung Transplant 2010;29:1119-1128.) *(See Expert Consult site for color version.)*

from 9.5 years for the period 1982 to 1989, to 11.7 years for the period 1990 to 1994, to 14.3 years for the period 1995 to 1999 (Fig. 50-8). Averaged over 15 years, an infant recipient would have an approximate 2% per year risk of mortality, whereas for older children, it remains approximately 4%, again indicating a longer-term survival advantage for younger cardiac transplant recipients.

The most predictive risk factors for 1-year mortality in the pediatric population remain congenital heart disease, donor age, pulmonary artery systolic pressure greater than 35 mm Hg, and the need for mechanical ventilation and hospitalization while awaiting transplantation. Among the most significant risk factors for 5-year mortality are dialysis, congenital heart disease, and female gender (Fig. 50-9). Causes of death include CAD,

acute rejection, lymphoma, graft failure, and infection. Retransplantations now account for 5% of all transplantation operations. Survival for retransplantation is decreased when the intertransplantation interval was less than 3 years and is relative to indication for primary transplantation (Fig. 50-10).[31,32]

Aside from survival, it has been demonstrated that transplanted hearts in children appear to grow normally, and the left ventricle increases muscle mass to maintain the normal left ventricular mass-to-volume ratio with time. Exercise testing in older children has shown peak heart rate and oxygen consumption to be consistently two thirds of that predicted in heart transplant recipients. Somatic growth appears to be normal in infants after heart transplantation, and neurologic development is generally preserved, although some neuro-

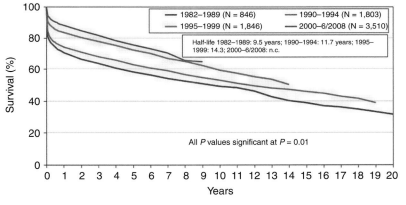

FIGURE 50-8 Survival analysis by era for transplantations performed January 1982 to June 2008. (From Kirk K, Edwards LB, Kucheryavaya AY, et al: The Registry of the International Society for Heart and Lung Transplantation: Thirteenth official pediatric heart transplantation report—2010. J Heart Lung Transplant 2010;29:1119-1128.) *(See Expert Consult site for color version.)*

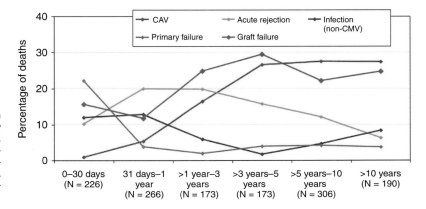

FIGURE 50-9 Relative incidence of leading causes of death for deaths occurring January 1998 to June 2009. CAV, coronary artery vasculopathy; CMV, cytomegalovirus. (From Kirk K, Edwards LB, Kucheryavaya AY, et al: The Registry of the International Society for Heart and Lung Transplantation: Thirteenth official pediatric heart transplantation report—2010. J Heart Lung Transplant 2010;29:1119-1128.) *(See Expert Consult site for color version.)*

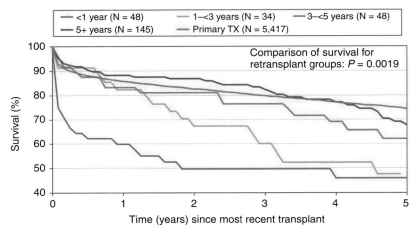

FIGURE 50-10 Survival rates for retransplantations, stratified by intertransplantation interval, for retransplantations performed January 1994 to June 2008. (From Kirk K, Edwards LB, Kucheryavaya AY, et al: The Registry of the International Society for Heart and Lung Transplantation: Thirteenth official pediatric heart transplantation report—2010. J Heart Lung Transplant 2010;29:1119-1128.) *(See Expert Consult site for color version.)*

logic abnormalities may be seen in up to 20% of neonatal recipients on long-term follow-up.

Conclusion

Despite further improvements in surgical technique, immunosuppression, perioperative management, and rejection surveillance, long-term results of pediatric heart transplantation have shown little change, with a 15-year survival rate of approximately 50%. Chronic rejection, graft CAD, and the long-term effects of steroids on growth continue to cloud the development of cardiac transplantation as the primary treatment of complex congenital heart disease. However, for many children with end-stage cardiomyopathy and structural heart disease not amenable to corrective surgery, transplantation is the only option. Future areas of research include the use of xenografts, ABO incompatibility, permanent mechanical support, and widening the bridge to transplantation with smaller and more adaptable assist devices.

The complete reference list is available online at www. expertconsult.com.

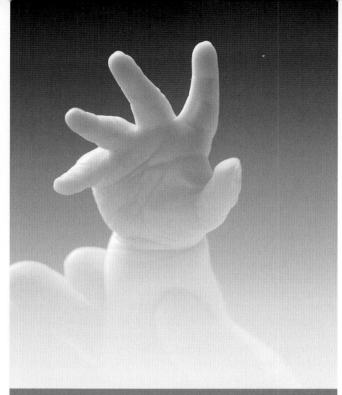

CHAPTER 51

Pediatric Lung Transplantation

Sanjiv K. Gandhi, Albert Faro,
and Charles B. Huddleston

The first reported attempt at lung transplantation occurred in 1963 and was performed by Dr. James Hardy at the University of Mississippi Medical Center.[1] The patient did not survive the hospitalization, dying 18 days after the transplant. There were a number of additional attempts at this during the next few years, with most failures related to poor healing of the airway anastomosis. Approximately 20 years after Dr. Hardy's ill-fated effort, the first truly successful lung transplant was performed in Toronto, Canada, by a team led by Dr. Joel Cooper. This patient had a single-lung transplant for pulmonary fibrosis and survived for more than 6 years, ultimately dying of renal failure.[2] During the subsequent years, and particularly in the late 1990s, pediatric lung transplantation has emerged as a viable treatment option for children with end-stage pulmonary parenchymal and vascular diseases. However, the number of children undergoing transplantations throughout the world since 1989 remains relatively small, representing only 4% of all lung transplantations performed.[3] In this chapter, pediatric lung transplantation is described as an isolated procedure, and heart-lung transplantation is not included.

Organ Allocation

In 2005, a new system to allocate lungs to recipients was established across the United States. Previously, lungs were allocated based on the amount of time the recipient had accrued on the waiting list (first come, first served). In an attempt to make distribution of lungs more equitable, a lung allocation score (LAS) was devised and implemented.[4] This score attempts to prioritize organs to patients on the list most in need of the organ (the sickest) as well as to those most likely to do well post-transplantation. This score is used in children 12 years and older. For those younger than 12 years, the old system still remains in effect at present.

Indications

Isolated lung transplantation is applicable to any child with life-threatening and progressive disability because of pulmonary parenchymal or vascular disease. In general, this treatment modality is indicated for increasing the duration of life and for improvement in the quality of life. The current long-term survival after lung transplantation is approximately 50% at 5 years. Thus the selection of patients for transplantation and the timing of the procedure are critically important. One would like to be able to predict when a child would be within 2 years of dying without any form of medical treatment. Obviously, this may be very difficult. The major diagnostic groups for pediatric lung transplantation are cystic fibrosis (CF), interstitial lung disease with pulmonary fibrosis, primary pulmonary hypertension, pulmonary hypertension associated with congenital heart disease, retransplantation, and a "miscellaneous" category (Table 51-1). Chronic obstructive lung disease, the most common indication for transplantation in adults, is remarkably absent from this list.[3]

CYSTIC FIBROSIS

This disease, the most common lethal hereditary disease in North America, comprises the largest diagnostic group of children younger than age 18 years who undergo lung transplantation. Although the median survival now exceeds 38 years, one eighth of the deaths from CF in 2008 still occurred in the pediatric age group. Without question, the most common cause of death is respiratory related. About 250 to 300 transplantations are performed annually in the United States for CF, and, although this number is growing slowly each year, donor availability still remains a major limiting factor.[5]

As with other diagnostic groups, timing of transplantation in the course of a chronic disease is a crucial issue. Kerem, in the early 1990s, demonstrated that a 1-second forced expiratory volume (FEV_1) less than 30% of predicted, a PaO_2 less than 55 mm Hg, and/or a PCO_2 greater than 50 mm Hg were associated with a survival beyond 2 years of less than 50%.[6] The impact of these factors is magnified in the pediatric age group, particularly in girls. However, more recent studies on the natural history of CF patients, once they have severely compromised lung function, show that an isolated measure of the FEV_1 alone may not be sufficiently predictive. The rate of

TABLE 51-1

Indications for Lung Transplantation in Children

Cystic fibrosis
Pulmonary fibrosis
Pulmonary vascular disease
Primary pulmonary hypertension
Eisenmenger syndrome
Bronchiolitis obliterans
Retransplantation
Other

decline in the FEV_1 may be a more accurate determinant of survival.[7,8] Other factors that may serve as relative indicators in deciding to proceed toward transplantation include the need for continuous supplemental oxygen, increased frequency of hospitalizations, and diminished weight for height (below the 80th percentile).[6] More recently, Liou and colleagues validated a formula that included microbiological data, body mass index measures, and presence of diabetes, in addition to lung function and gender, as important determinants in prognosticating 5-year survival.[9] The presence of antibiotic-resistant organisms in the sputum is a relative contraindication to lung transplantation. The synergistic effectiveness of antibiotic combinations is not useful in treating pulmonary exacerbations and is no longer readily available. Chronic infection with *Burkholderia cenocepacia,* pretransplantation, is associated with a particularly poor post-transplantation prognosis and therefore is of particular concern.[10,11] Portal hypertension with hepatic cirrhosis occurs in 5% to 10% of patients with CF. These children are at risk for variceal bleeding as well as derangements of synthetic function. In general, if the synthetic function is preserved, decompression of the portal venous system with percutaneous procedures will lower the risk to a level satisfactory for lung transplantation.[12] However, when there is also synthetic dysfunction of the liver, combined liver-lung transplantation may be the only appropriate option.[13,14] Diabetes mellitus is generally not considered a contraindication to transplantation unless there is evidence of vasculopathy, bearing in mind that control of serum glucose will be more difficult after transplantation.[15] As many as 10% to 15% of CF lung transplantation candidates will have had prior thoracotomies for either pneumothorax or pulmonary resection. Most centers do not consider this a contraindication to transplantation, although the resultant adhesions from these prior operations do increase the difficulty and the risk of bleeding.[16] Mechanical ventilation or presence of a tracheostomy are not in and of themselves contraindications to transplantation, but the overall medical condition of patients requiring this level of support must be carefully considered.[17]

PULMONARY VASCULAR DISEASE

This rather broad classification of patients includes those with primary pulmonary hypertension (PPH) and those with pulmonary hypertension associated with congenital heart disease (PH/CHD). The latter category includes patients with Eisenmenger syndrome but is not limited to this. These patients die of either progressive right-sided heart failure, arrhythmias, or a lethal episode of hemoptysis. It is difficult to predict when a patient might have a fatal arrhythmia or episode of hemoptysis. However, most patients with pulmonary vascular disease

will die of progressive right-sided heart failure over a protracted period of time.[18] In the past several years, a number of somewhat selective pulmonary vasodilators have become available for use in these patients. These include intravenous prostacyclin,[19] prostacyclin analogues iloprost (inhaled)[20] and betaprost (oral),[21] and bosentan,[22] an endothelin receptor antagonist. These drugs have enabled patients to delay the need for transplantation for years. In fact, the number of patients undergoing transplantation for pulmonary vascular disease has significantly dropped in recent years. The timing of transplantation for patients with pulmonary vascular disease is influenced significantly by the response to medical therapy and the underlying cause of the pulmonary vascular disease. Although primary pulmonary hypertension and Eisenmenger syndrome result in identical histologic changes in the pulmonary vascular bed, the latter of these two is associated with a much more favorable long-term prognosis. A retrospective analysis by Hopkins of 100 adults with severe pulmonary hypertension resulting from either Eisenmenger syndrome or PPH revealed that, in the former group, actuarial survival without transplantation was 97% at 1 year, 89% at 2 years, and 77% at 3 years. In contrast, survival was 77%, 69%, and 35% during the same respective time intervals in the PPH cohort.[23] It is presumed that the intracardiac defect allows the right ventricle to "decompress" via the defect when the afterload in the pulmonary vascular bed becomes prohibitively high. On the basis of this and other observations, atrial septostomy performed in the cardiac catheterization suite has been demonstrated to provide clinical benefit in patients with PPH.[24] Results from a multicenter study of patients with PPH performed before the advent of long-term intravenous prostacyclin therapy demonstrated a median survival from time of diagnosis of 2.8 years. In that study, a formula was developed incorporating hemodynamic variables to assist in predicting the 2-year mortality,[18] and it was recommended that patients should be listed when this figure is less than or equal to 50%. Studies regarding natural history in adults have been applied to children, but it is unclear whether this disease behaves the same in a younger population. Clabby and co-workers reviewed 50 patients from many centers to provide a means of estimating survival in children with PPH.[25] There was a direct correlation of mortality with the product of the mean right atrial pressure and the pulmonary vascular resistance.[25] With progress in the medical therapy of PPH to identify selective pulmonary vasodilators as well as the underlying mechanisms of this disease, these formulas predicting survival may be obsolete. The durability of medical therapy is unclear. How this therapy might be applied to secondary pulmonary hypertension, such as Eisenmenger syndrome, is speculative.

The two main issues in considering patients with Eisenmenger syndrome or PH/CHD for lung transplantation are the timing of listing and the complexity of the cardiac lesion to be repaired. As noted earlier, it is clear that, once the diagnosis is made, these patients can live much longer than those with PPH.[23] The mode of death in these patients is by progressive heart failure, pulmonary hemorrhage, stroke, or sudden death, presumably due to arrhythmias.[25] Patients should be listed when symptoms develop, when there has been a single pulmonary hemorrhage, or perhaps arbitrarily when they reach their late 30s. Most patients with PH/CHD have an atrial septal defect, ventricular septal defect, or patent ductus arteriosus. All of these require relatively simple cardiac repairs. However, there are patients with unrepaired atrioventricular canal defects, transposition of the great arteries, and truncus arteriosus who would require more complex procedures. An alternative for these patients would be heart-lung transplantation. The likelihood of obtaining a donor heart-lung block for anyone more than 40 kg is low because of the distribution policy for thoracic donor organs. In addition, the long-term survival after heart-lung transplantation is particularly poor (approximately 40% at 5 years post-transplantation).[3] These two issues must be factored into the decision as to whether one should perform the higher-risk procedure of lung transplantation in combination with repair of a complex cardiac lesion or heart-lung transplantation. Some patients with congenital heart disease who have undergone repair may not experience the expected decline in pulmonary vascular resistance after appropriate correction. Occasionally the repair has been performed relatively late in life, but there are children who have undergone timely repair and still present later with severe pulmonary hypertension. It is not clear how to classify these patients. In general, this is a less uniform group than either the patients with PPH or those with Eisenmenger syndrome. They seem to follow a clinical course similar to that seen in patients with PPH and should be treated in a similar fashion.[23]

Another diagnostic group with pulmonary vascular disease are patients with an inadequate pulmonary vascular bed. Examples of this include pulmonary atresia, ventricular septal defect and multiple aortopulmonary collaterals, and congenital diaphragmatic hernia, where there is primarily a general deficiency of pulmonary parenchyma. In the former group, complete correction (repair of the ventricular septal defect combined with reconstruction of the right ventricular outflow tract with a conduit to the unifocalized aortopulmonary collaterals) represents a high-risk but viable option for the majority of these patients. However, when the anatomy of the aortopulmonary collaterals is not amenable to unifocalization or when unifocalization has not produced satisfactory growth of the pulmonary vascular tree, the result is progressive cyanosis or progressive pulmonary hypertension or both. Lung transplantation with repair of the residual cardiac defect may be the only feasible option for survival. Children with congenital diaphragmatic hernias, despite having undergone a successful hernia repair, may still be left with inadequate pulmonary parenchyma and vascular bed to handle the full cardiac output. The resultant severe pulmonary hypertension is the usual cause of death in these infants and is an indication for transplantation. The problem here is that these infants often will require extracorporeal membrane oxygenation (ECMO) support during the perioperative period. This reduces the time that patients such as this can wait for a donor offer once listed for lung transplantation. It is possible that a single-lung transplant on the affected side would be sufficient in this circumstance. In this scenario, once the patient has grown, it may be possible to remove the transplanted lung altogether, leaving the patient with a presumably normal contralateral lung to maintain normal respiratory function. In reality, those patients with insufficient pulmonary reserve will have to be identified very early in the course for lung transplantation to be a realistic option. The mortality is quite high even when donor organs are identified.

In all the previous situations, isolated lung transplantation is appropriate only when left ventricular function is normal. Poor left ventricular function will result in elevated left ventricular end-diastolic pressure post-transplantation, which will add significantly to problems with pulmonary edema and early graft failure. Right ventricular function is frequently poor, particularly in the patient group with PPH. That should not be a deterrent to isolated lung transplantation, because the right ventricular function always returns to normal within a relatively short period of time.[26]

Although a prior thoracotomy is generally not a contraindication to lung transplantation in patients with pulmonary parenchymal disease, this is not true for those with pulmonary vascular disease, especially when secondary to congenital heart disease and associated with cyanosis. The adhesions that develop after a thoracotomy for palliation of cyanotic congenital heart disease are extremely vascular. Intercostal and internal mammary arteries will form direct connections through the pleura into the parenchyma of the lung in a compensatory attempt to enhance pulmonary blood flow. The bleeding that occurs during the recipient pneumonectomy portion of the transplantation procedure is often horrendous and life threatening.

PULMONARY FIBROSIS

These patients account for 5% to 10% of pediatric patients undergoing lung transplantation.[3] Placed in this category are those patients with "usual" interstitial fibrosis, radiation-induced fibrosis, bronchopulmonary dysplasia, and pulmonary fibrosis secondary to chronic aspiration. The progression of these disease processes is quite variable. Generally, patients should be listed when normal activities are markedly limited and minor viral illnesses lead to significant deterioration. Most patients will be oxygen dependent and may well have evidence of coexistent pulmonary hypertension. For those in whom aspiration is the underlying problem, the source of the aspiration must be eliminated.

The prognosis of children with idiopathic pulmonary fibrosis is not altogether clear. This may be because there is not a "usual interstitial pulmonary fibrosis" disease in children; the underlying causes are frequently unique and unusual. Decisions regarding listing for transplantation are somewhat difficult because of this. Pulmonary fibrosis presenting during infancy was once believed to have a poor prognosis; however, some studies have demonstrated improved survival with high doses of corticosteroid therapy.[27] The prognosis for adults with total lung capacity less than 60% predicted is still poor; nearly all are dead within 2 years.[28] It is difficult to translate this information into the pediatric experience. Pulmonary hypertension frequently accompanies this disease as it progresses. These patients should be evaluated and listed for transplantation when they become symptomatic. If there is a favorable response to corticosteroids, they can be followed with standard (age > 5 years) or infant (length < 90 centimeters) pulmonary function tests. One problem with managing this disease is that patients with progression of their disease tend to remain on relatively high doses of corticosteroids and come to transplantation in a rather cushingoid state. This should not exclude them from transplantation.

BRONCHIOLITIS OBLITERANS AND RETRANSPLANTATION

Bronchiolitis obliterans is not a specific disease but rather a histologic description characterized by the obstruction and destruction of the distal airways. It may occur as a consequence of any severe lung injury, including viral pneumonia, graft-versus-host disease after bone marrow transplantation, autoimmune diseases, chemical injury, Stevens-Johnson syndrome, and others. Of course, it is a relatively common late complication of lung transplantation (see later). The underlying etiology is unknown. "Primary" bronchiolitis obliterans (not related to prior lung transplantation) is a perfectly legitimate indication for lung transplantation: It is a slowly progressive disease in virtually all cases with no known effective treatment. When this disorder occurs as a consequence of an isolated lung injury, transplantation is a fairly straightforward decision process. However, those patients with prior bone marrow transplantations (usually for leukemia) offer special considerations.[29] Although the standard definition of "cure" is remission of the malignancy for more than 5 years, most of these patients present within 2 or 3 years of treatment. Another problem is the deranged immune competency seen after bone marrow transplantation and how the immunosuppressant agents used after lung transplantation might further affect this. We have found that these patients have less acute rejection than most other lung transplantation recipients but may be more prone to opportunistic infections.[29] However, the number of patients transplanted in this setting is low. For patients who acquire bronchiolitis obliterans through other immunologic injuries, such as autoimmune disorders, there are concerns about the likelihood of recurrence in transplanted lungs. One would have to ascertain that the primary process has completely abated before transplantation.

Retransplantation for acute graft failure after transplantation has an extremely poor prognosis.[30] Retransplantation for bronchiolitis obliterans is a controversial issue. Bronchiolitis obliterans accounts for the majority of deaths occurring more than 90 days post-transplantation.[3] This figure is borne out in our pediatric series.[31] Although early mortality after retransplantation is higher than for "first-time" lung transplantations, those who do survive this early phase have long-term survival similar to the non-redo transplantations.[30] Risk factors for poor early outcome include nonambulatory status, short period of time since the first transplantation, transplantation at a center with limited experience, and dependence on mechanical ventilation. We have further noted that a low glomerular filtration rate is an independent risk factor. Because patients continue to die on the waiting list, one could argue that no patient should ever be retransplanted because this might deprive an otherwise lower-risk patient from receiving organs in a timely fashion. At present this issue is unresolved. One can only advise use of proper judgment in selecting only the best candidates when the issue of retransplantation arises.

MISCELLANEOUS

A variety of diagnoses fall into this group. Congenitally based pulmonary parenchymal diseases constitute one of the more interesting broad categories. Typically, these full-term newborns present with severe respiratory distress and no obvious cause, such as meconium aspiration, sepsis, or persistent fetal circulation. The diagnoses falling into this category include surfactant protein B deficiency, other forms of pulmonary alveolar proteinosis, alveolar-capillary dysplasia, pulmonary dysmaturity, congenital interstitial pneumonitis, and others. These infants usually have severe respiratory failure and require a high level of ventilatory support. Often extracorporeal membrane oxygenation has been or is currently being used. An open-lung biopsy is often necessary to either make the diagnosis or to exclude other diagnoses. Surfactant protein (SP) B or C deficiency and the ABCA 3 mutation can now be diagnosed by looking for the specific genetic mutation in peripheral blood or cheek swabs and assaying tracheal effluent for the presence of this surfactant protein.[32] All children will survive less than 3 months even with aggressive therapy. Abnormalities in SP-C and ABCA3 can have more varied presentations. Additionally, because the surfactant proteins are expressed only in the lungs, extrapulmonary organ dysfunction is rare.[33] Until other therapies become available, lung transplantation is the only viable therapeutic option. In general, the waiting time for an organ offer is relatively short in infants. Therefore one might realistically believe that an infant with a 3-month life expectancy could undergo transplantation and survive. When an infant is on ECMO, every effort should be made to wean from it, using whatever means possible, including a high-frequency oscillating ventilator and/or nitric oxide. Although ECMO is not an absolute contraindication to transplantation, one should be very cautious in this setting because of the relatively high incidence of other organ dysfunction.

Contraindications

Contraindications to transplantation in children are also based on experience obtained in adults (Table 51-2). Absolute contraindications include systemic disease with major extrapulmonary manifestations or severe dysfunction of other organ systems. Thus widespread malignancy, collagen vascular disease, human immunodeficiency virus infection, and severe neuromuscular disease are absolute contraindications. The acceptable degree of renal insufficiency is open to some interpretation. Given the nephrotoxicity of cyclosporine and tacrolimus, the drugs that form the basis of nearly all immunosuppressant regimens, a serum creatinine value greater than 2.0 mg/dL and a probable need for post-transplantation dialysis are clinical parameters that would mitigate strongly against proceeding with transplantation. A glomerular

TABLE 51-2
Contraindications to Lung Transplantation

Absolute

Malignancy
Human immunodeficiency virus infection
Multisystem organ failure
Left ventricular dysfunction
Active collagen vascular disease
Severe neuromuscular disease

Relative

Renal insufficiency
Liver function impairment
Malnutrition
Resistant organisms in the sputum
Poorly controlled diabetes mellitus
Osteopenia
Prior thoracotomies in the presence of pulmonary vascular disease
Prior pneumonectomy with mediastinal shift
Extreme prematurity
Inadequate psychosocial support system
Poor compliance

filtration rate less than 50 mL/min has been associated with a poor outcome in some patients. Significantly deranged hepatic synthetic function precludes transplantation unless concomitant liver transplantation is also being undertaken. More complex issues include severe malnutrition, poorly controlled diabetes mellitus, osteopenia, vertebral compression fractures, and the need for mechanical ventilation. None of these factors in and of themselves serves as an absolute contraindication. Nonetheless, all such concerning aspects of the clinical presentation must be evaluated and carefully considered in the scope of the patient's overall state of health to assess the likelihood for successful recovery after transplantation. Chronic administration of corticosteroids before transplantation is considered to be undesirable, and, when possible, one should reduce the total daily dose or change to an every-other-day dosage schedule. Previously, corticosteroids were believed to have a significant negative impact on airway healing, particularly in the case of double-lung transplantation with a tracheal anastomosis. Bilateral sequential lung transplantation with bronchial anastomoses has obviated this problem to a large degree. Severe psychiatric disorder in either the patient or, in the case of a young child, the care provider, is a strong relative contraindication. Finally, a history of poor compliance with either a medical regimen or in keeping follow-up appointments is considered by most to be a strong relative contraindication to transplantation. Graft failure due to lack of proper care not only results in death to the recipient involved, but also results in either a delayed or denied transplantation for a more appropriate candidate.[34]

SPECIAL CIRCUMSTANCES

Some infants born extremely prematurely survive the early days of their lives only to develop severe bronchopulmonary dysplasia with respiratory failure within the first year of life. The incidence of significant cerebral injury in this group is high; approximately 50% of those surviving have some disability.[35] We can only assume that the incidence is higher in those with severe residual lung disease requiring transplantation. It is often difficult to assess the neurologic status in these infants because of their small size and often the need for sedation and neuromuscular paralysis for maintenance of satisfactory ventilation. It is probably unwise to submit an infant born at less than 28 weeks' estimated gestational age to lung transplantation, unless there has been an opportunity for an accurate neurologic examination. Imaging studies may offer some reassurance but are inconclusive. Another unusual situation that arises where lung transplantation may be considered appropriate is the child with severe acute respiratory distress syndrome. Those children still in the acute phase of this illness often have other organ dysfunction, and their condition is too unstable for them to wait the obligatory time once listed for transplantation, given the current organ allocation system for children less than 12 years of age. Those who survive the early phase of acute respiratory distress syndrome and are left with fibrotic lungs and stable ventilatory requirements should be evaluated. Finally, occasionally a patient with a history of prior pneumonectomy will be referred for lung transplantation. After pneumonectomy in children, the mediastinum shifts to the affected side. This distorts the hilar structures to the point that bilateral or single lung transplantation is virtually impossible. When possible, a patient undergoing pneumonectomy who might require lung transplantation in the future should have a prosthetic spacer placed in that side of the chest to maintain normal mediastinal geometry.

Donor Evaluation and Organ Procurement

Donor availability remains a major limitation to the applicability of transplantation for end-stage lung disease. Donors must be matched by ABO blood type compatibility and within a reasonable size range of the recipient. Height is used as the most accurate correlate to lung size. Height that falls within 15% to 20% of the recipient height is probably suitable. Extending this range upward is certainly feasible, because it is not difficult to reduce the size of the lungs by trimming off the edge or even using only the lower lobes. However, extending the lower limit should be done with great caution, because the transplanted lungs may not fill the chest and may be more prone to pulmonary edema. Donors are excluded in the presence of positive HIV serology, active hepatitis, history of asthma, tuberculosis, or other significant pulmonary disease. A history of limited cigarette smoking is probably acceptable if other parameters of the evaluation fall within the guidelines. In general, the upper limit of donor age is approximately 55 years. The chest radiograph should be free of infiltrates, and the arterial oxygen tension should be more than 300 mm Hg on an inspired oxygen fraction of 1.0 with an appropriate tidal volume and 5 cm H_2O positive end-expiratory pressure. Mild pulmonary contusions and subsegmental atelectasis would not necessarily exclude a donor as long as these criteria are met. Flexible bronchoscopy should be performed to examine the airways for erythema suggestive of aspiration of gastric contents. In addition, this provides an opportunity to assess the nature and quantity of pulmonary secretions. The presence of purulent secretions that do not clear well with suctioning should exclude the donor even if the chest radiograph is clear and the oxygenation is adequate.

The surgical part of the procurement process is performed through a median sternotomy. Both pleural spaces are opened widely to allow visual inspection of the lungs and also the topical application of cold saline and slush. The trachea is dissected out between the superior vena cava and aorta. It may be helpful to develop the interatrial groove, also, to allow a more accurate division of the left atrial tissue that must be shared with the cardiac donor team in most situations. The principles of the procurement process beyond this are (1) anticoagulation with high-dose (300 units/kg) heparin; (2) bolus injection of prostaglandin E_1 (50 to 70 mcg/kg) directly into the main pulmonary artery; (3) decompressing the right side of the heart by incising the inferior vena cava; (4) decompressing the left side of the heart by amputating the left atrial appendage; (5) high-volume (50 mL/kg), low-pressure flush of cold (4° C) pulmonary preservation solution of choice; (6) topical application of cold saline and slush to the lungs; and (7) continued ventilation of the lungs with low volumes and low pressures using an Fio_2 of 0.4. When all the preservation solution has been administered, the lungs are excised en bloc. The trachea is divided while the lungs are held in gentle inflation (pressure of $\approx$ 20 cm H_2O) with the Fio_2 at 0.4. The lungs are then extracted, placed in a bag containing the preservation solution used for the flush, and then placed in cold storage for transport.

Much research has been devoted to finding the "ideal" preservation solution to extend potential ischemic times and avoid reperfusion injury.[36] A full discussion of this complex topic goes beyond the scope of this chapter. The most commonly used preservation solutions at this time are modified Euro-Collins solution, University of Wisconsin solution, Perfadex, and Celsior. None of these is clearly superior to the others, and all work reasonably well. However, none reliably allows for preservation times greater than 8 hours, and none completely avoids reperfusion injury.

Technique of Transplantation

The surgical technique used for children is like that for adults, except that virtually all children will require cardiopulmonary bypass, whereas that is not always necessary in adults. Transplantation without cardiopulmonary bypass would require single-lung ventilation during the procedure. Maintaining single-lung ventilation in these small children is extremely difficult, because the airways are too small to accommodate double-lumen endobronchial tubes. Bilateral lung transplantation is performed for nearly all children because of concerns over the growth potential of the transplanted lungs. Trans-sternal bilateral anterior thoracotomy incision (the so-called "clamshell incision") through the fourth intercostal space provides excellent exposure of the heart and hilar regions. Though absorbable suture theoretically provides the greatest potential for growth, some surgeons use nonabsorbable suture material for the anastomoses.[37] We recommend a simple end-to-end rather than a telescoping anastomosis for the airway because of the high incidence of stenosis in the latter.[38,39] If the patient requires concomitant repair of an intracardiac lesion (e.g., with Eisenmenger syndrome), that is best performed after the recipient pneumonectomies and before implanting the donor lungs. Many of these patients have significant aortopulmonary collaterals resulting in significant pulmonary venous return to the heart while on cardiopulmonary bypass. After the recipient lungs have been removed, the absence of pulmonary venous return to the heart from bronchial arteries and other collateral vessels will allow for a bloodless operative field for the intracardiac repair. The subsequent period during which allograft implantation is performed provides sufficient time for cardiac reperfusion before weaning from cardiopulmonary bypass.

Living donor lobar transplantation and the use of cadaveric lobes, has become less commonplace as an alternative to standard cadaveric "whole lung" transplantation, since implementation of the LAS.[40] Although the upper lobes have been used, lower lobes seem better suited anatomically, with each lobe serving as an entire lung. When lobes come from a living donor, there is less bronchial and vascular tissue with which to work and thus longer cuffs of the bronchus, pulmonary artery, and pulmonary vein of the recipient will facilitate the procedure. A technique has been devised whereby a single left lung can be partitioned such that the upper lobe is used on the right and the lower lobe on the left.[41] The circumstances under which one might use this technique would be quite unusual—a single left lung from a large donor being made available to a desperately ill child. Nonetheless, it is another attempt at solving the ongoing problem of inadequate donor organ supply.

Immunosuppression

Although the precise protocols differ from one center to another, most use the so-called triple-drug immunosuppression approach (Table 51-3). Combinations of these immunosuppressant drugs allow for a better overall effect with a relatively less toxic dose of any one agent. Drug regimens generally include cyclosporine or tacrolimus in combination with azathioprine or mycophenolate mofetil (MMF) and prednisone. Most pediatric lung transplantation centers now use tacrolimus because of the cosmetic advantages it offers versus cyclosporine and therefore perhaps improving adherence, especially among adolescent recipients. The use of induction cytolytic therapy using antithymocyte globulin is somewhat controversial because of the potential of infectious complications associated with their use. Basiliximab, a specific monoclonal antibody to interleukin 2, is an alternative to cytolytic agents to "induce" tolerance.[42] Rather than being cytolytic, these drugs work by blocking a critical pathway in the activation of lymphocytes involved in cellular rejection. The low infection rate using these monoclonal antibodies has stimulated the reemergence of induction therapy early after lung transplantation.[43] The initial target trough cyclosporine blood level is 300 to 400 ng/mL by whole blood monoclonal assay. When tacrolimus is used, that target trough level is 10 to 15 ng/mL. The initial corticosteroid dose is 0.5 mg/kg daily of prednisone or methylprednisolone. MMF is given at a dose of 600 mg/m^2 twice daily while azathioprine is given in a dose of 2.5 to 3.0 mg/kg daily. Acute rejection is treated with 3 consecutive days of intravenous methylprednisolone at a dose of 10 mg/kg/day. Rejection refractory to methylprednisolone is treated with antithymocyte globulin for 7 to 10 days. Recurrent (greater than three) bouts of acute rejection may also prompt a change of the baseline immunosuppression. Although the corticosteroid dose is gradually tapered with

TABLE 51-3	
Immunosuppressant Agents	
Class of Drug	*Side Effects*
Interleukin-2 Synthesis Inhibitors	
Cyclosporine	Hypertension, seizures, nephrotoxicity, hirsutism, gingival hyperplasia
Tacrolimus	Hyperglycemia, seizures, nephrotoxic
Lymphocyte Proliferation Inhibitors	
Azathioprine	Leukopenia, nausea
Mycophenolate mofetil	Leukopenia, nausea, diarrhea, elevated liver enzymes
Sirolimus	Hypertriglyceridemia, delayed wound healing
Corticosteroids	Hypertension, hyperglycemia, cushingoid appearance
Induction Agents	
Antithymocyte globulin	Fever, chills, leukopenia, cytomegalovirus infections, post-transplantation lymphoproliferative disorder
OKT3	Fever, chills, cytomegalovirus infections, post-transplantation lymphoproliferative disorder
Daclizumab, basiliximab	Nausea, diarrhea

time, we do not believe it is appropriate to stop this drug altogether. The side effects of immunosuppressive drugs in children are similar to those seen in adults. Sirolimus (rapamycin) is chemically similar to tacrolimus but inhibits the proliferative response of lymphocytes to interleukin-2.[44] It does not share the nephrotoxic potential of tacrolimus. It is currently reserved for situations of failure of other immunosuppressant drugs. Some caution should be exercised in using sirolimus as initial immunosuppression early after transplantation because there has been evidence of impaired wound and airway healing resulting in serious complications.[45]

All patients receive prophylaxis against pneumocystis jiroveci pneumonia with either sulfamethoxazole-trimethoprim orally 3 times per week or when sulfa allergy or intolerance is present one may consider monthly treatment with aerosolized pentamidine or daily therapy with atovaquone. Prophylaxis against mucocutaneous *Candida* infections is also used.

Post-transplantation Surveillance

Surveillance after transplantation is based on periodic spirometry and bronchoscopy with biopsies and bronchoalveolar lavage. Before discharge from the hospital, patients are provided with a home spirometer and are asked to perform spirometry at least once daily. A decrease in FEV_1 of greater than 10% from baseline is considered an indication for evaluation. All patients, regardless of size, undergo regularly scheduled surveillance bronchoscopy to diagnose lower respiratory infections, subclinical graft rejection, and airway anastomotic complications. Virtually all episodes of suspected rejection should be confirmed with transbronchial biopsies. The main challenge occurs in small infants in whom a miniforceps is used through either the 2.8-mm or the 3.5-mm pediatric flexible fiberoptic bronchoscope. However, obtaining an adequate specimen with these forceps can be challenging. Recently a 4.0 mm bronchoscope with a 2.2-mm suction channel was introduced into clinical practice, thus allowing the use of adult-sized forceps for many young children. At our institution, bronchoscopy with biopsy is performed at 7 to 10 days and at 1, 2, 3, 6, 9, 12, and 18 months after transplantation as a surveillance procedure. Worsening pulmonary function, infiltrates on a chest radiograph, or deterioration in clinical status, such as fever or an oxygen requirement, also prompt bronchoscopy and biopsy. Bronchoalveolar lavage is performed at these procedures for quantitative bacterial, routine viral, and fungal cultures.

Post-transplantation Complications

AIRWAY ANASTOMOTIC COMPLICATIONS

Anastomotic complications can involve either the airway or the vascular anastomoses. Airway dehiscence was the major source of postoperative morbidity and mortality in the early days of lung transplantation when tracheal anastomoses were performed. Not until this problem was solved by using an omental wrap for the airway anastomosis could clinical lung transplantation progress.[46] Currently, dehiscence is rare in spite of the fact that most surgeons do not use the omental wrap any longer, but rather approximate donor and recipient peribronchial tissue over the anastomosis. Dehiscence of the airway may be either partial or total. Partial dehiscence can usually be treated expectantly but puts the airway at increased risk of late stenosis.[47] Complete dehiscence requires emergent therapy and is generally a lethal complication. Although reanastomosis should be attempted when possible, it is associated with a high rate of failure, and transplantation pneumonectomy is required. Smaller airway size in children prompted concerns about whether the incidence of bronchial anastomotic stenosis would be higher and also whether the anastomoses would grow. Current evidence suggests that the airways at the anastomoses grow and that the incidence of bronchial stenosis is not affected by age or size at the time of transplantation.[48,49] Bronchial stenosis is usually treated with dilatation initially with either progressively larger rigid bronchoscopes or with an angioplasty balloon. Balloon dilatation of a stricture may be preferable, because it is less likely than a rigid bronchoscope to injure the distal airway. Repeat bronchoscopy 10 to 14 days after initial dilatation of a bronchial stenosis is necessary to judge the overall effectiveness and to assess the likelihood of recurrence. Depending on the severity of the initial stricture or the rapidity with which it recurs, one might consider placing a stent. There are two basic types of stents applicable to this situation: Silastic and wire mesh. In general, wire mesh stents are easier to insert but much more difficult to remove, and Silastic stents are harder to place and easier to remove. Alternatives to stent placement include sleeve resection (of the bronchus or upper lobe) or retransplantation. Resection has been performed with good results in adults but would be a very difficult procedure in children.[50] Retransplantation should be reserved for situations in which the stricture extends beyond the bronchial bifurcation on either side and cannot be managed with either endobronchial techniques or local resection.

VASCULAR ANASTOMOTIC COMPLICATIONS

Problems with either the arterial or venous anastomoses are rare. In most instances, a stenosis in either of these is secondary to excessive length on the donor pulmonary artery or left atrial cuff or torsion of either of these structures when performing the anastomosis. Stenosis in one of the pulmonary artery anastomoses may or may not be manifest by right ventricular hypertension. Because pulmonary artery catheters are not often placed in children, one should check the right ventricular pressure by direct puncture once off cardiopulmonary bypass. If elevated, the pressure distal to each anastomosis should be checked also by direct puncture. Unilateral mild to moderate pulmonary arterial anastomotic stenosis may not result in significant elevation of right ventricular pressure. A perfusion lung scan is routinely performed within 24 hours of the transplantation to screen for technical problems with the vascular anastomoses. Any significant discrepancy between right- and left-sided perfusion should be immediately evaluated with either direct visualization in the operating room or angiography. Stenosis in either or both pulmonary venous anastomoses is manifest by pulmonary hypertension, profuse pink frothy sputum, and diffuse infiltrates on a chest radiograph. These findings may also be present with a severe reperfusion injury or diffuse alveolar damage. However, the pulmonary capillary wedge pressure is generally normal in the latter two instances and elevated with a stenosis in the pulmonary venous anastomosis. Transesophageal echocardiography is particularly helpful in the diagnosis of pulmonary venous anastomotic problems. Confirmation of the diagnosis usually requires direct measurement of the pulmonary venous and left atrial pressures, particularly in small children. Early correction is mandatory.

BLEEDING

A number of factors place these patients at increased risk for bleeding after transplantation. Nearly all transplantations in children require prolonged cardiopulmonary bypass for recipient pneumonectomies and implantation of donor organs. Additionally, many of these patients have undergone prior thoracotomies or sternotomies. Patients with cyanotic heart disease and a prior thoracotomy have the greatest risk of serious bleeding, as mentioned earlier.

PHRENIC NERVE INJURY

This complication occurs in about 20% of lung transplantations and is secondary to trauma because of stretch while retracting to expose the hilar regions; it is more common on the right side.[51] Recovery of diaphragmatic function within 6 months of transplantation is the general rule. The reason for the right side being injured more commonly probably relates to the proximity of the nerve to the pulmonary artery and the superior vena cava on that side. The superior vena cava (and thus the phrenic nerve) must be retracted to expose the proximal right pulmonary artery. Prior thoracotomy puts the nerve at greater risk for injury, because it may be obscured by adhesions.

HOARSENESS

Vocal cord paralysis caused by recurrent laryngeal nerve injury has an incidence of approximately 10%. This diagnosis is made at the time of flexible fiberoptic bronchoscopy with direct examination of the cords. In most cases, anatomic asymmetry improves without directed therapy within 6 months of transplantation. The left vocal cord is nearly always the one involved, and the injury presumably occurs as a result of dissection of the left pulmonary artery in the region of the ligamentum arteriosum.

GASTROINTESTINAL COMPLICATIONS

Many centers now routinely assess for the presence of gastroesophageal reflux because of its potential association with the development of bronchiolitis obliterans (BO).[52] Since instituting routine 24-hour pH probe monitoring at the 2-month post-transplantation evaluation, we have found that almost 70% of our patients have evidence of acid reflux. The etiology of this high incidence of gastroesophageal reflux is not clear but may be due to injury to the vagus nerves bilaterally in the process of performing the recipient pneumonectomies. Decreased intestinal motility is also a common problem in all age groups. Patients with CF are at risk for distal intestinal obstruction syndrome. This can be avoided by aggressively treating with osmotic cathartics after transplantation. Gastrografin enemas may be necessary if there is no response to oral cathartics.

ATRIAL FLUTTER

Atrial arrhythmias are relatively common with significant episodes of atrial flutter occurring in 10% of pediatric lung transplantation recipients. Many require long-term treatment.[53] Investigation into this entity using a model of lung transplantation has shown that the suture lines for the left atrial anastomoses provide sufficient substrate for the maintenance of atrial flutter when initiated by programmed extrastimulus.[54]

GRAFT COMPLICATIONS

Reperfusion injury manifesting as graft failure with diffuse infiltrates on chest radiography, frothy sputum, and poor oxygenation is the most common graft complication early after lung transplantation, occurring in 20% to 30% of transplantation recipients.[55] It is the most common cause of death within the first 30 days after transplantation.[3] The underlying cause is probably multifactorial, with both donor and recipient conditions contributing to this problem. The best preventive measures include careful evaluation and procurement of the donor organs as well as having a recipient free of active infection or other acute problems. A well-conducted transplantation procedure is also of utmost importance. The treatment of reperfusion injury is mostly supportive, although nitric oxide[56] and prostaglandin E_1[57] may be of some primary benefit.

Rejection is a common occurrence after lung transplantation, perhaps more so than in other solid organ transplantations (Fig. 51-1). The lung has a much larger endothelial surface than other organs. Because the major histocompatibility antigen expression on endothelial surfaces is the primary signal for local immune recognition, the lung would seem to be the least easily camouflaged organ in the body. In addition, the lung graft comes with its own parenchymal bronchial lymphocytes and macrophages. Gradually, these are replaced by the recipient lymphocytes and macrophages. This rather intense immunologic activity adds to the risk of rejection. Acute graft rejection early after transplantation presents in such a nonspecific fashion that each suspected episode should be documented with histologic evidence obtained by either transbronchial biopsy or open-lung biopsy. The great majority of episodes of acute rejection occur in the first 6 months after transplantation. Although the incidence of acute rejection in all children is about the same as that seen in adults, it appears that infants have a much lower incidence.[58,59] The precise reason for this is unclear but may have to do with the relative immaturity of the immunologic system in infants.

Antibody-mediated rejection (AMR) is now recognized as a serious and relatively common complication of lung transplantation. With the advent of better detection assays, one can now quantitate the amount of circulating donor-specific antibody in the recipient. However, it is also becoming increasingly clear that non–human leukocyte antigen (HLA) antibodies may also be responsible and that, in fact, autoantibodies to previously sequestered antigens may play a vital role

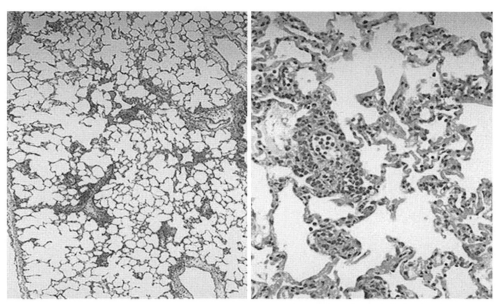

FIGURE 51-1 Acute rejection. Multiple lymphocytes are present in a perivascular position involving many blood vessels, which can be seen better on higher power. This was interpreted as grade A2 acute rejection.

in the development of bronchiolitis obliterans. Increasing experience with C4d immunostaining of biopsy specimens and C4d and C3d immunofluorescence permit histologic confirmation of AMR. The exact frequency of this complication in lung transplantation recipients is not yet known. AMR has shown itself to be fairly refractory to therapy. We use a protocol that includes plasmapheresis, intravenous bortezomib, intravenous immunoglobulin (IVIG), and rituximab.

Bronchiolitis obliterans is viewed by most clinicians to be a manifestation of chronic rejection and occurs in nearly 50% of all long-term survivors.[60] The precise cause is unknown, although donor ischemic time, episodes of early acute rejection, and history of lymphocytic bronchitis have been identified as risk factors.[61,62] Bronchiolitis obliterans presents as a significant fall in FEV_1 without other obvious cause. The chest radiograph is generally clear, and the computed tomographic examination of the chest usually demonstrates evidence of air trapping with mosaicism and occasionally bronchiectasis. Ventilation/perfusion lung scanning may demonstrate air trapping with xenon retention. Bronchoscopy with transbronchial biopsy and bronchoalveolar lavage should be done as part of the evaluation to rule out other potential causes, such as acute rejection or infection, and to assess the degree of active lymphocytic infiltration of the airways. The histologic picture of bronchiolitis obliterans is one of dense scarring of the membranous and respiratory bronchioles (Fig. 51-2). It may be inferred by the absence of identifiable bronchioles on biopsy material. Diagnosis of bronchiolitis obliterans by histologic examination of transbronchial biopsy material may be very difficult, however, and many do not consider it necessary to establish the diagnosis. A staging system has been established based on the degree of decline of FEV_1 or forced expiratory flow $(FEF)_{25-75}$ from the peak value: post-transplantation stage 0p = 10% (FEV_1) or 25% (FEF_{25-75}), stage 1 = 20% to 35%, stage 2 = 35% to 50% decline, and stage 3 = more than 50% decline.[63] The usual treatment for bronchiolitis

obliterans in the United States is to augment immunosuppression, usually beginning with antithymocyte globulin daily for 7 to 10 days; the clinical response has been variable. A change in the maintenance immunosuppression may also be appropriate. Antiproliferative agents may provide a more effective approach, but that has yet to be proved. Results from small studies suggest that azithromycin may be effective in stabilizing and perhaps even improving lung function.[64,65] Researchers at Duke University demonstrated that fundoplication in patients with BO and gastroesophageal reflux may potentially improve BO grade if performed early.[52] Total lymphoid irradiation and photopheresis are other modalities that have been proposed.[66] Patients not responding to these measures may be suitable candidates for retransplantation. As mentioned earlier, this is a somewhat controversial topic, because there is a shortage of donor organs, and the results with retransplantation overall are not quite as good as with first-time transplantations. However, if the candidates are ambulatory, not ventilator dependent, and at an experienced lung transplantation center, the survival results are not significantly different from first-time transplantations.[30]

Post-transplantation lymphoproliferative disease (PTLD) occurs in 10% to 19% of pediatric patients undergoing lung transplantation. PTLD occurs more frequently in association with a primary Epstein-Barr virus (EBV) infection.[67] Children may be somewhat more prone to this complication, because they are frequently seronegative for EBV infection at the time of transplantation and are therefore likely to acquire a primary EBV infection during their post-transplantation life. Reduction in immunosuppression is the mainstay of early therapy, although this may be insufficient and not uncommonly leads to the subsequent development of bronchiolitis obliterans. Rituximab, an anti-CD20 monoclonal antibody, has been used effectively in the treatment of PTLD.[60] Other treatment modalities include conventional chemotherapy,[68] irradiation, and infusion of human leukocyte antigen–matched T lymphocytes.[69]

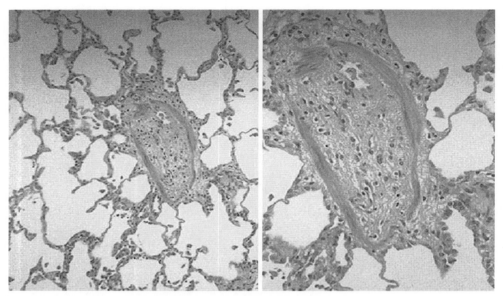

FIGURE 51-2   Histologic slide taken from the lung of a patient undergoing retransplantation for bronchiolitis obliterans. Small airways are obliterated by fibrous tissue.

INFECTION

Although infection is generally common after any solid organ transplantation, lung transplantation recipients are at greater risk. Donors are all on mechanical ventilation, resulting in colonization of the airway with bacteria from an intensive care unit. The lung is the only solid organ constantly in contact with the nonsterile outside world. An endotracheal tube necessary early after the transplantation bypasses some of the natural defenses available to the respiratory tract. Obligate denervation of the lung that occurs with transplantation results in the cough reflex being markedly diminished or absent altogether. These and numerous other factors demand that the caregivers maintain constant vigilance in the diagnosis and treatment of respiratory infections and also emphasize to the recipient the importance of pulmonary toilet.

All potential candidates are screened for the presence of organisms in the airway and evidence of previous infections. Evidence of prior viral infections is evaluated by serologic testing for antibodies to cytomegalovirus; herpes simplex virus; varicella; EBV; hepatitis A, B, and C; and human immunodeficiency virus. Viral serologic screening is less informative in young infants whose immunoglobulin pool reflects passively transferred maternal antibodies. The initial antimicrobial therapy given in the early post-transplantation period is directed in part by the results of pretransplantation studies. Ganciclovir is given at a dose of 5 mg/kg/day for 6 weeks for any positive donor or recipient serology for cytomegalovirus. If patients have evidence of present or past *Aspergillus* infection, antifungal therapy with either intravenous anidulafungin or voriconazole followed by oral voriconazole is used, depending on the clinical situation.

A number of viral respiratory infections are quite common in pediatric patients. Adenovirus and parainfluenza viruses are particularly bothersome in children. As for cytomegalovirus, primary disease is generally more likely to be severe than reactivation disease.[2] As mentioned earlier, primary infection with EBV is an important risk factor for the development of PTLD.

Fungal infections are uncommon but potentially devastating. Nystatin oral suspension is employed to reduce the risk of infection from *Candida* species. Virtually all infections caused by *Candida* species can be successfully treated with oral or intravenous triazole antifungal agents. Invasive *Aspergillus* infections, however, are much more difficult to treat and may result in widespread dissemination if appropriate antifungal therapy is delayed.

Bacterial infections are common after lung transplantation. Bacterial lower respiratory tract infections, which include both purulent bronchitis and pneumonia, occur in most patients at some point after transplantation. Patients with CF are more likely to experience this complication, with the organism usually the same as that colonizing the airway before transplantation. Prophylaxis against lower respiratory tract infections in CF lung transplantation recipients may be accomplished by administering aerosolized antibiotics (tobramycin or colistin) just as one might for end-stage CF.

OTHER COMPLICATIONS

Hypertension is a common problem after transplantation and is presumably due to treatment with the calcineurin inhibitors cyclosporine and tacrolimus, as well as prednisone. Renal insufficiency occurs with increasing time after transplantation and is also related to treatment with cyclosporine and tacrolimus. Diabetes mellitus occurs in approximately 15% of patients after transplantation, primarily in patients with CF.[2] Tacrolimus predictably increases the likelihood for the development of hyperglycemia.

Survival

The 3- and 5-year actuarial survival for children undergoing lung transplantation is approximately 54% and 45%, respectively, according to the International Society for Heart and

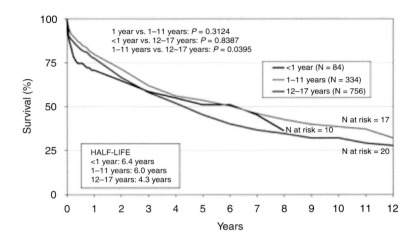

1 year vs. 1–11 years: $P = 0.3124$
<1 year vs. 12–17 years: $P = 0.8387$
1–11 years vs. 12–17 years: $P = 0.0395$

<1 year (N = 84)
1–11 years (N = 334)
12–17 years (N = 756)

N at risk = 17
N at risk = 10
N at risk = 20

HALF-LIFE
<1 year: 6.4 years
1–11 years: 6.0 years
12–17 years: 4.3 years

Survival (%)

Years

FIGURE 51-3 Kaplan-Meier survival curve for pediatric lung transplantation. (From Aurora P, Edwards LB, Kucheryavaya AY, et al: The Registry of the International Society for Heart and Lung Transplantation: Thirteenth Official Pediatric Lung and Heart/Lung Transplantation Report—2010. J Heart Lung Transplant 2010;29:1129-1141.)

Lung Transplantation registry (Fig. 51-3).[3] Acute graft failure accounts for the majority of deaths in the first 30 days. Infection is the cause of death in approximately 50% of those dying in the first year beyond the transplantation hospitalization. Bronchiolitis obliterans is the cause of death in 50% of patients beyond 1 year after transplantation and is clearly the major impediment to long-term survival.[30]

Pulmonary Function and Growth

It is unclear whether transplanted lungs grow in terms of number and size of alveoli, and experimental data are inconclusive.[70,71] Measurement of lung growth is fraught with a number of complicating factors. One cannot use pulmonary function tests and lung volume size as measured by either chest radiograph or computed tomography, because there are a number of elements that affect these studies that would not accurately reflect the number or size of alveoli. The impact of lung growth is particularly critical in small infants, because their transplanted lungs will have to grow substantially over the rest of their lives to handle the physiologic load presented to them. Those children in our series too young to undergo standard pulmonary function testing underwent infant pulmonary function tests that provide a measurement of functional residual capacity, a reasonable surrogate for lung volume. The average functional residual capacity per centimeter in height at 3 months after transplantation was 2.3 mL/cm and remained between 2.1 and 2.8 mL/cm through 15 months after transplantation. During this time, substantial somatic growth occurred in these infants.[72] Thus in the absence of central or peripheral airway obstruction, these data suggest that lung growth appropriate for size is occurring. However, we do not

know whether this represents an increase in the number of alveoli and/or an increase in the size of existing alveoli.

Future Considerations

Factors that limit the success of lung transplantation in children are similar to those in adults: donor shortage, balance of immunosuppression and prevention of infection, and development of bronchiolitis obliterans. Xenotransplantation may eventually offer another solution, but realistically, this is many years from application. Transplantation across ABO blood groups, now commonplace in infant cardiac transplantation, is another possibility in small children, though the overall impact of this would be minor. Newer immunosuppressive agents aimed at more specific areas of the immune response involved with organ recognition are necessary. Bronchiolitis obliterans remains the "Achilles heel" of long-term survival after lung transplantation. Although still not completely characterized as to its precise cause, most investigators ascribe this development to airway injury leading to chronic rejection. To that end, clinical and basic research aimed at understanding the vectors of injury and disease progression in bronchiolitis obliterans are of paramount importance to the field of lung transplantation. Because the airway as the site of injury is accessible for assessment and therapy, bronchiolitis obliterans may provide a model system whereby chronic rejection, which also affects long-term success in heart, kidney, and liver transplantation, can be understood and overcome.

The complete reference list is available online at www.expertconsult.com.

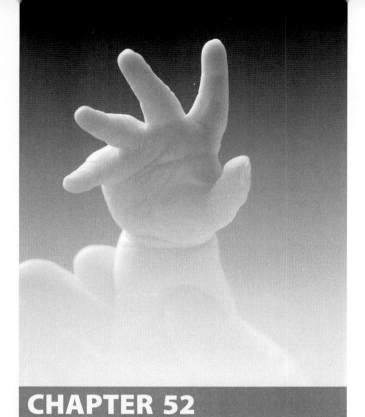

CHAPTER 52

Surgical Implications Associated with Pediatric Bone Marrow Transplantation

Thomas E. Hamilton and Robert C. Shamberger

Fifty-three years after the seminal report of hematopoietic stem cell transplantation (HSCT) in children and adolescents by Thomas and colleagues,[1] pediatric surgeons have retained an important role in successful implementation of this therapy. The expansion of HSCT to a variety of malignant and nonmalignant diseases has grown based on successful use of multiple stem cell sources and innovative conditioning regimens.[2] A fundamental understanding of these processes will assist pediatric surgeons when called upon for access or complications associated with patients undergoing HSCT.

Stem cells can be derived primarily from bone marrow, umbilical cord blood, or peripheral blood stem cells (PBSC). Along with advances in infection prophylaxis and supportive care, the switch to PBSC has led to mortality rates of less than 5% for autologous transplantation in many studies. One of the major advances of PBSC compared with autologous marrow is more rapid engraftment of the recipient. Faster hematopoietic recovery results in an abbreviated period of neutropenia, thrombocytopenia, and anemia, resulting in lower rates of infection and hemorrhage, less risk of transfusions, and earlier discharge. Harvest and storage of a patient's own hematopoietic stem cells (HSC), followed by reinfusion after high-dose chemotherapy (HDC), is commonly referred to as autologous HSCT or stem cell rescue. HDC is generally administered beyond the tolerance of the patient's marrow (myeloablative), meaning no recovery is possible without stored HSC.[3]

The transplantation process is divided into five phases: (1) conditioning, (2) stem cell infusion, (3) neutropenia, (4) engraftment, and (5) postengraftment phase. The conditioning phase involves intensive chemotherapy with or without total body irradiation to eliminate the disease. This period lasts between 7 and 10 days. The stem cell processing and infusion time varies based upon the size of the patient and source of the stem cells. The neutropenic phase lasts 2 to 4 weeks and is an interval when the patient is extremely vulnerable to infections because of the lack of an effective immune system. Wound healing is impaired, and empiric antibiotics are generally administered to minimize infectious complications. Mucus membranes are rapidly dividing tissues, and therefore susceptible to ulceration and the risk for nosocomial infections is high. Total parenteral nutrition is widely used in children during this phase.

The engraftment phase takes several weeks as transplanted cells incorporate into recipient tissues. The development of graft versus host disease (GVHD) and viral infections are the greatest clinical obstacles of this phase. The postengraftment phase lasts months to years as the gradual development of tolerance, weaning of immunosuppression, and immune reconstitution occur.[4] Pediatric surgeons are consulted frequently for access or associated complications in all phases of the transplantation process.

Stem Cell Harvest and Vascular Access

Multiple ports of access are required for peripheral stem cell harvest. Unlike adults, where large-bore antecubital catheters can be used for both harvest and infusion, pediatric patients generally require indwelling central venous catheters. The extracorporeal separation of blood components from patients or donors has spawned an entire field termed apheresis. As technologies of separation evolve, the one constant is the need for adequate access to withdraw and return blood components. Standard Broviac catheters collapse with the negative pressure required for apheresis (approximately 1 to 2 mL/kg/minute). Specially designed apheresis catheters allow faster flow rates because of larger-diameter stiffer walls and shorter catheter length. Most apheresis catheters are dual lumen offset with multiple ports to avoid mixing processed and unprocessed blood. Children weighing more than 10 kg will accommodate 8-Fr or larger (MedComp, Harleysville, Pa.) catheters. When children weigh less than 10 kg, temporary femoral or subclavian catheters may be used.[3] Because of the larger size and stiffness of the apheresis catheters and dilators, fluoroscopic guidance and respect for tissue is paramount. As one of my surgical mentors always said, "placing the line in is never as interesting to the surgeon as taking out the tumor, but it is just as important to the care of the child."

Complications of Immune System Ablation and Immunosuppression

INTESTINAL COMPLICATIONS

Abdominal pain and diarrhea are common post-HSCT. A substantial component of the initial inflammatory cascade is thought to occur in the gastrointestinal tract, and patients with higher volumes of diarrhea at the time of the preparative regimen have an increased risk of acute GVHD.[5] Barker and associates[6] performed a retrospective study of 132 consecutive pediatric HSCT patients, and diarrhea occurred in 67% of patients. Common etiologic agents included GVHD (27%), viral (6%), *Clostridium difficile* (8%), and unknown (28%). When stool cultures are negative, endoscopy is considered to differentiate infectious etiologies from GVHD. Gastric antral biopsies and small bowel biopsies may be preferred, because duodenal hematomas have been reported by Ramakrishna and Treem.[7] They recommended avoiding the duodenum if possible and maintaining platelet counts greater than 55,000/mm[3] for 48 hours postbiopsy when a duodenal biopsy is necessary. A prospective multicenter study of pediatric bone marrow transplantation (BMT) patients who underwent 1120 small bowel biopsies did not report hematoma as a complication.[8,9] Silbermintz and co-workers[10] reported successful identification of small bowel graft versus host disease by capsule endoscopy in a child with refractory hemorrhage, when upper and lower endoscopies were nondiagnostic. Identification of small intestinal cytomegalovirus (CMV) disease has also been reported by capsule endoscopy.[11] The future role for capsule endoscopy is increasing as the intestinal complications after HSCT predominate in the small intestine.[12] Accurate visualization may help guide the need for more intensive immunosuppressive therapy or to avoid immunosuppressive therapy.

Neutropenic enterocolitis (typhlitis) is characterized by necrotizing inflammation of the colon in a severely immunocompromised patient (Table 52-1). Clinically, fever, abdominal pain, tenderness, and neutropenia are present (Fig. 52-1). The incidence is low in children after HSCT. Barker's retrospective review of 132 consecutive pediatric HSCT patients reported an incidence of 3.5%.[6] Early experience with neutropenic enterocolitis was marked by controversy regarding the timing of surgical intervention, and mortality exceeded 50%.[13–16] Delineation of the criteria for surgical intervention reserved for clearly identified surgical complications has contributed to a substantial decrease in mortality and morbidity.[15,17]

Multiple contemporary series now report excellent outcomes using a strategy of bowel rest, prompt institution of appropriate intravenous fluid resuscitation, broad-spectrum antibiotics and antifungal therapy, nutritional support with total parenteral nutrition (TPN), and the use of granulocyte

TABLE 52-1
Neutropenic Enterocolitis: Criteria for Appropriate Surgical Intervention
1. Persistent gastrointestinal bleeding after resolution of neutropenia and thrombocytopenia and correction of clotting abnormalities
2. Evidence of free intraperitoneal perforation
3. Clinical deterioration requiring support with vasopressors or large volumes of fluid, suggesting uncontrolled sepsis
4. Development of symptoms of an intra-abdominal process, in the absence of neutropenia, which would normally require surgery

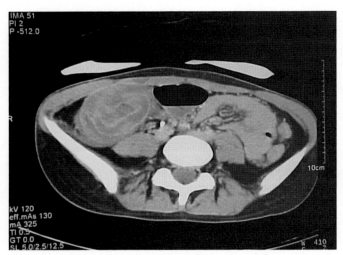

FIGURE 52-1 Typhlitis in a teenager with acute myelocytic leukemia who had undergone bone marrow transplantation (BMT). Note the thickened, onionskin appearance of the cecal wall and the pinpoint lumen. This patient underwent right hemicolectomy with ileostomy and mucous fistula; 1 year later, still in clinical remission from her leukemia, her condition was successfully reversed. Most cases of typhlitis are handled nonoperatively.

colony-stimulating factor (GCSF).[18–21] In 2002, Otaibi reported a series of 142 HSCT transplantations performed in Alberta Children's Hospital. Ninety-seven patients developed abdominal pain, and only five developed radiographically proven typhlitis. No patients required surgical intervention.[20] Mullassery, from The Royal Liverpool Children's Hospital reported a 5-year retrospective series in 2009 in which 18 of 596 patients had radiographically confirmed typhlitis and three required surgical intervention. One child, each, had extensive colonic necrosis, perforated gastric ulcer, and perforated appendix. A single mortality was also reported from fulminant gram-negative sepsis without intervention.[19]

HEPATOBILIARY COMPLICATIONS

Abnormal liver function studies are commonly identified in HSCT patients. An extensive 40-year review of hepatobiliary complications in HSCT has recently been published by McDonald.[22] Liver complications have become far less frequent as the understanding of how to prevent and treat severe hepatobiliary problems has emerged. Surgeons are frequently consulted to discern whether abnormal liver function studies are secondary to obstruction or parenchymal dysfunction. Biliary obstruction occurs secondary to calculous disease.

Safford and colleagues[23] reported a series of 575 patients, of which 235 received ultrasonography of the abdomen for pain, jaundice, sepsis, or metastases. Cholelithiasis was identified in 20 cases (8.5%). The overall incidence of cholelithiasis reported in the study was far greater than the 0.13% to 0.21%. incidence in children.[24] When the reason for HSCT was considered in Safford's series, 27% of patients who had HSCT for bone marrow failure versus 7.4% for neoplasia developed cholelithiasis ($P < 0.01$). This suggests a role for hemolysis. Despite the high incidence of cholelithiasis, 85% of children did not require surgical intervention. Nine (45%) died from primary disease, five (25%) showed sonographic resolution, and three (15%) had nonoperative follow-up for persistent cholelithiasis. Surgical interventions included one cholecystostomy, one open cholecystectomy, and one laparoscopic cholecystectomy in three (15%) patients who developed acute cholecystitis, with a mean time to operative intervention of 1.9 years without complication. There was no morbidity or mortality associated with conservative management of cholelithiasis in any child.[23]

Hepatic veno-occlusive disease (VOD), also known as sinusoidal obstruction syndrome (SOS) is a serious and frequent complication after HSCT. It is clinically heralded by a triad of (1) painful hepatomegaly, (2) hyperbilirubinemia, and (3) unexplained fluid retention. Milder cases resolve spontaneously, but severe cases may become rapidly fatal. Prognosis varies with extent of injury and the development of multiorgan system failure.[25] The pathogenesis involves sinusoidal endothelial cell and hepatocyte damage from high-dose alkylating chemotherapeutic agents.[22,25] Plasminogen activator inhibitor (PAI-1) serum levels have both diagnostic and prognostic value as a marker for VOD.[26] The intensity of the conditioning regimen and type of transplantation are important determinants for risk of VOD. Pediatric patients younger than 6.5 years at transplantation appear to be at increased risk of hepatic VOD.[27] Defibrotide (DF) is a polydisperse mixture of single-stranded oligonucleotide with local antithrombotic, anti-ischemic, and anti-inflammatory activity that has clinical efficacy in severe VOD. DF appears to modulate endothelial cell injury without enhancing systemic bleeding and protects the hepatic sinusoids without compromising the antitumor cytotoxic effects of therapy.[28] Ho and associates[25] reviewed hepatic VOD and multiple clinical trials with DF, where 30% to 60% complete remission rates are reported, even in patients with severe VOD and multiorgan system failure. Corbacioglu and colleagues[29] reported that 34 (76%) patients with severe VOD post-HSCT, treated with DF, achieved a complete response, and in multivariate analysis, early intervention (1 day vs. 5.5 days in nonresponders) was the only significant factor. Richardson and coworkers[30] recently reported a phase II multicenter randomized trial in adult and pediatric patients that established the safety and efficacy of defibrotide. Early stabilization or decreased bilirubin was associated with better response and day +100 post-HSCT survival, and decreased plasminogen activator inhibitor type 1 (PAI-1) during treatment was associated with better outcome; changes were similar in both treatment arms. A dosage of 25 mg/kg/day was selected for ongoing phase III trials of the treatment of VOD.

Focal nodular hyperplasia following pediatric HSCT has been identified in 17 of 137 patients prospectively studied, with a median delay of 6.4 years from a series reported by Sudour and associates.[31] The authors postulate an iatrogenic vascular origin, because 16 patients received myeloablative preconditioning, and only three had evidence of SOS. No complication or malignant transformation was reported; clinical and diagnostic imaging follow-up is recommended.

HEMORRHAGIC CYSTITIS

Hemorrhagic cystitis (HC) occurs in 10% to 20% of pediatric HSCT patients. Decker and colleagues[32] have recently reviewed the pediatric experience. HC is characterized by diffuse vesical bleeding which ranges from microscopic hematuria to gross hemorrhage with clot formation and urinary obstruction requiring instrumentation for evacuation. With severe HC, prolonged hospitalization with significant morbidity may occur. High-dose chemotherapy and immunosuppression that accompany HSCT make the pediatric patient particularly susceptible. Investigations point to a multifactorial pathophysiology of HC. Damage to the transitional epithelium by radiation, chemotherapy, and infectious agents have been postulated. BK virus is now a known pathogen with increasing evidence for a major role in HC. High-dose cyclophosphamide and bisulfan are well studied alkylating agents used in conditioning protocols for HSCT that are known to cause HC. Three main strategies for HC prophylaxis include mesna, hyperhydration with forced diuresis, and continuous bladder irrigation (CBI). Three-way catheter drainage is often difficult in pediatric populations and may require a suprapubic tube. Ultrasonography may underestimate the clot burden, and cystoscopy provides visualization with the opportunity for clot evacuation and fulguration of the bladder epithelium. Escalation to more intensive therapies, such as instillation of drugs into the bladder (intravesical therapy), carry increased risk. Many agents, including aluminum potassium sulfate, prostaglandins, and ε-aminocaproic acid and cidofovir have been used for intravesical therapy, but none are well studied in a pediatric population. HC is a self-limiting condition once engraftment and immune reconstitution occur, effective defense barriers of the bladder mucosa are reconstituted, and viral replication is controlled. More intensive therapies should be undertaken under the auspices of a multidisciplinary team.[33]

PULMONARY COMPLICATIONS

Opportunistic infections are common in HSCT patients. Pneumonia is the most common infectious complication but must be distinguished from noninfectious causes, such as bronchiolitis obliterans, diffuse alveolar hemorrhage (DAH), and a constellation of noninfectious fever accompanied by either skin rash, pulmonary infiltrates, or diarrhea—termed engraftment syndrome.[34] Early recognition and treatment of post-HSCT pneumonia favorably impacts survival.[35,36] A recent article from Shannon and co-workers[37] from M.D. Anderson Cancer Center has examined the utility of early versus late fiberoptic bronchoscopy (FOB) with bronchoalveolar lavage (BAL) post-HSCT in 501 consecutive adult patients. Five hundred and ninety-eight fiberoptic bronchoscopies (FOB) with bronchoalveolar lavage (BAL) were performed for the evaluation of pulmonary infiltrates. The overall diagnostic yield was 55%. The diagnostic yield was 2.5-fold higher when the FOB was performed within the first 4 days and highest (75%) when performed within 24 hours of clinical presentation. The rates of adjustment in antimicrobial therapy were not different with early versus late treatment (51%); however, late FOB-guided antibiotic adjustments were associated with 30-day pulmonary-associated deaths that were threefold higher (6% vs. 18%, P = 0.035). The authors conclude early referral for FOB may yield a higher diagnostic yield and favorably impact survival in adult patients.

The utility of lung biopsy in pediatric patients post-HSCT is controversial. Shorter and colleagues[38] reported a 10-year experience of 126 HSCT patients from Children's Hospital of Philadelphia from 1976 to 1986. Twenty-one patients had open lung biopsies; 14 showed no causative organisms. One patient had CMV, and three patients had *Pneumocystis carinii*. Thirteen patients died because of continued deterioration postbiopsy. Hayes-Jordan and associates[39] reported a retrospective series of 528 patients post-HSCT from St. Jude's Children's Research Center from 1991 to 1998. Eighty-three patients developed pulmonary infiltrate within 6 months; 43 (52%) had BAL and 19 (23%) had open lung biopsies, 6 (7%) underwent needle biopsy, and 5 (7%) underwent transbronchial biopsy. Histology identified infections in 6 (30%), bronchiolitis obliterans organizing pneumonia (BOOP) in 5 (26%), interstitial pneumonia in 4 (21%), gangliosidosis in 1, and lymphocytic infiltrate in 1. Despite changing the clinical plan, based on histology in 17 of 19 (90%) patients, improvement in outcome was only seen in 8 (47%). Postoperative morbidity at 30 days was 47%, including prolonged intubation (7 patients), pneumothorax (2 patients), and pleural effusion (1 patient). Thirty-day survival was 63.2%, and no patient with multiorgan system failure, ventilator dependence, or postoperative complication survived post–open lung biopsy. Careful patient selection and consideration of less-invasive modalities should be strongly considered in these extremely high-risk patients. Minimally invasive surgical techniques have been applied both diagnostically and therapeutically in childhood cancer;[40] however, the decrease in pulmonary compliance and increase in cardiac afterload is often prohibitive for thoracoscopic techniques in the post-HSCT patient population.

Invasive pulmonary aspergillosis (IPA) is a common infection in the HSCT population. A potentially lethal complication of HSCT is pulmonary hemorrhage secondary to the angioinvasive nature of this agent. IPA is one specific opportunistic infection where surgical therapy remains beneficial. Gow and colleagues[41] reported on 43 patients with invasive pulmonary aspergillosis, spanning 9 years, from St. Jude's Children's Cancer Research Hospital. Eighteen patients had surgical intervention, (16 thoracotomies [89%] and 2 thoracoscopies). Fourteen had one operation; 4 patients had two. Surgical resection of the affected parenchyma significantly improved survival (P < 0.001). The four survivors had disease amenable to wedge resection, the longest interval at the time of report being 43.5 months. When feasible, a surgical approach should be strongly considered, because, left untreated, invasive pulmonary aspergillosis is almost always fatal.

SOFT TISSUE INFECTIONS

Necrotizing soft tissue infections are rapidly progressive and carry a significant mortality and morbidity without prompt surgical intervention. Neutropenia makes the clinical picture even more challenging. As opposed to the otherwise healthy child, who typically has a solitary organism after a traumatic event, immunocompromised patients may have enteric translocation of gram-negative organisms. Extreme pain (often out of proportion to physical findings), fever, and tachycardia are the hallmarks of soft tissue infection. Johnston and colleagues[42] presented a retrospective series over an 11-year period, where seven neutropenic patients with deep soft tissue infections were identified. The median number of days postinitiation of chemotherapy was 14, pain was present in all patients, and 86% had fever and tachycardia. The pathogenic organism was from the gastrointestinal tract in four of seven patients. Five patients survived and were treated with urgent surgical debridement, intravenous antibiotics, GCSF, and hyperbaric oxygen. Butterworth and associates[43] reported an 11-year retrospective series of 19 patients with necrotizing soft tissue infections in healthy and immunocompromised children. An interesting finding in this series was that the immunocompromised patients were less likely to have severe tenderness and more likely to have polymicrobial perineal/buttock infections. When diagnostic uncertainty exists, judicious use of magnetic resonance imaging (MRI) may prove beneficial if tolerated by the patient's clinical status.

Post-transplantation Malignancies

As survival increases post-HSCT, attention has become directed toward late effects, including post-tranplant malignancies (PTMs). New malignancies post-HSCT fall into three broad categories: post-tranplant lymphoproliferative disorders (PTLD), hematologic malignancies (primarily treatment-related myelodysplastic syndrome and acute myeloid leukemia [MDS/AML]) and solid tumors. Baker and co-workers,[44] from the University of Minnesota, reported 147 PTMs in 137 pediatric and adult patients of 3,372 patients post–stem cell transplantation. The majority of PTMs were PTLD (44), with MDS/AML in 36 patients. Sixty-two solid tumors were reported in 57 patients. A significant finding was the risk of solid tumor malignancy continues to increase with each successive year of follow-up. The cumulative incidence of developing a solid tumor did not plateau and was 3.8% (95% confidence interval [CI], 2.2 to 5.4) at 20 years post-HSCT. The most common solid tumors reported were 11 basal cell and 8 squamous cell carcinomas of the skin, 4 breast, 5 carcinoma in situ, 8 melanoma, and 4 soft tissue sarcomas. Age greater than or equal to 20 years at the time of HSCT was the only significant predictor for development of a solid tumor (relative risk [RR] 2.0; 95% CI, 1.1 to 3.5; P = 0.03).[44] Forty-two percent of patients died from their post-transplantation solid tumor. Future efforts at long-term surveillance are warranted.

Conclusion

HSCT has evolved into a well-established clinical modality with increasing utility for multiple malignant and nonmalignant disease processes in children. Pediatric general surgeons are integral members of the multidisciplinary team required for HSCT because of the multitude of organ systems involved.

Pulmonary, gastrointestinal, hepatic, genitourinary, and soft tissues are all subject to surgical complications. Vascular access will continue to be required for medications, apheresis, and transfusions. Pediatric surgeons must have knowledge of the HSCT process and the surgical complications during all phases of transplantation, including long-term survivors, in order to provide expert advice for treatment and to contribute to the understanding of this rapidly expanding field.

The complete reference list is available online at www.expertconsult.com.

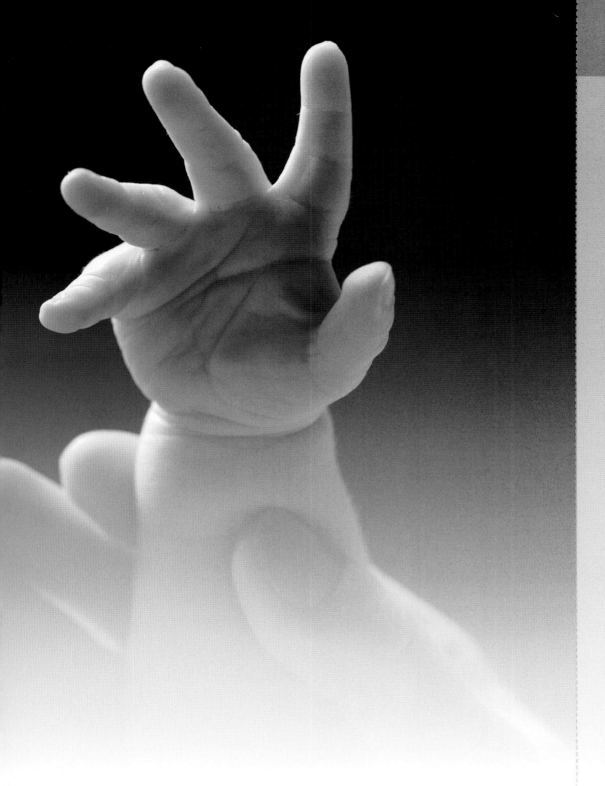

Part V

HEAD AND NECK

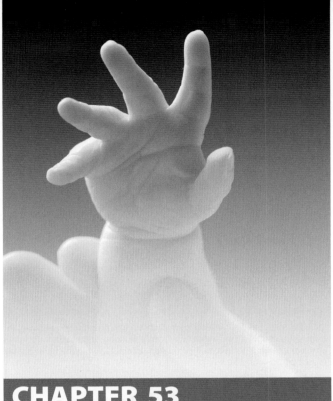

CHAPTER 53

Craniofacial Anomalies

Jason J. Hall and H. Peter Lorenz

In 1967, Dr. Paul Tessier presented his modifications of Gilles' previously little known and underutilized techniques to correct congenital or post-traumatic bony anomalies to the International Society of Plastic Surgeons in Rome. Over the next 30 years, his teachings formed the basis of a new subspecialty of plastic surgery—craniofacial surgery. Tessier developed precisely placed osteotomies, autologous nonvascularized bone and soft tissue grafts, and intracranial approaches to the facial skeleton. His techniques gave children and adults with previously "unfixable" craniofacial anomalies a chance for a more normal appearance. Currently, most major medical centers have a multidisciplinary team dedicated to the care of this special subset of patients. The craniofacial anomaly teams span many different specialties, which include plastic surgery, pediatric otolaryngology, pediatric neurosurgery, speech pathology, audiology, oral surgery, dentistry and orthodontics, social work, pediatrics, and genetics.

Fortunately, many of the anomalies discussed in this chapter are relatively rare, but for surgeons in a pediatric tertiary care center, these patients are seen as daily occurrences. This chapter is not meant as a definitive tome on the diagnosis and treatment of these disorders, but is meant to paint a picture of the spectrum of craniofacial anomalies with broad brushstrokes.

The first two sections discuss two of the more common skeletal anomalies treated by craniofacial surgeons: craniosynostosis and jaw anomalies that require orthognathic surgical correction. The final section deals with facial asymmetry and hypoplasia disorders that are rare and complex to treat.

The Craniosynostoses

Craniosynostosis refers to the premature closure of one or more cranial sutures and encompasses a wide range of anatomic derangements. Isolated, premature fusion of a single suture causes a predictable cranial deformity that can typically be recognized without the need for radiologic imaging by an experienced practitioner. However, complex craniosynostosis, consisting of multiple suture fusions, can be difficult to diagnose without radiologic imaging. Despite the wide range of clinical presentation, treatment for craniosynostosis cases is similar to any other surgical problem in children: accurate diagnosis, appropriate treatment planning, proper timing of surgery with respect to current and future growth, and surgical technique that gives a predictable correction and minimizes adverse long-term sequelae.

ETIOLOGY AND PATHOLOGIC ANATOMY

The infant skull undergoes a period of rapid expansion during the first year of life, which is driven by brain growth. Bone growth at patent cranial sutures causes calvarial expansion in a distinct morphologic pattern. Typically, suture fusion occurs from anterior to posterior and lateral to medial.[1] The metopic suture, which normally closes by 8 to 9 months of age, is the only suture to close completely during infancy; the remaining sutures do not completely fuse until adulthood. Most patients presenting with craniosynostosis have prenatal onset of suture fusion. However, in severe cases of syndromic craniosynostosis, progressive, multiple suture fusion can occur over the first 3 to 4 years of life.[2] In this situation, the calvarial deformity is typically not detected at birth except when quite severe. After a few months of rapid growth, the deformity typically becomes more apparent.

In 1851, Virchow published his landmark paper that laid the foundation for our understanding of craniofacial deformities associated with craniosynostosis. He described the growth pattern of the skull as being restricted in a plane perpendicular to the fused suture while being amplified in a plane parallel to the direction of the suture. This compensatory growth pattern causes predictable deformities in patients with single suture synostosis. The growth constriction, however, is not confined to the cranial vault, but also affects the cranial base to varying degrees. Moss proposed that the cranial base pathology was the inciting event, and that the calvarial fusion occurred as a secondary phenomenon.[3] However, cranial base anomalies are not corrected by calvarial vault surgery and are now not thought to be the inciting event.

Recent research has focused on the role of the dura and its influence on suture patency in the growing skull. A number of dural-related cytokines, such as heparin-binding factor, fibroblast growth factors (FGFs), bone morphogenic proteins (BMPs), transforming growth factor(s)-β (TGF(s)-β), and transcription factors Msx2 and TWIST, have a role in the regulation and coordination of suture patency.[4] A mutation of the *TWIST* gene on chromosome 7p21 has been linked with Saethre-Chotzen syndrome.[5,4] FGF receptor mutations causing constitutive activation of the receptor occur in many of the human craniosynostosis syndromes, including Apert, Crouzon, Muenke, and Pfeiffer syndromes.[4] Interestingly, one mechanism of bony fusion across the suture occurring with the *FGF-R* mutation is the loss of Noggin expression in the involved suture mesenchyme. Noggin is a BMP-inhibitor that prevents bony fusion in the mesenchyme. When Noggin is not present, bone forms across the mesenchyme, and the suture fuses.[6] Most incidences of craniosynostosis are the result of sporadic genetic anomalies. Yet, a number of both autosomal dominant and autosomal recessive syndromes, whose most striking phenotype is the pattern of craniosynostosis, are known. Patients with a family history of craniosynostosis should thus be referred to a dedicated craniofacial team and be evaluated by a skilled geneticist, as new genetic mutations linked to the craniosynostosis syndromes are being discovered frequently.

The treatment for craniosynostosis is surgical calvarial vault remodeling, which is performed to avoid future adverse sequelae. Chief among these is the avoidance of intracranial hypertension, which has been linked to brain damage, optic nerve compression, and cognitive impairment.[7] Early surgical correction (between 3 to 6 months of age) has the advantages of prevention of elevated intracranial pressure and its attendant consequences, improved reossification of calvarial bone defects, and the need for a less extensive surgical correction. Correction at a more advanced age (6 to 9 months) is reported to have more stable long-term results and lower rates of reoperation. These factors are taken into account by the craniofacial surgeon and pediatric neurosurgeon during the treatment planning process.

Common Patterns of Single Suture Craniosynostosis

The most common form of craniosynostosis is sagittal synostosis, with an incidence of approximately 2 per 10,000 live births. In concordance with Virchow's law, premature fusion of the sagittal suture leads to compensatory growth in the anteroposterior dimension, resulting in *scaphocephaly* (Fig. 53-1).

Unilateral coronal synostosis is less common, with an incidence of approximately 0.9 per 10,000 live births. The growth pattern in unicoronal synostosis is more complex, albeit leading to a stereotypical calvarial phenotype. Ipsilateral to the fused coronal suture, the supraorbital rim is flattened and recessed, and the forehead is flattened. As calvarial growth occurs, the contralateral forehead becomes bossed and the nasal bridge starts to twist, producing a C-shaped facial deformity (Fig. 53-2).

Premature fusion of the metopic suture results in constriction of growth in an axial plane centered on the caudal forehead. A palpable bony ridge is present in the midline of the forehead (described as a "keel-shaped forehead" or *trigonocephaly*). The forehead is narrow and pointed. The medial orbital rims are consequently closer to the midline, giving the appearance of hypotelorism. Bilateral lateral brow recession and temporal hollowing also occurs and exaggerates this appearance.

The least common form of single suture craniosynostosis affects the lambdoid suture. Common findings are posterior

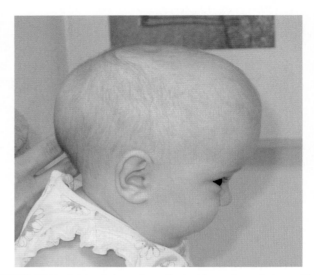

FIGURE 53-1 A lateral view of a patient with scaphocephaly resulting from sagittal synostosis. Note the frontal bossing, elongation along the anteroposterior (AP) axis, and prominent occiput, all of which are characteristic of this condition.

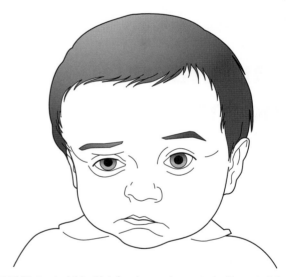

FIGURE 53-2 A child with left unicoronal synostosis. Characteristic findings include ipsilateral fronto-orbital retrusion, prominent contralateral forehead bossing, and nasal root deviation toward the affected side. The C-shaped facial deformity is notable here.

plagiocephaly, ipsilateral mastoid bossing, and both anterior and inferior ipsilateral ear displacement. A posterior skull base cant and contralateral forehead bossing occur in more advanced cases.

Multiple suture craniosynostoses are rare, and may present with a variety of skull-shaped deformities.

Syndromic Craniosynostosis

Children born with craniofacial dysostosis syndromes require multiple staged procedures to correct their bony deformities during their childhood years and extending into early adulthood. These patients have a higher relapse rate because multiple affected midface and skull base sutures are usually present. The syndromic craniosynostoses carry a greater risk of intracranial hypertension, as well.

Many of the craniofacial dysostosis syndromes are inherited in an autosomal dominant pattern and are the result of mutations in the *FGF*-receptor genes, which alter the signaling pathway. Although penetrance is complete in most syndromes, the expression of the mutation is highly variable. Examples of these include Crouzon, Apert, and Pfeiffer syndromes, the three most common craniofacial dysostosis syndromes, all of which have mutations in the *FGF*-receptor genes.

Crouzon syndrome is the most common syndromic craniofacial dysostosis, with an estimated incidence of 1 in 25,000 live births.[8] Crouzon syndrome is caused by a mutation in the *FGFR2* gene, causing increased receptor activation.[9] The syndrome is characterized by the triad of bicoronal craniosynostosis, exorbitism, and midface retrusion (Fig. 53-3). Exorbitism is the feature of this syndrome, which results in prominent globes. As such, ocular protection is a key feature the clinician must keep in mind when assessing these children. Exposure keratitis and conjunctivitis may prompt earlier surgical intervention to avoid permanent visual impairment.

Apert syndrome has an incidence of 1 per 160,000 live births and is also caused by an *FGFR2* mutation.[10] Unlike Crouzon syndrome, the genetic defect in Apert syndrome is a missense mutation, and the vast majority of Apert patients are the result of a sporadic mutation. The triad of bicoronal craniosynostosis, midface hypoplasia, and syndactyly of the hands and feet characterize Apert syndrome. The craniofacial findings include bicoronal suture fusion, a large anterior fontanelle, midface retrusion, and varying degrees of exorbitism.

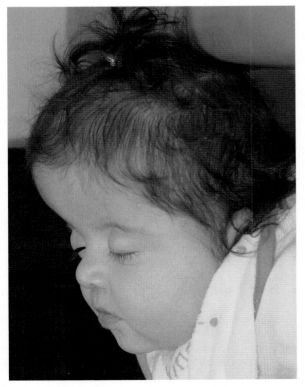

FIGURE 53-3   Brachycephaly, exorbitism, and midface retrusion, which are common findings in both Apert and Crouzon syndromes.

Neonatal respiratory distress from a narrowed nasal vault, sometimes severe enough to warrant tracheostomy, may occasionally occur.[11] A specialist in congenital hand anomalies typically addresses complex syndactyly of the hands and feet. Unlike Crouzon syndrome, mental retardation is common, and affects nearly 50% of children with Apert syndrome.

Other craniofacial dysostosis syndromes include Pfeiffer syndrome, Saethre-Chotzen syndrome, and Carpenter syndrome. These are much less common than either Crouzon or Apert syndrome and share varying degrees of craniosynostosis, midface retrusion, digital anomalies, and mental retardation. Management priorities in these children are similar to that of children with either of the previously mentioned syndromes.

DIAGNOSIS

A thorough history and physical examination is the cornerstone of diagnosing synostosis of the calvarial sutures. Single suture fusion results in the characteristic patterns of calvarial morphology described previously and are readily diagnosed by physical examination.

Measurement of head circumference with plotting on a standard growth curve gives an indication of head growth relative to the child's body. Physical examination should accurately define asymmetries in the infant skull. Head shape should be assessed from anterior, posterior, and top-down views to identify areas of relative bossing or recession. Ear position in both anterior-posterior and craniocaudal planes should be examined. Lateral examination of the forehead and face will identify forehead bossing and the position of the midface and orbits. Facial examination is especially important in identifying children with the craniofacial syndromes that have midface retrusion as part of their phenotype. Stigmata of intracranial hypertension should be investigated. For infants, these include a history of irritability, "burrowing" behavior, or repetitive head slapping.

Since the advent in the early 1990s of the American Academy of Pediatrics "Back to Sleep" campaign, designed to decrease the incidence of sudden infant death syndrome (SIDS), a sharp increase in the incidence of *positional plagiocephaly* has occurred. Positional plagiocephaly is the deformation of the calvarium despite the presence of widely patent cranial sutures. This condition may be difficult to differentiate from unilateral coronal or lambdoid craniosynostosis, which both result in forms of plagiocephaly. Usually, an experienced craniofacial surgeon can make the correct diagnosis based on physical examination findings alone. However, sometimes computed tomography (CT) imaging is needed. The correct diagnosis is critical, however, because children with positional plagiocephaly are treated with changes in sleeping position or, in more severe cases, a custom orthotic molding helmet.

Children who are suspected of having craniosynostosis should be referred to a craniofacial team for evaluation. This evaluation includes detailed cranial measurements and a thorough physical examination. CT scanning is rarely needed for diagnosis, but is obtained by many craniofacial surgeons prior to calvarial vault remodeling to assess for intracranial abnormalities. Given the additional cost, risks of sedation, and potential harmful effects of ionizing radiation on the growing child, radiologic imaging should be undertaken on a case-by-case basis as determined by the craniofacial surgeon.[12]

In addition to findings of suture fusion, stigmata of intracranial hypertension, such as a "moth-eaten" appearance of the calvarium on CT images or a "copper-beaten" appearance on plain radiographs will be seen. Papilledema may be seen on fundoscopic examination and is an indication for urgent cranial vault expansion.

TREATMENT

The mainstay of treatment for premature fusion of cranial sutures is surgical cranial vault remodeling. The two goals of surgery are to release the involved suture through resection and reconstruction of the cranial vault to a more normal shape. Surgery is a combined procedure between a craniofacial plastic surgeon and a pediatric neurosurgeon. In general, the pediatric neurosurgeon performs the initial craniotomy, and the craniofacial surgeon performs the bony reshaping. However, the procedure is mainly "bone surgery" and not "brain surgery." Cranial vault remodeling is accomplished by removing the abnormally shaped calvarial bones and recontouring them. The plasticity of the infant calvarium is utilized as the bones are bent and shaped to a more anatomic contour. Barrel stave osteotomies are commonly performed to expand the cranial vault. Wedge osteotomies are done to reduce the vault in areas of bony excess or bossing. Except in cases of isolated sagittal or lambdoid synostosis, the orbits are deformed, which necessitates advancement of the supraorbital rim in addition to reshaping of the forehead and anterior cranial vault. Bones are fixed into their new position with resorbable hardware consisting of polyglactic/polyglycolic acid plates and screws. This type of hardware undergoes degradation over the course of a year, and is not prone to intracranial migration, which can occur with traditional titanium hardware. After initial reconstruction in infants, bony defects remain after surgery. The unique osteogenic potential of the dura and overlying periosteum in infants results in primary bone formation and complete healing of these large bone defects. Bone defects that remain after 2 years of age typically require secondary bone grafting. Endoscopic techniques have been described for correction of both sagittal and coronal synostosis.[13,14] Although resection of the involved suture is performed, these techniques rely on a long period of postoperative molding helmet therapy to achieve final head shape. Despite their reported benefit of reduced blood loss and transfusion requirements, endoscopic techniques have not gained wide acceptance, primarily due to their poor head shape outcomes.

Timing of surgery is somewhat controversial among craniofacial surgeons. Some surgeons advocate "early" correction at 3 to 6 months of age, believing that the rapidly growing brain will assist in remodeling the skull if the fused suture is released and the calvarium reshaped. This theoretically reduces the amount of correction that needs to be performed in the operating room. Delaying surgery until 9 to 12 months of age allows the infant skull growth to begin to plateau prior to surgery. Although this reduces the amount of intrinsic bone shape normalization resulting from brain growth, the thicker calvarial bone may provide a more stable skeletal correction with less relapse. In reality, a large window exists when the surgery can be performed with acceptable risks and outcomes. Children who present late for corrective surgery present unique challenges to the craniofacial surgeon. Bone in these children is typically thicker and more difficult to contour with bone-bending forceps and simple barrel stave osteotomies. The asymmetric skull base is more developed and resistant to normalization, which increases the chances of a permanent deformity. Also, the diploic space between the inner and outer table has begun to form, subjecting the child to increased blood loss during surgical exposure and bony resection. The entire reconstructive procedure is more extensive, as even subcentimeter bone defects must be grafted in order to heal. Extracranial bone grafts (rib and/or iliac) are needed when the diploic space has not yet formed (before 5 years of age).

In children with syndromic craniosynostosis and midface retrusion, further reconstruction is frequently needed. A midface advancement consisting of either a Le Fort III or a monobloc osteotomy is performed between the ages of 5 and 8 years, unless the need for ocular protection forces earlier correction. The choice between procedures depends on forehead projection—a subcranial Le Fort III is performed if forehead projection is adequate, whereas a monobloc frontofacial advancement is needed if forehead retrusion has occurred. At the age of skeletal maturity (typically between the ages of 14 and 16), a Le Fort I maxillary osteotomy, with or without mandibular osteotomies, is usually needed to formally correct any malocclusion that commonly exists in these patients.

Orthognathic Surgery

The term *orthognathic* is derived from the Greek "orthos," meaning to straighten, and "gnathos" meaning jaw. Orthognathic surgery is a discipline that crosses the boundaries of many different specialties, principally oral and maxillofacial surgery and craniofacial surgery (a distinct subspecialty of plastic surgery). Orthognathic surgery repositions the dentofacial skeleton to correct either congenital or acquired malocclusions and restore a harmonious balance to the underlying bony facial form. These movements can involve both the maxilla and the mandible, either in segments or in conjunction with varying portions of the craniofacial skeleton. Certain procedures mandate the assistance of a pediatric neurosurgeon, because they require intracranial osteotomies to fully mobilize the bony segments for repositioning. An orthodontist who is familiar with the necessary dental movements is also needed to prepare a patient for surgery. The orthodontist also "fine-tunes" the dental occlusal relationships postoperatively, which is imperative for a successful outcome.

Although secondary trauma can lead to orthognathic surgery, the field predominantly addresses congenital and developmental deformities leading to malocclusion that cannot be corrected orthodontically. Nearly 25% of all patients who have undergone correction of a cleft lip and palate will develop severe maxillary hypoplasia that warrants surgical correction. Whether this is due to an intrinsic growth disturbance or restriction of growth of the midface due to postcleft surgical scarring is a hotly debated topic among craniofacial surgeons.

The age at which orthognathic procedures are performed is an important consideration in planning subsequent surgeries. Any skeletal facial advancement procedure performed prior to the age of bony maturity carries a significant rate of relapse as the remainder of the face grows; merely advancing the hypoplastic segments will not "unlock" their growth potential. For this reason, definitive orthognathic procedures are carried out in mid- to late adolescence, once the majority of facial skeletal growth is complete. Thus orthognathic surgery is usually done between 14 and 16 years for girls and 15 and 17 years for boys. Epiphyseal closure on anteroposterior hand radiographs is a good indicator of overall skeletal maturity.

Preoperative evaluation of patients with congenital dentofacial deformities usually occurs in the setting of a cleft/craniofacial team visit. An orthodontist is present for discussion of treatment options and will be intimately involved in both the preoperative and postoperative care of these patients. The patient's occlusion is determined according to the Angle classification, with class 1 being a "normal" occlusal relationship, class 2 as the typical "overbite," and class 3 being an "underbite." The facial profile and aesthetics are analyzed with special attention paid to the soft tissue bony landmarks. A lateral cephalometric radiograph, which is a standardized view with the head aligned in the neutral position, is used for treatment planning. The positions of the maxilla and mandible are determined with respect to the cranial base. Dental models are cast and mounted on an articulator in their anatomic relationship. Model surgery is performed wherein the models are precisely moved to place the teeth in proper planned postoperative occlusion. An acrylic splint is made from the models after each jaw is repositioned, which will be wired into place in the operating room to assure the bony segments are in proper position. This splint can be a final interdental splint for wear postoperatively.

In 1901, René Le Fort, a French surgeon and anatomist, carried out a series of rather grotesque experiments and defined a classification system for facial fractures that bears his name.[15,16] These "fault lines" of the facial bony skeleton were then subsequently adapted for use in elective orthognathic surgery and have become the mainstay of therapy to correct midfacial skeletal anomalies. The most common is the *Le Fort I osteotomy*, which repositions the tooth-bearing segment of the maxilla in either the anteroposterior or craniocaudal planes, or both. This osteotomy can be modified to divide the maxilla into two or three tooth-bearing segments, which can be moved independently to provide a functional, Angle class 1 occlusion and correct both sagittal and transverse maxillary deficiency. The Le Fort I osteotomy is used to correct cleft lip and palate-related maxillary hypoplasia. It is also used to correct vertical maxillary excess or rotational abnormalities of the maxilla.

Another commonly used corrective procedure in craniofacial surgery is the *bilateral sagittal split osteotomy* (BSSO). In this technically demanding procedure, the mandible is split in the sagittal plane from midramus to proximal body, sparing the inferior alveolar nerve on both sides. The BSSO movements can be adjusted to correct mandibular asymmetry, level the occlusal plane, or correct overall facial disharmony caused by overgrowth or undergrowth of the mandible. The BSSO is often combined with the Le Fort I osteotomy to correct larger mandibular–maxillary discrepancies. *Genioplasty* refers to reduction, advancement, or lateral movements of the bony chin point. It is generally considered a purely aesthetic procedure that can be added to enhance the facial skeletal balance.

Although not usually considered an orthognathic procedure, but rather a "craniofacial" procedure, the *Le Fort III osteotomy* is performed to reposition the midface (maxilla and zygomas) relative to the cranial base. In this procedure, osteotomies are created across the ascending portion of the zygoma, the zygomatic arch, orbital floor and both medial and lateral walls, frontonasal junction, and pterygomaxillary junction. The nasal septum is divided in the coronal plane. This allows for complete separation of the facial skeleton from the cranial base and subsequent advancement of the Le Fort III segment to correct midface hypoplasia. The Le Fort III advancement is used to correct severe malocclusion or upper airway obstruction from overall midface growth restriction. The majority of patients who undergo a Le Fort III osteotomy have a named syndrome (Crouzon, Apert, and Pfeiffer being the most common), and have their first midface advancement at age 5 or 6 years. Because the growth of the midface is not complete until mid- to late adolescence, a second advancement is frequently necessary. When midface retrusion is accompanied by growth restriction of the supraorbital rim and forehead, a *monobloc frontofacial advancement* may be necessary. This is an intracranial and extracranial procedure and requires both a pediatric neurosurgeon and a craniofacial surgeon for intracranial access. A monobloc advancement is similar to a Le Fort III osteotomy, except that the supraorbital rim and forehead are advanced along with the midface. This procedure has fallen out of favor because of infectious complications arising from difficulty obtaining adequate separation of the intracranial space and nasal cavities.[17] Thus the monobloc is now usually performed as a staged procedure (fronto-orbital advancement, followed by a Le Fort III osteotomy a few months later) or is performed with the use of distraction osteogenesis to allow the soft tissues to grow along with bony skeletal expansion, which minimizes the risk of intracranial infectious complications.

Distraction osteogenesis was pioneered by Ilizarov (a Russian orthopedist) in 1958, and adapted for use in the mandible by McCarthy in 1992.[18,19] It is now commonly used for a number of applications in craniofacial surgery. The principle behind distraction osteogenesis is that gradual expansion of the bony skeletal gap left by a surgically placed osteotomy will allow lengthening of the bone by gradual osteoblastic activity and ingrowth of new bone. This results in lengthening of the skeleton in the direction of the vector of expansion. Distraction is useful in situations that would require extensive bone grafting to obtain adequate bone length, or in cases in which opposing soft tissue forces would result in skeletal relapse if the bone was rapidly advanced and grafted. Clinically, maxillary distraction is most commonly applied when a large discrepancy exists between the maxilla and mandible as a result of a complete cleft lip and palate and resultant maxillary hypoplasia. Scarring from the numerous previous procedures makes maxillary advancement alone prone to relapse; by applying the principle of distraction, the bone and soft tissue are gradually expanded, and the cleft maxilla can be advanced into a normal occlusal relationship (Angle class 1) with minimal chances of relapse resulting from soft tissue resistance. Distraction is also useful to correct severe mandibular hypoplasia accompanying conditions such as hemifacial microsomia or Pierre Robin sequence, which will be discussed in subsequent sections of this chapter.

Craniofacial Clefts

Dr. Paul Tessier, the father of the field of craniofacial surgery, also developed a classification system for craniofacial clefts that is arguably the most widely used of those available today.

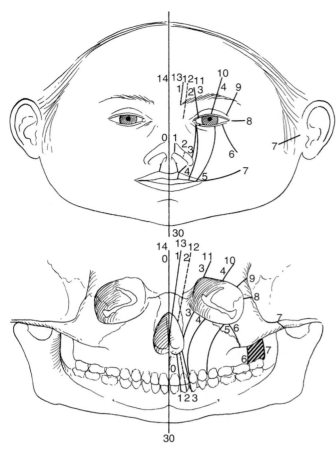

FIGURE 53-4 Tessier's pre-computed tomography classification system of rare craniofacial clefts. The lower image represents the cleft location of the bony skeleton, while the upper illustrates the cutaneous manifestations of the various bony clefts.

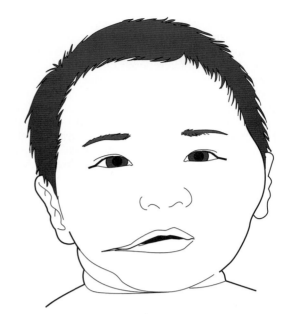

FIGURE 53-5 A child with a typical Tessier number 7 soft tissue cleft.

The Tessier system is based on specific anatomic derangements that fall along embryonic lines of fusion within the face (although these were not known at the time they were initially described) (Fig. 53-4). Tessier's classification system is notated 0 to 14, with clefts 0 to 7 describing facial clefts and clefts 8 to 14 describing cranial vault clefts. Each cleft has unique soft tissue and bone lines of clefting. Also, the facial and cranial clefts coincide such that the sum of the two components is 14 (i.e., 0 and 14 clefts coincide, as do 3/11 and 5/9, etc.). A thorough search along the meridian of the cleft will usually elucidate subtle (or not-so-subtle) findings.

The majority of craniofacial clefts are rare and will be seen infrequently during an individual surgeon's career. As such, the remainder of this section of the chapter will be spent dealing with those more common Tessier clefts.

CLEFT NUMBER 7

A number 7 cleft can be protean in physical manifestation and is known by a number of different names. Hemifacial microsomia, oculoauriculovertebral syndrome (OAV), first and second branchial arch syndrome, and otomandibular dysostosis syndrome all refer to the physical findings associated with a number 7 cleft. The number 7 cleft is thought to have an incidence of between 1 in 3000 and 1 in 5642[20] live births. A number 7 cleft is usually unilateral, but approximately

10% of affected children will have symmetric, bilateral involvement.[21]

The derivatives of the first and second branchial arch are abnormal, albeit to varying degrees. Macrostomia is a common finding, with the commissure of the lip being displaced laterally toward the affected side, resulting in an enlarged oral opening (Fig. 53-5). Preauricular "ear tags," embryologic remnants of the developing ear, are present anterior to the external auditory canal and contain small "stalks" of cartilage remnants (Fig. 53-6). The external ear can likewise be affected and can range from mild hypoplasia to near complete absence. A conductive hearing loss on the ipsilateral side is commonplace. The mandible is commonly affected, and the defect of the ascending ramus and condyle may range from mild hypoplasia to complete absence (Fig. 53-7). The facial nerve may be affected to varying degrees, as well, which in turn contributes

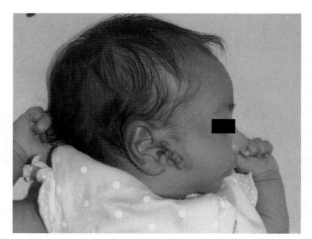

FIGURE 53-6 Multiple accessory external ear tags as seen in Tessier 7 clefts.

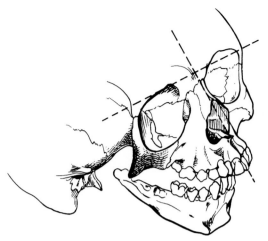

FIGURE 53-7 Skeletal findings in hemifacial microsomia. Note the absence of the ascending ramus and condyle of the mandible.

to weakness and underdevelopment of the muscles of facial expression that they supply.

Given that the manifestations of the number 7 cleft vary, so do the treatment options. In general, more severely affected children require earlier and more significant reconstruction. Cutaneous manifestations—macrostomia and branchial arch remnants—are usually treated with excision and local flap reconstruction during infancy. Underlying bony anomalies are treated based on severity. Children with mild hypoplasia of the ramus and condyle are followed throughout growth, and will usually develop an occlusal cant (Fig. 53-8) as they age. These children can be treated with orthognathic surgery after cessation of skeletal growth to reposition the hypoplastic mandible and maxilla with the combination of a Le Fort 1 osteotomy, bilateral sagittal split osteotomies, and an osseous genioplasty to align the chin point. Those with more severely hypoplastic rami will undergo distraction osteogenesis of the ramus during childhood, but will usually need formal orthognathic correction during late adolescence.[22] Children who are born with complete absence of an ascending ramus need an extensive reconstruction to achieve normal function of their mandible and a normal occlusal relationship. This is typically accomplished through the use of a free costochondral rib graft, which is performed around 7 years of age. Ear reconstruction with costal cartilage is performed at the same age, when necessary.

TREACHER COLLINS SYNDROME

First described in 1847,[23] Treacher Collins syndrome (or mandibulofacial dysostosis) is a relatively common syndrome made up of Tessier clefts 6, 7, and 8. Its incidence is estimated at 1 in 10,000 live births. Treacher Collins is caused by a mutation on chromosome 5q31.3-33.3 (the *TCOF1* gene) and is an autosomal dominant disorder with variable penetrance.

Treacher Collins patients manifest bilateral anomalies of the eyelids, zygomas, maxilla, mandible, and ears (Fig. 53-9). There is typically an antimongoloid slant to the palpebral fissures, with lower lid notching present. Eyelashes are often absent on the medial two thirds of the lower eyelid. The zygomas are severely hypoplastic or absent. The maxilla is hypoplastic with a shortened vertical height, which can impede or block nasal airflow. Shortening of both the length and height of the mandible results in narrowing of the posterior pharyngeal airway and can contribute to upper airway obstruction in these children, which in the past necessitated placement of a tracheostomy. Within the past 20 years, however, distraction osteogenesis has been applied to these patients to relieve early upper airway obstruction and avoid the need for long-term tracheostomy dependence. Severe microtia is often accompanied by atresia of the middle and inner ear; placement of bone-anchored hearing aids (BAHA) is commonly necessary to allow for improved hearing and speech development. As is the case with either isolated or syndromic microtia, reconstruction of the external ears is usually undertaken at age 7 or 8 with autologous costal cartilage grafts. At around this same time, onlay bone grafting of the maxilla and zygoma is performed to add projection and give a more normal midfacial profile. Correction of the eyelid notching with local tissue transfers is also performed at this age should it not be needed earlier because of corneal protection issues. Definitive orthognathic surgical correction of the associated deformities of the occlusal plane is performed in late adolescence.

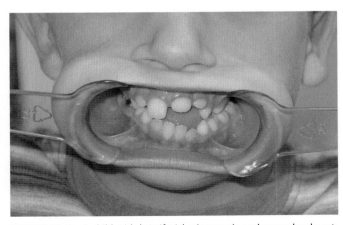

FIGURE 53-8 A child with hemifacial microsomia and an occlusal cant. Note the upward slant of the mandible caused by right-sided ramus hypoplasia.

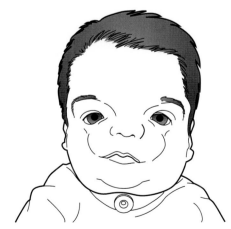

FIGURE 53-9 Typical findings in a patient with Treacher Collins syndrome. Down-slanting palpebral fissures, malar hypoplasia, and microtia are common hallmarks of this syndrome. This child lacks true colobomas of the lower eyelid but has loss of lower eyelid support and excess scleral show.

Acknowledgments

Special thanks to Henry K. Kawamoto, Jr., DDS, MD, for Figures 53-4 and 53-7.

The complete reference list is available online at www. expertconsult.com.

SELECTED READINGS

Bentz ML, Bauer BS, Zucker RM, eds. Principles and Practice of Pediatric Plastic Surgery. St Louis: Quality Medical Publishing; 2007.

Mathes SJ, ed. Plastic Surgery. Pediatric Plastic Surgery. Vol 4. Philadelphia: Saunders; 2005.

Posnick JC. Craniofacial and Maxillofacial Surgery in Children and Young Adults. Philadelphia: Saunders; 2000.

Thaller SR, Bradley JP, Garri JI, eds. Craniofacial Surgery. New York: Informa Healthcare; 2008.

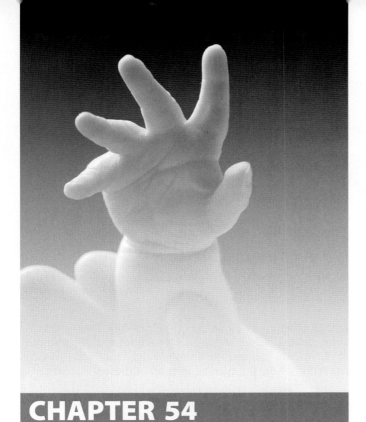

CHAPTER 54

Understanding and Caring for Children with Cleft Lip and Palate

James Y. Liau, John A. van Aalst, and
A. Michael Sadove

Epidemiology

The incidence of orofacial clefting varies among racial backgrounds. Because of the close association between cleft lip and palate, the presence of cleft lip is often described as being with or without cleft palate. Worldwide prevalence of cleft lip and palate is 1 per 700 live births.[1] People of African descent have the lowest incidence of cleft lip with/without cleft palate at 0.5 per 1000 live births, followed by whites (1 per 1000 live births), and Asians (1.3 per 1000 per live births). Overall, an isolated cleft lip makes up approximately 21% of all patients with cleft lip and palate. Unilateral clefts are roughly 9 times more prevalent than bilateral cleft lips, and males are more affected than females. The U.S. incidence of cleft palate alone ranges from 0.3 to 0.5 per 1000 live births.[2] A child with a cleft lip with or without cleft palate has an approximately 30% chance of having an associated syndrome; interestingly, a child with an isolated cleft palate has a 50% incidence of an associated syndrome.[2,3] Because of this association, genetic

workup and counseling is mandatory, as is heightened suspicion for other physical and physiologic anomalies.

Etiology

Genetic and environmental factors have both been associated with clefting. If other family members are affected by a cleft, offspring have an increased chance of being affected. For example, if a family already has a child with a cleft, or one parent has a cleft, the chance that the next child will have a cleft is 4%; with two affected children, the chance that a third child will have a cleft increases to 9%. The probability increases to 17% in a family if both a child and parent have a cleft.[4] This increase in frequency is seen in spontaneous clefting not associated with syndromes. There are some syndromes in which clefting can be passed down in an autosomal dominant fashion, such as van der Woude syndrome, where presence of the cleft palate is an autosomal dominant trait.

Environmental causes of clefting include the use of anticonvulsants, including phenytoin, which is associated with 10-fold increase in clefting; maternal smoking increases the incidence twofold. Other environmental influences, such as alcohol use, the use of retinoic acid, and dietary causes, including zinc and folate deficiencies, can cause syndromes with clefting; however, these are not directly linked to isolated cleft lip/palate. People with certain genotypes are more susceptible to certain environmental exposures; hence, women with less efficient methyl tetrahydrofolate reductase enzymes are more prone to clefting in the face of folic acid deficiency.[5-12]

Embryology

Basic understanding of midface and palatal embryologic development helps elucidate the pathoanatomy of cleft lip with or without palate. Orofacial clefting occurs when there is failure of fusion of maxillofacial structures migrating from lateral to medial during the initial 4 to 10 weeks of embryonic development. A key anterior–posterior embryologic and anatomic landmark in understanding clefts is the incisive foramen. The structures that form anterior to the foramen ultimately develop into the nose, lip, and alveolus; embryologically, these structures form first and are designated as the primary palate. The structures that form posterior to the foramen become the hard palate and soft palate, and are referred to as the secondary palate, because they fuse secondarily. Clefting of the lip (primary palate) occurs when the nasomedial and nasolateral prominences of the frontonasal prominence do not meet with the maxillary prominence (Fig. 54-1, *A*). Clefting of the palate (secondary palate) occurs when the lateral palatine shelves do not elevate and fuse at the midline to each other or to the primary palate (Fig. 54-1, *B*). Because the development of this craniofacial area is complex, deformities can occur at multiple points along the embryologic time line, resulting in a full spectrum or combination of anomalies.

Anatomy

UNILATERAL CLEFT LIP

A cleft lip affects the anatomy of the lip, philtrum, nose, as well as the alveolus, depending on the severity of the defect. Microform clefts are the mildest form of clefting, involving

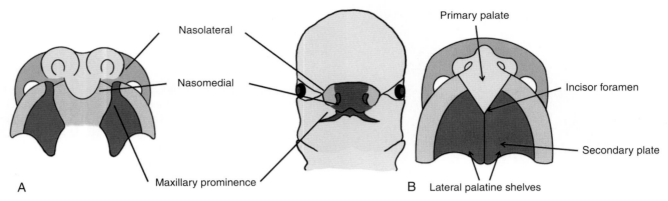

FIGURE 54-1   A, The nasolateral and nasomedial prominence fuse to make the lip and nose. Lack of fusion between the maxillary nasal prominence with the nasomedial prominence will yield a cleft lip. **B,** The lateral palatine shelves fuse in the midline, thus forming the secondary palate. The primary palate fuses posteriorly with the palatine shelves to form a complete palate. *(See Expert Consult site for color version.)*

the vermillion and white roll, and can be quite subtle (Fig. 54-2, *A*). Incomplete clefts are associated with absence of skin, mucosa, and orbicularis muscle but have a retained webbing of skin across the floor of the nasal aperture, referred to as a Simonart band (Fig. 54-2, *B*). A complete unilateral cleft involves the alveolus, and can be associated with a cleft of the palate (Fig. 54-2, *C*).

The most obvious deformity involving a cleft lip is discontinuity of the lip itself. However further analysis of the defect demonstrates deviation of the nasal septum and columella, as well as widening or flattening of the cleft-side nasal cartilage. Other defects include the lack of nasal floor and discontinuity of the lip, muscle, and the alveolar ridge. Successful surgical correction of the lip must address all of these structures.

BILATERAL CLEFT LIP

Bilateral clefts have a two-sided discontinuity of the lip, with a central portion, the premaxilla, which is discontinuous from either of the lateral segments. The premaxilla contains

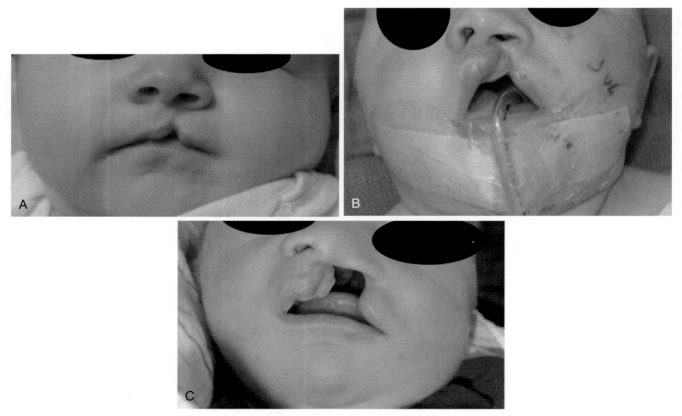

FIGURE 54-2   A, Microform cleft can be seen with mild notching of the lip's vermilion along with the minimal distortion of the nose. **B,** Incomplete cleft has some webbing across the cleft with some retention of the lateral nose; however, the skin across the cleft is devoid of orbicularis oris muscle and is functionless. This skin is also called a Simonart band. **C,** Complete cleft lip has lateralization of the lip and lateral nasal element. Notice the deviation of the nasal columella and philtrum away from the cleft, and the flattened nose on the cleft side. This picture also demonstrates the clefting of the palate, which allows an unobstructed view into the nasal airway.

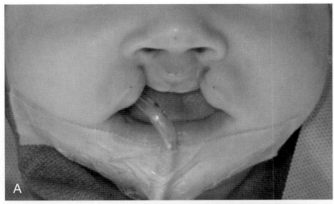

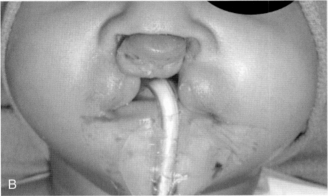

FIGURE 54-3   A, Bilateral cleft lip with a Simonart band transversing both clefts. **B,** Complete bilateral cleft lip. The midline protuberance is called the premaxilla and is much more protruding than an incomplete bilateral cleft; tethering of the Simonart bands help in keeping the premaxilla in a more anatomic position. Absence, or shortening of the columella, widening of the alar bases, and anterior projection of the premaxilla are all trademarks of bilateral cleft lips.

elements of skin, mucosa and bone, which can be asymmetrically deviated to one side or the other, and can be anteriorly positioned, depending on the severity of the deformity. Bilateral clefts can be incomplete with Simonart bands (Fig. 54-3, *A*), or complete with defects that proceed through the alveolar ridges (Fig. 54-3, *B*). A central feature of the bilateral cleft lip deformity is depression of the nasal tip, a shortened columella, and widely splayed alae.

CLEFT PALATE

Clefts of the palate can exist with clefts of the lip or may be present alone. Anatomically, the hard palate begins immediately posterior to the incisive foramen, with embryologic fusion of the palate from anterior to posterior. Hence, an isolated cleft of the soft palate may exist; however, an isolated cleft of the hard palate cannot. A complete cleft of the secondary palate includes both the hard and soft palate, extending anteriorly from the incisive foramen to the uvula, and this can be bilateral as well (Fig. 54-4). The primary function of the palate is to separate the oral cavity from the nasal cavity. This function is lost in the presence of a cleft. The function of the soft palate is primarily speech related and dependent on five paired muscles, the two most important of which are the levator veli palatini and the tensor veli palatini. Ordinarily, these muscles form a transverse sling enabling the palate to rise and move posteriorly to close the oropharynx from the nasopharynx. In a cleft palate, these muscles abnormally insert onto the posterior shelf of the hard palate, and as a consequence, the palate is deficient in its ability to seal off the oropharynx from the nasopharynx.

A submucous cleft is the most minor expression of the clefting spectrum. The soft palate mucosa is actually intact, but split posteriorly, resulting in a bifid uvula; there is a midline lucency in the soft palate, referred to as a zona pellucidum, which is a muscle diastasis, and a notch at the midline, posterior edge of the hard palate.[13] As in a full cleft, the levator and tensor veli palatine abnormally insert onto the posterior hard palate, preventing the soft palate from moving appropriately during speech, potentially leading to nasal sounding speech. The incidence of submucous clefts is roughly 1 in 1,200 to 2,000; however, this is likely an underestimation, because many patients may not seek treatment or even know of their submucous cleft unless there is functional speech deficit.[14]

Treatment Protocols

The timing for cleft lip repair in the United States is generally between 3 to 6 months of age. Depending on the severity of the deformity, various forms of presurgical orthopedics can be used to prepare the child for lip surgery. In general, the goals of these techniques are to improve the alignment of the alveolar segments, decrease the size of the soft tissue cleft, and to

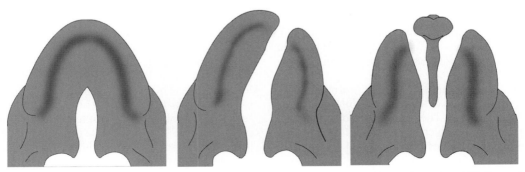

FIGURE 54-4 The figure on the *left* depicts a cleft of the secondary palate only; there is an intact hard palate. The *middle* figure depicts a complete unilateral cleft. The figure on the *right* depicts a complete bilateral cleft.

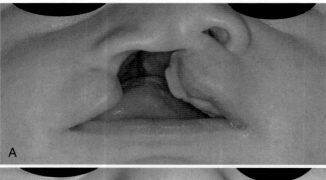

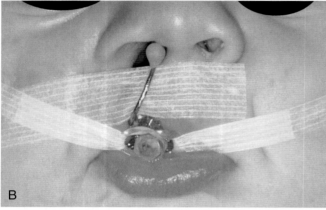

FIGURE 54-5   **A,** A unilateral cleft lip prior to nasoalveolar molding (NAM) has a wide alveolar cleft, slumping of the nasal cartilage on the cleft side, and lateralization of the alar base of the cleft side. **B,** Nasoalveolar molding assists in realigning the alveolar segments, reshaping the slumping nasal cartilage of the cleft side, and medializing the alar base of the cleft side.

improve the symmetry of the nose. The simplest form is a taping regimen (literally from cheek to cheek) that helps to pull the two sides of the clefts together, with the goal of narrowing the cleft and realigning the tissues in an anterior-posterior dimension. Some centers also use a technique termed nasoalveolar molding (NAM) to address the three major components of the cleft deformity (Fig. 54-5). NAM addresses the slumping of the nasal alar cartilage, helps realign the alveolar ridges, and brings the soft tissue of the lips into closer proximity.[15,16]

CLEFT LIP SURGICAL REPAIR

Unilateral

There are multiple surgical techniques for cleft lip repair. A recent survey of U.S. cleft surgeons found three predominant surgical techniques for unilateral cleft lip repair: the Millard rotation-advancement technique (46%), the Millard rotation-advancement technique with modifications (38%), and triangular flap techniques (9%).[17] Techniques for bilateral cleft lip repair include variations of techniques introduced by Millard and by Mulliken.[18]

In a unilateral cleft lip, there is absence of central tissue of the lip and philtrum, as well as of the nasal columella, depending on the severity of the cleft. The overall goals of surgery are restoration of lip continuity, which starts with functional orbicularis oris muscle reapproximation, establishing symmetry of the lip (especially at the central cupid's bow) and nose, with aesthetic placement of scars in anatomic subunits. The rotation-advancement repair, as described by Dr. Ralph Millard

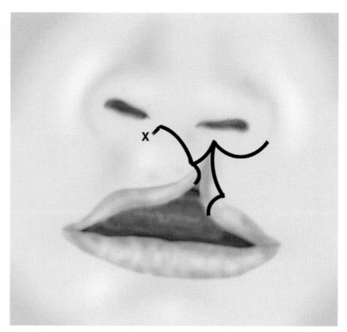

FIGURE 54-6   Markings for the rotation-advancement lip repair (Millard lip repair).

in 1976, addresses all of these goals (Fig. 54-6). Because there is a paucity of tissue medial to the cleft, the downward *rotation* of the remaining philtrum helps to provide adequate tissue that matches the contralateral, noncleft side. *Advancement* of the lateral tissue reconstructs the affected philtrum, thus providing lip continuity. Medialization of the base of the nose, as well as further soft tissue dissection of the nose, results in a symmetric reconstruction. Reapproximation of the orbicularis oris muscle provides oral competence. Further soft tissue arrangement in the nasal floor allows final closure of the lip and nose. Surgical details are found in several references.[19–21] A potential shortcoming of the rotation-advancement technique is the inability to provide adequate philtral length despite aggressive downward rotation of this tissue. This may result in the high point of the cupid's bow on the cleft side being located in a position higher than on the noncleft side.

Some of the more commonly used modifications of the rotation-advancement technique are the Mohler repair, the Noordoff vermilion flap, and the triangular advancement flap, although the details of these techniques are beyond the scope of this chapter (see the referenced articles for more complete descriptions).[22–24]

Another technique for unilateral cleft lip repair is the triangular flap technique (also known as the Tennison repair), introduced by Charles Tennison in 1952. Tennison approached the lack of central soft tissue of the cleft in a very different fashion than Millard. In this technique lip length is achieved by designing a triangular flap of the lateral, cleft side, which then inserts into a cut of the medial, noncleft side, thus providing the extra tissue for appropriate lip height. The muscle is repaired, as in the rotation-advancement technique, followed by reconstruction of the floor of the nose (full surgical details are found in the references).[25,26] Shortcomings of the Tennison repair include placement of the scar in a nonanatomic location, thus drawing attention to the repair, as well as an overly long lip, depending on the size of the triangular flaps.

Bilateral Cleft Lip Repair

Bilateral cleft lip repairs are especially challenging because of a central lack of soft tissue, and the anterior displacement of the premaxilla, which functionally increases the transverse width of cleft defect. Many surgeons use presurgical orthopedics to decrease premaxillary protrusion, thus increasing the columellar length and nasal tip projection. This technique also decreases the distance of the cleft, potentially making surgical repair easier for the surgeon (Fig. 54-7). The primary goals of surgery include lip and nasal symmetry, which is achieved through the creation of a philtral column, including the cupid's bow, reapproximation of the orbicularis oris, repositioning the nasal alar cartilages, lengthening the columella, and closure of the nasal floor (Fig. 54-8). The absence of the philtral column and cupid's bow is especially problematic since these structures are difficult to replicate in a repair. Postoperatively, these imperfections can be quite noticeable at conversational distances.[27] Realistically, patients with bilateral cleft lips will ultimately require revisional surgeries to correct the secondary stigmata of the repair, which include a shortened columella, blunted nasal tip, widened nasal ala, and a widened philtrum.

CLEFT PALATE SURGICAL REPAIR

Following surgical repair of the lip, repair of the palate is generally performed between 9 to 12 months of age. The choice of techniques for palate repair depends on the type of cleft. Recent surveys show that the most commonly used techniques are the Bardach two-flap palatoplasty (45%) (Fig. 54-9) and the Furlow palatoplasty (42%) (Fig. 54-10); the Veau-Ward-Kilner (VWK) pushback (Fig. 54-11) and the von Langenbeck (Fig. 54-12) techniques, although less common, are also used.[28] The common denominators for all of these techniques are repair in three layers (nasal mucosa, muscle layer of the soft palate, and the oral mucosa), and anatomic repositioning of the soft palate musculature. Bilateral cleft palate repair is similar in principle in that a three-layer repair is achieved (Fig. 54-13). See the references for complete descriptions of these techniques.[29]

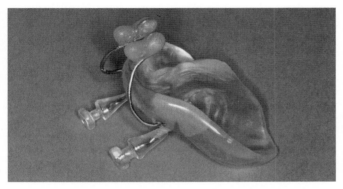

FIGURE 54-7 Nasoalveolar mold (presurgical orthopedics) for bilateral cleft lip, designed to align the alveolar segments, as well as realign the premaxilla into a more anatomic position.

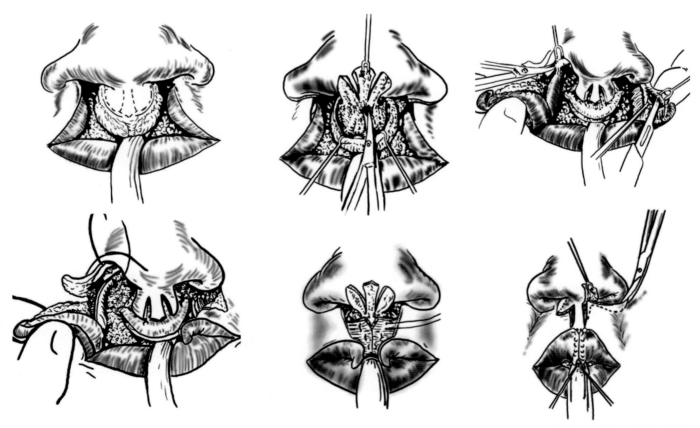

FIGURE 54-8 Schematic of the steps involved with a bilateral cleft lip repair. Re-creation of the columella, dissection of the muscle in the lateral lip elements, re-creation of the nasal floor, reapproximation of the lateral lip muscle, and insetting of the nasal alar bases with trimming of skin for final closure are all integral parts of bilateral cleft lip repair.

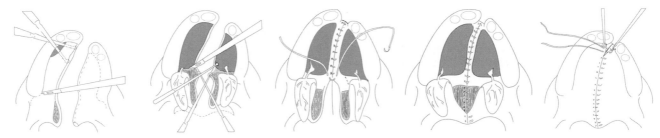

FIGURE 54-9 The Bardach two-flap palatal reconstruction consists of elevating the palatal mucosa off the hard palate bone as a flap, elevation of the nasal mucosa, and closure of these two layers separately for the hard palate. Pedicles for the mucosal flaps come from the greater palatine arteries posteriorly. Closure of the soft palate is a three-layer repair, including a nasal mucosal layer, muscle layer (levator veli palatini and tensor veli palatini realignment), and oral mucosal layer.

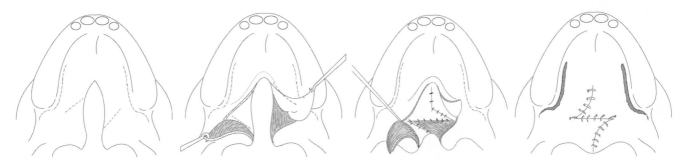

FIGURE 54-10 The double opposing Z-plasty, (Furlow palatoplasty) of the soft palate includes realignment of the levator and tensor veli palatine muscles in the form of Z-plasty. One flap has oral mucosa only, whereas the contralateral side has oral mucosa and muscle. The nasal layer consists of a separate nasal mucosal layer, which is on the side with oral mucosa and muscle flap, and the contralateral side has nasal mucosa and muscle. Closure of both layers in a double opposing Z-plasty assists in elongating the soft palate, which should subsequently improve palatal speech function.

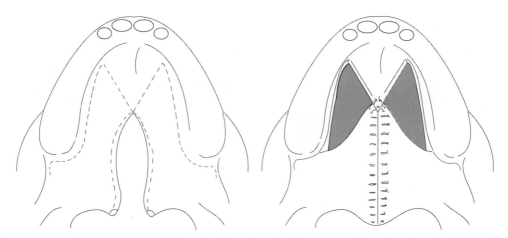

FIGURE 54-11 The Veau-Ward-Kilner repair consists of advancing the oral mucosal flaps posteriorly to allow closure of the hard palate. Muscle realignment of the soft palate assists in palatal function.

Muscle repair is integral to the palate's primary function, namely speech. Any repair that does not address the muscle will fail in the development of normal speech.[30] As previously noted, the levator veli palatine and the tensor veli palatine are the two most integral muscles in producing a functional palate. Detaching these muscles from their abnormal insertions to the remnant shelves of the posterior hard palate, and then reapproximating them to each other in a transverse palatal sling, is referred to as an intravelar veloplasty. Failure to perform this step will result in a nonfunctional palate.

Multidisciplinary Care

Patients with orofacial clefts require multidisciplinary care that is provided by plastic surgeons, otolaryngologists, dentists, orthodontists, oral surgeons, geneticists, audiologists, and speech and language pathologists. This team approach yields more comprehensive and coordinated care, which benefits the patient.[31–33] Longitudinal follow-up in a team environment is mandatory, because many issues, including the ability

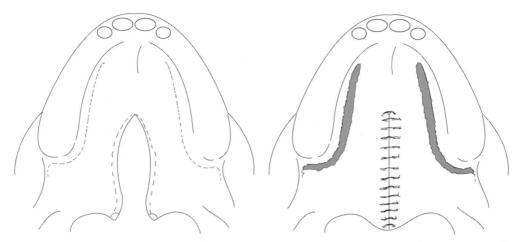

FIGURE 54-12 The von Langenbeck repair consists of relaxing incisions on the lateral palate with subsequent advancement to midline, allowing a palatal repair of both mucosa and muscle layers. Benefits include keeping a bipedicled flap; however, the advancement can be limited and inadequate with wider cleft defects.

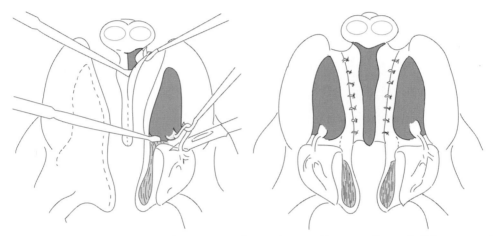

FIGURE 54-13 Closure of bilateral cleft palate follows in the same principles. Nasal mucosal layers are dissected off the vomer and palatine shelves and closed. Dissection of the hard palate oral mucosa allows closure separately, thus providing a two-layer closure. The soft palatal muscles are dissected and realigned to provide palatal function.

to produce normal speech, and dental eruption, continue to evolve as the patient grows.

Care of the cleft patient begins prenatally when a screening ultrasound makes the initial diagnosis. Ideally, counseling with the family begins during the perinatal period, and focuses on potential feeding concerns postnatally, the time line for surgical repair of the clefts, and team-centered care. In the neonatal period, feeding is the primary concern, especially in children with clefts of the palate. Appropriate weight gain must be monitored, as well as the family's overall psychological comfort with the child's cleft. A genetic evaluation, looking for evidence of associated anomalies and syndromes, and further counseling within a cleft team, prepare the family for the ongoing care of their child.

Secondary Cleft Management

Although patients with cleft lip and palate undergo initial repair of their clefts in the first 12 to 18 months of life, these patients will ultimately require further surgical interventions. Nasal and lip revision, if needed, can be pursued at 5 years of

age, which coincides with greater self-awareness of physical differences, and exposure to an expanding group of peers in school.

Between the ages of 7 and 9 years, during the period of mixed dentition (when the adult lateral incisor is ready to erupt through the area of the alveolar cleft), a bone graft generally harvested from the hip, is required in the alveolar cleft. The new bone allows eruption of the lateral incisor, and completes the continuity of the maxilla. Both before and after the bone graft, additional dental and orthodontic work may be required to align the teeth in normal anatomic position.

At facial skeletal maturity, generally at 15 years of age for females and 17 to 19 years of age for males, orthognathic surgery, with surgical movement of the maxilla, mandible, or both, may be required to achieve normal occlusion, overall facial appearance and profile. During the teenage years, further revisions of the lip and nose may be required to give these patients the desired aesthetic outcome that prepares them for adult life.

Velopharyngeal insufficiency (VPI) is the condition in which the repaired cleft palate is physically incapable of isolating the nasopharynx from the oropharynx, resulting in air escape through the nose during speech. The patient with VPI has a nasal quality to his or her speech. Usually the most affected sounds are plosives, /p/ and /b/, in words such a "papa" and "buggy." In a patient with VPI, the pressure is dissipated through the nose, making these sounds more nasal in quality: "mama" and "muggy." Depending on the severity of the condition, VPI can range from being barely audible to rendering speech unintelligible. VPI usually occurs in patients whose palates are short and scarred or who have an inadequately functioning soft palate muscle sling. The advent of VPI is usually noticed as children become more verbal, between 3 and 5 years of age. Another time period during which VPI may arise is during tonsillar and adenoid regression. As these tissues atrophy, the nasopharyngeal and oropharyngeal spaces enlarge; a marginally functional soft palate may no longer be able to seal the nasopharynx from the oropharynx, resulting in VPI. Because of these ongoing changes, vigilance for VPI must be maintained throughout a child's growth and development.

In patients suspected of VPI, evaluation by a speech therapist is vital in determining whether additional speech therapy or surgical intervention is required. Nasoendoscopy and video-fluoroscopy may be required to determine the degree of soft palate incompetence, which in turn helps to determine the optimal surgical technique to correct the child's VPI.

Conclusions

Cleft lip and palate can be visually and functionally devastating to a child. Multispecialty and interdisciplinary team care is both ideal and necessary for the care of these children because of the complexity of the anomalies and the longitudinal nature of cleft care. Establishing rapport with patients and their families, as well as among team specialists, can lead to life-changing differences in patients with clefts, allowing them to lead normal, productive lives, as well as making the formidable problems of cleft care rewarding to treat.

The complete reference list is available online at www. expertconsult.com.

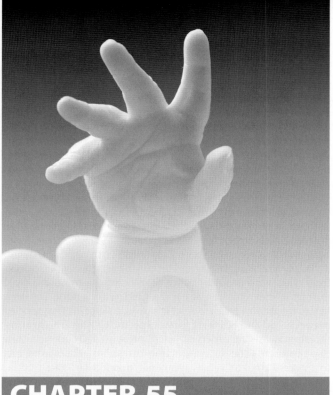

CHAPTER 55

Otolaryngologic Disorders

Lisa M. Elden, Ralph F. Wetmore,
and William P. Potsic

This chapter is divided according to anatomic structures: the ear, the nose, the oral cavity and pharynx, the larynx, and the neck. In each section we review anatomy, embryology, and examination, before discussing congenital and acquired disorders, including infections, trauma, and tumors.

Ear

ANATOMY

The ear is divided into three anatomic and functional areas: the external ear, the middle ear, and the inner ear. The external ear consists of the auricle, external auditory canal, and the lateral surface of the tympanic membrane. The auricle is a complex fibroelastic skeleton that is covered by skin and subcutaneous tissue that directs sound into the external ear canal.

The external auditory canal is oval with the long axis in the superior to inferior direction. In neonates, the external canal is almost entirely supported by soft, collapsible cartilage. As the temporal bone grows over several years, the bony portion of the canal enlarges to comprise the inner one third, leaving the outer two thirds supported by firm cartilage. Hair and cerumen glands are present in the outer two thirds of the external canal.

The ear canal is lined by skin that is continuous with the lateral surface of the tympanic membrane, and it is innervated by cranial nerves V, VII, IX, and X and by the great auricular nerve.

The tympanic membrane separates the external ear canal from the middle ear. It has three layers: an outer layer of squamous epithelium (skin); a middle layer of fibrous tissue that is attached to the malleus, the most lateral middle ear ossicle; and an inner layer of mucosa that is continuous with the mucosa lining the middle ear. The fibrous layer is also attached to a thick fibrous annulus that anchors the tympanic membrane to the temporal bone.

The middle ear is an air-filled space within the temporal bone of the skull that is lined by ciliated, columnar respiratory epithelium. The middle ear communicates with the mastoid air cell system posteriorly and is lined by the same mucosa. It also communicates with the nasopharynx anteriorly through the eustachian tube. The mucociliary transport system of the middle ear moves mucus and debris into the nasopharynx, where it is swallowed. Secretory cells are not evenly distributed throughout the middle ear and mastoid complex and are more numerous anteriorly near the eustachian tube.

Three ossicles are present in the middle ear—the malleus, incus, and stapes—that transmit sound from the vibrating tympanic membrane to the stapes footplate. Stapes movement creates a fluid wave in the inner ear that travels to the round window membrane and is dissipated by reciprocal motion to the stapes.

There are two striated muscles in the middle ear. The tensor tympani muscle lies parallel to the eustachian tube, and its tendon attaches to the medial surface of the malleus. The stapedius muscle lies along the vertical portion of the facial nerve in the posterosuperior part of the middle ear. Its tendon attaches to the head of the stapes. These muscles stiffen the ossicular chain in the presence of sustained loud noise.

The facial nerve traverses the middle ear with its horizontal portion lying superior to the stapes. Posterior to the stapes, the facial nerve turns inferiorly in a vertical fashion to exit the stylomastoid foramen deep to the tip of the mastoid. The chorda tympani nerve is a branch of the facial nerve that innervates taste to the anterior two thirds of the tongue. It exits the facial nerve in the vertical segment and passes under the posterosuperior surface of the tympanic membrane, crossing the middle ear lateral to the long process of the incus and medial to the malleus. The facial nerve lies within a protective bony canal throughout its course in the middle ear. However, the bony canal may be absent (in the horizontal portion) in as many as 8% to 30% of patients.[1] Cranial nerve IX supplies sensation to the floor of the middle ear.

The inner ear consists of the cochlea, semicircular canals, and vestibule. The cochlea is a coiled fluid-filled tube consisting of 2½ to 2¾ turns surrounded by dense bone. It contains the membranes that support the organ of Corti and has hair cells that detect the fluid wave from vibration of the stapes footplate. The hair cells create the neural impulses that are transmitted from the auditory nerve (cranial nerve VIII) to the brain, providing the sensation of hearing.

The three paired semicircular canals (horizontal, superior, and inferior) are also fluid-filled tubes surrounded by dense bone. The semicircular canals each have a hair cell–containing structure (the ampulla) that detects motion. The utricle and saccule of the vestibule also have hair cell structures that detect acceleration.[2]

EMBRYOLOGY

The external ear develops during the sixth week of gestation and is completely developed by the 20th week. Six hillocks fuse to form the basic units of the pinna. Defects in the fusion of the hillocks lead to preauricular tags and sinuses. The external auditory canal develops from the first branchial cleft. A solid epithelial plug forms during the beginning of the third month of gestation and canalizes in the seventh month to form the external auditory canal.

The middle ear space develops from the first pharyngeal pouch. The ossicles develop from the first and second pharyngeal arches. The inner ear arises from neuroectodermal tissue within the otic placode that forms the otic pit.[2]

Any combination of anomalies may occur. Abnormalities of the development of the ear may create anomalies of the pinna, external auditory canal, middle ear structures, and inner ear. One of the anomalies that involves the external and middle ear is aural atresia (absence of the external auditory canal). Absence of the external canal may occur with a deformed or normal external ear. The ossicles may be deformed and are usually fused to each other as well as the bony plate representing the undeveloped tympanic membrane. The facial nerve may also be altered in its course through the temporal bone. Reconstruction of the atretic canal, removal of the bony tympanic plate, release of the fused ossicles, and reconstruction of a new eardrum is a complex surgical procedure that may improve hearing. Rarely, there is incomplete development of the inner ear structures. The most common of these is dysplasia of the cochlea, and it may vary in severity. Dysplasia is associated with sensorineural hearing loss in most cases.[3,4]

EXAMINATION

The examination of the ear should always start with inspection of the outer ear and surrounding structures. Deformities of the outer ear structure may suggest the presence of other anomalies, such as a first branchial cleft sinus. A first branchial cleft sinus usually presents below the ear lobe near the angle of the jaw. The sinus tract may connect to the ear canal or, rarely, the middle ear.

The external auditory canal and tympanic membrane are best examined with a handheld otoscope that has a bright fiberoptic light source and a pneumatic bulb attached to its head. The largest speculum that comfortably fits in the external canal should be used to maximize visualization and minimize pain. A very small speculum may be inserted deeply, but it might lacerate the ear canal as well as limit visibility of the tympanic membrane. The otoscope permits visualization of the ear canal and tympanic membrane. A translucent tympanic membrane will also permit visualization of the contents of the middle ear.

A healthy middle ear contains air and is ventilated via the eustachian tube that connects to the nasopharynx. Insufflation of air into the ear canal via the pneumatic bulb should cause the tympanic membrane to move if the middle ear is normal (aerated) and fail to move if it is filled with effusion (mucus or pus). Cerumen may be encountered in the ear canal that obstructs the view of the tympanic membrane or fails to allow insufflation to occur with pneumatic otoscopy. Removal of cerumen may be performed by using an operating otoscope head and an ear curette. However, the use of a headlight, such

as the Lumiview (Welch Allyn, Skaneateles, NY) or operating microscope, permits the use of both hands and superior visualization. Care should be taken to secure the child to prevent sudden movement, and the ear curette should be used gently to avoid causing pain and a laceration of the ear canal. A mechanical test of tympanic compliance (tympanometry) may also be useful to help determine if the middle ear is normally aerated (type A, peaked tracing), fluid-filled (type B, flat tracing), or has negative pressure because it is poorly ventilated, suggesting eustachian tube dysfunction (type C, negative pressure tracing). Examination of a child with an apparent or suspected ear condition often requires objective assessment of hearing by audiometry. Current technology and expertise makes it possible to test a child at any age.

Behavioral audiometry can usually be accurately performed for a child who is older than 6 months of age by sound-field testing. Older children are presented with a tone through insert earphones and are tested across a range of frequencies between 250 and 8000 Hz for ear-specific testing. The hearing thresholds are recorded at each presented frequency, and this represents the air conduction threshold. The sound has to traverse the ear canal, tympanic membrane, and middle ear. The inner ear must respond by creating electrical impulses that are transmitted to the brain. Normal thresholds are less than 20 dB for children.

Bone conduction thresholds test the sensorineural component of hearing. A bone oscillator is used to test a range of frequencies by vibrating the skull, which stimulates the inner ear directly, bypassing the external and middle ear. Normally, air conduction thresholds require less energy than bone conduction thresholds. If bone conduction thresholds require less sound intensity to be heard than air conduction, the child has a conductive hearing loss. If air conduction and bone conduction thresholds are elevated but the same, the child has a sensorineural hearing loss. Most sensorineural hearing loss in children is a result of hair cell dysfunction in the organ of Corti. Hearing loss may be conductive, sensorineural, or mixed. Objective electrophysical tests, such as brainstem auditory-evoked response and sound emission tests that measure the intrinsic sounds from the inner ear (otoacoustic emissions), may be used in young infants and children who cannot participate in behavioral audiometry. All of these tools are used by pediatric audiologists.[5]

For purposes of describing hearing loss, a threshold of 20 to 40 dB is considered mild, 40 to 65 dB is moderate, 55 to 70 dB is moderately severe, 70 to 90 dB is severe, and greater than 90 dB is profound. Four of 1000 children are born with a hearing loss, and 1 of those children is born with a severe to profound hearing loss.

Conductive hearing loss may be corrected with otologic surgery. Hearing aids and frequency modulation (FM) amplification systems may be helpful to children with both conductive and sensorineural hearing loss. Assistance may be needed through auditory training, speech language therapy, and education to maximally develop communication skills. When a child has a sensorineural hearing loss that is too severe to be helped with hearing aids, a cochlear implant may be considered.

A cochlear implant is an electrical device that is implanted under the scalp behind the ear. Its processor converts sound to electrical impulses. A cable travels through the mastoid and facial recess to reach the middle ear, and the electrode array is inserted into the scala tympani of the cochlea through an opening that is made in the cochlea.

Cochlear implants stimulate the neural elements of the cochlea directly and bypass the hair cells. Because the vast majority of sensorineural hearing loss in children is due to hair cell dysfunction, nearly all children get sound perception from a cochlear implant. Rare conditions, such as an absent auditory nerve or an absent cochlea, preclude the use of a cochlear implant.

A multidisciplinary evaluation by a cochlear implantation team is required to evaluate a child and determine family expectations before performing a cochlear implantation. A temporal bone computed tomographic (CT) scan and/or magnetic resonance imaging (MRI) is performed to assess the cochlea and auditory nerves.

Children who are born deaf and are younger than the age of 3 years, as well as children who have already developed communication skills, language, and speech before losing their hearing, derive the greatest benefit from cochlear implants. Cochlear implantation is approved for children 12 months of age or older by the U.S. Food and Drug Administration. Children with cochlear implants should be vaccinated against *Streptococcus pneumoniae,* according to high-risk schedules, and against *Haemophilus influenzae,* according to standard schedules, because the implant wire crosses from the middle ear into the cochlea, increasing the risk of meningitis if the child gets otitis media. After a cochlear implant is performed, considerable auditory oral training is required to maximize a child's benefit to develop skills of audition, speech, and language. A child who has been deaf and without sound perception for several years is expected to benefit to a lesser degree.[6]

OTITIS MEDIA WITH EFFUSION AND INFLAMMATORY DISORDERS

Otitis media with effusion is the most common chronic condition of the ear during childhood. All children are born with small and horizontally oriented eustachian tubes that may at times be unable to clear mucus that is secreted in the mastoid and middle ear normally and when the child has an upper respiratory tract infection. The excess mucus usually clears within a few weeks as the upper respiratory tract infection resolves. Younger children (infants to 3 years of age) and children with craniofacial anomalies, such as cleft palate and Down syndrome, are more prone to having persistent middle ear effusions; there is no medication that is consistently effective in resolving such effusions.

Persistent effusion may cause a conductive hearing loss in the range of 20 to 40 dB. A middle ear effusion may also function as a culture medium and predispose children to recurrent acute otitis media (AOM).

When fluid persists in the middle ear for 3 to 4 months, causing a hearing loss or is associated with AOM, myringotomy and tympanostomy tube placement is helpful to resolve the hearing loss and reduce the frequency and severity of infection.

Myringotomy and placement of a tube is performed under general anesthesia using an operating microscope. A small incision is made in any quadrant of the tympanic membrane except the posterosuperior quadrant, where there would be risk of injuring the ossicles. The mucus is suctioned from the ear, and a Silastic tube is placed in the myringotomy to provide prolonged ventilation of the middle ear. The tube will usually extrude and the tympanostomy will heal in 6 months to 1 year. When the ear is no longer ventilated by a tube, the eustachian tube must ventilate the middle ear. If fluid recurs and persists, a repeat procedure may be needed. Most children outgrow this problem as their eustachian tube grows. Occasionally, adenoid tissue in the nasopharynx may contribute to the persistence of middle ear effusion and may also be removed at the time that a tube is placed. Children who have had multiple sets of tubes are candidates for adenoidectomy.

ACUTE OTITIS MEDIA

Acute otitis media is the most common infection of childhood except for acute upper respiratory tract infections. It is the most common bacterial infection for which children seek medical care from their primary care physician. Usual pathogens causing AOM include *Streptococcus pneumoniae, Haemophilus influenzae,* and *Moraxella catarrhalis.*[7]

AOM usually causes severe deep ear pain, fever, and a conductive hearing loss in the affected ear. The purulence in the middle ear is also present in the mastoid air cells because they are connected.

To prevent the overuse of antibiotics, the American Academy of Pediatrics (AAP) and the American Academy of Family Practitioners (AAFP) developed guidelines in 2004 to improve accuracy of diagnosis of AOM.[8] Three components should be present to diagnose AOM, including history of acute onset of symptoms within 48 hours of presentation, presence of middle ear effusion confirmed by pneumatic otoscopy or tympanometry, and signs of middle ear inflammation. The tympanic membrane typically is reddened and bulging, with obliteration of normal landmarks.[8]

Once an accurate diagnosis is made, the AAP/AAFP guidelines offer options for treatment in otherwise healthy children. They advocate that a period of observation (48 to 72 hours) is justified because AOM spontaneously resolves in many children (80% of episodes of AOM resolve within 2 to 7 days of symptom onset). Very young children (less than 6 months old) and those with Down syndrome, immune disorders, craniofacial anomalies, or chronic medical conditions should not be considered candidates for observation, because they are at higher risk of developing complications such as mastoiditis or meningitis.

Table 55-1 describes specific recommendations for treatment in otherwise healthy children aged 6 months to 12 years,

---

TABLE 55-1

AAFP/AAP Guidelines for Treatment of Acute Otitis Media in Children Younger Than 12 Years

Child Age	Certain Diagnosis	Uncertain Diagnosis
Younger than 6 months	Antibiotics	Antibiotics
6 months to 2 years	Antibiotics	Antibiotic if severe illness*; observe if nonsevere illness†
> 2 years to 12 years	Antibiotic if severe illness*; observe if nonsevere illness†	Observe

*Severe illness: fever > 39° C and/or moderate to severe otalgia.
†Nonsevere illness: fever < 39° C and/or mild otalgia.
AAFP, American Academy of Family Practitioners; AAP, American Academy of Pediatrics.

based on age, certainty of diagnosis, and severity of symptoms. All affected children should be given pain control, and children who are treated with observation should be followed up in 48 to 72 hours and treated if they continue to manifest symptoms.

Recommended first-line antibiotic therapy is higher-dose amoxicillin (80 mg per kilogram per day in two divided doses for 5 to 10 days). Higher dose therapy can effectively cover even intermediate and some highly resistant strains of *S. pneumoniae*. Infections caused by this organism are most likely to cause more serious complications and are least likely to spontaneously resolve. Azithromycin, erythromycin, or clarithromycin can be used as alternatives in patients with type 1 allergy (anaphylaxis or hives to amoxicillin). Second-line antibiotics should be considered in patients who fail to improve after several days of first-line antibiotics and includes higher-strength amoxicillin-clavulanate (90 mg per kilogram per day in two divided doses for 10 days) or oral cefdinir, cefuroxime, cefpodoxime, clindamycin, and, less commonly, intravenous or intramuscular ceftriaxone.

Occasionally, AOM does not respond as expected to standard antibiotic therapy. When this occurs, culture and sensitivity testing can be obtained by tympanocentesis. After sterilizing the ear canal with alcohol, a 22-gauge spinal needle can be placed through the posterior or anterior inferior quadrant of the tympanic membrane and fluid can be aspirated with a small syringe.

Complications of AOM are uncommon if appropriate antibiotic therapy is used. The conductive hearing loss resolves as the middle ear effusion clears. However, infection may necrose the tympanic membrane, causing a spontaneous perforation. Small perforations usually heal in less than 7 days, but larger perforations may persist, cause a conductive hearing loss, and require a tympanoplasty for closure. The ossicular chain may also be disrupted by necrosis of the long process of the incus requiring ossicular reconstruction to restore hearing.

Acute coalescent mastoiditis occurs when infection erodes the bony mastoid cortex and destroys bony septae within the mastoid. A subperiosteal abscess may also develop over the mastoid process. There is usually postauricular erythema and edema over the mastoid area. The auricle is displaced laterally and forward (Fig. 55-1). Otoscopy reveals forward displacement of the posterior superior skin of the ear canal.

In addition to antibiotics, treatment should include a wide-field myringotomy from the anterior inferior quadrant to the posterior inferior quadrant, a tympanostomy tube placement for middle ear drainage, and a postauricular mastoidectomy to drain the subperiosteal abscess and the mastoid.

Facial nerve paralysis may occur from inflammation of that portion of the facial nerve that is exposed in the middle ear during AOM. Treatment with parenteral antibiotics and ototopical antibiotic drops applied in the ear canal through a tympanostomy tube almost always results in complete recovery of facial function. A short course of oral steroids may also be helpful. Facial nerve recovery may take a few weeks to several months.

Intracranial complications of AOM include meningitis, epidural abscess, brain abscess, otitic hydrocephalus, and lateral sinus thrombosis. Meningitis is the most common intracranial complication of AOM and may be associated with profound sensorineural hearing loss and loss of vestibular function. Treatment of the intracranial complications of AOM is focused

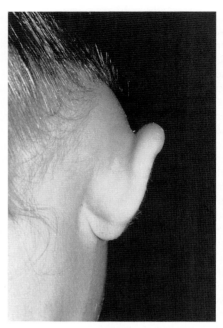

FIGURE 55-1 Acute mastoiditis. Extension of the acute inflammatory process from the middle ear and mastoid air cell systems to the overlying soft tissues displaces the auricle in an inferior and lateral direction from the side of the head. Fluctuance may be palpated over the mastoid cortex, and a defect in the cortical bone can frequently be appreciated. Surgical drainage with mastoidectomy is required.

on appropriate treatment of the intracranial process, in addition to a wide-field myringotomy and tympanostomy tube placement in the affected ear.[9]

OTITIS MEDIA WITH EFFUSION/CHRONIC OTITIS MEDIA/CHRONIC SUPPURATIVE OTITIS MEDIA

Otitis media with effusion is a descriptive term that refers to persistent middle ear effusion that usually is serous or mucoid in nature. Chronic otitis media is a term used to describe the effusion if it lasts longer than 3 months. Otitis media with effusion may occur following an ear infection, but can occur spontaneously, especially when the nose has been congested. It may be associated with hearing loss and the child may or may not be symptomatic with pain, irritability, or poor balance. Most effusions resolve spontaneously within weeks, and most children affected are younger than 5 years of age.

In otherwise healthy children, hearing tests or hearing screens should be performed once the effusion has been present for more than 3 months, and sooner if significant hearing loss is suspected or if the child is at high risk for developing significant speech and language delays. The associated hearing loss usually falls in the mild range (30 dB), but even in normal children, may contribute to the development of speech and language delays. Speech and language tests should be considered if hearing loss is documented. Children should be evaluated for surgical treatment with bilateral myringotomy and tube placement if they have ongoing pain or irritability attributable to the effusion, structural changes to the tympanic membrane (such as thinning or deep retractions), documented speech and language delays, or those who are at high risk for complications if observed (Down syndrome, those with existing speech delay, autism, or neurocognitive delays). Adenoidectomy would be considered as well if the adenoids are found to be enlarged, especially if the child has symptoms of heavy snoring, sleep apnea, or chronic nasal congestion.[10]

Chronic suppurative otitis media occurs when otorrhea (drainage of pus or mucous) persists for more than 3 months, either through a perforation of the tympanic membrane or through a tube in the tympanic membrane. A cholesteatoma of the middle ear may also be present in patients who have perforated tympanic membranes. A cholesteatoma is a squamous epithelial-lined cyst that may be congenital or acquired. Congenital cholesteatomas are caused by epithelial rests that persist in the middle ear during temporal bone development. They present behind an intact tympanic membrane and appear as a white, smooth mass, most often located in the anterior superior quadrant of the middle ear. They expand over time and are filled with squamous debris and may erode the ossicular chain and extend into the mastoid.

Acquired cholesteatomas develop from skin entering the middle ear after a tympanic membrane perforation or a retraction pocket from eustachian tube dysfunction and are usually located in the posterior-superior quadrant of the middle ear space. Cholesteatomas are usually painless, cause a conductive hearing loss, and, in acquired cases, often present as otorrhea. The otorrhea should be treated with ototopical antibiotic eardrops, but the only treatment of cholesteatomas is complete surgical excision by tympanomastoid surgery and ossicular reconstruction.[11] The potential complications of cholesteatomas are the same as those for acute suppurative otitis media (ASOM).

TRAUMA

Objects stuck deeply into the ear canal, such as a cotton-tipped applicator, may perforate the tympanic membrane. This usually causes acute pain, bleeding, and a conductive hearing loss. If the ossicular chain is not disrupted, the vast majority of these perforations will heal spontaneously in about 2 weeks. If the tympanic membrane is perforated and the middle ear is contaminated with water, topical antibiotics should be given.

Lacerations of the auricle should be cleaned to prevent tattooing and repaired by careful approximation of the skin and soft tissue to restore the contours of the ear. The cartilage itself does not usually need to be sutured. Partially or totally avulsed tissue should be replaced. If necrosis of tissue occurs, it can be debrided as needed. In severe injuries of the auricle, oral antibiotic treatment to cover *S. aureus* and *Pseudomonas* species is helpful to prevent chondritis and loss of the cartilage framework.

Blunt trauma to the ear is commonly seen in wrestlers, in children with poor neuromuscular tone, or in children with self-injurious behaviors. Blood or serum collects between the periosteum and the auricular cartilage. If the cartilage is fractured, the collection may occur on both sides of the ear. Evacuation of the collection is required to restore the contours of the ear, prevent infection, and prevent scarring with formation of a "cauliflower ear." Aspiration of the fluid and placement of a mastoid dressing for compression may be tried but is most often unsuccessful. Incision and drainage provides for complete evacuation of the blood or serum. Cotton dental rolls placed on each side of the auricle and held in place with bolster mattress sutures is the most effective management. The dental rolls should be left in place for 7 to 10 days while the patient also continues with a course of oral antibiotics. No outer dressing is required except in a child with cognitive impairment, who may pick at the bolsters.[11]

Blunt head trauma may disrupt the inner ear membranes causing sensorineural hearing loss and vertigo. No treatment is required, and the injury and symptoms may resolve spontaneously, but the sensorineural hearing loss may persist. Severe head trauma may cause fracture of the temporal bone of the skull. Temporal bone fractures can be classified as longitudinal, transverse, or mixed (Fig. 55-2) but are often

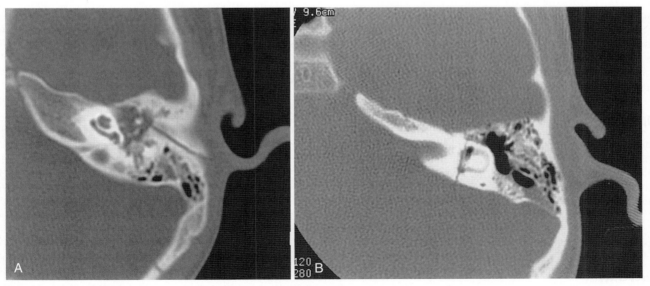

FIGURE 55-2   A, Longitudinal temporal bone fracture. These fractures run parallel to the petrous pyramid. The otic capsule is generally not affected by the fracture lines. Balance, hearing, and facial function are generally preserved. **B,** Transverse temporal bone fracture. These fractures generally extend through the cochlea and facial canal and result in deafness, vertigo, and facial nerve paralysis of immediate onset. Facial nerve exploration with repair should always be considered in these cases.

complex and do not neatly fit into one category or another. A high-resolution, thin-section CT scan of the temporal bone will define the extent of the fracture. The middle ear and mastoid are filled with blood when a fracture is present. The blood causes a conductive hearing loss that resolves when the ear clears.

Otoscopic evaluation of a child with a temporal bone fracture may reveal a laceration of the ear canal and tympanic membrane. Blood is usually present in the ear canal, and the tympanic membrane appears to be dark blue because the middle ear is filled with blood. There is often ecchymosis of the mastoid area (Battle's sign).

It is important during evaluation of a skull and temporal bone fracture to note and record the function of the facial nerve if the patient is not unconscious. Facial nerve paralysis may be immediate or delayed in onset. Delayed facial nerve paralysis has a good prognosis for spontaneous recovery. Immediate complete facial paralysis may indicate disruption of the nerve or compression by bone fragments. Immediate facial nerve paralysis requires exploration and repair once the patient is stable and sufficiently recovered from any associated trauma. The facial nerve should be decompressed in the mastoid, middle ear, and middle cranial fossa. Bone chips impinging on the nerve should be removed, and the nerve should be sutured or grafted if needed. All patients with temporal bone fractures should have an audiogram once their condition has stabilized. If the fracture disarticulates the ossicles, a conductive hearing loss will persist after the blood has cleared from the middle ear and mastoid.

Fractures of the temporal bone may transverse the cochlea and vestibular apparatus. These fractures usually cause a severe sensorineural hearing loss and loss of vestibular function on the affected side. Most children compensate for vestibular injuries within weeks, but sensorineural hearing loss is less likely to improve. A concussive injury of the cochlea may also simultaneously be present in the opposite ear in severe head trauma.

Temporal bone fractures may permit leakage of cerebrospinal fluid (CSF) into the middle ear and mastoid. CSF may also drain through the lacerated tympanic membrane, causing CSF otorrhea. These leaks usually stop spontaneously, but persistent CSF otorrhea may require a lumbar drain to reduce the pressure and permit healing. Rarely, tympanomastoid exploration is required to close the leak. Persistent CSF leaks in the ear are associated with meningitis.

TUMORS

Benign and malignant tumors of the ear are rare. Glomus tympanicum tumors and neuromas of the facial nerve may present in the middle ear. Also, eosinophilic granuloma and rhabdomyosarcoma may involve the structures of the temporal bone.[12,13]

Nose

ANATOMY

The nose can be divided into three anatomic sections. The bony vault is the immobile portion of the nose. It consists of the paired nasal bones, the frontal process of the maxillary bone, and the nasal process of the frontal bone. The cartilaginous vault is supported by the upper lateral cartilages and the cartilaginous nasal septum. The nasal lobule is supported by the lower lateral cartilages and the cartilaginous septum. The nasal septum is formed by the quadrilateral cartilage anteriorly. The posterior septum is composed of bone from the vomer, perpendicular plate of the ethmoid, nasal crest of the maxillary bone, and palatine bone.

Both the internal and external carotid artery systems supply blood to the nose. The roof and lateral wall of the internal nasal cavity are supplied by the anterior and posterior ethmoidal arteries, sphenopalatine artery, and greater palatine artery. The septum is supplied by the anterior and posterior ethmoidal arteries, palatine artery, and the superior labial artery. The convergence of these vessels in the anterior segment of the nose is referred to as the Kiesselbach plexus or the Little area. Venous drainage is accomplished mainly by the ophthalmic, anterior facial, and sphenopalatine veins.

The olfactory bulb is positioned high in the roof of the nasal cavity and is responsible for the sense of smell. Sensory information is transported by nerves that penetrate the cribriform plate and traverse cranial nerve I (the olfactory nerve) to the brain. Smell is also an important component of what is perceived as taste.

Bony projections, called turbinates, form the lateral nasal wall and significantly increase the surface area of the nose, allowing for more efficient humidification and warming of the air to 36° C. Three turbinates are usually present (i.e., inferior, middle, and superior). A supreme turbinate, which is essentially a flap of mucosa, is occasionally present. The turbinates contribute to the turbulent airflow that creates approximately 50% of the total airflow resistance to the lungs.

Cleaning of air is accomplished through the nasal hairs (vibrissae) and the mucosal surface. Anteriorly, the nose is lined with stratified squamous epithelium, which changes to respiratory epithelium immediately anterior to the turbinates. Trapped debris is transported in a posterior direction into the nasopharynx by a mucociliary transport mechanism.

Speech is affected by nasal anatomy and pathologic conditions. Hyponasality from nasal obstruction or hypernasality from an excessive air leak can affect voice quality and intelligibility of speech.

EMBRYOLOGY

The nose serves as a drainage port for the paranasal sinuses. The meati are spaces between the lateral aspect of the nasal turbinates and the medial aspects of the lateral nasal wall. Each meatus is named for the turbinate that surrounds it. The maxillary, frontal, and anterior ethmoidal sinuses drain into the middle meatus. The posterior ethmoidal sinuses drain into the superior meatus. The sphenoidal sinus drains into an area known as the sphenoethmoidal recess that is located posterior and superior to the superior turbinate. The nasolacrimal duct drains into the inferior meatus.

The nasal cavities develop from the nasal pits in the 4-week embryo. These pits deepen and move medially to form the nasal cavity. The oronasal membrane that separates the nose from the mouth resolves in the seventh week to permit communication between the nose and nasopharynx.

The paranasal sinuses develop from an outpouching of the lateral nasal walls during the third and fourth months of development. The maxillary and ethmoidal sinuses are present at birth. The frontal and sphenoidal sinuses develop several years after birth. The frontal sinus begins to develop at 7 years of age but is not fully aerated until adulthood.[14]

INFLAMMATORY CONDITIONS

Viral rhinosinusitis (the common cold) accounts for the majority of nose and sinus infections. It is caused by many strains of viruses and is a self-limited infection. Symptoms of fever, nasal congestion, headache, and clear rhinorrhea usually resolve over 5 to 7 days. Treatment is symptomatic.

BACTERIAL RHINOSINUSITIS

Acute bacterial rhinosinusitis may often follow an acute viral upper respiratory tract infection. The most common bacteria causing rhinosinusitis are *Streptococcus pneumoniae, Haemophilus influenzae,* and *Moraxella catarrhalis.* Acute rhinosinusitis causes malaise, headache, and nasal congestion. There may also be pain localized to the sinus region or pain on palpation over the maxillary or frontal sinuses. Chronic sinus infection may persist after the acute phase, and symptoms often last longer than 30 days.

The gold standard for diagnosing sinusitis is CT of the sinuses, but a thorough history and nasal examination is usually sufficient to diagnose acute rhinosinusitis. The nasal cavity can be visualized by using a large speculum on an otoscopic head. The posterior nasal cavity can be visualized with either a straight-rod endoscope or a flexible fiberoptic nasopharyngoscope.

The treatment of rhinosinusitis includes oral antibiotics, short-term use of topical nasal decongestants (e.g., oxymetazoline), and saline nasal sprays. Topical nasal corticosteroid sprays may be helpful for the treatment of both acute and chronic sinusitis.

Chronic sinusitis in a child may be exacerbated by gastroesophageal reflux disease, immunodeficiencies, mucociliary dysfunction, and, more commonly, upper respiratory allergy. These predisposing conditions should be managed while treating the sinus infection. If the signs and symptoms of chronic sinus infection persist, a sinus CT is required to evaluate the condition of the sinus mucosa and the drainage pathways. Endoscopic sinus surgery may be necessary to open the involved sinuses to provide drainage.

Chronic inflammation of the nasal and sinus mucosa may lead to nasal and sinus polyp formation that chronically obstructs the nose and sinuses. Antrochoanal polyps are large polyps that originate from the walls of the maxillary sinus and extend through the nasal cavity into the nasopharynx. Nasal polyps may be removed endoscopically, but a large antrochoanal polyp may require removal through an open maxillary sinus procedure. Nasal polyps in a child should always prompt an evaluation for cystic fibrosis.

COMPLICATIONS OF SINUSITIS

The sinuses surround the orbit so a common complication of acute rhinosinusitis in children is orbital cellulitis with erythema and edema of the eyelids. Chemosis (edema of the ocular conjunctiva) is usually absent. However, if a periorbital subperiosteal abscess forms adjacent to an infected sinus, there may be proptosis, chemosis, ophthalmoplegia, and loss of vision. Infection in the ethmoidal sinuses most commonly results in this complication. Subperiosteal periorbital abscess is demonstrated best by sinus CT (with axial and coronal cuts). Initial treatment should include intravenous antibiotics. Endoscopic or external drainage may be required in some cases.

Intracranial complications of sinusitis include cerebritis, meningitis, cavernous sinus thrombosis, as well as epidural, subdural, and brain abscesses. Treatment of impending or confirmed intracranial complications requires surgical drainage of the involved sinus and concurrent treatment of the intracranial lesion by a neurosurgeon.[15]

FUNGAL SINUSITIS

Fungal sinusitis may occur in immunocompromised children, specifically severe diabetics, children undergoing chemotherapy, and bone marrow transplant recipients. The more common invasive fungi include *Mucor* and *Aspergillus* species. The treatment of fungal sinusitis involves surgical drainage and intravenous antifungal agents.

However, a chronic form of fungal sinusitis is allergic fungal sinusitis. The presence of fungi causes inflammatory cells to proliferate in the sinuses, causing symptoms of nasal plugging and facial pain, along with discharge or polyps. These patients usually have other signs of allergy, such as asthma. The treatment of this condition is corticosteroids and debridement of the involved sinuses. The diagnosis is made by sinus CT findings and the presence of eosinophils as well as fungi in the sinus secretions that are removed at the time of surgery.[16]

CONGENITAL MALFORMATIONS

Pyriform Aperture Stenosis

Congenital stenosis of the anterior bony aperture causes partial nasal obstruction that may be severe enough to cause difficulty feeding, respiratory distress, and failure to thrive. Anterior rhinoscopy demonstrates a very constricted nasal opening bilaterally. CT of the nose shows marked narrowing of the pyriform aperture.

Neonates are obligate nasal breathers, and severe stenosis must be surgically corrected. Because the stenotic segment is very anterior and the remainder of the nasal cavity is normal, removal of the constricting bone with drills is done through a sublabial approach. The nasal openings are stented with 3.0-mm endotracheal tube stents that are sutured in place and removed after a few days.

Choanal Atresia

Choanal atresia may be unilateral or bilateral. The obstructing tissue is usually a bony plate, but a few cases will have only membranous atresia. Unilateral choanal atresia presents as chronic unilateral rhinorrhea. There is no significant respiratory distress. Because neonates are obligate nose breathers, bilateral choanal atresia is associated with severe respiratory distress, difficulty feeding, and failure to thrive. The diagnosis is suspected if catheters cannot be passed through the nose and into the pharynx. The obstruction may be visualized with a narrow flexible nasopharyngoscope after the nasal cavity has

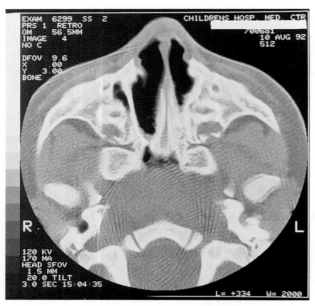

FIGURE 55-3   Choanal atresia. This disorder frequently presents at birth with respiratory distress.

been suctioned of mucus and the nasal mucosa has been constricted with a nasal decongestant (e.g., oxymetazoline). The diagnosis is best made with CT of the nasal cavity. CT will demonstrate the atresia, define the tissue (bony or membranous), and show the configuration of the entire nasal cavity.

Choanal atresia may be successfully treated by removing the obstructing tissue transnasally. Curettes, lasers, microdebriders, bone punches, and drills may all be effective to remove the atresia plate. However, when the bony plate is very thick and there is an extremely narrow posterior nasal cavity, a transpalatal repair is more direct. A transpalatal repair provides better access for more effective removal of the bony plate and posterior septum (Fig. 55-3). Stents fashioned from endotracheal tubes are placed and secured with sutures to the septum. They are removed after several weeks. The stents must be moistened with saline and suctioned several times daily to prevent mucus plugging and acute respiratory distress. Transpalatal repair of choanal atresia has a lower incidence of restenosis.[11]

Nasal Dermoid

Nasal dermoid cysts or sinuses present in the midline of the nasal dorsum (Fig. 55-4). They usually appear as a round bump or a pit with hair present in the pit (Fig. 55-5). They also may become infected. Nasal dermoid sinuses may extend through the nasal bones into the nasofrontal area and have an intracranial component. Both CT and MRI may be necessary to demonstrate the extent of the dermoid. Surgical removal is required to prevent infection and recurrence. This may be done between ages 3 and 5 years if prior infection has not occurred. Dermoids confined to the nose are resected completely using a midline incision with an ellipse around the sinus tract. The tract is followed to its termination, and the nasal bones may need to be separated to reach the end of the tract.[11] If an intracranial component is present, a combined craniotomy and nasal approach with a neurosurgeon is recommended.

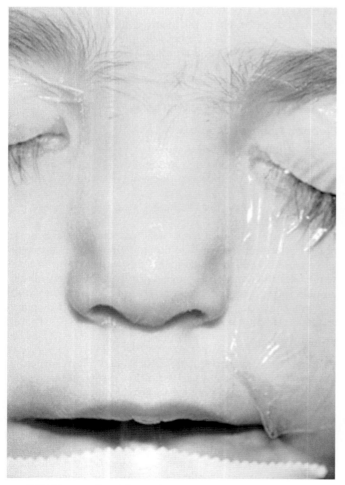

FIGURE 55-4   Nasal dermoid presenting in the midline as a pit.

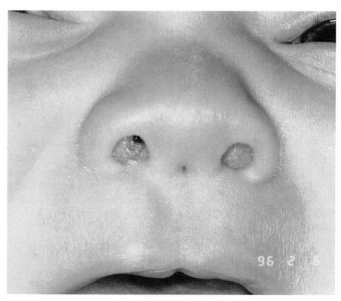

FIGURE 55-5   Nasal dermoid. These lesions typically present on the nasal dorsum as a single midline pit, often with a hair extruding from the depths of the pit. The pits may also be found on the columella. The dermoid will then tract through the septum toward the cranial base.

Nasal Glioma and Encephalocele

A nasal glioma presents as an intranasal mass and may be confused with a nasal polyp. The mass contains dysplastic brain tissue and may have an intracranial connection. CT and MRI are important to define the extent of the glioma and intracranial component as well as to plan the surgical approach.

An encephalocele presents as a soft compressible mass and may also be confused with a nasal polyp or a nasal dermoid. Intranasal encephaloceles extend through a defect in the skull at the cribriform plate. CT and MRI define the extent of the encephalocele and are necessary to design the surgical approach. Surgical removal often includes a frontal craniotomy. Nasal encephaloceles may be associated with CSF rhinorrhea and meningitis.

TRAUMA

Anosmia

Head trauma can lead to temporary or permanent anosmia (lack of sense of smell). In one large study of head trauma patients ($n = 190$), 11% reported loss of sense of smell that persisted after their initial recovery and later was confirmed by smell tests. Those at higher risk had trauma that led to intracranial hematoma and/or hemorrhages or injury near the skull base.[17]

Nasal Fracture

An infant may be born with the soft nasal bones and the septum deviated to one side either as a result of a difficult delivery or from persistent intrauterine compression of the nose. The nasal structures can most often be returned to the midline with digital manipulation. If the nasal deformity is partially reduced, the nose usually straightens with growth during the first 12 to 18 months of age.

Nasal bone and nasal septal fractures in older children usually occur from a blow to the face during sports. There is usually a brief period of epistaxis and deviation of the nasal dorsum to one side. Swelling occurs rapidly, and the degree of the cosmetic deformity or the need for fracture reduction may not be easily determined. At the fourth to sixth day after injury, the edema subsides and the need for reduction can be determined. Nasal bone radiographs are of little help in making this judgment; so, the need for nasal fracture reduction is usually based solely on clinical examination. Effective closed nasal fracture reduction may be done up to 2 weeks after the injury. Closed reduction under general anesthesia is the method of choice. Oral antibiotics prevent infection and are essential if nasal packing is used to support the nasal bone.

Although nasal fracture reduction is not urgent, a septal hematoma from a fractured septum should be excluded by the initial physician seeing the child. A septal hematoma that remains untreated may cause cartilage necrosis and loss of nasal support, with a resulting saddle-nose deformity. Treatment of a septal hematoma is with incision and evacuation of the clot. The mucoperichondrial flap should then be sutured in place by bolster sutures through the septum. A small rubber band drain may be required and, if used, should remain in place for 12 to 24 hours, and antibiotics be given for 10 to 14 days to prevent secondary infection while a drain is in place.

Epistaxis in children usually occurs in Little's area of the anterior septum and frequently results from digital trauma (nose picking). The bleeding usually stops with pressure by squeezing the nasal ala. Infrequently, cauterization of the vessels under general anesthesia is needed to reduce the frequency of bleeding. In cases that fail to stop with pressure, the nose should be packed with absorbable materials (such as Gelfoam or cellulose) or nonabsorbable gauze. Finally, in severe cases, embolization or emergent surgery has been used to control bleeding from the internal maxillary and anterior ethmoid arteries, which are the primary sources of nose bleeds. Hematology consultation should be considered in severe or recurrent cases to evaluate for coagulopathies.

Nasal Foreign Bodies

Children may be observed inserting a foreign body into their nose, or they may inform their parents of the event. Most children, however, present with a foul-smelling unilateral purulent nasal discharge and deny putting anything into their nose.

Most nasal foreign bodies are painless and do no harm to the nose but cause a foul nasal discharge. Disc batteries, on the other hand, cause very rapid alkali burns of the nasal cavity and pain. Batteries must be removed from the nose quickly because the chemical burn occurs in minutes to hours. If extensive tissue necrosis occurs, it may cause a nasal stenosis or septal perforation.

Removal of a nasal foreign body is aided by decongesting the nasal mucosa and using a headlamp to visualize the foreign body. A variety of forceps or hooks may be used. If the object is deep in the nose, the removal is best performed under general anesthesia. The endotracheal tube prevents aspiration of the object into the tracheobronchial tree if it is pushed back into the nasopharynx. One must remember that multiple foreign bodies may be present on one or both sides of the nose.

Nasal Lacerations

Nasal lacerations should be closed with care to match edges and restore the contours of the nose. Standard wound closure technique is used. The nasal mucosa does not need to be sutured unless a large flap is displaced.

NASAL/NASOPHARYNGEAL TUMORS

Rhabdomyosarcoma, lymphoma, squamous cell carcinoma, and esthesioneuroblastoma may occur in the nose and sinuses of children. Fortunately, these malignant tumors are very rare in children. The treatment of children with malignant tumors of the nose and sinuses usually involves a multidisciplinary, multimodal approach.

Juvenile nasopharyngeal angiofibroma is a benign tumor of adolescent males that originates from the lateral wall of the nose and nasopharynx. The tumor may completely obstruct the nose and fill the nasopharynx. This type of angiofibroma may also extend intracranially through the base of the skull. Patients with these tumors present with nasal obstruction, recurrent epistaxis, and rhinorrhea.

The tumor may be seen with a flexible fiberoptic nasopharyngoscope or a rod lens telescope after decongesting the nasal mucosa. It appears as a smooth reddish mass. Biopsy of the mass should be avoided because of the potential for severe bleeding. CT and MRI define the extent and location of the tumor. On imaging, the mass originates in the pterygopalatine fossa within the aperture of the pterygoid (vidian) canal. It causes anterior bowing of the posterior wall of the maxillary sinus and erosion of the greater wing of the sphenoid as it grows into the nose and nasopharynx. MR angiography helps to delineate the blood supply, which may originate from both the internal and external carotid arteries. Contrast angiography may be reserved for presurgical planning and embolization of the copious blood supply that is often present.

The treatment of juvenile nasopharyngeal angiofibroma is complete surgical resection after preoperative embolization. Depending on the material used, the embolization may be effective for days to weeks. A variety of surgical approaches may be used, including endoscopic resection of small tumors using instruments to reduce blood loss, such as suction cautery or coblation tools. Extensive tumors may require a combined midfacial and craniotomy approach.[18]

Some authors have proposed radiation therapy as the primary treatment of juvenile nasopharyngeal angiofibroma, but many surgeons are concerned about the long-term effects of radiation in children, including the induction of malignant tumors.

Nasopharyngeal carcinoma can occur in adolescents and is more common in those of Asian or African descent. It arises from the epithelium of the nasopharynx and histologically is composed of lymphoepithelial cells of variable stages of differentiation. Epstein-Barr viral infection has been implicated as a possible cause in some cases, but genetic factors appear to make some individuals more susceptible to developing this tumor. Most children present with advanced disease and tend to have undifferentiated subtypes. They usually have a history of unilateral nasal plugging and otalgia or hearing loss caused by a blocked eustachian tube. They may also present with metastasis in the posterior triangle lymph nodes. Treatment consists of radiotherapy and, in some cases, adjuvant chemotherapy.

Oral Cavity/Pharynx

ANATOMY

The boundaries of the oral cavity include the lips anteriorly, the cheeks laterally, and the palate superiorly. The posterior boundary is a plane that extends from the soft palate to the junction of the anterior two thirds and posterior one third of the tongue. The oral cavity is composed of the vestibule, the space between the lips and cheeks and alveolar ridges, and the oral cavity proper. The vestibule and oral cavity proper are separated by the alveolar ridge and teeth. The vestibule is divided in the midline by the frenula of the upper and lower lips. The alveolar ridge is contiguous superiorly with the hard palate. The parotid ducts (Stensen ducts) enter the vestibule opposite the second maxillary molars. The submandibular ducts (Wharton ducts) enter the floor of mouth near the lingual frenulum.

The palate is formed by a fusion of the primary palate anteriorly and medial growth of the palatal processes that form the secondary palate. The hard palate divides the nasal and oral cavities and is formed by the premaxilla and the horizontal plates of the palatine bones. The soft palate is formed by a muscular aponeurosis of the tensor veli palatini tendon. Five muscles insert into this aponeurosis and include the tensor veli palatini, levator veli palatini, palatoglossus, palatopharyngeus, and the musculus uvulae. Defects in formation of the hard and/or soft palate result in clefting. The sensory and motor innervation of the palate is through the trigeminal nerve and pharyngeal plexus.

The circumvallate papillae divide the tongue into the anterior two thirds that lies in the oral cavity and the posterior one third lying in the oropharynx. The innervation and vascular supply to the two major divisions of the tongue reflect their differences in origin—the anterior two thirds of the tongue being a first branchial arch derivative (trigeminal), whereas the posterior one third being a combination of third and fourth arch derivatives (pharyngeal plexus). The hypoglossal nerve supplies motor innervation to the intrinsic musculature. In addition to the intrinsic tongue musculature, the action of four extrinsic muscles combine to provide mobility. The genioglossus protrudes and depresses, the hyoglossus retracts and depresses, the styloglossus retracts, and the palatoglossus elevates. In addition to the circumvallate papillae, other taste buds on the tongue surface include conical, filiform, fungiform, and foliate papillae.

The pharynx is a fibromuscular tube that extends from the skull base to the level of the cricoid cartilage of the larynx and can be divided into three levels. The nasopharynx extends from the skull base to the level of the soft palate, the oropharynx extends from the soft palate to the tongue base, and the hypopharynx extends from the tongue base to the cricoid cartilage. Three muscular constrictors combine to form the muscular portion of the pharynx: superior, middle, and inferior constrictors. The Passavant ridge is a muscular segment of the superior constrictor that is involved in velopharyngeal closure. Lower fibers of the inferior constrictor help to form the upper esophageal sphincter. The motor and sensory innervation of the pharynx is from the glossopharyngeal and vagus nerves via the pharyngeal plexus.

A collection of lymphoid tissue within the pharynx forms the Waldeyer's ring, which includes the palatine tonsils, the adenoids (pharyngeal tonsil), and lymphoid follicles lining the lateral and posterior pharyngeal walls.

ACUTE PHARYNGOTONSILLITIS

In addition to the acute onset of sore throat, viral pharyngitis typically presents with fever and malaise. Signs include erythema of the pharynx and cervical lymphadenopathy. Depending on the viral agent, associated symptoms of nasal obstruction and rhinorrhea may also be present. Rhinovirus, coronavirus, parainfluenza virus, respiratory syncytial virus, adenovirus, and influenza virus are agents responsible for viral pharyngitis.

Primary herpetic gingivostomatitis, caused by herpes simplex virus types 1 or 2, presents as fever, adenopathy, and vesicles and ulcers on the lips, tongue, buccal mucosa, soft palate, and pharyngeal mucosa. Herpangina and Coxsackie virus (hand-foot-and-mouth disease) are viral infections that involve the oropharynx. Epstein-Barr virus (EBV) infection (infectious mononucleosis) presents as acute pharyngotonsillitis (often with white sloughing debris on the tonsils), fever, generalized adenopathy, malaise, and splenomegaly. Although EBV infection is suspected by the appearance of 10% or more atypical lymphocytes on a complete blood cell count and the presence of a positive Monospot test, the definitive diagnosis is confirmed by elevated titers of EBV. A short course of corticosteroids has been proven to reduce the lymphoid hypertrophy that can cause acute airway obstruction.

Group A beta-hemolytic streptococci (GABHS, i.e., *S. pyogenes*) commonly infect the pharynx. In addition to sore throat, associated symptoms include fever, headache, and abdominal pain. Associated signs include pharyngeal erythema, halitosis, tonsillar exudates, and tender lymphadenopathy. Lack of cough helps differentiate it from other upper respiratory tract infections. Diagnosis may be confirmed initially with a rapid streptococcal antigen test. Because rapid antigen testing is more sensitive than formal plating on blood agar, a negative test does not need confirmation, but positive rapid streptococcal tests should be confirmed with formal plating. Other bacterial pathogens that cause acute pharyngitis include *Haemophilus influenzae* and groups C and G beta-hemolytic streptococci. Occasionally, concurrent infection with penicillin-resistant *Staphylococcus aureus* may interfere with treatment of a GABHS infection.[19] Although many cases of GABHS infections respond to treatment with penicillin V or amoxicillin, emerging resistance to oropharyngeal pathogens mandates treatment of recalcitrant cases with an antibiotic having known effectiveness against beta-lactamase–producing organisms. In cases in which a lack of compliance is suspected, intramuscular benzathine penicillin or ceftriaxone may be used.

Acute pharyngitis may also be associated with acute bacterial infections of the nose, nasopharynx, and sinuses. These infections may be caused by a variety of viral and bacterial pathogens; in addition to a sore throat, symptoms include fever, mucopurulent nasal drainage, nasal obstruction, and facial pain.

RECURRENT PHARYNGOTONSILLITIS

Recurrent infection of the pharynx may be either viral or bacterial. GABHS are the most worrisome bacterial organisms, because recurrent infection may lead to complications such as scarlet fever, acute rheumatic fever, septic arthritis, and acute glomerulonephritis. In addition to a history of multiple positive cultures for *S. pyogenes*, elevated antistreptolysin-O (ASO) titers may identify patients with chronic infection who are at risk for developing complications. Some asymptomatic children may be chronic carriers of GABHS, and elevated ASO titers may not be a reliable indicator for distinguishing between an active infection and the carrier state.

Treatment of recurrent streptococcal infection or the child who is a carrier should include a trial course of an antibiotic shown to reduce carriage (e.g., clindamycin, vancomycin, or rifampin). Children with recurrent pharyngotonsillitis unresponsive to medical therapy or those who suffer a complication should be considered for surgical management. Whereas treatment of each child should be individualized, suggested guidelines for surgical candidates include seven infections in 1 year, five or more infections per year for 2 years, or three or more infections per year for 3 years.[20] Other factors to be considered in using a surgical option include severity of infection, response to antibiotic therapy, loss of time from school, and need for hospitalization.

CHRONIC PHARYNGOTONSILLITIS

The pharynx and, specifically, the tonsils may be the target of chronic infection. Affected children complain of chronic throat pain, halitosis, and production of white particles or tonsilliths. Signs include erythema of the tonsils, cryptic debris, and chronically enlarged cervical lymphadenopathy. A variety of viral and bacterial agents can be blamed for chronic infection of the pharynx. Cultures may or may not be positive in these patients because surface cultures may be negative while core tissue is positive. Antibiotic therapy directed at oral anaerobes or *S. aureus* may be helpful in resistant cases. Children with infections unresponsive to medical management are candidates for tonsillectomy.

Periodic fever, aphthous ulcers, pharyngitis, and cervical adenitis (PFAPA) is a syndrome that occurs most commonly in young children (mean age 39 months). The cause is unknown. It is characterized by recurrences of fevers that usually last 3 to 7 days, along with aphthous stomatitis, pharyngitis, cervical adenitis, and headache. The recurrences occur in cycles of every 1 to 2 months, and the child is well between episodes. Throat cultures are negative. Antibiotics are not effective in treating this condition, but steroids (prednisone 1 mg per kilogram in a single dose) have been shown to reduce the duration of fever in individual episodes (from 4 days to 1 day in one study); however, sometimes steroids may also reduce the duration of intervals between infections. Most children have spontaneous resolution of these fevers over several years (mean time to resolution is 32 months). Tonsillectomy has been shown to be effective in significantly reducing the duration of this syndrome and frequency of episodes.[21,22]

ORAL TRAUMA

Injuries to the oropharynx and palate are relatively common in children, usually occurring when a child runs with a toy or stick in his mouth. Most result in mucosal lacerations that spontaneously heal, but larger lacerations may require sedation or anesthesia to repair. Use of prophylactic antibiotics is reserved for larger wounds. Although rare, blunt (and less often penetrating) injuries can occur when the object strikes the jugular vein or the carotid artery that can result in immediate neurovascular injury and poor neurologic outcomes. However, more subtle injuries to the intima of the carotid can lead to pseudoaneurysms that may later develop emboli. These emboli can cause brain infarcts with severe neurologic sequelae over the following several days. Ideally, if a vascular injury has been identified, then aspirin, or, less often, anticoagulant therapy could be used to prevent these emboli from forming. Unfortunately, no specific clinical factors (including size or location of wound) have been shown to correlate with the presence of a subtle vascular injury. Computed tomography angiography (CTA) has been used to rule out a significant vascular injury, but benefit from CTA remains controversial, because only 2.8% of studies are positive.[23]

PERITONSILLAR CELLULITIS/ABSCESS

Localized extension of tonsillar infection may result in peritonsillar cellulitis. The same pathogens that cause acute pharyngotonsillitis are responsible for peritonsillar cellulitis. In addition to a severe sore throat, symptoms and signs include drooling, trismus, muffled voice, ipsilateral referred otalgia, and tender lymphadenopathy. The affected tonsil is usually displaced in a medial and inferior position. Peritonsillar cellulitis may progress to frank abscess formation (quinsy).

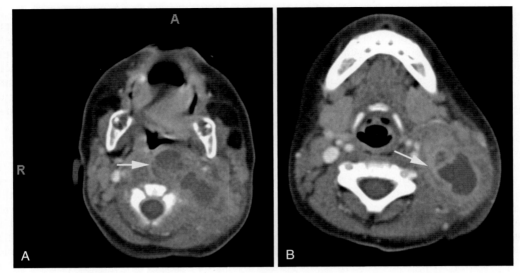

FIGURE 55-6   **A,** Retropharyngeal abscess. Computed tomography of the cervical area demonstrates fluid loculated in the retropharyngeal space. The abscess is typically unilateral and frequently extends into the medial aspect of the peripharyngeal space. In the absence of associated complications, drainage can be done intraorally (*arrow*). **B,** Lateral neck abscess on the left side (*arrow*).

Early cases of peritonsillar cellulitis may respond to oral antibiotics, such as the penicillins, cephalosporins, erythromycins, or clindamycin. Unresponsive cases of cellulitis or abscess should be treated with intravenous antibiotics. In children with suspected abscess formation, a variety of surgical drainage procedures can be performed. Needle aspiration or incision and drainage have been shown to be equally effective.[24] In persistent cases or in those children who will require general anesthesia for drainage, consideration should be given to performing a tonsillectomy (quinsy tonsillectomy).

RETROPHARYNGEAL/PARAPHARYNGEAL SPACE INFECTIONS

Signs and symptoms of deep neck space (retropharyngeal/ parapharyngeal) infections that involve the pharynx typically are as fever, drooling, irritability, decreased oral intake, torticollis, and/or trismus. Often there is a history of a preceding viral illness. Stridor or symptoms of upper airway obstruction may be seen in half of patients.[25] A neck mass or enlarged cervical nodes may be present, depending on the location of the infection. Usual pathogens include coagulase-positive staphylococci and GABHS. Anaerobic bacteria have been found in as many as 50% of cases.[25] Complications of deep neck space infections include airway obstruction, bacteremia, rupture of the abscess into the pharynx with aspiration, mediastinal extension of infection, jugular thrombosis, and carotid artery rupture.

In suspected cases, the diagnosis of a retropharyngeal/ parapharyngeal space infection is confirmed with either contrast medium–enhanced CT or MRI. Widening of the retropharynx on a lateral neck radiograph suggests a retropharyngeal infection. Although ultrasonography can detect the presence of an abscess cavity, CT or MRI are most helpful in demonstrating the extent of infection and the location of surrounding structures of importance, specifically the great vessels. Contrast medium–enhanced CT is particularly useful in distinguishing a phlegmon (cellulitis) from cases of frank suppuration. Demonstration of a hypodense region with surrounding rim enhancement has been shown to correlate with an abscess in 92% of cases (Fig. 55-6).

The initial management of a deep neck infection should begin with intravenous antibiotics, including clindamycin, cefazolin, beta-lactamase penicillins, or a combination thereof. Sixty-seven percent of children with these infections (including those presenting with cellulitis or early abscess) require eventual drainage. Surgical drainage should be reserved for those children who present with airway symptoms along with obvious abscess and for those who fail to show clinical improvement or progress to frank abscess formation on CT after 48 to 72 hours of intravenous (IV) antibiotics. The usual approach to surgical drainage is intraoral, if the abscess points medial to the great vessels, or extraoral, if the infection points lateral to the great vessels.

Complications of deep neck infections should be treated aggressively. Mediastinal spread requires prompt surgical drainage in most cases. An infected jugular thrombosis (Lemierre syndrome) can be a source of metastatic spread of infection as septic emboli. Signs and symptoms include spiking chills and fever (picket-fence fevers) and a neck mass despite appropriate antibiotic therapy. Anticoagulation or excision of the infected thrombus may be required to eradicate the infection.

SLEEP-DISORDERED BREATHING

In the past decade, the impact of sleep-disordered breathing (SDB) on the health of children has been well described, beginning with the report of normative sleep data by Marcus and colleagues.[26] Children appear to have briefer but more frequent episodes of partial (hypopnea) and complete (apnea) obstruction. Because an apnea of less than 10 seconds may represent several missed breaths in a child, an apnea of any duration is abnormal. In most cases the site of obstruction during sleep is in the pharynx. In contrast to adults with this disorder, in whom the pharyngeal impingement is due to adipose tissue surrounding the pharyngeal musculature, the major cause of airway obstruction in children results from adenotonsillar hypertrophy.

The apnea index (AI) represents the number of apneas in an hour, with a normal value being less than 1 in children. Because most children have an increased frequency of partial obstructions compared with adults, a measure of hypopneas may be more significant. A hypopnea is variably described as a reduction in airflow or respiratory effort or oxygen desaturation or combination thereof. The apnea/hypopnea index (AHI) is a measure of both apneas and hypopneas in an hour and may be a better reflection of SDB in children. An AHI greater than 5 is abnormal in adults, whereas, an AHI greater than 1.0 to 1.5 is abnormal in children. The upper airway resistance syndrome represents obstructed breathing with normal respiratory indices but with sleep fragmentation and electroencephalographic arousals that indicate disordered sleep.

The major group at risk for SDB includes children with adenotonsillar hypertrophy secondary to lymphoid hyperplasia (Figs. 55-7 and 55-8). Whereas the age of affected children ranges from 2 years through adolescence, the prevalence mirrors the age of greatest lymphoid hyperplasia, 2 to 6 years, the age the tonsils and adenoids are largest in size. Other at-risk groups include syndromic children with Down syndrome who also have relative macroglossia and tend to have larger tonsils and adenoids, children with craniofacial disorders, and patients with cleft palate or storage diseases (Hunter and Hurler syndromes). Adverse effects of obstructive sleep apnea on children include poor school performance, failure to thrive, facial and dental maldevelopment, and, rarely, severe cardiac impairment, including systemic hypertension, cardiac arrhythmias, and cor pulmonale with heart failure.

Daytime symptoms include noisy mouth-breathing, nasal obstruction and congestion, hyponasal speech, and dyspnea

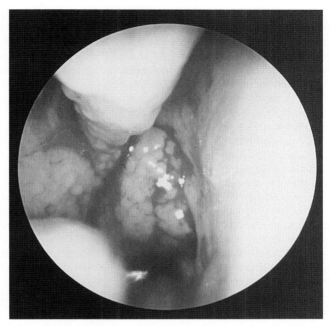

FIGURE 55-8 Adenoid hypertrophy. Hypertrophy of the adenoids may cause the nasopharynx to be obstructed with tissue. Smaller amounts of tissue are also able to obstruct nasal respiration by growing into the posterior choana as shown in this photograph.

on exertion. In contrast to adults, hypersomnolence is uncommon in children because of the lower incidence of gas exchange abnormalities, specifically hypercarbia. Children may complain of headaches, seem irritable, and perform poorly in school. Nighttime symptoms are more obvious and include snoring, gasping, and choking respirations, apnea, coughing, and a variety of other behaviors, including sleepwalking, sleep-talking, rocking, head banging, and bruxism. Enuresis may appear in children with airway obstruction and then resolve after surgical treatment. In addition to enlarged tonsils, signs include the presence of a posterior pharyngeal flap in cleft palate patients, a craniofacial disorder, adenoid facies, and, rarely, evidence of right-sided heart failure.

The diagnosis of SDB is suggested by history and physical examination. Confirmation of obstruction and apnea may be made with overnight pulse oximetry and video or audio monitoring of sleep. The gold standard in the diagnosis of obstructive sleep apnea remains formal polysomnography, including measures of nasal and oral airflow, transcutaneous oxygen and carbon dioxide, chest wall movements, electrocardiography, extraocular muscle movements, electroencephalography, leg movements, and gastric pH monitoring in selected cases. Depending on the suspected site of obstruction, adjuvant studies, such as a lateral neck radiograph, MRI of the head and neck, and flexible upper airway endoscopy, might be helpful.

The nonsurgical management of SDB consists of weight loss in obese patients and treatment of underlying allergies and gastroesophageal reflux. Nasal and dental appliances to maintain airway patency that may be useful in adults are usually poorly tolerated in children. Nasal continuous positive airway pressure, the mainstay of treatment in adults, is tolerated in many children and should be considered as a treatment option, especially in patients in whom other therapies have been exhausted or proven ineffective.

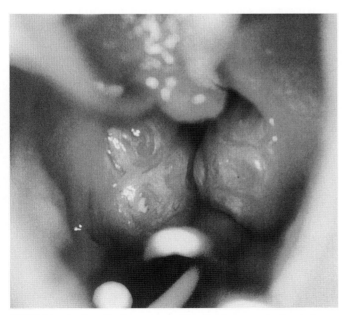

FIGURE 55-7 Tonsillar hypertrophy. Tonsillar hypertrophy is rated on a scale of 1 to 4. Grade 1+ tonsils are hypertrophic, grade 2+ tonsils extend slightly beyond the tonsillar pillars, grade 3+ tonsils extend in a medial direction beyond the anterior tonsillar pillars, and grade 4+ tonsils touch in the midline.

The initial surgical treatment for most children with SDB remains a tonsillectomy and adenoidectomy, a therapy that is usually curative. In patients with documented sleep apnea or a sleep disorder, both procedures should be used even if the tonsils appear small. Tonsillectomy and adenoidectomy techniques that have been standard for decades have been supplanted in some institutions by new technology, including use of coblation, harmonic scalpel, and the microdebrider. Efficacy of these newer techniques versus established methods remains unproven.

Complications after tonsillectomy and adenoidectomy usually consist of respiratory compromise and acute or delayed bleeding. Since the advent of modern pediatric anesthesia, respiratory complications, such as aspiration with resultant pneumonia and lung abscess, are rare. Humidification, intraoperative corticosteroids, and antibiotics have all been shown to improve the postoperative course after tonsil and adenoid surgery. Young children are most vulnerable to complications, and, in most institutions, children younger than 3 to 4 years of age are observed overnight for signs of dehydration and respiratory compromise.

Adjuvant surgery in the management of SDB includes craniofacial repair or posterior flap revision surgery in appropriate patients. Midface, mandibular, and hyoid advancement have proved useful in selected patients, along with nasal surgery such as septoplasty, partial inferior turbinectomy, or nasal polypectomy. Tracheostomy remains the treatment of last resort in patients who fail to respond to other forms of therapy.

ANKYLOGLOSSIA

Ankyloglossia or tongue-tie is a common congenital disorder involving the lingual frenulum (Fig. 55-9). Neonates with diminished tongue mobility resulting from a foreshortened frenulum may have problems in sucking and feeding. Because the frenulum is thin and relatively avascular in neonates and young infants, it can often be incised as an office procedure. In older children the greatest effect of ankyloglossia is on speech and it can lead to dental caries because it may be difficult to clean the lower teeth. Because the tip of the tongue curls under on protrusion and has limited lateral and superior movement, speech articulation may be affected. Surgical treatment in these patients may require a short general anesthetic because the frenulum is thicker and more vascular, requiring surgical correction that includes simple division either with or without a Z-plasty repair.

MACROGLOSSIA

Macroglossia is uncommon. Generalized macroglossia, as seen in association with Beckwith-Wiedemann syndrome, with glycogen storage diseases (Hunter and Hurler syndromes) or hypothyroidism, is rare. Relative macroglossia can be seen normally on occasion but is most common in Down syndrome. The most serious complication of this condition is airway obstruction. In infants, macroglossia should be distinguished from focal enlargement of the tongue seen in patients with a lymphatic malformation or hemangioma. Glossoptosis, posterior displacement of a normal-sized tongue, is seen in association with cleft palate and micrognathia in infants afflicted with the Pierre Robin sequence. The airway symptoms in most of these infants usually improve over the first year or two of life; so, supportive care is most often recommended (including oral airways and upright positioning with feeding). Infants with severe airway obstruction secondary to an enlarged or displaced tongue may require tongue reduction or a temporary tongue-to-lower lip adhesion suture, respectively. Tracheostomy is reserved for the worst cases. Macroglossia in older children that affects cosmesis, interferes with speech, or causes drooling may be treated with a variety of other tongue reduction techniques.

BENIGN LESIONS

Epulis is a congenital granular cell tumor that typically presents as a soft, pink submucosal mass on the anterior alveolar ridge of the maxilla (Fig. 55-10). Females are more

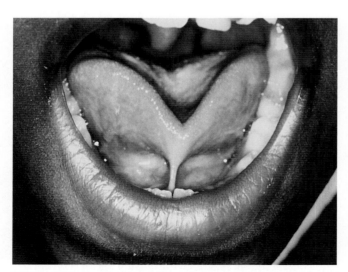

FIGURE 55-9 Ankyloglossia. Abnormal development of the lingual frenulum that limits extension of the tongue tip beyond the mandibular incisors frequently causes articulation disorders and should be corrected.

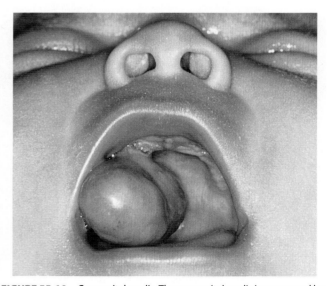

FIGURE 55-10 Congenital epulis. The congenital epulis is an unusual benign lesion that frequently arises from the anterior maxillary alveolar ridge. Airway and feeding difficulties may develop secondary to large lesions. Surgical excision is required.

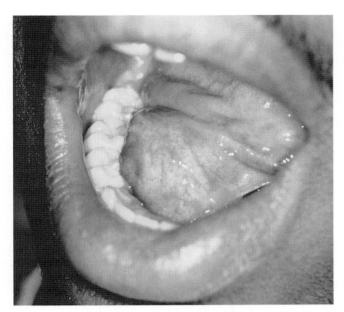

FIGURE 55-11 A ranula is a pseudocyst caused by obstruction of a sublingual gland. It generally presents as a unilateral, painless swelling in the floor of the mouth.

commonly affected, and symptoms are usually confined to feeding problems. Surgical excision is curative.

Ranula is a pseudocyst located in the floor of the mouth that may occur congenitally or result from intraoral trauma (Fig. 55-11). Large ranulas may extend through the mylohyoid musculature and present in the neck as a "plunging ranula." Treatment of ranulas is by excision or marsupialization of the pseudocyst, often in conjunction with excision of the sublingual gland. Mucoceles are also pseudocysts of minor salivary gland origin and frequently rupture spontaneously. Recurrent or symptomatic mucoceles respond to surgical excision.

Hemangioma is a proliferative endothelial lesion found commonly in the head and neck. Their growth characteristics include enlargement during the first year of life, followed by spontaneous resolution. Surgical excision or treatment with corticosteroids may be necessary in lesions that cause ulceration and bleeding, airway obstruction, cardiovascular compromise, or platelet-trapping coagulopathy (Kasabach-Merritt syndrome). Longer-term systemic treatment with propranolol has recently been found to effectively reduce the size of symptomatic hemangiomas and may work by promoting vasoconstriction and downregulation of certain growth factors.[27] Vascular malformations, including venous, arterial, or arteriovenous malformations, rarely occur in the oral cavity and pharynx and necessitate intervention only if they cause pain, bleeding, ulceration, or heart failure. Management of complicated cases is by surgical excision or sclerotherapy for low-flow lesions (venous) and angiographic embolization for high-flow lesions. Lymphatic malformation, formerly known as lymphangioma or cystic hygroma, is congenital and usually presents before 2 years of age. Histologically, lymphatic malformations consist of multiple dilated lymphatic channels or may contain either capillary or venous elements (venolymphatic malformations). Lymphatic malformations have been characterized as microcystic, macrocystic, or mixed based on their histologic patterns. Lymphatic malformations

can occur anywhere in the neck and may cause extensive cosmetic deformity and functional problems in cases with involvement of the tongue, floor of mouth, mandible, or larynx. Deep and macrocystic disease may be controlled with aspiration and sclerotherapy performed by interventional radiologists, whereas treatment of microcystic or more superficial disease usually is surgical. Surgical resection of lymphatic malformations may be fraught with difficulty because they lack a capsule and are infiltrative. During surgical excision, care should be taken to avoid damaging nearby vital structures, and debulking is an acceptable option to total radical excision in many cases. Postoperative suction drains can be helpful in preventing the recurrence of lymphatic drainage under skin flaps. Coblation therapy and carbon dioxide laser therapy have been used in superficial lymphatic malformations of the tongue.

Foregut cysts are true cysts, lined with respiratory epithelium, that present in the floor of mouth and should be distinguished from dermoid cysts, lined with stratified squamous epithelium and skin appendages, which may also be found in this location. A thyroglossal duct cyst may rarely present in the base of the tongue. Likewise, aberrant thyroid tissue, lingual thyroid, presents as a purple mass in the tongue base. Thyroid tissue in this location is usually hypofunctioning, and affected children require thyroid supplementation. Other aberrant rests of tissue, choristomas, consist of gastric, enteric, or neural tissue of normal histology in an abnormal location.

Second branchial cleft derivatives will rarely present as a cystic mass near the superior pole of the tonsil. Their extent and associated tracts can be demonstrated on MRI. A Tornwaldt cyst is a blind pouch in the nasopharynx that represents a persistence of an embryonic connection between the primitive notochord and the pharynx. Other benign nasopharyngeal masses include nasopharyngeal teratomas, dermoid lesions (hairy polyp), and nasopharyngeal encephaloceles. Most of these lesions are best evaluated by CT and/or MRI to determine their extent and the presence of an intracranial connection. Surgical excision is curative in most cases.

Squamous papillomas are benign slow-growing lesions typically found on the soft palate, uvula, and tonsillar pillars and are the result of infection with serotypes 6 and 11 of the human papillomavirus (HPV). Because of concern that these lesions could spread to the larynx or trachea, complete surgical excision is usually recommended. Pleomorphic adenoma (mixed tumor) is a benign neoplasm of minor salivary glands with a predilection for the palate, although it may also be found in the lip and buccal mucosa. Treatment is with surgical excision.

MALIGNANT LESIONS

Rhabdomyosarcoma, the most frequent soft tissue malignancy of childhood, typically occurs in the 2- to 6-year-old group and is derived from embryonic skeletal muscle.[28,29] In the oral cavity and oropharynx, it presents as a rapidly growing mass in the tongue, palate, and uvula or cheek. These tumors metastasize early to local lymph nodes, lung, and bone. Surgical therapy is limited to biopsy, excision of small lesions, or surgical salvage of treatment failures. The usual therapy includes a combination of chemotherapy and radiation therapy.

Lymphoma of the oral cavity and oropharynx typically involves the lymphoid tissue of the Waldeyer ring and presents as a mass of the tonsil or in the nasopharynx.[30] The diagnosis may be suspected by evidence of involved adenopathy in the neck but is confirmed by surgical biopsy. Treatment is with a combination of chemotherapy and radiation therapy.

Other rare malignant neoplasms of the oral cavity and pharynx include malignant salivary gland tumors (mucoepidermoid carcinoma) and epidermoid or squamous cell carcinoma. This latter tumor has been reported in organ transplant patients and adolescents who use snuff or chewing tobacco.[31] Treatment is usually surgical depending on the site and extent of involvement.

Larynx

ANATOMY

With the exception of the hyoid bone, the major structural framework of the larynx consists of cartilage and soft tissue. The hyoid bone lies superior to the larynx and is attached to it by the thyrohyoid membrane and strap muscles. The hyoid bone is derived from the second and third branchial arches. The cartilaginous structures of the larynx are composed of hyaline cartilage, with the exception of the epiglottis, which is composed of elastic cartilage. The cartilaginous structures of the larynx develop from the fourth, fifth, and sixth branchial arches. There are nine laryngeal cartilages, three that are single (thyroid, cricoid, and epiglottis) and six that are paired (arytenoid, cuneiform, and corniculate). The thyroid cartilage consists of two quadrilateral cartilages that form the anterior framework of the larynx. The cricoid cartilage is the only completely cartilaginous structure in the airway and provides posterior stability and a base of support for the cricoarytenoid and cricothyroid joints.

The cricothyroid muscles are paired extrinsic laryngeal muscles that serve to tilt the larynx down and forward, tensing the vocal folds. Paired intrinsic muscles—the thyroarytenoid, thyroepiglottic, and aryepiglottic muscles—act as a sphincter to close the larynx. The vocalis muscle comprises the internal fibers of the thyroarytenoid muscle and attaches to the vocal ligament. Action of this muscle serves to regulate the pitch of the vocal ligament. The other set of paired muscles includes the posterior cricoarytenoid, lateral cricoarytenoid, and interarytenoid muscles. The posterior cricoarytenoid muscles serve to abduct the vocal folds, whereas the cricoarytenoid and interarytenoid muscles adduct the vocal folds.

The quadrangular membrane is a connective tissue covering of the superior larynx that ends in a free margin along the vestibular ligament of the false cord. The conus elasticus is a membrane of elastic tissue that extends superiorly from the cricoid cartilage to form the paired vocal ligaments, the supporting structures of the vocal folds.

The blood supply of the larynx arises from the superior and inferior laryngeal arteries. The former is a branch of the superior thyroid artery, whereas the latter is a branch from the thyrocervical trunk. The intrinsic muscles of the larynx are innervated by the recurrent laryngeal nerve, which also supplies sensory branches to the inferior larynx. The superior laryngeal nerve has two branches: The external branch innervates the cricothyroid muscle, while the internal branch supplies sensation to the superior larynx.

The larynx has multiple functions within the upper airway. During respiration, it regulates airflow by opening during inspiration. The posterior cricoarytenoid muscle contracts with each inspiration to abduct the cords just before activation of the diaphragm. The protective function of the larynx produces two reflexes: cough and closure. Cough is important to expel mucus and foreign objects. The closure reflex serves to prevent aspiration of foreign matter. In addition to closure, the larynx elevates during swallowing. Both closure and elevation occur simultaneously along with relaxation of the cricopharyngeus muscle during the swallow of a bolus. Finally, the larynx plays an important role in speech production by generating sound. Vibration of the mucosa covering the vocalis structures produces sound whose pitch and register is altered by changes in tension, length, and mass of the underlying vocalis muscle and ligament.

The larynx of an infant sits much higher than that of an adult. The cricoid is located at the level of C4, whereas the tip of the epiglottis is at C1. The close approximation of the epiglottis to the soft palate makes the infant an obligate nose breather. By 2 years of age, the larynx has descended to the level of C5 and reaches the adult level of C6 to C7 by puberty. The glottis of the newborn is 7 mm in the anteroposterior dimension and 4 mm in the lateral dimension. The narrowest area of the infant airway, the subglottis, is approximately 4 mm in diameter.

UPPER AIRWAY ASSESSMENT

Symptoms of acute airway obstruction include dyspnea, cough, vocal changes, dysphagia, and sore throat. Dyspnea and rapid or labored breathing are indications of inadequate ventilation and may be triggered by changes in PCO_2 and PO_2. A stimulus anywhere in the airway may produce cough. It is difficult to localize the site of the stimulus from the quality of the cough. Changes in the child's vocal character, such as hoarseness or a muffled or weak cry, may help in localizing the area of obstruction. Dysphagia for solids and/or liquids is often associated with airway obstruction. Depending on the cause of airway obstruction, affected patients may complain of sore throat.

The child's overall appearance is the first sign to be assessed in airway obstruction, because airway status often dictates how quickly further evaluation and intervention need to be performed. The level of consciousness should be determined, because the unconscious or obtunded patient may need immediate airway management. Along with cyanosis in a patient without cyanotic heart disease, the presence of anxiety, restlessness, and diaphoresis are all ominous signs of impending airway compromise. Other symptoms of airway obstruction include tachypnea and substernal retractions. The child with airway obstruction is often tachycardic. The presence of bradycardia is a late indicator of severe hypoxia. The presence of a muffled cry often suggests obstruction at the level of the pharynx, whereas a barking cough is associated with laryngeal inflammation and edema. Stertor is a snorting sound whose origin is often in the pharynx. Stridor is noise produced by turbulent airflow in the laryngeal or tracheal airway. Inspiratory stridor suggests turbulence at or above the glottis. Expiratory stridor results from turbulent airflow in the distal trachea or bronchi. Biphasic stridor suggests a tracheal or subglottic source. A barking or croupy cough usually occurs when the subglottic trachea is involved. The degree and loudness of the sound is not always indicative of the severity of obstruction, because stridor can become softer just before complete obstruction. Other important signs of airway obstruction include drooling and use of accessory respiratory muscles.

In addition to determination of the child's physical status, assessment of the degree of airway obstruction should include an evaluation of the ventilatory status. Pulse oximetry provides an immediate record of arterial oxygenation, while transcutaneous monitoring of carbon dioxide is a good indicator of ventilation. The lateral neck radiograph remains the best study for the initial evaluation of a child with airway obstruction, because it demonstrates the anatomy from the tip of the nose to the thoracic inlet. It can demonstrate findings of retropharyngeal or subglottic swelling from edema or infection and identify free air in the soft tissue spaces. The anteroposterior view of the neck is also helpful, specifically in defining areas of narrowing, such as a steeple sign associated with subglottic edema. A chest radiograph is also important in the initial assessment to identify foreign bodies or other conditions such as unilateral emphysema, atelectasis, or pneumonia that may account for the child's respiratory compromise. If time permits, a barium swallow or airway fluoroscopy may provide additional information.

Additional airway evaluation may include a brief flexible endoscopic examination. The nose is first sprayed with a combination of 2% lidocaine and oxymetazoline, and the child is gently restrained. The airway can be examined from the nares to the glottis. Attempts to pass a flexible scope through the glottis in a child with airway obstruction should be avoided. Likewise, flexible endoscopy should be avoided in a child with supraglottitis because of the possibility of precipitating complete obstruction. Children with suspected airway pathology distal to the glottis or those in whom the possibility that flexible endoscopy could compromise the airway should undergo any airway examination in the operating room where rigid endoscopes and other airway equipment is immediately available to secure the airway if necessary.

Nonsurgical intervention in the child with acute airway obstruction may begin with just observation alone in a high surveillance unit. Humidified oxygen administered by face mask will improve PO_2 and clearance of secretions. Racemic epinephrine administered by nebulizer acts to reduce mucosal edema and is useful in conditions such as laryngotracheobronchitis (infectious croup). Because its length of action lasts 30 to 60 minutes, treated patients should be observed for signs of rebound for 4 to 6 hours after administration. Corticosteroids have been shown to have value in the management of postintubation croup, adenotonsillar hypertrophy that results from EBV infection, allergic edema, and spasmodic and viral croup. Corticosteroids and propranolol have been used successfully in infants to treat subglottic hemangiomas.[32,33]

Other adjuvant therapies include antibiotics and inhalation of helium/oxygen mixture (heliox). Although viral agents are often responsible for inflammation in the larynx and trachea, bacterial superinfection is also common. Because of the prevalence of penicillin-resistant organisms, broad-spectrum antibiotics, including a higher-generation cephalosporin, penicillinase-resistant penicillin, or beta-lactamase penicillin, are useful in preventing or eradicating infection. Heliox is a mixture of gas in which helium is used to replace nitrogen. The advantage of the helium-oxygen mixture is that its low density reduces air turbulence and gas resistance, allowing improved delivery of oxygen in patients with airway obstruction.

Nonsurgical airway management may include use of nasal or oral airways, endotracheal intubation, and, rarely, transtracheal ventilation. Nasal airways of rubber or other synthetic material can be easily inserted into the nose of most children after adequate lubrication with a water-soluble lubricant. Their best use is in cases where the pharynx is the site of obstruction. Oral airways are not as readily tolerated by children and only serve as a brief solution to an airway problem. During the 1970s, endotracheal intubation with polyvinyl chloride tubes revolutionized the management of supraglottitis, and even today intubation remains the mainstay of initial airway therapy in most children with severe airway obstruction. The size of the endotracheal tube used correlates with the age of the child. The subglottis, the narrowest part of the infant airway, typically admits a 3.5- or 4.0-mm inner-diameter tube. The tube used in children older than 1 year can be roughly estimated by using the following formula: tube size = (age in years/4) + 4. Once the airway has been established, the tube should be carefully secured and the child appropriately sedated and/or restrained, if necessary, to avoid accidental self-extubation. Another method of airway management should be considered in children with an unstable cervical spine or in whom oral or neck trauma makes visualization difficult. Transtracheal ventilation, insertion of a 16-gauge needle through the cricothyroid membrane for the delivery of oxygen, should be reserved for emergencies and used only until a more stable airway can be obtained.

The surgical management of the child with acute airway obstruction should begin with endoscopy. The larynx can be visualized with one of a variety of pediatric laryngoscopes and the airway secured with a rigid pediatric ventilating bronchoscope of appropriate size. Once the airway is secured, a more stable form of airway management can be used. Rarely, in a child with acute airway obstruction, an airway cannot be established, and a cricothyrotomy may need to be performed. As in adults, this procedure avoids some of the risks of bleeding and pneumothorax inherent in a formal emergency tracheostomy. A small endotracheal or tracheostomy tube can be inserted through the incision in the cricothyroid membrane, but conversion should be made to a more stable airway as soon as possible. Tracheostomy remains the preferred airway in cases of acute obstruction in which a translaryngeal approach is unsuccessful or must be avoided. The emergent tracheostomy should be avoided if at all possible to lessen complications of bleeding, pneumothorax, pneumomediastinum, subcutaneous emphysema, or damage to surrounding structures. The incidence of these complications can be reduced by careful attention to surgical technique, good lighting, and adequate assistance.

CONGENITAL LARYNGEAL ANOMALIES

Laryngomalacia is the most common cause of newborn stridor and is caused by prolapse of the supraglottic structures (arytenoid cartilages, aryepiglottic folds) during inspiration (Fig. 55-12). Symptoms typically appear at birth or soon thereafter and include high-pitched inspiratory stridor, feeding difficulties, and, rarely, apnea or signs of severe airway obstruction. Gastroesophageal reflux disease (GERD) is common in children with laryngomalacia and tends to worsen the

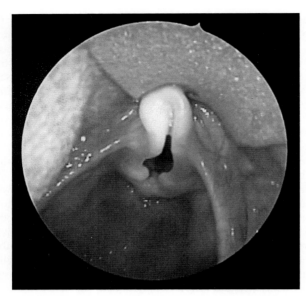

FIGURE 55-12 Laryngomalacia. This disorder classically presents as an omega-shaped epiglottis. The arytenoid mucosa is redundant, and the aryepiglottic folds are foreshortened. The result is a hooding of tissue over the glottic inlet that leads to airway obstruction on inspiration.

airway symptoms, because it creates swelling of the posterior cricoid region of the larynx. The diagnosis of laryngomalacia is confirmed by flexible endoscopy of the larynx, and other airway pathology can be excluded with lateral neck, chest, and airway fluoroscopy. Barium swallow radiography is helpful to identify the presence of GERD. In most cases, laryngomalacia is self-limited and resolves by 18 months of age. Changes in positioning and feeding, treatment of reflux, and, in some neonates, use of monitoring may be necessary. In severe cases, surgical intervention with either a supraglottoplasty (surgical division with or without partial resection of the aryepiglottic folds) or a tracheostomy may be necessary.

Tracheobronchomalacia is defined as collapse of the tracheobronchial airway. It may be congenital or acquired (from long-standing intubation and infection) and may be segmental or involve the entire tracheobronchial tree. Depending on the extent and location, symptoms include low-pitched biphasic or expiratory stridor and signs of respiratory compromise. The diagnosis is usually made with endoscopy, although fluoroscopy of the airway may often demonstrate it. Treatment ranges from observation in most cases to airway management with a tracheostomy tube and positive-pressure ventilation in severe cases. Tracheomalacia may be localized, especially when associated with esophageal atresia, and aortopexy is occasionally the treatment of choice if due to extensive compression from vessels (see Chapter 69). Tracheal stents have also been used for more extensive tracheomalacia.

Vocal fold paralysis is the second most common congenital laryngeal anomaly (after laryngomalacia) and may be unilateral or bilateral. Congenital vocal fold paralysis may be caused by neurologic abnormalities (hydrocephalus, Arnold-Chiari malformation), birth trauma, or, rarely, in association with neoplasms of the larynx or neck. Acquired vocal fold paralysis may result from trauma or from neoplasms of the chest or neck, or it may be iatrogenic, typically after surgery of the neck, esophagus, or arch of the aorta. The risk of vocal cord paralysis is higher in premature babies who have surgery

before they reach normal birth weights. Neonates with bilateral involvement typically present with high-pitched inspiratory or biphasic stridor but a good cry. Respiratory compromise and feeding difficulties may accompany the stridor because the vocal cords cannot abduct and the resultant airway is narrow. However, compensatory extralaryngeal muscles can help adduct the cords to produce a strong voice. In infants with unilateral involvement, the airway may be adequate because the affected vocal cord remains partly lateralized at rest. Unlike the case of bilateral vocal cord paralysis, the extralaryngeal muscles cannot cause the cord to adduct upon vocalization or during a swallow. As a result, these infants are at increased risk of aspiration and often have breathy, weak voices. The diagnosis of unilateral or bilateral vocal fold paralysis is confirmed with flexible or rigid endoscopy. Additional studies in the evaluation of patients with vocal fold paralysis include lateral neck and chest radiography, barium swallow, and CT or MRI of the head and neck. Most children with unilateral involvement can be observed. As they grow, they may be candidates for vocal cord medialization procedures, whereby, agents such as Gelfoam or Teflon are injected lateral to the cord to improve vocalization. Another treatment option is ansa cervicalis–to–recurrent laryngeal nerve anastomosis to reinnervate the affected cord. This increases the tone, bulk, and tension of the cord, but does not restore normal mobility.[34] Infants with bilateral vocal fold paralysis often require a tracheostomy. In addition, infants with associated feeding difficulties may need a gastrostomy. In older children (4 or 5 years of age) with bilateral vocal cord paralysis, a more permanent solution, such as a cordotomy or arytenoidectomy, can be considered to improve the glottic airway and to allow for decannulation of the tracheotomy tube.

Congenital subglottic stenosis is the third most common congenital laryngeal anomaly and is defined as a neonatal larynx in a term baby without a history of prior instrumentation or intubation who fails to admit a 3.5-mm endotracheal tube (Fig. 55-13). The underlying abnormality is a cricoid cartilage that is either small or deformed. Children with Down syndrome are at higher risk for this condition. Infants with congenital subglottic stenosis present with inspiratory

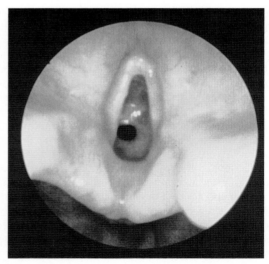

FIGURE 55-13 Subglottic stenosis. Congenital and acquired stenosis create airway obstruction, depending on the severity and type of stenosis. Various forms of reconstruction are available (see Chapter 65).

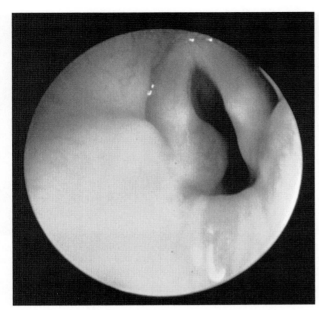

FIGURE 55-14 Subglottic hemangiomas typically arise from the posterior lateral aspect of the larynx. Small lesions may be managed conservatively, whereas lesions with aggressive growth patterns that do not respond to propranolol or steroids require tracheotomy to bypass the laryngeal obstruction.

or biphasic stridor, barking cough, and other symptoms of airway obstruction. The diagnosis is often suggested by narrowing of the subglottis on a lateral neck radiograph and confirmed by endoscopy. Treatment depends on the severity of symptoms and ranges from observation to laryngeal reconstruction to tracheostomy.

A child with a subglottic hemangioma presents with the onset of progressive stridor during the first few months of life (Fig. 55-14). Hemangiomas are proliferative endothelial lesions that can form in the submucosa of the posterior and lateral subglottis. Occasionally, they may involve the subglottis in a circumferential pattern. Associated cutaneous hemangiomas may be found in approximately 50% of patients, but only 1% of patients with cutaneous lesions have airway lesions. Symptoms are dependent on the amount of airway compromise and include biphasic stridor, barking cough, difficulty feeding, and other symptoms and signs of airway obstruction. The diagnosis may be suggested on a lateral neck radiograph but is confirmed with endoscopy. Nonsurgical management of infants with a subglottic hemangioma includes observation or treatment with systemic corticosteroids or propranolol. Surgical therapy includes laser excision, open excision through a laryngofissure, or a tracheostomy.

A laryngocele is an air-filled dilatation of the saccule of the larynx that communicates with the laryngeal airway. It may present internally into the posterior superior false cord region or externally through the thyrohyoid membrane. A saccular cyst is fluid filled and protrudes between the true and false vocal folds. The diagnosis of this lesion is confirmed endoscopically, and CT of the larynx is helpful in assessing its extent and if it is fluid or air filled. Treatment is with endoscopic marsupialization or excision through a laryngofissure.

INFLAMMATORY DISEASE OF THE UPPER AIRWAY

Laryngotracheobronchitis (viral croup) is an inflammation of the subglottic airway caused by a variety of parainfluenza and influenza viral agents. The infection may involve the entire glottis and extend into the trachea and bronchi. Affected children fall typically into the 1- to 3-year-old group; males are more commonly affected than females. Symptoms and signs of viral croup include biphasic stridor, barking cough, and hoarseness, often in association with a prodromal viral upper respiratory tract infection. The diagnosis of croup is made clinically, but endoscopic examination may help to exclude other pathologic processes. Care should be taken not to instrument the subglottis, causing more swelling and inflammation and precipitating acute obstruction. Lateral neck radiography demonstrates subglottic narrowing, whereas anteroposterior neck films show a "steeple sign," the result of subglottic edema. Treatment of viral croup is typically supportive with humidification. Treatment with nebulized racemic epinephrine in the emergency department or hospital setting often relieves symptoms; however, rebound of signs may occur several hours later, and children should be monitored accordingly. A meta-analysis of randomized controlled trials has shown treatment with glucocorticoids is effective in improving symptoms within 6 hours, for up to 12 hours, with significant improvement in croup scores, shorter hospital stays, and less use of epinephrine.[35] Severely affected children may require intubation for respiratory failure (less than 5% of affected patients). A smaller than normal tube should be chosen to avoid edema and scarring. In rare cases, a tracheostomy may be required if the inflammation fails to resolve.

A child younger than 1 year of age with recurrent bouts of "croup" should be suspected of having either congenital subglottic stenosis or a hemangioma. Spasmodic croup is the recurrence of crouplike symptoms in a child who is otherwise well. Fever is rarely present, and the attacks frequently occur at night. Gastroesophageal reflux disease has been suggested as a possible inciting process. Treatment of spasmodic croup is usually observant, although corticosteroids or antireflux medications may prove beneficial.

Supraglottitis (epiglottitis) is an infectious disease that involves the supraglottic larynx. In children, the most common pathogen is *Haemophilus influenzae* type B (HIB), followed by *S. pneumoniae* and *S. aureus*. The incidence of supraglottitis in children has diminished markedly since the introduction of the conjugated HIB vaccine in the early 1990s.[36] However, HIB-related supraglottitis continues to occur in children who have been vaccinated, with a reported 2% vaccine failure rate. Alternatively, *S. pneumoniae, S. aureus,* and viruses are more likely to cause supraglottitis in adolescents and adults.

Children who develop supraglottitis are somewhat older than those seen with croup in the 2- to 6-year-old group. Symptoms and signs have a rapid onset, progress quickly to frank airway obstruction, and include stridor, dysphagia, fever, muffled voice, and signs of systemic toxicity. Affected children frequently sit and assume the "sniffing" position in an attempt to maximize their airway. Intraoral or endoscopic examination should be avoided in suspected patients because of concern for precipitating complete obstruction. Lateral neck radiography demonstrates a classic "thumbprint sign" of the epiglottis but should only be obtained if facilities are present in close proximity to secure the airway.

Prompt airway management is essential in children with supraglottitis. In severe cases, the child's airway should be secured in either the emergency department or operating room with team members, including a pediatrician, anesthesiologist, critical care physician, otolaryngologist, or pediatric surgeon or others familiar with the pediatric airway. After inducing the child with general anesthesia, the airway should be intubated. Examination of the supraglottis may be made, and cultures of the larynx and blood are obtained. Equipment to perform a tracheostomy should be readily available. The child should remain intubated for 24 to 72 hours and should be supported with intravenous fluids and antibiotics that treat antibiotic-resistant *H. influenzae, S. pneumoniae,* and *S. aureus* (third-generation cephalosporins or ampicillin-sulbactam).

Bacterial tracheitis (membranous croup) often occurs as a complication of another infection, such as measles, varicella, or other viral agents. The most common organisms include *S. aureus,* GABHS, *M. catarrhalis,* or *H. influenzae.* It can occur in any age child and present with stridor, barking cough, and low-grade fever. Symptoms and signs then progress to include high fever and increasing obstruction and toxicity. The diagnosis may be suspected by diffuse narrowing of the tracheal air shadow on chest radiograph but is confirmed by endoscopic examination in the operating room. Purulent debris and crusts can be removed at this time. Cultures of secretions and crusts may be helpful in guiding intravenous antibiotic therapy that should be aimed initially at the usual pathogens. The airway should be secured with an endotracheal tube or, rarely, a tracheostomy. Repeat endoscopic examination of the airway may be warranted to continue debridement and to determine the feasibility of extubation.

CHRONIC AIRWAY OBSTRUCTION

The chronic management of subglottic stenosis and other prolonged airway disorders is discussed in Chapter 65.

BENIGN LARYNGEAL NEOPLASMS

Recurrent respiratory papillomatosis (RRP) is the most common benign neoplasm of the larynx in children. Squamous papillomas involve the larynx and, occasionally, the trachea and lower respiratory tract as exophytic lesions. Because of its recurrent nature, RRP causes morbidity and, rarely, mortality resulting from malignant degeneration. Patients may be almost any age, but the disease is more aggressive in children. Human papillomavirus (HPV) subtypes 6, 11, 16, and 18 have all been identified within papilloma tissue. The first two subtypes have been associated with genital warts, whereas the latter two have been associated with cervical and laryngeal cancers. The exact mechanism of HPV infection in the larynx remains unknown. In most cases, transmission of virus to the child is thought to occur via vaginal birth in a mother with cervical HPV infection or warts. However, children can still get RRP even when born by cesarean section.

Children afflicted with RRP present initially with hoarseness but may also have symptoms and signs of airway obstruction, including stridor. Lateral neck radiography may suggest laryngeal involvement, but the diagnosis is confirmed by direct laryngoscopy and biopsy (Fig. 55-15). In addition to the trachea and bronchi, squamous papillomas may also be found in the oral cavity.

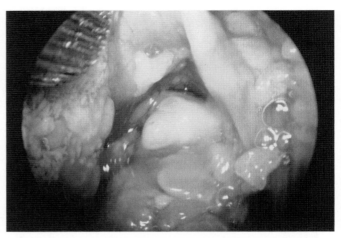

FIGURE 55-15   Recurrent respiratory papillomatosis. Severe papillomatosis may completely obstruct the larynx. Papillomas are characterized by malignant degeneration and aggressive growth patterns.

Surgical excision is the mainstay of therapy in patients with RRP. In the past, papillomas were excised using the carbon dioxide laser. More recently, the laryngeal microdebrider has become the preferred method of excision in many centers. In aggressive cases with swift recurrence and accompanying airway obstruction, tracheostomy may be necessary for airway management, although tracheostomy has been implicated in the spread of disease to the trachea and lower respiratory tract. Medical adjuvant therapy that has been used with mixed results includes interferon, photodynamic therapy with dihematoporphyrin ether, indole-3-carbinol, or antiviral agents such as cidofovir.

Other benign laryngeal neoplasms are rare and include connective tissue tumors such as chondromas or fibromas, neurogenic tumors such as neurofibromas, or granular cell tumors and other cell types such as hamartomas or fibrous histiocytomas. Malignant tumors of the larynx are also rare and include squamous cell carcinoma and a variety of epithelial and connective tissue malignancies, such as spindle cell carcinoma, rhabdomyosarcoma, mucoepidermoid carcinoma, and chondrosarcoma. Metastatic tumors and lymphoma may also rarely involve the larynx in children. Diagnosis is suspected by the sudden appearance of stridor, hoarseness, and airway obstruction and confirmed by biopsy. Treatment is dependent on cell type and may include surgical excision, radiation therapy, and/or chemotherapy.

Neck

ANATOMY

The surgical anatomy and embryology of the neck is discussed in Chapter 59.

CLINICAL EVALUATION

The initial examination of a disease or disorder of the neck begins with a thorough history. A detailed history can often serve to focus the differential diagnosis of a neck disorder. The age of the child is an important first consideration. The appearance of a neck mass in an infant often suggests a congenital disorder, whereas the sudden appearance of a mass in an adolescent might suggest a malignant process. Inflammatory diseases of the neck may occur in any age group but typically mirror the incidence of upper respiratory tract infections in children. Growth and temporal relationships are often important clues to a diagnosis. Neck masses that grow rapidly suggest either an inflammatory or malignant process, whereas slow-growing masses are typically benign. A history of systemic infection elsewhere in the body or recent travel or exposure to farm animals often points to an infectious origin. A history of trauma to the neck may explain the sudden appearance of a neck mass. Likewise, changes in the size of a neck mass with eating may suggest a salivary gland origin. Vascular lesions enlarge with straining or crying. Finally, systemic symptoms of fever, weight loss, night sweats, or fatigue in association with the sudden development of a neck mass may indicate a malignant process.

The physical examination of a child with a neck mass should begin with a comprehensive examination of the entire head and neck. Because the vascular, neural, and lymphatic patterns of the head drain into the neck, the source of neck disorders may be found in the head. Depending on the differential diagnosis, a physical examination of the entire body, including an assessment of lymph nodes in the groin and axillae and the presence of an enlarged spleen or liver, is essential. Palpable lymph nodes in the neck of children are a common finding, but lymph nodes larger than 2 cm fall outside the range of normal hyperplastic nodes and should be either monitored or investigated. The sudden appearance of large nodes in either the posterior cervical or supraclavicular regions may suggest a malignancy, especially if unilateral.[37] The consistency of a neck mass is also important in narrowing the differential diagnosis. Hard masses tend to be associated with either infection or malignancy. Fixation of a neck mass to skin or nearby structures is also suggestive of a malignancy. Cysts or abscesses tend to have a characteristic feel on palpation and are usually ballotable, and the overlying skin may be inflamed if infected. Depending on the differential diagnosis after a history and physical examination, radiologic studies may be useful. A lateral neck radiograph may demonstrate an abnormality of the nasopharynx, retropharynx, or cervical spine. Likewise, a chest radiograph may identify a malignancy, sarcoidosis, or tuberculosis. Infection or a neoplastic process in the sinuses may appear on a sinus series. CT and MRI are useful in the evaluation of a neck mass. Demonstration of hypodensity on CT suggests an inflammatory or necrotic process. Ring enhancement of a hypodense region on a contrast CT scan is indicative of an abscess. MRI is excellent for distinguishing fine detail within soft tissue and in the evaluation of vascular lesions of the neck. Finally, ultrasonography is helpful in distinguishing solid and cystic masses and may be the only imaging modality required in the assessment of neck masses. Use of ultrasonography preoperatively in patients with a thyroglossal duct cyst is also a simple and economic way to assess the presence of normal thyroid tissue when it is not easily felt. Ultrasonography should be used in the assessment of any thyroid mass, while thyroid scanning is now thought to be of limited value in the pediatric age group.

Selected laboratory studies may be helpful in the evaluation of a child with a neck disorder. A complete blood cell count with differential may identify patients with either a malignancy or systemic infection. Serologic testing for EBV or cytomegalovirus infection, toxoplasmosis, or cat-scratch disease may be diagnostic. Thyroid function testing is essential in any child with a suspected thyroid disorder. Finally, collection of urine for catecholamine metabolites (vanillylmandelic acid) may assist in the diagnosis of neuroblastoma.

If the diagnosis remains in doubt at this point, incisional or excisional biopsy may be indicated. Biopsy provides material for pathologic examination, culture, and other more sophisticated testing if necessary. Fine-needle aspiration of a neck mass in children for suspected malignancy is not as reliable as in adults.

CONGENITAL TRACTS AND CYSTS

Congenital sinuses and cysts are discussed in Chapter 59.

INFLAMMATORY AND INFECTIOUS MASSES

Viral adenitis is the most common infectious disorder to involve the neck in children. Enlarged or hyperplastic lymph nodes are frequently the result of viral upper respiratory tract illnesses. Common pathogens include rhinovirus, adenovirus, and enterovirus, but measles, mumps, rubella, varicella, EBV, and cytomegalovirus may also cause lymphadenopathy. The diagnosis is often suspected by other findings in the history or physical examination and can be confirmed by serologic testing. Acute human immunodeficiency virus infection may present, as do other viral syndromes, with fever, headache, malaise, gastrointestinal symptoms, and a neck mass.

The usual source of bacterial cervical adenitis is the pharynx. Causative organisms are often streptococcal or staphylococcal species. Patients present with systemic symptoms of fever and malaise in addition to a neck mass that is diffusely swollen, erythematous, and tender. In contrast to viral adenitis, which is frequently bilateral, bacterial infections of the neck are usually unilateral. CT with contrast medium enhancement may be helpful in the evaluation of large infectious neck masses that may contain an abscess cavity (Fig. 55-6, *B*), although ultrasound examination can provide similar information without radiation. Needle aspiration of suspected infectious masses may provide material for culture and decompress the mass.

Most children with bacterial cervical adenitis respond to oral antibiotics chosen to cover group A streptococci and *S. aureus,* but those who fail to improve require IV antibiotics. The initial choice of antibiotic is important. A recent study has shown a predominance of *S. aureus* (63%) compared with *Streptococcus* group A isolates (22%) obtained from those abscesses requiring surgical drainage. Of those with *S. aureus* infections, 27% were methicillin-resistant *Staphylococcus aureus* (MRSA), and all of these were sensitive to clindamycin and trimethoprim-sulfamethoxazole. Of the methicillin-sensitive *Staphylococcus aureus* (MSSA) isolates; 100%, 86%, and 82% were sensitive to trimethoprim-sulfamethoxazole, clindamycin, and ciprofloxacin, respectively.[38]

Cat-scratch disease is caused by *Bartonella henselae* infection. The clinical picture includes the sudden appearance of unilateral lymphadenopathy after a scratch from a cat. Fever and malaise may be accompanying symptoms in many cases. Serologic testing for antibodies to *Bartonella* is diagnostic. Cat-scratch disease is usually self-limited, although some benefit has been described with the use of erythromycins and other antibiotics.[39]

In the past, most mycobacterial infections have been caused by atypical organisms, such as *Mycobacterium avium-intracellulare, M. scrofulaceum, M. bovis,* or *M. kansasii.* These organisms are commonly found in the environment in dirt, dust, water, and sometimes in food. In the past decade or so, mycobacterial tuberculosis has made a resurgence as the pathogen responsible for a neck infection. A chest radiograph should be obtained if *M. tuberculosis* is suspected. *M. tuberculosis* is usually associated with abnormal chest radiograph and the presence of a positive tuberculous skin test. Tuberculosis should be treated with appropriate antituberculous chemotherapy.

Children with nontubercular (NTM) or atypical mycobacterial infections have weakly positive or negative skin tests and present with a typical indolent course consisting of slowly growing, nontender nodes in the preauricular, intraparotid, submandibular, or posterior triangle regions that do not respond to antibiotics. Systemic symptoms are rare. After several days to weeks, the skin overlying the node typically assumes a violet color, and the area may become fluctuant and tender to palpation. The diagnosis is mainly clinical, because the organism will often take several weeks to grow in culture, and acid-fast bacilli are not always demonstrated. The treatment is surgical and consists of excision of the involved node(s). Combination therapy using clarithromycin and rifabutin may be effective but requires a prolonged course; it is generally reserved for recurrences or nodes that are not safely accessible by surgical approach.

Rarely, the neck may be involved with infections such as tularemia, brucellosis, actinomycosis, plague, histoplasmosis, or toxoplasmosis. Inflammatory disorders that may affect the neck include Kawasaki syndrome, sarcoidosis, sinus histiocytosis (Rosai-Dorfman disease), Kikuchi-Fujimoto disease, and PFAPA syndrome (periodic recurrent fever).

MALIGNANT NEOPLASMS

Thyroid malignancies are discussed in Chapter 58, and malignant lymphadenopathies in Chapters 38 and 57.

Neurofibromatosis is a benign disorder that in some forms (plexiform) may infiltrate surrounding tissues. For this reason, CT and/or MRI are vital in the preoperative evaluation of these lesions. When the tumors are multiple and extensive, surgical resection is reserved for symptomatic lesions, because complete excision is usually impossible without compromising neurovascular structures. Neuroblastoma is a malignancy that develops from neural crest cells and may present as a solitary tumor or as lymphadenopathy. Clinical staging determines the mode of therapy that includes surgery, chemotherapy, and radiation therapy.

Rhabdomyosarcoma rarely presents as a primary tumor in the neck, more often being found as a primary tumor in the orbit, temporal bone, or nasopharynx. The diagnosis is made by biopsy, and patients are staged according to involvement. Treatment includes surgery, chemotherapy, and radiation therapy.

Malignancies of almost any type and location in the body can metastasize to the neck. The most common are thyroid malignancies. In adolescents, carcinomas, especially those arising in the nasopharynx, may spread to the neck lymphatics.

The complete reference list is available online at www. expertconsult.com.

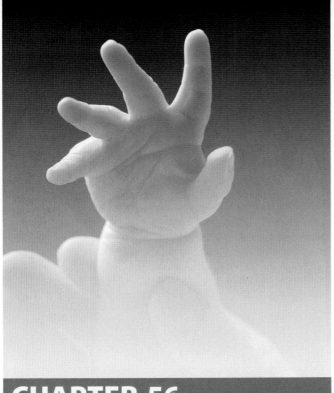

CHAPTER 56

Salivary Glands

Douglas Sidell and Nina L. Shapiro

Salivary gland disorders are rare in children. They often present as a painful or, less commonly, a painless swelling in the affected gland. Disease processes may be of infectious, inflammatory, systemic, autoimmune, congenital, neoplastic, or traumatic origin.[1] Treatment is guided by the medical or surgical nature of the specific disease process.

Classification

Salivary glands may be divided into major and minor categories. The former category includes the parotid, submandibular, and sublingual glands, all of which are paired structures with their own well-defined anatomy, including blood supply and ductal drainage. Their function is augmented and facilitated by the minor salivary glands, which include the mucus-secreting tissues in the buccal mucosa, palate, mucosal surfaces of the lips, and floor of the mouth.

Embryology

In the sixth week of gestation, solid epithelial buds of ectoderm from the developing mouth invaginate into the surrounding mesenchyme. A groove from this invagination develops into a tunnel, which subsequently forms branches of salivary ductal tissue. The mesenchymal tissue forms the capsule and connective tissue of the salivary glands. This process is similar for all of the major salivary gland embryogenesis.[2] During early gestation, the parotid ductules begin to grow around the facial nerve and its branches. This is of great clinical and surgical significance, because the facial nerve may be compressed or invaded by parotid gland lesions, or its branches may be injured during parotid gland surgery.[3]

Anatomy and Physiology

The parotid gland is located in the space between the external auditory canal and the mandible. Its main duct (Stensen duct) crosses the masseter muscle and opens in the buccal mucosa at the level of the second maxillary molar. The deep lobe of the parotid gland lies medial to the facial nerve branches and the mandible. Deep lobe parotid gland masses may extend to the parapharyngeal space and present as intraoral growths. The parotid gland is the only salivary gland containing lymph nodes, which may become apparent during certain pathologic processes, such as atypical mycobacterial adenitis (see Chapter 57). Accessory parotid tissue is present in some children and in approximately 20% of adults. It can occur superficial to the masseter and is often mistaken for a neoplasm.[4] The submandibular gland is located in the submandibular triangle of the neck. The main submandibular duct (Wharton duct) exits the gland at a right angle and enters the mouth just lateral to the midline lingual frenulum. The sublingual gland is located at the lateral aspect of the floor of the mouth.[1]

The salivary glands serve to lubricate the mouth for hygiene, speech, and deglutition; to moisten food for taste and mastication; and to initiate early starch digestion with α-amylase.[1] These processes may be initiated by various stimuli, including cerebral, visual, olfactory, or gustatory.

Pathology

The majority of salivary masses in children are congenital vascular lesions, with hemangiomas seen in 50% to 60% of salivary gland masses and lymphatic malformations in approximately 25%.[5] Acquired lesions are of inflammatory, infectious, autoimmune, traumatic, or neoplastic origin. Salivary gland swelling is characteristic of nearly all glandular pathologic processes, and may be accompanied by pain, tenderness, or abnormal ductal discharge.[4] Advanced stages of disease may lead to cranial nerve involvement with resultant paresis or paralysis.

Diagnosis

HISTORY

A careful history should focus on the duration of the lesion, its bilateral or unilateral presentation, and whether there is any symptom fluctuation associated with eating. A complete medical history is essential, because the salivary glands may be involved in several systemic conditions.

PHYSICAL EXAMINATION

The physical examination should include careful inspection of the overlying skin, both local and distant, to evaluate for any cutaneous hemangiomas, as well as of the intraoral mucosa to evaluate for intraoral extension of the mass. Longitudinal duct massage will assess for duct obstruction or purulent material in the saliva. Benign salivary lesions tend to be mobile, soft, and spongy, whereas malignant and infectious lesions are more often fixed and firm on palpation.

DIAGNOSTIC IMAGING

Plain radiographs of the salivary glands are helpful in detecting salivary duct calculi or diffuse glandular calcification.[1] Sialography is useful in identifying strictures, sialectasis, calculi, or saccular dilatation (Fig. 56-1).[6] High-resolution ultrasonography is a useful, noninvasive technique in the diagnosis of sialectasis and salivary gland calculi.[7] The addition of color-flow Doppler imaging can provide accurate information regarding the consistency of the lesion and its vascular pattern (Fig. 56-2).[8]

Computed Tomography

Computed tomography (CT) is an excellent diagnostic modality for assessing both the pathology and anatomy of the salivary glands. It can aid in distinguishing intrinsic or extrinsic lesions. Use of an intravenous contrast agent can help detect an abscess or delineate the vascularity of congenital and acquired vascular lesions.[1] These features help in both medical and surgical planning.[9,10]

Magnetic Resonance Imaging

Magnetic resonance imaging (MRI) provides the best soft tissue detail of the salivary glands, and it is the only imaging technique that can delineate the facial nerve anatomy within the parotid glands. Signal intensity variations (T1- and T2-weighted images) provide additional valuable information regarding the nature of the mass.[11,12]

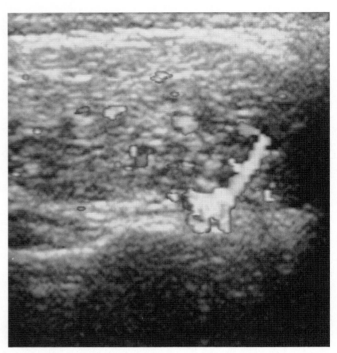

FIGURE 56-2   Doppler ultrasound study shows vascular pooling in a parotid hemangioma.

BIOPSY

Fine-needle aspiration (FNA) biopsy is an excellent tool in the diagnostic evaluation of salivary gland masses.[13,14] The overall diagnostic accuracy is 84%, with a sensitivity and specificity approaching 92% for parotid lesions.[15–17] Obtaining an adequate needle biopsy specimen may preclude the necessity for surgical therapy or aid in surgical planning. Understandably, the accuracy and dependability of FNA rely heavily on the expertise of the cytopathologist and may vary based on institution or clinical setting.[13] For deeper salivary gland tumors, fine-needle aspiration may be performed under image guidance. Open excisional biopsy is the definitive tool for investigation and may be curative. If the size and location of the lesion are favorable, the entire tumor may be resected intact with a clear surrounding cuff of normal tissue. The diagnosis of Sjögren syndrome may be obtained by incisional biopsy of the minor salivary glands of the labial mucosa, or, alternatively, of the parotid gland.[18]

SIALENDOSCOPY

Sialendoscopy involves semirigid endoscopy and microinstrumentation to evaluate and treat certain disorders of the parotid and submandibular glands. Although relatively new, this technique is increasing in popularity and has been demonstrated to effectively classify and treat ductal lesions, such as stricture and calculi. Sialendoscopy has been reported to produce a greater sensitivity in detecting salivary calculi than conventional radiography, MRI, or ultrasonography. Duct marsupialization and intraductal calculi retrieval have been demonstrated, allowing for the early treatment of some lesions without the requirement for open surgery.[19,20]

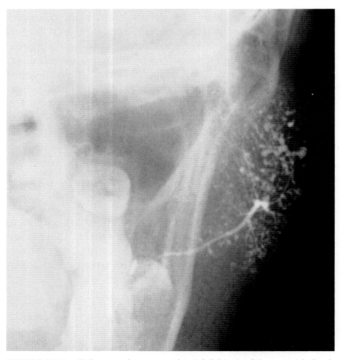

FIGURE 56-1   Sialogram shows saccular sialolithiasis of the parotid gland.

Inflammatory Disease

VIRAL SIALADENITIS

Acute inflammation of the salivary glands may be viral in up to 85% of cases, and the majority of viral sialadenitis involves the parotid glands. Viral infections are characterized by a benign self-limiting course over 2 to 3 weeks. Antipyretics, analgesics, and anti-inflammatory agents may be given for relief of symptoms. Causative organisms include coxsackievirus A and echovirus. Before the nearly universal implementation of the mumps vaccine in 1967, mumps virus (paramyxovirus) was the most common cause of acute parotid inflammation in children.[21–24] Other potential causes include cytomegalovirus (CMV), which is most commonly seen as a component of disseminated CMV infection in infants and young children,[25] and Epstein-Barr virus (EBV), which in healthy children is associated with infectious mononucleosis and in chronically ill children may be associated with human immunodeficiency virus (HIV) infection.[26,27]

BACTERIAL SUPPURATIVE SIALADENITIS

Acute suppurative sialadenitis most often presents as rapidly developing pain, swelling, and occasional ductal discharge, with associated fever and poor oral intake. It is primarily seen in the parotid glands and less commonly in the submandibular or sublingual glands. The causative organisms are usually *Staphylococcus aureus* and *Streptococcus viridans*.[28] Acute sialadenitis often occurs in dehydrated patients because of decrease in salivary flow and dry oral mucosa.[29] Most cases will respond to antistaphylococcal antibiotics, with careful attention to hydration, oral hygiene with mouthwashes, warm local compresses, and sialogogues, such as sour lemon drop candies, to stimulate salivary flow. Rarely, despite treatment, the infected tissue will coalesce to form an abscess. Treatment of a salivary gland abscess includes intravenous antibiotics and surgical drainage.[30] If an abscess develops in the parotid gland, fascial incisions parallel to the course of the facial nerve are made to drain the abscess. If the facial nerve is paretic preoperatively, abscess drainage will usually facilitate resolution of nerve function.[1]

CHRONIC SIALADENITIS

Chronic sialadenitis is the most common cause of inflammatory salivary gland disease in children and may lead to structural changes in the gland and acinar destruction (Fig. 56-3). There are obstructive and nonobstructive causes of this condition. Obstruction is caused by ductal stenosis, which may be congenital, caused by a stone, or result from chewing or biting the ductal opening. In such cases, the duct should be probed and stented for continuous drainage. Nonobstructive chronic sialadenitis may occur in conjunction with metabolic disorders, such as Sjögren syndrome, or chronic granulomatous disease, such as sarcoidosis, tuberculosis, or atypical mycobacterial disease.

The treatment of obstructive sialadenitis is initially conservative, with warm compresses and anti-inflammatory medications. Ductal dilatation or marsupialization may be necessary for recalcitrant disease. Gland excision is rarely required.

Sialolithiasis (salivary gland or duct calculi) is rare in children and occurs in the submandibular gland in 80% of cases. When the stone is located at the distal salivary duct, it may be excised by a simple incision at the ductal orifice. Temporary stent placement may be necessary. Rarely, a large calculus will be located in the proximal salivary duct or salivary gland parenchyma and may require complete gland excision with the stone-containing duct.

Cystic Disease

Cystic disease may be acquired, congenital, or traumatic. Congenital cystic disease may occur in the salivary glands, but it is not of salivary gland origin. Work type I and type II first branchial cleft cysts may present as parotid gland masses, and depending on the orientation of the tract, may have accompanying otorrhea.[31,32] Congenital lymphatic malformations may also present in the parotid, submandibular, or sublingual glands. Large, bilateral intraparotid lymphoepithelial cysts are characteristic of HIV infection.[1] Small mucous retention cysts may present in the minor salivary glands of the labial or buccal mucosa; these cysts usually result from single or

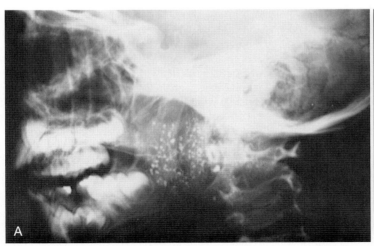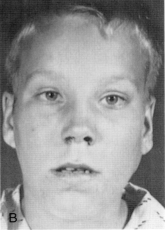

FIGURE 56-3 A, Sialogram of patient with history of recurrent parotid swelling. Note normal ductal system with early diffuse punctate sialectasis. **B,** Parotid gland swelling between acute attacks of inflammation.

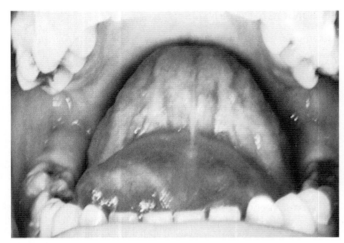

FIGURE 56-4 Floor of mouth ranula with posterosuperior lingual elevation.

repeated local trauma to the minor salivary glands and may lead to recurrent local mucosal swellings. If they do not resolve spontaneously, they will require complete excision. Local drainage or marsupialization will result in recurrence.

RANULA

A ranula is a mucus extravasation cyst of the sublingual gland. Initial presentation is a bluish, cystic mass at the floor of mouth, which may lead to lingual elevation or difficulty with deglutition. They may extend to the neck through the mylohyoid (plunging ranula) (Fig. 56-4). Surgical management is controversial and ranges from simple transoral marsupialization to combination transoral-transcervical approaches.[33,34] Despite controversy, recurrence rates as high as 67% have been described with marsupialization alone. Recent evidence, derived from the largest review to date, suggests that the excision of the ipsilateral sublingual gland produces the lowest incidence of recurrence.[35] During sublingual gland excision, care must be taken to avoid Wharton duct injury, and it can be avoided by placing a lacrimal probe in the duct intraoperatively. The lingual nerve must also be meticulously dissected just deep to the sublingual gland.

Neoplasms

Salivary gland neoplasms are extremely rare in children and comprise less than 1% of all pediatric neoplasms.[5,28,36,37] Less than 5% of salivary gland neoplasms occur in patients younger than 16 years of age.[38,39] However, when present, a pediatric salivary tumor must be assessed to rule out malignancy.[40–42] In the pediatric population, greater than 90% of salivary neoplasms occur in the parotid gland.[43] Caution should be exercised when evaluating adolescents, because imaging characteristics change over time as the gland is replaced with fat. Occasionally, this can cause benign disease to be mistaken for an infiltrative tumor on CT.[4]

BENIGN NEOPLASMS AND MALFORMATIONS

Benign neoplasms account for 60% of salivary tumors in children and are most commonly vascular in origin.[5] Vascular lesions include hemangiomas and lymphatic malformations, which are both congenital in origin (Fig. 56-5).

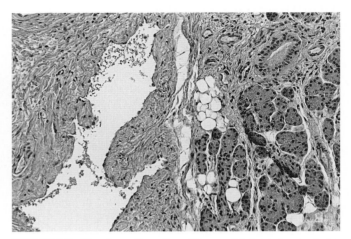

FIGURE 56-5 Vascular malformation of the parotid gland, showing large, irregular vascular spaces. (Hematoxylin-eosin stain, ×50.)

Hemangiomas

Hemangiomas are one of the most common salivary (primarily intraparotid) neoplasms in children, with infantile hemangiomas comprising greater than 90% of all salivary lesions in children less than 1 year of age.[4] Hemangiomas usually present in infancy as a soft, nontender parotid swelling, with or without associated pigmented cutaneous lesions.[44] Diagnosis is usually confirmed with ultrasonography, which demonstrates a lobulated, hypervascular mass, with arterial and venous signals visible on color-flow Doppler.[4,45] MRI may also be useful but is rarely required. Parotid hemangiomas often resolve spontaneously and do not require treatment. If they are rapidly growing or are causing functional impairments, such as facial nerve weakness, external auditory canal obstruction, or cutaneous breakdown, systemic therapy such as corticosteroids, propranolol, or interferon alfa-2a or alfa-2b are viable options to inhibit vascular growth and promote involution of the tumor.[46–49]

Lymphatic Malformations

Lymphatic malformations are less common than hemangiomas. They do not undergo spontaneous involution, are usually present at or soon after birth, and grow with the growth of the child.[44] They are not true salivary lesions, but they are commonly seen in the submandibular and parotid region in infants and young children.[50] Lymphatic malformations are susceptible to infection, with potential for cellulitis, intralesional bleeding, abscess formation, or lymphangiomatous extension to the floor of mouth or trachea with airway compromise. Treatment modalities have been an area of much investigation. Surgical resection must be complete to obviate recurrence. This is often difficult, because of the fragility of the tumor lining, its infiltrative nature, and its proximity to major vessels and branches of the facial nerve.[51,52] In an effort to avoid surgical morbidity, success with intralesional sclerotherapy has been demonstrated, resulting in reduction in tumor size and minimal scarring or recurrence.[53]

Pleomorphic Adenoma

Pleomorphic adenomas (benign mixed tumors) are the most common nonvascular benign salivary tumors in children (Fig. 56-6).[42,54] They present as firm, rubbery masses, most often in the parotid gland, with an average age at presentation of 9.5 years within the pediatric population.[54,55] The tumor

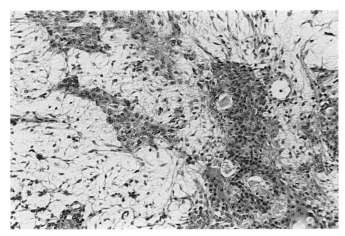

FIGURE 56-6 Pleomorphic adenoma (mixed tumor) of the parotid gland. Epithelial areas are mixed with myxomatoid and chondroid stroma. (Hematoxylin-eosin stain, ×50.)

presents as a painless, slowly growing mass and is rarely infiltrative.[56] They have variable echogenicity on imaging, with increased heterogenicity seen in larger lesions secondary to necrosis or cystic changes.[4] Treatment of superficial lobe tumors includes superficial parotidectomy with facial nerve dissection and preservation. Recurrence rates have been reported to be up to 40%; so, long-term follow-up is recommended.[57,58] Simple excisional biopsy should be avoided, because it is associated with a higher recurrence rate. Rarely, recurrent pleomorphic adenomas may undergo malignant degeneration.[59]

Monomorphic Adenomas

Monomorphic adenomas are rare in children. Histologically, they may resemble adenoid cystic carcinoma, a highly aggressive malignant salivary tumor.[60] Treatment includes complete surgical resection and close long-term follow-up.

Papillary Cystadenoma Lymphomatosum (Warthin Tumor)

These tumors are most commonly seen in men and are often bilateral parotid lesions. They may rarely present as benign parotid tumors in children.[1] Treatment is similar to that for pleomorphic adenomas.

MALIGNANT NEOPLASMS

Malignant salivary neoplasms are rare in children. When present, they are often low-grade lesions, located most commonly in the parotid gland, and have a female preponderance.[54] Diagnostic evaluation should include CT or MRI and fine-needle aspiration biopsy. Treatment is surgical, with complete tumor excision with clear margins. Invasive malignancies may require sacrifice of the facial nerve branches. Postoperative radiation therapy is recommended for high-grade lesions.[61,62]

Mucoepidermoid Carcinoma

Mucoepidermoid carcinoma is the most common pediatric salivary malignancy and is most commonly low grade and located in the parotid gland. Surgery is usually curative.[39,63] For high-grade mucoepidermoid carcinomas, or those

involving the submandibular or minor salivary glands, concomitant neck dissection and adjuvant radiation therapy is recommended by many institutions.[36,64,65]

Acinic Cell Carcinoma

Acinic cell carcinomas present in a similar fashion as mucoepidermoid carcinomas. They tend to be low grade, and treatment is similar to that of mucoepidermoid carcinoma (Fig. 56-7).

Adenoid Cystic Carcinoma

Adenoid cystic carcinoma is a rare, high-grade salivary gland tumor. Perineural invasion may result in cranial nerve deficits. There is a high incidence of regional nodal metastases, as well as distant metastases to the lungs, liver, and bone. Treatment includes wide surgical resection, neck dissection, and adjuvant radiation therapy.[61]

Rhabdomyosarcoma

Rhabdomyosarcoma may present as a parotid mass. Histologic variants include undifferentiated and embryonal types (Fig. 56-8). Treatment and outcomes depend on tumor stage and may include wide local surgical resection with radiation and chemotherapy.

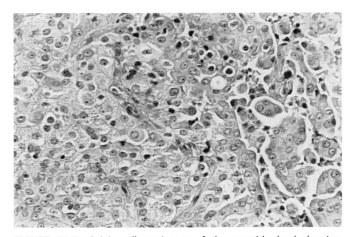

FIGURE 56-7 Acinic cell carcinoma of the parotid gland showing invasive proliferation. (Hematoxylin-eosin stain, ×100.)

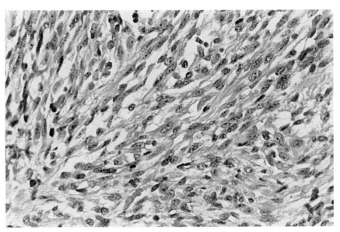

FIGURE 56-8 Rhabdomyosarcoma of the parotid gland showing spindle cell sarcoma with myogenous differentiation. (Hematoxylin-eosin stain, ×100.)

Surgical Considerations

PAROTID GLAND

An S-shaped incision is made, beginning in the preauricular crease and extending in a curvilinear fashion to the postauricular region, followed by an inferior extension to 2 finger-breadths below the angle of the mandible (Fig. 56-9). Skin flaps are elevated, and the greater auricular nerve and posterior facial vein will be identified and may need to be sacrificed to expose the posterior border of the parotid gland. Blunt dissection along the tragal pointer and mastoid process, following the posterior belly of the digastric muscle, will allow visualization of the main trunk of the facial nerve as it emerges from the stylomastoid foramen. Meticulous dissection along the facial nerve branches in an anterior direction will elevate

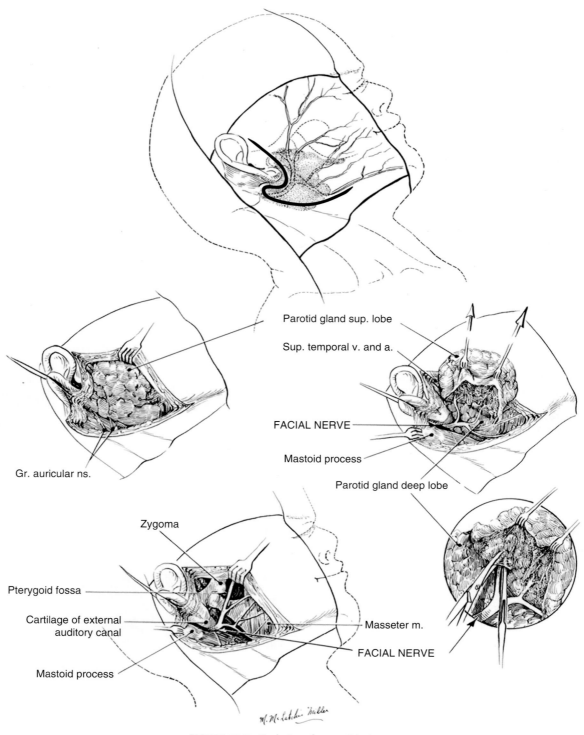

Parotid gland sup. lobe

Sup. temporal v. and a.

FACIAL NERVE

Mastoid process

Parotid gland deep lobe

Gr. auricular ns.

Zygoma

Pterygoid fossa

Cartilage of external auditory canal

Masseter m.

FACIAL NERVE

Mastoid process

FIGURE 56-9 Technique for parotidectomy.

the superficial lobe of the parotid gland. Careful blunt dissection, with use of the bipolar cautery and facial nerve monitor, will maximize excellent surgical results with minimal morbidity.[64,67]

SUBMANDIBULAR GLAND

For submandibular gland resection, a horizontal skin incision is made in a natural skin crease approximately two fingerbreadths inferior to the body of the mandible. The dissection plane is carried to the investing fascia of the submandibular gland. Exposure should reveal the mylohyoid muscle anteriorly, the sternocleidomastoid muscle posteriorly, and the digastric muscle inferiorly. Identification and division of the anterior facial vein, just deep to this fascia, will facilitate protection of the facial nerve. Anterior retraction of the mylohyoid muscle and downward retraction on the submandibular gland will enable identification of the lingual nerve and Wharton duct. Division of the duct will free the lingual nerve from the gland and allow complete blunt dissection of the gland.[66]

Conclusion

Although salivary gland disorders are rare in childhood, knowledge of the anatomy of the major salivary glands and understanding of both systemic and neoplastic physiology is critical. Neoplasms of the salivary glands are very rare in children and are commonly benign.[31,68] Evaluation and management should be tailored to the specific entity. A multitude of diagnostic tools are available and may include radiologic or pathologic studies.

Inflammatory and infectious disorders are often treated medically, whereas neoplastic disorders require surgical intervention. Patients and families must be counseled regarding potential short-term and long-term complications of facial nerve injury.

Despite the rigorous demands of parotid and submandibular gland surgery, in experienced hands, with adequate monitoring and meticulous dissection and hemostasis, surgical results are excellent.[67]

The complete reference list is available online at www. expertconsult.com.

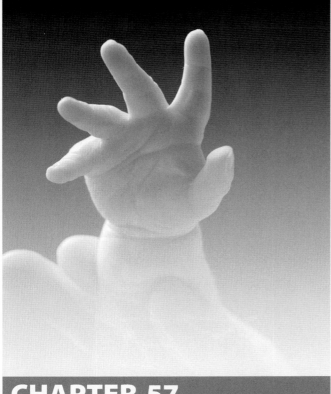

CHAPTER 57

Lymph Node Disorders

Faisal G. Qureshi and Kurt D. Newman

Lymphadenopathy is defined as an enlargement or a change in the character of a lymph node. Pathologic lymphadenopathy is usually a symptom of infectious, noninfectious conditions, or, in rare cases, malignant disease. Lymphadenopathy, especially cervical lymphadenopathy, is quite common in childhood, with a reported prevalence of 28% to 55% in otherwise normal infants and children.[1,2] In addition, children have palpable nodes in most of the superficial lymphatic basins, including cervical, axillary, and inguinal regions that are non-pathologic; there is progressive increase in lymphoid mass from birth until early adolescence. This lymphoid tissue then normally diminishes throughout puberty.[3]

Many lymph nodes are palpable in children, and generally, cervical nodes less than 2 cm, axillary nodes less than 1 cm, and inguinal nodes less than 1.5 cm are considered physiologic in young children. Palpable epitrochlear and supraclavicular nodes should, however, be viewed with suspicion and trigger investigations.

The primary goal of a consulting surgeon is to determine the need for a tissue diagnosis. A key consideration is to resolve the family's fears of malignancy in an efficient and cost-effective manner. This chapter focuses primarily on lymphadenopathy in the cervical region. Some comments are made about other regions.

Anatomy

The regional lymph node groups of the head and neck are shown in Figure 57-1. The precise borders for these groups have been classified by the American Head and Neck Society and are shown in Figure 57-2.[4] Drainage to lymphatic basins usually follows predictable, anatomic routes, with the nomenclature reflecting the site of the lymph nodes. The face and oropharynx drain predominantly to the preauricular, submandibular, and submental nodes; the posterior scalp drains to the occipital nodal group; and the mouth, tongue, tonsils, oropharynx, and nasopharynx drain to superficial and deep chains of the anterior cervical nodes. Significant lymphatic collateralization exists.

Differential Diagnosis

Most lymphadenopathy is benign in nature and is generally associated with a short duration of symptoms. Table 57-1 shows a list of differential diagnoses. Generalized lymphadenopathy is defined as enlargement of more than two noncontiguous lymph node groups.

MALIGNANCY

Malignancy accounts for 11% to 24% of the diagnoses, depending on the nature of the group reporting their result. The higher rates are reported in series from oncology practices.[5,6] Malignant processes are more common in the age group of 2 to 12 years old and very rare in the age group of less than 2 years old. Malignancy as a cause is also more common in children with chronic generalized lymphadenopathy, nodes greater than 3 cm in diameter, and nodes in the supraclavicular region. Associated symptoms of night sweats, weight loss, and hepatosplenomegaly also increase the chance of malignancy. Finally abnormal laboratory and radiologic evaluation are associated with increased malignancy rates.[7] Soldes and colleagues reviewed predictors of malignancy in children with peripheral lymphadenopathy and determined that increasing node size, increasing number of sites of adenopathy, and age were associated with an increasing risk of malignancy ($P < 0.05$).[8] In addition, supraclavicular adenopathy, an abnormal chest radiograph, and fixed nodes were all significantly associated with malignancy.

The most common malignancies as a cause of lymphadenopathy are Hodgkin and non-Hodgkin lymphomas, leukemia, and metastatic disease.

Evaluation

A careful history, physical examination, appropriate laboratory evaluation, and targeted imaging will usually help in deciding the need for tissue sampling. Persistent or progressive new-onset lymphadenopathy of greater than 4 to 6 weeks duration usually triggers a workup by the referring pediatrician. Indeed, most children with acute lymphadenopathy are rarely ever evaluated by pediatric surgeons. Most will improve with antibiotic therapy initiated by their pediatrician or the lymphadenopathy will resolve spontaneously when related to viral illnesses.

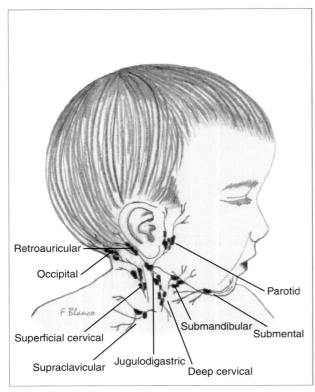

FIGURE 57-1 Regional lymph node groups of the head and neck.

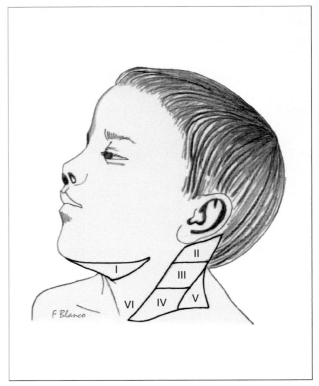

FIGURE 57-2 Lymphatic node levels of the neck. Level I: submental and submandibular; level II: superior jugular; level III: middle jugular; level IV: inferior jugular; level V: supraclavicular or posterior; and level VI: central or anterior.

TABLE 57-1	
Differential Diagnosis of Lymphadenopathy in Children	
Generalized lymphadenopathy: infectious	Viral: CMV, HIV, rubella, varicella, measles, EBV, herpes, hepatitis Bacterial: typhoid, tuberculosis, mycobacterial, syphilis, LGV, leptospirosis, brucellosis Protozoal: for instance, toxoplasmosis, leishmaniasis Fungal: for instance, coccidioidomycosis, *Cryptococcus*, histoplasmosis Other: syphilis, Lyme disease
Generalized lymphadenopathy: malignant	Lymphoma, leukemia, neuroblastoma, thyroid tumor, metastasis (e.g., osteosarcoma, glioblastoma)
Generalized lymphadenopathy: others	Autoimmune disorders: for instance, JRA, SLE, drug reactions, CGD, lymphohistiocytosis, LCH, dermatomyositis Storage disorders: for instance, Gaucher disease, Niemann-Pick disease Miscellaneous: Addison disease, Castleman disease, Churg-Strauss syndrome, Kawasaki disease, Kikuchi disease, lipid storage disease, sarcoidosis
Localized lymphadenopathy: infectious	*Staphylococcus aureus*, group A *Streptococcus* (e.g., pharyngitis), anaerobes (periodontal disease), acute bacterial lymphadenitis, cat-scratch disease, tularemia, bubonic plague, diphtheria, chancroid, viral URI, mononucleosis, tuberculosis/atypical mycobacterium
Localized lymphadenopathy: malignant	Lymphoma, leukemia, neuroblastoma, rhabdomyosarcoma, parotid tumor, nasopharyngeal tumor, solid tumor metastasis
Localized lymphadenopathy: site specific	Cervical: Kawasaki disease Occipital: tinea capitis, pediculosis capitis Preauricular: cat-scratch disease, chronic eye infections Supraclavicular: histoplasmosis, coccidioidomycosis Mediastinal: sarcoidosis, cystic fibrosis, histoplasmosis, Axillary: local infection, brucellosis, immunization reactions, JRA Inguinal: syphilis, LGV, diaper rash
Localized cervical masses: non-nodal masses	Mumps, thyroglossal duct, branchial cleft cyst, sternocleidomastoid tumor, cervical ribs, lymphatic malformation, hemangiomas, laryngocele, dermoid cyst

CGD, chronic granulomatous disease; CMV, cytomegalovirus; EBV, Epstein-Barr virus; HIV, human immunodeficiency virus; JRA, juvenile rheumatoid arthritis; LCH, Langerhans cell histiocytosis; LGV, lymphogranuloma venereum; SLE: systemic lupus erythematosus; URI, upper respiratory infection.

Once a child is referred to a surgeon, important historical questions include duration, progression, location, and associated symptoms, such as pain, fever, weight loss, and night sweats. Additional clinical information includes recent illnesses, especially upper respiratory tract symptoms, infections, trauma, bites, and dental problems. Drug use and sexual activity are important questions, especially in adolescents. Recent immunizations, especially bacillus Calmette-Guérin (BCG) should be evaluated. Social history, including recent travel, animal exposure, and exposure to tuberculosis and tropical diseases should be sought.

Once a general physical examination is completed, including a search for organomegaly, specific evaluation of the enlarged lymph nodes and other nodal basins should be performed. The skin and subcutaneous tissue that is drained by the affected lymph nodes should be evaluated; the characteristics of the lymph node should be noted. Normal nodes are usually soft, mobile, small, and nontender. Lymphadenopathy secondary to infections is also usually soft and can be mobile. However, on occasion, bacterial invasion of lymph nodes can result in erythema, tenderness, and fluctuance. With time, infected nodes can become adherent and have no inflammatory signs. Firm, fixed, nontender rubbery nodes can indicate a neoplastic process in older children.[8]

A thorough history and physical examination usually help separate local from generalized processes and help guide further evaluation, including laboratory and radiologic evaluation.

INVESTIGATION

Laboratory Studies

Most patients have had a laboratory evaluation prior to referral to surgery. These tests usually include a complete blood count (CBC) with manual differential, sedimentation rate, and C-reactive protein. However, these are not always helpful in determining the specific etiology of the disease process. Pancytopenia can be seen in leukemia; lymphocytosis is seen with mononucleosis, cytomegalovirus (CMV), and toxoplasmosis.

Based on the history and physical examination, more specific tests for Epstein-Barr virus (EBV), CMV, toxoplasmosis, brucellosis, histoplasmosis, syphilis, bartonellosis, and coccidioidomycosis should be considered. Tests for human immunodeficiency virus (HIV) should also be considered, based on the history as well as the tuberculin skin test.

Serum lactate dehydrogenase should be assayed when suspecting leukemia or lymphoma as a byproduct of high cell turnover.

Radiologic Evaluation

Diagnostic imaging can be used to determine the characteristic of the lymphadenopathy, identify potential sources of infection, identify mediastinal and abdominal masses, and to help differentiate enlarged lymph nodes from other pathology. Chest radiographs, ultrasonography with Doppler, and computer tomography have all been used in the evaluation of adenopathy.

In children with long-term lymphadenopathy, a two-view chest radiograph is helpful to rule out mediastinal masses that may compress the airway with or without significant symptoms. A chest radiograph should be performed prior to any operative intervention, including biopsies done under general anesthesia. Patients with large mediastinal masses compressing the airway should not undergo general anesthesia, because this could result in airway collapse (see Chapter 38).[9]

Ultrasonography (US) is helpful when the nodes are difficult to palpate and to help differentiate nodes from other structures, such as thyroglossal duct cysts and dermoid cysts in the neck, and undescended testis and inguinal hernias in the groin, US may also be helpful in determining the characteristics of the node. Fluctuance and abscess formation will help guide therapies such as needle aspiration or incision and drainage.

Attempts have been made to use ultrasonography and Doppler characteristics to differentiate neoplastic from nonneoplastic etiologies. Reactive lymphadenopathy is associated with central necrosis, central hyperechogenicity, long to short–axis ratio (>2.0), hilar vascularity, and low pulsatility index.[10–14] However, these modalities are not sensitive or specific enough to primarily rule out neoplastic processes. The decision to delay biopsy diagnosis should not be dependent on US/Doppler findings.

Computed tomography (CT) is useful in patients with mediastinal masses and suspected intra-abdominal malignancies. Airway compromise may be best evaluated by chest CT. Interventional radiologists sometimes use CT scans to help guide biopsies from mediastinal masses.

Diagnostic Procedures

The decision to proceed with obtaining tissue from the involved lymph node is made in conjunction with the referring physician and after appropriate physical, laboratory, and radiologic evaluation as required. Often, the child has been observed for several weeks prior to referral to a surgeon. Small, soft, mobile nodes should not undergo biopsy, because these are most likely benign unless they are in the supraclavicular region. Tissue diagnosis is helpful when lymph nodes persist or enlarge after adequate antibiotic therapy, when they are associated with signs or symptoms of malignancy, and, finally, if the diagnosis is questioned.

Most authors recommend waiting at least 4 to 6 weeks before obtaining tissue samples. Earlier biopsy should be considered for nodes in the supraclavicular or epitrochlear region, nodes greater than 3 cm in diameter, and for children with a history of malignancy, weight loss, night sweats, fever, or hepatosplenomegaly. Similarly, physical characteristics of the lymph node may also indicate earlier biopsy.[15,16]

Fine-Needle Aspiration   Fine-needle aspiration (FNA) has been used extensively in adults, with practical advantages, including its simplicity, speed in the outpatient setting without sedation, as well as its cost effectiveness. In addition, the sensitivity and specificity reaches more than 90%.

The use of FNA in children has increased, especially in countries where tuberculosis is prevalent.[17–20] Aspirates should be sent for Gram stain, acid-fast stain, and cultures for aerobic/anaerobic bacteria, mycobacteria, and fungi.

However, the use of FNA in children has not become universal, because the aspirate usually provides a small sample, which limits the ability to perform flow cytometry, chromosomal analysis, and electron microscopy. Most pediatric hematologists and pathologists prefer excisional biopsy, because it allows the assessment of nodal architecture and permits the use of special stains. In addition, some children will not permit FNA without some sedation, which negates a primary benefit of FNA. Aspirates may also have a higher rate of false-negative rates in the diagnosis of Hodgkin disease, a common malignant condition in children. Finally, the risk of seeding the needle site tract with malignant cells, although small, is a legitimate concern of physicians and parents alike.[21]

Excisional Biopsy Excisional biopsy provides enough tissue to perform flow cytometry, chromosomal analysis, electron microscopy, and the use of special stains. Indications for an excisional biopsy include
1. Lymph nodes that are hard/matted
2. Lymph nodes fixed to surrounding tissue
3. Progressively enlarging nodes without response to antibiotic therapy
4. Presence of abnormally enlarged nodes after 4 to 6 weeks
5. Supraclavicular, epitrochlear lymph nodes
6. Hepatosplenomegaly
7. Mediastinal or hilar masses
8. Laboratory anomalies, especially anemia, leukocytosis, leucopenia, and thrombocytopenia
9. Symptoms such as fever, weight loss, and night sweats
10. Suspicion of atypical mycobacterial adenitis
11. Diagnostic dilemma

Most excisional biopsies are done under general anesthesia or sedation and, very rarely, under local anesthesia. The biopsy should be coordinated with pathology so that the lymph node can be sent as a fresh specimen. The nodes should not be fixed in formalin. As discussed earlier, a chest radiograph should be obtained to rule out a mediastinal mass that may compromise the airway prior to exposing children to general anesthesia or sedation.

In a recent review, Oguz et al. reviewed their experience with 457 children (2 months to 19 years old) with lymphadenopathy who were referred to their oncology group; 346 (75.7%) had benign processes, and 111 (24.3%) had malignant disease. Of these, 134 patients underwent excisional biopsy for indications highlighted previously. Table 57-2 highlights the findings on excisional biopsy and compares them to findings by other authors.[7]

TABLE 57-2

Excisional Biopsy Results

Excisional Biopsy Results	Oguz et al, 2006[7] (n = 134)	Moore et al, 2003[5] (n = 1332)	Yaris et al, 2006[21a] (n = 38)
Malignant	79.8%	11.8%	50%
Hodgkin lymphoma	40.2%	6%	
Non-Hodgkin lymphoma	29.1%	2.1%	
Nasopharyngeal cancer	3.7%		
Thyroid cancer	2.2%		
Miscellaneous	4.2%	3.9%	
Benign	20.1%	88.2%	50%
Chronic lymphadenitis	5.9%	11.3%	
Hyperplasia	5.9%	47.8%	25%
Tuberculosis	2.9%	25%	15.7%
Reactive	2.2%		
Miscellaneous	3.2%	4.1%	

As can be seen, the pathologic diagnosis varied depending on the reporting group and the associated referral pattern, with higher malignant rates documented by oncology groups[7,21a] and higher infectious rates reported by authors in developing countries.[5]

Management of Adenopathy

Darville and colleagues have suggested a helpful algorithm for the management of cervical lymphadenopathy (Fig. 57-3).[22] This algorithm is a useful tool to help surgeons determine their role in the management of enlarged lymph nodes. As suggested elsewhere in this chapter, most of the medical evaluation and management has usually been performed by the referring physician; however, it is the surgeon's responsibility to review each case prior to intervention.

SURGICAL MANAGEMENT

Surgical management is usually limited to diagnostic FNA, excisional biopsy, incision and drainage, and total excision. Further details are provided under the specific conditions discussed later.

ACUTE LYMPHADENITIS

The most common cause of self-limiting, acute, inflammatory lymph node is a viral infection.[23] Acute bilateral cervical adenopathy is most often caused by a viral respiratory tract infection (rhinovirus, parainfluenza virus, influenza virus, respiratory syncytial virus, coronavirus, adenovirus, reovirus) and is usually hyperplastic in nature.[24] Viral-associated adenopathy does not suppurate and usually resolves spontaneously.

Unilateral lymphadenitis is usually caused by streptococcal or staphylococcal infection in 40% to 80% of the cases.[25] These are usually large (>2 cm), solitary, and tender in the preschool child.[26] The submandibular, upper cervical, submental, occipital, and lower cervical nodes are affected in decreasing order of frequency.[27] Suppurative adenitis is associated with group A streptococcal or penicillin-resistant staphylococci. *Staphylococcus* infection leading to lymphadenitis seems to occur more commonly in infants.[28] Other less frequent causal organisms include *Hemophilus influenzae* type B, group B streptococci, and anaerobic bacteria. Community-acquired methicillin-resistant *Staphylococcus aureus* (MRSA) is now more commonly being isolated from superficial abscesses and suppurative lymphadenitis in children. Clindamycin is an appropriate agent to use under these circumstances.[25,29]

Suppurative lymphadenitis presents with local inflammatory signs, including unilateral tender adenopathy involving the submandibular or deep cervical nodes draining the oropharynx. Erythema, fever, malaise, and signs of systemic illness may occur. The primary infection in the head and neck regions should be looked for with careful attention to the oropharynx and middle ear. Appropriate treatment should be started, usually an empirical 5- to 10-day course of an oral β-lactamase–resistant antibiotic. Intravenous antibiotics should be started if systemic signs are present or in very young infants. A response should be observable within 72 hours, and failure of therapy usually necessitates additional diagnostic testing. This is usually fine-needle aspiration or ultrasonography.

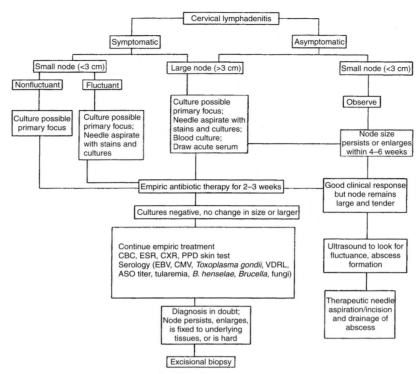

FIGURE 57-3   Evaluation and treatment algorithm. ASO, antistreptolysin titer; CBC, complete blood count; CMV, cytomegalovirus; CXR, chest radiograph; EBV, Epstein-Barr virus; ESR, erythrocyte sedimentation rate; PPD, purified protein derivative; VDRL, Venereal Disease Research Laboratory. (Reprinted with permission from Elsevier.[22])

Aspirate culture by FNA can guide further organism-specific antibiotic treatment, including clindamycin if MRSA is encountered. If no fluid is aspirated, sterile saline can be injected and then aspirated to obtain material for culture.[26] In addition, repeated aspiration together with antibiotics is an effective treatment for fluctuant lymphadenitis.[30] As stated previously, however, FNA may require sedation or anesthesia in young children.

Ultrasonography may help to differentiate between solid and cystic masses and can identify fluid that may require operative drainage. Incision and drainage is a more definitive surgical approach to suppurative fluctuant lymphadenitis. Gauze packing has been used to prevent early skin closure and achieve hemostasis; however, the use of minimal incisions, with vessel loops functioning as drains, has been gaining wider acceptance recently.[31]

PERSISTENT LYMPHADENITIS

Persistent lymphadenitis that does not resolve despite 2 to 4 weeks of appropriate therapy warrants additional diagnostic workup. Some common causes of persistent lymphadenitis are discussed in this section.

Atypical Mycobacterial Adenitis

The genus *Mycobacterium* is characterized on light microscopy to be bacilli distinguished by their dense lipid capsules. The lipid capsules resist decolorization by acid alcohol after staining and thus are termed *acid-fast bacilli*. In the United States, 70% to 95% of mycobacterial lymphadenitis cases are caused by atypical mycobacteria (nontuberculous strains).

The most common agents include *M. avium-intracellulare, M. scrofulaceum, M. fortuitum,* and *M. chelonei.*[32] In contrast to tuberculous adenitis, atypical (or nontuberculous) mycobacterial adenitis is generally considered a local infectious process, without systemic involvement in immunocompetent hosts. Disseminated disease is more commonly observed in patients with underlying acquired or congenital immunodeficiency states. Atypical mycobacterial adenitis is not contagious, and the portal of entry in otherwise healthy children is the oropharynx.[33]

Atypical mycobacterial adenitis usually occurs in young children between 1 and 5 years of age. The common clinical presentation is focal, unilateral involvement of the jugulodigastric, preauricular, or submandibular nodal group. There is rapid onset of nodal enlargement, and the skin gradually develops a pink or red hue; with time, the overlying skin becomes thin.[26] In contrast to acute suppurative lymphadenitis, there is no response to first-line antibiotics, and the clinical course is described as indolent, with the involved nodal group being minimally tender, firm, and rubbery to palpation, well circumscribed, and sometimes adherent to underlying structures. Although remarkably nontender, these lesions develop a draining sinus tract in 10% of patients.[34,35] Signs of systemic illness or inflammation are usually minimal or nonexistent. Chest radiographs are usually normal.

Differentiating atypical mycobacterial and mycobacterial tuberculous cervical lymphadenitis can occasionally be challenging, based purely on epidemiologic and clinical features. Age (<5 years), race (white), place of residence (rural), bilaterality (rare) all point toward atypical mycobacterial infection. Purified protein derivative (PPD) skin testing in children with atypical mycobacterial lymphadenitis can result in an intermediate reaction because of cross reactivity, usually less than 15 mm. Blood interferon-gamma release assay is emerging as the discriminating test of choice; it was originally described for pulmonary disease but is now being used for nodal disease as well.[36] Other criteria that point toward a diagnosis of tuberculous lymphadenitis are (1) a positive PPD, (2) abnormal chest radiograph, and (3) contact with a person with infectious tuberculosis. Spyridis and colleagues have shown that fulfilling two of three criteria results in diagnosis of tuberculous lymphadenitis with a 92% sensitivity.[37]

Unlike tuberculous adenitis, atypical mycobacterial adenitis generally does not respond to chemotherapy. The treatment of choice is complete surgical excision with primary wound closure. In a literature review of the surgical treatment of atypical mycobacterial cervicofacial adenitis in children, excision, incision and drainage, curettage, and needle aspiration were compared across 16 studies. The cure rates were 92%, 10%, 86%, and 41%, respectively.[38] Incision and drainage should be avoided, because it often results in a chronically draining sinus. There have been reports of adequate medical treatment of atypical mycobacterial lymphadenitis; however, in a recent multicenter randomized trial comparing surgical excision and antibiotics, surgical excision was superior, with a 96% cure rate compared with 66% with antibiotic therapy.[39] Multidrug antibiotic therapy, usually including clarithromycin and rifabutin, may be used as an adjunct for unresectable or recurrent disease.[40] Surgical treatment should include elliptic excision of the overlying skin when it is thinned out, debridement of subcutaneous granulation tissue, and complete excision of the involved node(s) with closure of the overlying skin; formal lymph node dissection is not required. Curettage is recommended only if surgical excision is not possible because of unacceptable cosmetic outcomes or risk of injuries to adjacent nerves. A nerve stimulator may be helpful for lesions at the angle of the mandible to avoid injury to branches of the facial nerve.

Mycobacterial Adenitis

In developed countries, tuberculous adenitis or scrofula is almost exclusively caused by *M. tuberculosis*. Before control of bovine tuberculosis, the predominant cause of tuberculous adenitis was *M. bovis*. Occasional cases of *M. bovis* are observed from underdeveloped regions in which consumption of contaminated raw meat occurs. Patients proven to have human tuberculous adenitis often report previous exposure to a known carrier of tuberculosis, but most patients do not have active disease on a chest radiograph.[37] Differentiation between tuberculosis and atypical mycobacterial adenitis has been highlighted previously. Tuberculous adenitis is considered to be a local manifestation of a systemic disease and not an initial primary focus of tuberculous infection.[41]

Clinically, children with tuberculous adenitis are usually older and present with nonsuppurative lymphadenitis, which may be bilateral.[42] A retrospective review of 24 immunocompetent children with tuberculous lymphadenitis showed that no patient had bilateral disease, and the submandibular (29%) and the anterior cervical (71%) sites were the only areas of involvement.[37] However, posterior triangle nodal involvement does occur.

The diagnosis of tuberculous adenitis can be made on the criteria established by Spyridis and colleagues[37] and positive acid-fast bacteria on stain or culture of nodal tissue. Diagnostic confirmation may be aided by FNA with aspirate culture and cytologic examination.[43] Rapid diagnosis of tuberculous adenitis by DNA amplification of nodal material using polymerase chain reaction (PCR) has been reported.[44] Blood testing and PPD are also used. A negative tuberculin PPD test essentially excludes the diagnosis of tuberculous adenitis. If a diagnostic dilemma persists, surgical excisional biopsy is warranted. Incisional biopsy or incision and drainage should be avoided to prevent development of chronic, draining sinus tracts.[23,45] Fistula and cheloid formation can be seen in up to 100% of patients who undergo incision and drainage of tuberculous infected lymph nodes.[37]

Tuberculous adenitis generally responds to medical management that consists of multiple-agent chemotherapy. The World Health Organization recommends directly observed short-course therapy, including isoniazid, rifampin, ethambutol, and pyrazinamide for the first 2 months, followed by isoniazid and rifampin for an additional 4 months.[46] Nodal regression usually occurs within 3 months. Although antituberculous chemotherapy remains essential, the role of complete surgical excision of involved nodes is more controversial.[47] Complete excision of involved nodes is prudent when biopsy is required for diagnosis, when a chronically draining sinus tract evolves during medical treatment, or when optimal medical management fails.

CAT-SCRATCH DISEASE

Cat-scratch disease is a common cause of lymphadenitis in children, with an estimated incidence in the United States of 9.3 per 100,000 ambulatory pediatric and adult patients per year.[48] The highest age-specific incidence is among children younger than 10 years of age.[2] Current microbiologic and PCR-directed DNA analysis demonstrates that the pleomorphic, gram-negative bacillus *Bartonella henselae* (formerly *Rochalimaea*) is the causative organism of cat-scratch disease.[49] Most cases can be directly related to contact with a cat, and the usual site of inoculation is an extremity. Subsequent adenitis occurs at regional lymphatic drainage basins (inguinal, axillary, epitrochlear nodes) 5 days to 2 months later.[50] Similarly, cervical lymphadenopathy is observed with scratches in the head and neck region. Although the primary manifestation of *Bartonella henselae* infection is lymphadenopathy, some series report up to 25% of cases resulting in severe systemic illnesses.[51]

Initial infection occurs at the portal of entry in the skin, such as a scratch or bite. Papule formation may be observed at the site of inoculation in 3 to 5 days, with development of subacute lymphadenopathy at regional nodal drainage beginning within 1 to 2 weeks. Early systemic symptoms of fever, malaise, myalgia, and anorexia are commonly reported.

Although most cases involve the lymph nodes of limbs, approximately 25% of cases involve the cervical nodes.[50] Diagnosis is based on a history of exposure to cats, presence at a site of inoculation, and regional lymphadenopathy. Identification of *Bartonella henselae* from involved lymph nodes using Warthin-Starry silver impregnation stain has traditionally been used for diagnosis, but the stain has been found to be unreliable and lacking specificity. PCR for *Bartonella henselae* using paraffin sections from lymph nodes or other tissue is more reliable and specific.[52] To confirm diagnosis without obtaining tissue, many centers use serologic testing, which has been available for several years; it has a low sensitivity but is highly specific.[53]

Lymphadenitis associated with cat-scratch disease is usually benign, self-limiting, and resolves within 6 to 8 weeks without specific treatment.[54] Antibiotic treatment has thus been controversial, although azithromycin has been associated with rapid resolution of the adenitis.[55] Suppuration is unusual; however, if it occurs, needle aspiration may provide symptomatic relief. Excisional biopsy is generally unnecessary but may be warranted if a draining sinus tract develops or if the diagnosis is uncertain and the potential for malignancy cannot be excluded.

MISCELLANEOUS LESIONS

Various other infectious and inflammatory conditions can produce lymphadenopathy in infants and children. Most patients with these disorders do not require surgical management or, in particular, excisional biopsy of the lesions. A systematic approach to evaluation of these patients, as outlined previously, generally leads to the correct diagnosis. Surgical management of these lesions should be directed to patients who present diagnostic dilemmas and have nodal disease in suspicious areas, or have persistent adenopathy despite adequate medical therapy.

Infectious Lymphadenopathy

Lymphadenopathy caused by infectious agents include toxoplasmosis (caused by *Toxoplasma gondii*), tularemia (caused by *Francisella tularensis),* and mononucleosis (caused by Epstein-Barr virus). Infection with *Actinomyces israelii* in the head and neck may lead to cervicofacial actinomycosis that is characterized by a woody indurated cervical mass and development of chronic, draining fistulas. Direct involvement of the lymph nodes is uncommon, but the induration can make the clinical differentiation difficult.[56] Infection with HIV can produce general lymphadenopathy in infants and children.[57]

Inflammatory Disorders

Inflammatory disorders include Kawasaki disease, Kikuchi disease, Castleman disease, and Rosai-Dorfman disease.

Kawasaki disease, or mucocutaneous lymph node syndrome, is a febrile disorder of childhood that is characterized in part by the abrupt onset of erythematous changes in the oropharyngeal mucosa, acute vasculitis, and extensive nonsuppurative, nontender cervical adenopathy.[58] Diagnosis is made on clinical grounds, and the resolution of the nodal disease occurs relatively quickly in the course of the disease.

Kikuchi disease, or histiocytic necrotizing lymphadenitis, may present as cervical lymphadenopathy that resolves spontaneously. It typically presents in the older child with bilateral, painful cervical nodes. There are associated fevers, night sweats, splenomegaly, leucopenia with atypical lymphocytosis, and elevated erythrocyte sedimentation rate (ESR). This disease can be clinically confused with malignant disease, and the patients often appropriately undergo excisional biopsy for definitive diagnosis.[59]

Castleman disease, also called angiofollicular or giant lymph node hyperplasia may also occasionally present as a solitary, enlarged cervical lymph node. The enlarged node appears hypervascular on US/Doppler or CT scan. Surgical excision is curative in the localized form.[60] The multicentric form of the disease, often accompanied by visceral involvement, is considered a type of lymphoproliferative disorder and requires systemic therapy.

Rosai-Dorfman disease, or sinus histiocytosis with massive lymphadenopathy, is a rare disorder affecting predominantly African-American children in the first decade of life. Disease progresses from unilateral cervical adenopathy to massive bilateral cervical involvement and extension to other nodal groups or extra nodal sites. The disorder is benign but has a slow rate of resolution spanning 6 to 9 months. Excisional biopsy may aid diagnosis.[61]

MALIGNANT DISORDERS

Although lymphoma is the most common malignant disorder manifested by cervical adenopathy, neuroblastoma and thyroid carcinoma are other childhood cancers that can present as enlarged cervical lymph nodes.

Lymphomas are one of the more common malignant conditions in children. They may present as primary neck adenopathy that does not resolve with antibiotics or is enlarging. Patients with congenital or acquired immunodeficiency states, including HIV infection, are at greater risk for developing malignant lymphoproliferative conditions. Excisional biopsy is often used to help diagnose lymphomas.

In *neuroblastoma,* adenopathy is usually bilateral. These patients often have stage 4 disease, and if the primary is not evident on examination and radiologic evaluation, excisional biopsy is performed for initial diagnosis of neuroblastoma.

Metastatic thyroid carcinoma may present with unilateral cervical lymph node enlargement that should not be mistaken for ectopic thyroid gland. If a thorough neck examination does not reveal a thyroid nodule, and a history of neck irradiation or other high-risk factors is obtained, thyroid ultrasonography should be performed as part of the evaluation of neck lymphadenopathy.

Summary

Most adenopathy in children is nonpathologic and spontaneously resolves. Pathologic lymphadenopathy has a large differential diagnosis, with viral lymphadenitis being the most common. Surgical consultation is often obtained when the lymph nodes do not spontaneously resolve, if there is concern for malignancy, or if there is a diagnostic dilemma. Most of the investigation is usually performed prior to surgical consult, but the surgeon must be aware of an adequate workup prior to intervention. The surgeon's role is usually limited to excisional biopsy, incision and drainage, and, rarely, aspiration in children, depending on the pathology suspected. FNA for diagnosis has a more limited role in children but may be useful in selected cases.

The complete reference list is available online at www.expertconsult.com.

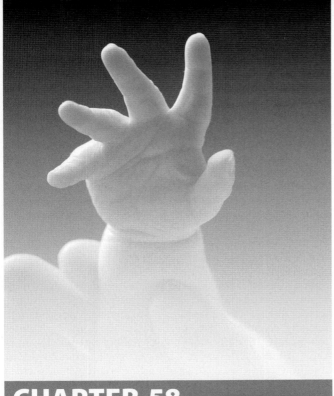

CHAPTER 58

Childhood Diseases of the Thyroid and Parathyroid Glands

Hannah G. Piper and Michael A. Skinner

Diseases of the thyroid and parathyroid glands are relatively uncommon in the pediatric population. The incidence of thyroid nodules is estimated to be 20 per 1000 children, and the incidence of hyperparathyroidism is approximately 4 per 100,000 children.[1,2] However, although rare, there is a wide range of pathology, both benign and malignant, with which pediatric surgeons must remain familiar. Surgery plays a central role in the management of many of these disorders, including thyroid nodules, parathyroid adenomas, and, occasionally, goiter and hyperthyroidism.

Thyroid Embryology and Physiology

The thyroid begins to form 24 days after fertilization and is both the first and the largest of the endocrine glands in the developing embryo. The thyroid commences as an endodermal outpouching on the floor of the primordial pharynx and becomes the thyroid diverticulum. This diverticulum then descends from the pharynx, passing anterior to the hyoid bone and maintains a connection to the base of the tongue, known as the thyroglossal duct. The migration is usually complete by 7 weeks of gestation, at which point the thyroglossal duct is obliterated. Initially, the thyroid diverticulum is hollow but then becomes solid cellular parenchyma with both a right and left lobe. The cells are arranged in spherical units called follicles, which are filled centrally with proteinaceous colloid. Parafollicular cells, or C cells, derived from neural crest cells, are found between the follicles and are the source of calcitonin. In approximately 50% of people, a pyramidal lobe extends superiorly from the isthmus. Infrequently, there will be an ectopic thyroid gland found along the normal route of descent. A lingual thyroid is the most common ectopic location, representing 90% of cases.[3] When present, a lingual thyroid is usually the only thyroid tissue and can sometimes be mistaken for accessory thyroid tissue or a thyroglossal duct cyst. Ectopic tissue will often produce insufficient amounts of hormones and can become secondarily enlarged; therefore care must be taken to avoid inadvertent removal of the only viable thyroid tissue.[4,5] Accessory thyroid tissue can also be found anywhere along the normal pathway of thyroid descent, as seen in Figure 58-1, but these remnants are usually insufficient in size to have any normal function.

Thyroid follicular cells are responsible for the synthesis of thyroid hormones. This begins when tyrosine molecules within thyroglobulin are iodinated to form monoiodotyrosine (MIT) and diiodotyrosine (DIT), neither of which is biologically active. Active hormone synthesis occurs when either two DIT molecules couple to form thyroxine (T_4), accounting for 90% of excreted hormone, or one DIT and one MIT molecule combine to form triiodothyronine (T_3), accounting for about 9% of excreted hormone. Thyroid-stimulating hormone (TSH) is the main stimulus for hormone production and release and is produced by the anterior pituitary gland. TSH release, in turn, is controlled by thyrotropin-releasing hormone (TRH) produced in the hypothalamus. Circulating thyroid hormone is reversibly bound to carrier proteins, most commonly thyroxine binding globulin (TBG) and has a wide range of physiologic effects. Children with congenital hypothyroidism are at risk for significant neurologic impairment, delayed bone development, and decreased metabolism. In contrast, infants and children with hyperthyroidism may have tachycardia with increased cardiac output, excessive sweating, weight loss, and tremors.

The parafollicular cells produce calcitonin, a 32–amino acid polypeptide. Calcitonin lowers serum calcium and phosphate by inhibiting bone resorption and likely plays a role in calcium deposition after a postprandial serum rise. Interestingly, there are no known definitive complications in humans from either excess or deficient calcitonin.

Evaluation of the Thyroid Gland

Proper evaluation of a child with potential thyroid disease begins with a focused history inquiring about symptoms of hyperthyroidism or hypothyroidism as well as any family history of thyroid disease or multiple endocrine neoplasia. This is followed by a detailed examination of the neck. The thyroid should be palpated to evaluate size, consistency, symmetry, and whether there are any nodules or associated enlarged

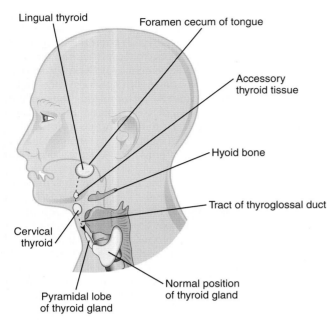

FIGURE 58-1 Usual sites of ectopic thyroid tissue. The broken line demonstrates the path of normal thyroid descent. (Reprinted from The Pharyngeal (Branchial) Apparatus: In Moore K, Persaud TVN: The Developing Human: Clinically Oriented Embryology, ed 6. Philadelphia, WB Saunders, 1998, p 233; with permission from WB Saunders.) *(See Expert Consult site for color version.)*

lymph nodes. Certain features on physical exam are suggestive of specific disease processes. For example, diffuse enlargement can be seen in Graves' disease and Hashimoto and endemic goiter. A tender gland can be found with an acute inflammatory process, multiple nodules are more common in a metabolic or inflammatory process, and a single nodule is more likely to be neoplastic. Other worrisome signs suggestive of a neoplasm are rapid growth, hardness, fixation to surrounding structures, and enlarged cervical nodes.

Useful laboratory tests include measurement of TSH, which when elevated, suggests hypofunction and when suppressed suggests elevated hormone circulation. To estimate circulating thyroid hormone, a plasma free T_4 level can be measured. Plasma total T_4 and T_3 can be measured along with thyroglobulin to properly calculate unbound, active hormone.

Finally, thyroid imaging may be necessary. Ultrasonography (US) can be used to evaluate cysts and nodules and can be helpful in following these lesions over time. In addition, US can be used to help guide FNA for diagnostic purposes. Features on US suggestive of malignancy include hypoechogenicity, microcalcifications, irregular margins, and hypervascularity.[6] Radionuclide scintigraphy is also occasionally useful for thyroid imaging. In patients with suppressed TSH iodine-131 (^{131}I) or technetium-99m (^{99m}Tc) can be used to identify hyperfunctioning areas of the thyroid gland. Scintigraphy can also be used to assess for recurrent disease or metastatic disease in the setting of malignancy. An emerging imaging technique is single-photon emission computed tomography (SPECT), which gives a more three-dimensional view of increased uptake. This can also be combined with traditional CT (SPECT/CT) to add anatomic detail, increasing both the sensitivity and specificity over conventional scintigraphy,[7] as seen in Figure 58-2.

Non-neoplastic Thyroid Conditions

GOITER

A goiter is an enlargement of the thyroid gland that can be diffuse or nodular in nature, and patients can be euthyroid, hypothyroid, or hyperthyroid. The most common cause worldwide is iodine deficiency, resulting in hypertrophy secondary to substrate deficiency. However, in locations with

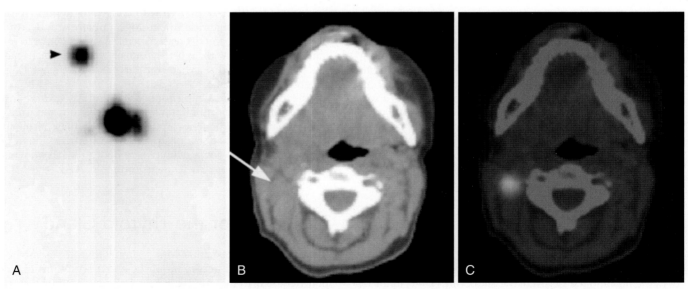

FIGURE 58-2 SPECT/CT for nodal localization: cervical nodal metastasis in a 12-year-old girl. **A,** Planar image shows a single focus in the right upper neck *(arrowhead)* and two foci of activity in the central neck. **B** and **C,** Computed tomography (CT) and fused single-photon emission computed tomography (SPECT)/CT localizes the right upper neck focus to an enlarged lymph node *(arrow).* (Reprinted from Wong KK, Zarzhevsky N, Cahill JM, et al: Hybrid SPECT-CT and PET-CT imaging of differentiated thyroid cancer. Br J Radiol 2009;82:860-876, 2009; with permission from the British Journal of Radiology.) *(See Expert Consult site for color version.)*

adequate dietary iodine intake, most patients will have simple colloid goiter and maintain normal thyroid function. For the most part, this type of goiter requires no specific therapy, because the rate of regression is no different whether or not the patient is treated with hormone suppression.[8] Surgery is indicated if the goiter grows so large that there is significant airway compression or if there is a nodule that is concerning for possible malignancy.

THYROIDITIS

Inflammation of the thyroid gland can have several different etiologies, including autoimmune, viral, bacterial, or an infiltrative fibrous process. The most common type of thyroiditis in children is chronic lymphocytic or Hashimoto thyroiditis. Hashimoto thyroiditis is an autoimmune process in which antibodies against thyroid antigen are produced, resulting in a lymphocytic infiltrate within the gland. It often occurs in association with other autoimmune disorders, such as type I diabetes, Addison disease, systemic lupus and juvenile arthritis, as well as in children with Down and Turner syndromes. Initially, patients may be euthyroid or hyperthyroid, but this can be transient, and eventually hypothyroidism may ensue. Usually, the management is expectant with about 30% of patients, demonstrating resolution over time. Exogenous thyroid hormone should be provided to patients who are hypothyroid but does not seem to have any meaningful effect on reducing the size of the goiter or decreasing progression of disease in euthyroid patients.[9]

Other forms of thyroiditis, although rare, can also be seen in children, as listed in Table 58-1. Subacute thyroiditis is thought to be viral in nature, and patients often present with fever and gland tenderness in the setting of a recent upper respiratory infection. Initially, there may be excessive hormone release, followed by transient hypothyroidism. About 10% of patients develop permanent hypothyroidism. In most cases, nonsteroidal anti-inflammatory medication or low-dose corticosteroids is the only treatment required. Acute suppurative thyroiditis is bacterial in origin, can present with hard nodules, and be diagnosed on ultrasonography or with fine-needle aspiration (FNA). Treatment is with antibiotics, drainage if necessary, and, very rarely, thyroid lobectomy. Many cases formerly called acute suppurative thyroiditis are the result of a third or fourth branchial pouch remnant, also called pyriform sinus fistula. This should be suspected, especially when the infection presents in the left superior pole (see Chapter 59). Ideally, treatment is with antibiotics, followed by excision of the fistula tract to the pyriform sinus.[10]

HYPOTHYROIDISM

The primary cause of congenital hypothyroidism is abnormal thyroid gland development rather than from a problem with the hypothalamic-pituitary-thyroid axis. Most commonly, it is secondary to either thyroid dysgenesis or agenesis and, less commonly, from defects in thyroid hormone synthesis or from the transfer of maternal thyroid blocking antibodies. Dietary iodine deficiency in utero can also lead to hypothyroidism, and in those cases, a palpable goiter may be appreciated. T_4 is essential for myelinization of the central nervous system during the first 3 years of life. Deficiencies in T_4 can lead to intellectual disability, which is completely preventable if recognized.[11] Newborn screening for hypothyroidism is essential and involves measuring TSH. Some states also require measuring T_4, which will allow for rare cases of central hypothyroidism to be detected. However, if these tests are normal but symptoms persist, it is important to maintain a high index of suspicion, because up to 50% of cases of central hypothyroidism will have a normal newborn screen.[12] In older children with acquired hypothyroidism, presenting signs and symptoms include a decline in linear growth, fatigue, constipation, and poor school performance. Preteens or teenagers may complain of dry skin, thin hair, weight gain, and menstrual irregularities. The most common causes of pediatric hypothyroidism can be seen in Table 58-2.

HYPERTHYROIDISM

Graves' disease, or diffuse toxic goiter, is the most common cause of hyperthyroidism in children, with an incidence of 0.02%,[13] and it is approximately 5 times more common in girls than in boys. Thyroid gland hypertrophy occurs because antibodies against the TSH receptor bind and mimic the effect of TSH. Patients usually present with a firm, smooth goiter and symptoms of hyperthyroidism. Occasionally, there can be fibroblast deposition in the eyes, leading to exophthalmos, or in the skin, leading to pretibial myxedema, although these findings are less common in children. Severe hyperthyroidism is sometimes seen with associated hyperthermia and tachycardia, referred to as thyroid storm, and initial treatment includes active cooling and propanolol.

Usually, first-line therapy for Graves' disease is antithyroid medication (methimazole or propylthiouracil), and improvement in symptoms can occur within 1 month of treatment. Treatment is maintained for 12 to 18 months, during which time thyroid function is monitored routinely.[14] Remission is achieved in 30% of children after the first course of medication, and risk factors for relapse include young age and severe

TABLE 58-1
Types of Thyroiditis

Histopathology	Eponym	Etiology	Goiter	TSH	T₄	Thyroid Function
Chronic lymphocytic	Hashimoto	Autoimmune	Yes	Variable	Variable	Hyper or hypo
Subacute granulomatous	De Quervain	Viral (mumps, Coxsackie virus, EBV)	Variable	Low	High	Hyper then hypo
Subacute lymphocytic	Silent	Autoimmune	Yes	Low	High	Hyper then hypo
Acute suppurative	Bacterial	Bacterial, fungal, parasitic	Variable	Normal	Normal	Variable
Invasive fibrous	Reidel	Unknown	No	Normal or low	Normal or low	Hypothyroid

EBV, Epstein-Barr virus; T₄, thyroxine; TSH, thyroid-stimulating hormone.
Data from Arici C, Clark OH: Thyroiditis: Cameron J (ed): Current Surgical Therapy, ed 7. Philadelphia, Elsevier, 2001, p 597, with permission from Elsevier.

TABLE 58-2

Pediatric Causes of Hypothyroidism

| No Goiter | Newborn to childhood Adolescence | Gland dysgenesis Deficiency of the hypothalamic/ pituitary axis Postsurgical |
| Goiter | Newborn Childhood to adolescence | Inborn error in hormone synthesis Maternal ingestion (propylthiouracil, methimazole, iodides) Severe endemic iodine deficiency Ingestion of goiter-inducing drugs Inborn error in hormone synthesis Hashimoto thyroiditis Infiltrative disease (lymphoma) |

biochemical hyperthyroidism at the time of diagnosis.[15,16] Because of the relatively low remission rate, some advocate the use of radioactive iodine (I^{131}). The radioactive iodine is ingested and then incorporated into the thyroid. The radiation to thyroid cells leads to gland ablation over the following 6 to 18 weeks. However, this is not recommended for children less than 5 years of age, and most patients will be made hypothyroid after treatment requiring hormone replacement therapy.

Surgery is also an option for some children with Graves' disease, usually for those who have very large goiters, are unable to take antithyroid medication, or cannot tolerate radioactive iodine. Surgery is also the treatment of choice if there is any concern of underlying malignancy in the gland. The preferred operation continues to be debated. In a large meta-analysis looking at more than 7000 adult patients, there were no cases of recurrent disease after total thyroidectomy versus an 8% recurrence rate after subtotal thyroidectomy. The incidence of other complications, including injury to the recurrent laryngeal nerve or hypoparathyroidism, did not differ between the two groups.[17]

Neoplastic Thyroid Conditions

MANAGEMENT OF THYROID NODULES

Thyroid nodules are less common in children than in adults, with an incidence of 1% to 2%.[2] However, when found, there is a 16% to 27% chance that the nodule will be malignant, which is far greater than the estimated 5% in the adult population.[18,19] In general, discrete lesions that are distinct from the surrounding thyroid tissue and are equal to 1 cm should be investigated. This begins with a history and physical exam, as well as measuring serum T_4 and TSH levels. The utility of imaging is less clear, especially in children. Some advocate that if a nodule

is functional on scintigraphy, no further workup is required; however, this must be practiced with caution because, although rare, functional nodules can still harbor malignancy. Ultrasonography can be useful for measuring the size of a nodule, determining if it is solid or cystic, and locating it within the gland. Certain features on ultrasonography can raise or lower the suspicion of malignancy; for example, an entirely cystic lesion has a very low probability of being malignant. However, ultrasonography cannot definitively make the diagnosis of a malignancy.[6] The use of FNA for cytologic evaluation is now the most accurate diagnostic intervention in adult patients[20] and is standard in the workup of a thyroid nodule. FNA is also commonly used in children and adolescents, with the goal of trying to reduce diagnostic thyroid surgery for benign lesions. The question that is raised is whether this test has a low enough false-negative rate to justify its use in the pediatric population. Most would agree that for adolescents FNA can be used reliably, because it has an accuracy of at least 90%, and any potential delay in diagnosis will not likely result in decreased survival. Because younger children have a higher incidence of malignancy in any thyroid nodule, there has been some reservation in relying on FNA.[21] However, FNA results are useful for planning a resection (thyroidectomy versus hemithyroidectomy) in this population. A recent meta-analysis supporting the use of FNA included 12 studies collectively reviewing 183 patients with malignant nodules and 347 patients with benign nodules, the age range being 1 to 21 years. The analysis found that FNA has a sensitivity of 94% and specificity of 81% for detecting malignancy.[22] A selection of individual studies included in the analysis can be seen in Table 58-3.[18,23–27] In part, FNA is not very specific because when the cytology reveals follicular cells, malignancy cannot be determined because the diagnosis hinges on the presence of capsular invasion, which can only be seen on histology.[28,29] Overall, FNA is a useful tool in the workup of pediatric patients with thyroid nodules but should not overshadow other important clinical information, such as a history of radiation or prior malignancy; the family history; enlarging, fixed nodules; or associated cervical lymphadenopathy.

If FNA is performed, the results are reported as benign, malignant, or indeterminate. Resection is indicated for malignant or indeterminate nodules, or for benign nodules that continue to grow or have other worrisome features on follow-up.

WELL-DIFFERENTIATED THYROID CARCINOMA

Well-differentiated thyroid cancer (WDTC) includes papillary and follicular cell tumors, accounting for approximately 1% of malignancies in prepubertal children and up to 7% in

TABLE 58-3

Sensitivity and Specificity of FNA in Children and Adolescents

Study	Type of Study	Age Range (Years)	No. of Patients	Minimum Follow-up	Sensitivity	Specificity
Chang and Joo, 2006	Retrospective	2-21	37	23 months	100%	85.7%
Amrikachi et al, 2005	Retrospective	10-21	31	24 months	100%	64.7%
Arda et al, 2001	Prospective	Children	44	24 months	100%	95%
Khurana et al, 1999	Retrospective	9-20	57	24 months	92.9%	81.4%
Raab et al, 1995	Retrospective	1-18	63	24 months	88.9%	92.6%
Gharib and Goellner, 1993	Retrospective	<17	41	24 months	90%	96.8%

Data from Stevens C, Lee JK, Sadatsafavi M, Blair GK: Pediatric thyroid fine-needle aspiration cytology: A meta-analysis. J Pediatr Surg 2009;44:2184-2191; with permission from Elsevier.

adolescents, making it the most common endocrine cancer in the pediatric population.[13] Thyroid cancer occurs at least 4 times as often in females as males and is most common in white patients.[30] The overall incidence does appear to be increasing in children at a rate of approximately 1.1% per year. This is potentially because of a rise in the use of radiotherapy for other malignancies.[31] Head and neck radiation has been widely recognized as a significant risk factor for the development of WDTC. Patients exposed to as little as 50 cGy prior to the age of 4 years have presented 10 to 30 years later with thyroid cancer.[32] Malignancies with the strongest correlation with a secondary thyroid cancer include Hodgkin and non-Hodgkin lymphoma, neuroblastoma, and Wilms' tumor.[33] It is therefore important to provide careful follow-up for children who have been successfully treated for cancer.

On a molecular level, there is increasing evidence that the *RET* (rearranged during transfection) proto-oncogene plays a role in WDTC. The *RET* proto-oncogene is a tyrosine kinase receptor that, when exposed to radiation, can fuse to another gene to form a hybrid oncogene (*RET/PTC*), resulting in increased tyrosine kinase activity.[34] Even more common is for WDTC to be caused by an activating mutation in the B isoform of the Raf kinase (BRAF). These cancers tend to be larger at the time of presentation and may have a poorer prognosis.[35]

Papillary cancer is the most common type of thyroid cancer seen in children but also has the best survival, with estimates of 98% at 5 years. Follicular cancer is about 6 times less common, with approximately 96% survival at 5 years.[30,36]

In general, the treatment of WDTC in children is similar to that of adults. However, it must be taken into consideration that children often present with larger tumors, are more likely to have metastatic spread to cervical nodes, have a higher recurrence rate, and have a longer overall survival.[37] The primary therapy is surgical resection of the gland with or without lymph node dissection, depending on whether there is clinical evidence of nodal disease.[38] There continues to be some debate regarding how much of the gland should be resected. The surgical options include total thyroidectomy, near-total thyroidectomy (leaving less than 1 g of tissue near the ligament of Berry), subtotal thyroidectomy, and hemithyroidectomy. The argument for more aggressive resection revolves around decreased recurrence rates, the ability to treat residual disease with radioiodine ablation therapy, and the ability to assess for recurrence by following thyroglobulin levels. In addition, some surgeons prefer total or near-total thyroidectomy in the setting of malignancy, because at least 50% of children will have bilateral or multifocal disease.[39] In a retrospective review of 68 children who were less than 19 years of age and undergoing thyroid surgery for malignancy, 75% had a total thyroidectomy, 9% had a lobectomy, and 6% had a subtotal thyroidectomy. Forty-four percent of patients who had less than a total thyroidectomy needed further surgery for recurrence compared with only 12% of patients who had a total thyroidectomy, which was a significant difference.[36] Similarly, a larger, recent review of 215 children with papillary thyroid cancer also found that recurrence rates were significantly higher in children having undergone lobectomy compared with total or near-total thyroidectomy (35% vs. 6%).[40] However, mortality from thyroid cancer in children is very low, with 98.8% overall survival at 10 years, and therefore it is unclear whether the increased recurrence rate affects mortality.

Support for less-than-total thyroidectomy is based upon minimizing potential morbidity from the operation. Estimates of complications after total thyroidectomy vary widely, depending on the series and the time frame of the study, ranging anywhere from 12% to 20%.[36,41,42] Two of the most significant complications are injury to the recurrent laryngeal nerves and permanent hypoparathyroidism. For an experienced surgeon, the incidence of recurrent laryngeal nerve injury is less than 1%, and it is less than 2% for permanent hypoparathyroidism.[43] However, a recent study found that incidental removal of parathyroid glands occurs in up to 21% of thyroid surgeries and is not clearly dependent on the extent of resection.[44] A retrospective review of 1200 children undergoing thyroid and parathyroid surgery found that hypocalcemia accounted for 68% of the complications, and voice disturbances accounted for another 6%. Interestingly, they also found that the complication rates were age dependent: 22% in children less than 6 years, 15% in children aged 7 to 12 years, and 11% in children aged 13 to 17 years, and these differences were statistically significant.[45] It does appear that surgeons with more experience and a higher case volume of thyroid surgery have fewer complications. In a study by Tuggle and colleagues,[46] surgeons were classified as high volume (>30 cases per year), pediatric (>90% of cases were children), or other. A total of 607 patients were included in the study, and the authors found that high-volume surgeons, on average, performed 72 thyroid procedures per year, pediatric surgeons performed 2 thyroid procedures per year, and other surgeons performed 7 thyroid procedures per year. The complication rates were 8.7%, 13.4%, and 13.2%, respectively.

One strategy to reduce the incidence of hypoparathyroidism is to autotransplant one or two of the glands into the sternocleidomastoid, which can be done immediately during the dissection if the blood supply is thought to be compromised.[47] To minimize injury to the recurrent laryngeal nerve, intraoperative nerve stimulation can be used, which can help identify its course during dissection.[48,49]

Unfortunately, the recurrence rate for thyroid cancer in children after surgical resection is up to 32% when followed for 40 years.[40] For this reason, long-term follow-up for these children is required. Current recommendations for children who have had a total or near-total thyroidectomy include a ^{131}I whole-body scan 6 weeks after thyroid resection to assess for any residual disease, and treatment with the radionuclide can be administered as needed, at this time, for remnant ablation.[50] These children can then be monitored for recurrence by checking annual plasma thyroglobulin and antithyroglobulin antibody levels, as well as obtaining an annual neck ultrasound scan. Further whole-body radionuclide scanning is unnecessary for children with low-risk tumors, undetectable thyroglobulin levels, and negative neck US. Annual scans can be considered for patients with intermediate- or high-risk tumors but should be done with a low-activity radionuclide.[51]

There is now evidence that radiation exposure from radioiodine remnant ablation (RRA) may predispose children to other malignancies. This potential risk must be carefully considered given the low mortality (<2%) associated with thyroid cancer. In a recent review of 215 patients less than 21 years of age with papillary thyroid cancer, there were no disease-associated deaths within the first 20 years following surgery. In addition, none of the patients with distant metastases died of their disease. It was found that recurrence rates of local and

TABLE 58-4

ATA Risk Category Guidelines for Prophylactic Thyroidectomy and Screening for Medullary Thyroid Cancer

ATA Risk Level	Age at RET Testing	Age at First US	Age at First Serum Calcitonin	Age of Prophylactic Surgery
D	Within first year	Within first year	6 months unless already postoperative	Within first year
C	<3-5 years	>3-5 years	>3-5 years	Before age 5 years
B	<3-5 years	>3-5 years	>3-5 years	Consider before age 5 years; may delay*
A	<3-5 years	>3-5 years	>3-5 years	May delay after age 5 years*

*Criteria for delay must be met: normal basal and stimulated calcitonin, normal annual neck US, less aggressive MTC family history.
ATA, American Thyroid Association; MTC, medullary thyroid cancer; RET, rearranged during transfection (proto-oncogene); US, ultrasonography.
Adapted from Kloos RT, Eng C, Evans DB, et al: Medullary thyroid cancer: Management guidelines of the American Thyroid Association. Thyroid. 2009;19:565-612; with permission from Mary Ann Liebert, Inc.

distant disease were lower in patients treated with RRA, but this did not reach statistical significance. Interestingly, they did report a statistically higher mortality rate from secondary malignancy compared with an aged-matched control group. Of the patients in the study who died of a secondary malignancy, 73% had received RRA. This does not prove the association, but it does raise some concern.[40]

MEDULLARY THYROID CANCER

Medullary thyroid cancer (MTC) arises from the parafollicular cells of neuroectodermal origin and accounts for approximately 5% of thyroid cancers. MTC that arises sporadically usually involves only one lobe, whereas cases of familial inheritance usually involve both lobes. Inherited MTC includes the multiple endocrine neoplasia type 2 syndromes (MEN2A and MEN2B) as well as familial medullary thyroid cancer. In general, hereditary medullary thyroid cancer begins with parafollicular cell hyperplasia and then progresses to invasive microcarcinoma, followed by macroscopic disease if left untreated. The RET proto-oncogene also plays an important role in medullary thyroid cancer, including not only familial but also 40% of sporadic cases,[52-55] and RET testing is used to make the diagnosis of MEN2. When there is a germline RET mutation, the aberrant protein is expressed in all of the tissues in which it is produced, leading to MEN2 or familial medullary thyroid cancer. Sporadic MTC occurs when there is a somatic mutation with aberrant protein expression only in the thyroid.[56] Although essentially all patients with MEN2A will eventually develop medullary thyroid cancer, MTC in MEN2B tends to develop earlier and is in general more aggressive.[35] Because of this, when families are known to carry the RET mutation, genetic testing should be performed before 5 years of age in families with MEN2A and even earlier for MEN2B. Less clear is the age at which to perform prophylactic thyroidectomy. On the one hand, the goal is to perform thyroidectomy well before the onset of metastatic disease, after which point cure can be difficult,[56] but on the other hand it is also important to minimize the risks to the recurrent laryngeal nerve and parathyroid glands, which are at higher risk in smaller children. Determining the ideal age for thyroidectomy has been based upon numerous criteria, including the age of the youngest family member to develop cancer, the mean age of onset for a particular genotype, and yearly neck ultrasound findings.[57-59] It is known that for MEN2A, microinvasive carcinoma can be seen in children as young as 5 years of age.[60] The most current recommendations have been established by the American Thyroid Association (ATA) and are guided by the fact that the risk of developing MTC correlates with specific RET mutations where different codons are known to have different clinical behavior.[61] There are four risk categories—ATA-A having the lowest risk and ATA-B through ATA-D almost always resulting in MTC.[62] Specific recommendations based on these risk categories are seen in Table 58-4. In general, a central neck node dissection is not necessary during prophylactic thyroidectomy for children, unless there is evidence of nodal disease.[63] For patients with a suspicion of sporadic medullary thyroid cancer, serum calcitonin levels are useful for screening.[62] Treatment after the diagnosis of established medullary cancer includes total thyroidectomy with central node dissection of all nodal tissue from the hyoid bone to the sternal notch and to the carotid sheaths laterally. Preoperative neck ultrasonography is recommended for all children with medullary thyroid cancer to assess for nodal disease.[64] Children can then be followed with serum calcitonin and carcinoembryonic antigen (CEA) levels, which reliably correlate with disease recurrence. Survival in patients with established medullary thyroid cancer has been most recently reported as 96% at 5 years and 86% at 15 years.[30] Novel therapy in adults with metastatic medullary thyroid cancer includes the use of an oral RET inhibitor that blocks kinase signaling. There is evidence that the inhibitor may halt disease progression in the adult population.[65] To date, similar studies have not been done in children.

Parathyroid Embryology and Physiology

The parathyroid glands arise from the third and fourth pharyngeal pouches, which are paired endoderm-lined structures between the branchial arches. By the sixth week of gestation, the dorsal aspects of the third and fourth pouches differentiate into the inferior and superior parathyroids, respectively. The ventral aspects of the third pouches form the thymus and the ventral aspects of the fourth pouches develop into the ultimobranchial body, which eventually fuses with the thyroid to supply the parafollicular cells that produce calcitonin. The thymus and parathyroid glands then lose their connection to the pharynx and descend into the neck. Typically the parathyroid glands migrate to the posterior aspect of the thyroid gland, where they obtain their blood supply from the thyroid capsule. However, there is significant variability in the eventual location of the parathyroid glands, as seen in Figure 58-3. They are variable in both location and number and can be found anywhere in the vicinity of the thyroid or thymus. The superior glands tend to be more consistent in their location than the inferior glands.

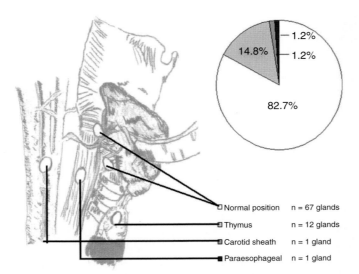

- □ Normal position n = 67 glands
- ◪ Thymus n = 12 glands
- ▨ Carotid sheath n = 1 gland
- ■ Paraesophageal n = 1 gland

FIGURE 58-3 Location of parathyroid glands found and removed during primary parathyroidectomy. (Reprinted from Schlosser K, Schmitt CP, Bartholomaeus JE, et al: Parathyroidectomy for renal hyperparathyroidism in children and adolescents. World J Surg 2008;32:801-806; with permission from Springer.)

The parathyroid glands regulate calcium and phosphorous by secreting parathyroid hormone (PTH). PTH is an 84–amino acid protein with a very short half-life that is primarily metabolized by the liver and kidney. PTH secretion is normally stimulated by a drop in circulating calcium and is then inhibited by a negative feedback loop. An increase in serum phosphorus also indirectly stimulates PTH secretion by lowering serum calcium. PTH also acts directly on bones by increasing osteoclast activity, on the kidneys by increasing renal calcium absorption, and on the gastrointestinal (GI) tract by increasing vitamin D activation.

Disorders of the Parathyroid Glands

DiGEORGE SYNDROME

DiGeorge syndrome is a congenital disorder characterized by athymia or thymic hypoplasia and absence of the parathyroid glands due to failure of the third and fourth pharyngeal pouches to differentiate. Infants are hypocalcemic and also have increased susceptibility to infection. Additional associated characteristics can include shortened philtrum, low set ears, nasal clefts, thyroid hypoplasia, and cardiac anomalies, especially truncus arteriosus. Treatment is largely symptomatic and includes supplementation with calcium and vitamin D. Emerging therapies include replacement with synthetic PTH[66] and thymus transplantation for children with severe immunodeficiency.[67]

HYPERPARATHYROIDISM

There are several forms of hyperparathyroidism, all of which lead to excessive PTH secretion. In the case of primary hyperparathyroidism, this results from one or more abnormal parathyroid glands. In secondary hyperparathyroidism, elevated PTH is in response to hypocalcemia, and in tertiary hyperparathyroidism, PTH remains elevated despite correction of the hypocalcemia. Both secondary and tertiary types are seen in the setting of renal disease. Neonatal severe hyperparathyroidism (NSHPT) is a rare disorder that presents with severe hypercalcemia resulting from a homozygous loss-of-function mutation with four-gland hyperplasia. Treatment has traditionally been with a three and one half–gland parathyroidectomy or total parathyroidectomy with autotransplantation. More recently, there has also been some success with medical management with bisphosphonates.[68]

In general, hyperparathyroidism presents clinically with symptoms related to elevated calcium or is suspected when hypercalcemia is found incidentally. However, the differential diagnosis of hypercalcemia in children is quite broad, and this must be kept in mind during the initial evaluation, as outlined in Table 58-5. For example, familial hypocalciuric hypercalcemia is an autosomal dominant condition resulting from a mutation in the calcium sensing receptor. Children have elevated serum calcium but can be distinguished from having hyperparathyroidism by detecting decreased 24-hour urinary calcium levels. PTH levels are often within the normal range. Usually these children are completely asymptomatic, and no specific treatment is required. This condition should be excluded prior to considering parathyroid resection for hypercalcemia.

The incidence of primary hyperparathyroidism in children is estimated to be 2 to 5 per 100,000.[69] In contrast to adults, children may present with more serious effects of hypercalcemia, including renal failure, cardiac arrhythmias, and osteopenia.[2] When suspected, the diagnosis can be confirmed by measuring serum calcium and PTH. Most commonly, there will be a solitary parathyroid adenoma, and there are several localization studies that can be used to identify the abnormal gland. The imaging options include ultrasonography,

TABLE 58-5

Causes of Hypercalcemia in Children

Endocrine
  Primary hyperparathyroidism
  Secondary hyperparathyroidism
  Tertiary hyperparathyroidism
  Thyrotoxicosis
  Familial hypocalciuric hypercalcemia
  Neonatal severe hyperparathyroidism
  Ectopic parathyroid hormone production
Granulomatous disease
  Sarcoidosis
  Tuberculosis
  Fungal infection
Pharmacologic
  Vitamin D
  Vitamin A
  Thiazide diuretics
  Theophylline
  Milk alkali
  Lithium
Immobilization
Subcutaneous fat necrosis

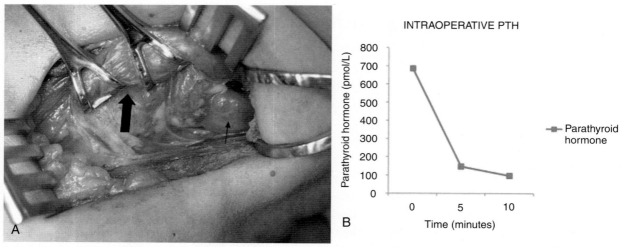

FIGURE 58-4 **A**, Parathyroid adenoma in the setting of hypercalcemia. The small arrow demonstrates the parathyroid adenoma, and the large arrow demonstrates the retracted thyroid gland. **B**, Intraoperative PTH monitoring for the patient seen in **A** demonstrating the fall in PTH over 10 minutes after removal of the parathyroid gland. *(See Expert Consult site for color version.)*

[99m]Tc-sestamibi planar scintigraphy, SPECT, SPECT/CT, and/or magnetic resonance imaging (MRI). Because of the rarity of parathyroid adenomas in children, most of the studies used to compare techniques have been done in adults. In one study by Munk and colleagues,[70] ultrasonography and ^{99m}Tc-sestamibi scans were in agreement 70% of the time and, when in agreement, identified the correct gland in 97% of cases. When these tests were not in agreement, MRI was used, and if consistent with either an ultrasound or ^{99m}Tc-sestamibi scan, the correct gland was identified 100% of the time. There were six patients (11%) in whom there was no definitive agreement among the three tests. More advanced scintigraphy is now being used (SPECT), which allows for a three-dimensional reconstruction, and this can also be combined with traditional CT (SPECT/CT), allowing for more anatomic detail.[71] However, whether the added detail improves accurate localization is still debated.[72] If localization is successful, a directed resection can then be used instead of the traditional four-gland exploration. However, in the hands of an experienced surgeon, this remains a very reliable approach. To confirm resection of the adenoma, intraoperative PTH measurement can be used. The half-life of PTH is approximately 3 to 4 minutes, and at least a 50% decrease from baseline should be observed to confirm removal of the abnormal parathyroid.[73] An example of a typical decline can be seen in Figure 58-4. It is important to follow the PTH level far enough out to ensure the decline is not temporary, which can be seen with multiple-gland disease.[74] If the PTH remains elevated, a complete cervical exploration should be pursued. If a normal parathyroid is resected or devascularized during thyroid surgery, the gland should be autotransplanted into the forearm or sternocleidomastoid.[75] Hyperparathyroidism is also seen in the setting of multiple endocrine neoplasia and is usually the result of four-gland hyperplasia.

The surgical options include resection of only visibly enlarged glands, three and one half–gland parathyroidectomy, or total parathyroidectomy with autografting.[76,77]

Secondary and tertiary hyperparathyroidism are most commonly seen with end-stage renal disease and affect all four glands. Usually, this can be managed with dietary modifications, dialysis, phosphate binders, and vitamin D. However, vitamin D analogs and calcimimetics have not been approved for long-term use in children because of concern for interference with longitudinal growth and the possible impact on timing of puberty.[78] There is some debate as to whether the optimal surgical management is total parathyroidectomy with autotransplantation or subtotal parathyroidectomy, but the preferred management in the United States tends to be the former.[75,79]

Parathyroid Carcinoma

Parathyroid carcinoma is exceedingly rare in children, with only seven case reports in the literature to date. In all cases, the patients presented with a neck mass and severe hypercalcemia with extremely elevated PTH (3 to 10 times normal). The first step in management is to control the hypercalcemia, followed by surgical excision if appropriate. The recommended resection includes en-bloc hemithyroidectomy, parathyroidectomy, and lymph node dissection. If completely resected, 90% long-term survival can be achieved. However, with incomplete resection, the recurrence rate is up to 50%.[80]

The complete reference list is available online at www.expertconsult.com.

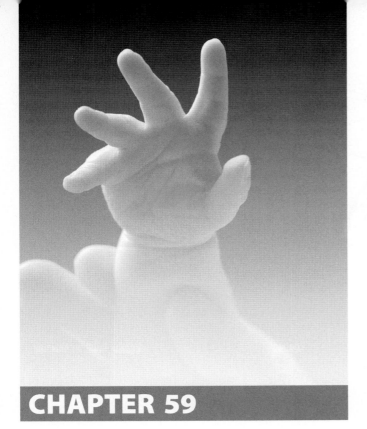

CHAPTER 59

Neck Cysts and Sinuses

Craig Lillehei

Cysts and sinuses of the neck represent a wide variety of anomalies, both congenital and acquired. The focus of this chapter is on those of congenital origin. It is a fascinating opportunity to apply our understanding of embryologic development to the spectrum of malformations seen and to guide appropriate management. The most common lesions arise from thyroglossal duct or branchial anomalies (particularly from the second cleft). Nonetheless, one must be cognizant of the range of usual variants as well as the broad differential diagnosis. Lymphatic and vascular malformations will be addressed elsewhere (see Chapter 125). Although present at birth, congenital lesions may not become evident for weeks, months, or even years. However, there are recognizable patterns. Accurate diagnosis guides appropriate intervention. Proper identification is aided by careful history and physical examination. Age at presentation, evolution, anatomic location, and associated drainage are often important diagnostic clues. Radiographic studies, such as ultrasonography or cross-sectional imaging (computed tomography [CT], magnetic resonance imaging [MRI]), may be helpful in selected cases. Although the exact identity is not always evident preoperatively, an awareness of differential diagnostic possibilities will guide the prepared mind and improve prospects for optimal outcomes. The emphasis is total excision of the lesions to minimize the risks of recurrence, infection, or malignancy. Knowledge of the relevant local anatomy and adjacent structures is crucial to safe surgical dissection.

Embryology

During the fourth week of gestation, neural crest cells migrate into the future head and neck region. A series of six paired branchial or pharyngeal arches begin to develop (Fig. 59-1). In humans the fifth arch, if present, is only very short lived. Their mesoderm is covered externally by ectoderm and lined internally by endoderm. Each arch contains a distinct artery, nerve, cartilage rod, and muscle. These arches are separated by depressions that are referred to as clefts on their external ectodermal surface, and pouches on their internal endodermal surface. These swellings may give rise to normal cervical structures, leave pathologic remnants, or involute entirely. In fish and amphibians, the closing membranes that separate the branchial pouches and clefts regress with the resultant connections forming gills.[1]

Each branchial arch and its components can be traced to the formation of future anatomic structures as outlined in Table 59-1. The first branchial arch forms the mandible and a portion of the maxilla. It is also involved in structures of the inner ear. The first cleft and pouch connect to form the eustachian tube/middle ear, tympanic membrane, and external auditory canal. The other branchial cleft components usually regress. However, it is important to note that during development the second, third, and fourth branchial clefts share a common external opening, the cervical sinus of His (Fig. 59-2, A). For this reason the location of the external opening of a persistent sinus or fistula from these clefts cannot be used to distinguish between them.

The remaining pouches give rise to normal glandular structures (Fig. 59-2, B). The palatine tonsil and supratonsillar fossa originate from the second pouch. The tonsils are the only structures to remain at their pouch of origin. The third pouch gives rise to the thymus and inferior parathyroid glands, while the fourth pouch is responsible for the superior parathyroid glands. It is believed that the calcitonin-producing cells of the thyroid gland arise from the ultimobranchial body, probably a remnant of the ventral portion of the caudal pharyngeal complex formed by the fourth and vestigial fifth pouch (see Fig. 59-2).

The thyroid gland arises from an endodermal thickening in the floor of the primitive pharynx called the tuberculum impar (see Fig. 59-1). A bilobate diverticulum develops between the anterior and posterior muscle complex of the tongue. As the embryo elongates this anlage descends anterior to or through the eventual location of the hyoid bone and fuses with elements of the fourth and fifth branchial pouches to form the thyroid gland. This descending median thyroid anlage gives rise to the thyroglossal duct, which usually obliterates by the fifth week of gestation.[2] The proximal remnant of this pathway is the foramen cecum at the base of the tongue, whereas the distal remnant is represented by the pyramidal lobe of the thyroid gland (Fig. 59-3). Cystic remnants or accessory thyroid tissue can remain anywhere along this tract (Fig. 59-4).

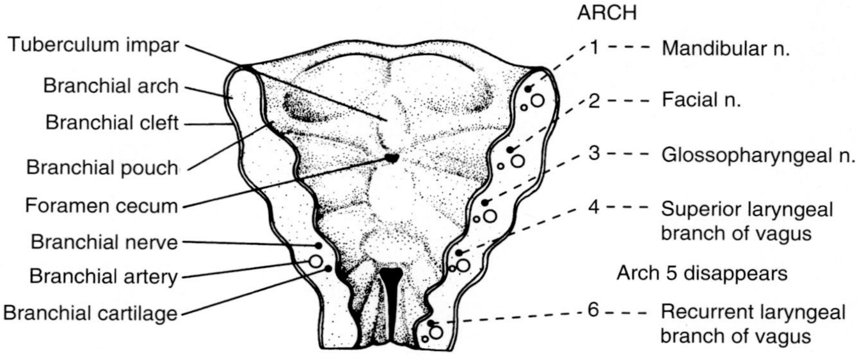

FIGURE 59-1 Early development of branchial apparatus. (From Donegan JO: Congenital neck masses. In Cummings CW, Fredrickson JM, Harker LA, et al [eds]: Otolaryngology—Head and Neck Surgery, ed 2. St Louis, Mosby-Year Book, 1993.)

TABLE 59-1

Derivatives of Branchial Arches, Clefts, and Pouches

		Dorsal	*Ventral*	*Midline Floor of Pharynx*
I				
Arch		Incus body	Meckel cartilage	Body of tongue
	External maxillary artery	Malleus head	Malleus	
	Nerve V	Pinna		
Cleft		External auditory canal		
Pouch		Eustachian tube		
		Middle ear cavity		
		Mastoid air cells		
II				
Arch		Stapes	Styloid process	Root of tongue
	Stapedial artery		Hyoid (lesser horn and part of body)	Foramen cecum
	Nerves VII and VIII			Thyroid gland's median anlage
Pouch		Palatine tonsil		
		Supratonsillar fossa		
III				
Arch			Hyoid (greater horn and part of body)	
	Internal carotid artery		Part of epiglottis	
	Nerve IX		Thymus	
Pouch		Inferior parathyroid		
		Piriform fossa		
IV				
Arch			Thyroid cartilage	
	Arch of aorta (L)		Cuneiform cartilage	
	Part of subclavian artery (R)		Part of epiglottis	
	Nerve X			
Pouch		Superior parathyroid (lateral anlage of thyroid gland)	Thymus (inconstant)	
V				
Arch				
Pouch		Ultimobranchial body (lateral anlage of thyroid gland)		
VI				
Arch			Cricoid	
	Pulmonary artery		Arytenoid	
	Ductus arteriosus (L)		Corniculate cartilage	
	Nerve X (recurrent laryngeal)			

From Skandalakis JE, Gray SW, Todd NW: The pharynx and its derivatives. In Skandalakis JE, Gray SW (eds): Embryology for Surgeons, ed 2. Baltimore, Williams & Wilkins, 1994.

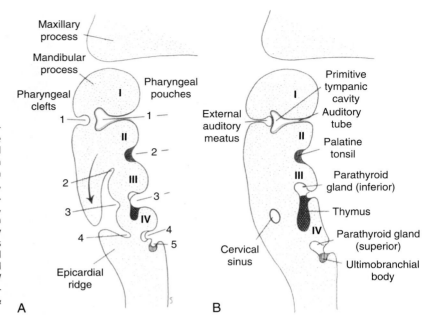

FIGURE 59-2 **A,** Schematic representation of the development of the pharyngeal (or branchial) clefts and pouches. Note that the second arch grows over the third and fourth arches, thereby burying the second, third, and fourth pharyngeal clefts. **B,** Remnants of the second, third, and fourth pharyngeal clefts form the cervical sinus, which is normally obliterated. Note the structures formed by the various pharyngeal pouches. (From Sadler TW: Head and neck. In Langman J, Sadler TW (eds): Langman's Medical Embryology, ed 7. Baltimore, Williams & Wilkins, 1995.)

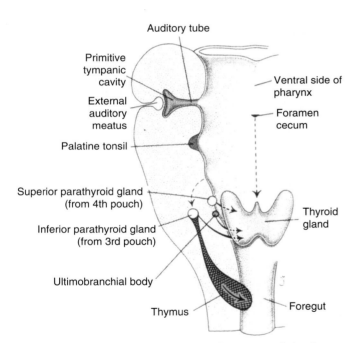

FIGURE 59-3 Schematic representation of migration of the thymus, parathyroid glands, and ultimobranchial body. The thyroid gland originates in the midline at the level of the foramen cecum and descends to the level of the first tracheal ring. (From Sadler TW: Head and neck. In Langman's Medical Embryology, ed 7. Baltimore, Williams & Wilkins, 1995.)

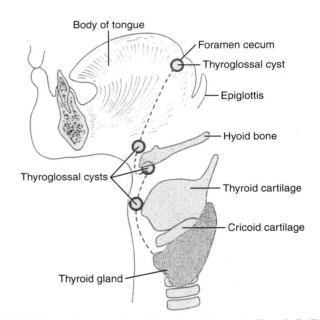

FIGURE 59-4 Various locations of thyroglossal duct cysts. (From Sadler TW: Head and neck. In Sadler TW (ed): Langman's Medical Embryology, ed 11. Baltimore, Lippincott Williams & Wilkins, 2010.)

Thyroglossal Duct Cysts

Thyroglossal duct remnants are clearly the most common midline congenital cervical anomalies. As described, they occur along the path of thyroid descent from the foramen cecum at the base of the tongue to the lower neck. The remnants usually lie in close proximity to the hyoid bone. Given this relationship one can appreciate why the cysts often move cephalad with swallowing or tongue protrusion. Although classically described as midline, up to 40% may lie just lateral to the midline. Most lesions present as cystic masses, but up to 25% have a draining sinus.[7] Because the thyroglossal duct

Although the exact incidence varies between different pediatric series, thyroglossal duct remnants are typically the more common etiology of congenital neck cysts or sinuses, followed closely by branchial cleft remnants.[3–5] In general, thyroglossal duct lesions lie close to the midline, whereas branchial remnants present more laterally in the neck, although atypical locations have been described.[6]

does not communicate with ectoderm during development, the sinus is either the result of spontaneous rupture, infection, or a prior drainage procedure. Approximately 60% of thyroglossal duct cysts are adjacent to the hyoid bone, 24% lie above the hyoid, and 13% lie below.[8] The remaining 8% of cysts are intralingual and may pose a risk for acute airway obstruction, particularly in the neonate.[9] Most thyroglossal duct cysts present during the first 5 years of life.[2]

In view of the potential communication with the oral cavity, it is not surprising that the cysts may fluctuate in size or that approximately one third of patients present with an active infection of the cyst or history of prior infection.[2] Some patients may actually report noticing a foul taste. The most common pathogens are *Haemophilus influenzae, Staphylococcus aureus,* and *Staphylococcus epidermidis*.[7,10]

The thyroglossal duct remnants are lined by ductal epithelium and may contain solid thyroid tissue. In fact, in roughly 1% to 2% of patients with presumed thyroglossal duct cysts, the actual lesion is a median ectopic thyroid.[8] It may represent their only functional thyroid tissue in which case excision would be problematic. Further evaluation may be obtained with a screening thyroid-stimulating hormone (TSH) level and neck ultrasonography. If there is evidence of hypothyroidism or the mass appears solid without a visible normal thyroid gland, one might wish to obtain a thyroid scan to determine whether there is any additional thyroid tissue. Such patients are often hypothyroid with an elevated TSH, which is responsible for the hypertrophy of the ectopic tissue. In the setting of hypothyroidism, hormonal supplementation would be appropriate and might promote shrinkage of the hypertrophic thyroid tissue, thereby obviating the need for surgery.

SURGICAL MANAGEMENT

The primary indication for excision of thyroglossal duct remnants is to avoid problems with recurrent infection. However, malignancy within thyroglossal duct remnants is also well described.[11] Such tumors usually present as papillary carcinoma in adults, but pediatric cases are reported, and multiple cell types have been encountered.[12–14]

Appropriate surgical management of uncomplicated thyroglossal duct disease involves complete resection of the cyst and its tract in continuity with the central hyoid bone, as described by Sistrunk.[15] One should be aware that in young children the hyoid bone may override the thyroid notch, potentially placing the larynx at risk. The patient is positioned supine with the head elevated and neck extended. A transverse cervical incision is used to carefully mobilize the cyst along with its tract. The underlying hyoid bone is divided about 1 cm from the midline on either side after dividing the attachments of the mylohyoid and hyoglossus muscles from its superior border. En-bloc resection is completed with suture ligation of the proximal tract, prior to removal of the specimen (Fig. 59-5). Elegant studies of resected surgical specimens by Horisawa and colleagues, as depicted in Figure 59-6, demonstrate the importance of this strategy to achieve complete excision, thereby reducing the likelihood of recurrence.[16]

In the setting of acute infection, initial efforts are aimed to control the infection. If antibiotics alone are insufficient, aspiration or incision and drainage of the cyst/abscess may be required. Once the infection is well-controlled, the described Sistrunk procedure can be performed using an elliptic skin

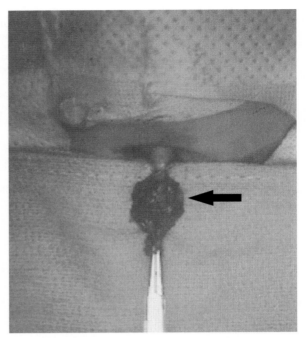

FIGURE 59-5   Sistrunk procedure: intraoperative photograph of resection of thyroglossal duct cyst in continuity with central hyoid bone *(arrow)*. *(See Expert Consult site for color version.)*

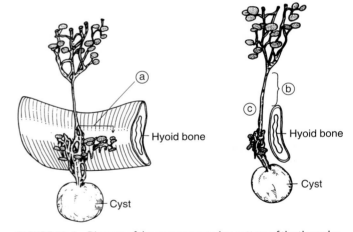

FIGURE 59-6   Diagram of the common running pattern of the thyroglossal duct based on anatomic reconstruction. *a,* Horizontal distance from midline to the most distant thyroglossal duct; *b,* length of the single duct above the hyoid bone; *c,* point where the diameter of the duct is measured. (From Horisawa M, Niinomi N, Ito T: What is the optimal depth for core-out toward the foramen cecum in a thyroglossal duct cyst operation? J Pediatr Surg 1992;27:710-713.)

incision around the cutaneous opening to permit excision of this tract in continuity with the remainder of the specimen.

Recurrences after thyroglossal duct excisions may occur in up to 10% of cases.[17,18] The most likely cause is incomplete excision of the tract or intraoperative rupture. An association with preoperative infection has been suggested,[19,20] but not confirmed in more recent analyses. Postoperative infection is clearly associated with recurrence, but it is uncertain whether this development represents cause or effect.[18] Excision of a recurrent thyroglossal duct remnant has a 20% to 35% risk of failure.[10,21] Wider resection is recommended, including the pyramidal lobe if present, central strap muscles, additional hyoid bone, and residual tissue up to the foramen cecum.[17,22]

Branchial Anomalies

Most branchial cleft anomalies arise from the second cleft/pouch, with a much smaller proportion from the first. Remnants of the third or fourth pouches are rare. It is the internal opening of branchial sinuses that best defines their embryologic origin. The anomalies may present as fistulae, cysts, sinus tracts, or cartilaginous remnants and are thought to arise from incomplete obliteration during embryogenesis. To clarify, cysts have mucosal or epithelial lining, but no external openings. Sinuses may communicate either externally with the skin or internally with the pharynx, whereas fistulae connect to both. When an external tract is present, branchial anomalies are usually diagnosed within the first decade of life. However, when there is no external opening the diagnosis may be delayed into adulthood. Up to 10% of these lesions are bilateral as depicted in Figure 59-7.[23,24] The presence of preauricular pits in patients with branchial anomalies should raise the suspicion for the branchio-oto-renal (BOR) and branchio-oculo-facial (BOF) syndromes. Both are autosomal dominant conditions with associated hearing loss, ear malformations, and renal anomalies in the BOR syndrome, while BOF includes eye anomalies, such as microphthalmia and obstructed lacrimal ducts, and facial anomalies consisting of cleft or pseudocleft lip/palate.[24,25]

It is worth mentioning that short sinus tracts, pedunculated skin appendages or subcutaneous cartilaginous remnants are often encountered in the anterior neck and upper chest. These structures are probably branchial remnants, but cannot usually be ascribed to a specific arch. Lesions presenting below the clavicles are more likely epidermoid or dermoid cysts rather than branchial remnants. Most often elective excision is used.

SECOND BRANCHIAL ANOMALIES

Second branchial cleft anomalies typically lie somewhere between the lower anterior border of the sternocleidomastoid (SCM) muscle and tonsillar fossa of the pharynx. They may be in close proximity to the glossopharyngeal and hypoglossal nerves as well as carotid vessels as the tract travels through the carotid bifurcation and over the nerves to enter the lateral pharyngeal wall as depicted in Figure 59-8.

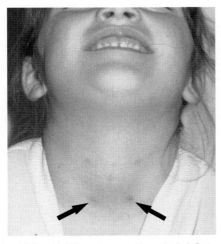

FIGURE 59-7 Child with bilateral second branchial cleft sinuses *(arrows)*. *(See Expert Consult site for color version.)*

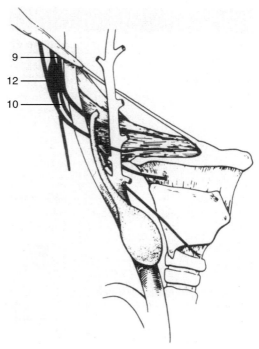

FIGURE 59-8 Second branchial cleft cyst and sinus tract. (From Donegan JO: Congenital neck masses. In Cummings CW, Fredrickson JM, Harker LA, et al [eds]: Otolaryngology—Head and Neck Surgery, ed 2. St Louis, Mosby-Year Book, 1993.)

The branchial anomalies are lined by epithelium. Overall cystic lesions are more common than fistulae, but usually present later (e.g., second decade).[7] Cysts most often present as nontender soft tissue masses beneath the SCM muscle. However, they may present with acute infection. Change in size during upper respiratory infections is noted in up to 25%.[26] The anomalies have been classified into four types.[5] Type 1 are superficial, but located deep to the platysma and cervical fascia, along the anterior border of the SCM muscle. Type 2 anomalies are the most common. They course deep to the SCM muscle and either anterior or posterior to the carotid artery. Type 3 lesions pass between the carotid bifurcation and lie adjacent to the pharynx. Type 4 lesions are medial to the carotid sheath and in close approximation to the pharynx, usually at the level of the tonsillar fossa.

The most common presentation in infants and young children is a second branchial cleft sinus with drainage from a small cutaneous pit along the anterior border of the lower sternocleidomastoid muscle. On occasion, a subcutaneous tract is palpable more cephalad. Less common symptoms include stridor, dysphagia, odynophagia, or cranial nerve palsies. Branchiogenic carcinoma has been diagnosed in adults.[27]

Given the risks of infection, further enlargement or malignancy, elective excision is recommended once the diagnosis has been made. There is typically no urgency; so, one can defer excision beyond 3 to 6 months of age or to allow treatment of an acute infection. Systemic antibiotics and aspiration are generally preferable to incision and drainage, which might produce more distortion of the surgical planes; however, when diagnosis is unclear, the latter allows biopsy of the cyst wall, which can help to distinguish between an infected branchial cleft cyst and simple bacterial lymphadenitis.

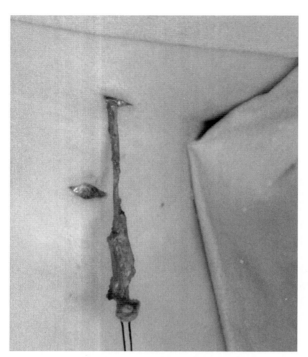

FIGURE 59-9 Intraoperative photo showing excision of second branchial cleft sinus/fistula using second parallel ("step-ladder") cervical incision. *(See Expert Consult site for color version.)*

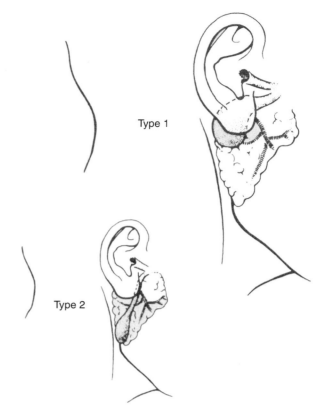

FIGURE 59-10 Type I and type II first branchial cleft abnormalities. (From Donegan JO: Congenital neck masses. In Cummings CW, Fredrickson JM, Harker LA, et al [eds]: Otolaryngology—Head and Neck Surgery, ed 2. St Louis, Mosby-Year Book, 1993.)

The goal is complete excision of the tract without injury to surrounding nerves or vascular structures. A transverse cervical incision in a skin crease directly over the cyst will aid to optimize the future cosmetic result. In the case of a sinus or fistula, precise identification may be facilitated by gently inserting a probe, catheter, or monofilament suture into the tract. A lacrimal probe dipped in methylene blue has also been used to stain the tract and make it easier to identify should it break during dissection. Excision is best accomplished by dissection directly on the surface of the lesion. The tract may be very thin-walled; so, one must be careful to avoid avulsion with possible loss of the proximal lumen. If the tract is long, exposure may be improved by a second (so-called "stepladder") incision along a skin crease more cephalad (Fig. 59-9). Second branchial anomalies presenting as pharyngeal cysts can be excised by an intraoral approach.[28,29]

FIRST BRANCHIAL ANOMALIES

First branchial cleft anomalies are rare, but more common in females. Accurate diagnosis is difficult and may be quite delayed.[30] Remnants may persist anywhere between the external auditory canal and submandibular area. They should be distinguished from preauricular pits and sinuses, which arise from failure of the auricular hillocks to fuse. The first cleft anomalies often lie in close association to the parotid gland and facial nerve. In 1972, Work classified first branchial anomalies into types 1 and 2 (Fig. 59-10).[31] Type 1 lesions are rarer and considered duplications of the membranous external auditory canal. They are of ectodermal origin and generally course lateral to the facial nerve. Type 2 lesions contain both ectodermal and mesodermal elements, which may include cartilage. These anomalies pass medial to the facial nerve but may present

in preauricular, infraauricular, or postauricular locations. Sinuses may present with external drainage below the angle of the mandible or otorrhea, which may become infected. Cysts present as soft tissue masses in this region which may also become secondarily infected. A communication with the external auditory canal may be present. A careful otologic examination is important to define the pathology.

Complete surgical excision is once again recommended, but great care must be taken given the proximity of the facial nerve. In infants and children, the nerve is probably even more susceptible given that it is smaller and more superficial without well-developed landmarks.[32] Many authors recommend initial exposure of the main trunk of the facial nerve and its peripheral branches with superficial parotidectomy to reduce the risk of facial nerve injury.[33,34] Prior infection may distort accurate tissue dissection planes. It is necessary to excise the involved skin and cartilage of the external auditory canal. Furthermore, if the tract extends medially to the tympanic membrane a second operation may be required to remove this segment.[35,36]

THIRD AND FOURTH BRANCHIAL ANOMALIES

Third and fourth branchial anomalies are very rare and almost always occur on the left side of the neck. Most present as sinuses or infected cysts rather than congenital fistulae and drain into the piriform sinus. Although sometimes combined

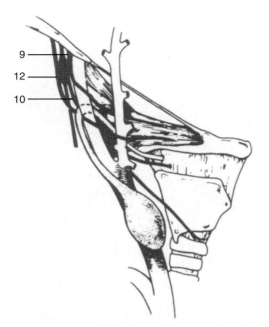

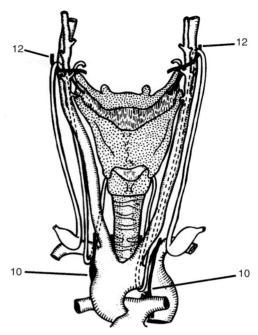

FIGURE 59-11 Third branchial cleft cyst and sinus tract. Note that these occur much more frequently on the left side (approximately 90%); also, during surgery the tract is often seen to go straight up from the left upper thyroid lobe area toward the thyroid cartilage, without passing behind the carotid artery as the embryologic development would suggest. (From Donegan JO: Congenital neck masses. In Cummings CW, Fredrickson JM, Harker LA, et al [eds]: Otolaryngology—Head and Neck Surgery, ed 2. St Louis, Mosby-Year Book, 1993.)

FIGURE 59-12 Anatomic relationships of theoretical course of fourth branchial fistula. Such a complete fistula has never been described in humans. (From Liston SL: Fourth branchial fistula. Otolaryngol Head Neck Surg 1981;89:520-522.

generically as piriform sinus tracts, distinction is possible. As noted in Figure 59-1 the superior laryngeal nerve represents the nerve to the fourth branchial arch. Third pouch anomalies enter the piriform sinus above the superior laryngeal nerve, whereas fourth pouch anomalies enter below this nerve. A third branchial cleft fistula theoretically would extend from the anterior border of the SCM, traversing deep to the internal carotid artery and glossopharyngeal nerve, piercing the thyroid membrane above the internal branch of the superior laryngeal nerve and entering the pharynx at the piriform sinus as depicted in Figure 59-11. A fourth branchial fistula would course around the subclavian artery on the right or aortic arch on the left to ascend back up over the hypoglossal nerve and enter the piriform apex or cervical esophagus (Fig. 59-12). A complete fourth branchial fistula has yet to be identified in humans,[5] and most third branchial fistulae described appear to have been secondary to infection or repeated surgery.[37]

Presentation of piriform sinus tracts may be quite subtle and their diagnosis very challenging. Noncommunicating or noninfected communicating cysts may present as cold thyroid nodules, which may be partly or totally intrathyroid.[37] A history of repeated upper respiratory tract infections and sore throats, hoarseness or pain, and tenderness of the thyroid gland should raise suspicion. Infection may result in suppurative thyroiditis[38]; any thyroid abscess in a child should raise the suspicion of a branchial remnant, particularly if closely related to the left upper pole of the thyroid gland. Acute respiratory compromise in neonates has been described.[39] Needle aspiration may be required to temporarily relieve respiratory symptoms. A contrast esophagogram after resolution of the acute infection may demonstrate the tract from the piriform

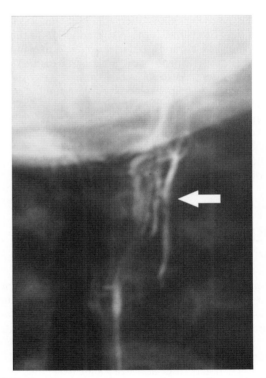

FIGURE 59-13 Contrast esophagogram demonstrating contrast within piriform sinus tract *(arrow). (See Expert Consult site for color version.)*

sinus as depicted in Figure 59-13. Other imaging has been successful if air is visualized within the cyst or tract originating from the piriform fossa opening.[40] Combinations of ultrasonography, CT, MRI, and thyroid scan may help in establishing a diagnosis.[37]

Once again, complete excision is necessary to avoid continued difficulties. Often several previous operations have been performed before the correct pathology is recognized.[41,42] Direct laryngoscopy or rigid pharyngoscopy, using a Hopkins rod-lens telescope, is recommended for accurate diagnosis as well as endoscopic cannulation of the opening into the piriform sinus, if possible, to facilitate accurate dissection.[37,43] A standard collar incision is used with identification of the recurrent laryngeal nerve. Partial or total ipsilateral thyroid lobectomy with excision of the tract to the piriform sinus is usually required. Partial resection of the thyroid cartilage may also be necessary to remove the entire tract.[44] Cauterization of the internal opening has been described.[45,46]

Dermoid Cysts

Cervical dermoid cysts are thought to arise from elements trapped during fusion of the anterior branchial arches. They are composed of ectodermal and mesodermal elements, but in contrast to teratomas, do not contain any endodermal derivatives.[35] These lesions are typically midline and well-circumscribed. They are lined by squamous epithelium and usually contain sebaceous debris, which can become secondarily infected. Although they appear echogenic rather than cystic on ultrasound examination, imaging is useful to differentiate submental dermoids from benign reactive lymph nodes. The overlying skin is often adherent, and a small cutaneous pit may be visible. If the cyst is adherent to the underlying fascia or lies within the strap muscles, it may move with swallowing or tongue protrusion, making the distinction from a thyroglossal duct cyst impossible. Complete excision is appropriate. A yellowish appearance at surgery and the sebaceous cyst content allow distinction from a thyroglossal duct cyst, which more often contains a clear viscous fluid. If the cyst lies adjacent to the hyoid bone and a diagnostic doubt exists, a formal Sistrunk procedure with in continuity excision of the central hyoid bone is recommended to ensure complete removal of the pathology.

Congenital Midline Cervical Clefts

Congenital midline cervical clefts are very rare anomalies thought to arise from failure of anterior fusion of the first two branchial arches.[47,48] They typically present as a longitudinal area of thinned or atrophic skin along the anterior midline of the neck. Characteristically, there are skin tags at the upper end and small sinus tracts at the inferior aspect. Secretions may be noted from accessory salivary glands draining into the cleft.[49,50] Early complete excision is recommended, both for cosmesis as well as to avoid limitations to neck extension and mandibular growth. Wound closure is accomplished using a series of Z-plasties, to avoid a contracting linear scar (Fig. 59-14).[51,52]

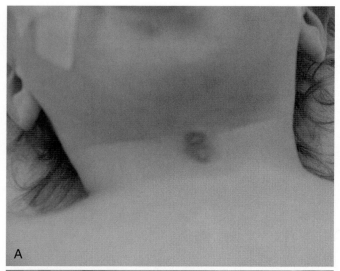

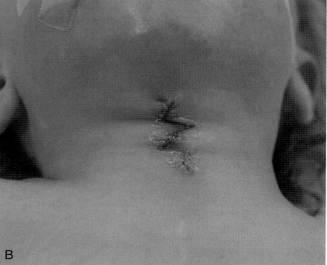

FIGURE 59-14   Photographs of infant with midline cervical cleft (**A**) and Z-plasty reconstruction after excision (**B**). *(See Expert Consult site for color version.)*

Cervical Thymic Cysts

Thymic cysts are usually seen within the chest and mediastinum. However, given that the thymus arises from the third, and sometimes fourth, branchial pouches, one can appreciate the possibility for a cervical location. Cervical thymic cysts typically present in the anterior triangle, more commonly on the left than the right. They occur more frequently in males, with peak onset at age 5 to 7 years.[53] They may be difficult to distinguish preoperatively from more common cystic lesions, such as branchial cleft cysts or lymphatic malformations. They can be unilocular or multilocular. Extension into the mediastinum is common and accounts for the often-described physical finding of enlargement with a Valsalva maneuver. The precise diagnosis is usually made postoperatively when elements of thymus are identified within the cyst wall. The fluid within these cysts is typically brownish in color. The lesions are almost always benign. Surgical excision is generally quite straightforward, although one needs to be cognizant of potentially adherent vessels (e.g., carotid artery, jugular vein) or nerves (e.g., phrenic, recurrent laryngeal). Although the aim is to completely remove the cyst, one should be careful in very young children, to avoid removing the entire thymus, which might have untoward immunologic consequences.

Although the focus of this chapter has been congenital lesions, the differential diagnosis for neck cysts and sinuses must be much broader. A wide variety of acquired conditions, including infections and tumors, should also be considered. The distinction between infection of a congenital cervical remnant and a primary cervical infection with the development of an abscess or draining sinus may not always be straightforward. Nonetheless, an awareness of the congenital possibilities and their likely anatomic locations will assist the astute clinician.

The complete reference list is available online at www. expertconsult.com.

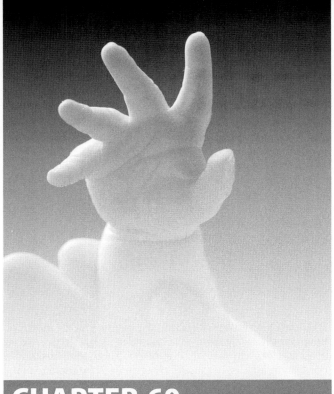

CHAPTER 60

Torticollis

Spencer W. Beasley

There are many causes of torticollis in childhood (Table 60-1), but most are rare. The most common cause of torticollis is tightness and shortening of one sternomastoid muscle, a condition that occurs in about 0.4% of all births. Typically, at about 3 weeks of age, a visible or palpable swelling develops in part or all of the muscle; this swelling is called a sternomastoid tumor. It affects the right side in about 60%,[1] is bilateral in 2% to 8%,[2,3] and often persists for up to 1 year. Older children may present with a fibrotic, shortened sternomastoid muscle, which is presumed in many to be the legacy of a previously unrecognized sternomastoid tumor.

History

Alexander the Great may have had torticollis, according to Plutarch.[4] Antyllus is said to have performed tenotomies in 350 AD, but the first authenticated division of the sternocleidomastoid was by Minnus in Amsterdam in 1641.[5] A sternocleidomastoid tumor was described by Heusinger in 1826.[6] Torticollis was also a subject of interest to Dupuytren.[7]

Etiology

Although often referred to as "congenital torticollis," the sternomastoid mass and the torticollis are rarely noticeable at birth. Little is known about the etiology of sternomastoid

fibrosis, although several theories have been put forward to explain the condition. It may be due to an idiopathic intrauterine embryopathy[8] or could be the manifestation of an intrauterine positional disorder producing sternocleidomastoid compartment syndrome.[9] The high incidence of obstetric difficulties, such as breech presentation and the need for assisted delivery,[10,11] may be the result rather than the cause of the shortened sternomastoid muscle, as was initially thought. There is no report of a sternomastoid tumor detected by antenatal ultrasonography.[12] Concomitant hip dysplasia is common.[10]

Pathology

The basic abnormality on histology is fibrous replacement of muscle bundles.[13] The lesion, called fibromatosis colli, is often classified with other types of fibromatoses, such as the Dupuytren contracture and plantar fibromatosis. Jones[8] has described endomysial fibrosis involving the deposition of collagen and fibroblasts around individual muscle fibers that undergo atrophy. The sarcoplasmic nuclei are compacted to form giant cells that appear to be multinucleated. The maturity of the fibrous tissue in neonates suggests that the disease may begin before birth[8,14,15] and may therefore contribute to the frequency of obstetric difficulties during delivery. The reported incidence of breech deliveries is about 20% to 30%[16]—much higher than the normal incidence. About 60% of affected infants are involved in a complicated birth,[16] which suggests that the fibrosis may affect the position of the fetus in utero and perhaps even prevent normal engagement of the head in the maternal pelvis.

The natural history of untreated sternomastoid fibrosis is complete resolution in 50% to 70% of patients at 6 months of age. In about 10%, the tumor and sternomastoid shortening persist beyond 12 months of age.[2,17] The severity and distribution of the fibrosis within the sternomastoid muscle is variable and has led to a variety of classifications based either on a palpable localized sternomastoid tumor or thickening and shortening of the whole muscle or on the basis of ultrasonographic findings.[18,19] The systems of classification have some prognostic significance in that localized lesions within the sternomastoid (clinically or ultrasonographically) are more likely to resolve spontaneously than those involving the whole muscle. In older children with torticollis, the appearance of degenerating fibers is more consistent with disuse atrophy produced by limitation of movement caused by the fibrosis.

Clinical Features

STERNOMASTOID TORTICOLLIS

The tumor is a hard, spindle-shaped, painless, discrete swelling usually about 1 to 3 cm in diameter within the substance of one sternomastoid muscle. Almost always, it first becomes evident at about 3 weeks after birth. Obvious head tilt or torticollis tends to develop later.[12] In infants, the head is rotated to the side opposite the tumor, with only slight flexion of the head to the affected side (Fig. 60-1).

In other patients, the sternomastoid tumor is less discrete, and the sternomastoid appears to be thickened and tightened along its whole length. The shortening of the muscle restricts rotation and lateral flexion of the head (Fig. 60-2).

TABLE 60-1

Causes of Torticollis in Infants and Children

Cause	Comment
Sternomastoid "tumor"	Common; appears at 3 weeks of age
Abnormal position in utero	Tends to improve with age
Cervical hemivertebrae	Structural; confirmed on plain radiograph
Cervical lymphadenitis/abscess	Acute; usually occurs in first 2 years of life
Retropharyngeal abscess[31,58] and pyogenic cervical spondylitis[59]	Acute; signs of toxicity, cervical pain
Posterior fossa tumors[61]	A rare cause; headaches, vomiting, and other neurologic signs present[61]
Acute atlantoaxial subluxation	May occur after tonsillectomy[30]
Atlantoaxial rotatory subluxation	Significance disputed[58,59]; diagnosed on dynamic CT
Spasmodic with Sandifer syndrome[59]	Due to gastroesophageal reflux
Congenital absence of sternomastoid	Unilateral, extremely rare[60]
Postural	Familial

CT, computed tomography.

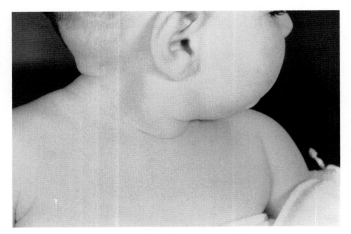

FIGURE 60-1   Appearance of a right sternomastoid tumor in infancy; the head is turned to the contralateral side.

The rotational component of the action of the sternomastoid is easy to measure. It is assessed by standing behind the child's head and passively rotating the head while it is held between both hands. The sternomastoid muscle is stretched to its maximum length by rotation to the side of the affected muscle. Where the muscle is fibrotic, it cannot be stretched to its full length, and rotation to the ipsilateral side is restricted.

Older children with torticollis compensate for the more pronounced tilt by elevating one shoulder to enable the eyes to keep as level as possible (Fig. 60-3). Such compensation is not seen in infants, because there is no need for them to maintain their eyes in a horizontal plane until they stand up.[20] Moreover, older children do not turn their heads to the contralateral side as much, because they tend to compensate by twisting the neck and back to keep their eyes pointing forward.

DIFFERENTIAL DIAGNOSIS

Initial clinical assessment must establish whether the wry neck is caused by shortness of one sternomastoid muscle or by some other condition. In sternomastoid fibrosis, the anterior border of the muscle stands out as a tight band, although in some small infants in whom the neck is relatively short, the muscle may be difficult to see readily. For this reason, the full length of the muscle must be palpated to determine whether there is an area of thickening or fibrosis along part or all of its length. In about two thirds, there is a definite localized swelling (tumor) in the muscle; in the remainder, the whole muscle appears to be affected. There is no role for plain radiography where the sternomastoid is tight or shortened.[21] Although not required for diagnosis, appearance on ultrasonography may help predict (to a degree) the likelihood of spontaneous resolution.[1,19,22] Inexperienced ultrasonographers, worried by the infiltrative and ill-defined appearance, may recommend

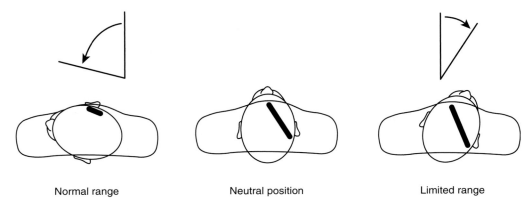

Normal range   Neutral position   Limited range

FIGURE 60-2   Restriction of rotation of the head secondary to shortening of the sternomastoid muscle as viewed from above the head. The black bars represent the right sternomastoid muscle and show that its inability to lengthen limits rotation to that side.

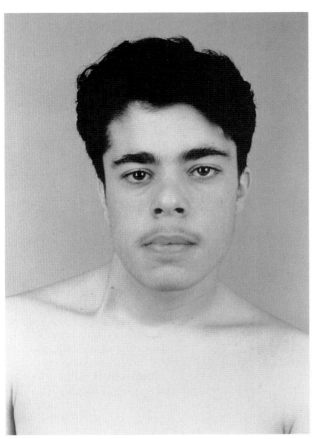

FIGURE 60-3 Appearance of torticollis as a result of sternomastoid fibrosis in an older child. The eyes are kept horizontal, but the shortened sternomastoid muscle causes compensatory elevation of the shoulder. (From Beasley SW, et al: Pediatric Diagnosis. London, Chapman & Hall, 1994, with permission.)

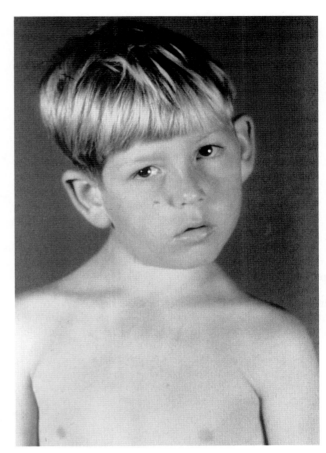

FIGURE 60-4 Torticollis caused by atlanto-occipital subluxation after tonsillectomy. Notice that there is no tightness of the sternomastoid muscle on either side. (From Beasley SW, et al: Pediatric Diagnosis. Chapman & Hall, London, 1994, with permission.)

further imaging or biopsy of the "tumor"; this is not indicated in the presence of the typical palpable mass within the sternomastoid and torticollis. It is possible to diagnose a sternomastoid torticollis on magnetic resonance imaging (MRI)[22,23] and computed tomography (CT),[24] but neither alters management and should not be performed routinely.[23,25]

An obvious mass or fibrosis of the muscle may not always be noticeable in idiopathic torticollis, but in such instances, alternative diagnoses must be sought (see Table 60-1 and Fig. 60-4).[20,26]

A squint may cause head tilt from imbalance in rotation of the eyes. The squint may not be obvious at first because the tilt compensates for the abnormal position of the eyes. When the head is straightened passively, the squint becomes apparent. Occasionally, sternomastoid fibrosis may occur coincidentally with ocular torticollis.

Posterior fossa tumors may compress the brainstem at the foramen magnum and produce acute stiffness of the neck that causes it to be held to one side. The neck is frozen in this position and is difficult to move actively or passively. The presence of a central nervous system tumor may be known already, but occasionally, acute torticollis is the first manifestation. Careful neurologic examination may show abnormalities of the lower cranial nerves and cerebellar function, and the causative lesion is demonstrated on CT or MRI.

Hemivertebrae involving the cervical spine may produce a tilt of the head that is evident from birth and does not progress. Vertebral lesions can be identified clinically by inspection and palpation of the dorsal cervical spines and confirmed on plain radiographs of the neck.

Acute torticollis has been attributed to atlantoaxial rotatory subluxation as determined on dynamic CT,[27,28] but others doubt the existence or significance of these findings and suggest that CT scans are not necessary at the initial examination.[29] Atlantoaxial subluxation has been reported after tonsillectomy.[30] Acute torticollis can also result from inflammatory conditions of the neck, including retropharyngeal abscess,[31] and can be a symptom of acute lymphoblastic leukemia.[32]

Secondary Effects of Torticollis

Table 60-2 lists the secondary effects of torticollis.

TABLE 60-2	
Secondary Effects of Torticollis	
Infants	Plagiocephaly
	Hemifacial hypoplasia
Older children	Compensatory scoliosis

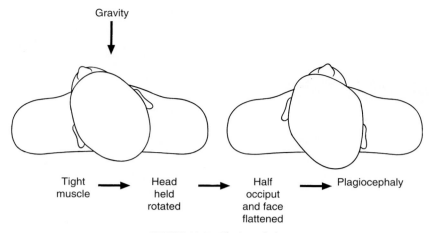

Gravity

Tight muscle → Head held rotated → Half occiput and face flattened → Plagiocephaly

FIGURE 60-5   Plagiocephaly.

PLAGIOCEPHALY

In small infants with torticollis and fixed rotation of the head, gravity deforms the relatively soft head as it lies in the same position for a prolonged period. Flattening of one occiput leads to secondary flattening of the contralateral forehead (Fig. 60-5). This asymmetric skull deformity is called plagiocephaly and develops in the first few months of life.[33] It is best observed from above the head. Once the child begins to sit up or the torticollis resolves, the plagiocephaly tends to resolve as well.[34] It may take several years to disappear, and a few children have a slight permanent deformity. It is possible that many children with plagiocephaly have had unrecognized torticollis during infancy.[35]

HEMIFACIAL HYPOPLASIA

Progressive facial deformity is seen when one sternomastoid muscle immobilizes the face for a long time. The malar eminence on the side of the face limited by the fibrotic muscle grows more slowly than the normal side does[9] and causes progressive asymmetry (Fig. 60-6). This inhibition of growth of the mandible and

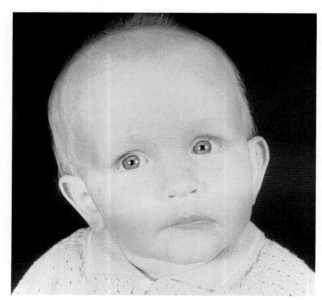

FIGURE 60-6   Hemifacial hypoplasia on the right side.

maxilla embodies an important principle of pediatrics: Normal growth of bones depends on normal muscular movement.

The degree of hypoplasia of one side of the face can be determined by the angle between the plane of the eyes and the plane of the mouth. Normally these lines are parallel, but they form an angle to each other when the face is asymmetric. The development of hemifacial hypoplasia is one indication for surgery; division of the tight sternomastoid muscle allows resolution of the skeletal abnormality and subsequent normal growth.[9]

Significant hemifacial hypoplasia takes about 8 months to develop[8] but is more often recognized at about 3 to 4 years of age.[17] It becomes less obvious with ongoing growth once the torticollis has resolved.

POSTURAL COMPENSATION

When children are old enough to walk, the eyes are kept horizontal to facilitate balance and horizontal eye movement. The child compensates for the short fibrous sternomastoid by elevating the ipsilateral shoulder (see Fig. 60-3). In addition, there may be compensatory cervical and thoracic scoliosis. Adjacent muscles, such as the trapezius, may be wasted because of relative inactivity.[8]

Conservative Management

Sternomastoid fibrosis resolves spontaneously in the vast majority of infants. Therefore surgery is required only rarely, in those in whom the torticollis has not resolved. The value of manipulation of the head and neck has not been proven,[12] although it is widely used and may have some benefit in the first year of life.[36] Physiotherapy and regular neck exercises appear to be safe[36] and may make the parents feel that "something is being done" for their infant. Unintentional snapping during manipulation has been reported with no apparent deleterious effect on outcome.[37] Some clinicians advocate early institution of intensive passive neck range-of-motion stretching exercises and have reported high rates of resolution,[9,38–40] while others believe that there is no convincing evidence that these measures alter the natural history of the condition.

Others consider it important to encourage parents to place toys and other desirable objects on the ipsilateral side to encourage the infant to turn toward the affected side.[8] Again, this strategy probably helps the parent more than the infant, but is unlikely to do any harm. Attempts to put the infant to sleep with the head facing toward the affected side tend to fail, particularly if the muscle is tight. Botulinum toxin injection appears to be ineffective in patients presenting in late childhood or adulthood,[41] but results are more encouraging in younger children.[42]

In most cases, reassurance is all that is required. The passage of time is probably as effective as the various manipulations when torticollis is due to sternomastoid fibrosis.

Operative Treatment

INDICATIONS FOR SURGERY

Indications for surgery include
1. Persistent sternomastoid tightness limiting head rotation in children more than 12 to 15 months of age[43]
2. Persistent sternomastoid tightness with progressive hemifacial hypoplasia
3. Diagnosis in children older than 1 year[44]

OPERATIVE TECHNIQUE

The procedure is performed under general anesthesia with laryngeal or endotracheal intubation, according to the expertise and preference of the pediatric anesthetist. The child is placed supine with the shoulders elevated and the neck rotated to the contralateral side. The muscle is best divided at its lower end,[4,9] although division at its upper end,[45] at both ends,[46–48] or in its midportion[8,49] have all been described. Endoscopic tenotomy of the muscle is also feasible[50–53] including through a transaxillary approach.[54,55]

A 3- to 4-cm transverse incision is made in a skin crease about 1 cm above the sternal and clavicular heads of the affected sternomastoid (Fig. 60-7). The platysma is divided with diathermy so that no bleeding occurs in the line of the incision. The external jugular vein can be retracted if it is within the field of view. The tight fibrosis of the two heads of sternocleidomastoid are divided with diathermy near their lower end. Tightness of the cervical fascia between the sternomastoid and trapezius is usually palpable once the sternomastoid has been divided, and this

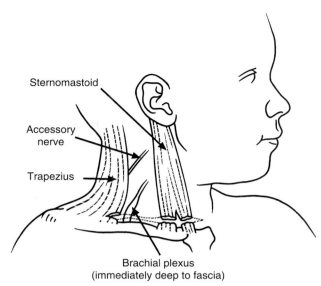

FIGURE 60-8 Division of the sternomastoid and investing cervical fascia to the anterior border of the trapezius.

fascia also should be divided (Fig. 60-8). This is done under direct vision to avoid damage to other structures, particularly the spinal accessory nerve and brachial plexus.

The wound is infiltrated with bupivacaine or other local anesthetic agent. The platysma is closed with continuous 4-0 absorbable suture and the skin with subcuticular 5-0 Monocryl absorbable suture. No drains are required.

The procedure can be performed as a day case, and no postoperative restriction of movement is necessary. Full range of the neck is normally achieved within 1 week of surgery. Physiotherapy is usually unnecessary, although some advocate an extended period of physiotherapy postoperatively.[46] In older children, restoration of a full range of movement may take longer, and the final cosmetic appearance is less certain.[56]

COMPLICATIONS

A hematoma may develop if hemostasis was inadequate at the time of surgery. Diathermy dissection keeps blood loss to a minimum. Larger superficial veins may require ligation and division if they cannot be retracted.

Incomplete division of both heads of the sternocleidomastoid muscle or failure to divide the cervical fascia over the posterior triangle of the neck may produce persistent torticollis. Careful inspection and palpation of the neck for residual tightness and bands at the time of surgery should prevent this complication from occurring. Recurrent torticollis is rare after surgical treatment and is seen in less than 3% of patients.[57]

FOLLOW-UP

Patients should be monitored until (1) the torticollis has resolved completely, (2) there is full range of movement of the head and neck, and (3) the sternomastoid muscle feels normal. In an older child with secondary scoliosis, follow-up, including radiologic studies, if required, should continue until the scoliosis has resolved.

The complete reference list is available online at www. expertconsult.com.

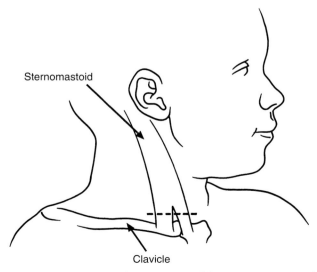

FIGURE 60-7 Skin incision for low division of the sternomastoid muscle.

Index

Page numbers followed by *f* indicate figures and *t* indicate tables.

B

B cell(s), in host defense, 147
B-cell lymphoma, 485, 523, 523t, 524–525, 524f
Baby Doe law, 240
Back pain, in spinal epidural abscess, 1697
Backboard, 335f, 357
Baclofen, for gastroesophageal reflux disease, 953
Bacterial infection
    in ascites, 1171
    in community-acquired pneumonia, 855–858, 856f
    in necrotizing enterocolitis, 1194–1195, 1197
    in renal transplant patient, 651t
Bacterial overgrowth
    methods to decrease, 1206–1207
    in short bowel syndrome, 1140
Bacterial toxins, 150
Bacterial virulence, 149–150
Ballard score for gestational age, 89, 90f
Balloon dilatation
    for Crohn strictures, 1214
    esophageal. See Esophagus, dilatation of.
    for laryngotracheal stenosis, 846, 846f
Bannayan-Riley-Ruvalcaba syndrome, 1630
Bardach two-flap palatoplasty, 703, 704f
Bardet-Biedl syndrome, 1592
Bariatric surgery in adolescents, 1041–1054
    clinical pathway for, 1049–1050
    cognitive developmental concepts related to, 1044–1045, 1045t
    compliance following, 1044–1045, 1045t
    ethical considerations in, 241–242
    guidelines for, 1048–1049
    historical perspective on, 1041–1042
    nutritional and metabolic consequences of, 1046–1048
    obesity science related to, 1042
    outcome of, 1041
    patient selection for, 1048, 1048t
    procedures for, 1045–1048, 1045t, 1047f
    psychological factors related to, 1043–1044, 1049
    regionalization of, 1041
    team approach to, 1048–1049
    timing of, 1049
    training for, 1045
Barium enema. See also Enema, contrast.
    in alimentary tract duplications, 1158f
    in appendicitis, 1257
    in constipation, 1314
    hydrostatic, in intussusception, 1104, 1104f
    intestinal perforation with, 1108, 1108f
    in intussusception, 1101
    in megacystis-microcolon-intestinal hypoperistalsis syndrome, 1286, 1286f
    in ulcerative colitis, 1221, 1221f
Barium meal, in achalasia, 945, 945f
Barium swallow
    in motility disorders, 941
    in pyloric atresia, 1035, 1035f
    in thoracic enteric duplications, 1158–1159, 1159f
Barlow test, 1700
Barotrauma
    with emphysema, 828
    with mechanical ventilation, 122
Barrett esophagus, in gastroesophageal reflux disease, 483, 956, 956f
    after caustic injury, 924
    after esophageal atresia repair, 913
Bartonella henselae infection, 727–728
Bartsocas-Papas syndrome, 977t
Basal cell carcinoma, sebaceous nevus and, 1714
Basal cell nevus syndrome, 529
Basal ganglia, tumors of, 593–594
Basal metabolic rate, 97
Basement membrane, 370
Basiliximab
    in liver transplantation, 650t
    in lung transplantation, 676–677, 676t
    in renal transplantation, 624
BB gun injuries, 348
Bcl-2 gene, in neuroblastoma, 449
Beardmore, H., 7, 7f
Becker nevus, of breast, 773

Beckwith-Wiedemann syndrome, 405
    abdominal wall defects in, 977, 977t
    adrenocortical tumors in, 561
    hepatoblastoma in, 466–467
    umbilical defects in, 969
    Wilms' tumor in, 424–425, 427
Bell-clapper anomaly, 1014
Bell necrotizing enterocolitis staging criteria, 1187, 1188t, 1199
Beneficence principle, 237
    bariatric surgery and, 242
Bentec bag, in gastroschisis reduction, 982
Benzodiazepines, for burns, 382–383
Bernard-Soulier syndrome, 171
Best Evidence, 233
Best interests standard, 241
Beta blockers
    in burn injury, 380–381
    for congestive heart failure, 135, 137t
    for pheochromocytoma, 560
    for variceal hemorrhage, 1362–1363
Beta-catenin mutation, in hepatoblastoma, 467
Betamethasone
    for labial adhesions, 1558
    maternal, for cystic lung lesions, 826
Bias
    in case-control studies, 229
    in case reports, 227–228
    identification of, 233–234
Biatrial anastomosis, in heart transplantation, 664, 664f, 665
Bicaval anastomosis, in heart transplantation, 664–665, 666f
Bicycle injury, prevention of, 259
Bier block, 221–222
Bifid nipples, 772
Bifid scrotum, 1583–1584, 1586f
Bile cysts, post-traumatic, 462
Bile duct
    common, 1371
        anomalies of, 1372
    cystic dilatation of. See Choledochal cyst.
    development of, 1332
    trauma to, 299, 300f
Bile lake, 464, 465f
Bile reflux, 882
Bilhaut-Cloquet procedure, 1723
Biliary ascites, 1173–1174
Biliary atresia, 1321–1332
    choledochal cyst with, 1333–1334
    classification of, 1321–1322, 1322f
    clinical presentation in, 1323–1324, 1323f
    embryogenesis of, 1322
    epidemiology of, 1321–1322
    etiology of, 1322, 1322t
    historical perspective on, 1321
    liver biopsy in, 1324
    nutritional complications of, 1328
    nutritional support in, 197, 197t
    outcomes with, 1327–1328
    pathology of, 1322–1323, 1323f
    scintigraphy in, 1324, 1334–1335
    treatment of, 1324–1327
        complications of, 1328–1329
        liver transplantation in, 644, 644f, 1326, 1327, 1329
        postoperative care in, 1327, 1327t
        preoperative care in, 1324
        steroid controversy in, 1327, 1327t
        surgical controversies in, 1326
        surgical technique for, 1324–1326, 1325f, 1326f
Biliary dyskinesia, 1343
Biliary stent, in bile duct injury, 299, 300f
Biliary tract
    carcinoma of, 1333, 1339
    embryology of, 1332
    rhabdomyosarcoma of, 480, 497
Biliopancreatic diversion, 1046
Bilirubin
    in choledochal cyst, 1334
    in intestinal failure–associated liver disease, 1139
Billroth, endothelial cords of, 1385
Bioartificial liver device (BAL), 33

Biobrane, in burn care, 377–378, 378f, 384
Biochemical markers
    of sepsis, 153–154
    of ureteropelvic junction obstruction, 1419–1420
Biochemical screening, in prenatal diagnosis, 77
Bioelectrical impedance analysis, 180
Bioethics. See Ethics.
Biofeedback program, for dysfunctional elimination syndromes, 1463–1464
Biologic materials, 1712
Bioluminescent imaging, 47–48
Biopsy, 417–423
    of bone tumors, 582, 583f
    of brain tumors, 593
    of burn wound, 372
    of chest wall tumors, 573
    core needle, 418–420, 419f, 419t
    fine-needle aspiration, 418. See also Fine-needle aspiration.
    laparoscopy with, 420
    liver
        in biliary atresia, 1324
        in portal hypertension, 1361–1362
    lung, 875–876, 875f, 876f
    open incisional, 422
    percutaneous needle, 418
    rectal
        in Hirschsprung disease, 1267–1268, 1268f
        in intestinal neuronal dysplasia, 1280, 1281f
        in isolated hypoganglionosis, 1282, 1283f
    of rhabdomyosarcoma, 493–494
    salivary gland, 730
    specimen handling for, 417–418
    stereotactic, of brain tumors, 593
    thoracoscopy with, 420–422, 421f
Birth, transitional circulation at, 112, 135
Birth injuries, 391–393
    fractures in, 391–392
    neurologic, 392
    soft tissue, 391
    thoracoabdominal, 392–393, 392f
Birth weight
    gestational age and, 89, 91f
    hypospadias and, 1536–1537
    necrotizing enterocolitis and, 1135–1136, 1188–1189, 1203
    subgroups for, 89
Bishop-Koop enterostomy, 1080–1081, 1080f
Bite injuries, 340–341
BK virus infection, in renal transplant patient, 628
Black widow spider bite, 341
Bladder
    adenocarcinoma of, after bladder exstrophy repair, 1523–1524
    anatomic relationships of, 320
    capacity of, 1454
    compliance of, 1457, 1458f, 1467
    drainage of, for posterior urethral valves, 1556
    neuropathic, 1467, 1469–1470, 1470f
        in cerebral palsy, 1460–1461
        detrusor-sphincter dyssynergy in, 1455–1456, 1458f
        megaureter with, 1497, 1498
        in myelodysplasia, 1457–1459, 1458f, 1459f
        in sacral agenesis, 1460, 1460f
        in spinal cord tethering, 1459–1460
        treatment of, 1459, 1459f
        urinary tract infection and, 1428
        voiding cystourethrography in, 1454, 1455f
    overactive, 1464
    pressure in, 1454–1455, 1456f, 1458f
    rhabdomyosarcoma of, 498
    stones in, 1438. See also Urolithiasis.
    suspensory ligament of, 1303
    trauma to, 312, 313, 320–322, 321f
        causes of, 320
        classification and definitions of, 320–321
        diagnosis of, 321
        grading of, 314t
        management of, 321–322
        pelvic fracture with, 321, 321f
    valve, 1468, 1468f
    wall thickening in, imaging of, 1429–1430, 1429f

Cardiac arrhythmias, in neonate, 138–139, 139t
Cardiac catheterization
    in heart transplantation, 662
    in patent ductus arteriosus, 1648
Cardiac evaluation, in heart transplantation, 662
Cardiac failure. *See* Heart failure.
Cardiac index, in pectus excavatum, 783
Cardiac output
    in burn injury, 371
    left ventricular end-diastolic pressure and, 133–134, 134f
Cardiac surgery, antibiotic prophylaxis and, 1647
Cardiac tissue engineering, 30–31
Cardiac tissue viability, positron emission tomography of, 46
Cardiac transplantation. *See* Heart transplantation.
Cardiac valves
    injury to, 281, 281f
    tissue-engineered, 30–31
Cardiomyopathy, heart transplantation for, 660–661, 660f, 661f
Cardiopulmonary bypass, for aortic injury, 283
Cardiopulmonary dysfunction, after radiation therapy for Hodgkin lymphoma, 522
Cardiopulmonary indices, in congenital diaphragmatic hernia, 816
Cardiopulmonary resuscitation
    extracorporeal life support for, 123–136. *See also* Extracorporeal life support.
    in lung transplantation, 676
Cardiovascular death, in renal transplant patient, 629
Cardiovascular disorders. *See also* Heart disease, congenital.
    neonatal, 135–140
        arrhythmias as, 138–139, 139t
        congenital heart disease as, 139–140
        congestive heart failure as, 135–138, 137t
    obesity and, 1042–1043
    in renal transplant patient, 629
Cardiovascular physiology, neonatal, 133–134, 134f
Cardioversion, for supraventricular tachycardia, 138
Carney-Stratakis syndrome, 484
Carney triad, 484, 567
Carnitine, in parenteral nutrition, 191–192
Caroli disease, 1331–1332, 1335, 1336
Carotid artery
    aneurysm of, 1644–1645, 1645f
    coiling of, 1644, 1644f
    dissection of, 1644
    in extracorporeal life support, 127, 127f
    injury to, 717
    occlusion of, 1644
Carpenter syndrome, 693
Cartilage, tissue engineering of, 29–31, 30f
Case-control studies, 228–229
Case reports, 227–228
Caspase 8, 410
Casting
    for clubfoot, 1705
    for developmental dysplasia of hip, 1702
    for knee dislocation, 1706
Castleman disease, cervical lymphadenopathy in, 743
Cat-scratch disease, 727–728
    hepatic, 1351
    lymphadenitis in, 742–743
Catecholamine-resistant shock, 159t, 160–161
    persistent, 161
Catecholamines
    adrenal regulation of, 558
    in burn injury, 380
    in neuroblastoma, 444–445
    in pheochromocytoma, 559
    postoperative elevation of, 105
Catheterizable channels, continent, 1462, 1479–1480, 1481f, 1493–1494, 1493f, 1494f
Catheterization
    arterial, 116–117, 214
    cardiac
        in heart transplantation, 662
        in patent ductus arteriosus, 1648
    central venous
        for intraoperative monitoring, 214
        venous thromboembolism with, 175

Catheterization (*Continued*)
    epidural, 225
    infections related to
        with parenteral nutrition, 193–194
        in short bowel syndrome, 1139–1140
    pulmonary artery, 117
    radial artery, 116–117
    umbilical, 116–117, 1634–1635, 1635f
    urinary. *See* Urinary catheterization.
    vascular injuries during, 366
    venous, for parenteral nutrition, 188–189
Caudal block, 224–225, 224f
    in hypospadias repair, 1551
    in inguinal hernia repair, 988–989
Caustic injury. *See* Esophagus, caustic injury to.
Cavitation devices, 50
CCAM volume ratio (CVR), 85
CD11b/CD18, in neutrophil adhesion, 146
CD30, in Hodgkin lymphoma, 519, 519f
CD44, in neuroblastoma, 449
Cecal volvulus, 1117, 1124, 1252
Cecocolic loop, 1113, 1113f, 1114f
Cecostomy
    continent, 1482, 1482f
    tube, 1237, 1240
Celecoxib, for familial adenomatous polyposis, 488
Celiac artery, stenosis of, 1639–1641, 1640f
Cell cycle, 398
Cell death, programmed, 399
Cell differentiation
    extracellular matrix in, 29
    multipotent, 28–29, 28f
Cell-mediated immunity, 146–148
Cell physiology, normal, 398–402
Cellulitis
    orbital, 713
    peritonsillar, 717–718
Central nervous system. *See also* Brain; Spinal cord.
    anomalies of, with cloacal exstrophy, 1527
    formation of, 1673–1674, 1674f, 1675f
    injuries to, 343–364
        in birth trauma, 392
    suppurative infections of, 1693–1697
Central venous catheter
    for intraoperative monitoring, 214
    venous thromboembolism with, 175
Central venous parenteral nutrition, 189, 193–194
Cephalosporins, for urinary tract infection, 1431–1432
Cerebellar ataxia, in neuroblastoma, 443
Cerebellum
    astrocytoma of, 594, 595f
    tumors of, 594
Cerebral contusion, 344, 345–346, 345f
Cerebral palsy, 392
    neuropathic bladder in, 1460–1461
    nutritional support in, 199, 199t
Cerebral perfusion pressure, in trauma patient, 268–269
Cerebrocostomandibular syndrome, 807–808, 977t
Cerebrospinal fluid
    absorption of, 1681
    formation of, 1681
    leakage of
        in basilar skull fracture, 352–353
        after myelomeningocele repair, 1676
        in temporal bone fracture, 712
    obstruction of, hydrocephalus from, 1681
    shunting of
        complications of, 1683–1686
        for hydrocephalus, 1683
Cerebrovascular disease, 1643–1645, 1643f, 1644f, 1645f
Cerebrovascular injuries, 346–347, 353
Cerumen, removal of, 708
Cervical adenitis, 727. *See also* Lymphadenitis.
Cervical clefts, midline, 760, 760f
Cervical dermoid cyst, 760
Cervical ectopia cordis, 803
Cervical esophagus, duplications of, 1158
Cervical lymphadenopathy, 737–746
    anatomy of, 737, 738f
    differential diagnosis of, 737, 738t
    evaluation of, 740, 740t

Cervical lymphadenopathy (*Continued*)
    infectious, 743
    in inflammatory disorders, 743
    in malignant disorders, 743
    management of, 740–743, 741f
Cervical spine
    control of, in trauma patient, 263–265, 264f
    hemivertebrae involving, 765
    injury to, 335, 335f, 354, 356–357, 356t, 358–359, 358f
        in birth trauma, 392
Cervical thymic cysts, 760–761
Cervical torso vascular injuries, 363
Cervical tumors, in Peutz-Jeghers syndrome, 1184
Cervicofacial teratoma, 516
Cervicomedullary astrocytoma, 597
Cervix, adenocarcinoma of, 1609
Cesarean delivery
    for conjoined twins, 1733
    defects managed by, 78t
CFTR gene. *See* Cystic fibrosis transmembrane regulator (*CFTR*) gene.
Cheatle slit, 1067, 1068f
Chédiak-Higashi syndrome, 529
Chemical burns, 383
Chemical exposure, hypospadias and, 1537
Chemoattractants, 149
Chemoembolization, hepatic arterial (transarterial)
    for hepatoblastoma, 475
    for hepatocellular carcinoma, 479–480
Chemotaxins, in neutrophil diapedesis, 146
Chemotherapy
    for bone tumors, 583
    for colorectal cancer, 490
    common agents for, 406, 407t
    for Ewing sarcoma family/primitive neuroectodermal tumors of chest wall, 575, 575f
    for fibrosarcoma of chest wall, 575–576
    for hepatoblastoma, 470, 471–472
    for hepatocellular carcinoma, 477–478
    for Hodgkin lymphoma, 520
    hyperthermic intraperitoneal, 503, 504f
    for hypothalamic/chiasmatic astrocytoma, 598
    for neuroblastoma, 456
    for non-Hodgkin lymphoma, 525–526
    for primitive neuroectodermal tumors, 594–596
    principles of, 405–410, 407t
    for pulmonary blastoma, 569–570
    radiation therapy with, 412
    for rhabdomyosarcoma, 495–496
    risk stratification in, 406
    for sacrococcygeal teratoma, 512–513, 515f
    side effects of, 406, 407t
    targeted, 406–410
    terminology in, 406
    for testicular tumors, 556, 556t
    for tuberculosis, 742, 857
    for Wilms' tumor, 434–435, 435t
Chest
    examination of, in thoracic trauma, 273
    flail, 275
    funnel. *See* Pectus excavatum.
    trauma to. *See* Thoracic trauma.
Chest radiography. *See* Radiography, chest.
Chest tube
    breast deformity from, 771, 772f
    for chylothorax, 878
    complications related to, 874
    for empyema, 872
    for hemothorax, 277
    for pneumothorax, 275, 276f, 872–873
        care and removal of, 874
        in neonate, 873–874, 874f
        in older child, 875
    size of, guide for, 875, 875t
    in trauma patient, 265–266, 266f
Chest wall
    congenital deformities of, 779–812
        in diffuse skeletal disorders, 805–808, 807f, 808f
        involving depression. *See* Pectus excavatum.
        involving protrusion. *See* Pectus carinatum.

G

Galactorrhea, 774, 774f
Galeazzi sign, 1700
Gallbladder. *See also* Chole- *entries*.
   carcinoma of, 1339
   disorders of, 1341–1349
   hydrops of, 1342
   polyps of, 1343
Gallbladder-ventriculo shunt, 1343
Gallstones. *See* Cholelithiasis.
Ganglioglioma, 599–600, 599f
   seizures in, 1687–1688, 1688f, 1692
Ganglion cell(s). *See also* Aganglionosis.
   in Hirschsprung disease, 1265, 1267, 1274–1276
   in hypertrophic pyloric stenosis, 1021
   in intestinal neuronal dysplasia, 1280, 1281f
   in isolated hypoganglionosis, 1282, 1283f
   in megacystis-microcolon-intestinal
      hypoperistalsis syndrome, 1286
Ganglion cell tumors, 591
Ganglioneuroblastoma, 448
Ganglioneuroma, 447–448
Gangliosides, in neuroblastoma, 449
Gangrene
   intestinal
      in necrotizing enterocolitis, 1195, 1195f, 1200
         predictors of, 1200
      umbilical, 964
      vasospasm and, 366–367
GANT (gastrointestinal autonomic nerve tumor), 484
GAP (glans approximation procedure), 1540–1541,
   1542f
Gardner syndrome, 487, 1182
Gartner duct, 1441–1443
   cysts of, 1558, 1608
Gas exchange
   extreme modes of, 119–120
   pulmonary, 114–115, 115f
   structural development related to, 109–110, 110f
Gastrectomy
   laparoscopic sleeve, 1046
   for stress ulcers, 1034–1035
Gastric. *See also* Stomach.
Gastric acid
   secretion of, 1030
   ulcers and, 1030
Gastric aspiration, lung abscess from, 868
Gastric banding, laparoscopic adjustable,
   1041–1042, 1046
Gastric bypass surgery, 1041–1042, 1046, 1047f
Gastric decompression
   for gastric volvulus, 1037–1038
   in trauma patient, 268
Gastric duplications, 1036, 1156–1157,
   1159–1160
Gastric emptying, delayed, gastroesophageal reflux
   disease with, 957
Gastric feedings, 186
Gastric lymphoma, MALT, 522–523
Gastric mucosa
   heterotopic, in Meckel diverticulum, 1086–1087,
      1087f
   ischemia of, stress ulcers and, 1031
Gastric outlet obstruction, congenital, 1035–1036,
   1035f, 1036f
Gastric reflux, into colonic interposition, 932
Gastric teratoma, 516
Gastric transposition, for esophageal replacement,
   907, 908f, 929t, 934–938, 936f, 937t
Gastric tube, for esophageal replacement, 907, 929t,
   932–934, 933f, 934f, 934t
Gastric ulcer. *See* Peptic ulcer disease.
Gastric varices. *See also* Varices.
   injection therapy for, 1363
Gastrin, in Zollinger-Ellison syndrome, 1034
Gastrinoma, 1383
Gastritis. *See also* Peptic ulcer disease.
   bleeding in, 1149–1150
   causes of, 1030t
   clinical findings in, 1031t
   stress, 1149
Gastrocystoplasty, 1475, 1475f, 1492
   complications of, 1484–1485
Gastroduodenostomy, for pyloric atresia, 1036

Gastroesophageal reflux disease, 947–961
   apneic spells and, 950–951, 951t
   Barrett esophagus in, 483, 956, 956f
   in caustic esophageal stricture, 923, 924f
   in congenital anomalies and diseases, 957–958
   in congenital diaphragmatic hernia, 822, 822f
   with delayed gastric emptying, 957
   diagnostic studies in, 952–953, 952f, 953f
   epidemiology of, 947
   in esophageal atresia
      preoperative, 912
      after repair, 913, 957–958
   esophagoscopy in, 882, 882f, 883f
   hiatal hernia and, 957
   with laryngomalacia, 723–724
   with laryngopharyngeal reflux, 840
   laryngotracheal stenosis and, 846
   after lung transplantation, 678
   in neurologically impaired children, 956–957
   pathophysiology of, 948–949
   primary, 944–945
   recurrent, 955–956
   symptoms of, 949–951, 951f, 951t
   treatment of
      conservative, 953
      endoluminal, 57, 957
      surgical, 954, 954f. *See also* Fundoplication.
Gastrografin enema, for meconium ileus, 1078–1079
Gastroileal pouch, 1494–1495
Gastrointestinal anomalies
   with anorectal malformations, 1290
   with cloacal exstrophy, 1526
   with esophageal atresia, 897
   Meckel diverticulum as. *See* Meckel diverticulum.
Gastrointestinal atresia, familial, 1060–1061, 1061t,
   1065, 1066f
Gastrointestinal autonomic nerve tumor, 484
Gastrointestinal bleeding, 1147–1155
   evaluation of, 1147–1148, 1148t, 1149f, 1150f
   in gastrointestinal vascular malformations, 1154
   lower
      in anal fissure, 1151
      in anorectal trauma, 1153, 1153f
      diagnostic algorithm for, 1150f
      evaluation of, 1153, 1153f
      in juvenile polyps, 1152, 1152f
      in Meckel diverticulum, 1089–1091,
         1151–1152, 1151f, 1152f
      sources of, 1148t, 1151–1152
   novel techniques for identification of, 1154
   in peptic ulcer disease, 1032, 1033–1034
   in portal hypertension, 1358–1360. *See also* Varices.
   resuscitation for, 1147
   versus swallowed maternal blood, 1148
   upper
      diagnostic algorithm for, 1149f
      in esophageal varices, 1150
      esophagoscopy in, 883
      in gastritis, 1149–1150
      in hemorrhagic disease of newborn, 1148–1149
      nonvariceal, 1150–1151
      sources of, 1148–1151, 1148t
Gastrointestinal peptides, in hypertrophic pyloric
   stenosis, 1022
Gastrointestinal tissue engineering, 32
Gastrointestinal tract
   as barrier to infection, 145–146, 145f
   in burn injury, 371
   contrast studies of, in conjoined twins, 1733
   duplications of. *See* Alimentary tract duplications.
   functional abnormalities of, after bladder
      augmentation or replacement, 1484–1485,
      1495–1496
   hemangioma of, 1616
   polypoid disease of, 486–487
   trauma to, 305–308, 307f
      imaging of, 307–308
      intestinal stricture after, 1133
      seat-belt sign in, 307, 307f
   tumors of, 483–493
      carcinoid, 485–486
      colorectal cancer as, 486. *See also* Colorectal
         cancer.
      esophageal, 483

Gastrointestinal tract (*Continued*)
      gastric, 483
      intestinal, 485
      stromal, 484–485
   venous malformation of, 1625
Gastrointestinal vascular malformations, bleeding,
   1154
Gastrojejunal feeding tube
   in neurologically impaired children with reflux,
      956–957
   in short bowel syndrome, 1138
Gastrojejunostomy
   intussusception around tube in, 1098
   pyloric exclusion with, 300–301, 303f
Gastropathy, in portal hypertension, 1359, 1368
Gastroschisis
   antenatal considerations in, 977–978
   associated conditions with, 979, 979t
   complicated, 973–974, 982, 984
   complications of, 983
   cryptorchidism in, 1004–1005
   at delivery, 975–976, 976f, 978–979
   description of, 973–974, 974f, 974t
   embryogenesis of, 975–976, 976f
   fetal interventions for, 87–88
   historical perspective on, 973
   incidence of, 979
   jejunoileal atresia and stenosis with, 1060,
      1068–1069, 1241, 1241f
   outcome of, 983–984
   treatment of, 982, 982f
   umbilical hernia versus, 974–975
Gastrostomy, 186. *See also* Enterostoma.
   in cricopharyngeal disorders, 942
   endoscopic placement of, 884–885
   for esophageal atresia, 893, 907–908, 909f
   esophageal dilatations through, 884
   intussusception around, 1098
   percutaneous endoscopic, in neurologically
      impaired children with reflux, 956
Gaucher disease, splenectomy for, 1387
GD2
   antibodies against, 411
      for neuroblastoma, 457–458
   in neuroblastoma, 449
GDNF gene, in Hirschsprung disease, 21t
Gefitinib, 410
Gender assignment
   in 46,XX DSD, 1573
   in 46,XY DSD, 1573–1574
   in cloacal exstrophy, 1528
   in penile agenesis, 1585
Gender assignment surgery
   female, 1577
      clitoroplasty in, 1578–1579, 1578f, 1579f
      labioplasty in, 1579, 1579f, 1580f
      planning and timing of, 1578
      postoperative care in, 1582
      single-stage, 1578
      vaginoplasty in, 1580–1582, 1580f, 1581f,
         1582f, 1583f
   male, 1582–1583, 1584f
      hypospadias repair in, 1582–1583, 1585f
      müllerian duct remnants and, 1585, 1587f,
         1588f
      penile agenesis and, 1585–1586, 1588f, 1589f
      penoscrotal transposition and, 1583–1584,
         1586f
Gene chips, 48
Gene therapy, 23–26
Gene transfer
   challenges in, 25–26
   current status of, 26
   viral vectors for, 23–25, 23f, 24t
Genetic counseling, molecular genetics and, 22
Genetic disease
   monogenic, 20, 20f
   oligogenic, 20–21, 21t
   polygenic or complex, 21–22
   reconceptualization of, 19–20, 20f
Genetic screening, for cancer, 405
Genetics, molecular. *See* Molecular genetics.
Genital defects, in bladder exstrophy, 1516–1517,
   1517f, 1518f

Insulin-like growth factor 3, in testicular descent, 1003
Insulin resistance syndrome, 1042–1043
Insulinoma, 1383
Integra, in burn care, 378
Intensity-modulated radiation therapy, 413
Intensive care unit, neonatal, 8
Intercellular adhesion molecule-1, in neutrophil adhesion, 146
Intercostal drainage. *See* Chest tube.
Interferon-α, 411
    for infantile hemangioma, 1616
    for subglottic hemangioma, 850
Interferon-γ, 149
    in atypical mycobacterial lymphadenitis, 741–742
Interleukin(s), in stress response, 104
Interleukin-1, 149
    in necrotizing enterocolitis, 1190t, 1191
Interleukin-2, 149
Interleukin-2 receptor antibodies, in transplantation
    heart, 665–666
    liver, 650t
    renal, 624
Interleukin-4, in necrotizing enterocolitis, 1190t, 1191
Interleukin-6, 149
    in necrotizing enterocolitis, 1190t, 1191
Interleukin-8, 149
    in necrotizing enterocolitis, 1190t, 1191
Interleukin-10, in necrotizing enterocolitis, 1190t, 1191–1192
Interleukin-11, in necrotizing enterocolitis, 1190t, 1192
Interleukin-12, 149
    in necrotizing enterocolitis, 1190t, 1191
Interleukin-18, in necrotizing enterocolitis, 1190t, 1191
Intermittent mandatory ventilation, 118
    synchronized, 118
Intermittent positive-pressure ventilation, 117
International Neuroblastoma Pathology Classification (INPC), 446–447, 447f
International Society of Pediatric Oncology (SIOP) staging system for Wilms' tumor, 423, 424t, 429–430
Intersex. *See* Disorders of sex development (DSD).
Interstitial cells of Cajal, deficiency of, in internal anal sphincter achalasia, 1284
Intestinal adaptation, promotion of, in short bowel syndrome, 1141
Intestinal aganglionosis, near-total, 1272–1274
Intestinal atresia and stenosis
    colonic, 1247, 1248f
    duodenal, 1051–1060. *See also* Duodenal atresia and stenosis.
    familial, 1060–1061, 1061t, 1065, 1066f
    genetics of, 1248
    jejunoileal. *See* Jejunoileal atresia and stenosis.
Intestinal conservation, in short bowel syndrome, 1141
Intestinal dysmotility. *See also* Constipation; Hirschsprung disease.
    in intestinal rotation and fixation, 1124
    intestinal transplantation for, 653, 654f
    after pull-through, 1275–1276
    in short bowel syndrome, 1140
Intestinal failure. *See also* Short bowel syndrome.
    causes of, 653, 654f
    definition of, 1135
    liver disease with, 1138–1139
    management of, 653
    nutritional support for, 1137–1138
    transplantation for, 653–659
Intestinal ischemia, in necrotizing enterocolitis, 1194
Intestinal lengthening procedures, in short bowel syndrome, 1141–1144, 1142f, 1143f, 1144f
Intestinal loops, persistent dilated, in necrotizing enterocolitis, 1198–1199, 1201
Intestinal neuronal dysplasia, 1250, 1277–1278, 1279–1282
    clinical presentation in, 1280
    diagnosis of, 1280–1282, 1281f
    history and pathogenesis of, 1279–1280
    incidence of, 1280

Intestinal neuronal dysplasia (*Continued*)
    outcome of, 1282
    treatment of, 1282
Intestinal obstruction. *See also* Meconium ileus; Volvulus.
    adhesions with
        inflammatory, 1130
        postoperative, 1127–1129, 1128f, 1129f
    in ascariasis, 1133
    causes of, 1127–1135
    distal, 1082
    in duplication cysts, 1133
    embryology of, 1127
    after foreign body ingestion, 1133
    gastrointestinal lesions with, 1132–1133
    hernias with, 1130–1131, 1130f, 1131f
    in Hirschsprung disease, 1266
    after ileoanal pouch procedure, 1228
    in inflammatory pseudotumor, 1133
    in intussusception, 1093–1094
    in Meckel diverticulum, 1090–1091, 1090f, 1091f
    in mesenteric and omental cysts, 1133, 1166–1167, 1167f
    postoperative
        adhesive, 1127–1129, 1128f, 1129f
        after appendectomy, 1262
        ileus and, 1129
        intussusception and, 1130
        after pull-through for Hirschsprung disease, 1274–1277, 1274t, 1275f
    spectrum of disorders causing, 1127
Intestinal perforation
    diagnosis of, 290
    with intussusception reduction, 1107–1108, 1108f
    primary peritoneal drainage for, 1201
    in utero, 87
Intestinal pseudoobstruction, 1133–1134, 1134t
    chronic, 1250
    esophageal dysmotility in, 944
Intestinal rotation and fixation, 1111–1127
    disorders of. *See also* Volvulus.
        anomalies associated with, 1115
        asymptomatic, 1116
        atypical, 1114–1115, 1120, 1120f, 1124
        classification of, 1114–1115, 1120, 1120f
        clinical manifestations of, 1115–1116, 1116f
        complications of, 1124–1125
        growth disorders in, 1114
        with heterotaxia, 1115, 1120, 1122f
        historical perspective on, 1111
        management of
            laparoscopic versus open reduction in, 1122–1123
            operative, 1120–1122, 1123f
            postoperative, 1124–1125
            preoperative, 1120
            resection and second-look procedures in, 1124
        with mesocolic hernia, 1117, 1118f, 1120, 1124
        radiologic findings in, 1117–1120, 1119f, 1120f, 1121f, 1122f
        reversed, 1115
            with colonic obstruction, 1117, 1117f, 1124
        terminology in, 1114–1115, 1115f
    normal, 1111–1117, 1115f, 1119f
        cecocolic loop in, 1113, 1113f, 1114f
        duodenojejunal loop in, 1111, 1112f
        fixation in, 1114–1115, 1115f
        side and direction of, 1112
        simultaneous rotation of both ends and entire intestinal tract in, 1113–1114, 1114f
Intestinal stoma. *See* Enterostoma.
Intestinal stricture
    in Crohn disease, 1210, 1210f
        balloon dilatation for, 1214
        surgery for, 1213–1214, 1213f, 1214f
    after ileoanal pouch procedure, 1228
    in necrotizing enterocolitis, 1203, 1249, 1250f
    posttraumatic, 1133
Intestinal transplantation, 653–659
    abdominal wall closure after, 655, 656f
    assessment and preparation for, 654
    complications of, 656
    immunosuppressive therapy for, 655–656

Intestinal transplantation (*Continued*)
    indications for, 653–654, 654f
    operative procedures in, 654–655, 655f
    postoperative care in, 655–656
    results of, 656–658, 657f
    in short bowel syndrome, 1145
    timing of, 653–654
Intestinal tumors, 485
    in Peutz-Jeghers syndrome, 1184
Intestinal vaginoplasty, 1596–1598, 1597f
Intestine. *See also* Colon; Gastrointestinal *entries;* Small intestine.
    bacterial overgrowth in
        methods to decrease, 1206–1207
        in short bowel syndrome, 1140
    distention of, in necrotizing enterocolitis, 1188f, 1198
    echogenic, fetal, 87
    invagination of. *See* Intussusception.
    mucosal gland abnormalities of, in meconium ileus, 1074
    stretching of, 1144
    tissue-engineered, 32, 1144
Intra-abdominal pressure
    measurement of, 298
    in trauma patient, 298–299, 299f
Intra-abdominal testis, 1005, 1005f
Intracellular fluid, in neonates, 91–92
Intracerebral hematoma, traumatic, 346
Intracranial aneurysm, traumatic, 353
Intracranial hematoma
    in birth trauma, 392
    removal of, 351, 351f, 352f
Intracranial hemorrhage, with extracorporeal life support, 129
Intracranial hypotension, from overshunting, 1685–1686
Intracranial infections, 1693–1697, 1694f, 1695f
Intracranial lesions, stereotactic radiosurgery for, 53–54
Intracranial pressure. *See also* Hydrocephalus.
    increased
        in brain tumors, 591
        in craniosynostosis, 692
        management of, 350–351, 351t
    monitoring of
        in epilepsy surgery, 1689–1690
        after shunt implantation, 1686
        in traumatic brain injury, 350
    in trauma patient, 268–269
Intrahepatic duct cysts, dilatation of, 462
Intrahepatic hematoma, 464, 465f
    in birth trauma, 392, 392f
Intraosseous line, in trauma patient, 266, 267
Intraperitoneal fluid. *See also* Ascites.
    free, 1171
        computed tomography of, 308
    in necrotizing enterocolitis, 1198
Intraspinal infections, 1697
Intrathoracic access and procedures, 873–876
Intrauterine growth restriction, 89–90
Intravenous anesthesia, 201, 202f, 211–212, 212f
Intravenous immunoglobulin
    for immune thrombocytopenic purpura, 170, 1387
    for necrotizing enterocolitis, 1205
    for sepsis, 162
Intraventricular hemorrhage, 347–348, 347f
Introital cysts, 1608
Introital masses, 1606
Intubation, endotracheal. *See* Endotracheal intubation.
Intussusception, 1093–1114
    anatomic, 1098
    definition of, 1093
    diagnosis of, 1095f, 1099
        clinical, 1095f, 1099
        radiologic, 1099–1101, 1100f, 1101f
    epidemiology of, 1094
    future expectations for, 1109–1110
    historical perspective on, 1093
    idiopathic, 1095f, 1096–1097
    ileocolic, 1098, 1098f, 1107

Tumorigenesis, 399–400, 400t, 401f
Tunica albuginea, 1537
Turbinates, 712
Turcot syndrome, 487, 1182
Turkey, pediatric surgery in, 15
Twin reversed arterial perfusion sequence (TRAP sequence), 88
Twin-twin transfusion syndrome, fetal interventions for, 87
Twinning, partial or abortive, in alimentary tract duplications, 1155
Twins, conjoined. See Conjoined twins.
Two-hit mechanism of carcinogenesis, 399
Tympanic membrane, 707
  perforation of, 711
Tympanometry, 708
Tympanostomy tube, 709
Tyrosinemia, hepatocellular carcinoma and, 476

U

Ulcer(s). See also Peptic ulcer disease.
  acute upper gastrointestinal bleeding from, 1150–1151
  aphthous, in Crohn disease, 1210
  cutaneous, hemangioma with, 1616
  rectal, solitary, 1319
Ulcerative colitis, 1217–1234
  clinical examination in, 1219–1221, 1220f, 1221f, 1221t
  clinical manifestations of, 1219, 1220f
  colorectal cancer in, 489, 1219
  epidemiology of, 1218
  etiology of, 1218
  exacerbations of, 1222
  medical management of, 1221–1222
  pathology of, 1218–1219, 1218f
  postoperative care in, 1226
  surgical management of, 1222–1224
    complications and outcomes of, 1227–1229
    historical perspective on, 1217
    ileoanal pouch procedure in, 1223–1224, 1223f, 1224f, 1225f, 1226f
    ileoanal pull-through in, 1223
    J pouch in, 1224, 1225, 1226–1227, 1227f
    laparoscopic, 1225–1226, 1226f
    protective ileostomy in, 1226–1227
    stooling after, 1226–1227, 1227f
    straight pull-through in, 1223, 1225–1227, 1225f, 1227f
Ulnar defects, 1722
Ulnar nerve, injury to, 337–338, 338f
Ultimobranchial body, 755f
Ultrasonography, 38–40
  in alimentary tract duplications, 1157, 1157f
  in anorectal malformations, 1294
  in appendicitis, 1257–1258
  in ascites, 1172, 1173f
  in biliary atresia, 1323–1324
  in bladder dysfunction, 1454, 1455f
  in cervical lymphadenopathy, 739
  before cholecystectomy, 1344–1345, 1345t
  in choledochal cyst, 1334
  in conjoined twins, 1731
  contrast-enhanced, 40, 40f
  in developmental dysplasia of hip, 1700, 1700f
  in disorders of sex development, 1575, 1576f
  Doppler, 38
    of burns, 372
    in cervical lymphadenopathy, 739
    after renal transplantation, 623
    of salivary glands, 730, 730f
  in ectopic ureter, 1446
  FAST (focused abdominal sonography for trauma), 290, 290f, 308, 313
  fetal surgery and, 40
  in gallbladder disease, 1343
  harmonic, 40, 41f
  in hepatic abscess, 1350–1351, 1350f
  in hypertrophic pyloric stenosis, 1023, 1023f
  in inguinal hernia, 987–988, 988f
  in intestinal rotation and fixation disorders, 1118, 1119f

Ultrasonography (Continued)
  in intussusception, 1100–1101, 1100f, 1101f, 1103, 1106
  in mesenteric and omental cysts, 1168, 1168f
  in multicystic dysplastic kidney, 1400–1401, 1400f, 1401f
  in musculoskeletal trauma, 331–332
  of neck mass, 727
  in necrotizing enterocolitis, 1199
  of ovarian tumors, 532–533, 532f
  in pancreatitis, 1373, 1375
  percutaneous needle biopsy guided by, 418
  in pheochromocytoma, 559–560
  in portal hypertension, 1361
  prenatal
    of abdominal wall defects, 977–978
    in alimentary tract duplications, 1157
    in bladder exstrophy, 1517–1518
    in bronchopulmonary sequestration, 827–828, 827f
    in choledochal cyst, 1333
    in congenital diaphragmatic hernia, 813–814, 814f
    in congenital lobar emphysema, 828–829
    in conjoined twins, 1730–1731, 1731f
    diagnostic, 78, 79f
    in duodenal atresia and stenosis, 1053, 1053f
    in jejunoileal atresia and stenosis, 1061
    in megacystis-microcolon-intestinal hypoperistalsis syndrome, 1285
    of ovarian tumors, 532, 532f
    in ureteropelvic junction obstruction, 1413–1414, 1413f
  in renal injury, 313
  in renal vein thrombosis, 1439
  of simple renal cyst, 1403, 1403f
  of testicular tumors, 550
  therapeutic use of, 49
  in thoracic trauma, 273–274
  three-dimensional, 38–39, 39f
  of thyroid gland, 746
  of thyroid nodules, 748
  in ureterocele, 1448, 1448f
  in ureteropelvic junction obstruction, 1415–1416, 1415f, 1420–1421
  in urinary tract infection, 1429–1430, 1429f, 1430f
  in vascular trauma, 363
  of Wilms' tumor, 427
Umbilical artery
  cannulation of, 970–971
  catheterization of, 1634–1635, 1635f
  embryology of, 962f, 963t
  single, 967
Umbilical hernia, 963, 968–970
  anatomy of, 968–969
  bladder exstrophy with, 1516, 1516f
  description of, 974–975, 974f
  embryogenesis of, 976
  giant, 971
  incidence of, 969
  natural history of, 969
  surgical management of, 969–970, 970f
  treatment of, 982
Umbilical-placental circulation, 134–135, 136f
Umbilical vein, 1355, 1356f
  cannulation of, 970–971
  embryology of, 962f, 963t
Umbilicoplasty
  for abdominal wall defects, 971–972, 972f
  for giant umbilical hernia with redundant skin, 971
Umbilicus, 959–974
  acquired abnormalities of, 964, 968t
  appearance of, aesthetics of, 961
  at birth, 963–964
  catheterization of, 116–117
  congenital malformations of, 961, 964–968, 965f, 966f
  dysmorphology of, 967
  embryology of, 961–963, 962f, 963t
  granuloma of, 964
  infection of, 964
  lint in, 968
  new, creation of, 971–972, 972f

Umbilicus (Continued)
  piercing of, 967–968
  protrusions at, 967
  reconstruction and preservation of, 971–972
  use of, 970–971
Undiversion, 1487
Unicameral bone cyst, 578–579, 579f
  injection therapy for, 584
  location of, in relation to physis, 579f
Unicornuate system, 1603–1604, 1603f, 1604f
Unicornuate uterus, 1487
United Kingdom, pediatric surgery in, 10–11, 11f, 12f
United Network for Organ Sharing, 620
United States, pediatric surgery in, 4–6, 4f, 5f, 6f
Upper gastrointestinal series
  in duodenal atresia and stenosis, 1054, 1054f
  in gastroesophageal reflux disease, 952
  in hypertrophic pyloric stenosis, 1023, 1023f
  in intestinal rotation and fixation disorders, 1120, 1120f
  in necrotizing enterocolitis, 1199
Urachal remnants, 966–967, 966f
Urachus
  embryology of, 961–963, 962f, 963t
  patent, 966, 966f
  tumors arising from, 967, 967t
Ureter. See also Megaureter.
  blind-ending, 1443
  ectopic, 1445–1447, 1446f
    megaureter with, 1497
  inverted Y, 1443
  for Mitrofanoff neourethra, 1480
  reimplantation of, for megaureter, 1499–1501, 1500f, 1502–1503, 1504f
  stones in, 1438. See also Urolithiasis.
  trauma to, 313, 314t, 319–320
  Wilms' tumor extension to, 431–432
Ureteral anastomosis, in renal transplantation, 622–624
Ureteral buds, 1405
Ureteral duplication, 1441–1454
  embryogenesis of, 1441–1444, 1442f
  types of, 1441
Ureteral stent
  after pyeloplasty, 1425
  for urolithiasis, 1437
Ureterectomy, partial nephrectomy with, 1444, 1445f, 1447
Ureteric bud, 1395, 1411–1412
Uretero-ureteral reflux (yo-yo reflux), 1444
Uretero-ureterostomy, 1444, 1445, 1447
Ureterocele, 1447–1451
  classification of, 1447–1448, 1447t
  clinical presentation in, 1448
  definition of, 1441
  diagnosis of, 1448–1450, 1448f, 1449f
  imaging of, 1429–1430, 1430f
  megaureter with, 1497
  prolapse of, 1448, 1449f, 1558
  prolapsed ectopic, 1607, 1608f
  treatment of, 1450
  vesicoureteral reflux and, 1450, 1451
Ureterocystoplasty, 1475, 1476f, 1477f
Ureteroneocystostomy, 1445
  in bladder exstrophy repair, 1522–1523, 1524f
Ureteropelvic junction, injury to, 319
Ureteropelvic junction obstruction, 1411–1429. See also Hydronephrosis.
  clinical features of, 1412–1414
    antenatal, 1413–1414, 1413f, 1413t
    postnatal, 1414, 1414t
  crossing vessels in, 1420
  diagnosis of, 1414–1420
    biochemical markers in, 1419–1420
    intravenous urography in, 1414
    magnetic resonance urography in, 1417–1418, 1418f
    pressure-flow study (Whitaker test) in, 1419, 1419f
    retrograde pyelography in, 1418, 1419f
    scintigraphy in, 1416–1417, 1416f, 1417f, 1418f
    ultrasonography in, 1415–1416, 1415f
    voiding cystourethrography in, 1417